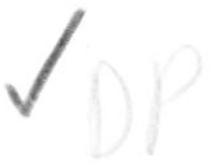

MW00359081

Perioperative Care of the Cancer Patient

Carin A. Hagberg, MD

Chief Academic Officer
The University of Texas MD Anderson Cancer Center;
Division Head
Anesthesiology, Critical Care & Pain Medicine
The University of Texas MD Anderson Cancer Center
Houston, TX, USA;
Bud Johnson Clinical Distinguished Chair

Vijaya N. R. Gottumukkala, MBBS, MD(Anes), FRCA

Professor
Anesthesiology & Perioperative Medicine
The University of Texas MD Anderson Cancer Center
Houston, TX, USA

Bernhard J. Riedel, MD, MBA, PhD

Professor
Anesthesiology, Perioperative and Pain Medicine
Peter MacCallum Cancer Centre
Melbourne, Victoria, Australia

Joseph L. Nates, MD, MBA, CMQ, MCCM

Professor, Deputy Chair
Director Surgical and Medical Intensive Care Units
Critical Care Department
Division of Anesthesiology, Critical Care & Pain Medicine
The University of Texas MD Anderson Cancer Center
Houston, TX, USA

Donal J. Buggy, DSc, MD, MSc, DME, FRCPI, FFSEM, FRCA, FCAI

Professor
Anaesthesiology & Perioperative Medicine
Mater Misericordiae University Hospital, School of Medicine, University College Dublin;
Consultant
Anaesthesiology
Mater Misericordiae University Hospital Dublin,
Dublin, Ireland

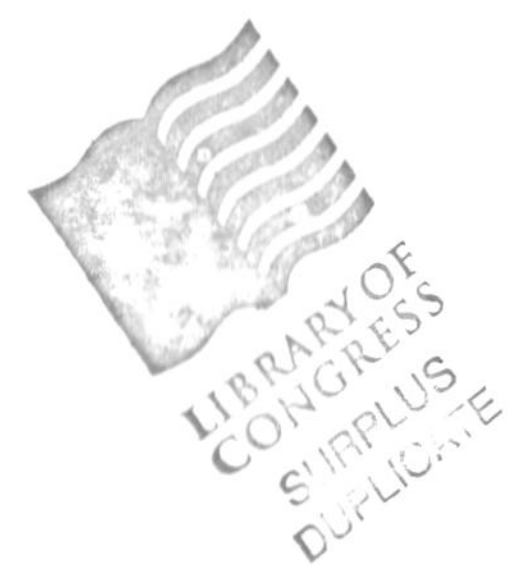

ELSEVIER

Elsevier

1600 John F. Kennedy Blvd.
Ste 1800
Philadelphia, PA 19103-2899

PERIOPERATIVE CARE OF THE CANCER PATIENT ISBN: 978-0-323-69584-8

Library of Congress Control Number: 2021947605

Publisher: Sarah Barth
Senior Content Development Manager: Somodatta Roy Choudhury
Senior Content Development Specialist: Malvika Shah
Publishing Services Manager: Shereen Jameel
Senior Project Manager: Manikandan Chandrasekaran
Design Direction: Julia Dummitt

Printed in India
Last digit is the print number: 9 8 7 6 5 4 3 2 1

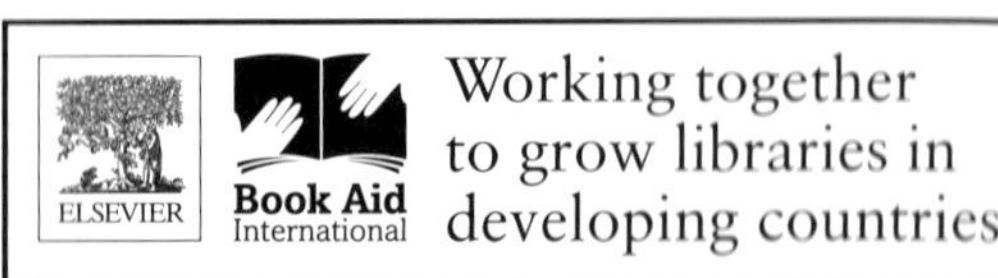

We dedicate this issue to all of our cancer patients and their loved ones. We find inspiration for our ongoing clinical, research, and educational efforts from their fighting spirit, courage, strength, and hope for a cure.

Contributors

Salahadin Abdi, MD, PhD
Professor and Chair
Pain Medicine
The University of Texas MD Anderson Cancer Center
Houston, TX, USA

Anoushka M. Afonso, MD
Associate Attending
Department of Anesthesiology & Critical Care
Memorial Sloan Kettering Cancer Center
New York, NY, USA

Thomas A. Aloia, MD
Professor of Surgery
Surgical Oncology
The University of Texas MD Anderson Cancer Center
Houston, TX, USA

Gabriele Baldini, MD, MSc
Assistant Professor, Anesthesiologist
Anesthesia
McGill University Health Centre, Montreal General Hospital
Montreal, Quebec, Canada

Jose Banchs, MD
Associate Professor
Cardiology
The University of Texas MD Anderson Cancer Center
Houston, TX, USA

Daniel T. Baptista-Hon, BSc, MSc, PhD
Assistant Professor
Faculty of Medicine
Macau University of Science and Technology
Macau, SAR, China;
Honorary Lecturer
School of Medicine
University of Dundee
Dundee, United Kingdom

Karen Basen-Engquist, PhD
Professor
Department of Behavioral Science
Division of Cancer Prevention and Population Sciences
The University of Texas MD Anderson Cancer Center
Houston, TX, USA

Rosalind S. Bello, MA, CPHQ
Director
Cancer Control Health Policy
The University of Texas MD Anderson Cancer Center
Houston, TX, USA

Shamgar Ben-Eliyahu, PhD
Sagol School of Neuroscience and School of Psychological Sciences
Tel-Aviv University
Tel-Aviv, Israel

Celena Scheede Bergdahl, MSc, PhD
Professor
Department of Kinesiology and Physical Education
McGill University
Montreal, Quebec, Canada

Sushma Bhatnagar, MD
Professor and Head
Department of Onco-Anesthesia and Palliative Medicine
Institute Rotary Cancer Hospital and National Cancer Institute
All India Institute of Medical Sciences
New Delhi, India

Joshua Botdorf, DO, FACP, CMQ
Assistant Professor
Critical Care and Respiratory Medicine
The University of Texas MD Anderson Cancer Center
Houston, TX, USA

Christelle Botha, FANZCA
Consultant Anatesthetist
Department of Cancer Anaesthesia
Perioperative and Pain Medicine, Peter MacCallum Cancer Centre
Melbourne, Victoria, Australia

David L. Brown, MD
Chief Executive Officer
Curadux Inc.
Austin, TX, USA

Donal J. Buggy, DSc, MD, MSc, DME, FRCPI, FFSEM, FRCA, FCAI
Professor
Anaesthesiology & Perioperative Medicine
Mater Misericordiae University Hospital, School of Medicine, University College Dublin;
Consultant,
Anaesthesiology
Mater Misericordiae University Hospital Dublin
Dublin, Ireland

Kate L. Burbury, MBBS(Hons), FRACP, FRCPA, DPhil
Deputy Chief Medical Officer
Executive
Peter MacCallum Cancer Centre;
Consultant Haematologist
DHMO
Peter MacCallum Cancer Centre
Melbourne, Victoria, Australia

Joseph Butler, PhD, FACS, FRCS
Consultant Spine Surgeon
National Spinal Injuries Unit
Mater Misericordiae University Hospital
Dublin, Ireland

Ronan Cahill, MB, BAO, BCh, FRCS, MD
UCD Centre for Precision Surgery
Surgery
University College Dublin
Surgery
Mater Misericordiae University Hospital
Dublin, Ireland

Franco Carli, MD, MPhil
Professor
Anesthesia
McGill University
Montreal, Quebec, Canada

Meghan Carton, BM, BS
Doctor
Anaesthetics
Mater Misericordiae University Hospital
Dublin, Ireland

Juan P. Cata, MD
Professor
Department of Anesthesiology and Perioperative Medicine
The University of Texas MD Anderson Cancer Center
Houston, TX, USA

Cara Connolly, MB, BCh, BAO, LRCP & SI (Hons), MSc, FCAI
Consultant Anaesthetist
Department of Anaesthesia
Mater Misericordiae University Hospital
Dublin, Ireland

German Corrales, MD
Department of Anesthesiology and Perioperative Medicine
The University of Texas MD Anderson Cancer Center
Houston, TX, USA

Jose Cortes, MD
Assistant Professor
Pediatrics
The University of Texas MD Anderson Cancer Center
Houston, TX, USA

Kimberly D. Craven, MD
Clinical Assistant Professor
Department of Anesthesiology
Perioperative Care & Pain Management
NYU Langone – Brooklyn
Brooklyn, NY, USA

John Wilson Crommett, MD
Associate Professor
Critical Care Medicine
The University of Texas MD Anderson Cancer Center
Houston, TX, USA

Kristin P. Crosby, MD
Fellow
Pediatric Critical Care Medicine
New York Presbyterian Hospital – Weill Cornell Medicine
New York, NY, USA

Luis Felipe Cuellar Guzman, MD
Anesthesiologist in Oncological Patient and Pain Medicine Specialist
Anesthesiology Department Head, National Institute of Cancer Mexico;
Onco Anesthesia
National Institute of Cancer Mexico
Mexico City, Mexico;
Professor Course Cancer Anesthesia Fellowship Program
National Institute of Cancer Mexico
Anesthesiology Department
National Institute of Cancer
Mexico

Anahita Dabo-Trubelja, MD, FASA
Associate Attending
Anesthesiology and Critical Care
Memorial Sloan Kettering Cancer Center
New York, NY, USA

Anh Quynh Dang, MD
Associate Professor
Anesthesiology and Preoperative Medicine
The University of Texas MD Anderson Cancer Center
Houston, TX, USA

Alessandro R. De Camilli, MD
Assistant Attending, Anesthesiology and Critical Care Medicine
Anesthesiology and Critical Care
Memorial Sloan Kettering Cancer Center
New York NY, USA

Madhavi D. Desai, DA, DNB
Assistant Professor and Consultant
Department of Anaesthesia, Critical Care and Pain
Tata Memorial Hospital and Homi Bhabha National Institute
Mumbai, Maharashtra, India

Jugdeep Dhesi, BSc, PhD, FRCP
Consultant Geriatrician
Ageing and Health
Guy's and St Thomas' NHS Trust
London, United Kingdom;
Hon. Reader
Kings College London
London, United Kingdom;
Hon. Associate Professor
University College London
London, United Kingdom

Jeson R. Doctor, MD, DNB, MNAMS, MBBS
Professor and Consultant Anaesthesiologist
Department of Anaesthesiology
Critical Care and Pain Tata Memorial Hospital
Homi Bhabha National Institute
Mumbai, Maharashtra, India

Jennifer S. Downs, MMed, FCS(SA)
Surgical Oncology Fellow
Cancer Surgery
Peter MacCallum Cancer Centre
Melbourne, Victoria, Australia

Julia A. Dubowitz, MBBS
Specialist Anaesthetist
Department of Anaesthetics, Perioperative and Pain Medicine
Peter MacCallum Cancer Centre;
Clinical Fellow
Department of Critical Care
University of Melbourne
Parkville, Melbourne, Australia

German Echeverry, MD
Attending Physician
Department of Anesthesiology and Critical Care Medicine
Memorial Sloan Kettering Cancer Center
New York, NY;
Attending Physician
Department of Anesthesia
Mount Sinai Medical Center
Miami Beach, FL, USA

Mats Enlund, MD, PhD
Associate Professor
Centre for Clinical Research-Västerås
Uppsala University
Västerås, Sweden;
Senior Consultant
Department of Anaesthesia & Intensive Care
Central Hospital
Västerås, Sweden

Linette Ewing, DO, MPH
Assistant Professor
Pediatric Critical Care
The University of Texas MD Anderson Cancer Center
Houston, TX, USA

Dylan Finnerty, FCAI, FJFICMI, EDICM
Research Fellow
Anaesthesiology & Perioperative Medicine
Mater Misericordiae University Hospital University College Dublin
Dublin, Ireland

Joël Fokom Domgue, MD, MPH
Research Scientist
Epidemiology
The University of Texas MD Anderson Cancer Center
Houston, TX, USA

John Frenzel, MD, MS
Director, Learning Health System
Institute for Cancer Care Innovation
The University of Texas MD Anderson Cancer Center
Houston, TX, USA

Colleen M. Gallagher, PhD, FACHE, HEC-C
Executive Director
Section of Integrated Ethics
The University of Texas MD Anderson Cancer Center;
Professor
Department of Critical Care Medicine
The University of Texas MD Anderson Cancer Center
Houston, TX, USA;
Research Scholar
UNESCO Chair in Bioethics and Human Rights
Rome, Italy

Dorian Yarih García-Ortega, MD, MSc, FACS
Master in Musculoskeletal Tumors
Surgeon Oncologist
Skin, Soft Tissue and Bone Tumors Department
National Cancer Institute
Mexico City, Mexico

Michelle Gerstman, MBBS, FANZCA, MD
Consultant Anaesthetist
Anaesthetics, Perioperative Medicine and Pain Medicine
Peter MacCallum Cancer Centre
Melbourne, Victoria, Australia

Arunangshu Ghoshal, MD, MRes
Assistant Professor
Palliative Medicine
Tata Memorial Hospital
Homi Bhaba National Institute
Mumbai, Maharashtra, India

Vijaya N. R. Gottumukkala, MBBS, MD(Anes), FRCA
Professor
Anesthesiology & Perioperative Medicine
The University of Texas MD Anderson Cancer Center
Houston, TX, USA

Michael P. W. Grocott, MB, BS, MD, FRCA, FRCP, FFICM
Professor
Respiratory and Critical Care Research Theme
Southampton NIHR Biomedical Research Centre
University Hospital Southampton NHS Foundation Trust/ University of Southampton
Southampton, United Kingdom;
Anaesthesia, Perioperative and Critical Care Medicine Research Unit
University Hospital Southampton NHS Foundation Trust
Southampton, United Kingdom

Carlos E. Guerra-Londono, MD
Department of Anesthesiology, Pain Management, and Perioperative Medicine
Henry Ford Health System
Detroit, MI, USA

Sushan Gupta, MD
Department of Internal Medicine
Carle Foundation Hospital
Champaign, IL, USA

David E. Gyorki, MBBS, MD, FRACS
Surgical Oncologist
Division of Cancer Surgery
Peter MacCallum Cancer Centre
Melbourne, Victoria, Australia

Tim G. Hales, BSc, PhD
Professor of Anaesthesia
Institute of Academic Anaesthesia
University of Dundee, Dundee, Scotland
United Kingdom

Ernest Hawk, MD, MPH
Vice President and Division Head
Division of Cancer Prevention and Population Sciences
T. Boone Pickens Distinguished Chair for Early Prevention of Cancer
The University of Texas MD Anderson Cancer Center
Houston, TX, USA

Alexander G. Heriot, MB BChir, MA, MD, MBA, FRACS, FRCS(Gen.), FRCSEd, FACS, FASCRS, GAICD
Director of Surgery
Division of Cancer Surgery
Peter MacCallum Cancer Centre
Melbourne, Victoria, Australia

Joseph M. Herman, MD
Director of Clinical Research
Northwell Health
New Hyde Park, NY, USA

Jonathan G. Hiller, MBBS, GCEpi, MAICD, FANZCA, PhD
Division of Surgical Oncology
Anaesthesia
Peter MacCallum Cancer Centre
Parkville, Victoria, Australia;
Central Clinical School
Medicine, Nursing and Health Sciences
Monash University
Prahran, Victoria, Australia

Ruth E. Hubbard, BSc, MBBS, MRCP, MSc, MD, FRACP
Professor
Centre for Health Services Research
University of Queensland
Brisbane, Queensland, Australia

Hilmy Ismail, MD, FRCA, FANZCA
Consultant Anaesthetist
Anaesthesia and Preoperative Medicine
PeterMacCallum Cancer Center
Melbourne, Victoria, Australia;
Senior Lecturer
Anaesthesia
University of Melbourne
Melbourne, Victoria, Australia

Nelda Itzep, MD
Assistant Professor
Pediatrics
The University of Texas MD Anderson Cancer Center
Houston, TX, USA

Emily Jasper, MBBS (Hons)
Research Registrar
Ageing and Health
Guy's and St Thomas' NHS Foundation Trust
London, United Kingdom;
Senior Registrar/Advanced Trainee
Department of Rehabilitation and Aged Care
North Metropolitan Health Service
Perth, Western Australia, Australia

Saba Javed, MD
Assistant Professor
Department of Anesthesiology
University of Texas Medical School at Houston
Houston, TX, USA

Bhawna Jha, MD, MRCPsych
Interventional Pain Physician
Medical Director–Bundle Payment For Care Improvement
Physician Advisor–Utilization Management and Review
University of Arkansas for Medical Sciences (UAMS)
Little Rock, AR, USA

Shaman Jhanji, MB ChB, MRCP, FRCA, FFICM, PhD
Consultant in Intensive Care Medicine and Anaesthetics
Department of Anaesthesia, Perioperative Medicine, Pain and Intensive Care
Royal Marsden Hospital
London, United Kingdom;
Team Leader/Honorary Clinical Senior Lecturer
Division of Cancer Biology
Institute of Cancer Research
London, United Kingdom

Daryl Jones, BSc(Hons), MB BS, FRACP, FCICM, MD, PhD
Consultant Intensive Care specialist
Austin Health and Warringal hospital;
Acting Deputy Director
Austin Department of Intensive Care;
Adjunct Professor
University Melbourne;
Adjunct Professor (Research)
DEPM Monash University;
Medical Director
Critical Care Outreach Austin Hospital;
Past President
International Society of Rapid Response Systems
Melbourne, Victoria, Australia

Ravish Kapoor, MD
Associate Professor
Department of Anesthesiology and Perioperative Medicine
The University of Texas MD Anderson Cancer Center
Houston, TX, USA

Faraz Khan, MB, BCh, BAO, MRCS, MD, MSc
Specialist Surgical Lecturer
Colorectal Surgery
Mater Misericordiae University Hospital
Dublin, Ireland

James S. Killinger, MD
Medical Director, Pediatric Intensive Care Unit
Pediatrics
Memorial Sloan Kettering Cancer Center
Associate Professor of Clinical Pediatrics
Pediatrics
Weill Cornell Medicine
New York, NY, USA

Samantha Koschel, BMed MD, GradDipAnat
Urology Registrar
Cancer Surgery
Peter MacCallum Cancer Centre
Melbourne, Victoria, Australia

Alan Kotin, MD
Attending Anesthesiologist
Anesthesiology
Memorial Sloan Kettering Cancer Center
New York, NY, USA

Atul Prabhakar Kulkarni, MBBS, MD (Anesthesiology)
Professor and Head
Division of Critical Care Medicine
Tata Memorial Hospital
Homi Bhabha National Institute
Mumbai, Maharashtra, India

Adam La Caze, BPharm, BA (Hons), PhD
Senior Lecturer
School of Pharmacy
The University of Queensland
Brisbane, Queensland, Australia

Nathan Lawrentschuk, MBBS, FRACS Urol, PhD
Professor
Director of Urology
Royal Melbourne Hospital
Parkville, Victoria, Australia

Lauren Adrienne Leddy, MB, BCh, BAO
Medical Student
Medicine
University College Dublin
Dublin, Ireland

Celia R. Ledet, MD
Assistant Professor
Department of Surgical Oncology
The University of Texas MD Anderson Cancer Center
Houston, TX, USA

Denny Z. H. Levett, MA, BM BCh, PhD
Anaesthesia and Critical Care Research Area
Southampton NIHR Biomedical Research Centre
University Hospital Southampton NHS Foundation Trust;
Integrative Physiology and Critical Illness Group
Clinical and Experimental Sciences
Faculty of Medicine
University of Southampton
Southampton, United Kingdom

Debra Leung, MBBS Hons, BMedSci, FANZCA
Specialist Anaesthetist
Department of Anaesthesia, Perioperative and Pain Medicine
Peter MacCallum Cancer Centre;
Senior Clinical Fellow
Centre for Integrated Critical Care
The University of Melbourne
PhD candidate
The Sir Peter MacCallum Department of Oncology
The University of Melbourne
Melbourne, Victoria, Australia

Hui-Shan Lin, FRACP, MPhil
Geriatrician
Geriatric Medicine
The Royal Brisbane and Woman's Hospital
Brisbane, Queensland, Australia

Alexandra L. Lewis, MD, MPH
Assistant Attending
Anesthesiology and Critical Care
Memorial Sloan Kettering Cancer Center
New York, NY, USA

Daqing Ma, MD, PhD, FRCA, MAE
Professor of Anaesthesia
Anaesthetics, Pain Medicine and Intensive Care
Imperial College London, Chelsea & Westminster Hospital
London, United Kingdom

Kevin Madden, MD
Assistant Professor
Palliative, Rehabilitation, and Integrative Medicine
The University of Texas MD Anderson Cancer Center
Houston, TX, USA

Anirban Maitra, MBBS
Professor and Scientific Director
Sheikh Ahmed Pancreatic Cancer Research Center
The University of Texas MD Anderson Cancer Center
Houston, TX, USA

Karen Colbert Maresso, MPH
Program Director, Division of Cancer Prevention and Population Sciences
The University of Texas MD Anderson Cancer Center
Houston, TX, USA

Jennifer Mascarenhas, MD, MA
Doctor
Anesthesiology
Memorial Sloan Kettering Cancer Center
New York, NY, USA

K. A. Kelly McQueen, MD, MPH
Chair and Professor
Anesthesiology
University of Wisconsin Madison
Madison, WI, USA

Rodrigo Mejia, MD
Professor
Pediatrics
Section Chief, Pediatric Critical Care
The University of Texas MD Anderson Cancer Center
Houston, TX, USA

Lachlan F. Miles, MBBS (Hons.), PGCertCU, PhD, FANZCA
Honorary Principal Fellow
Department of Critical Care
The University of Melbourne;
Deputy Head of Research
Department of Anaesthesia
Austin Health
Melbourne, Victoria, Australia

Sana Mohiuddin, MD
Fellow
Pediatrics
The University of Texas MD Anderson Cancer Center
Houston, TX, USA

Daniela Molena, MD
Surgical Director of Esophageal Cancer Surgery Program
Thoracic Surgery
Memorial Sloan Kettering Cancer Center
New York, NY, USA

Tracy-Ann Moo, MD
Breast Service, Department of Surgery
Memorial Sloan Kettering Cancer Center
New York, NY, USA

Karen Moody, MD, MS
Associate Professor of Pediatrics
Director, Palliative and Supportive Care
Pediatrics
The University of Texas MD Anderson Cancer Center
Houston, TX, USA

Declan G. Murphy, MB, BCh, BaO, FRCS, FRACS
Professor
Division of Cancer Surgery
Peter MacCallum Cancer Centre
Melbourne, Victoria, Australia

Sheila Nainan Myatra, MD, FCCM, FICCM
Professor
Department of Anesthesiology, Critical Care and Pain
Tata Memorial Hospital
Homi Bhabha National Institute
Mumbai, Maharashtra, India

Joseph L. Nates, MD, MBA, CMQ, MCCM
Professor, Deputy Chair
Director Surgical and Medical Intensive Care Units
Critical Care Department
Division of Anesthesiology, Critical Care & Pain Medicine
The University of Texas MD Anderson Cancer Center
Houston, TX, USA

Jonas A. Nelson, MD
Plastic and Reconstructive Surgery Service, Department of Surgery
Memorial Sloan Kettering Cancer Center
New York, NY, USA

Aisling Ní Eochagáin, MB, BCh, BAO, FCAI, MSc, DLM, DEcon, CLC
Clinical research fellow
Mater Misericordiae University Hospital
Dublin, Ireland

Ellen O'Connor, MBBS, DipSurgAnat
Urology Research Fellow
Division of Cancer Surgery
Peter MacCallum Cancer Centre
Melbourne, Victoria, Australia;
Urology Research Fellow
Department of Surgery
University of Melbourne, Austin Health
Heidelberg, Victoria, Australia

Regina Okhuysen-Cawley, MD
Associate Professor
Pediatrics
Baylor College of Medicine
Houston, TX, USA

Pascal Owusu-Agyemang, MD
Professor
Anesthesiology and Perioperative Medicine
The University of Texas MD Anderson Cancer Center
Houston, TX, USA

Gouri H. Pantvaidya, MS, DNB, MRCS
Professor
Surgery
Tata Memorial Centre
Mumbai, Maharashtra, India

Pamela C. Papadopoulos, PhD
Associate Director, Research Planning and Development
Moon Shots Program
The University of Texas MD Anderson Cancer Center
Houston, TX, USA

Marie-Odile Parat, PharmD, PhD
Associate Professor
School of Pharmacy
University of Queensland
Brisbane, Queensland, Australia

Judith Partridge, MSc, PhD, FRCP
Consultant Geriatrician
Perioperative Medicine for Older People Undergoing Surgery
Guy's and St Thomas' NHS Foundation Trust
London, United Kingdom

Sephalie Patel, MD
Associate Member
Vice Chair, Department of Anesthesiology
H. Lee Moffitt Cancer Center
Tampa, FL, USA

Vikram B. Patel, MD, DABA, FIPP, DABIPP
Director
Pain Medicine
Phoenix Interventional Center for Advanced Learning
Algonquin, IL, USA

Nicholas Perry, BSc, MBBS, PhD
Specialist Registrar in Anaesthesia
Imperial School of Anaesthesia
London, United Kingdom

Thais O. Polanco, MD
Plastic and Reconstructive Surgery Service, Department of Surgery
Memorial Sloan Kettering Cancer Center
New York, NY, USA

Shannon M. Popovich, MD, CMQ
Associate Professor of Anesthesiology
Anesthesiology & Perioperative Medicine
The University of Texas MD Anderson Cancer Center
Houston, TX, USA

George Poulogiannis, BSc, MSc, MPhil, PhD
Team Leader in Signalling & Cancer Metabolism
Cancer Biology
Institute of Cancer Research
London, United Kingdom

Perez-Gonzalez Oscar Rafael, MD
Onco Anesthesiologist
Oncological Anesthesia
National Cancer Institute
Mexico City, Mexico;
Professor
Anesthesiology
Hospital General
Quintana Roo, Mexico

Sanketh Rampes, MBBS, MA (Cantab)
Doctor
Faculty of Medicine & Life Sciences
King's College London
London, United Kingdom

Krithika S. Rao, MBBS, MD
Assistant Professor
Department of Palliative Medicine and Supportive Care
Kasturba Medical College, Manipal Manipal Academy of Higher Education
Manipal, Karnataka, India

Sally Radelat Raty, MD, MHA
Professor
Anesthesiology and Perioperative Medicine
The University of Texas MD Anderson Cancer Center
Houston, TX, USA

Shehla Razvi, MD
Assistant Professor
Pediatric Critical Care
The University of Texas MD Anderson Cancer Center
Houston, TX, USA

Natasha Reid, PhD, GradCert ClinEpi, BSc
Research Fellow
Centre for Health Services Research
The University of Queensland
Brisbane, Queensland, Australia

Itay Ricon-Becker, MA
Neuroimmunology Research Unit
School of Psychological Sciences
Tel-Aviv University
Tel-Aviv, Israel

Bernhard J. Riedel, MD, MBA, PhD
Professor
Anesthesiology, Perioperative and Pain Medicine
Peter MacCallum Cancer Centre
Melbourne, Victoria, Australia

Emily B. Roarty, PhD
Associate Vice President
Strategy and Impact
The University of Texas MD Anderson Cancer Center
Houston, TX, USA

Maria Alma Rodriguez, MD
Director, Survivorship Programs
Office of the Chief Medical Officer
The University of Texas MD Anderson Cancer Center
Professor
Lymphoma and Myeloma
The University of Texas MD Anderson Cancer Center
Houston, TX, USA

Suzanne Russo, MD
Clinical Associate Professor
Case Western Reserve University School of Medicine
University Hospitals of Cleveland
Cleveland, OH, USA

Iqira Saeed, BPharm (hons)
Student
School of Pharmacy
University of Queensland
Brisbane, Queensland, Australia

Sunil K. Sahai, MD, FAAP, FACP, SFHM
Professor & Division Chief – General Medicine
Department of Internal Medicine
The University of Texas Medical Branch
Galveston, TX, USA

Naveen Salins, MD
Professor
Palliative Medicine and Supportive Care
Kasturba Medical College
Manipal, Karnataka, India

Niranjan Sathianathen, MD
Urology Registrar
Urology
Peter MacCallum Cancer Centre
Melbourne, Victoria, Australia

Shveta Seth, BPT, MPT
Department of Onco-Anaesthesia and Palliative Medicine, Dr. B. R. Ambedkar Institute Rotary Cancer Hospital, AIIMS
New Delhi, India

Paul N. Shaw, BSc(Hons), PhD
Associate Dean (Academic)
Faculty of Medicine
The University of Queensland
Brisbane, Queensland, Australia

Aislinn Sherwin, MSc, BSc, MD, BCh, BAO, FCAI, MCAI
Anaesthesiology Fellow
Department of Anaesthesia and Pain Medicine
Mater Misericordiae University Hospital
Dublin, Ireland

Sanjay Shete, PhD
Betty B. Marcus Chair in Cancer Prevention
Professor of Biostatistics and Epidemiology
Deputy Division Head, Cancer Prevention and Population Sciences
The University of Texas MD Anderson Cancer Center,
Houston, TX, USA

Qiuling Shi, MD, PhD
Professor
School of Public Health and Management
Chongqing Medical University
Chongqing, China

Conor Shields, BSc, MD, FRCSI
Professor
Surgery
Mater Misericordiae University Hospital
Dublin, Ireland

Jo-Lynn Tan, MD
Urology Registrar
Urology
St Vincent's Hospital Melbourne
Melbourne, Victoria, Australia

Hanae K. Tokita, MD, FASA
Director of Anesthesia
Josie Robertson Surgery Center;
Associate Attending
Department of Anesthesiology & Critical Care Medicine
Memorial Sloan Kettering Cancer Center
New York, NY, USA

Tom Wall, FCAI, MRCPI, FJFICMI
Research Fellow
Department of Anaesthesiology and Perioperative Medicine
Mater Misericordiae University Hospital
Dublin, Ireland;
Clinical Lecturer
School of Medicine
University College Dublin
Dublin, Ireland

Ronald S. Walters, MD, MBA, MHA, MS
Associate Head
Institute Cancer Care Innovation
The University of Texas MD Anderson Cancer Center
Houston, TX, USA

Xin Shelley Wang, MD, MPH
Professor
Department of Symptom Research
The University of Texas MD Anderson Cancer Center
Houston, TX, USA

Phil Ward, MBBS, MRCP, FRCA, FFICM
Consultant in Intensive Care Medicine & Anaesthesia
Intensive Care
University College London Hospitals NHS Foundation Trust
London, United Kingdom

Anna Louise Waylen, BMedSci, FANZCA
Specialist Anaesthetist
Auckland City Hospital
Auckland, New Zealand

Laurence Weinberg, MBBCH, BSc, MRCP, FANZCA, DPCritCareEcho, MD
Assistant Professor
Anaesthesia
Austin Health
Melbourne, Victoria, Australia

Matthias Wilhelm Wichmann, MD, FRACS
Assistant Professor
Rural School of Medicine
Flinders University
Adelaide, South Australia, Australia;
Assistant Professor
Division of Surgery – The Queen Elizabeth Hospital
University of Adelaide
Adelaide, South Australia, Australia;
Consultant General Surgeon
General Surgery
Mount Gambier General Hospital
Mount Gambier, South Australia, Australia

Timothy Wigmore, BM, BCh, MA, FRCA, FFICM, FCICM
Consultant
Anaesthesia and Intensive Care
The Royal Marsden
London, United Kingdom

Syed Wamique Yusuf, MBBS, FACC, FRCPI
Professor
Department of Cardiology
The University of Texas MD Anderson Cancer Center
Houston, TX, USA

Wafik Zaky, MBBCh
Associate Professor
Pediatric
The University of Texas MD Anderson Cancer Center
Houston, TX, USA

Gang Zheng, MD
Faculty Anesthesiologist, & Certification of American Board of Anesthesiology (ABA)
Professor
Anesthesiology & Preoperative Medicine
The University of Texas MD Anderson Cancer Center
Houston, TX, USA

Preface

Cancer is a major global public health concern that affects all citizens and communities across the world. The incidence of cancer is increasing rapidly due to environmental factors, lifestyle and behavioral choices, and longer life expectancies. Globally, the incidence of cancer is predicted to increase by 50% by the year 2030; and during the same period, cancer-related mortality is projected to increase by 60% to 13.1 million deaths worldwide. This increasing trend in cancer-related mortality is despite a slow but steady decline in cancer-related death rates since the early 1990s in the United States and the western world. This dichotomy is mainly due to the increasing incidence of cancer and cancer-related mortality in the developing world and the overall increase in global population, particularly the relatively marked increase in the population over the age of 60 years.

There are more than 20 million cancer survivors currently living in the United States alone. Of the nearly 20 million new cancer cases worldwide in 2021, over 80% of cases will need surgery, some several times as curative resection is essential for global cancer control, particularly for those with solid tumors. It is estimated that by 2030, over 45 million surgical procedures will be needed globally for cancer control. Furthermore, patients with cancer and cancer survivors alike will continue to need the services of our specialty in the perioperative setting well beyond their primary cancer care. Some of the unique challenges for clinicians managing these patients in the perioperative setting include the need to understand the epidemiology, biology, and rapidly evolving therapeutics of cancer, as well as their effects on the physiologic and functional status of patients. The critical care and pain management needs of this patient population are also unique. Therefore, it is essential for anesthesiologists, surgeons, nurses, perioperative (e.g., ICU, pain, palliative), and integrative medicine specialists to understand and master these fields.

Our understanding of perioperative factors that contribute to tumor spread and recurrence (from minimal residual disease, circulating tumor cells, or micro metastatic disease) is rapidly evolving with the potential to influence long-term cancer outcomes positively. The perioperative period is a pathophysiological state characterized by intense emotional and physiological (surgical) stress, pain, inflammation, immune suppression, negative nitrogen balance, and insulin resistance. The combined effect of this neuroinflammatory signaling in the perioperative period can lead to immune suppression and altered immune responses, a vital prerequisite for wound healing and recovery from surgery. However, these pathways are also an integral component of the inflammatory-immune responses leading to an immunosuppressive microenvironment in tumor stromal tissue, particularly in the presence of postoperative complications. In the surgical cancer patient, effective perioperative strategies should, therefore, not only aim to provide effective anesthesia and analgesia, minimize preventable complications and enhance functional recovery, but also attenuate the surgical stress response to positively modulate the inflammatory-immune response for improved oncological outcomes.

This unique multidisciplinary textbook on "Perioperative Care of the Cancer Patient" highlights key topics of cancer epidemiology, cancer biology, cancer therapeutics and their effects on the physiologic and functional status of patients, and the unique challenges of cancer patients and survivors in the perioperative/periprocedural setting, which directly influence patient outcomes. Finally, special considerations of childhood cancers; unique intensive care needs of patients with cancer; cancer pain management; rehabilitative, palliative care, and integrative medicine interventions in the cancer patient; value proposition; and research opportunities and challenges in perioperative cancer care are also addressed. Each of the chapters is authored by international experts in the field and discusses the current understanding and practices, current controversies and unanswered questions, and the direction for future studies. This exercise, we hope, will highlight the need for ongoing scientific study on key areas to further enhance perioperative and periprocedural care of our patients with cancer and cancer survivors.

We believe this is an exciting time for Anesthesiology and Perioperative Medicine, as we continue to partner with our oncology, internist, intensivist, pain management, rehabilitative-palliative care-integrative medicine specialists, proceduralist colleagues, and research teams to break down silos and work together as "one team" to improve postoperative outcomes, enhance the quality of recovery and life for our patients, and offer improved disease-free survival. This patient-centered, multidisciplinary, disease-focused, value-based approach should enhance the perioperative experience and disease-free survival for our patients with cancer while reducing health care costs.

We would like to express our sincere gratitude to the international panel of authors who contributed to this important educational initiative despite the challenges of the COVID-19 pandemic. Our sincere thanks to the publishing team for their patience and for working with us through the delays and challenges related to COVID-19.

Sincerely,

Carin A. Hagberg, Vijaya N. R. Gottumukkala,
Bernhard J. Riedel, Joseph L. Nates, Donal J. Buggy

Contents

Section 1: Basic Principles (Epidemiology; Cancer Biology; Overview of Cancer Therapies)

Section 2: Inflammatory-Immune Responses, Perioperative Period, and Cancer Outcomes

Section 3: Perioperative/Periprocedural Care in the Cancer Patient

Section 4: Acute Postoperative and Intensive Care of the Cancer Patient

SECTION 1

Basic Principles (Epidemiology; Cancer Biology; Overview of Cancer Therapies)

1

Cancer Epidemiology, Prevention, and Survivorship

KAREN COLBERT MARESSO, KAREN BASEN-ENGQUIST, AND ERNEST HAWK

Introduction

Cancer epidemiology provides the tools and methods to understand the cancer problem in any given population, from the local level up to the global level. Incidence, prevalence, and mortality are the most commonly used measures to assess the cancer burden. Examining temporal trends in these measures or comparison of these measures between states, regions, or countries can uncover important causes of cancer. The study of cancer from an epidemiological perspective has uncovered numerous causes of cancer and has hence paved the way towards prevention and early detection. Perhaps the most well-known accomplishment of cancer epidemiology was the identification of tobacco as a cause of lung cancer in 1964.[1] This finding revolutionized our understanding of cancer, as it was the first time that a common, modifiable behavior—tobacco smoking—was shown to result in cancer, and subsequently led to the development and implementation of a wide range of preventive measures throughout the second half of the 20th century that have demonstrably reduced both the use of tobacco and deaths from lung cancer.[2,3] This chapter reviews and summarizes the latest data on the most basic measures of the global cancer burden and then briefly describes cancer prevention and early detection recommendations, as well as survivorship care.

Cancer Epidemiology

Cancer incidence and *mortality* are defined as the number of new cancer cases and deaths, respectively, that occur in a given population over a specified time period. The selection of the time period is arbitrary, although often these measures are expressed as an absolute number of new cases or deaths per year. While this may be helpful for planning health services in a given population, this simplified expression does not provide risk information, and it does not allow for comparisons of incidence and mortality to be made among different populations. For these uses, incidence and mortality are generally expressed as a rate or proportion of the number of new cancer cases or deaths over the number of persons at risk of developing or dying from cancer during a specified time period per 1000, 10,000, or 100,000 individuals. Often, incidence and mortality will be reported as an "age-standardized rate" (ASR) to facilitate comparisons among populations that have different age distributions.

The number of new cancer cases and deaths are captured by population-based cancer registries oriented toward a geographic or geopolitical area, such as a country, although these registries typically capture just a small proportion of the global population. Coverage also varies by country. Population coverage is typically greater for mortality than for incidence. Sometimes incidence and mortality rates are estimated in cohort studies. Cancer incidence and reporting can be influenced by the screening practices, diagnostic intensity, and primary prevention programs in the population under study. Cancer mortality data are influenced by the adequacy of death certification, including autopsy rates, by changes in cancer treatment effectiveness, and by the availability of prevention programs in the population under study.

Cancer prevalence is defined as the number of cancer cases in a population at a specific point in time over the number of persons in the population at that time point. Unlike the incidence rate, prevalence is not a measure of cancer risk. Nevertheless, it can be useful for planning health services. Ascertaining the prevalence of cancer can be done through population-based cancer registration or estimated from cross-sectional studies. Determinants of cancer prevalence include the incidence and prognosis of the cancer in question, as well as mortality from other competing causes.

Cancer survival is defined as the proportion of cancer patients surviving for a specified time after diagnosis. Despite numerous limitations, it is considered the best available measure for evaluating the effectiveness of cancer treatments. Survival is influenced by the natural history of the disease, the stage at diagnosis, and therapeutic efficacy. Survival data require long-term follow up of large number of patients, are sensitive to both the misclassification of the cause of death and to lead-time bias, and provide no insight into the quality of life lived. There are various measures of survival, each serving a different purpose and each with its own limitations. Observed survival is the probability of surviving for a specific time period, generally starting at the date of cancer diagnosis, and considers all causes of death. Corrected or cause-specific cancer survival excludes deaths due to causes other than the cancer of interest and therefore is a more valid estimate of the excess death due to a cancer. Relative cancer survival compares the observed survival of a group of cancer patients to the expected survival of a group from the general population with the same age and sex distribution.

Cancer Burden in the World

Cancer is a leading cause of death around the world. In 2018, there were an estimated 18.1 million (including non-melanoma skin cancer) new cancer cases and 9.6 million (including non-melanoma skin cancer) cancer deaths.[4] Fig. 1.1 illustrates the distribution of these cases and deaths among the 10 most common cancers in 2018. Lung cancer is the most commonly diagnosed cancer worldwide, accounting for nearly 12% of all cancer cases in men and women combined. Unsurprisingly, it is also the leading cause of global cancer mortality, accounting for just over 18% of all cancer deaths. Lung, breast, colorectal, and prostate are the top four most common cancers, accounting for a combined 40.5% of all new cases worldwide. Lung, colorectal, stomach, and liver are the top four causes of cancer mortality, accounting for a combined 44% of global cancer deaths. Of note is the significant burden of liver and stomach cancer mortality among men. Also notable, cervical cancer, which is almost entirely preventable through cervical screening and HPV vaccination, remains a leading cause of cancer and cancer death among women.

Worldwide, men experience higher cancer incidence and mortality than women. Incidence for all cancers combined is 20% higher in men (218.6 vs. 182.6 per 100,000), and all-site mortality is 50% higher in men (122.7 vs. 83.1 per 100,000).[4] There is substantial variation in these rates by world region. This variation reflects differences in risk factor exposures and in the availability of preventive, early detection, and treatment resources that exist across populations. In turn, risk factor exposures and access to treatment and resources are driven by a country's level of socioeconomic development, or its human development index (HDI), a composite measure of income, education, and life expectancy.[4] Both incidence and mortality are higher in high-income countries than in lower-income countries. Furthermore, in countries with a low HDI, infection-related cancers, such as cervical, stomach, and liver predominate. As a country transitions to higher levels of HDI, infection-related cancers typically decrease and lifestyle-related cancers, such as breast and colorectal, emerge.

Figs. 1.2 and 1.3 highlight the variation in cancer incidence and mortality around the world. A few patterns can be discerned from these maps. First, cancer incidence varies more for men than for women. Breast cancer was the top cancer in women in at least 154 countries, while cervical cancer was the most common cancer in 28 countries, mainly those in sub-Saharan Africa. Among men, there are 10 different cancers that claim the top spot across 185 countries. Second, cancer mortality varies more than cancer incidence. Among women, cervical cancer is the leading cause of cancer mortality in sub-Saharan Africa, while lung cancer leads cancer mortality in more developed countries, such as the United States and Canada, northern and eastern Europe, Australia, and China. Stomach cancer mortality predominates in parts of South America and liver cancer mortality predominates in Mongolia, Cambodia, and Guatemala. Among men, stomach cancer is the leading cause of cancer mortality in the Middle East and parts of South America, while liver cancer is the leading cause of cancer mortality in Egypt, parts of western Africa and southeast Asia. Deaths due to lip and oral cancer are the most common type of cancer mortality in India and Pakistan, and Kaposi sarcoma and leukemia lead cancer mortality in eastern and southern Africa.

Data from both high- and low-income countries suggest that mortality from cancer has decreased globally by approximately 1% annually between 2000 and 2010.[5] Data from various regional studies and from Globocan confirm this. While declines have been observed in most countries for the most common cancers (lung [men only], breast, prostate, stomach, colorectal, and uterine), mortality rates are rising for liver cancer, and lung cancer in women, in many countries.

Projections from Globocan indicate that cancer incidence and mortality will rise rapidly worldwide over the next few decades due to the aging and growth of the population. By 2040, it is projected that there will be nearly 30 million new cases of cancer, with nearly 17 million deaths, occurring annually. Yet, many of these cases and deaths are preventable with knowledge we already have. However, additional investment in both research and cancer control, particularly in low- and middle-income countries, is urgently needed to address the current and even greater future burden of cancer.

Cancer Prevention and Early Detection

An estimated one-third to one-half of cancer occurring today in western (or "westernized") populations is preventable through adoption of healthy lifestyles,[6] including avoidance of known risk factors and adherence to screening recommendations.

Lifestyle Prevention

Established modifiable lifestyle risk factors for cancer around the world are tobacco (including exposure to secondhand smoke); excess body weight; alcohol intake; consumption of red and processed meats; low consumption of fruits, vegetables, dietary fiber, and dietary calcium; physical inactivity; ultraviolet radiation (including tanning beds); and six cancer-associated infections (HIV, HPV, HBV, HCV, *H. pylori*, and HHV8). Recent data analyzed and published by the American Cancer Society suggest that as much as 42% of

Both Genders

A

Incidence

Mortality

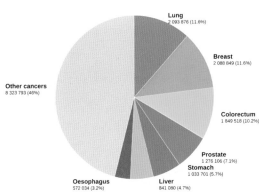

Lung
2 093 876 (11.6%)
Breast
2 088 849 (11.6%)
Colorectum
1 849 518 (10.2%)
Prostate
1 276 106 (7.1%)
Stomach
1 033 701 (5.7%)
Liver
841 080 (4.7%)
Oesophagus
572 034 (3.2%)
Other cancers
8 323 793 (46%)

Total : 18 078 957

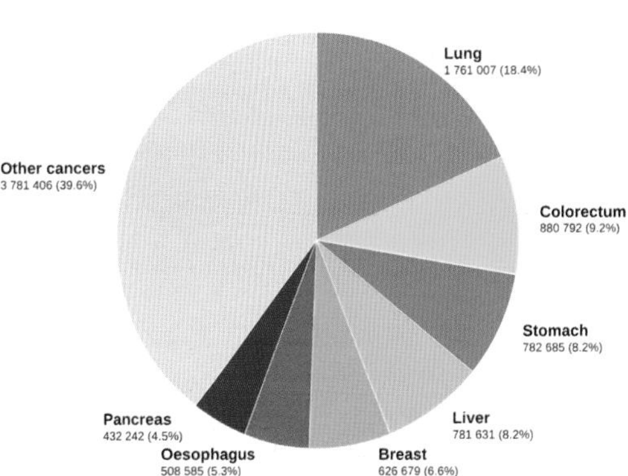

Total : 9 555 027

Females

B

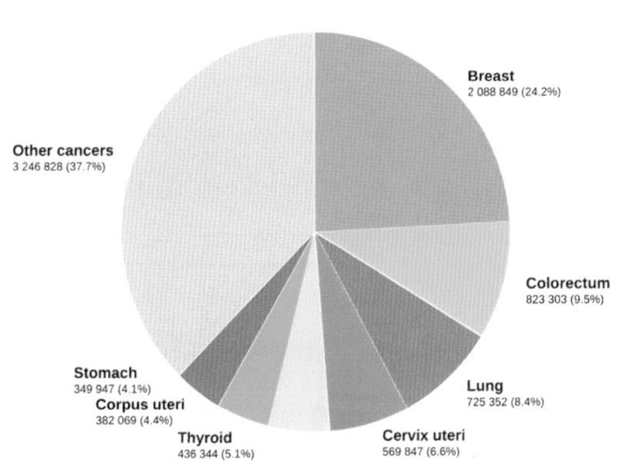

Total : 8 622 539

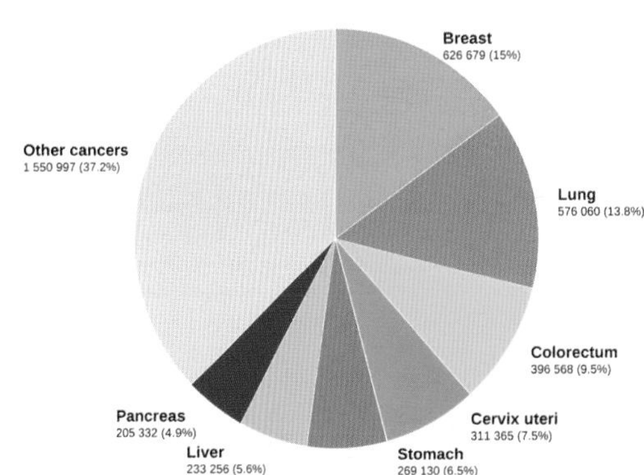

Total : 4 169 387

Males

C

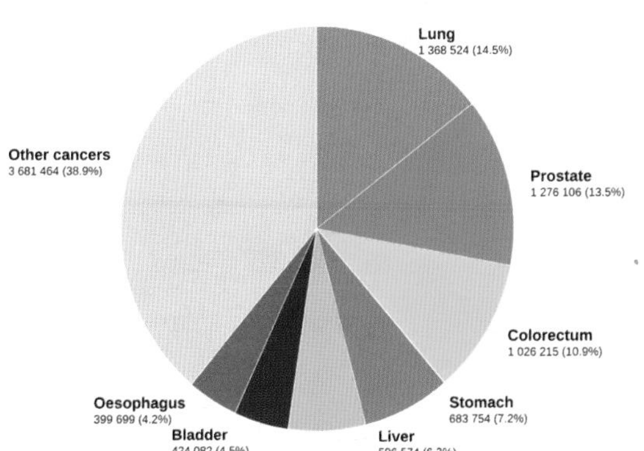

Total : 9 456 418

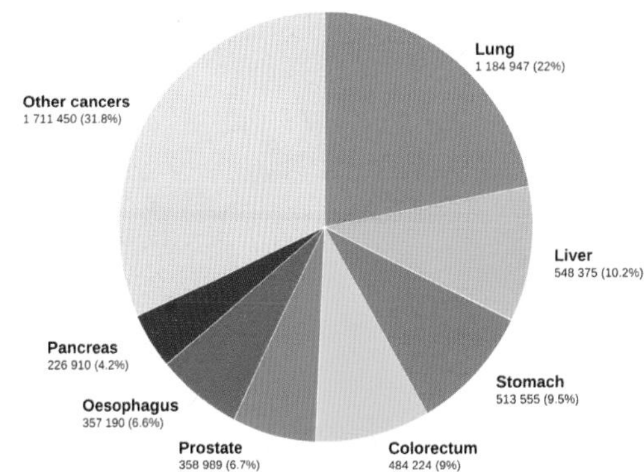

Total : 5 385 640

• **Fig. 1.1** Distribution of incidence (*left*) and mortality (*right*) by cancer site for the top 10 most common cancers worldwide by (A) both sexes combined, (B) females, and (C) males. Non-melanoma skin cancer is included in the "Other" category. (Source: Globocan 2018.)

A

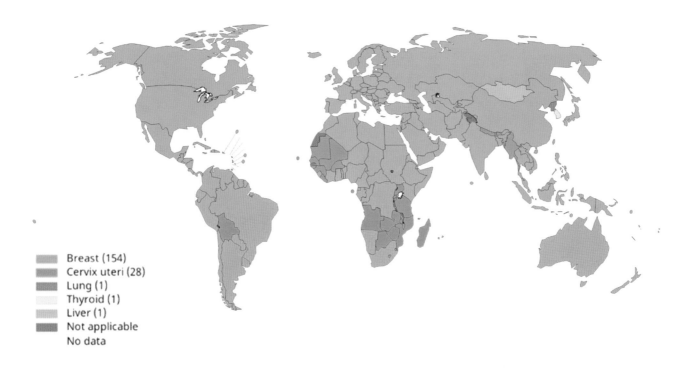

B

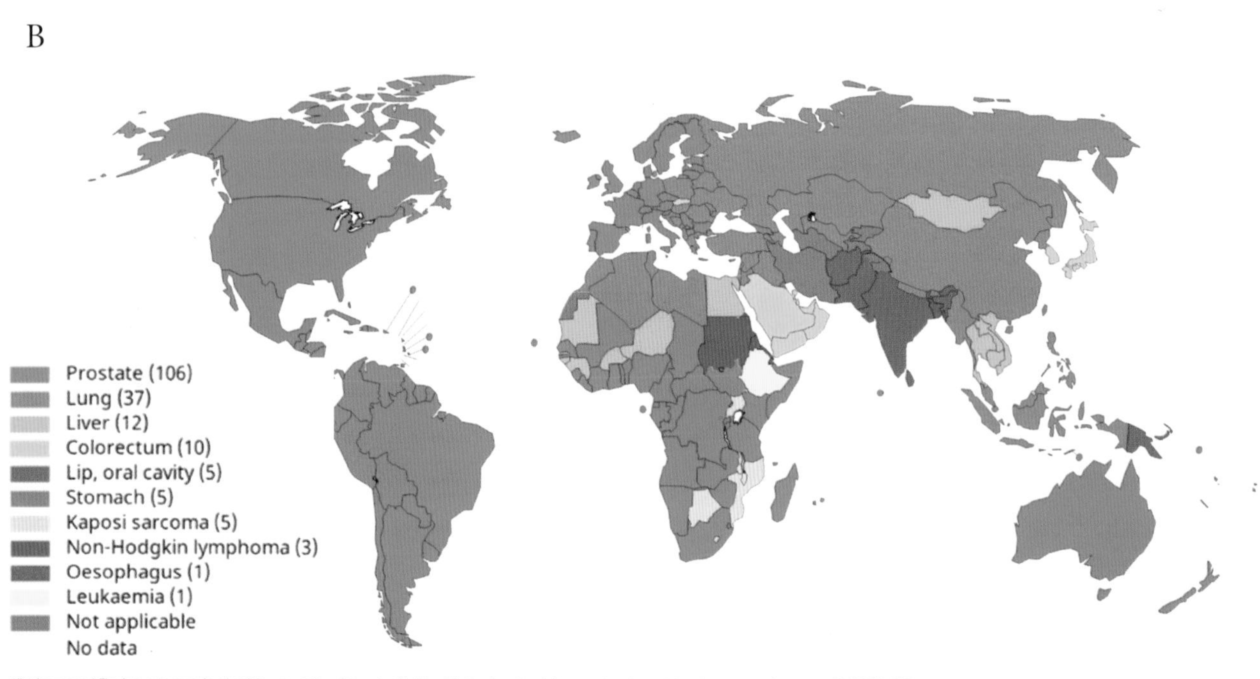

Data source: GLOBOCAN 2018
Graph production: IARC
(http://gco.iarc.fr/today)
World Health Organization

• **Fig. 1.2** Map illustrating the most common cancers by country for (A) females and (B) males. The number of countries included in each cancer site is shown in the legend. (Source: Globocan 2018.)

A

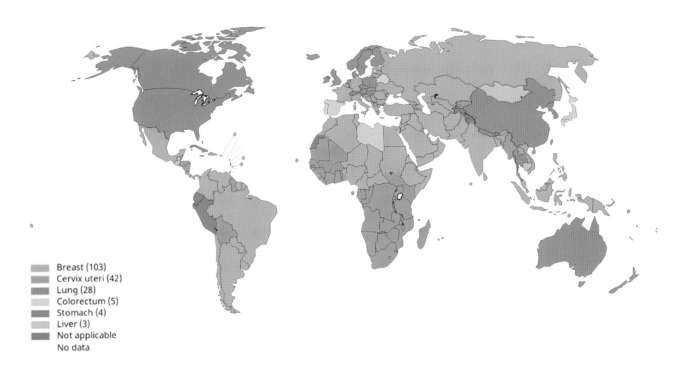

B

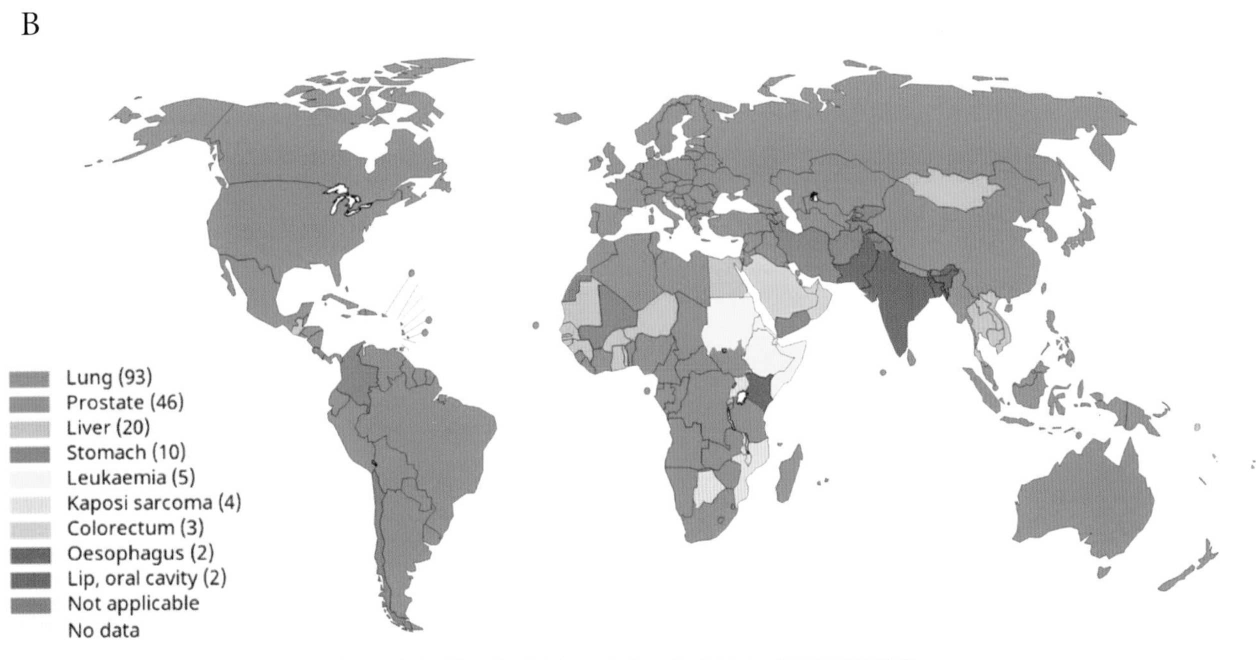

Data source: GLOBOCAN 2018
Graph production: IARC
(http://gco.iarc.fr/today)
World Health Organization

• **Fig. 1.3** Map illustrating the most common cause of cancer mortality by country for (A) females and (B) males. The number of countries included in each cancer site is shown in the legend. (Source: Globocan 2018.)

cancer cases and 45% of cancer deaths in the United States are attributable to the above modifiable risk factors.[7] While the proportions of cancer cases and deaths attributable to any one or a combination of risk factors vary around the world as the prevalence of risk factors varies geographically, a significant proportion of cancer can be prevented through personal lifestyle choices.

Despite the well-established harms of tobacco, it continues to be the predominant cancer risk factor throughout much of the world. In 2017, tobacco accounted for nearly one-quarter of all cancer deaths globally.[8] Infectious agents also remain an important cause of cancer in many parts of the world. HPV in sub-Saharan Africa is a particular problem, where its prevalence is estimated at 21% among women.[8] Obesity, already an epidemic in high-income countries, is rapidly growing in prevalence around the world as low- and middle-income countries transition to higher levels of economic development and increasingly adopt "westernized" lifestyles.

Evidence-based comprehensive tobacco control strategies have been shown to reduce the prevalence of tobacco use and lead to reductions in the incidence and mortality of lung cancer.[3] Such strategies include antitobacco mass media campaigns, tobacco taxation, marketing bans and plain packaging, smoke-free policies to protect nonsmokers, and promoting and ensuring access to cessation resources (e.g., through national quit lines). Many middle- and low-income countries struggle to fund and implement comprehensive tobacco control programs. The World Health Organization's Framework Convention on Tobacco Control (FCTC) and MPOWER measures provide a foundation for these countries to implement effective tobacco control interventions. Approximately 63% of the world's population is now covered by at least one MPOWER tobacco control measure.[9] Newer tobacco products, such as electronic cigarettes (i.e., e-cigs), will need to be evaluated for their short- and long-term health effects but may represent a threat to decades of progress on controlling the tobacco epidemic. Prophylaxis against cancer-associated infectious agents, when available, can lead to significantly improved cancer outcomes. Administration of the HPV vaccine through national programs has resulted in significantly reduced risks of precancerous cervical lesions.[10] Unfortunately, uptake of the vaccine is extremely low in most countries where the infection is highly prevalent.[8] And while obesity is rising around the globe, there are few evidence-based strategies to mitigate its negative health effects, including cancer. Eating a plant-based diet, limiting sedentary activities, and moving more are important ways to maintain a healthy weight throughout life.

Both the American Cancer Society (ACS)[11] and the World Cancer Research Fund (WCRF)[12] have published cancer prevention recommendations for nutrition and physical activity that are based on regularly updated reviews of the evidence (Table 1.1). These recommendations are in addition to avoiding tobacco, preventing overexposure to UV radiation, and adhering to age-appropriate cancer screening and vaccination schedules. Large observational studies[13,14]

TABLE 1.1 ACS (2020) and WCRF (2018) Cancer Prevention Recommendations for Nutrition and Physical Activity

ACS	WCRF
Achieve and maintain a healthy weight throughout life.	Be a healthy weight.
Be physically active (Adults: 150-300 minutes of moderate-intensity or 75-150 minutes of vigorous-intensity activity each week. Reaching or exceeding the upper limit of 300 minutes is ideal).	Be physically active.
Follow a healthy eating pattern at all ages. (Include foods that are high in nutrients, a variety of vegetables and fruits, and whole grains. Limit red and processed meats, sugar-sweetened beverages, highly processed foods and refined grain products).	Eat a diet rich in wholegrains, vegetables, fruit and beans. Limit consumption of red and processed meats, fast foods, other processed foods high in fat, starches or sugars. Limit consumption of sugar sweetened drinks.
It is best not to drink alcohol. (People who choose to drink alcohol should have no more than 1 drink per day for women or 2 drinks per day for men).	Limit alcohol consumption.
	Do not use supplements for cancer prevention. For mothers: breastfeed your baby, if you can. After a cancer diagnosis, follow each of these recommendations regarding healthy lifestyles, if you can.

ACS: Reprinted by the permission of the American Cancer Society, Inc. www.cancer.org. *WCRF:* This material has been reproduced from the World Cancer Research Fund/American Institute for Cancer Research. Diet, Nutrition, Physical Activity and Cancer: a Global Perspective. Continuous Update Project Expert Report 2018. Available at dietandcancerreport.org.

ACS, American Cancer Society; *WCRF*, World Cancer Research Fund.

ACS recommendations available at: https://www.cancer.org/healthy/eat-healthy-get-active/acs-guidelines-nutrition-physical-activity-cancer-prevention/guidelines.html

WCRF recommendations available at: dietandcancerreport.org.

and a systematic review[15] indicate that following the ACS or WCRF cancer prevention recommendations in a comprehensive manner significantly reduces the risks of developing and dying from cancer. Because lifestyle choices are influenced by one's background and surrounding physical and social environment, implementation of evidence-based cancer control strategies that seek to make the healthy choice the default choice through policy, education, and delivery of community-based clinical services is greatly needed to prevent more cancers.

Screening/Early Detection

The goal of cancer screening is to detect cancer early, before symptoms occur, when it is more easily treated. Wilson and Junger first published several criteria for a screening test to be useful.[16] The three primary criteria are (1) the test must detect the disease earlier than routine methods, (2) earlier treatment must lead to improved outcomes, and (3) the benefits of screening must be greater than the risks of any subsequent diagnostic and therapeutic treatments. Because screening programs are resource-intensive and require extensive health services infrastructure, they should only be undertaken when their efficacy has been clearly demonstrated, optimally through well-designed randomized controlled trials (RCTs). When RCTs are not available or feasible, as in the case of colonoscopies for colorectal cancer screening, observational data and/or meta-analyses are often relied upon as evidence of screening effectiveness. The ideal measure of the efficacy of a screening test is a reduction in cancer mortality among those being screened in comparison with those who do not undergo screening. Evaluations of screening tests may suffer from self-selection bias (i.e., the tendency for healthier individuals to attend screening exams compared with those who are less healthy), lead time bias (i.e., the perceived increase in survival time attributed to a screening test which accelerates the time of diagnosis compared with the onset of a symptomatic presentation, but without actually lengthening the time to cancer mortality), and length time bias (i.e., slower-growing cancers are more likely to be detected by screening than faster-growing, more aggressive cancers since they have a longer detectable preclinical phase), which can lead to over-diagnosis and over-treatment. Over-diagnosis is finding cancers that would never become clinically relevant in an individual's lifetime, and over-treatment is the treatment of those cancers with the potential for causing important side effects. This has been an issue mainly in breast and prostate cancer screening.

Implementation of screening programs for common cancers, specifically cervical, breast, prostate, lung, and colorectal, have been shown to reduce the mortality associated with these cancers. However, implementation of these tests has been inconsistent around the world, and screening programs vary greatly among countries in the manner in which they are conducted. Some countries such as Australia, Finland, and the UK that can systematically call and recall target populations offer organized screening programs on a national level. Other countries without this ability, like the United States, France, and Germany have unorganized or opportunistic screening programs in place, which reach fractions of the recommended populations.

As lung cancer is the number one cause of cancer and cancer death worldwide, there has been long-standing interest in developing a screening test for this highly prevalent and lethal cancer. In 2011, the National Lung Screening Trial demonstrated an approximate 20% reduction in lung-cancer mortality in heavy smokers through the annual use of low-dose computed tomography (LDCT).[17] More recently, the NELSON trial results suggest an even greater mortality benefit of 26% in high-risk men and 61% in high-risk women.[18] However, concerns over the potentially high false-positive rate of the test provide justification for the application of informative risk prediction models to identify those who would most benefit from LDCT screening for early detection while minimizing false positives. This is an active area of research in lung cancer screening. Screening in the United States is opportunistic and rates are extremely low at 3.9% (in 2015).[19] No country to date has implemented an organized lung cancer screening program, although many countries in Europe and east Asia have started small trials or regional demonstration projects to determine the feasibility of lung screening in their respective countries.[20]

Screening for cervical cancer through use of the pap smear is one of the most successful tests ever offered in medicine, as observational data show that it has resulted in decreases of cervical cancer incidence and mortality on the order of 75%–90% in high-income countries where large-scale, population-based cervical screening programs have been in effect since the middle of the 20th century.[21] Much of the developing world has yet to see such cervical screening programs implemented due to low availability of the health services resources needed for screening, follow up, and subsequent treatment for screen positives. Hence, cervical cancer continues to be a leading cause of cancer and cancer death in areas such as sub-Saharan Africa. The HPV test is beginning to replace the pap smear for cervical screening. Several RCTs demonstrate that HPV testing is superior to pap testing in reducing incidence of cervical precancers and cancers.[22] Although not yet adopted in the United States, primary HPV testing for cervical screening has already been implemented in some countries such as Australia and the Netherlands or is in the process of being implemented in others throughout Europe. Visual inspection with ascetic acid (VIA) was shown to result in a 31% mortality reduction among screened women in India in a large RCT[23] and can be offered in low-resource settings when primary HPV testing is unavailable.[24] HPV vaccination is an important component of cervical cancer prevention, but does not remove the need for routine cervical cancer screening according to age and clinical history.

Systematic reviews of RCTs of screening mammography have demonstrated an approximate 20% mortality reduction in women ages 40–74 years,[25,26] although most of the RCTs were initiated prior to or in the early 1980s and so are limited by the quality of mammography available at the time the trials were conducted, with many cancers having to be 1 cm or greater to be detected. Observational data are believed to better reflect contemporary screening practices in which the detection of sub-centimeter tumors is commonplace. These data suggest a 48% reduction in breast cancer mortality with modern screening mammography.[27] This is supported by modeling studies that estimate a 29%–54% mortality reduction.[28] Although the age to start screening (40 vs. 50 years) and the frequency with which to screen (annual vs. biennial) may differ by the organization making the recommendation, all agree that there is a mortality benefit to beginning screening at age 40 years and that annual screening results in fewer breast cancer deaths than does biennial screening. Large-scale breast cancer screening programs relying upon mammography are again limited to higher-income countries in North and South America, Europe, Australia, and New Zealand. Although evidence supporting the use of clinical breast examination alone for screening is mixed, it is encouraged in specific situations in basic- and limited-resource settings.[29]

Numerous tests exist for colorectal cancer screening. The gold standard test is colonoscopy because of its high sensitivity and specificity for the identification of adenomas and its ability to both diagnose and reduce risks associated with biopsied precancerous lesions. Although there is no evidence from RCTs supporting the use of colonoscopy, there is observational evidence from the Nurses' Health Study and the Health Professionals Follow-up Study demonstrating a 68% reduction in colorectal cancer mortality[30] Flexible sigmoidoscopy, while not typically offered in the United States, is offered in other countries and is supported by RCTs showing a 26%–31% reduction in colorectal cancer mortality.[31,32] Use of guaic-based stool tests is supported by several RCTs, with mortality reductions of up to 32%. Stool-based fecal immunohistochemical tests (FIT) are more accurate than the guaic-based stool tests although RCT evidence of any mortality benefit associated with their use is lacking. A FIT test that includes DNA markers is also available, but again, data supporting a mortality benefit are lacking. Two newer screening tests are virtual colonoscopy (CT [computed tomography] colonography) and a blood test that detects circulating methylated *SEPT9* DNA, a marker for colorectal cancer.[33] These tests are still evolving and the balance between benefits and harms for each of these tests remains unclear. As with cervical and breast cancer screening, large-scale colorectal cancer screening programs are limited to high-income countries.

Screening for prostate cancer with the prostate-specific antigen (PSA) test has been highly controversial and recommendations for the test have changed repeatedly. An initial RCT conducted in the United States did not suggest a mortality benefit but results were called into question when it was determined that there was a high rate of PSA testing in the control arm of the trial.[34,35] A second trial in Europe did find a significant 20% reduction in prostate-cancer mortality as a result of PSA screening.[36] However, there was a high risk of over-diagnosis of prostate cancer in subjects lacking clinical symptoms. And while the 12- to 14-year follow up results from the Swedish and Netherlands sites of the ERSPC trial found enhanced benefit of PSA screening,[37] the 12- to 15-year follow-up results from the Finland and Spanish sites failed to demonstrate significant effect on prostate-cancer mortality.[38,39] The latest evidence suggests that the benefits and harms of screening are more closely matched than previously thought.[40] Consequently, most organizations now recommend individualized decision-making for men ages 55–69 years.

Going forward, genomic- and proteomic-based approaches have the potential to refine risk assessment and stratification, allowing for more tailored screening and early detection strategies.[41] However, the use of such approaches is still in its early stages.

Chemoprevention

Cancer chemoprevention is the use of drugs, vaccines, and natural compounds to inhibit, reverse, or delay the onset of carcinogenesis.[42] This approach may also be referred to as molecular prevention,[43] or in the case of established precancers, cancer interception.[44] Table 1.2 lists medications that have been FDA-approved for the treatment of precancerous lesions and/or cancer risk reduction. Almost half of the agents are for treatment of precancerous skin lesions (i.e., actinic or solar keratosis). This is due, at least in part, to the accessibility and visibility of the target organ. Tamoxifen, approved for reducing the risk of invasive breast cancer, was initially approved for use in advanced breast cancer. Its use in women at high risk of breast cancer nearly halves the risk of invasive disease.[45] Despite this, uptake of the drug among eligible women has been poor due to concerns over potential toxicity. Celecoxib, a nonsteroidal antiinflammatory (NSAID), was approved to reduce the number of colorectal adenomas in adults at very high risk of colorectal cancer due to familial adenomatous polyposis (FAP). However, given concerns over reported cardiovascular toxicity associated with the use of celecoxib in RCTs at the time, the labeling indication was voluntarily withdrawn by Pfizer. Experiences with both tamoxifen and celecoxib highlight the importance of the balance between risks and benefits for preventive agents. Despite the early concerns with celecoxib, NSAIDs in general remain a promising class of agents for cancer chemoprevention and continue to be actively investigated for the prevention of colorectal and numerous other cancers. Aspirin is perhaps the most promising and well-studied NSAID. Aspirin has been shown to reduce the incidence and mortality of colorectal cancer in randomized trials of cardiovascular disease prevention.[46,47] While it has yet to be approved for general population use to prevent or reduce the risk of cancer, the United States Preventive Services Task Force (USPSTF) has recognized colorectal cancer prevention as a benefit of aspirin use in those aged 50–59 years who are at increased risk of cardiovascular disease.[48] Enhancing our

TABLE 1.2 **Approved Agents for the Treatment of Precancerous Lesions or Cancer Risk Reduction, 2019**

Agent	Targeted Cohort	Indication
Tamoxifen	Women with ductal carcinoma in situ (DCIS) following breast surgery and radiation	Reduce the risk of invasive breast cancer.
	Women at high risk for breast cancer	Reduce the incidence of breast cancer.
Raloxifene	Postmenopausal women at high risk for invasive breast cancer	Reduction in risk of invasive breast cancer.
Cervarix	Females aged 9–25 years	Prevention of the following, caused by HPV types 16 and 18: • cervical cancer • cervical intraepithelial neoplasia (CIN) grade 2 or worse and adenocarcinoma in situ (AIS) • CIN grade 1
Gardasil 9	Females aged 9–26 years	Prevention of the following diseases caused by HPV types included in the vaccine: • cervical, vulvar, vaginal, and anal cancer caused by types 16, 18, 31, 33, 45, 52, and 58 • genital warts caused by HPV types 6 and 11 And the following precancerous or dysplastic lesions caused by types 6, 11, 16, 18, 31, 33, 45, 52, and 58: • CIN grade 2/3 and cervical AIS • CIN grade 1 • vulvar intraepithelial neoplasia (VIN) grades 2 and 3 • vaginal intraepithelial neoplasia (VaIN) grades 2 and 3 • anal intraepithelial neoplasia (AIN) grades, 1, 2, and 3
Gardasil 9	Males aged 9–15 years	Prevention of following diseases caused by HPV types included in vaccine: • anal cancer caused by HPV types 16, 18, 31, 33, 45, 52, and 58 • genital warts caused by HPV types 6 and 11 And the following precancerous or dysplastic lesions caused by HPV types 6, 11, 16, 18, 31, 33, 45, 52, and 58: • AIN grades 1, 2, and 3
Photodynamic therapy (PDT) with Photofrin	Males and females with high-grade dysplasia in Barrett's esophagus.	Ablation of high-grade dysplasia (HGD) in Barrett's esophagus patients who do not undergo esophagectomy.
Celecoxib[a]	Males and females aged ≥18 years with familial adenomatous polyposis (FAP)	Reduction in the number of adenomatous colorectal polyps in FAP, as an adjunct to usual care (e.g., endoscopic surveillance, surgery).
Bacillus-Calmette-Guerin (BCG)	Males and females with *carcinoma in situ* (CIS) of the urinary bladder	Intravesical use in the treatment and prophylaxis of CIS of the urinary bladder and for the prophylaxis of primary or recurrent stage Ta and/or T1 papillary tumors following transurethral resection (TUR).
Valrubicin	Males and females with Bacillus-Calmette-Guerin (BCG)-refractory CIS	Intravesical therapy of BCG-refractory CIS of the urinary bladder in patients for whom immediate cystectomy would be associated with unacceptable morbidity or mortality.
Fluorouracil	Males and females with multiple actinic or solar keratosis	Topical treatment of multiple actinic or solar keratosis.
Diclofenac sodium	Males and females with actinic keratosis	Topical treatment of actinic keratosis.
PDT with 5-aminolevulinic acid	Males and females with actinic keratosis of the face or scalp	Topical treatment of minimally to moderately thick actinic keratosis of the face or scalp.
Masoprocol[b]	Males and females with actinic (solar) keratosis	Topical treatment of actinic keratosis.

Continued

TABLE 1.2 Approved Agents for the Treatment of Precancerous Lesions or Cancer Risk Reduction, 2019—cont'd

Agent	Targeted Cohort	Indication
Imiquimod	Immunocompetent adults	Topical treatment of clinically typical, nonhyperkeratotic, nonhypertrophic actinic keratosis on the face or scalp.
Ingenol mebutate	Those with actinic keratosis on the face, scalp, trunk and extremities	Topical treatment of actinic keratosis.

[a]*FDA* labeling voluntarily withdrawn by Pfizer; February, 2011.
[b]Withdrawn from US market; June, 1996.

understanding of the type, timing, and sequence of molecular changes that underlie the development and progression of precancerous lesions, as is being facilitated by efforts to map various precancerous genomes,[49] will help drive the identification of novel chemopreventive agents. Additionally, a reverse migration strategy, where drugs approved for treatment against established cancers are tested earlier in the carcinogenic process (as happened with tamoxifen), offers another potential pathway to making this strategy a reality. Of course, any potential chemopreventive or interceptive agent must undergo rigorous evaluation in Phase I–IV trials to define the most safe and effective dosing regimen. Potential agents for molecular cancer prevention currently under investigation include COX-2 inhibitors, retinoids, HER2 receptor kinase inhibitors, IGF inhibitors, metformin, statins, PARP inhibitors, and innovative vaccine and inflammation- and immunoprevention-based approaches.

Cancer Survivorship

Earlier diagnosis and improved treatment success rates for many cancers has resulted in an increasing number of cancer survivors. The number of individuals living with a previous diagnosis of cancer has greatly increased. In the United States, it is estimated that 15.5 million people are cancer survivors, comprising approximately 4.7% of the population. This number is expected to rise dramatically, with projections estimating that there will be 20 million cancer survivors in the United States by 2026.[50] Globally, the number of people alive 5 years or more after a cancer diagnosis is estimated at 43.8 million.[51] In low- and middle-income countries, data on cancer survivorship are sparse, but as cancer treatment improves in these countries, increases in the number of survivors can also be expected.

While higher survival rates are indeed good news for individuals diagnosed with cancer, many of the treatments used to treat cancer have lasting and long-term effects that can influence survivors' health and ability to return to their usual activities. Cancer survivors across multiple types of cancer frequently report problems with fatigue, anxiety (particularly with regard to fear of recurrence), and exhibit decreased physical functioning.[52-55] These problems affect quality of life and may interfere with survivors' ability to return to work, family roles, and valued leisure time activities. An inability to return to work can exacerbate the financial toxicity that often accompanies cancer diagnosis and treatment.[56] Cancer treatment can have long-term effects on multiple organ systems, including the cardiovascular, pulmonary, and central and peripheral nervous systems. For example, the common chemotherapeutic agent doxorubicin can be cardiotoxic, and survivors who receive this treatment may experience heart failure many years after their initial treatment.[57] Many survivors exhibit a premature aging syndrome, in which they experience certain chronic diseases (e.g., cardiovascular disease) and disability (e.g., declines in physical and cognitive functioning) at younger ages than expected.[53,58] Furthermore, cancer survivors are at elevated risk of developing second primary cancers,[59] which may be related to their treatment, risk behaviors, or genetic susceptibility.

Interventions to ameliorate the after-effects of cancer have been the subject of research over the past 20 years. For example, psychosocial support and self-management interventions have been shown to help survivors cope with anxiety, depression, and fear of recurrence.[60-62] Numerous studies have shown that exercise reduces survivors' fatigue and improves their physical functioning, and there are currently national guidelines for cancer survivors related to exercise, diet, and weight management (ACS, American College of Sports Medicine [ACSM]).[63,64] The ACSM recently reviewed the evidence on exercise for cancer survivors and found (1) strong evidence that exercise improves fatigue, anxiety, depressive symptoms, physical functioning, and quality of life in people who have been diagnosed with cancer; and (2) moderate evidence that exercise improves bone health and sleep.[63] In addition, observational studies of breast, colorectal, and prostate cancer patients have shown that survivors who are physically active after cancer have lower cancer-specific and overall mortality than those who are sedentary.[65]

In addition to diet and physical activity, tobacco cessation should be an important priority for cancer survivors who continue to smoke or use tobacco products after diagnosis. Continued tobacco use after a cancer diagnosis is associated with poorer cancer-specific and overall survival, and increases the risk of recurrence, poor treatment response, and treatment toxicity.[2] Because of the clear benefits of tobacco cessation for cancer patients, National Cancer Institute–designated cancer centers have been encouraged to make tobacco use treatment part of the standard of care for patients. Some of these programs have shown considerable gains in helping survivors to become tobacco-free.[66]

References

1. Smoking and Health–Report of the. Advisory Committee to the Surgeon General of the Public Health Service. U.S. Department of Health, Education, and Welfare; 1964.
2. National Center for Chronic Disease Prevention and Health Promotion, Office on Smoking and Health. *The Health Consequence of Smoking–50 Years of Progress: A Report of the Surgeon General*. Atlanta, GA: Centers for Disease Control and Prevention (US); 2014.
3. King B, Pechacek T, Mariolis P, National Center for Chronic Disease Prevention and Health Promotion (U.S.). *Best Practices for Comprehensive Tobacco Control Programs – 2014*. U.S Department of Health & Human Services; 2014.
4. Bray F, Ferlay J, Soerjomataram I, Siegel RL, Torre LA, Jemal A. Global cancer statistics 2018: GLOBOCAN estimates of incidence and mortality worldwide for 36 cancers in 185 countries. *CA Cancer J Clin*. 2018;68:394–424.
5. Hashim D, Boffetta P, La Vecchia C, et al. The global decrease in cancer mortality: trends and disparities. *Ann Oncol*. 2016;27:926–933.
6. Colditz GA, Wolin KY, Gehlert S. Applying what we know to accelerate cancer prevention. *Sci Transl Med*. 2012;4:127.
7. Islami F, Goding Sauer A, Miller KD, et al. Proportion and number of cancer cases and deaths attributable to potentially modifiable risk factors in the United States. *CA Cancer J Clin*. 2018;68:31–54.
8. Jemal A, Torre L, Soerjomataram I, Bray F. *Cancer Atlas*. American Cancer Society; 2019. 3rd ed.
9. World Health Organization. *WHO Report on the Global Tobacco Epidemic, 2017: Monitoring Tobacco Use and Prevention Policies*: World Health Organization; 2017.
10. Arbyn M, Xu L, Simoens C, Martin-Hirsch PP. Prophylactic vaccination against human papillomaviruses to prevent cervical cancer and its precursors. *Cochrane Database Syst Rev*. 2018;5:CD009069.
11. Kushi L, Doyle C, McCullough M, et al. American Cancer Society Guidelines on nutrition and physical activity for cancer prevention: reducing the risk of cancer with healthy food choices and physical activity. *CA Cancer J Clin*. 2012;62:30–67.
12. World Cancer Research Fund/American Institute for Cancer Research. *Diet, Nutrition, Physical Activity, and Cancer: A Global Perspective*: Continuous Update Project Expert Report; 2018.
13. Kabat GC, Matthews CE, Kamensky V, Hollenbeck AR, Rohan TE. Adherence to cancer prevention guidelines and cancer incidence, cancer mortality, and total mortality: a prospective cohort study. *Am J Clin Nutr*. 2015;101:558–569.
14. McCullough ML, Patel AV, Kushi LH, et al. Following cancer prevention guidelines reduces risk of cancer, cardiovascular disease, and all-cause mortality. *Cancer Epidemiol Biomarkers Prev*. 2011;20:1089–1097.
15. Kohler LN, Garcia DO, Harris RB, Oren E, Roe DJ, Jacobs ET. Adherence to diet and physical activity cancer prevention guidelines and cancer outcomes: a systematic review. *Cancer Epidemiol Biomarkers Prev*. 2016;25:1018–1028.
16. Wilson J, Jungner G. *Principles and Practice of Screening for Disease*. World Health Organization; 1968.
17. Aberle DR, Adams AM, et al.National Lung Screening Trial Research Team. Reduced lung-cancer mortality with low-dose computed tomographic screening. *N Engl J Med*. 2011;365:395–409.
18. De Koning H, Van Der Aalst C, Ten Haaf K, Oudkerk M. Effects of volume CT lung cancer screening: mortality results of the NELSON randomised-controlled population based trial. *J Thorac Oncol*. 2018;13.
19. Jemal A, Fedewa SA. Lung cancer screening with low-dose computed tomography in the United States – 2010 to 2015. *JAMA Oncol*. 2017;3(9):1278–1281.
20. Pinsky PF. Lung cancer screening with low-dose CT: a worldwide view. *Transl Lung Cancer Res*. 2018;7(3):234–242.
21. Scarinci IC, Garcia FAR, Kobetz E, et al. Cervical cancer prevention: new tools and old barriers. *Cancer*. 2010;116:2531–2542.
22. Koliopoulos G, Nyaga VN, Santesso N, et al. Cytology versus HPV testing for cervical cancer screening in the general population. *Cochrane Database Syst Rev*. 2017;8(8):CD008587. doi:10.1002/14651858.CD008587.pub2.
23. Shastri SS, Mittra I, Mishra GA, et al. Effect of VIA screening by primary health workers: randomized controlled study in Mumbai, India. *J Natl Cancer Inst*. 2014;106:dju009.
24. Jeronimo J, Castle PE, Temin S, et al. Secondary prevention of cervical cancer: ASCO resource-stratified clinical practice guideline. *J Glob Oncol*. 2017;3:635–657.
25. Marmot MG, Altman DG, Cameron DA, Dewar JA, Thompson SG, Wilcox M. The benefits and harms of breast cancer screening: an independent review. *Br J Cancer*. 2013;108:2205–2240.
26. Myers ER, Moorman P, Gierisch JM, et al. Benefits and harms of breast cancer screening: a systematic review. *JAMA*. 2015;314:1615–1634.
27. Broeders M, Moss S, Nyström L, et al. The impact of mammographic screening on breast cancer mortality in Europe: a review of observational studies. *J Med Screen*. 2012;19(Suppl 1):14–25.
28. Mandelblatt JS, Cronin KA, Bailey S, et al. Effects of mammography screening under different screening schedules: model estimates of potential benefits and harms. *Ann Intern Med*. 2009;151:738–747.
29. Yip CH, Smith RA, Anderson BO, et al. Guideline implementation for breast healthcare in low- and middle-income countries: early detection resource allocation. *Cancer*. 2008;113:2244–2256.
30. Nishihara R, Wu K, Lochhead P, et al. Long-term colorectal-cancer incidence and mortality after lower endoscopy. *N Engl J Med*. 2013;369:1095–1105.
31. Atkin WS, Edwards R, Kralj-Hans I, et al. Once-only flexible sigmoidoscopy screening in prevention of colorectal cancer: a multicentre randomised controlled trial. *Lancet*. 2010;375:1624–1633.
32. Schoen RE, Pinsky PF, Weissfeld JL, et al. Colorectal-cancer incidence and mortality with screening flexible sigmoidoscopy. *N Engl J Med*. 2012;366:2345–2357.
33. Inadomi JM. Screening for colorectal neoplasia. *N Engl J Med*. 2017;376:149–156.
34. Andriole GL, Crawford ED, Grubb RL, et al. Mortality results from a randomized prostate-cancer screening trial. *N Engl J Med*. 2009;360:1310–1319.
35. Andriole GL, Crawford ED, Grubb RL, et al. Prostate cancer screening in the randomized prostate, lung, colorectal, and ovarian cancer screening trial: mortality results after 13 years of follow-up. *J Natl Cancer Inst*. 2012;104:125–132.

36. Schröder FH, Hugosson J, Roobol MJ, et al. Screening and prostate-cancer mortality in a randomized European study. *N Engl J Med*. 2009;360:1320–1328.
37. Roobol MJ, Kranse R, Bangma CH, et al. Screening for prostate cancer: results of the Rotterdam section of the European randomized study of screening for prostate cancer. *Eur Urol*. 2013;64:530–539.
38. Kilpeläinen TP, Tammela TL, Malila N, et al. Prostate cancer mortality in the Finnish randomized screening trial. *J Natl Cancer Inst*. 2013;105:719–725.
39. Luján M, Páez A, Angulo JC, et al. Prostate cancer incidence and mortality in the Spanish section of the European Randomized Study of Screening for Prostate Cancer (ERSPC). *Prostate Cancer Prostatic Dis*. 2014;17:187–191.
40. Fenton JJ, Weyrich MS, Durbin S, Liu Y, Bang H, Melnikow J. Prostate-specific antigen-based screening for prostate cancer: evidence report and systematic review for the US Preventive Services Task Force. *JAMA*. 2018;319:1914–1931.
41. Cohen JD, Li L, Wang Y, et al. Detection and localization of surgically resectable cancers with a multi-analyte blood test. *Science*. 2018;359:926–930.
42. Sporn MB, Dunlop NM, Newton DL, Smith JM. Prevention of chemical carcinogenesis by vitamin A and its synthetic analogs (retinoids). *Fed Proc*. 1976;35:1332–1338.
43. Maresso KC, Tsai KY, Brown PH, Szabo E, Lippman S, Hawk ET. Molecular cancer prevention: current status and future directions. *CA Cancer J Clin*. 2015;65:345–383.
44. Blackburn EH. Cancer interception. *Cancer Prev Res (Phila)*. 2011;4:787–792.
45. Fisher B, Costantino JP, Wickerham DL, et al. Tamoxifen for prevention of breast cancer: report of the National Surgical Adjuvant Breast and Bowel Project P-1 Study. *J Natl Cancer Inst*. 1998;90:1371–1388.
46. Rothwell PM, Wilson M, Elwin CE, et al. Long-term effect of aspirin on colorectal cancer incidence and mortality: 20-year follow-up of five randomised trials. *Lancet*. 2010;376:1741–1750.
47. Flossmann E, Rothwell PM. Effect of aspirin on long-term risk of colorectal cancer: consistent evidence from randomised and observational studies. *Lancet*. 2007;369:1603–1613.
48. Bibbins-Domingo K, U.S. Preventive Services Task Force. Aspirin use for the primary prevention of cardiovascular disease and colorectal cancer: U.S. Preventive Services Task Force recommendation statement. *Ann Intern Med*. 2016;164:836–845.
49. Srivastava S, Ghosh S, Kagan J, Mazurchuk R, National Cancer Institute's HTAN Implementation. The making of a precancer atlas: promises, challenges, and opportunities. *Trends Cancer*. 2018;4:523–536.
50. Miller KD, Siegel RL, Lin CC, et al. Cancer treatment and survivorship statistics, 2016. *CA Cancer J Clin*. 2016;66:271–289.
51. Cancer IAfRo. *Latest global cancer data: cancer burden rises to 18.1 million new cases and 9.6 million cancer deaths in 2018*: International Agency for Research on Cancer/World Health Organization; 2018.
52. Jefford M, Ward AC, Lisy K, et al. Patient-reported outcomes in cancer survivors: a population-wide cross-sectional study. *Support Care Cancer*. 2017;25:3171–3179.
53. Leach CR, Bellizzi KM, Hurria A, Reeve BB. Is it my cancer or am I just getting older?: Impact of cancer on age-related health conditions of older cancer survivors. *Cancer*. 2016;122:1946–1953.
54. Winters-Stone KM, Medysky ME, Savin MA. Patient-reported and objectively measured physical function in older breast cancer survivors and cancer-free controls. *J Geriatr Oncol*. 2019;10:311–316.
55. Yabroff KR, Lawrence WF, Clauser S, Davis WW, Brown ML. Burden of illness in cancer survivors: findings from a population-based national sample. *J Natl Cancer Inst*. 2004;96:1322–1330.
56. Gordon LG, Merollini KMD, Lowe A, Chan RJ. A systematic review of financial toxicity among cancer survivors: we can't pay the co-pay. *Patient*. 2017;10:295–309.
57. Curigliano G, Cardinale D, Dent S, et al. Cardiotoxicity of anticancer treatments: epidemiology, detection, and management. *CA Cancer J Clin*. 2016;66:309–325.
58. Ness KK, Kirkland JL, Gramatges MM, et al. Premature physiologic aging as a paradigm for understanding increased risk of adverse health across the lifespan of survivors of childhood cancer. *J Clin Oncol*. 2018;36:2206–2215.
59. Curtis RE, Freedman DM, Ron E, et al. *New malignancies among cancer survivors: SEER cancer registries, 1973–2000*: National Cancer Institute; 2006.
60. Kim SH, Kim K, Mayer DK. Self-management intervention for adult cancer survivors after treatment: a systematic review and meta-analysis. *Oncol Nurs Forum*. 2017;44:719–728.
61. Dawson G, Madsen LT, Dains JE. Interventions to manage uncertainty and fear of recurrence in female breast cancer survivors: a review of the literature. *Clin J Oncol Nurs*. 2016;20:E155–E161.
62. Duncan M, Moschopoulou E, Herrington E, et al. Review of systematic reviews of non-pharmacological interventions to improve quality of life in cancer survivors. *BMJ Open*. 2017;7:e015860.
63. Campbell KL, Winters-Stone KM, Wiskemann J, et al. Exercise guidelines for cancer survivors: consensus statement from international multidisciplinary roundtable. *Med Sci Sports Exerc*. 2019;51:2375–2390.
64. Rock CL, Doyle C, Demark-Wahnefried W, et al. Nutrition and physical activity guidelines for cancer survivors. *CA Cancer J Clin*. 2012;62:243–274.
65. Friedenreich CM, Neilson HK, Farris MS, Courneya KS. Physical activity and cancer outcomes: a precision medicine approach. *Clin Cancer Res*. 2016;22:4766–4775.
66. Cinciripini PM, Karam-Hage M, Kypriotakis G, et al. Association of a comprehensive smoking cessation program with smoking abstinence among patients with cancer. *JAMA Netw Open*. 2019;2:e1912251.

2

Global Cancer Surgery—The *Lancet* Commission

K. A. KELLY McQUEEN AND ANAHITA DABO-TRUBELJA

Introduction

Since 1991, the global burden of disease has shifted from communicable to noncommunicable disease (NCDs), primarily due to prevention, mitigation, and treatment of infectious disease in low- and middle-income countries (LMICs). This epidemiological shift has impacted global mortality rates and other important health indicators,[1] and there has been a simultaneous increase in disability and death primarily due to cancer. The increase in cancer has especially impacted low-income countries (LICs), specifically those in sub-Saharan Africa. Economic progress and the westernization of lifestyle have led to increased exposure to cancer risk factors, including tobacco use, sedentary lifestyle, and diet changes to include more processed foods. Overall, Asia and Africa have a 50% higher cancer incidence and higher mortality in relation to the number of new cancer cases.[2] This trend is likely due to a triad of causes: higher frequency of cancer types associated with poorer prognosis, limited access to diagnosis, and limited access to treatment.[3,4] Globocan cancer statistics for 2018[5] estimated that there are 8.8 million global cancer-related deaths annually—approximately 17% of all global deaths—with 70% of these cancer deaths occurring in LICs. Without investment in early diagnosis and access to treatment, including surgery, the number of cancer-related deaths might rise to 13.2 million by 2030.[4,5]

Cancer is a diverse group of diseases, impacting every anatomic and physiologic system during every stage of life. To positively impact cancer and its effect on disability and mortality, health care systems must focus on early diagnosis and access to treatment. Effective cancer mitigation and cure has been accomplished in most high-income countries (HICs) but is rare in LICs. The inflection point for cancer diagnosis often includes surgical intervention in the form of biopsy or resection. The treatment of many cancers is also surgical, and so the increase in cancer burden in LICs has emphasized the role of surgery and safe anesthesia in LICs. The critical lack of access to surgery and safe anesthesia in LICs has negatively impacted cancer diagnosis and treatment, and continues to hinder the progress in LMICs. There is an urgent need for timely access to surgical services, the implementation of screening programs, and a focus on the risk factors.[6]

The World Health Organization (WHO)'s adoption of the global surgery agenda proposed by the *Lancet*,[7] with commitments by national Ministries of Health (MOH) and local health care systems, will improve access to timely, effective, and safe surgical and anesthesia care, and cancer diagnosis and management programs, thereby socially and economically impacting individuals, families, communities, and countries alike. This agenda aims to achieve a 25% reduction in premature mortality from cancer-related deaths by the year 2025.

The global surgery initiative comprises four essential pillars of cancer treatment and care to engage cancer services worldwide that best fit specific national needs:

- Improve cancer data for public health use
- Improve patient early access and detection—frequently surgical
- Provide timely and accurate treatment—often surgical
- Provide primary and supportive palliative care—may also have a surgical component

The Global Surgical and Anesthesia Crisis

The contribution of communicable disease to the global burden of disease mandated the focus on this disease group in LMICs during much of the last century.[6,8–11] This mandate resulted in a neglect of surgery, except for emergency surgery, and played down the importance of safe anesthesia. However, the shift in epidemiology from communicable to NCDs that began in the 1990s led to a greater surgical disease burden. In most, if not all LICs, surgical systems had atrophied due to the necessary focus on communicable disease, and there were limited efforts to train future anesthesiologists and surgeons. Consistent with the focus on infectious disease were the global public health perceptions that surgery is a "luxury" that is too complicated for the limited health care systems in LICs, and "too expensive."

During the important shift in opinion toward the greater burden of NCD, little infrastructure and few resources[12,13] were available for the growing need for surgery and safe anesthesia.

This reality was recognized by a few internationally focused surgeons and anesthesiologists and their local counterparts, but was not acknowledged by the global public health community until 2015.

Emergence of Global Surgery

In 2015, three important initiatives came to fruition. The Disease Control Priorities in Developing Countries 3rd Edition (DCP3), a publication of the World Bank that is published approximately every 5 years with the intention of setting health priorities in LMICs, focused on Essential Surgery for the first time in the history of the publication. The first volume of DCP3, Essential Surgery, focused on the global burden of surgical disease, estimating that more than 30% of the global disease burden could be averted with appropriate surgical intervention and safe anesthesia. Further, the authors and editors proposed a list of 44 cost-effective and essential surgical interventions, inclusive of appropriate anesthesia techniques, to address the global burden of surgical disease in district hospitals in all LMICs. A month after the DCP3 publication in March 2016, the *Lancet* Commission on Global Surgery (LCoGS) was published. This landmark publication built on the foundations of DCP3 and furthered the global surgery agenda through modeling, suggesting that 5 billion people lacked access to surgery and safe anesthesia when needed. The key *Lancet* indicators include access to essential surgery and safe anesthesia within 2 h, an increase in overall surgical volume in LMICs, an increase in surgical, anesthesia, and obstetrical providers per 100,000 population, tracking of the perioperative mortality rate (POMR), and a focus on decreasing impoverishing and catastrophic expenditures related to emergency and essential surgery. These two pivotal publications were followed in May 2015 by the annual World Health Assembly, which unanimously resolved to support and improve access to safe, timely, and affordable surgical, obstetric, and anesthesia care, to optimize health outcomes through the World Health Assembly Resolution #68.15.[7,14,15] In summary, these documents and the resolution concluded with a moral and economic imperative to include emergency and essential surgery and safe anesthesia in primary health care in LMICs. They paved the way to improving surgical care for the 5 billion citizens without access to this basic health care need.

The events of 2015 and the initiatives that have followed, including the National Surgical, Obstetric, and Anesthesia Plans (NSOAPs),[16] have led to more generous support for surgery and anesthesia and ongoing plans to scale up and provide 44 essential surgeries in all district hospitals in LMICs. The plan focuses on access to surgery and safe anesthesia, previously unprioritized in most national health care plans. A surgical assessment tool (SAT) is used to evaluate critical components of a surgical system—infrastructure, service delivery, workforce, information management, and financing—and to inform the NSOAP (Fig. 2.1).

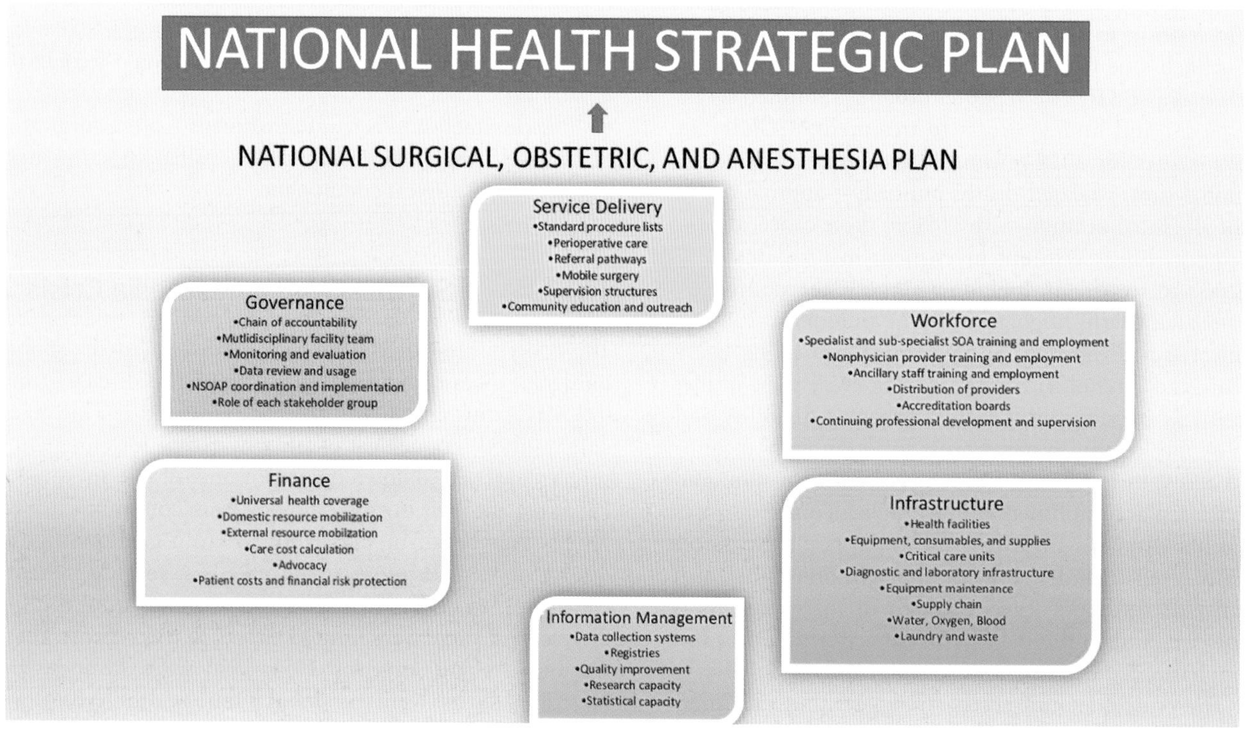

• **Fig. 2.1** National Surgery, Obstetric, and Anesthesia Plans (NSOAPs).

The NSOAP process is a framework for the planning, delivery, and management of quality surgical, obstetric, and anesthesia services at all levels of health delivery systems by incorporating three steps:

1. Expansion of the workforce and infrastructure at the district level
2. Increase health management information systems
3. Develop financing mechanisms and strong leadership.

The NSOAP is an ambitious plan and to date has only been implemented in a few countries. Zambia was the first to report success. The plan aligns with current health care policies and has seen a modest 3% increase in health care costs. The development of the plan in Zambia can serve as a model to other countries that wish to develop similar surgical services and research strategies for better perioperative outcomes.[17]

Perioperative Management

The perioperative period, from preoperative evaluation to postoperative management and outcomes, is a relatively new commitment in HICs. As such, and because of the related resource requirement, it has not become a commitment in LMICs. In fact, many LMICs are struggling to adequately provide comprehensive preoperative evaluation and related testing.

While this phase of surgical care has yet to be realized in low-resource settings, where the scale-up to safe anesthesia and surgery has just begun, it is important to the future of anesthesia and surgical outcomes in LMICs. Pain management is an important part of the perioperative process. Uncontrollable postoperative pain increases the incidence of chronic pain.[18,19] Pain medications are often unavailable, even though they are on the WHO list of essential medications. Deficits in the perioperative workforce have shifted the tasks of health care workers to those less qualified. This task shifting is a controversial subject among health care professionals as concerns regarding training and patient safety exist.[20,21] The level of professional care in the perioperative period is unknown in LICs, and family members are often the direct caregivers in the immediate postoperative period. This contributes to higher-than-expected perioperative morbidity and mortality.[22]

Few studies have addressed the issue of postoperative mortality in LICs. The high rates of postoperative mortality reported are commonly due to unrecognized hypoxia and hypovolemia. Inadequate equipment, especially pulse oximetry, lack of trained anesthesia and perioperative personnel, and inadequate supervision contribute to this high mortality rate.[23–25] There is also a lack of postoperative follow up once the patient is discharged home. This results in mortality rates 100–1000 times higher in LICs compared with those in HICs.[26,27] Improvement in surgical and anesthesia resources will lead to a reduction in POMRs in LICs. The POMR will be shifted toward patients with increased comorbidities and greater acuity of illnesses.[22]

Perioperative patient management is one focus of the NSOAP process. For example, in Uganda, implementation of the NSOAP process has resulted in a better understanding of surgical services, partnerships within different levels of care to improve access to safe surgery and the first country-wide quality metrics. An example would be a retrospective analysis of surgical volume and perioperative mortality as recorded in a simple logbook. POMR is a good indicator of a healthy surgical service.[28] Surgical societies, regional organizations, professional societies, and MOH engage and work together at every level from local to national to provide essential surgical services. These coordinated efforts strengthen the health care system and contribute to overall social and economic well being and lead to the meaningful exchange of ideas and resources.[29,30]

Cancer Anesthesia and Surgery

Surgical Access

Access to surgery and safe anesthesia is essential to the diagnosis and treatment of cancer in LMICs. Limited by workforce, infrastructure, necessary equipment, and medicines in LMIC, the support of the LCoGS and the practical process of NSOAPs are just the beginning. National MOH ultimately must invest in the resources necessary for the success of the NSOAP process, and thereafter in a system-wide commitment to a surgical program that is accessible, scalable, safe, and trusted by the population. The growth of surgical programs will take time; these must be practical and acknowledge local strengths and challenges. Recommendations from the NSOAPs include increasing education and training, task shifting to nonphysician providers, building and equipping surgical facilities, and purchasing equipment for surgery and anesthesia, including safety monitoring equipment.[31]

Safe Anesthesia

Anesthesia must be emphasized as an integral part of every health care system and as essential for surgical programs. This seems obvious, but anesthesia continues to be a challenge, even an afterthought, in many resource-constrained settings. The historical and current underresourcing of anesthesia has resulted in poor anesthesia outcomes in many LICs.[32] While multifactorial, this reality is primarily due to a lack of education and training for nonphysician anesthesia providers, as well as limited access to essential medicines, including oxygen and absent or underutilized safety monitoring equipment.[33,34]

Patient safety initiatives in HICs have resulted in better patient outcomes[32,35–37]; however, limited emphasis and advances in patient safety in LICs contribute to poor anesthesia outcomes.[38–50] This has not gone unnoticed by the international community. Efforts to provide training for anesthesia providers, access to essential medicines, guidelines, and support have been ongoing for many years.[51–71]

The global health initiative for safe surgery and anesthesia[7,14] has prioritized access to safe anesthesia and surgery and emphasized that this is a fundamental human right for proper health care. International standards, developed by the WHO and the World Federation of Societies of Anesthesiologists, provide guidance to MOH and health care systems to improve quality of care and patient safety.[72] However, such guidelines have little impact without investment from governments. It is estimated that 32 million people worldwide receive anesthesia, oxygen, and critical monitoring from unqualified anesthesia providers,[73–76] and for these patients, it is imperative that basic patient safety practices be embraced. A bare minimum approach is possible, entailing the use of a precordial stethoscope, pulse oximetry, and oxygen, and being vigilant to the clinical signs of color, pupils, and pulse.[77–79]

Pain Management

Pain management is recognized as a fundamental right in health care as part of the Universal Declaration of Human Rights[80] and is an essential part of anesthetic management. Pain medicines, opioids, and multimodal therapies are often unavailable in LICs, despite their low costs and inclusion on the WHO list of essential medications (Table 2.1).[81–83] In addition to a lack of available pain medications, there is a shortage of trained personnel in regional anesthesia, outside of spinal anesthesia. Equipment to perform regional procedures is often nonexistent. Currently, pain management in the postoperative period is often left to the family to administer.[84–91] As the WHO mandates essential surgery availability in LICs, it is important to focus on intraoperative and acute postoperative pain management.

TABLE 2.1 The World Health Organization's List of Essential Medicines for Anesthesia and Pain Management 2013

Medication Class	Medication
Inhalational gas	Oxygen, halothane, isoflurane, nitrous oxide
Muscle relaxant	Atracurium, suxamethonium
Sedative/hypnotic	Ketamine, propofol or thiopental, midazolam, diazepam
Narcotic	Morphine, codeine
Local anesthetic	Lidocaine, bupivacaine
Nonsteroidal antiinflammatory	Ibuprofen, paracetamol
Antiemetic	Ondansetron
Chronic pain medication	Amitriptyline
Muscle relaxant reversal	Neostigmine
Narcotic antidote	Naloxone
Adrenergic system modulators	Epinephrine, atropine, ephedrine

In 2012, the first WHO global survey on the availability and barriers to access of opioid analgesics to patients in pain was conducted in 81 countries, in collaboration with 17 leading cancer and palliative organizations worldwide. A majority of the global medical opioid consumption occurs in HICs, and only 7% occurs in LICs.[92–94] Globally, there are 5.5 million patients with terminal cancer and an estimated 80% experience moderate-to-severe pain due to inadequate access to medicines.[95,96] The survey identified the following barriers:

1. Essential opioids are not available. Of the seven on the WHO mandatory list for cancer pain management, only morphine and codeine are on national lists.
2. Legal and regulatory restrictions limit access to health care providers and discourage their ability to prescribe them.
3. Administrative overregulation and costs passed on to the patient discourage patients from seeking pain relief, regardless of pain levels.
4. Inadequate clinical education, misconceptions, social stigma, and fear of addiction are persistent barriers that most urgently need addressing.

There has been an international effort by the WHO to address cancer pain treatment. Morphine was included on the WHO essential medicine list back in 1977, and the three-step analgesic ladder for cancer pain in 1986 incorporated multimodal therapies, all of which are on the WHO list of essential medications (Table 2.1).

In 2008, the Global Year Against Cancer Pain Initiative implemented an educational program based on local needs with a detailed budget at minimal social cost for LMICs.[97] This initiative created a system of pain centers to act as regional hubs for education and training in pain management. They also coordinate with local governments for the expansion of programs. Several reviews have led to significant improvement in clinical management and pain education.[98–100]

Palliative Pain Management

As the burden of cancer increases in the developing world, a high number of cases will be incurable at the time of diagnosis. Furthermore, it is estimated that 80% of cancer patients will experience moderate-to-severe pain in their cancer journey. In many LMICs, cultural norms, societal attitudes, and personal beliefs accept pain as part of the disease process. In addition, in many of these countries, few doctors and nurses have adequate knowledge of the pain management and treatment options available.[101–105] Lack of adequate and timely assessment provides little information about the actual incidence and prevalence of acute postoperative pain or chronic pain conditions.[106,107] The WHO Essential Medications List for pain management includes lidocaine, bupivacaine, morphine, codeine, ketamine, ibuprofen, paracetamol, and amitriptyline. This list informs the MOH about what should be available to treat acute and chronic pain, but in many LMICs, these medications are only sporadically available or not available at all. The basic treatment of postoperative pain, as well as chronic pain and palliative care, will need to be the focus of all medical personnel, including anesthesia providers and general practitioners, for the adequate treatment of cancer in LMICs. To date, there is limited literature on the incidence and prevalence of postoperative and chronic pain in LMICs. Cancer pain and postoperative pain may lead to disability from chronic pain, which is known to have economic consequences in LMICs.[7,108,109]

Implementing policies on evidence-based measures and monitoring progress toward alleviating the burden of pain must use a rigorous research agenda. This endeavor would primarily be supported through nongovernmental and international funding agencies and societies.[110–113]

Future Advances for the Surgical and Anesthesia Management of Cancer Patients in Low-Income Countries

Advancing surgery and safe anesthesia in LMICs will improve cancer care in these settings. The qualities of a successful surgical program are inherent to health care systems in general, and improving surgical and anesthesia care results in improvements elsewhere in the health care system, including critical care and pain management.

Advancing the surgical agenda and adding modern paradigms to the perioperative care process is likely to provide additional improvements to comprehensive cancer care in these settings. In addition, applying the Enhanced Recovery After Surgery (ERAS) principles of care is likely to benefit cancer patients and surgical outcomes in LMICs. Discussions regarding ERAS for LICs are underway, and it is recognized that applying ERAS standardization may improve overall cost-effectiveness and outcomes as LIC surgical systems scale up.[114,115]

Factors, such as nutritional status, comorbidities, prevalence of HIV, and the burden of disease, should be taken into account when developing an ERAS protocol.[116]

A modified approach to ERAS has shown to provide some benefit in limited resource health care systems (Fig. 2.2). However, more piloting and outcomes analysis are necessary in the short term. Standardization, guidelines, and protocols that are inherent in ERAS success in HICs must be embraced by all health system stakeholders for success and impact on perioperative care and surgical and anesthesia outcomes. Protocols should focus on all elements of ERAS: preoperative evaluation and optimization, cost-effective antibiotics, regional anesthesia, multimodal pain therapy, early removal of drains, and early mobilization. Implementation of modified ERAS protocols is possible at district-level hospitals for all 44 essential surgical procedures and is likely to prove cost-effective and efficient, and improve perioperative outcomes.[114,117,118]

As implementation of scale-up to universal access of surgical care and safe anesthesia continues to advance globally, the need for data collection, including POMR and other outcomes, is increasingly important.[119,120] Infection rates, time to discharge, and POMR are important indicators in LMICs, although such data have not been routinely collected.[121,122] POMR and infection rates are endorsed by the WHO as two of the 100 health indicators for all settings.[119] This endorsement is essential for moving the collection of these outcome indicators forward, and the collection and reporting of these indicators will support the development of a culture of safety and improved patient outcomes related to surgery and anesthesia.

Recommendations

The role of anesthesia in the global burden of surgical disease in LMICs is essential, and its mission critical to every hospital system. The scope of anesthesia care encompasses preoperative preparation to intraoperative management and from resuscitation and pain management to critical and palliative care. Cancer care in LMICs and reducing the burden of surgical disease in LMICs will not be possible without adequate access to safe anesthesia, and improving outcomes is dependent on a team approach that includes the anesthesia team. We recommend prioritizing anesthesia education and professionalization in LMICs, including anesthesia in all efforts aimed at improving surgical care, emphasizing the continuum of care from preoperative preparation to pain management, and focusing on patient safety in all settings. Consistent with the success of cancer management in HICs, a team approach in LMICs that includes primary care, surgery, anesthesia, and nursing teams is recommended.

Conclusions

Cancer is a growing concern in LMICs and a significant contributor to disability and premature death. Anesthesia is central to the care of cancer patients in LMICs, providing intraoperative care, acute and chronic pain management, and critical care management. Improving anesthesia in LICs will significantly impact cancer patients' surgical care and improve outcomes over time. Strategies for acute and chronic pain management, as well as palliative care, are likely to be driven by anesthesiologists and nonphysician providers in LICs. Comprehensive perioperative care of cancer patients in LICs will improve cancer outcomes in LICs and are likely to improve the quality of life for these patients and their families.

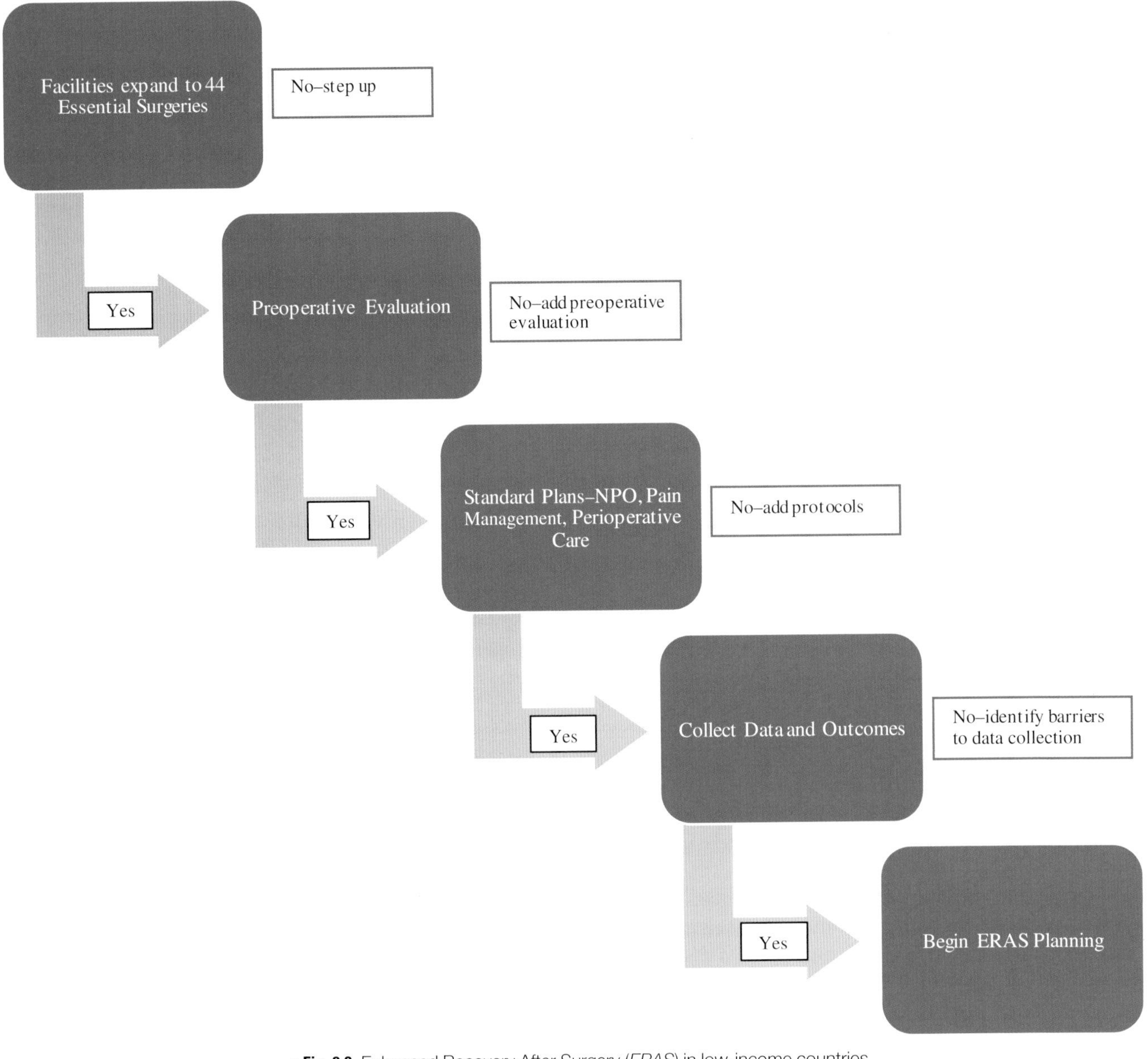

• **Fig. 2.2** Enhanced Recovery After Surgery (*ERAS*) in low-income countries.

References

1. Bray F. Soerjomataram I. The changing global burden of cancer: transitions in human development and implications for cancer prevention and control. In: Gelband H., Jha P., Sankaranarayanan R., Horton S., eds. Cancer: Disease Control Priorities. Washington, DC: The International Bank for Reconstruction and Development / The World Bank; 2015: Ch. 2., 3rd ed. 3.
2. Popat K, McQueen K, Feeley TW. The global burden of cancer. *Best Pract Res Clin Anaesthesiol.* 2013;27(4):399–408.
3. Maule M, Merletti F. Cancer transition and priorities for cancer control. *Lancet Oncol.* 2012;13:745–746.
4. World Health Organization. Global Health Observatory. Geneva: World Health Organization; 2018. Available at https://www.who.int/gho/database/en/.
5. Ferlay J, Colombet M, Soerjomataram I, et al. *Global and Regional Estimates of the Incidence and Mortality for 38 Cancers: GLOBOCAN 2018*: International Agency for Research on Cancer/World Health Organization; 2018.
6. Lopez AD, Mathers CD, Ezzati M, Jamison DT, Murray CJ. Global and regional burden of disease and risk factors, 2001: systematic analysis of population health data. *Lancet.* 2006;367:1747–1757.
7. Meara JG, Leather AJ, Hagander L, et al. Global surgery 2030: evidence and solutions for achieving health, welfare, and economic development. *Lancet.* 2015;386(9993):569–624.
8. Debas H, Gosselin R, McCord C, Thind A. Surgery. In: Jamison D, ed. *Disease Control Priorities in Developing Countries.* 2nd ed.: Oxford University Press; 2006.
9. Daar AS, Singer PA, Persad DL, et al. Grand challenges in chronic non-communicable diseases. *Nature.* 2007;450:494–496.
10. Lozano R, et al. Global and regional mortality from 235 causes of death for 20 age groups in 1990: a systematic analysis for the Global Burden of Disease Study 2010. *Lancet.* 2012.

11. Murray CJ, Vos T, Lozano R, et al. Disability-adjusted life years (DALYs) for 291 diseases and injuries in 21 regions, 1990–2010: a systematic analysis for the Global Burden of Disease study 2010. *Lancet*. 2012;380(9859):2197–2223.
12. Bickler S, Spiegel D, Hsia R, Dunbar P, McQueen K, Jamison D. Key concepts for estimating the burden of surgical conditions and the unmet need for surgical care. *World J Surg*. 2010;34(3):374–380.
13. United Nations Development Programme. *Human Development Report 2016: Human Development for Everyone*: United Nations Development Programme; 2016.
14. Jamison D, Gelbend H, Horton S, Jha P, Laxminarayan R., Mock C. Priorities in Developing Countries. International Bank for Reconstruction and Development/The World Bank; 2018. 3rd ed.
15. Spiegel DA, Abdullah F, Price RR, Gosselin RA, Bickler SW. World Health Organization Global Initiative for Emergency and Essential Surgical Care: 2011 and beyond. *World J Surg*. 2013;37(7):1462–1469. doi:10.1007/s00268-012-1831-6.
16. Price R, Makasa E, Hollands M. World Health Assembly Resolution WHA68.15: "Strengthening Emergency and Essential Surgical Care and Anesthesia as a Component of Universal Health Coverage"—Addressing the Public Health Gaps Arising from Lack of Safe, Affordable and Accessible Surgical and Anesthetic Services. *World J Surg*. 2015;39(9):2115–2125. doi: 10.1007/s00268-015-3153-y. PMID: 26239773.
17. Peck GL, Hanna JS. The National Surgical, Obstetric, and Anesthesia Plan (NSOAP): recognition and definition of an empirically evolving global surgery systems science comment on "Global surgery – informing national strategies for scaling up surgery in sub-Saharan Africa". *Int J Health Policy Manag*. 2018;7(12):1151–1154. doi:10.15171/ijhpm.2018.87.
18. Perkins FM, Kehlet H. Chronic pain as an outcome of surgery. *Anesthesiology*. 2000;93:1123–1133.
19. Macrae WA. Chronic post-surgical pain: 10 years on. *Br J Anaesth*. 2008;101:77–86.
20. WHO. Task Shifting Global Recommendations and Guidelines. 2008. Available at http://www.who.int/healthsystems/TTR-Task-Shifting.pdf.
21. Chu K, Rosseel P, Gielis P, Ford N. Surgical task shifting in sub-Saharan Africa. *PLoS Med*. 2009;6(5):e1000078. doi:10.1371/journal.pmed.1000078.
22. McQueen K, Coonan T, Ottaway A, et al. Anesthesia and perioperative care. Essential Surgery. World Bank Group; 2015:263–277. In: Debas HT, Donkor P, Gawande A, Jamison DT, Kruk ME, Mock CN, eds. Disease Control Priorities, Vol. 1. 3rd ed.
23. Enohumah KO, Imarengiaye CO. Factors associated with anaesthesia-related maternal mortality in a tertiary hospital in Nigeria. *Acta Anaesthesiol Scand*. 2006;50(2):206–210.
24. Glenshaw M, Madzimbamuto FD. Anaesthesia associated mortality in a district hospital in Zimbabwe: 1994 to 2001. *Cent Afr J Med*. 2005;51(3–4):39–44.
25. Zoumenou E, Gbenou S, Assouto P, et al. Pediatric anesthesia in developing countries: experience in the two main University Hospitals of Benin in West Africa. *Paediatr Anaesth*. 2010;20(8):741–747.
26. Kushner AL, Cherian M, Noel L, Speigel DA, Groth S, Etienne C. Addressing the millennium development goals from a surgical perspective: essential surgery and anesthesia in 8 low- and middle-income countries. *Arch Surg*. 2010;145(2):154–159.
27. Hansen D, Gausi SC, Merikebu M. Anaesthesia in Malawi: complications and deaths. *Trop Doct*. 2000;30(3):146–149.
28. Watters DA, Hollands MJ, Gruen RL, et al. Perioperative mortality rate (POMR): a global indicator of access to safe surgery and anesthesia. *World J Surg*. 2015;39(4):856–864. doi:10.1007/s00268-014-2638-4. PMID: 24841805.
29. Anderson GA, Ilcisin L, Abesiga L, et al. Surgical volume and postoperative mortality rate at a referral hospital in Western Uganda: measuring the Lancet Commission on Global Surgery indicators in low-resource settings. *Surgery*. 2017;161(6):1710–1719. doi:10.1016/j.surg.2017.01.009.
30. Bruno E, White MC, Baxter LS, et al. An evaluation of preparedness, delivery and impact of surgical and anesthesia care in Madagascar: a framework for a national surgical plan. *World J Surg*. 2017;41(5):1218–1224. doi:10.1007/s00268-016-3847-9.
31. Johnson W, Lin Y, Mukhopadhyay S, Meara J. Surgical Care Systems Strengthening Developing National Surgical, Obstetric and Anaesthesia Plans. World Health Organization; 2017.
32. Bainbridge D, Martin J, Arango M, Cheng D. Perioperative and anaesthetic-related mortality in developed and developing countries: a systematic review and meta-analysis. *Lancet*. 2012;380(9847):1075–1081.
33. Steffner, KR, McQueen KA, Gelb AW. Patient safety challenges in low-income and middle-income countries. *Curr Opin Anesthesiol*. 2014;27:623–630.
34. Beringer RM, Eltringham RJ. The Glostavent: evolution of an anaesthetic machine for developing countries. *Anaesth Intensive Care*. 2008;36(3):442–448.
35. Eichorn JH. Prevention of intraoperative anesthesia accidents and related severe injury through safety monitoring. *Anesthesiology*. 1989;70:572–577.
36. Merry AF, Cooper JB, Wilson IH, Eichhorn JH. International standards for a safe practice of anesthesia 2010. *Can J Anaesth*. 2010;57(11):1027–1034.
37. Mackay P, Cousins M. Safety in anaesthesia. *Anaesth Intensive Care*. 2006;34(3):303–304.
38. Hodges SC, Mijumbi C, Okello M, McCormick BA, Walker IA, Wilson IH. Anaesthesia services in developing countries: defining the problems. *Anaesthesia*. 2007;62(1):4–11.
39. Walker IA, Obua AD, Mouton F, Ttendo S, Wilson IH. Paediatric surgery and anaesthesia in South-Western Uganda: a cross-sectional survey. *Bull World Health Organ*. 2010;88(12):897–906.
40. Bosenberg AT. Pediatric anesthesia in developing countries. *Curr Opin Anaesthesiol*. 2007;20(3):204–210.
41. Weiser TG, Haynes AB, Molina G, et al. Size and distribution of the global volume of surgery in 2012. *Bull World Health Organ*. 2016;94(3):201–209F. doi:10.2471/BLT.15.159293.
42. Walker I, Wilson I, Bogod D. Anaesthesia in developing countries. *Anaesthesia*. 2007;62(Suppl 1):2–3.
43. Jochberger S, Ismailova F, Lederer W, et al. Anesthesia and its allied disciplines in the developing world: a nationwide survey of the Republic of Zambia. *Anesth Analg*. 2008;106(3):942–948.
44. Vo D, Meena CN, Bianchi S, et al. Anesthesia capacity in low- and middle-income countries. *J Anesth Clin Res*. 2012;3(4):207.
45. Linden AF, Sekidde FS, Galukande M, Knowlton LM, Chackungal S, McQueen KA. Challenges of surgery in developing countries: a survey of surgical and anesthesia capacity in Uganda's public hospitals. *World J Surg*. 2012;36(5):1056–1065. doi:10.3421007/s00268-012-1482-7 343.
46. Heywood AJ, Wilson IH, Sinclair JR. Perioperative mortality in Zambia. *Ann R Coll Surg Engl*. 1989;71(6):354–358.
47. McKenzie AG. Mortality associated with anaesthesia at Zimbabwean teaching hospitals. *S Afr Med J*. 1996;86(4):338–342.

48. Ouro-Bang'na Maman AF, Tomta K, Ahouangbévi S, Chobli M. Deaths associated with anaesthesia in Togo, West Africa. *Trop Doct.* 2005;35(4):220–222.
49. Vasdev GM, Harrison BA, Keegan MT, Burkle CM. Management of the difficult and failed airway in obstetric anesthesia. *J Anesth.* 2008;22(1):38–48.
50. Cherian M, Choo S, Wilson I, et al. Building and retaining the neglected anaesthesia health workforce: is it crucial for health systems strengthening through primary health care? *Bull World Health Organ.* 2010;88(8):637–639.
51. World Health Organization. Emergency an essential surgical care programme. 2014. Available at http://www.who.int/surgery/en/.
52. Chowdhury S, Chowdhury Z. Tubectomy by paraprofessional surgeons in rural Bangladesh. *Lancet.* 1975;2:567–569.
53. Bergström S, McPake B, Pereira C, Dovlo D. Workforce innovations to expand the capacity for surgical services. In: Debas HT, Donkor P, Gawande A, Jamison DT, Kruk ME, Mock CN, eds. Essential Surgery. World Bank; 2015:307–316. *Disease Control Priorities.* 3rd ed. Vol 1.
54. WHO. Optimising health worker roles to improve access to key maternal and newborn health interventions through task shifting. 2012. Available at http://www.optimisemnh.org.
55. Greene NM. Anesthesia in underdeveloped countries: a teaching program. *Yale J Biol Med.* 1991;64(4):403–407.
56. Enright A, Wilson IH, Moyers JR. The World Federation of Societies of Anaesthesiologists: supporting education in the developing world. *Anaesthesia.* 2007;62(Suppl 1):67–71.
57. Dubowitz G, Evans FM. Developing a curriculum for anaesthesia training in low- and middle-income countries. *Best Pract Res Clin Anaesthesiol.* 2012;26(1):17–21.
58. Kinnear JA, Bould MD, Ismailova F, Measures E. A new partnership for anesthesia training in Zambia: reflections on the first year. *Can J Anaesth.* 2013;60(5):484–491.
59. Twagirumugabe T, Carli F. Rwandan anesthesia residency program: a model of north-south educational partnership. *Int Anesthesiol Clin.* 2010;48(2):71–78.
60. Newton MB, Bird P. Impact of parallel anesthesia and surgical provider training in Subsaharan Africa: a model for a resource-poor setting. *World J Surg.* 2010;34(3):445.
61. Burn SL, Chilton PJ, Gawande AA, Lilford RJ. Peri-operative pulse oximetry in low-income countries: a cost-effectiveness analysis. *Bull World Health Organ.* 2014;92(12):858–867. doi:10.2471/BLT.14.137315.
62. Beringer RM, Eltringham RJ. The Glostavent: evolution of an anaesthetic machine for developing countries. *Anaesth Intensive Care.* 2008;36(3):442–448.
63. Thoms GM, McHugh GA, O'Sullivan E. The global oximetry initiative. *Anaesthesia.* 2007;62(Suppl 1):75–77.
64. WHO. WHO Guidelines for Safe Surgery. Safe Surgery Saves Lives. Geneva, Switzerland: World Health Organization; 2009.
65. WHO Press: World Health Organization, Geneva. http://whqlibdoc.who.int/publications/2009/9789241598552_eng.pdf 39133.
66. WHO. *Surgical Safety Checklist.* Geneva, Switzerland: World Health Organization; 2009.
67. WHO. *WHO Model Lists of Essential Medicines.* Geneva, Switzerland: World Health Organization; 2013.
68. WHO. *Surgical Care at the District Hospital.* Geneva, Switzerland: World Health Organization; 2003.
69. Hodges AM, Hodges SC. A rural cleft project in Uganda. *Br J Plast Surg.* 2000;53(1):7–11.
70. Henderson K. Lessons from working overseas. *Anaesthesia.* 2007;62(Suppl 1):113–117.
71. Hodges SC, Hodges AM. A protocol for safe anesthesia for cleft lip and palate surgery in developing countries. *Anaesthesia.* 2000;40155(5):436–441.
72. Gelb AW, Morriss WW, Johnson W, et al. International Standards for a Safe Practice of Anesthesia Workgroup. World Health Organization-World Federation of Societies of Anaesthesiologists (WHO-WFSA) International Standards for a Safe Practice of Anesthesia. *Anesth Analg.* 2018;126(6):2047–2055. doi:10.1213/ANE.0000000000002927.
73. Meara, J, Leather, A, Hagander, L. Lancet Commission on Global Surgery. *Lancet.* 2015;325(Special Issue 2)S1–S57.
74. Funk LM, Weiser TG, Berry WR, et al. Global operating theatre distribution and pulse oximetry supply: an estimation from reported data. *Lancet.* 2010;376(9746):1055–1061.
75. McQueen K. Oxygen: the missing element in LICs. *World J Surg.* 2016;40:249–250.
76. Finch LC, Kim RY, Ttendo S, et al. Evaluation of a large-scale donation of Lifebox pulse oximeters to non-physician anaesthetists in Uganda. *Anaesthesia.* 2014;69(5):445–451.
77. Haynes AB, et al. A surgical safety checklist to reduce morbidity and mortality in a global population. *N Engl J Med.* 2009;360(5):491–499.
78. Pugel AE, Simianu VV, Flum DR, Patchen Dellinger E. Use of the surgical safety checklist to improve communication and reduce complications. *J Infect Public Health.* 2015;8(3):219–225. doi:10.1016/j.jiph.2015.01.001.
79. McQueen K, Coonan T, Ottaway A, et al. The bare minimum: the reality of global anesthesia and patient safety. *World J Surg.* 2015. 39(9):2153–2160.
80. Dubowitz G, Evans FM. Developing a curriculum for anaesthesia training in low- and middle-income countries. *Best Pract Res Clin Anaesthesiol.* 2012;26(1):17–21.
81. Brennan F, Carr DB, Cousins M. Pain management: a fundamental human right. *Anesth Analg.* 2007;105:205–221.
82. Walters JL, Jackson T, Byrne D, McQueen K. Postsurgical pain in low- and middle-income countries. *Br J Anaesth.* 2016;116(2):153–155.
83. Tsang A, Von Korff M, Lee S, et al. Common chronic pain conditions in developed and developing countries: gender and age differences and comorbidity with depression-anxiety disorders. *J Pain.* 2008;9:883–891.
84. WHO. Universal Access to Emergency and Essential Surgical Care. Available at https://www.who.int/surgery/emergency-essential-surgical-care-2014.
85. McQueen KA. Pain management: a global perspective. *Br J Anaesth.* 2013;111:843–844.
86. Dubowitz G, Detlefs S, McQueen KA. Global anesthesia workforce crisis: a preliminary survey revealing shortages contributing to undesirable outcomes and unsafe practices. *World J Surg.* 2010;34:438–444.
87. Doohan NC, Derbew M, McQueen KA. Solutions for the global surgery crisis: the role of family medicine in surgery, obstetrics, and anesthesia. *Fam Med.* 2014;46:679–684.
88. Wang BS, Zhou LF, Coulter D, et al. Effects of caesarean section on maternal health in low-risk nulliparous women: a prospective matched cohort study in Shanghai, China. *BMC Pregnancy Childbirth.* 2010;10:78.
89. McGuire CI, Baigrie RJ, Theunissen D, Fernandes NL, Chapman LR. Outcome of laparoscopic inguinal hernia repair in a South African private practice setting. *S Afr J Surg.* 2012;50:115–158.

90. Malik AM, Jawaid A, Talpur AH, Laghari AA, Khan A. Mesh versus non-mesh repair of ventral abdominal hernias. *J Ayub Med Coll Abbottabad.* 2008;20:54–56.
91. Ebrahimzadeh MH, Hariri S. Long-term outcomes of unilateral transtibial amputations. *Mil Med.* 2009;174:593–597.
92. Lacoux PA, Crombie IK, Macrae WA. Pain in traumatic upper limb amputees in Sierra Leone. *Pain.* 2002;99:309–312.
93. Knaul FM, Farmer PE, Krakauer EI, et al. Alleviating the access abyss in palliative care and pain relief—an imperative of universal health coverage: The Lancet Commission report. *Lancet.* 2018; 391(10128):1391–1454.
94. United Nations. *Sustainable Development Goals. 17 Goals to Transform Our World.* United Nations; 2015.
95. International Narcotics Control Board. *Availability of Internationally Controlled Drugs: Ensuring Adequate Access for Medical and Scientific Purposes.* United Nations; 2016.
96. Odonkor CA, Addison W, Smith S, Osei-Bonsu E, Tang T, Erdek M. Connecting the dots: a comparative global multi-institutional study of prohibitive factors affecting cancer pain management. *Pain Med.* 2017;18(2):363–373.
97. Global Alliance to Pain Relief Initiative (GAPRI) Access to *Essential Pain Medicines Brief.* 2010.
98. WHO. Cancer Fact Sheet No. 297. 2015.http://www.who.int/mediacentre/factsheets/fs297/en.
99. The World Health Organization Briefing Note–February 2009. Access to Controlled Medications Programme: Improving access to medications controlled under international drug conventions. Available at https://www.who.int/medicines/areas/quality_safety/ACMP_BrNoteGenrl_EN_Feb09.pdf.
100. WHO Guidelines for the Pharmacological and Radiotherapeutic Management of Cancer Pain in Adults and Adolescents. Geneva: World Health Organization; 2018. ANNEX 5, Opioid Analgesics and International Conventions. Available at https://www.ncbi.nlm.nih.gov/books/NBK537494/.
101. Manjiani D, Paul DB, Kunnumpurath S, Kaye AD, Vadivelu N. Availability and utilization of opioids for pain management: global issues. *Ochsner J.* 2014;14(2):208–215.
102. Human Rights Watch. Global State of Pain Treatment: Access to Palliative Care as a Human Right. May 2011. Available at http://www.hrw.org/sites/default/files/reports/hhr0511W.pdf.
103. Jamison DT, Gelband H, Horton S, et al. Disease Control Priorities: Improving Health and Reducing Poverty: World Bank; 2017. 3rd ed. Volume 9.
104. WHO. *WHA67.19. Strengthening of palliative care as a component of comprehensive care throughout the life course*: World Health Organization; 2014.
105. Saini S, Bhatnagar S. Cancer pain management in developing countries. *Indian J Palliat Care.* 2016;22(4):373–377.
106. Cherny NI, Cleary J, Scholten W, Radbruch L, Torode J. The global opioid policy initiative (GOPI) project to evaluate the availability and accessibility of opioids for the management of cancer pain in Africa, Asia, Latin America and the Caribbean, and the Middle East: Introduction and methodology. *Ann Oncol.* 2013;24(Suppl 11):7–13.
107. Jemal A, Center MM, DeSantis C, Ward EM. Global patterns of cancer incidence and mortality rates and trends. *Cancer Epidemiol Biomarkers Prev.* 2010;19(8):1893–1907.
108. Poudel A, Kc B, Shrestha S, Nissen L. Access to palliative care: discrepancy among low-income and high-income countries. *J Glob Health.* 2019;9(2):020309. doi:10.7189/jogh.09.020309.
109. World Health Organization supports global effort to relieve chronic pain. *Indian J Med Sci.* 2004;58(10):451–452.
110. Missair A, Bollini C. Pain management in developing countries: an update. *ASA Monitor.* 2013;77(5):52–54.
111. Bond M. Pain education issues in developing countries and responses to them by the International Association for the Study of Pain. *Pain Res Manage.* 2011;16(6):404–406.
112. Bond M. Pain and its management in developing countries. *Pain Manag.* 2011;1(1):3–5.
113. Bosnjak S, Maurer MA, Ryan KM, Leon MX, Madiye G. Improving the availability of opioids for the treatment of pain: the international pain policy fellowship. *Support Care Cancer.* 2011;19(8):1239–1247.
114. McQueen K, Oodit R. Derbew M, et al. Enhanced recovery after surgery for low- and middle-income countries. *World J Surg.* 2018;42:950–952. https://doi.org/10.1007/s00268-018-4481-5. [Journal]; 2018.
115. Joliat GR, Ljungqvist O, Wasylak T, et al. Beyond surgery: clinical and economic impact of enhanced recovery after surgery programs. *BMC Health Serv Res.* 2018;18:1008. doi:10.1186/s12913-018-3824-0.
116. Plenge, Nortje MB, Marais LC, et al. Optimising perioperative care for hip and knee arthroplasty in South Africa: a Delphi consensus study. *BMC Musculoskelet Disord.* 2018;19:140doi:10.1186/s12891-018-2062-2.
117. Quezada F. Enhanced Recovery After Surgery (ERAS) protocols for low- and middle-income countries. *World J Surg.* 2018; 42:4125.
118. Oodit RL, Ljungqvist O, Moodley J. Can an enhanced recovery after surgery (ERAS) programme improve colorectal cancer outcomes in South Africa? *S Afr J Surg.* 2018;56(1):8–11.
119. McQueen K, Oodit R, Derbew M, Banguti P, Ljungqvist O. Enhanced recovery after surgery for low-and middle-income countries. *World J Surg.* 2018;42:950–952. doi:10.1007/s00268-018-4481-5.
120. Bhangu A. Prioritizing research for patients requiring surgery in low- and middle-income countries. NIH. Global Health Research Unit on Global Surgery. *Br J Surg.* 2019;106:e113–e120.
121. The World Health Organization. Report on the formal meeting of Member States to conclude the work on the comprehensive global monitoring framework, including indicators, and a set of voluntary global targets for the prevention and control of noncommunicable diseases. November 2012. Available at http://apps.who.int/gb/ebwha/pdf_files/EB132/B132_6-en.pdf.
122. Watters DA, Hollands MJ, Gruen RL, et al. Perioperative mortality rate (POMR): a global indicator of access to safe surgery and anaesthesia. *World J Surg.* 2015;39(4):856–864.

3

Cancer Biology and Implications for the Perioperative Period

NICHOLAS J.S. PERRY, SHAMAN JHANJI, AND GEORGE POULOGIANNIS

Introduction

In spite of the evident cytoreductive, potentially curative advantages of surgery, there has long been a suspicion that resecting primary tumors carries an intrinsic, paradoxical risk with respect to disease progression.[1,2] Anecdotal evidence prompted surgeons in the second half of the 19th century to draw comparisons between operative dissemination of cancer and of tuberculosis, seeking to understand how an apparently benign neoplasm might become malignant and disseminate so "astonishingly swiftly" after surgery.[1] Like tuberculosis, the phenomenon was assumed to have a mechanical etiology, resulting from "notoriously forceful" manipulations of the tumor, as it was examined and dissected out. However, analysis of autopsy data from 735 women with breast cancer soon revealed that other factors were also in play, since the distribution of distant growths could not be explained simply by chance or anatomical drainage patterns. Tumors appeared to show a predisposition to metastasize to certain organs over others, leading Stephen Paget to postulate in 1889 that metastasis involves favorable interactions between disseminating tumor cells and the sites to which they colonize.[3] This enduring "seed and soil" hypothesis continues to form the framework for exploring the biology of metastasis today and seems to be a particularly suitable metaphor for describing the risks of surgical dissemination and postoperative disease progression.

Except for some notable examples, much of our current insight into cancer pathogenesis has been shaped over the past 40 years–a revolutionary period propelled by remarkable developments in experimental tools and technology and a global will to invest in tackling this ever-more prevalent disease. Since the milestone discovery by Varmus and Bishop in 1976 that so-called "proto-oncogenes" within the normal cell genome have the capacity, when corrupted, to trigger the transformation of a healthy cell into the beginnings of a tumor,[4] a wealth of knowledge and detail has amassed regarding the molecular mechanisms that underpin the origins of cancer, drive its progression, and determine its response to therapy. This has enabled pioneering advances in diagnostics and targeted therapeutics that have translated into a number of clinical successes, where certain cancers are now considered largely curable and others now carry survival rates measured in years rather than months. Yet, the persistence of high mortality across many types of cancer clearly indicates that major challenges remain, particularly in terms of overcoming metastatic disease and therapy resistance.

Reductionism prevails in cancer research as a logical, pragmatic approach to managing its complexity, yet the pitfalls encountered over recent decades have reinforced the need to continually reevaluate the way in which we think about cancer. In the years following the Varmus-Bishop discovery, it became widely held that cancer was a disease of identifiable genes and that a logical solution would be found in deciphering a set of genetic rules common to all mammalian cells undergoing neoplastic transformation.[5] Yet, as the inventory of recognized oncogenes and tumor suppressor genes grew longer, it became clear that tumors follow variable and unpredictable genetic paths, even within the same tissues of origin.[6,7] Contemporary paradigms portray a more nuanced, less tumor-centric perspective of disease progression, where cancer genetics only partially determine the clinical course. Accordingly, cancers are no longer viewed as insular masses of genetically aberrant, incessantly proliferating cells, rather as a diverse catalog of diseases whose individual characteristics and clinical course are influenced by heterotypic and dynamic interactions among mutant genes, microenvironmental landscapes, systemic physiology, and host defenses.

With such changes in perspective, one might reason that the "cut, burn, and poison" approach that has formed the cornerstone of cancer treatment for much of the last century is outdated; after all, criticism is often leveled at such techniques for the indiscriminate way in which they are deployed against cancers of very different molecular background. However, while there have been notable and promising developments to improve clinical outcomes by moving toward so-called "personalized medicine"—where precision therapies are tailored to a tumor's individual molecular complexion and vulnerabilities, rather than simply its tissue of origin and broad histological subtype—the promise of many targeted biological therapies to drastically reform long-term survival outcomes has yet to be realized. The inconvenient reality of cancer heterogeneity, even within a single tumor, challenges the notion that drugs with narrow molecular targets may achieve lasting efficacy, particularly in advanced disease, while the associated cost burden to health economies is enormous. Surgery, radiotherapy, and cytotoxic chemotherapy therefore retain their place as essential, often highly effective tools in modern cancer care and are likely to remain so for the foreseeable future. Consequently, alongside ongoing efforts to pioneer the next revolutions and drug discoveries in clinical oncology, there is also clear impetus to continue to deliver evolutionary improvements to current clinical practices, especially where these are a common or even ubiquitous component of disease management.

The attention focused toward inadvertent surgical cooperation in disease progression now extends to a range of factors beyond the physical effects of tumor handling. These include the activation of evolutionarily conserved responses to tissue trauma, such as sympathetic nervous system activation and inflammation—aggravated further by postoperative infective or wound-healing complications—as well as a postoperative period of impaired immunological competence, in which antitumor immunity may be temporarily compromised.[8,9] There are also concerns about the impact of perioperative pharmacology, most prominently centering around anesthetic and analgesic drugs and their purported influence over cancer cell biology and host immunity.[10,11] In light of an improved awareness of the cancer cell–extrinsic factors that contribute to cancer pathogenesis, and the manner in which they do so, it is increasingly conceivable to appreciate how the inflammatory, immunological, and metabolic state of the surgical patient might relate to and impact upon conditions so prominently associated with tumor evolution and metastasis (Fig. 3.1).[8]

Much of the detail concerning individual components of perioperative care, their potential interplay with cancer pathogenesis, and their potential role in influencing disease outcomes will be explored in the chapters that follow. The goal of this chapter is to introduce the common biological themes applicable to solid cancers and to construct a conceptual framework that begins to relate these themes to the potentially influential events taking place within the perioperative period.

Development of a Tumor

The origins of more than 200 types of human cancers are diverse, but fundamentally are thought to concern a series of genetic, environmental, and host interactions that drive healthy somatic cells through a multistep process toward a neoplastic state. The defining, transformative event involves the corruption and unfaithful propagation of a cell's genetic code, with the chances of such events occurring now clearly understood to be influenced by a combination of hereditary and environmental factors. The principles of Darwinian natural selection govern the likelihood as to whether these mutations are carried forward through subsequent rounds of cell division,[12,13] with those attributable to phenotypes that confer some degree of survival, functional, or proliferative advantage tending to drive the emergence of a predominant clone that may eventually manifest as a tumor. The great majority of human tumors are benign; it is the acquisition of invasive or disseminative capabilities that determines malignancy, and it is the metastases spawned by these tumors that are responsible for 90% of cancer-related deaths.[14]

Cancer is a disease of clonal evolution[12,15] that explains both the process of carcinogenesis and the tendency for most advanced cancers to eventually acquire therapy resistance. For many years, the prevailing model of tumor development traced neoplasms to a single ancestral cell of origin, which acquired the necessary initiating genetic lesion(s) to transition from health to a cancer cell. In a linear fashion, its progeny would sequentially acquire and accumulate mutations that enabled an ever-more autonomous, inimical existence, culminating with the host-compromising capabilities of invasion, dissemination, and growth in distant sites. We now understand that most cancers exhibit a considerable degree of clonal and subclonal heterogeneity, comprising numerous genetically and phenotypically distinct subpopulations of cells that both compete and cooperate with each other (Fig. 3.2).[16–18] These arise from heritable and stochastic genetic and epigenetic changes over time, driven locally by microenvironmental variation across the three-dimensional architecture of a developing tumor, and systemically by factors such as nutrition, hormones, infection, and environmental exposures.[12] Furthermore, while metastasis has long been described in terms of a late event in the evolution of a primary tumor, there is increasing evidence that dissemination occurs early, in some cases even before the discernible manifestation of a primary tumor,[19] potentially leading to the parallel progression of secondary growths at distant sites that are remarkably distinct from each other and the primary tumor (Fig. 3.3).[20]

These observations have transformed thinking in cancer biology in recent years, lifting the horizons of research beyond cancer cell-autonomous paradigms of oncogenes and tumor suppressors towards the dynamic forces at play within the intratumoral and organismal ecosystem. They also point to the troubling reality that many tumors will have seeded distant organs with thousands of cancer cells by the time of diagnosis, where disparate ecologies provide the pressures for further clonal diversification. Thus, while disease may appear clinically localized, the likely existence of invisible micrometastases means that the systemic impact of surgery and anesthesia following complete resection of the primary tumor should never be discounted.

Nature of a Tumor

The biological complexities of tumors have been rationalized by Hanahan and Weinberg's widely acknowledged "Hallmarks of Cancer,"[21,22] which sets out the unifying themes and overarching phenotypic characteristics of

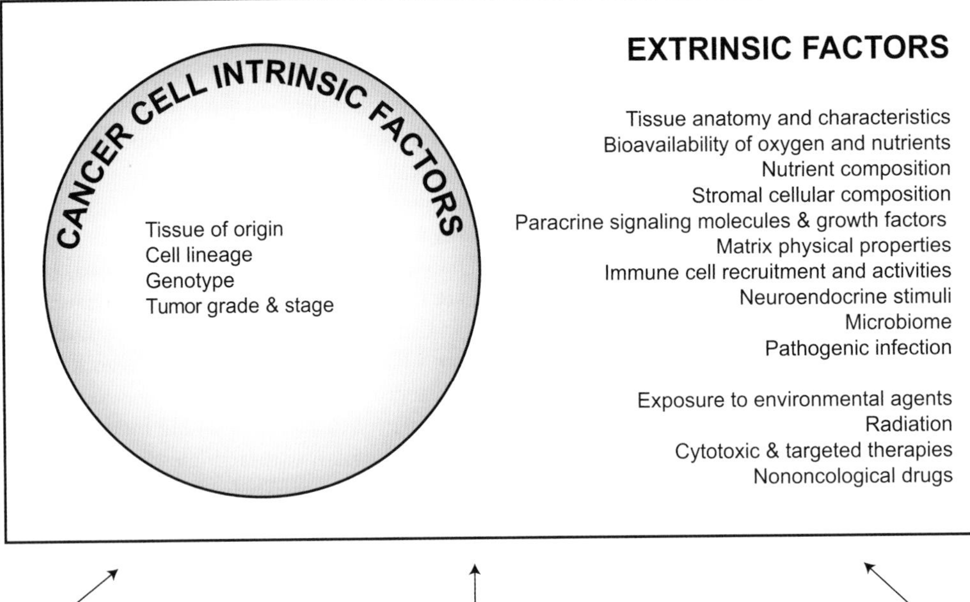

Preoperative

- Anxiety-driven SNS activation
- "Prehabilitation" / physiological optimisation
- Neoadjuvant therapy

Intraoperative

- Tumour handling
- Vascular dilatation
- SNS activation
  - SNS fibers
  - circulating catecholamines
- Inflammatory initiation
  - local wound healing
  - systemic response
- Anesthetics / analgesics
  - Volatiles vs TIVA
  - Opioids
  - NSAIDs
  - Local anaesthetics
  - Neuraxial / regional
- Blood products
- Stasis
- Nutritional / fluid status
- Local / systemic hypoxia
- Clotting / platelet activity

Postoperative

- Ongoing inflammatory and SNS responses
- Pain
- Analgesia
  - opioids
  - NSAIDs
  - adjuncts
- Blood products
- Complications
  - infections
  - wound breakdown
  - organ dysfunction
  - cardiovascular
  - thrombotic / bleeding
- Stasis
- Nutrition and metabolism
- Lifestyle
- Return to intended oncological therapy

• **Fig. 3.1** The intrinsic and extrinsic factors that determine cancer cell phenotypes and tumor progression. Cancer cell phenotypes reflect the cumulative influence of these factors over the course of carcinogenesis and treatment. Some dynamic factors may induce acute phenotypic changes, while extreme or sustained pressures may apply selective forces to an evolving neoplasm. It is postulated that a range of potentially modifiable perioperative factors may also extrinsically influence the course of disease. *NSAIDs*, Nonsteroidal antiinflammatory drugs; *SNS*, sympathetic nervous system; *TIVA*, total intravenous anesthesia

human tumors, as they evolve from healthy, somatic cells to malignant neoplasms capable of unrestricted and potentially disseminated growth. In keeping with the reductionist nature of cancer research, these hallmarks are often studied and therapeutically targeted in relative isolation from one another, although their codependency and complementarity is essential to bear in mind.

Proliferative Signaling and Cell-Cycle Deregulation

Probably the most prominent feature of a cancer cell is its capability to sustain proliferation. Proliferation is normally tightly controlled by a concert of growth signaling molecules and checkpoints in order to maintain normal tissue function, architecture, and repair capabilities throughout the mammalian lifespan, but defects in one or more nodes of these cellular systems can lead to progressive deregulation and autonomy of cell-cycle progression. There are a number of ways in which cancer cells have been shown to exploit the enabling mechanisms of proliferation, including overexpression of cell surface receptor proteins to render cells hyperresponsive to relatively low ligand bioavailability and autocrine stimulation via the self-production of growth factor ligands, as well as by engaging in reciprocal signaling with resident and infiltrating cells of the local

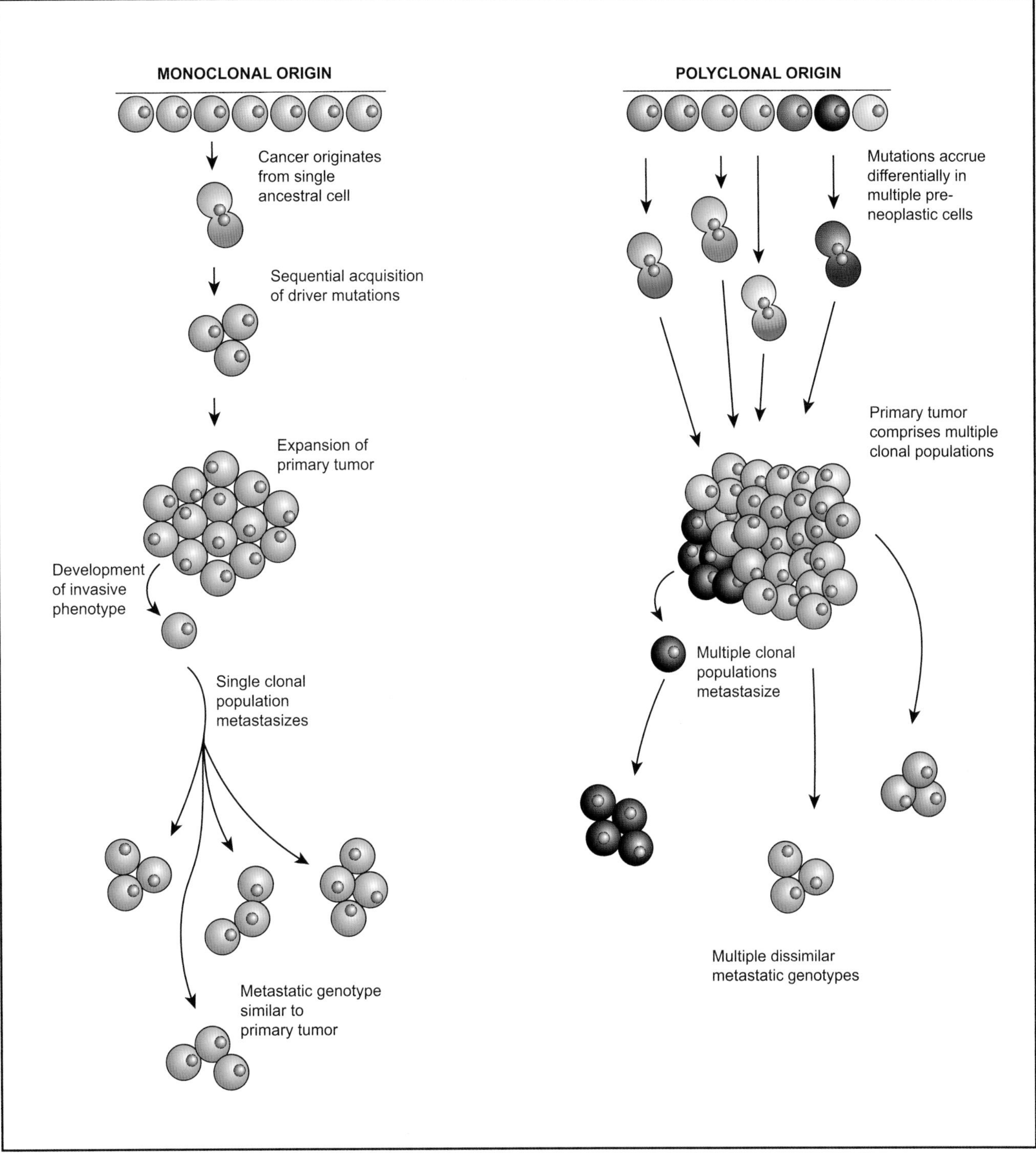
MONOCLONAL ORIGIN
Cancer originates from single ancestral cell
Sequential acquisition of driver mutations
Expansion of primary tumor
Development of invasive phenotype
Single clonal population metastasizes
Metastatic genotype similar to primary tumor
POLYCLONAL ORIGIN
Mutations accrue differentially in multiple pre-neoplastic cells
Primary tumor comprises multiple clonal populations
Multiple clonal populations metastasize
Multiple dissimilar metastatic genotypes

• **Fig. 3.2** Clonal evolution of tumors and metastases. The monoclonal theory of cancer evolution indicates that cancers originate from a single ancestral cell. The acquisition of mutations to proto-oncogenes or tumor suppressor genes initiates transition from a healthy cell to a cancer cell, giving rise to a tumor comprising a single clonal population. In this model, all tumor cells and metastatic descendants should harbor the same initiating lesion(s). Multiregion and paired primary-metastatic genome analyses have shown that considerable clonal heterogeneity can exist, which may be alternatively explained by polyclonal origin. Here, two or more cells acquire (potentially different) initiating mutations that each give rise to their own clonal population. This has implications for molecular stratification of tumors and therapeutic decision-making, since each clone may respond quite differently.

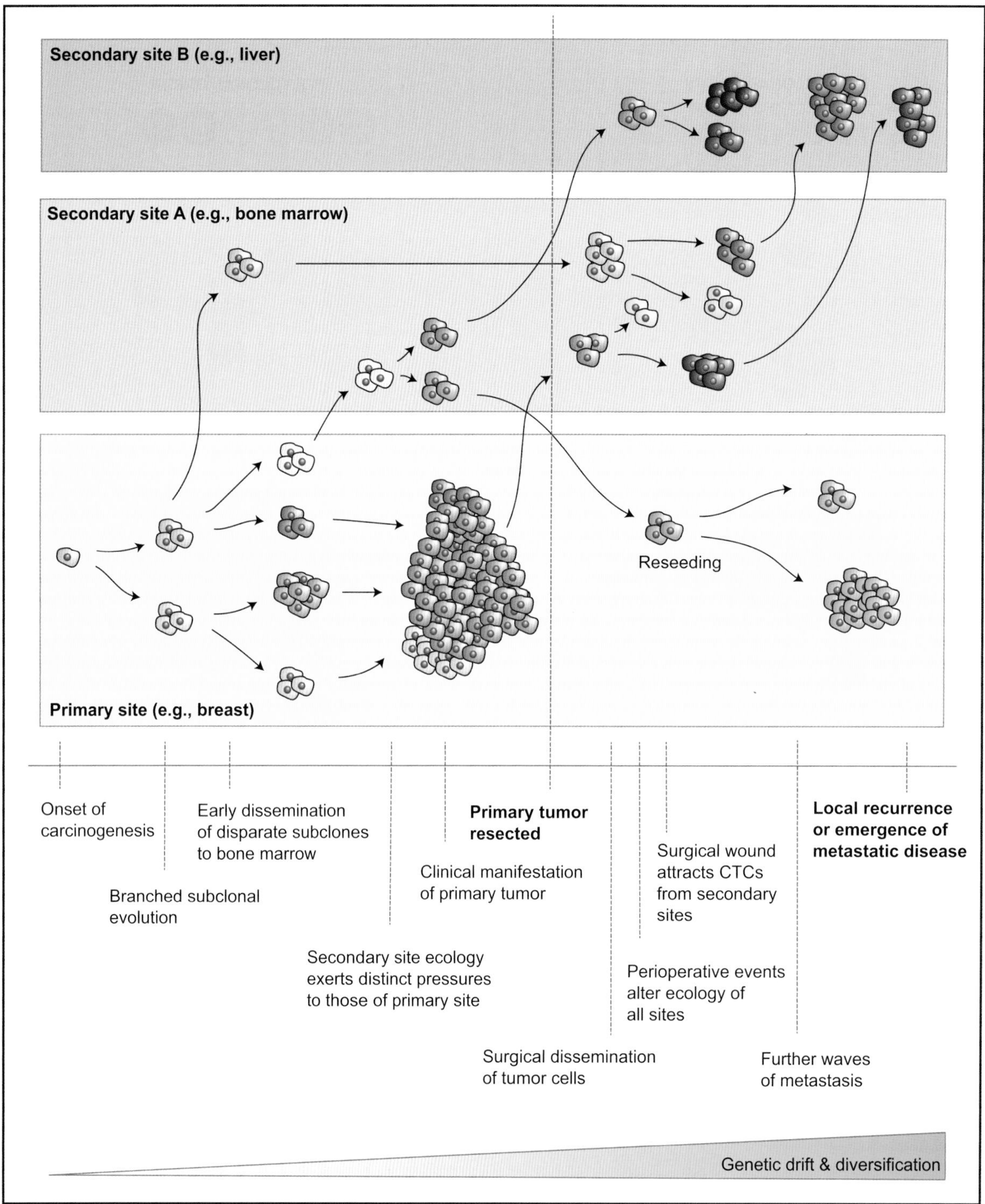

• **Fig. 3.3** Parallel progression of disseminated tumor cells. In contrast to the linear model of carcinogenesis where metastatic potential is said to be a late acquisition, cancer cells may disseminate early in the course of disease in response to extrinsic cues, potentially prior to the manifestation of a primary tumor. These disseminated cells evolve under disparate ecologies and selective pressures to those of the primary tumor, resulting in substantial genetic and phenotypic diversification. However, if quiescent or growth-restricted (for example, by the immune system), they might never clinically emerge. Systemic environmental influences such as perioperative stress, inflammation, or pharmacology could impact these populations, leading to overt metastatic outgrowth and/or further rounds of metastasis, including reseeding of the primary tumor site. *CTCs*, Circulating tumor cells

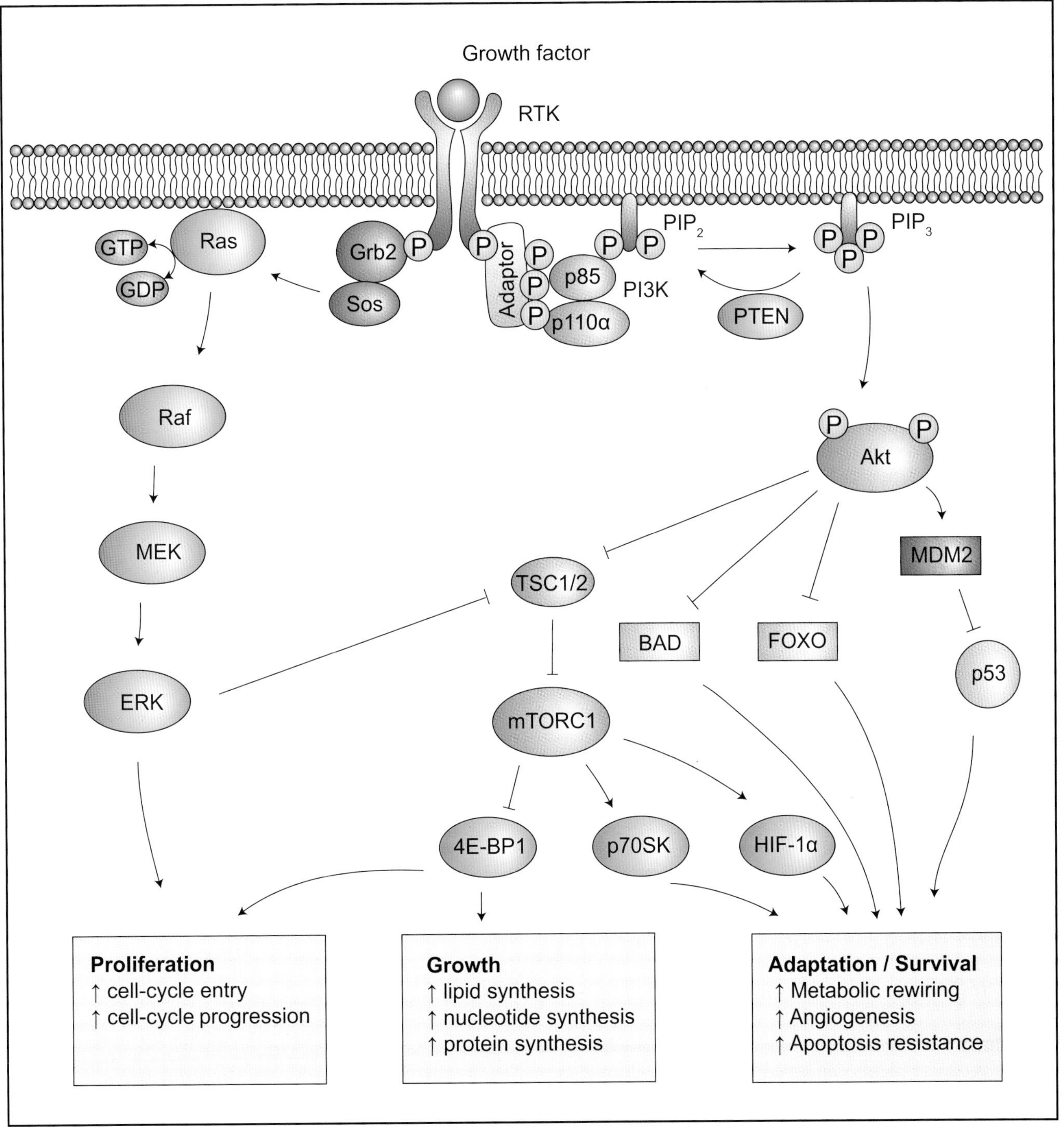

• **Fig. 3.4** Cancer cell signal transduction via the *PI3K/Akt/mTOR* and *RAS/RAF/MEK/ERK* pathways. Phosphoinositide 3-kinase (*PI3K*) is stimulated by diverse growth factor receptor tyrosine kinases or G-protein coupled receptors (not shown). PI3K catalytic and regulatory subunits (*p110α* and *p85*, respectively) are recruited to the plasma membrane by adaptor proteins that interact with activated receptors. PI3K phosphorylates phosphatidylinositol 4,5-bisphosphate (*PIP_2*) to generate phosphatidylinositol 3,4,5-trisphosphate (*PIP_3*). Phosphatase and tensin homolog (*PTEN*) reverse this reaction. PIP_3 is a second messenger that activates the pleiotropic Akt serine/threonine kinase (also known as protein kinase B, *PKB*). Akt phosphorylates the tuberous sclerosis proteins (*TSC*) 1 and 2, thereby dissociating the TSC1/2 complex and lifting its restriction of mammalian target of rapamycin complex 1 (*mTORC1*). Activation of mTORC1 upregulates lipid and protein synthesis, which supports cell growth and proliferation. Akt also phosphorylates BCL-2-associated agonist of cell death (*BAD*) and the Forkhead Box O (*FOXO*) transcription factors, leading to their inactivation, while phosphorylation of MDM2 negatively regulates p53, each increasing resistance to apoptosis. Meanwhile, docking proteins Grb2 and Sos associate with stimulated receptor tyrosine kinases and promote the active GTP-bound state of Ras. Active Ras initiates the downstream Raf/MEK/ERK cascade that culminates in promotion of cell-cycle entry and progression. ERK also reinforces mTORC1 activity by phosphorylating TSC1/2. Hyperactivation or growth factor autonomy commonly arises in tumors with mutations to one or more nodes in these pathways.

stroma. However, many tumors acquire growth factor independence through somatic mutations of key ligand receptors, enzymes, or transduction molecules comprised within mitogenic circuits (Fig. 3.4). Such pathways exist to mediate signals from cell surface receptors to the nucleus in order to permit the interpretation of and response to specific extracellular cues, such as the presence of growth factors, cytokines, and microenvironmental stress; however, their corruption may lead to inappropriate, constitutive activation in the absence of such cues. For example, activating mutations that affect the structure of the B-Raf serine/threonine kinase—which stimulates the extracellular signal-regulated kinase (ERK)/mitogen-activated protein kinase (MAPK) cascade—are known to exist in approximately 8% of all human cancers,[23] especially melanomas (50%).[24] Mutations of Ras—a binary molecular switch that cycles between active guanosine triphosphate (GTP)-bound and inactive guanosine diphosphate (GDP)-bound states, also upstream of the ERK/MAPK cascade—underlie approximately 90% of pancreatic cancers and 50% of colon cancers.[25] In such cases, Ras GTPase activity is compromised, leading to the impairment of an intrinsic negative feedback mechanism operating to ensure signal transmission is transient.

Phosphoinositide 3-kinase (PI3K) signaling is one of the most frequently dysregulated pathways in cancer[26] and exerts influence on many hallmark phenotypes besides proliferation. Aside from responding to increased oncogenic signals upstream, it may be hyperactivated directly by malignant transformations. These include gain-of-function mutations to the PI3K catalytic subunit (most commonly the *PIK3CA* oncogene encoding p110α) that phosphorylates phosphatidylinositol 4,5-bisphosphate (PIP_2) to generate phosphatidylinositol 3,4,5-trisphosphate (PIP_3), as well as inactivating mutations or loss-of-heterozygosity in tumor suppressor genes such as *PTEN*. PTEN is a 3′ phosphatase that counteracts PI3K by dephosphorylating PIP_3 back to PIP_2.[27] The net result of an overabundance of PIP_3 is the hyperactivation of multiple downstream effectors, including most notably, the pleiotropic serine/threonine kinase Akt (also known as protein kinase B).[28,29] Among the most highly conserved functions of Akt are its roles in promoting cell growth, via activation of mTOR complex 1 (mTORC1), and in supporting cell proliferation by the complementary phosphorylation of GSK3, TSC2, and PRAS40, which drive cell-cycle entry and progression, and the inactivation of the $p27^{Kip1}$ and $p21^{Cip1/WAF1}$ cyclin-dependent kinase inhibitors. Reflecting the advantageous nature of amplified PI3K-Akt signaling in tumorigenesis, a recent meta-analysis of cancer genome data from nearly 5000 tumor samples revealed that *PIK3CA* and *PTEN* represent the second- and third-most frequently mutated genes in human cancer.[30]

The most commonly mutated gene, accounting for approximately 50% of all human cancers, is the tumor suppressor, p53,[30,31] which illustrates the gain that also comes from circumventing antiproliferative safeguards. Accordingly, *TP53* is the most studied human gene in history[32] and is frequently referred to as the "guardian of the genome" in recognition of its central role in DNA damage response. In response to cellular insults and abnormalities, including genotoxic, metabolic, and replication stress, the stabilization and subsequent activity of this DNA-binding protein can arrest cell-cycle progression, instigate a raft of reparative and adaptive pathways, and govern cell-fate decisions such as apoptosis and senescence, with the overriding purpose of conserving genomic integrity.[33] Consistent with mediating its tumor-suppressive function through a transcriptional mechanism, the vast majority of cancer-associated *TP53* mutations occur in its DNA-binding domain.[34,35] Its role in cancer biology is appearing increasingly context-dependent, but in elementary terms, loss of p53 both lifts a major restriction on cell proliferation and promotes genome instability and phenotypic evolution by permitting the accumulation of oncogenic mutations through successive rounds of cell division.

Evading Cell Death

In addition to directing cell proliferation, both PI3K signaling and p53 (among many other players) are critically involved in determining cell survival. After sensing overwhelming stress or irreparable DNA damage, p53 transcriptionally activates a group of BCL-2 family proteins, including BAX, NOXA, and PUMA, which initiate apoptosis[36]—an orderly cascade beginning with mitochondrial outer membrane permeabilization (MOMP) and culminating in the proteolysis and self-destruction of a cell. Evidently, the acquisition of a loss-of-function mutation to p53 constitutes a major mechanistic opportunity for a renegade cell to evade death, as it navigates the numerous physiological stresses associated with hyperproliferation, tumorigenesis, or anticancer therapy. In tumors with functional p53, similar ends may also be achieved by alternative means to inhibit the activity of proapoptotic proteins or by overexpressing the counterbalancing, antiapoptotic members of the BCL-2 family, including BCL-2 itself, as well as $BCL\text{-}X_L$ and MCL-1. For instance, Akt can directly phosphorylate the proapoptotic BH3-only protein BAD,[37] thereby sequestering it from its target in the mitochondrial outer membrane and preventing its action in MOMP. Akt also phosphorylates the Forkhead Box O (FOXO) transcription factors,[38] leading to their displacement from the nucleus and suppression of FOXO target expression, including proapoptotic molecules such as BIM, PUMA, and Fas ligand (FasL). A third Akt-mediated survival mechanism returns us once more to p53, as Akt phosphorylates and promotes the nuclear translocation of MDM2—an E3 ubiquitin ligase and the main negative regulator of p53.[39,40]

The Tumor Microenvironment

Studying the genetic basis of cancer growth reveals the impact of chronically dysregulated signaling in mediating

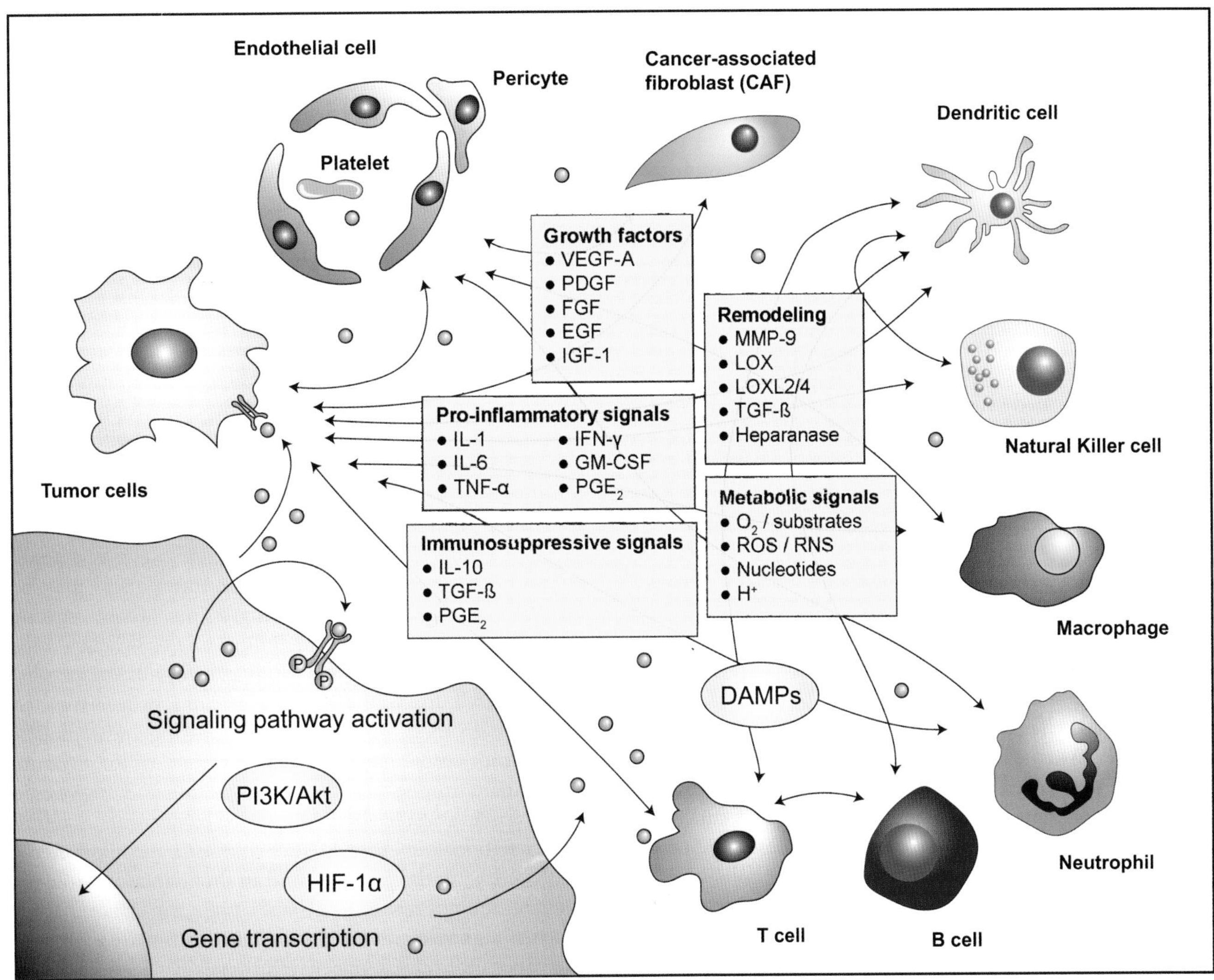

• **Fig. 3.5** Reciprocal signaling in the tumor microenvironment. Secretion of diverse signaling molecules promotes tumor cell and stromal cell activities in autocrine and paracrine fashions, leading to considerable crosstalk. Emerging neoplasms emit damage-associated molecular proteins (*DAMPs*) and other proinflammatory signals that initiate recruitment and activation of innate immune cells. In turn, these secrete further inflammatory cytokines and growth factors that both sustain the inflammatory response and reciprocally stimulate tumor cells. Simultaneously, secretion of angiogenic factors by tumor and stromal cells stimulates angiogenesis and endothelial activation, which further increases infiltration of circulating immune cells and alters the metabolic and physicochemical characteristics of the tumor. Chronic inflammation tends to promote differentiation of infiltrating immune cells into immunosuppressive, tumor-supportive phenotypes that contribute to immune evasion. Under the influence of soluble factors such as transforming growth factor beta (*TGF-β*), fibroblasts differentiate into cancer-associated fibroblasts that contribute their own growth factors and promote remodeling of the extracellular matrix. Metabolic factors such as oxygen and substrate availability and the secretion of by-products such as lactate and reactive oxygen/nitrogen species (*ROS/RNS*) exert significant stresses upon all cells, promoting adaptive behaviors through, for example, hypoxia Inducible factor 1 alpha (*HIF-1α*) and contributing to cell death and immune cell exhaustion. *EGF*, Epithelial growth factor; *FGF*, fibroblast growth factor; *GM-CSF*, granulocyte-macrophage colony-stimulating factor; H^+, protons; *IFN-γ*, interferon gamma; *IGF-1*, insulin-like growth factor-1; *IL*, interleukin; *LOX*, lysyl oxidase; *LOXL2/4*, lysyl oxidase-like 2/4; *MMP*, matrix metalloproteinase; *PDGF*, platelet-derived growth factor; *PGE_2*, prostaglandin E_2; *TNF-α*, tumor necrosis factor alpha; *VEGF-A*, vascular endothelial growth factor.

cancer cell phenotypes. Perhaps of greater interest to the perioperative physician is to know how, and to what consequence, these same oncogenic signaling pathways might be acutely perturbed by extrinsic events. After all, little can be done about tumor genotype by the time of presentation, whereas there may be an opportunity to modulate certain external influences that commonly cooperate in disease progression. Over the past decade, an abundance of work examining the conditions and other constituents of the tumor microenvironment (TME) has demonstrated the impact of such extrinsic factors on the growth and malignant potential of cancer cells, many of which can be closely compared with conditions and physiological processes engaged during the perioperative period.

In contrast to previous tumor-centric perspectives of cancer pathogenesis, we now know that an array of other specialized, nonmalignant cells—which comprise more than 50% of the mass of tumors—actively collaborate in promoting tumor growth and malignant progression (Fig. 3.5). These include fibroblasts and myofibroblasts, immune inflammatory cells, mesenchymal stem and progenitor cells, and vascular endothelial cells and pericytes. They are recruited and activated by danger-associated molecular patterns (DAMPs), cytokines, chemokines, and angiogenic factors emanating from emerging neoplasias, in much the same fashion as an acute inflammatory response to tissue trauma or infectious pathogens. Over time, transformed and nontransformed cells act in concert to form an increasingly reactive stroma, rich in soluble growth and inflammatory mediators, which sustains the inflammatory response, dynamically remodels the extracellular matrix, and reciprocally reinforces the malignant behavior of cancer cells.

Catecholamines emanating from the systemic circulation and infiltrating sympathetic neural fibers modulate transformed and nontransformed cells alike through activation of beta-adrenergic signaling. Adrenoceptors are often abundantly expressed at the sites of primary and metastatic tumors.[41] When stimulated by adrenaline or noradrenaline, the resulting cyclic AMP (cAMP) flux upstream of protein kinase A (PKA) and ERK/MAPK signaling pathways leads to an array of phenotypic responses in cancer cells and supporting stromal cells.[41,42] In addition to the aforementioned effects of MAPK signaling on cell growth and proliferation, these responses include cell metabolic, morphology, and motility changes, as well as inducing and sustaining angiogenesis, differentiation, and inflammation, which collectively remodel the TME.[41,43] Accordingly, in vivo cancer models show heightened sympathetic nervous system and beta-adrenergic signaling activation to accelerate tumor growth and metastasis,[43–49] while those models and epidemiological data from cancer patients point to the therapeutic potential of beta blockers.[50–52]

The biology of the TME is also substantially determined by its changing physical and chemical characteristics. Reflecting the increased metabolic activities of both tumor and stromal cells in conjunction with aberrant and underdeveloped vascularity, developing tumors are typified by hypoxia, acidosis, an accumulation of catabolic metabolites, and raised interstitial pressure. The extracellular matrix is also stiff and fibrotic in view of the increased collagen deposition by resident and recruited fibroblasts and frequent remodeling,[53,54] further exacerbating problems associated with hypoperfusion. These conditions invariably place substantial stresses upon all cells, invoking prosurvival adaptions in malignant cells and a state of exhaustion in tumoricidal immune cells, all the while perpetuating reactive changes in the stroma. In a perioperative context, it is worth considering how surgical disruption of local vasculature and lymphatics and the accompanying tissue edema, inflammation, and hypoxia may contribute to a wound microenvironment very similar to that of a growing tumor. Such stimulating conditions might support a residual fraction of cancer cells to reestablish a tumor or to disseminate, which could partially explain why surgical wound and inflammatory complications are associated with an increased risk of cancer recurrence.[55,56]

Tumor Immune Landscape

Infiltrating immune cells act in conflicting ways depending on tissue context or the balance of stimuli.[57,58] Many early tumors are rejected or kept in check by cell-mediated immune responses that sense altered-self cells and effect their elimination. In particular, the activities of natural killer (NK) cells, dendritic cells, M1-polarized macrophages, and cytotoxic $CD8^+$ T cells are strongly associated with a favorable prognosis.[59–63] $CD8^+$ T cells are supported by $CD4^+$ T helper 1 (T_H1) cells that produce interleukin (IL)-2 and interferon gamma (IFN-γ); an abundance of these is also associated with a good prognosis.[64] Conversely, as chronic inflammation ensues, a number of immune cells may be coopted to promote tumor progression. These include subpopulations of T cells, including $CD4^+$ T helper cells with a T_H2 orientation, as well as neutrophils, mast cells, M2-polarized macrophages, and myeloid progenitors. In keeping with their usual function in clearing and remodeling wounds, these latter types of immune cell contribute substantially to pools of growth-promoting and angiogenic factors such as EGF, FGF, and VEGF; invasion-enabling matrix remodeling enzymes such as matrix metalloproteinase (MMP)-9 and heparinase; and an abundance of cytokines and chemokines that amplify and sustain the inflammatory state through paracrine feedback loops with malignant cells and other infiltrates. Collectively, these have been shown to elicit and sustain multiple traits of high-grade malignancy and are associated with a poor prognosis.[57,65]

Cancer cells also exploit mechanisms to actively evade cell-mediated immunity, some of which may be driven by specific oncogenes such as BRAF and STAT3, but otherwise often arise through crosstalk with other stromal constituents.[66–68] For example, production of the eicosanoid prostaglandin E_2 impairs NK cell viability and cytolytic activity and subverts NK cell-mediated recruitment of dendritic cells into the TME resulting in immune escape[60,69]; this is in keeping with data showing correlations between poor NK cell abundance and function with local recurrence, metastasis, and reduced overall survival.[61,70,71] Similarly, expression of transforming growth factor (TGF)-β by both tumor cells and stromal cells promotes T-cell exclusion from tumors, inhibits the acquisition of an antitumor T_H1 phenotype, and stimulates the differentiation of immunosuppressive regulatory T (T_{reg}) cells, which at least partially explains why patients with elevated TGF-β levels tend to mount poor antitumor immune responses and derive less therapeutic benefit from immunotherapy.[72–74] T_{reg} cells crucially operate to maintain self-tolerance and immune homeostasis by competing for IL-2, secreting immunosuppressive cytokines (such as IL-10 and TGF-β), and suppressing antigen-presenting cell (APC)

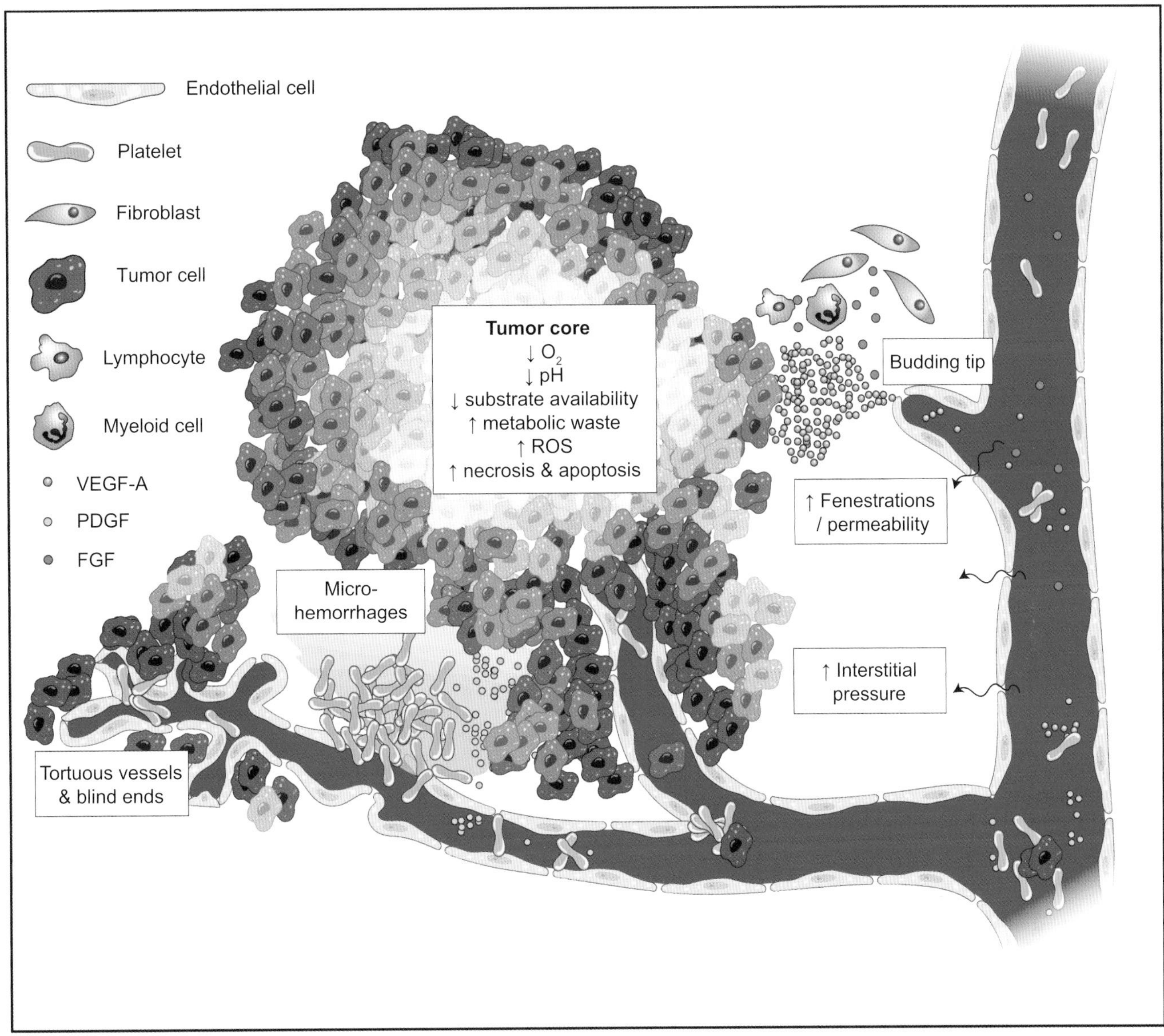

• **Fig. 3.6** Tumor angiogenesis. As proliferation continues, the expanding mass simultaneously grows further away from its blood supply while increasing its metabolic demands for oxygen and nutrients. A diffusion gradient is established across the tumor, where cells at the core find themselves increasingly starved of oxygen and metabolic substrates. Anoxic regions may become necrotic, but metabolic adaptations can allow cells to survive elsewhere in the tumor where oxygen tension and substrate availability is low. Secretion of angiogenic factors and matrix remodeling molecules by tumor and stromal cells stimulates sprouting of existing nearby vasculature and vasculogenesis toward and into the tumor to increase blood supply. Tumor vasculature is immature and dysfunctional, characterized by tortuosity, blind ends, and leakage. Activated platelets at sites of contact with vascular basement membrane or tumor stroma release stores of angiogenic and growth factors into the tumor microenvironment. The reactive stroma perpetuates endothelial activation and dysfunction, contributing further to interstitial edema and hypoperfusion. *FGF*, Fibroblast growth factor; *PDGF*, platelet-derived growth factor; *ROS*, reactive oxygen/nitrogen species; *VEGF-A*, vascular endothelial growth factor-A.

function by expressing cytotoxic T lymphocyte antigen 4 (CTLA-4), but their contribution in an oncological context only serves to antagonize effector lymphocytes, undermine host defense, and worsen clinical outcomes.[75,76]

Angiogenesis

As with any other tissue, tumors need to develop a vascular infrastructure to maintain delivery of sufficient oxygen and nutrients and to drain metabolic by-products. The sprouting and assembly of new blood vessels from the preexisting vascular network is usually a transient homeostatic process in health, but is a consistent and usually sustained feature of growing tumors that has been described in terms of tripping an "angiogenic switch." Often evident in histological slices of premalignant lesions such as dysplasia, it is also an early feature of tumor development,[77] becoming more robust and penetrating as the growing tumor develops a fuller stromal compartment and strives to satisfy its metabolic demands. Yet tumor-associated vasculature is typically structurally aberrant and dysfunctional, reflecting the excessive and disorderly proangiogenic signaling driving the process. It is characterized by excessive branching, fenestrations, blind ends, and discontinuous cellular architecture that contribute to a state of turbulent flow, impaired perfusion, excessive vascular permeability, and acute fluxes in oxygen tension and substrate availability (Fig. 3.6).[78]

Much attention has been directed toward the prototypical angiogenic factor vascular endothelial growth factor-A (VEGF-A) and the receptor tyrosine kinases that mediate its canonical effects on endothelial cell proliferation, migration, survival, and permeability. VEGF-A is secreted by most cancer cells, as well as surrounding stromal cells,[79] while the degree of expression correlates with invasiveness, metastasis, recurrence, and prognosis.[80] As a transcriptional target of hypoxia inducible factor (HIF)-1, its expression is prominently influenced by tumor hypoxia.[81] Similarly, oncogenic mutations that directly enhance HIF stability (such as VHL mutations commonly seen in clear cell renal carcinomas) or signaling pathway activity upstream of HIF-1, including PI3K/Akt signaling, also drive angiogenesis through VEGF-A.[82,83] However, its expression—along with other proangiogenic factors such as platelet-derived growth factor (PDGF) and fibroblast growth factor (FGF)—may also be induced and reciprocally reinforced in the stromal compartment by activated platelets, immune inflammatory cells, and fibroblasts, highlighting the importance of extrinsic regulation of angiogenesis by the TME.

Reprogramming Cellular Energy Metabolism

The rapid and sustained proliferative activities of a growing tumor must be accompanied by substantial adaptations to cellular metabolism, especially within a context of limited oxygen and nutrient bioavailability. Metabolic "reprogramming," a term widely used in recent cancer metabolism literature, describes the upregulation or suppression of conventional metabolic pathways undertaken to satisfy the heightened energy and biosynthetic requirements of tumors, improve cellular fitness, and support cell survival under stressful and nutrient-deprived conditions.[84,85]

The first observations on this were made by Otto Warburg, long before the discovery of oncogenes and tumor suppressors. Enhanced glycolysis is a normal physiological response to hypoxia, but Warburg noticed that cancer cells preferentially employ glucose metabolism over oxygen-consuming mitochondrial metabolism, leading to the production of substantial quantities of lactate regardless of oxygen availability (a phenomenon now known as the Warburg effect).[86–88] Indeed, a marked increase in glucose uptake and utilization is a characteristic of many tumors,[89] and it is this very phenotype that has been exploited in diagnostics for many years through use of a radiolabeled glucose analog (^{18}F-fluorodeoxyglucose, FDG) in positron emission tomography (PET). From a cellular energetics perspective, this state of "aerobic glycolysis" is ostensibly counterintuitive, since glycolysis is 18 times less efficient in yielding ATP per mole of glucose than oxidative phosphorylation. This led Warburg to reason that perhaps it was not adopted out of choice, but rather out of necessity to compensate for defects in the mitochondrial respiratory apparatus. However, while certainly true in some instances, numerous observations have since demonstrated that defective respiration is not a ubiquitous feature of malignant cells and that many cancers exhibit the Warburg effect while retaining functional mitochondrial respiration.[89] Moreover, enhanced expression of glucose transporters and rate-limiting glycolytic enzymes have now been extensively associated with activation of oncogenes such as KRAS[90] and MYC,[91–93] loss of tumor suppressors like p53,[94–96] or malignant cooption of physiological PI3K/Akt/mTOR[97] or HIF[98] signaling, suggesting that such a metabolic phenotype is actively selected for its capabilities in supporting tumorigenesis.[84,99] Indeed, we now understand that an overriding advantage of upregulating glycolysis in cancer is to enhance the flux of glycolytic intermediates through subsidiary pathways involved in macromolecular biosynthesis and redox homeostasis (Fig. 3.7A).

Substrates besides glucose also contribute to core bioenergetic, anabolic, and redox control pathways in cancer. One such example is the nonessential amino acid glutamine,[100] which contributes to tricarboxylic acid (TCA) cycle anaplerosis[101] (the replenishment of the cycle with carbon molecules extracted for macromolecule biosynthesis). The alternative carbon source that glutaminolysis provides is especially relied upon when the use of pyruvate-derived carbons through oxidative TCA cycle reactions is impaired by hypoxia or mitochondrial dysfunction (Fig. 3.7B). Such conditions would normally be growth limiting, but many cancers can continue to synthesize the lipids required for cell growth and division through reductive metabolism of glutamine.[102–104] Fatty acids,[105] branched-chain amino acids,[106] serine, and glycine[107] are other prominent examples of commonly utilized fuels, while in the event of severe nutrient or growth factor deprivation, cells make use of a number of catabolic and scavenging pathways to replenish the pool of vital metabolites. These include autophagy[108]—a highly regulated process of degrading and recycling intracellular macromolecules and organelles—and micropinocytosis,[109] which enables cells to engulf, internalize, and recycle extracellular debris. Collectively, these observations illustrate the potential for cancer cells to acquire remarkable metabolic plasticity, allowing them to call upon a multitude of fuels depending on prevailing nutrient availability and their chief biological requirements at any given time. This, in turn, empowers them to compete, survive, and grow within the harsh constraints of the TME or elsewhere.

Invasion and Metastasis

The vast majority of cancer deaths are caused by metastatic disease, yet this remains an area of cancer biology that is

A

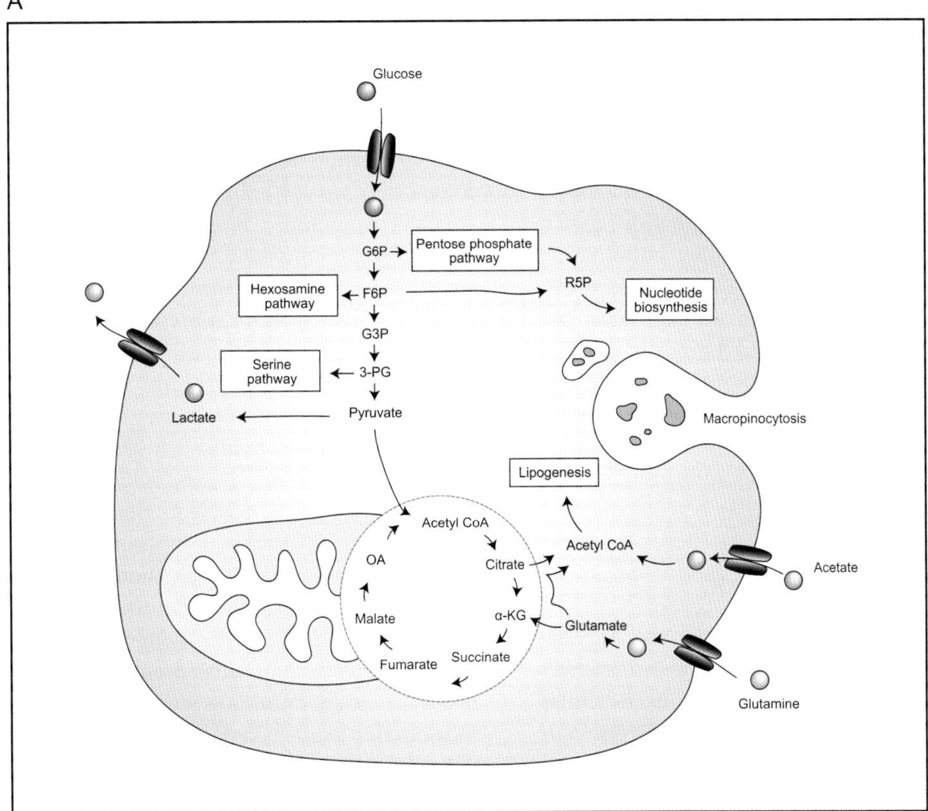

B

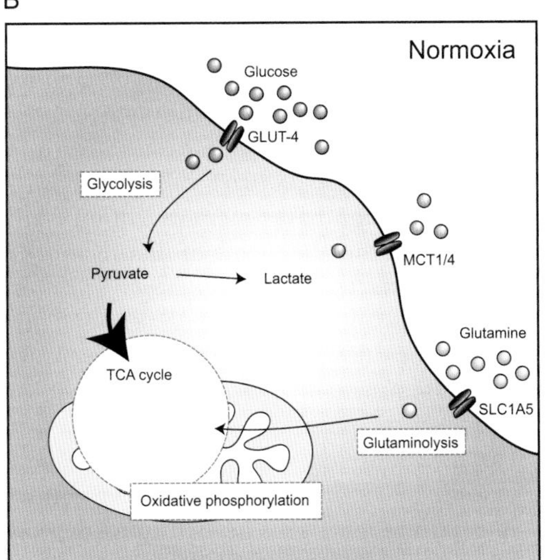

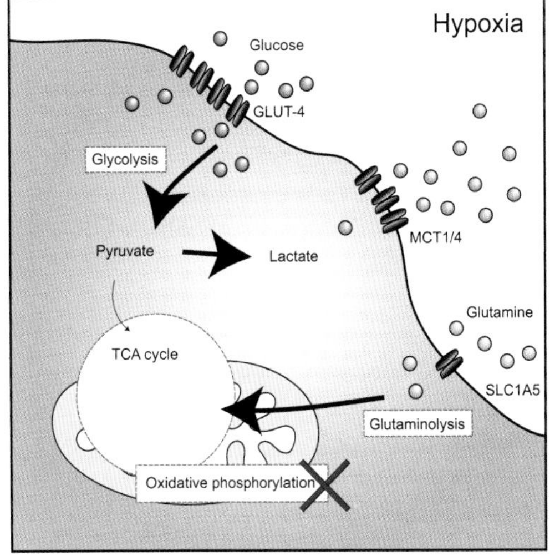

• **Fig. 3.7** Overview of cancer metabolism. **(A)** Cancer cells frequently upregulate glycolysis, even under aerobic conditions. Glucose metabolism can allow diversion of carbon toward subsidiary pathways including the hexosamine, serine, and pentose phosphate pathways. These play a role in generating the biomass required for ongoing cell growth and proliferation as well as maintaining antioxidant capacity. Pyruvate may be supplied to the tricarboxylic acid (*TCA*) cycle for oxidative metabolism or alternatively converted into lactate to help maintain energetic favorability for glycolysis. TCA cycle intermediates form precursors for other growth-enabling macromolecules, such as citrate for lipid synthesis. Glutamine may also supply a carbon to the TCA cycle in the form of alpha-ketoglutarate (αKG) that under reductive conditions can also generate citrate for fatty acid biosynthesis. Under severe nutrient-deprived conditions, cancer cells can also engulf extracellular debris and recycle macromolecules to support metabolism in a process known as macropinocytosis. **(B)** When oxygen tension is low, oxidative metabolism is impaired and cells must rely on glycolysis for energy. Sensors and regulators of hypoxia, including hypoxia inducible factor-1α, upregulate glucose uptake and glycolysis by increasing the expression of glucose transporters and glycolytic enzymes. Pyruvate is diverted away from mitochondria and metabolized predominantly into lactate to maintain glycolytic favorability, while intracellular pH is maintained by enhancing lactate efflux through monocarboxylate transporters. Reductive metabolism of glutamine-derived αKG maintains pools of key TCA cycle intermediates such as citrate to support continued lipid synthesis and growth under hypoxia.

poorly understood. At its most basic level, the dissemination of cancer cells and subsequent seeding of distant tumor colonies are portrayed as a multistep process known as the metastatic cascade.[110,111] This begins with the acquisition of a migratory and invasive phenotype, enabling cells to exit the primary site and gain access to blood and lymphatic vessels. Following a period of transit through the circulatory system, there is a progression through margination, arrest, and extravasation in distant organ capillaries, culminating in the colonization and outgrowth of new, secondary disease. However, as illustrated by the behavior of ovarian carcinomas that tend to disseminate transcoelomically through the peritoneum, the predilection of certain cancers for specific secondary sites, and the curious genotypic discrepancies between metastatic colonies and their parent tumors, the reality is considerably more complex and multifactorial than this schema depicts.

Epithelial-Mesenchymal Transition

The first stage of metastasis is expedited by the acquisition of properties that fundamentally alter a cancer cell's relationship with the primary tumor and the extracellular matrix. These properties—notably including morphological changes, increased motility, and a loss of cell-to-cell adhesion—are bestowed through the hijacking of a multifaceted developmental and tissue repair program known as epithelial-mesenchymal transition (EMT).[112,113] EMT is orchestrated by several transcription factors, including Slug, Twist, Snail, and Zeb1/2 that regulate the expression of overlapping sets of genes. One of the best characterized transcriptional responses involves the repressed expression of E-cadherin, a pivotal cell-to-cell adhesion glycoprotein that tethers adjacent epithelial cells by adherens junctions. Loss of E-cadherin facilitates the disaggregation and liberation of tumor cells from the primary tumor.[114] EMT also heightens expression of the matrix degradation enzymes necessary to enable invasive passage through surrounding tissue and enhances resilience against anoikis (a form of cell death that occurs following matrix detachment and during dissemination). As well as conspiring to promote metastasis, EMT has also been associated with increased resistance to chemotherapy and radiotherapy.

Although the terminology and its portrayal in the literature might create an impression that cancer cells tend to exist in one of two binary states, EMT may be activated transiently and to a spectrum of extents, granting cancer cells a certain plasticity to respond to their surrounding landscape and extrinsic events during the course of invasion and metastasis. To reinforce this point, while the induction of a fully mesenchymal state may favor certain aspects of invasion and dissemination, it has been indicated by recent studies to be dispensable for metastasis[115,116] and indeed for hindering the tumor-initiating capacity required to produce metastatic colonies.[117,118] Furthermore, E-cadherin, whose expression is repressed by EMT programs, has been shown to act as a necessary survival factor during the detachment, dissemination, and colonization phases of metastasis across multiple models of breast cancer.[119] This suggests that it is not the outright switch to a mesenchymal phenotype per se that promotes metastasis, rather it is the flexibility to reversibly express certain mesenchymal traits while retaining a selection of important others that are epithelial.[14]

EMT programs may be driven intrinsically by oncogenic signaling, but consistent with the notion of cellular plasticity in relation to the surrounding microenvironment, they are also activated in response to extrinsic metabolic factors and heterotypic signals arising from the surrounding stroma.[58] Classically, these include TGF-β, Wnt, and Notch, but additionally implicated are growth factors, such as epidermal growth factor (EGF), FGF, PDGF, hypoxia-induced signaling through HIF-1, and inflammatory molecules such as NF-κB, IL-1β, and TNF-α that derive from an array of infiltrating myeloid and lymphoid cells.[120–122] Critical observations from recent experimental models support this. First, signs of EMT have been found even in premalignant lesions, rendering cells competent to disseminate and form metastases seemingly without an opportunity to acquire the necessary driver mutations stochastically during primary tumor development.[19,123,124] Second, EMT, dissemination, and metastasis of developing pancreatic cancers are dramatically enhanced by iatrogenic acute pancreatitis,[19] while early metastasis of ductal carcinoma in situ (DCIS) lesions in breast is reliant upon signals emanating from macrophages,[125] thereby demonstrating the potent effects of inflammatory conditions to cancer cell phenotypes and metastatic potential. Finally, hypoxic preconditioning of neuroblastoma cells not only enhances their own capacity to metastasize but also enables hypoxia-naïve cells to follow, illustrating that cancer cells can have "memory" of an earlier environment and impart the phenotype of that memory on neighboring counterparts.[126]

Such examples indicate that the traits of high-grade malignancy do not develop in the exclusively cancer cell–autonomous manner once held. Moreover, they strongly allude to the possibility that nascent cancer cells might be empowered to negotiate the steps of the invasion-metastasis cascade by extrinsic factors alone; in other words, that acquisition of mutations beyond those that promote early tumor formation may not be a prerequisite for metastasis. The extrapolation of such a hypothesis to the surgical setting has yet to be robustly tested, but given the parallels between the reactive tumor-associated stroma and healing wounds, it is conceivable that the signals elicited by surgical wounding impinge on residual cancer cells to activate previously quiescent EMT programs. This, at least in some circumstances, might be sufficient to provoke the emergence of postoperative disease.

Circulating Tumor Cells

Elevated levels of circulating tumor cells (CTCs) indicate poor prognosis for several cancers,[127–129] reflecting

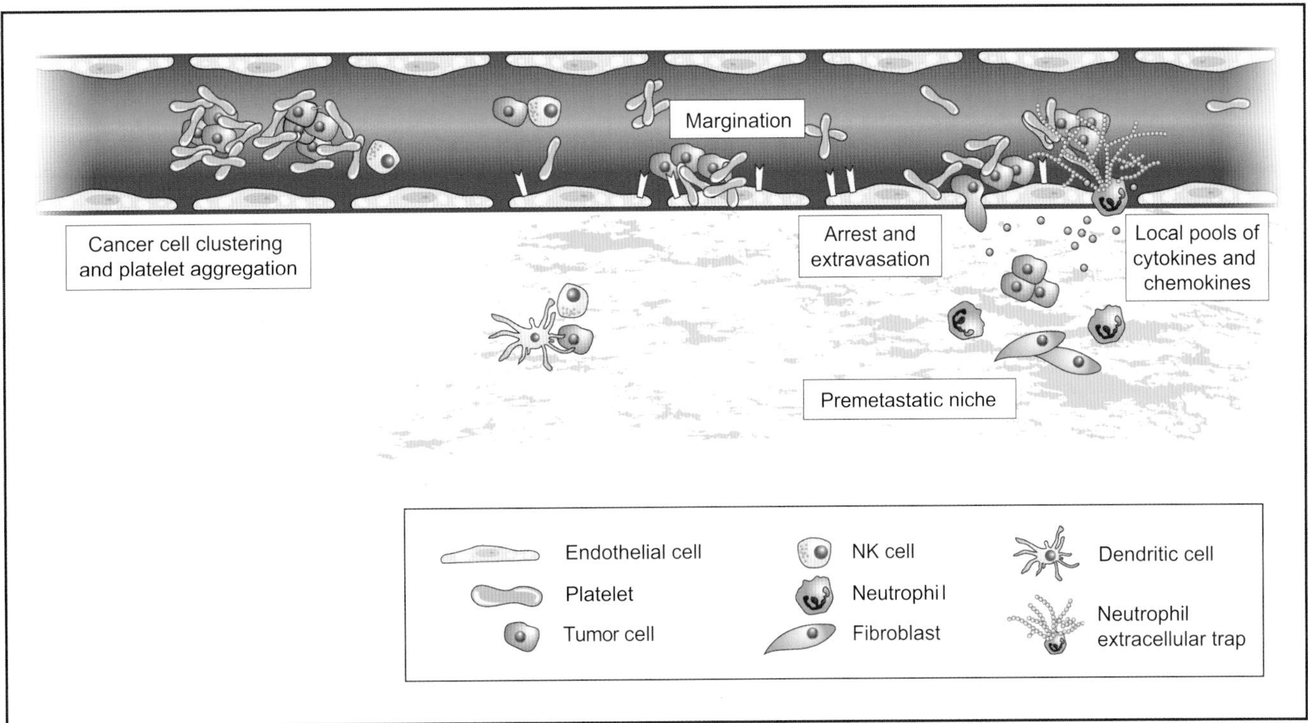

• **Fig. 3.8** Survival and extravasation of circulating tumor cells (CTCs). CTCs are exposed to harsh physical forces in the circulation and vulnerable to attack from circulating and marginated innate immune cells. Most will die, but some survive to reach the small-caliber capillary beds of distant organs. Formation of clusters with other CTCs or aggregates with platelets offers physical and biological protection from these threats. Activated platelets supply signaling molecules such as TGF-β to CTCs to maintain or tune a state of partial epithelial-mesenchymal transition (EMT). Larger aggregates may arrest by becoming physically lodged, but others may marginate in a fashion similar to that of immune cells, where expression of adhesion molecules on the surface of the endothelium attracts and holds cells to the vascular wall. In inflamed tissues, endothelial dysfunction exposes underlying basement membrane or collagen, where platelets form aggregates; meanwhile, activated neutrophils externalize DNA molecules to form neutrophil extracellular traps. Both help to trap CTCs and bring them into close contact with the vascular endothelium, through which they can migrate to reach the extravascular parenchyma.

the importance of the hematogenous route of dissemination and the notion that these cells stand as intermediaries between primary and metastatic disease. These relatively rare cells have historically proved difficult to study, but technical improvements in their isolation from blood samples and in molecular single-cell analysis promise novel opportunities, both in terms of understanding their biology and, perhaps, in tracking the influence of perioperative factors on their abundance and fate. Indeed, their behavior has emerged as a topic of interest in perioperative oncology in light of evidence that there is a spike in their number during and after surgery[130,131] and that detection of CTCs in the postoperative period has been identified as an independent prognostic marker of recurrence.[132]

CTCs are many times greater in number than that of clinically detectable metastases,[133,134] indicating that factors aside from quantity, such as survival and cell-intrinsic tumor initiation capacity, are important determinants of metastasis. Indeed, the extensive attrition of CTCs following direct injection into the bloodstream in experimental models illustrates the great inefficiency of the latter steps of the metastatic cascade.[135–138] Intravascular transit is replete with obstacles, and CTCs must first survive long enough to reach the small-caliber vessels of distant tissues, if they are to successfully seed new colonies. In addition to the cell-intrinsic stresses that are induced by loss of attachment and which often lead to anoikis,[139,140] CTCs are subjected to fluidic forces and shear stress to which they are naïve and are exposed to threats from circulating and marginalized innate immune effectors such as NK cells.[141–143] Traveling in clusters or as aggregates with activated platelets helps to physically shield them from such hazards,[144] while signaling cues from platelets serve to fine tune or sustain EMT programs while in transit (Fig. 3.8).[145] Metabolic adaptations further bolster anoikis resistance, in particular, by upregulating antioxidant pathways to tackle redox stress.[139,146,147]

Colonization

Colonization of secondary sites represents the most complex and rate-limiting step of metastasis, requiring CTCs to successfully extricate themselves from the vasculature, settle, and ultimately proliferate in a new host tissue. Many CTCs, particularly if traveling as clumps, become mechanically trapped in capillaries, but interactions with leukocytes and the vascular endothelium also facilitate margination and arr est.[145,146,148,149] Activated neutrophils play a prominent role here, sequestering CTCs in neutrophil extracellular traps (NETs),[150,151] which are web-like structures of externalized chromatin and antimicrobial granule proteins intended to ensnare circulating pathogens during infection.[152] Entangled CTCs are brought into closer contact with the vascular endothelium, to which they may adhere and traverse, and where they may be stimulated in paracrine fashion by localized chemokine pools (Fig. 3.8). Additionally contributing to microvascular thrombosis, organ dysfunction, and delayed wound healing,[153,154] NETs are increasingly recognized to play a role in a wide range of perioperative pathologies and have been highlighted as prominent candidates in mediating the links between surgical stress and postoperative metastatic progression.[155,156]

The vascular wall is an obvious physical barrier to colonization, and the fenestrated nature of sinusoids in the liver and bone marrow explains the high incidence of liver and bone metastasis.[157,158] However, model systems also highlight the importance of tumor-, platelet-, and leukocyte-derived mediators of endothelial disjunction and permeability, such as VEGF, cyclooxygenase (COX)2, and angiopoietin-like 4 (ANGPTL4), in overcoming this barrier,[159–162] implying that states of endothelial permeability arising from systemic inflammatory responses or postoperative microcirculatory dysfunction might also expediate metastatic colonization of cells disseminated during or shortly after surgery. In support of this, models of systemic inflammation induced by lipopolysaccharide (LPS) or cecal ligation have been shown to significantly enhance tumor cell extravasation and metastasis by inducing adhesive interactions and endothelial barrier disruption,[150,163] while oxidative stress associated with surgical trauma has been implicated in endothelial dysfunction, downregulation of tight junction proteins, exposure of subendothelial extracellular matrix, and increased postoperative liver metastasis in rats.[164]

Metastatic Outgrowth

The outgrowth and clinical manifestation of a metastatic colony in a distant organ represents the final stage in the malignant progression of a cancer, but this too is governed by a multitude of factors, many of which remain poorly understood. Even small tumors are capable of dispersing millions of cancer cells; many patients harbor disseminated cancer cells in their bone marrow for years, yet only about half of these patients develop metastases.[135,165] Similarly, most patients undergoing intentionally curative primary tumor resection, who go on to develop metastatic disease, do not show signs until months, years, or even decades after primary tumor resection.[14,135] Together, these observations indicate that for much of the time, single disseminated cells or small micrometastatic clusters lie dormant and clinically imperceptible—a state commonly referred to as minimal residual disease.

Just as the microenvironment and other non-transformed stromal constituents are integral to primary tumor development, so too do they appear crucial in determining the fate of disseminated cancer cells. The new ecologies these cells find themselves in are unfamiliar, devoid of the original stromal constituents, growth factors, and signals that had sustained and shaped them at the primary site, while stromally-derived paracrine factors such as TGF-β can actively induce proliferative quiescence and inhibit self-renewal.[166,167] Latency may therefore reflect an incapacity to proliferate in these new arenas, or a net equilibrium between proliferation and elimination where micrometastases are kept in check by immune surveillance or other such restraints.[168]

Again, an inflammatory etiology has been heavily connected with this final phase of metastatic outgrowth. Studies show the metastatic microenvironment to host a variety of bone marrow–derived cells that exhibit inflammatory features.[169–171] While the primary tumor has been shown in many cases to be responsible for priming these distant "premetastatic niches" through systemic release of cytokines and angiogenic factors to promote colony outgrowth spontaneously,[58,171] it is also clear that extrinsic triggers of inflammation and organ dysfunction elicit similar effects. For example, instillation of bacterial LPS into the respiratory tract to generate an organ-specific inflammatory microenvironment significantly enhances pulmonary metastatic outgrowth in mouse models.[172] In addition to expressing well-characterized inflammatory mediators of tumor progression, including TNF-α, IL-1β, IL-6, and COX-2, neutrophils recruited to the lungs were also found to release proteases that degrade thrombospondin-1, a potent antiangiogenic matrix glycoprotein that normally maintains a tumor-inhibitory microenvironment.[172] Furthermore, systemic cytokines generated in response to surgical wounding ultimately cooperate in releasing restrained micrometastases from CD8$^+$ cytotoxic T cell-mediated immune control by mobilizing inflammatory bone marrow–derived monocytes that differentiate into tumor-associated macrophages.[173] Taken together, these exemplify the potential impact of the systemic sequelae of surgery and its associated complications to the delicate immune equilibrium and composition of the metastatic microenvironment that might otherwise restrict the emergence of metastases.

Approaching Cancer Biology in Perioperative Medicine

In many ways, the evolution of paradigms in cancer biology over recent decades mirrors that of the disease becoming ever more detailed, diverse, and context-dependent.[5] In the face of such daunting complexity, how should perioperative medicine approach the underlying disease and what modifiable aspects of care are most likely to bear meaningful influence across a spectrum of patients, each with their own unique disease characteristics and comorbidities? A first step might be to identify the broad basis by which apparently

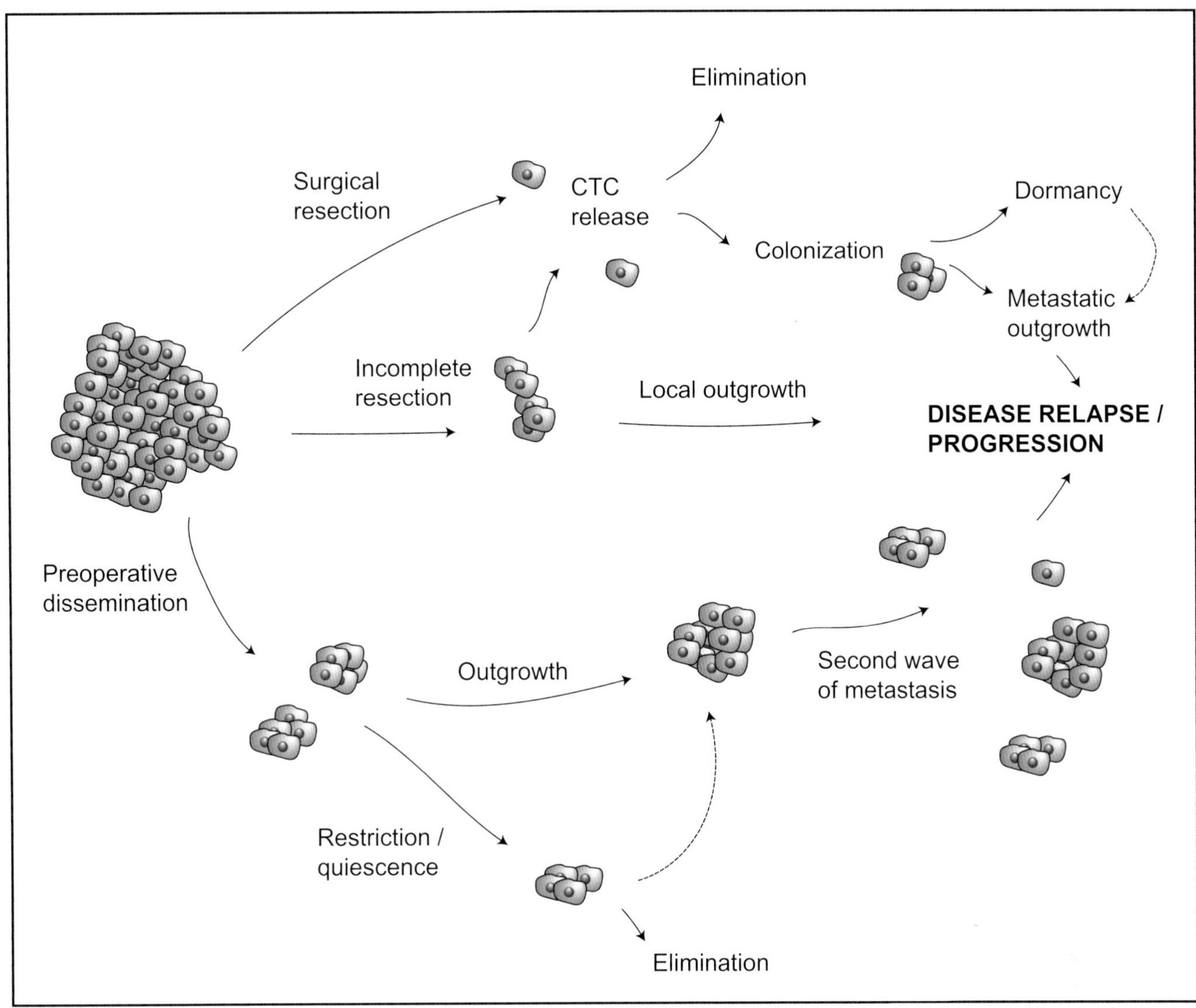

• **Fig. 3.9** Model of postoperative disease course. **(A)** Incomplete resection may lead to local recurrence and metastatic dissemination, which could be accelerated by surgical wounding responses and tissue disruption. **(B)** During surgical resection of the (ostensibly localized) primary tumor, tumor cells may be disseminated into the circulation or operative field. These may fail to colonize or be eliminated by the immune system, adjuvant therapies or other restrictive forces. Postoperative colonies may lie dormant in perpetuity, or begin to grow sometime after surgery—potentially following a long latency period—resulting in disease relapse. **(C)** Alternatively (or additionally), micrometastatic disease may have established prior to surgery. These may remain restricted or eventually eliminated, or may be influenced by systemic perioperative events to overcome their restrictions and emerge as new metastatic disease. *CTC*, Circulating tumor cell.

localized, surgically "curable" cancers can recur or progress (Fig. 3.9). This serves to reframe the potential risks of the perioperative period for all patients, irrespective of disease stage, and may help to explain the discrepant patterns and timing of postoperative relapse. Second, a systematic comparison of the fundamental elements of cancer evolution with the inherent physiological responses to surgery highlights a multitude of cellular and systemic similarities that seem to underlie observations dating back well over a century.[1,174] As the impact of extrinsic factors in shaping disease progression becomes clearer, there is certainly an abundance of logic in seeking to offset the acute dyshomeostasis brought about by surgical wounding, systemic stress and inflammation, infectious complications, anesthetic and analgesic drugs, altered nutritional, hematological and fluid balance status, and a host of other such factors. However, with much of the primary research still in its infancy and current opinions being shaped by secondary analyses and new interpretations of preexisting data, it is perhaps premature to resolve the collective, let alone individual contribution of each of these components at this time.

Since a substantial portion of patients harbor subclinical micrometastases with seemingly localized disease, an important research priority is to delineate the perioperative impact on the biology of disseminated tumor cells. As precursors of metastatic disease, these concealed populations pose a forbidding challenge to cancer therapeutics: their indolence allows them to escape much of the damage inflicted by cytotoxic chemotherapies that preferentially destroy actively proliferating cells, and the stark contrast in their behavior and signaling in comparison to actively cycling primary tumor cells are likely to render them insensitive to targeted therapies. Clearly, preventing dissemination is better than treatment, but where this precedes diagnosis, the hope is that their outgrowth remains restricted. Recent preclinical evidence indicates that the systemic inflammation and immune disequilibrium following surgical wounding lift such restrictions on disseminated cells,[173] highlighting a major host vulnerability, and potentially, a repurposed role for antiinflammatory drugs in the perioperative period.

As a rate-limiting step in the metastatic cascade, factors that influence survival and colonization of CTCs are also of interest. As highlighted by the experimental models of metastasis and acute inflammation presented earlier, these cells may be aided through physical interactions with activated platelets, neutrophils, and vascular endothelium, and temporarily endowed with a phenotypic plasticity that aids transit and extravasation. Colonization and outgrowth are further enhanced by supportive niches, which may be primed by factors arising either from the primary tumor or from systemic stress and inflammatory responses. By increasing the odds of CTC survival and colonization, perioperative events potentially cooperate in early disease progression or lay foundations for disease relapse ahead of a postoperative latency period. Prospective clinical evidence is currently limited, but concerted efforts to maintain physiological homeostasis alongside judicious use of antiinflammatory, antiplatelet, and antithrombotic adjuncts may plausibly help to counterbalance these risks.

Finally, it is worth considering the benefits that may come from attending to holistic, often-neglected aspects of perioperative health care, such as psychology and nutrition. Feelings of stress and anxiety about impending surgery and the disease itself, as well as postoperative pain, invoke neuroendocrine responses that can directly influence the molecular biology of cancer cells and stromal cells in the TME or premetastatic niche.[41] Emerging preclinical and clinical evidence suggests that the risk of cancer recurrence may be reduced by perioperatively modulating these responses by, for example, use of beta blockers.[175,176] Similarly, recent work from the field of cancer metabolism has begun to illuminate the metabolic addictions and vulnerabilities of cancer cells. Future research will need to establish how the systemic catabolic state of major surgery, as well as any associated dietary factors, may relate to the metabolic determinants of tumor progression, metastasis, and response to oncological therapies.

References

1. Gerster II AG. On the surgical dissemination of cancer. *Ann Surg.* 1885;2:98–109. doi:10.1097/00000658-188507000-00009.
2. Murthy SM, Goldschmidt RA, Rao LN, Ammirati M, Buchmann T, Scanlon EF. The influence of surgical trauma on experimental metastasis. *Cancer.* 1989;64:2035–2044.
3. Paget S. The distribution of secondary growths in cancer of the breast. *Lancet.* 1889;133:571–573. doi:10.1016/S0140-6736(00)49915-0.
4. Stehelin D, Varmus HE, Bishop JM, Vogt PK. DNA related to the transforming gene(s) of avian sarcoma viruses is present in normal avian DNA. *Nature.* 1976;260:170–173. doi:10.1038/260170a0.
5. Weinberg RA. Coming full circle-from endless complexity to simplicity and back again. *Cell.* 2014;157:267–271. doi:10.1016/j.cell.2014.03.004.
6. Stratton MR, Campbell PJ, Futreal PA. The cancer genome. *Nature.* 2009;458:719–724. doi:10.1038/nature07943.
7. Lipinski KA, Barber LJ, Davies MN, Ashenden M, Sottoriva A, Gerlinger M. Cancer evolution and the limits of predictability in precision cancer medicine. *Trends Cancer.* 2016;2:49–63. doi:10.1016/j.trecan.2015.11.003.
8. Hiller JG, Perry NJ, Poulogiannis G, Riedel B, Sloan EK. Perioperative events influence cancer recurrence risk after surgery. *Nat Rev Clin Oncol.* 2018;15:205–218. doi:10.1038/nrclinonc.2017.194.
9. Ben-Eliyahu S. The promotion of tumor metastasis by surgery and stress: immunological basis and implications for psychoneuroimmunology. *Brain Behav Immun.* 2003;17(Suppl 1):S27–S36 doi:S0889159102000636.
10. Tavare AN, Perry NJ, Benzonana LL, Takata M, Ma D. Cancer recurrence after surgery: direct and indirect effects of anesthetic agents. *Int J Cancer.* 2012;130:1237–1250. doi:10.1002/ijc.26448.
11. Perry NJS, Buggy D, Ma D. Can anesthesia influence cancer outcomes after surgery? *JAMA Surg.* 2019;154:279–280. doi:10.1001/jamasurg.2018.4619.
12. Greaves M, Maley CC. Clonal evolution in cancer. *Nature.* 2012;481:306–313. doi:10.1038/nature10762.
13. Merlo LM, Pepper JW, Reid BJ, Maley CC. Cancer as an evolutionary and ecological process. *Nat Rev Cancer.* 2006;6:924–935. doi:10.1038/nrc2013.
14. Lambert AW, Pattabiraman DR, Weinberg RA. Emerging biological principles of metastasis. *Cell.* 2017;168:670–691. doi:10.1016/j.cell.2016.11.037.
15. Nowell PC. The clonal evolution of tumor cell populations. *Science.* 1976;194:23–28. doi:10.1126/science.959840.
16. Marusyk A, Almendro V, Polyak K. Intra-tumour heterogeneity: a looking glass for cancer? *Nat Rev Cancer.* 2012;12:323–334. doi:10.1038/nrc3261.
17. Marusyk A, Tabassum DP, Altrock PM, Almendro V, Michor F, Polyak K. Non-cell-autonomous driving of tumour growth supports sub-clonal heterogeneity. *Nature.* 2014;514:54–58. doi:10.1038/nature13556.
18. Gerlinger M, Rowan AJ, Horswell S, et al. Intratumor heterogeneity and branched evolution revealed by multiregion sequencing. *N Engl J Med.* 2012;366:883–892. doi:10.1056/NEJMoa1113205.
19. Rhim AD, Mirek ET, Aiello NM, et al. EMT and dissemination precede pancreatic tumor formation. *Cell.* 2012;148:349–361. doi:10.1016/j.cell.2011.11.025.
20. Klein CA. Parallel progression of primary tumours and metastases. *Nat Rev Cancer.* 2009;9:302–312. doi:10.1038/nrc2627.
21. Hanahan D, Weinberg RA. Hallmarks of cancer: the next generation. *Cell.* 2011;144:646–674. doi:10.1016/j.cell.2011.02.013.

22. Hanahan D, Weinberg RA. The hallmarks of cancer. *Cell.* 2000; 100:57–70 doi:S0092-8674(00)81683-9.
23. Davies H, Bignell GR, Cox C, et al. Mutations of the BRAF gene in human cancer. *Nature.* 2002;417:949–954. doi:10.1038/nature00766.
24. Network CGA. Genomic classification of cutaneous melanoma. *Cell.* 2015;161:1681–1696. doi:10.1016/j.cell.2015.05.044.
25. Simanshu DK, Nissley DV, McCormick F. RAS proteins and their regulators in human disease. *Cell.* 2017;170:17–33. doi: 10.1016/j.cell.2017.06.009.
26. Engelman JA. Targeting PI3K signaling in cancer: opportunities, challenges and limitations. *Nat Rev Cancer.* 2009;9:550–562. doi:10.1038/nrc2664.
27. Fruman DA, Chiu H, Hopkins BD, Bagrodia S, Cantley LC, Abraham RT. The PI3K pathway in human disease. *Cell.* 2017;170:605–635. doi:10.1016/j.cell.2017.07.029.
28. Manning BD, Cantley LC. AKT/PKB signaling: navigating downstream. *Cell.* 2007;129:1261–1274. doi:10.1016/j.cell.2007.06.009.
29. Manning BD, Toker A. AKT/PKB signaling: navigating the network. *Cell.* 2017;169:381–405. doi:10.1016/j.cell.2017.04.001.
30. Lawrence MS, Stojanov P, Mermel CH, et al. Discovery and saturation analysis of cancer genes across 21 tumour types. *Nature.* 2014;505:495–501. doi:10.1038/nature12912.
31. Kandoth C, McLellan MD, Vandin F, et al. Mutational landscape and significance across 12 major cancer types. *Nature.* 2013;502:333–339. doi:10.1038/nature12634.
32. Dolgin E. The most popular genes in the human genome. *Nature.* 2017;551:427–431. doi:10.1038/d41586-017-07291-9.
33. Hafner A, Bulyk ML, Jambhekar A, Lahav G. The multiple mechanisms that regulate p53 activity and cell fate. *Nat Rev Mol Cell Biol.* 2019;20:199–210. doi:10.1038/s41580-019-0110-x.
34. Kastenhuber ER, Lowe SW. Putting p53 in context. *Cell.* 2017;170:1062–1078. doi:10.1016/j.cell.2017.08.028.
35. Follis AV, Llambi F, Ou L, Baran K, Green DR, Kriwacki RW. The DNA-binding domain mediates both nuclear and cytosolic functions of p53. *Nat Struct Mol Biol.* 2014;21:535–543. doi:10.1038/nsmb.2829.
36. Villunger A, Michalak EM, Coultas L, et al. p53- and drug-induced apoptotic responses mediated by BH3-only proteins puma and noxa. *Science.* 2003;302:1036–1038. doi:10.1126/science.1090072.
37. Datta SR, Dudek H, Tao X, et al. Akt phosphorylation of BAD couples survival signals to the cell-intrinsic death machinery. *Cell.* 1997;91:231–241. doi:10.1016/s0092-8674(00)80405-5.
38. Brunet A, Bonni A, Zigmond MJ, et al. Akt promotes cell survival by phosphorylating and inhibiting a Forkhead transcription factor. *Cell.* 1999;96:857–868. doi:10.1016/s0092-8674(00)80595-4.
39. Mayo LD, Donner DB. A phosphatidylinositol 3-kinase/Akt pathway promotes translocation of Mdm2 from the cytoplasm to the nucleus. *Proc Natl Acad Sci USA.* 2001;98:11598–11603. doi:10.1073/pnas.181181198.
40. Zhou BP, Liao Y, Xia W, Zou Y, Spohn B, Hung MC. HER-2/neu induces p53 ubiquitination via Akt-mediated MDM2 phosphorylation. *Nat Cell Biol.* 2001;3:973–982. doi:10.1038/ncb1101-973.
41. Cole SW, Sood AK. Molecular pathways: beta-adrenergic signaling in cancer. *Clin Cancer Res.* 2012;18:1201–1206. doi:10.1158/1078-0432.CCR-11-0641.
42. Zhang X, Odom DT, Koo SH, et al. Genome-wide analysis of cAMP-response element binding protein occupancy, phosphorylation, and target gene activation in human tissues. *Proc Natl Acad Sci USA.* 2005;102:4459–4464. doi:10.1073/pnas.0501076102.
43. Zahalka AH, Arnal-Estape A, Maryanovich M, et al. Adrenergic nerves activate an angio-metabolic switch in prostate cancer. *Science.* 2017;358:321–326. doi:10.1126/science.aah5072.
44. Kim-Fuchs C, Le CP, Pimentel MA, et al. Chronic stress accelerates pancreatic cancer growth and invasion: A critical role for beta-adrenergic signaling in the pancreatic microenvironment. *Brain Behav Immun.* 2014;40:40–47. https://doi.org/10.1016/j.bbi.2014.02.019.
45. Hassan S, Karpova Y, Baiz D, et al. Behavioral stress accelerates prostate cancer development in mice. *J Clin Invest.* 2013;123:874–886. doi:10.1172/jci63324.
46. Nagaraja AS, Dorniak PL, Sadaoui NC, et al. Sustained adrenergic signaling leads to increased metastasis in ovarian cancer via increased PGE2 synthesis. *Oncogene.* 2016;35:2390–2397. doi:10.1038/onc.2015.302.
47. Lucido CT, Callejas-Valera JL, Colbert PL, et al. Beta2-Adrenergic receptor modulates mitochondrial metabolism and disease progression in recurrent/metastatic HPV(+) HNSCC. *Oncogenesis.* 2018;7:81. doi:10.1038/s41389-018-0090-2.
48. Le CP, Nowell CJ, Kim-Fuchs C, et al. Chronic stress in mice remodels lymph vasculature to promote tumour cell dissemination. *Nat Commun.* 2016;7:10634. doi:10.1038/ncomms10634.
49. Sloan EK, Priceman SJ, Cox BF, et al. The sympathetic nervous system induces a metastatic switch in primary breast cancer. *Cancer Res.* 2010;70:7042–7052. doi:10.1158/0008-5472.Can-10-0522.
50. Barron TI, Connolly RM, Sharp L, Bennett K, Visvanathan K. Beta blockers and breast cancer mortality: a population- based study. *J Clin Oncol.* 2011;29:2635–2644. doi:10.1200/JCO.2010.33.5422.
51. Childers WK, Hollenbeak CS, Cheriyath P. Beta-blockers reduce breast cancer recurrence and breast cancer death: a meta-analysis. *Clin Breast Cancer.* 2015;15:426–431. doi:10.1016/j.clbc.2015.07.001.
52. De Giorgi V, Grazzini M, Benemei S, et al. Propranolol for off-label treatment of patients with melanoma: results from a cohort study. *JAMA Oncol.* 2018;4:e172908. doi:10.1001/jamaoncol.2017.2908(2018).
53. Gilkes DM, Bajpai S, Chaturvedi P, Wirtz D, Semenza GL. Hypoxia-inducible factor 1 (HIF-1) promotes extracellular matrix remodeling under hypoxic conditions by inducing P4HA1, P4HA2, and PLOD2 expression in fibroblasts. *J Biol Chem.* 2013;288:10819–10829. doi:10.1074/jbc.M112.442939.
54. Gilkes DM, Semenza GL, Wirtz D. Hypoxia and the extracellular matrix: drivers of tumour metastasis. *Nat Rev Cancer.* 2014;14:430–439. doi:10.1038/nrc3726.
55. Murthy BL, Thomson CS, Dodwell D, et al. Postoperative wound complications and systemic recurrence in breast cancer. *Br J Cancer.* 2007;97:1211–1217. doi:10.1038/sj.bjc.6604004.
56. McSorley ST, Watt DG, Horgan PG, McMillan DC. Postoperative systemic inflammatory response, complication severity, and survival following surgery for colorectal cancer. *Ann Surg Oncol.* 2016;23:2832–2840. doi:10.1245/s10434-016-5204-5.
57. Binnewies M, Roberts EW, Kersten K, et al. Understanding the tumor immune microenvironment (TIME) for effective therapy. *Nat Med.* 2018;24:541–550. doi:10.1038/s41591-018-0014-x.
58. Joyce JA, Pollard JW. Microenvironmental regulation of metastasis. *Nat Rev Cancer.* 2009;9:239–252. doi:10.1038/nrc2618.
59. Coca S, Perez-Piqueras J, Martinez D, et al. The prognostic significance of intratumoral natural killer cells in patients with colorectal carcinoma. *Cancer.* 1997;79:2320–2328. doi:10.1002/(sici)1097-0142(19970615)79:12<2320::aid-cncr5>3.0.co;2-p.

60. Böttcher JP, Bonavita E, Chakravarty P, et al. NK cells stimulate recruitment of cDC1 into the tumor microenvironment promoting cancer immune control. *Cell.* 2018;172:1022–1037. doi:10.1016/j.cell.2018.01.004.
61. Chiossone L, Dumas PY, Vienne M, Vivier E. Natural killer cells and other innate lymphoid cells in cancer. *Nat Rev Immunol.* 2018;18:671–688. doi:10.1038/s41577-018-0061-z.
62. Engblom C, Pfirschke C, Pittet MJ. The role of myeloid cells in cancer therapies. *Nat Rev Cancer.* 2016;16:447–462. doi:10.1038/nrc.2016.54.
63. Gentles AJ, Newman AM, Liu CL, et al. The prognostic landscape of genes and infiltrating immune cells across human cancers. *Nat Med.* 2015;21:938–945. doi:10.1038/nm.3909.
64. Bindea G, Mlecnik B, Tosolini M, et al. Spatiotemporal dynamics of intratumoral immune cells reveal the immune landscape in human cancer. *Immunity.* 2013;39:782–795. doi:10.1016/j.immuni.2013.10.003.
65. Fridman WH, Zitvogel L, Sautès-Fridman C, Kroemer G. The immune contexture in cancer prognosis and treatment. *Nat Rev Clin Oncol.* 2017;14:717–734. doi:10.1038/nrclinonc. 2017.101.
66. Sumimoto H, Imabayashi F, Iwata T, Kawakami Y. The BRAF-MAPK signaling pathway is essential for cancer-immune evasion in human melanoma cells. *J Exp Med.* 2006;203:1651–1656. doi:10.1084/jem.20051848.
67. Yu H, Kortylewski M, Pardoll D. Crosstalk between cancer and immune cells: role of STAT3 in the tumour microenvironment. *Nat Rev Immunol.* 2007;7:41–51. doi:10.1038/nri1995.
68. Vinay DS, Ryan EP, Pawelec G, et al. Immune evasion in cancer: Mechanistic basis and therapeutic strategies. *Semin Cancer Biol.* 2015;35(Suppl):S185–S198. doi:10.1016/j.semcancer.2015.03.004.
69. Pietra G, Manzini C, Rivara S, et al. Melanoma cells inhibit natural killer cell function by modulating the expression of activating receptors and cytolytic activity. *Cancer Res.* 2012;72:1407–1415. doi:10.1158/0008-5472.CAN-11-2544.
70. Tartter PI, Steinberg B, Barron DM, Martinelli G. The prognostic significance of natural killer cytotoxicity in patients with colorectal cancer. *Arch Surg.* 1987;122:1264–1268. doi:10.1001/archsurg.1987.01400230050009 (1987).
71. Barry KC, Hsu J, Broz ML, et al. A natural killer-dendritic cell axis defines checkpoint therapy-responsive tumor microenvironments. *Nat Med.* 2018;24:1178–1191. doi:10.1038/s41591-018-0085-8.
72. Tauriello DVF, Palomo-Ponce S, Stork D, et al. TGFβ drives immune evasion in genetically reconstituted colon cancer metastasis. *Nature.* 2018;554:538–543. doi:10.1038/nature25492.
73. Mariathasan S, Turley SJ, Nickles D, et al. TGFβ attenuates tumour response to PD-L1 blockade by contributing to exclusion of T cells. *Nature.* 2018;554:544–548. doi:10.1038/nature25501.
74. Budhu S, Schaer DA, Li Y, et al. Blockade of surface-bound TGF-β on regulatory T cells abrogates suppression of effector T cell function in the tumor microenvironment. *Sci Signal.* 2017;10:494. doi:10.1126/scisignal.aak9702.
75. Togashi Y, Shitara K, Nishikawa H. Regulatory T cells in cancer immunosuppression - implications for anticancer therapy. *Nat Rev Clin Oncol.* 2019;16:356–371. doi:10.1038/s41571-019-0175-7.
76. Schmidt A, Oberle N, Krammer PH. Molecular mechanisms of treg-mediated T cell suppression. *Front Immunol.* 2012;3:51. doi:10.3389/fimmu.2012.00051.
77. Hanahan D, Folkman J. Patterns and emerging mechanisms of the angiogenic switch during tumorigenesis. *Cell.* 1996;86:353–364. doi:10.1016/s0092-8674(00)80108-7.
78. De Palma M, Biziato D, Petrova TV. Microenvironmental regulation of tumour angiogenesis. *Nat Rev Cancer.* 2017;17:457–474. doi:10.1038/nrc.2017.51.
79. Apte RS, Chen DS, Ferrara N. VEGF in signaling and disease: beyond discovery and development. *Cell.* 2019;176:1248–1264. doi:10.1016/j.cell.2019.01.021.
80. Kerbel RS. Tumor angiogenesis. *N Engl J Med.* 2008;358:2039–2049. doi:10.1056/NEJMra0706596 (2008).
81. LaGory EL, Giaccia AJ. The ever-expanding role of HIF in tumour and stromal biology. *Nat Cell Biol.* 2016;18:356–365. doi:10.1038/ncb3330.
82. Turner KJ, Moore JW, Jones A, et al. Expression of hypoxia-inducible factors in human renal cancer: relationship to angiogenesis and to the von Hippel-Lindau gene mutation. *Cancer Res.* 2002;62:2957–2961.
83. Jiang BH, Zheng JZ, Aoki M, Vogt PK. Phosphatidylinositol 3-kinase signaling mediates angiogenesis and expression of vascular endothelial growth factor in endothelial cells. *Proc Natl Acad Sci USA.* 2000;97:1749–1753. doi:10.1073/pnas.040560897.
84. DeBerardinis RJ, Chandel NS. Fundamentals of cancer metabolism. *Sci Adv.* 2016;2:e1600200. doi:10.1126/sciadv.1600200.
85. Ward PS, Thompson CB. Metabolic reprogramming: a cancer hallmark even Warburg did not anticipate. *Cancer Cell.* 2012;21:297–308. doi:10.1016/j.ccr.2012.02.014.
86. Warburg O. On respiratory impairment in cancer cells. *Science.* 1956;124:269–270.
87. Warburg O. On the origin of cancer cells. *Science.* 1956; 123:309–314. doi:10.1126/science.123.3191.309.
88. Vander Heiden MG, Cantley LC, Thompson CB. Understanding the Warburg effect: the metabolic requirements of cell proliferation. *Science.* 2009;324:1029–1033. doi:10.1126/science.1160809.
89. Koppenol WH, Bounds PL, Dang CV. Otto Warburg's contributions to current concepts of cancer metabolism. *Nat Rev Cancer.* 2011;11:325–337. doi:10.1038/nrc3038.
90. Ying H, Kimmelman AC, Lyssiotis CA, et al. Oncogenic Kras maintains pancreatic tumors through regulation of anabolic glucose metabolism. *Cell.* 2012;149:656–670. doi:10.1016/j.cell.2012.01.058.
91. Dang C, Le A, Gao P. MYC-induced cancer cell energy metabolism and therapeutic opportunities. *Clin Cancer Res.* 2009; 15:6479–6483. doi:10.1158/1078-0432.CCR-09-0889.
92. Dang CV. MYC on the path to cancer. *Cell.* 2012;149:22–35. doi:10.1016/j.cell.2012.03.003.
93. Osthus RC, Shim H, Kim S, et al. Deregulation of glucose transporter 1 and glycolytic gene expression by c-Myc. *J Biol Chem.* 2000;275:21797–21800. doi:10.1074/jbc.C000023200.
94. Bensaad K, Tsuruta A, Selak MA, et al. TIGAR, a p53-inducible regulator of glycolysis and apoptosis. *Cell.* 2006;126:107–120. doi:10.1016/j.cell.2006.05.036.
95. Bensaad K, Vousden KH. p53: new roles in metabolism. *Trends Cell Biol.* 2007;17:286–291. doi:10.1016/j.tcb.2007.04.004.
96. Vousden KH, Ryan KM. p53 and metabolism. *Nat Rev Cancer.* 2009;9:691–700. doi:10.1038/nrc2715.
97. Dibble CC, Manning BD. Signal integration by mTORC1 coordinates nutrient input with biosynthetic output. *Nat Cell Biol.* 2013;15:555–564. doi:10.1038/ncb2763.
98. Semenza G. HIF-1: upstream and downstream of cancer metabolism. *Curr Opin Genet Dev.* 2010;20:51–56. doi:10.1016/j.gde.2009.10.009.

99. DeBerardinis RJ, Lum JJ, Hatzivassiliou G, Thompson CB. The biology of cancer: metabolic reprogramming fuels cell growth and proliferation. *Cell Metab.* 2008;7:11–20. doi:10.1016/j.cmet.2007.10.002.
100. Wise DR, Thompson CB. Glutamine addiction: a new therapeutic target in cancer. *Trends Biochem Sci.* 2010;35:427–433. doi:10.1016/j.tibs.2010.05.003.
101. Owen OE, Kalhan SC, Hanson RW. The key role of anaplerosis and cataplerosis for citric acid cycle function. *J Biol Chem.* 2002;277:30409–30412. doi:10.1074/jbc.R200006200.
102. Mullen AR, Wheaton WW, Jin ES, et al. Reductive carboxylation supports growth in tumour cells with defective mitochondria. *Nature.* 2011;481:385–388. doi:10.1038/nature10642.
103. Wise DR, Ward PS, Shay JE, et al. Hypoxia promotes isocitrate dehydrogenase-dependent carboxylation of α-ketoglutarate to citrate to support cell growth and viability. *Proc Natl Acad Sci USA.* 2011;108:19611–19616. doi:10.1073/pnas.1117773108.
104. Metallo CM, Gameiro PA, Bell EL, et al. Reductive glutamine metabolism by IDH1 mediates lipogenesis under hypoxia. *Nature.* 2011;481:380–384. doi:10.1038/nature10602.
105. Currie E, Schulze A, Zechner R, Walther TC, Farese RV. Cellular fatty acid metabolism and cancer. *Cell Metab.* 2013;18:153–161. doi:10.1016/j.cmet.2013.05.017.
106. Mayers JR, Wu C, Clish CB, et al. Elevation of circulating branched-chain amino acids is an early event in human pancreatic adenocarcinoma development. *Nat Med.* 2014;20:1193–1198. doi:10.1038/nm.3686.
107. Serine Locasale JW. glycine and one-carbon units: cancer metabolism in full circle. *Nat Rev Cancer.* 2013;13:572–583. doi:10.1038/nrc3557.
108. Galluzzi L, Pietrocola F, Levine B, Kroemer G. Metabolic control of autophagy. *Cell.* 2014;159:1263–1276. doi:10.1016/j.cell.2014.11.006.
109. Commisso C, Davidson SM, Soydaner-Azeloglu RG, et al. Macropinocytosis of protein is an amino acid supply route in Ras-transformed cells. *Nature.* 2013;497:633–637. doi:10.1038/nature12138.
110. Fidler IJ. The pathogenesis of cancer metastasis: the 'seed and soil' hypothesis revisited. *Nat Rev Cancer.* 2003;3:453–458. doi:10.1038/nrc1098.
111. Gupta GP, Massagué J. Cancer metastasis: building a framework. *Cell.* 2006;127:679–695. doi:10.1016/j.cell.2006.11.001.
112. Thiery JP. Epithelial-mesenchymal transitions in tumour progression. *Nat Rev Cancer.* 2002;2:442–454. doi:10.1038/nrc822.
113. Polyak K, Weinberg RA. Transitions between epithelial and mesenchymal states: acquisition of malignant and stem cell traits. *Nat Rev Cancer.* 2009;9:265–273. doi:10.1038/nrc2620.
114. Onder TT, Gupta PB, Mani SA, Yang J, Lander ES, Weinberg RA. Loss of E-cadherin promotes metastasis via multiple downstream transcriptional pathways. *Cancer Res.* 2008;68:3645–3654. doi:10.1158/0008-5472.CAN-07-2938.
115. Zheng X, Carstens JL, Kim J, et al. Epithelial-to-mesenchymal transition is dispensable for metastasis but induces chemoresistance in pancreatic cancer. *Nature.* 2015;527:525–530. doi:10.1038/nature16064.
116. Fischer KR, Durrans A, Lee S, et al. Epithelial-to-mesenchymal transition is not required for lung metastasis but contributes to chemoresistance. *Nature.* 2015;527:472–476. doi:10.1038/nature15748.
117. Ocaña OH, Córcoles R, Fabra A, et al. Metastatic colonization requires the repression of the epithelial-mesenchymal transition inducer Prrx1. *Cancer Cell.* 2012;22:709–724. doi:10.1016/j.ccr.2012.10.012 (2012).
118. Tsai JH, Donaher JL, Murphy DA, Chau S, Yang J. Spatiotemporal regulation of epithelial-mesenchymal transition is essential for squamous cell carcinoma metastasis. *Cancer Cell.* 2012;22:725–736. doi:10.1016/j.ccr.2012.09.022.
119. Padmanaban V, Krol I, Suhail Y, et al. E-cadherin is required for metastasis in multiple models of breast cancer. *Nature.* 2019;573:439–444. doi:10.1038/s41586-019-1526-3.
120. Lamouille S, Xu J, Derynck R. Molecular mechanisms of epithelial-mesenchymal transition. *Nat Rev Mol Cell Biol.* 2014; 15:178–196. doi:10.1038/nrm3758.
121. Scheel C, Eaton EN, Li SH, et al. Paracrine and autocrine signals induce and maintain mesenchymal and stem cell states in the breast. *Cell.* 2011;145:926–940. doi:10.1016/j.cell.2011.04.029.
122. Yang MH, Wu MZ, Chiou SH, et al. Direct regulation of TWIST by HIF-1alpha promotes metastasis. *Nat Cell Biol.* 2008;10:295–305. doi:10.1038/ncb1691.
123. Hüsemann Y, Geigl JB, Schubert F, et al. Systemic spread is an early step in breast cancer. *Cancer Cell.* 2008:1358–1368. doi:10.1016/j.ccr.2007.12.003 (2008).
124. Hosseini H, Obradovic MM, Hoffmann M, et al. Early dissemination seeds metastasis in breast cancer. *Nature.* 2016;540:552–558. doi:10.1038/nature20785.
125. Linde N, Casanova-Acebes M, Sosa MS, et al. Macrophages orchestrate breast cancer early dissemination and metastasis. *Nat Commun.* 2018;9:21. doi:10.1038/s41467-017-02481-5.
126. Herrmann A, Rice M, Lévy R, et al. Cellular memory of hypoxia elicits neuroblastoma metastasis and enables invasion by non-aggressive neighbouring cells. *Oncogenesis.* 2015;4:e138. doi:10.1038/oncsis.2014.52.
127. Cristofanilli M, Budd GT, Ellis MJ, et al. Circulating tumor cells, disease progression, and survival in metastatic breast cancer. *N Engl J Med.* 2004;351:781–791. doi:10.1056/NEJMoa040766.
128. Scher HI, Jia X, de Bono JS, et al. Circulating tumour cells as prognostic markers in progressive, castration-resistant prostate cancer: a reanalysis of IMMC38 trial data. *Lancet Oncol.* 2009;10:233–239. doi:10.1016/S1470-2045(08)70340-1.
129. Rahbari NN, Aigner M, Thorlund K, et al. Meta-analysis shows that detection of circulating tumor cells indicates poor prognosis in patients with colorectal cancer. *Gastroenterology.* 2010;138:1714–1726. doi:10.1053/j.gastro.2010.01.008.
130. Brown DC, Purushotham AD, Birnie GD, George WD. Detection of intraoperative tumor cell dissemination in patients with breast cancer by use of reverse transcription and polymerase chain reaction. *Surgery.* 1995;117:95–101.
131. Hashimoto M, Tanaka F, Yoneda K, et al. Significant increase in circulating tumour cells in pulmonary venous blood during surgical manipulation in patients with primary lung cancer. *Interact Cardiovasc Thorac Surg.* 2014;18:775–783. doi:10.1093/icvts/ivu048.
132. Peach G, Kim C, Zacharakis E, Purkayastha S, Ziprin P. Prognostic significance of circulating tumour cells following surgical resection of colorectal cancers: a systematic review. *Br J Cancer.* 2010;102:1327–1334. doi:10.1038/sj.bjc.6605651.
133. Nagrath S, Sequist LV, Maheswaran S, et al. Isolation of rare circulating tumour cells in cancer patients by microchip technology. *Nature.* 2007;450:1235–1239. doi:10.1038/nature06385.
134. Baccelli I, Schneeweiss A, Riethdorf S, et al. Identification of a population of blood circulating tumor cells from breast cancer patients that initiates metastasis in a xenograft assay. *Nat Biotechnol.* 2013;31:539–544. doi:10.1038/nbt.2576.

135. Massague J, Obenauf AC. Metastatic colonization by circulating tumour cells. *Nature*. 2016;529:298–306. doi:10.1038/nature17038.
136. Chambers AF, Groom AC, MacDonald IC. Dissemination and growth of cancer cells in metastatic sites. *Nat Rev Cancer*. 2002;2:563–572. doi:10.1038/nrc865.
137. Luzzi KJ, MacDonald IC, Schmidt EE, et al. Multistep nature of metastatic inefficiency: dormancy of solitary cells after successful extravasation and limited survival of early micrometastases. *Am J Pathol*. 1998;153:865–873. doi:10.1016/S0002-9440(10)65628-3.
138. Wong CW, Lee A, Shientag L, et al. Apoptosis: an early event in metastatic inefficiency. *Cancer Res*. 2001;61:333–338.
139. Jiang L, Shestov AA, Swain P, et al. Reductive carboxylation supports redox homeostasis during anchorage-independent growth. *Nature*. 2016;532:255–258. doi:10.1038/nature17393.
140. Simpson CD, Anyiwe K, Schimmer AD. Anoikis resistance and tumor metastasis. *Cancer Lett*. 2008;272:177–185. doi: 10.1016/j.canlet.2008.05.029.
141. Hanna N, Fidler IJ. Role of natural killer cells in the destruction of circulating tumor emboli. *J Natl Cancer Inst*. 1980;65:801–809. doi:10.1093/jnci/65.4.801.
142. Hanna N. Inhibition of experimental tumor metastasis by selective activation of natural killer cells. *Cancer Res*. 1982;42:1337–1342.
143. Melamed R, Rosenne E, Shakhar K, Schwartz Y, Abudarham N, Ben-Eliyahu S. Marginating pulmonary-NK activity and resistance to experimental tumor metastasis: suppression by surgery and the prophylactic use of a beta-adrenergic antagonist and a prostaglandin synthesis inhibitor. *Brain Behav Immun*. 2005;19:114–126. doi:10.1016/j.bbi.2004.07.004.
144. Nieswandt B, Hafner M, Echtenacher B, Männel DN. Lysis of tumor cells by natural killer cells in mice is impeded by platelets. *Cancer Res*. 1999;59:1295–1300.
145. Labelle M, Begum S, Hynes RO. Direct signaling between platelets and cancer cells induces an epithelial-mesenchymal-like transition and promotes metastasis. *Cancer Cell*. 2011;20:576–590. doi:10.1016/j.ccr.2011.09.009.
146. Labuschagne CF, Cheung EC, Blagih J, Domart MC, Vousden KH. Cell clustering promotes a metabolic switch that supports metastatic colonization. *Cell Metab*. 2019;30:720–734. doi:10.1016/j.cmet.2019.07.014 e725.
147. Piskounova E, Agathocleous M, Murphy MM, et al. Oxidative stress inhibits distant metastasis by human melanoma cells. *Nature*. 2015;527:186–191. doi:10.1038/nature15726.
148. Aceto N, Bardia A, Miyamoto DT, et al. Circulating tumor cell clusters are oligoclonal precursors of breast cancer metastasis. *Cell*. 2014;158:1110–1122. doi:10.1016/j.cell.2014.07.013.
149. Palumbo JS, Talmage KE, Massari JV, et al. Platelets and fibrin(ogen) increase metastatic potential by impeding natural killer cell-mediated elimination of tumor cells. *Blood*. 2005;105:178–185. doi:10.1182/blood-2004-06-2272.
150. Cools-Lartigue J, Spicer J, McDonald B, et al. Neutrophil extracellular traps sequester circulating tumor cells and promote metastasis. *J Clin Invest*. 2013; 123(8):3446–3458. doi:10.1172/JCI67484.
151. Spicer JD, McDonald B, Cools-Lartigue JJ, et al. Neutrophils promote liver metastasis via Mac-1-mediated interactions with circulating tumor cells. *Cancer Res*. 2012;72:3919–3927. doi:10.1158/0008-5472.CAN-11-2393.
152. Brinkmann V, Reichard U, Goosmann C, et al. Neutrophil extracellular traps kill bacteria. *Science*. 2004;303:1532–1535. doi:10.1126/science.1092385.
153. Papayannopoulos V. Neutrophil extracellular traps in immunity and disease. *Nat Rev Immunol*. 2018;18:134–147. doi:10.1038/nri.2017.105.
154. Cedervall J, Zhang Y, Olsson AK. Tumor-induced NETosis as a risk factor for metastasis and organ failure. *Cancer Res*. 2016;76:4311–4315. doi:10.1158/0008-5472.CAN-15-3051.
155. Tohme S, Yazdani HO, Al-Khafaji AB, et al. Neutrophil extracellular traps promote the development and progression of liver metastases after surgical stress. *Cancer Res*. 2016;76:1367–1380. doi:10.1158/0008-5472.CAN-15-1591.
156. Eustache JH, Tohme S, Milette S, Rayes RF, Tsung A, Spicer JD. Casting a wide net on surgery: the central role of neutrophil extracellular traps. *Ann Surg*. 2019. doi:10.1097/SLA.0000000000003586.
157. Budczies J, von Winterfeld M, Klauschen F, et al. The landscape of metastatic progression patterns across major human cancers. *Oncotarget*. 2015;6:570–583. doi:10.18632/oncotarget.2677.
158. Obenauf AC, Massagué J. Surviving at a distance: organ-specific metastasis. *Trends Cancer*. 2015;1:76–91. doi:10.1016/j.trecan.2015.07.009.
159. Padua D, Zhang XH, Wang Q, et al. TGFbeta primes breast tumors for lung metastasis seeding through angiopoietin-like 4. *Cell*. 2008;133:66–77. doi:10.1016/j.cell.2008.01.046.
160. Gupta GP, Nguyen DX, Chiang AC, et al. Mediators of vascular remodeling co-opted for sequential steps in lung metastasis. *Nature*. 2007;446:765–770. doi:10.1038/nature05760.
161. Harney AS, Arwert EN, Entenberg D, et al. Real-time imaging reveals local, transient vascular permeability, and tumor cell intravasation stimulated by TIE2hi macrophage-derived VEGFA. *Cancer Discov*. 2015;5:932–943. doi:10.1158/2159-8290.CD-15-0012.
162. Tichet M, Prod'Homme V, Fenouille N, et al. Tumor-derived SPARC drives vascular permeability and extravasation through endothelial VCAM1 signalling to promote metastasis. *Nat Commun*. 2015;6:6993. doi:10.1038/ncomms7993.
163. Chen MB, Hajal C, Benjamin DC, et al. Inflamed neutrophils sequestered at entrapped tumor cells via chemotactic confinement promote tumor cell extravasation. *Proc Natl Acad Sci USA*. 2018;115:7022–7027. doi:10.1073/pnas.1715932115.
164. Gül N, Bögels M, Grewal S, et al. Surgery-induced reactive oxygen species enhance colon carcinoma cell binding by disrupting the liver endothelial cell lining. *Gut*. 2011;60:1076–1086. doi:10.1136/gut.2010.224717.
165. Braun S, Vogl FD, Naume B, et al. A pooled analysis of bone marrow micrometastasis in breast cancer. *N Engl J Med*. 2005;353:793–802. doi:10.1056/NEJMoa050434.
166. Gao H, Chakraborty G, Lee-Lim AP, et al. The BMP inhibitor Coco reactivates breast cancer cells at lung metastatic sites. *Cell*. 2012;150:764–779. doi:10.1016/j.cell.2012.06.035.
167. Bragado P, Estrada Y, Parikh F, et al. TGF-β2 dictates disseminated tumour cell fate in target organs through TGF-β-RIII and p38α/β signalling. *Nat Cell Biol*. 2013;15:1351–1361. doi:10.1038/ncb2861.
168. Sosa MS, Bragado P, Aguirre-Ghiso JA. Mechanisms of disseminated cancer cell dormancy: an awakening field. *Nat Rev Cancer*. 2014;14:611–622. doi:10.1038/nrc3793.
169. Gao D, Joshi N, Choi H, et al. Myeloid progenitor cells in the premetastatic lung promote metastases by inducing mesenchymal to epithelial transition. *Cancer Res*. 2012;72:1384–1394. doi:10.1158/0008-5472.CAN-11-2905.
170. Hiratsuka S, Watanabe A, Sakurai Y, et al. The S100A8-serum amyloid A3-TLR4 paracrine cascade establishes a pre-metastatic phase. *Nat Cell Biol*. 2008;10:1349–1355. doi:10.1038/ncb1794.

171. Liu Y, Cao X. Characteristics and significance of the pre-metastatic niche. *Cancer Cell.* 2016;30:668–681. doi:10.1016/j.ccell.2016.09.011.
172. El Rayes T, Catena R, Lee S, et al. Lung inflammation promotes metastasis through neutrophil protease-mediated degradation of Tsp-1. *Proc Natl Acad Sci USA.* 2015;112:16000–16005. doi:10.1073/pnas.1507294112.
173. Krall JA, Reinhardt F, Mercury OA, et al. The systemic response to surgery triggers the outgrowth of distant immune-controlled tumors in mouse models of dormancy. *Sci Transl Med.* 2018;10. doi:10.1126/scitranslmed.aan3464.
174. Paget S. The distribution of secondary growths in cancer of the breast. *Cancer Metastasis Rev.* 1989;8:98–101.
175. Benish M, Bartal I, Goldfarb Y, et al. Perioperative use of beta-blockers and COX-2 inhibitors may improve immune competence and reduce the risk of tumor metastasis. *Ann Surg Oncol.* 2008;15:2042–2052. doi:10.1245/s10434-008-9890-5.
176. Goldfarb Y, Sorski L, Benish M, Levi B, Melamed R, Ben-Eliyahu S. Improving postoperative immune status and resistance to cancer metastasis: a combined perioperative approach of immunostimulation and prevention of excessive surgical stress responses. *Ann Surg.* 2011;253:798–810. doi:10.1097/SLA.0b013e318211d7b5.

4

Traditional Cancer Therapies and Perioperative Implications

SEPHALIE PATEL AND SUNIL K. SAHAI

Introduction

Preoperative cancer therapies such as chemotherapy and radiation can have direct implications on perioperative management during cancer surgery. Chemotherapy is intended to prevent proliferation of malignant cells (cytostatic) and cause death of tumor cells (cytotoxic). It can be given at various stages during cancer treatment, including before surgery (neoadjuvant), after surgical resection (adjuvant), or as palliative therapy to improve quality of life. Chemotherapy is usually administered in cycles every 2–3 weeks, which allows patients to recover from its toxic effects. In this chapter, we focus on reviewing traditional chemotherapeutic agents, their toxicities on organ systems, and how to mitigate these effects perioperatively. Most commonly, patients experience toxicities related to cardiac, pulmonary, gastrointestinal, and hematologic systems. A full discussion of the perioperative implications of the numerous classes of chemotherapy is beyond the scope of this chapter. We have attempted to summarize the perioperative implications of chemotherapy in Table 4.1. Radiation therapy has fewer systemic perioperative concerns, but patients do frequently present with late complications from therapy that may alter perioperative evaluation and management.

Cardiovascular

Cardiac toxicity from chemotherapy is common, with effects ranging from ECG abnormalities to congestive heart failure. These effects can continue for years after the cardiotoxic drug has been halted.[1] In practice, cardiotoxicity can manifest as multiple different conditions, including (1) cardiac dysfunction, (2) cardiac ischemia, (3) cardiac arrhythmias, and (4) fibrosis and pericarditis (Fig. 4.1).[2] Risk of cardiotoxicity increases with the presence of preexisting cardiovascular risk factors (smoking, hypertension, diabetes, etc.), female sex, age >70 years, use of multiple chemotherapies, and prior radiation therapy to the mediastinum.[2,3]

Anthracyclines belong to the antimetabolite class of chemotherapeutics and include doxorubicin, daunorubicin, epirubicin, idarubicin, mitoxanotrone, and valrubicin. Anthracycline-related cardiotoxicity ranges from 0.9% to 26% and depends on individual and cumulative doses.[2] Four types of adverse cardiac toxicities related to anthracyclines are recognized. Acute cardiotoxicity occurs during and immediately after administration of the drug. Side effects include hypotension, vasodilation, and arrhythmias. Acute cardiotoxicity can occur up to 1–3 days after drug administration and can manifest as pericarditis and myocarditis. Early chronic cardiotoxicity occurs up to 1 year after completing treatment. Symptoms include dilated cardiomyopathy, congestive heart failure, and left ventricular dysfunction. Delayed chronic cardiotoxicity occurs more than 1 year after completing treatment, and symptoms include restrictive cardiomyopathy, dilated cardiomyopathy, and congestive heart failure.[4,5] Anthracycline-mediated toxicity is also related to the cumulative dose received by a patient. Limiting the total dose to 400–450 mg/m^2 minimizes the risk of congestive heart failure to less than 5%.[1] Cardiotoxicity can be detected by a rise in troponin level immediately after administration; however, this is not monitored in routine practice.

Taxanes belong to the class of microtubule assembly inhibitors and include paclitaxel, docetaxel, and cabazitaxel. These medications can be cardiotoxic in up to 2.3%–8% of patients. Cardiac side effects include bradycardia and autonomic dysfunction, most often manifesting as asymptomatic sinus bradycardia.[6] When combined with anthracyclines, taxanes may induce cardiomyopathy by increasing the amount of anthracycline metabolites produced.[7]

Fluorouracil (5-FU) is the third most common chemotherapeutic agent used for treatment of solid tumors.[8] After anthracyclines, 5-FU is the second most common drug to cause cardiotoxicity manifesting as chest pain, atypical chest pain, and acute coronary syndrome, including myocardial infarction.[9]

Monoclonal antibodies are an emerging class of treatment and include trastuzumab and bevacizumab. Trastuzumab has been associated with a 3%–64% risk of cardiac dysfunction.[10] The risk is increased when administered

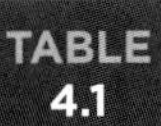

TABLE 4.1 **Chemotherapy and Perioperative Concerns**

Class	Agents	Common Perioperative Concerns
Alkylating Agents		
Nitrosoureas	Carmustine Lomustine	Pulmonary fibrosis
Methylating agents	Procarbazine	Edema Tachycardia
	Dacarbazine	Hepatic necrosis and occlusion Hepatic vein thrombosis
	Temozolomide	Seizure and gait abnormality Peripheral edema
Platinums	Cisplatin Carboplatin Oxaliplatin	Acute renal tubular necrosis Magnesium wasting Peripheral sensory neuropathy Paresthesias Ototoxicity
Nitrogen mustards	Cyclophosphamide Ifosfamide	Pericarditis Pericardial effusions Pulmonary fibrosis Hemorrhagic cystitis Water retention Anemia
	Melphalan	SIADH
	Chlorambucil	SIADH Seizures
Antimetabolites		
Anthracyclines	Doxorubicin Daunorubicin Epirubicin Idarubicin Mitoxantrone Valrubicin	Cardiomyopathy ECG changes
Antitumor antibiotics: Natural product	Bleomycin Mitomycin C	Pulmonary fibrosis Pneumonitis Pulmonary hypertension
Pyrimidine analogue	Capecitabine Cytarabine (Ara-C) Fluorouracil	Myocardial ischemia/infarction Coronary vasospasm
	Gemcitabine	Edema Proteinuria
Purine analogue	Thioguanine Pentostatin	Hepatotoxicity Pulmonary toxicity Deep vein thrombophlebitis Chest pain Edema AV block Arrhythmia Hypo- and hypertension
	Cladribine	Thrombosis Tachycardia Acute renal failure Tumor lysis syndrome
	Fludarabine	Cerebrovascular accident/transient ischemic attack Angina Thrombosis Arrhythmia Heart failure Acute renal failure Tumor lysis syndrome

Continued

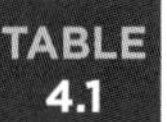

TABLE 4.1 Chemotherapy and Perioperative Concerns—cont'd

Class	Agents	Common Perioperative Concerns
	Mercaptopurine	Intrahepatic cholestasis and focal centrilobular necrosis
Folate antagonist	Methotrexate	Elevated liver enzymes Pulmonary edema Pleural effusions Encephalopathy Meningismus Myelosuppression
Substituted urea	Hydroxyurea	Seizure Edema
Microtubule Assembly Inhibitors		
Taxanes	Paclitaxel Docetaxel	Peripheral neuropathy Bradycardia Autonomic dysfunction Cardiomyopathy (combination with anthracyclines)
Alkaloids	Vinblastine	Hypertension Angina Cerebrovascular accident Coronary ischemia ECG abnormalities Raynaud's phenomenon SIADH GI bleed
	Vincristine	Paresthesias Recurrent laryngeal nerve palsy Autonomic dysfunction Orthostasis Hypo- and hypertension SIADH
Biologic Agents		
Monoclonal antibody	Alemtuzumab	Dysrhythmia/tachycardia/SVT Hypotension and hypertension
	Bevacizumab	Pulmonary bleeding Hypertension Thromboembolic events
	Cetuximab Rituximab	Cardiopulmonary arrest Tumor lysis syndrome Electrolyte abnormality
	Trastuzumab Pertuzumab Ofatumumab	Cardiomyopathy Thrombus formation Pulmonary toxicity Tachycardia Hypertension
	Daclizumab	Chest pain Hyper- and hypotension Thrombosis
	Ibritumomab Palivizumab Muromonab-CD3	Peripheral edema Arrhythmia Tachycardia Hyper- and hypotension
Immune Checkpoint Inhibitors		
	Ipilimumab (Yervoy) Nivolumab (Opdivo) Pembrolizumab (Keytruda) Atezolizumab (Tecentriq)	Immune-mediated adverse effects may affect numerous organ systems. Adverse effects may present as myocarditis, dermatitis, nephritis, encephalitis, pneumonitis, thyroiditis, hepatitis, hypophysitis, colitis, arthritidis, etc.

TABLE 4.1 Chemotherapy and Perioperative Concerns—cont'd

Class	Agents	Common Perioperative Concerns
	Avelumab (Bavencio) Durvalumab (Imfinzi) Cemiplimab (Libtayo)	A high clinical suspicion for late immune-mediated side effects needs to be present for patients with prior treatment of immune checkpoint inhibitors
Biological Response Modulators		
Interleukins	Aldesleukin Denileukin Diftitox	Capillary leak syndrome Peripheral edema Hypotension ECG changes
Interferon	Interferon Alfa-2b Interferon Alfacon-1	Arrhythmia Chest pain Pulmonary pneumonitis Ischemic disorders Hyperthyroidism Hypothyroidism Pulmonary infiltrates Ischemic disorders
	Peginterferon alfa-2a Peginterferon alfa-2b	Hyperthyroidism Hypothyroidism
Vascular Endothelial Growth Factor (VEGF) Inhibitors		
Tyrosine kinase inhibitors	Imatinib	Edema Left ventricular dysfunction
	Sorafenib	Cardiac ischemia and infarction Hypertension Thromboembolism Cardiac ischemia and infarction Thromboembolism
	Sunitinib	Adrenal insufficiency Pulmonary hemorrhage Hypertension Hypothyroidism Cardiomyopathy QT prolongation Torsade de pointes
	Dasatinib	Fluid retention Cardiomyopathy QT prolongation Pulmonary hemorrhage Platelet dysfunction
	Nilotinib	QT prolongation Hypertension Peripheral edema
Epidermal Growth Factor Receptor (EGFR) Inhibitors		
	Erlotinib	Deep venous thrombosis Arrhythmia Pulmonary toxicity Cerebrovascular accidents Myocardial ischemia Syncope Edema
	Lapatinib	Cardiomyopathy Pulmonary toxicity QT prolongation
	Panitumumab	Pulmonary fibrosis Peripheral edema
Angiogenesis inhibitors		
Immunomodulators	Thalidomide	Thromboembolism Edema Bradycardia
	Lenalidomide	Thromboembolism

Continued

TABLE 4.1 Chemotherapy and Perioperative Concerns—cont'd

Class	Agents	Common Perioperative Concerns
Enzymes		
	Asparaginase	Thrombosis Glucose intolerance Coagulopathy
Miscellaneous		
Topoisomerase I inhibitor	Irinotecan Topotecan Rubitecan	Neutropenia Diarrhea Cholinergic syndrome
Epipodophyllotoxin topoisomerase II inhibitor	Etoposide	Neutropenia Stevens-Johnson syndrome Toxic epidermal necrolysis Myocardial infarction Congestive heart failure
Selective Estrogen Receptor Modulators		
	Tamoxifen Toremifene	Thromboembolism
Aromatase inhibitors		
	Anastrozole Letrozole Exemestane	Perioperative implications Unknown/limited data
mTor inhibitors		
	Sirolimus Everolimus Temsirolimus	Dyslipidemia Hypertension Renal dysfunction Hyperglycemia/diabetes Interstitial lung disease
Hedgehog Pathway Inhibitors		
	Vismodegib	Perioperative implications Unknown/limited data
Androgen Targets		
	Abiraterone	Hypertension Hypertriglyceridemia Hyperglycemia Hypernatremia Hypokalemia QT prolongation
	Bicalutamide	Hepatoxicity Hyperglycemia Prolonged QT interval
Histone Deacetylase Targets		
	Romidepsin Vorinostat	Prolonged QT interval Hyperglycemia Prolonged QT interval
Folate Targets		
	Pralatrexate	Perioperative implications Unknown/limited data
Retinoic Acid Receptor Targets		
	Isotretinoin Acitretin	Hypertriglyceridemia

TABLE 4.1 Chemotherapy and Perioperative Concerns—cont'd

Class	Agents	Common Perioperative Concerns
Proteasome Targets		
	Bortezomib Carfilzomib	Peripheral neuropathy Heart failure Hepatoxicity Cardiac ischemia
Immunomodulatory Agents		
	Thalidomide Lenalidomide	Thromboembolism

AV, Atrioventricular; *GI*, gastrointestinal; *SIADH*, syndrome of inappropriate antidiuretic hormone; *SVT*, supraventricular tachycardia.

Both generic and brand names are used in this table. Some chemotherapy agents have Index names that are also used.

Adapted and updated from Sahai SK, Zalpour A, Rozner MA. Preoperative evaluation of the oncology patient. *Med Clin North Am*. 2010;94(2):403–419. With permission from Elsevier.

Updated using Lexicomp Online, Hudson, Ohio: Wolters Kluwer Clinical Drug Information, Inc.; 2019. Available at http://webstore.lexi.com/ONLINE

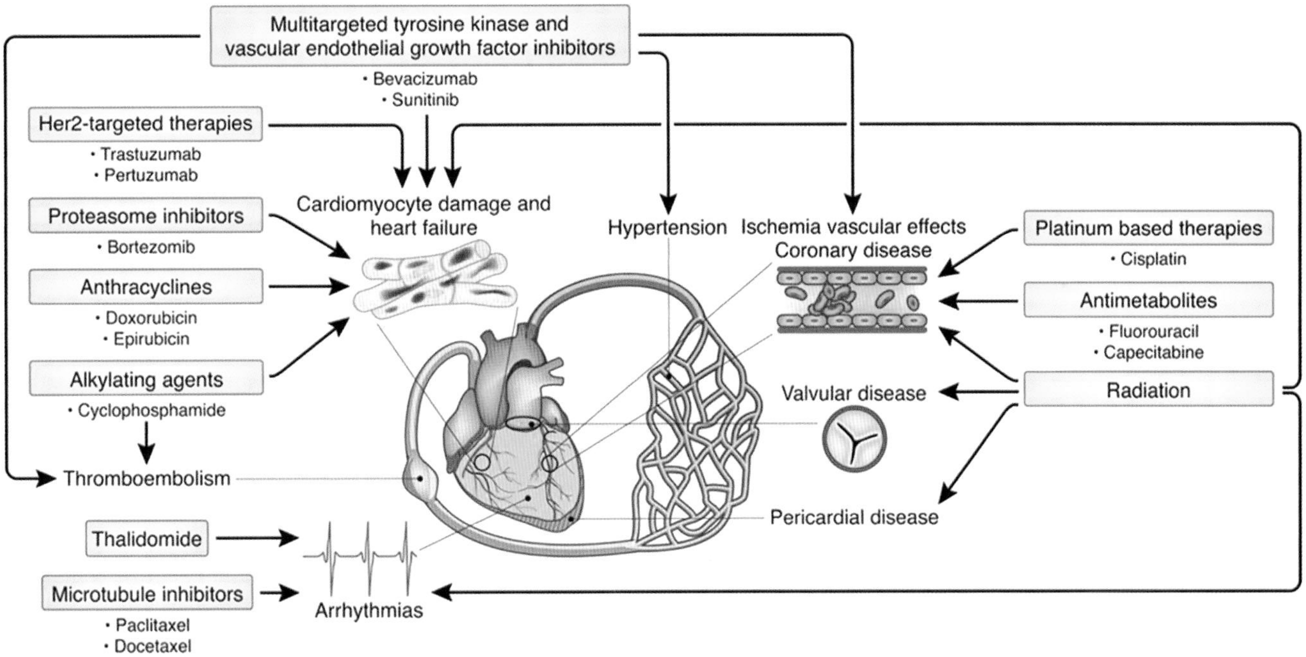

• **Fig. 4.1** Cardiovascular side effects of chemotherapy and radiation.
From Lenneman CG, Sawyer DB. Cardio-oncology: an update on cardiotoxicity of cancer-related treatment. *Circ Res*. 2016;118(6):1008–1020. With permission from Wolters Kluwer Health, Inc.

concomitantly with other chemotherapeutics and with a length of treatment longer than 6 months. Cardiotoxicity is usually reversed when treatment is halted or can be managed with cardiac therapy.[11] If cardiac dysfunction following therapy does not improve rapidly, treatment can include angiotensin converting enzyme (ACE) inhibitors and beta blockers.[6] Bevacizumab inhibits vascular endothelial growth factor (VEGF) receptors and is commonly associated with hypertension. Due to VEGF inhibition, a decrease in nitric oxide increases peripheral vascular resistance leading to an increase in blood pressure.[11] This can commonly be managed with ACE inhibitors and calcium channel blockers.

Tyrosine kinase inhibitors (sunitinib and sorafenib) were originally thought to be less toxic than other therapies due to their targeting of specific proteins. Their broad use has shown a variety of cardiac side effects, including hypertension, heart failure, QT prolongation, and myocardial ischemia. Hypertension has been reported in 15%–47% of patients on tyrosine kinase inhibitors and is much more likely in patients with renal cell carcinoma. Heart failure and left ventricular dysfunction occur more commonly with sorafenib (4%–8%), pazopanib (7%–11%), and sunitinib (2.7%–19%).[12]

In order to administer chemotherapeutics safely, cardiac evaluation is advised in all patients before initiation of these drugs for whom a suspicion of potential cardiotoxicity exists.[13] Left ventricular function can be monitored by cardiac MRI or echocardiography. Biomarkers such as troponins and nt-pro BNP can be used for detection of early cardiotoxicity if a clinical suspicion exists and may predict postoperative complications.[14,15] Interval monitoring of ECG is recommended for patients at risk for arrhythmias and QT prolongation. While most of the cardiotoxic effects of chemotherapy are reversible, anthracyclines can be associated with irreversible damage. Fortunately, perioperative management of chemotherapy-induced cardiomyopathy is consistent with ACC/AHA/HFSA guidelines for the management of heart failure.[16]

In terms of perioperative considerations, side effects from radiation therapy that affect the cardiovascular system are of concern. Radiation therapy to the chest may result in several different forms of cardiovascular disease that develop over several months to years. Radiation triggers endothelial proliferation, which accelerates atherosclerosis, and microvascular ischemia and fibrin deposition, which cause fibrosis of the pericardium, myocardium, conduction system, and cardiac valves. The perioperative clinician should pay particular attention to signs of pericarditis, new murmurs, and ECG changes.[17] Radiation therapy to the head and neck area can result in radiation-induced carotid stenosis.[18] Combining radiation with chemotherapeutic agents that also have cardiovascular side effects poses an additional risk for developing cardiovascular disease.

Patients with cardiovascular disease are frequently on antiplatelet, antithrombotic, or anticoagulant medications for primary or secondary prevention of adverse cardiac or vascular events. Patients with recent cardiac stents may be on dual antiplatelet therapy, while others with recent venous thromboembolic events may be on full-dose anticoagulation. As such, a detailed history and medical management plan for these agents in line with current evidence and local guidelines should be addressed in the perioperative evaluation consultation. Consideration of the risks and benefits of stopping and/or continuing antithrombotics/anticoagulants should be noted at the time of perioperative evaluation.

Pulmonary

Pulmonary complications from chemotherapy most commonly involve infection. Side effects may occur from direct cytotoxicity to the lungs, oxidative damage, or disruption of collagen synthesis.[19] Pulmonary toxicity can result from bleomycin, cyclophosphamide, nitrosoureas, mitomycin, busulfan, and methotrexate. Diagnosis of pulmonary toxicity can be difficult due to a large differential diagnosis of respiratory symptoms. Once pulmonary embolism, metastatic disease, and infection are ruled out, pulmonary toxicity needs to be considered. Methotrexate and cyclophosphamide are most commonly associated with pneumonitis.[20]

Bleomycin-related pulmonary toxicity is usually dose dependent and can occur in 6%–10% of patients, occasionally being fatal.[21] Patients exposed to a total of 270 mg have a 0%–2% chance of developing pulmonary toxicity, while patients receiving 360 mg have an incidence of 6%–18%.[22,23] Doses greater than 400 mg are avoided due to the increased rate of pulmonary complications. While pulmonary toxicity is most likely to occur in the first 6 months of treatment, the potential of exacerbating the condition with high oxygen concentrations remains throughout a patient's lifetime. Initial symptoms can include dry cough and shortness of breath and can progress to pneumothorax and pneumomediastinum in extreme cases. Radiographic findings include linear interstitial shadowing. Perioperatively, these patients should be maintained on minimal oxygen concentrations with use of positive end-expiratory pressure (PEEP) to optimize oxygenation. Postoperative care should include a comprehensive pain regimen, chest physiotherapy, and early mobilization. Although controversial, high inspired oxygen concentrations should be avoided in patients treated with bleomycin. While some studies have found high inspired oxygen concentration to be associated with acute respiratory distress syndrome (ARDS) and respiratory distress,[24] others have found no association between FIO_2 and development of ARDS.[25] Instead, fluid balance, blood loss, and transfusion have been found to be associated with an increased likelihood of postoperative pulmonary morbidity.[26] Conservative fluid management is recommended in this population.

While bleomycin is the most well-known agent that causes interstitial lung disease, other agents, such as the monoclonal antibodies (bevacizumab, trastuzumab), antimetabolites (capecitabine, 5-FU), and alkylating agents, are known to cause pneumonitis and fibrosis.[19] Patients who present with a history of dyspnea or shortness of breath should be evaluated for pulmonary compromise, and if needed, undergo further targeted testing for risk stratification. In most cases, asymptomatic patients need no further evaluation beyond a physical exam. Pleural effusions as a result of targeted therapy do occur with some frequency, and as such, preoperative thoracentesis may be needed to allow for adequate lung expansion, especially in the symptomatic patient. Docetaxel and tyrosine kinase inhibitors are known to have pleural effusions as side effects.[19,27]

Renal

Nephrotoxic effects of chemotherapy are most likely to be seen with the platinum subgroup of alkylating agents that include cisplatin, carboplatin, and oxaliplatin. Up to 30% of patients receiving cisplatin can develop nephrotoxicity.[28] Proximal tubules are selectively injured with this chemotherapy, manifesting in renal impairment, including hypomagnesemia, salt wasting, and anemia. Cisplatin is also associated with hypomagnesemia from urinary magnesium wasting. This condition may exacerbate cisplatin's nephrotoxic effects, and magnesium levels should therefore be monitored. Increased risk of cisplatin-related nephrotoxicity occurs with higher doses, preexisting renal impairment, and concurrent use of nephrotoxic agents. The peak plasma platinum level is directly correlated with nephrotoxicity, with a level greater than 400 ng/mL being associated with a 30% decrease in creatinine clearance.[29]

Nephrotoxicity can be minimized with lower doses of cisplatin, intensive hydration, and use of cisplatin analogues. Lower doses of cisplatin have been effectively used for palliative therapy without compromising efficacy and have minimized the toxic effects of cisplatin. Intensive hydrating regimens with normal saline are recommended to reduce the concentration of cisplatin in the renal tubules and decrease the likelihood of toxicity.[30] Finally, cisplatin analogues, such as carboplatin and oxaliplatin, should be considered, as they are less nephrotoxic and just as effective chemotherapeutics.

The syndrome of inappropriate antidiuretic hormone secretion (SIADH) occurs in 1%–2% of cancer patients. Chemotherapeutics, such as vincristine, vinblastine, and cyclophosphamide, are occasionally implicated.[31]

Nervous System

The chemotherapeutic groups of drugs most likely to cause nervous system toxicity manifesting as neuropathy include vinca alkaloids, cisplatin, and taxanes. Vinca alkaloids include vinblastine and vincristine, and are plant-derived cytotoxic agents with antimicrotubule activity. Vincristine doses are limited by toxicity that can lead to axonal neuropathy. Almost all patients on vincristine will develop a degree of neuropathy. Symptoms are usually noticed after a few weeks of treatment with cumulative doses between 30 and 50 mg.[32] Neuropathy related to vincristine is usually reversible with full recovery taking up to several months. In order to minimize side effects, a vincristine dose of 1.4 mg/m^2 is recommended. Vinblastine- and vinorelbine-related neuropathies are less likely and less severe than vincristine.

Patients using cisplatin have up to a 50% chance of developing paresthesia. If treatment is continued, severe complications, such as loss of deep tendon reflexes and sensory ataxia, can occur. Taxanes are also associated with a predominantly sensory neuropathy. The most significant risk factor for taxane-related neuropathy seems to be a cumulative dose with a neurotoxic threshold of 1000 mg/m^2 for paclitaxel and 400 mg/m^2 for docetaxel.[33]

Methotrexate can also contribute to central nervous system complications, including aseptic meningitis, leukoencephalopathy, transverse myelopathy, and acute/subacute encephalopathy. High doses of methotrexate (>1000 mg/m^2) are most likely to cause neurotoxicity.[34] Intrathecal methotrexate can be acutely associated with aseptic meningitis or as a delayed reaction causing leukoencephalopathy. Risk of methotrexate-related leukoencephalopathy increases with concurrent whole brain radiotherapy or prior treatment with methotrexate.

Gastrointestinal

Chemotherapy-related enterotoxicity could include diarrhea, constipation, and intestinal perforation. Diarrhea associated with chemotherapy is most often associated with the fluoropyrimidines and irinotecan. Diarrhea can be secretory or osmotic, or due to altered intestinal motility resulting from epithelial damage or ischemic mucosal damage that can occur with chemotherapy targeting VEGF. More severe complications such as neutropenic enterocolitis can occur in patients with leukemia undergoing induction therapy.[35] Liver dysfunction can be caused by methotrexate, plicamycin, streptozocin, 6-mercaptopurine, L-asparaginase, and cytosine arabinoside (ARA-C). In all cases, side effects of chemotherapy that disrupt the normal functioning of the gastro-intestinal tract and therefore nutritional status, can have profound perioperative concerns, such as increased perioperative morbidity and mortality and increased length of hospital stay.[36] In addition to traditional perioperative concerns regarding cardiac and pulmonary status prior to surgery, optimization of perioperative nutritional status must be considered.[37]

Hematologic

A full discussion regarding the hematologic malignancies associated with cancer treatment is beyond the scope of this chapter. Most chemotherapeutics lead to myelosuppression and pancytopenia. Myelosuppression is usually reversible after 1–6 weeks of ceasing therapy; however, it may persist longer in some patients. Coagulation and platelet survival may also be disturbed by chemotherapy. Careful monitoring of hematologic status is required throughout treatment. Implications for the perioperative period mostly reside in concerns regarding anemia and thrombocytopenia from treatment. There is a growing body of evidence that intravenous iron replacement therapy prior to surgery may reduce the need for perioperative transfusions and their associated complications.[38-40]

In addition to bleeding risks, the cancer patient remains uniquely susceptible to perioperative thromboembolism due to the nature of the disease. The hypercoagulable state of cancer, plus the inherent risks for postoperative thromboembolism place the cancer patient at elevated risk for postoperative clots.[41] Upon treatment with thalidomide, patients with multiple myeloma are at higher risk of developing thrombotic complications, and as such, many are on preventive anticoagulation therapy during treatment.[42]

Endocrine

Management of chemotherapy- or steroid-induced diabetes, or exacerbation of preexisting diabetes is beyond the scope of this chapter; however, optimization of diabetes prior to surgery is recommended. In practice, in view of the relatively short lead times to surgery, we do not recommend delaying surgery to optimize diabetes, as there may be a risk of tumor recurrence if the delay pushes the patient past the optimal surgical resection window. In the ideal perioperative environment, optimization of diabetes would begin at the time of diagnosis, with monitoring and therapeutic adjustments in the neoadjuvant period. Patients receiving steroids as part of their chemotherapy regimen may experience short-term adrenal insufficiency and as such, need to be managed along established guidelines[43,44] Patients that receive radiation therapy to the head and neck area are at risk of developing hypothyroidism, which may not manifest clinically, or symptoms attributed to chemotherapy-induced fatigue.[45] Hyponatremia, in the form of a paraneoplastic process such as SIADH, may occur from the tumor itself (small-cell lung cancer) or be a result of chemotherapy (cyclophosphamide, vincristine, cisplatin).[46,47]

Premature Aging

Cancer survivors have a higher rate of morbidity and mortality due to complications from prior treatment. Survivors have a higher incidence of chronic comorbid conditions that appear to manifest at an earlier age than their peers who do not have a history of cancer.[48] This syndrome has been described as premature aging, as research indicates that changes in the cellular biology of the cancer survivor bears a resemblance to the changes seen in the elderly.[49] Premature aging along with the multi-hit hypothesis of cancer frailty (prior cancer treatment, age, sarcopenia, medical comorbidities, sedentary lifestyle, and cancer fatigue) complicates the perioperative evaluation of the cancer patient and should be considered when making recommendations for perioperative care.[50] Please see Chapter 14: Preoperative Evaluation and Medical Optimization of the Cancer Patient for a more robust discussion of these issues.

Conclusion

In summary, the revolutionary advances in neoadjuvant chemotherapy and radiation therapy over the last 50 years have dramatically improved outcomes in cancer. With the number of chemotherapeutic agents increasing in number yearly, it is incumbent on the perioperative clinician to recognize that there may be side effects that affect perioperative evaluation and risk stratification. From traditional therapies such as anthracyclines with well-documented effects of cardiotoxicity to newer agents such as the tyrosine kinase inhibitors resulting in pleural effusions, the perioperative team must be cognizant of the varied side effects that may affect the cancer patient.

References

1. Ewer MS, Ewer SM. Cardiotoxicity of anticancer treatments. *Nat Rev Cardiol.* 2015;12(11):620.
2. Lenneman CG, Sawyer DB. Cardio-oncology: an update on cardiotoxicity of cancer-related treatment. *Circ Res.* 2016;118(6):1008–1020.
3. Pinder MC, Duan Z, Goodwin JS, Hortobagyi GN, Giordano SH. Congestive heart failure in older women treated with adjuvant anthracycline chemotherapy for breast cancer. *J Clin Oncol.* 2007;25(25):3808–3815.
4. Simunek T, Sterba M, Popelova O, Adamcova M, Hrdina R, Gersl V. Anthracycline-induced cardiotoxicity: overview of studies examining the roles of oxidative stress and free cellular iron. *Pharmacol Rep.* 2009;61(1):154–171.
5. Scully RE, Lipshultz SE. Anthracycline cardiotoxicity in long-term survivors of childhood cancer. *Cardiovasc Toxicol.* 2007;7(2):122–128.
6. Berardi R, Caramanti M, Savini A, et al. State of the art for cardiotoxicity due to chemotherapy and to targeted therapies: a literature review. *Crit Rev Oncol Hematol.* 2013;88(1):75–86.
7. Gianni L, Salvatorelli E, Minotti G. Anthracycline cardiotoxicity in breast cancer patients: synergism with trastuzumab and taxanes. *Cardiovasc Toxicol.* 2007;7(2):67–71.
8. Grem JL. 5-Fluorouracil: forty-plus and still ticking. A review of its preclinical and clinical development. *Invest New Drugs.* 2000;18(4):299–313.
9. Sara JD, Kaur J, Khodadadi R, et al. 5-fluorouracil and cardiotoxicity: a review. *Ther Adv Med Oncol.* 2018;10:1758835918780140.
10. de Forni M, Malet-Martino MC, Jaillais P, et al. Cardiotoxicity of high-dose continuous infusion fluorouracil: a prospective clinical study. *J Clin Oncol.* 1992;10(11):1795–1801.
11. Ng R, Better N, Green MD. Anticancer agents and cardiotoxicity. *Semin Oncol.* 2006;33(1):2–14.
12. Lee W-S, Kim J. Cardiotoxicity associated with tyrosine kinase-targeted anticancer therapy. *Mol Cell Toxicol.* 2018;14(3):247–254.
13. Chang H-M, Moudgil R, Scarabelli T, Okwuosa TM, Yeh ETH. Cardiovascular complications of cancer therapy. Best practices in diagnosis, prevention, and management: part 1. *J Am Coll Cardiol.* 2017;70(20):2536–2551.
14. Shen JT, Xu M, Wu Y, et al. Association of pre-operative troponin levels with major adverse cardiac events and mortality after noncardiac surgery: a systematic review and meta-analysis. *Eur J Anaesthesiol.* 2018;35(11):815–824.
15. Duceppe E, Patel A, Chan MTV, et al. Preoperative N-terminal pro-B-type natriuretic peptide and cardiovascular events after noncardiac surgery: a cohort study. *Ann Intern Med.* 2020;172:96–104. doi:10.7326/M19-2501.
16. Yancy CW, Jessup M, Bozkurt B, et al. 2017 ACC/AHA/HFSA focused update of the 2013 ACCF/AHA guideline for the management of heart failure: a report of the American College of Cardiology/American Heart Association Task Force on clinical practice guidelines and the Heart Failure Society of America. *Circulation.* 2017;136(6):e137–e161.
17. Sahai SK. Perioperative assessment of the cancer patient. *Best Pract Res Clin Anaesthesiol.* 2013;27(4):465–480.
18. Xu J, Cao Y. Radiation-induced carotid artery stenosis: a comprehensive review of the literature. *Interv Neurol.* 2014;2(4):183–192.
19. Becker A, Frauenfelder T. Pulmonale komplikationen in der chemotherapie. *Radiologe.* 2014;54(10):1023–1038.
20. Meadors M, Floyd J, Perry MC. Pulmonary toxicity of chemotherapy. *Semin Oncol.* 2006;33(1):98–105.
21. Keijzer A, Kuenen B. Fatal pulmonary toxicity in testis cancer with bleomycin-containing chemotherapy. *J Clin Oncol.* 2007;25(23):3543–3544.

22. Jules-Elysee K, White DA. Bleomycin-induced pulmonary toxicity. *Clin Chest Med.* 1990;11(1):1–20.
23. Culine S, Kramar A, Theodore C, et al. Randomized trial comparing bleomycin/etoposide/cisplatin with alternating cisplatin/cyclophosphamide/doxorubicin and vinblastine/bleomycin regimens of chemotherapy for patients with intermediate- and poor-risk metastatic nonseminomatous germ cell tumors: Genito-Urinary Group of the French Federation of Cancer Centers Trial T93MP. *J Clin Oncol.* 2008;26(3):421–427.
24. Goldiner PL, Schweizer O. The hazards of anesthesia and surgery in bleomycin-treated patients. *Semin Oncol.* 1979;6(1):121–124.
25. LaMantia KR, Glick JH, Marshall BE. Supplemental oxygen does not cause respiratory failure in bleomycin-treated surgical patients. *Anesthesiology.* 1984;60(1):65–67.
26. Donat SM, Levy DA. Bleomycin associated pulmonary toxicity: is perioperative oxygen restriction necessary? *J Urol.* 1998;160(4):1347–1352.
27. Ho MY, Mackey JR. Presentation and management of docetaxel-related adverse effects in patients with breast cancer. *Cancer Manag Res.* 2014;6:253–259.
28. Pabla N, Dong Z. Cisplatin nephrotoxicity: mechanisms and renoprotective strategies. *Kidney Int.* 2008;73(9):994–1007.
29. Reece PA, Stafford I, Russell J, Khan M, Gill PG. Creatinine clearance as a predictor of ultrafilterable platinum disposition in cancer patients treated with cisplatin: relationship between peak ultrafilterable platinum plasma levels and nephrotoxicity. *J Clin Oncol.* 1987;5(2):304–309.
30. Crona DJ, Faso A, Nishijima TF, McGraw KA, Galsky MD, Milowsky MI. A systematic review of strategies to prevent cisplatin-induced nephrotoxicity. *Oncologist.* 2017;22(5):609–619.
31. Berardi R, Mastroianni C, Lo Russo G, et al. Syndrome of inappropriate anti-diuretic hormone secretion in cancer patients: results of the first multicenter Italian study. *Ther Adv Med Oncol.* 2019;11:1758835919877725.
32. Postma TJ, Benard BA, Huijgens PC, Ossenkoppele GJ, Heimans JJ. Long-term effects of vincristine on the peripheral nervous system. *J Neurooncol.* 1993;15(1):23–27.
33. Grisold W, Cavaletti G, Windebank AJ. Peripheral neuropathies from chemotherapeutics and targeted agents: diagnosis, treatment, and prevention. *Neuro Oncol.* 2012;14(Suppl 4):iv45–iv54.
34. Schmiegelow K. Advances in individual prediction of methotrexate toxicity: a review. *Br J Haematol.* 2009;146(5):489–503.
35. Aksoy DY, Tanriover MD, Uzun O, et al. Diarrhea in neutropenic patients: a prospective cohort study with emphasis on neutropenic enterocolitis. *Ann Oncol.* 2007;18(1):183–189.
36. Braga M, Sandrucci S. Perioperative nutrition in cancer patients. *Eur J Surg Oncol.* 2016;42(6):751–753.
37. Huhmann MB, August DA. Perioperative nutrition support in cancer patients. *Nutr Clin Pract.* 2012;27(5):586–592.
38. Busti F, Marchi G, Ugolini S, Castagna A, Girelli D. Anemia and iron deficiency in cancer patients: role of iron replacement therapy. *Pharmaceuticals (Basel).* 2018;11(4):94.
39. Osorio J, Jerico C, Miranda C, et al. Perioperative transfusion management in gastric cancer surgery: analysis of the Spanish subset of the EURECCA oesophago-gastric cancer registry. *Cir Esp.* 2018;96(9):546–554.
40. Auerbach M. Intravenous iron in the perioperative setting. *Am J Hematol.* 2014;89(9):933.
41. Ivatury SJ, Holubar SD. Just do it: changing our culture to embrace optimal perioperative venous thromboembolism chemoprophylaxis for abdominal and pelvic cancer patients. *Ann Surg Oncol.* 2016;23(5):1420–1421.
42. Singh A, Gajra A. Thromboembolism with immunomodulatory agents in the treatment of multiple myeloma. *Cardiovasc Hematol Agents Med Chem.* 2011;9(1):7–13.
43. Axelrod L. Perioperative management of patients treated with glucocorticoids. *Endocrinol Metab Clin North Am.* 2003;32(2):367–383.
44. Kohl BA, Schwartz S. How to manage perioperative endocrine insufficiency. *Anesthesiol Clin.* 2010;28(1):139–155.
45. Miller MC, Agrawal A. Hypothyroidism in postradiation head and neck cancer patients: incidence, complications, and management. *Curr Opin Otolaryngol Head Neck Surg.* 2009;17(2):111–115.
46. Castillo JJ, Vincent M, Justice E. Diagnosis and management of hyponatremia in cancer patients. *Oncologist.* 2012;17(6):756–765.
47. Raftopoulos H. Diagnosis and management of hyponatremia in cancer patients. *Support Care Cancer.* 2007;15(12):1341–1347.
48. Armenian SH, Gibson CJ, Rockne RC, Ness KK. Premature aging in young cancer survivors. *J Natl Cancer Inst.* 2019;111(3):226–232.
49. Cupit-Link MC, Kirkland JL, Ness KK, et al. Biology of premature ageing in survivors of cancer. *ESMO Open.* 2017;2(5):e000250.
50. Sahai SK, Ismail H. Perioperative implications of neoadjuvant therapies and optimization strategies for cancer surgery. *Curr Anesthesiol Rep.* 2015;5(3):305–317.

5

Newer Cancer Therapies and Perioperative Implications

JOSEPH M. HERMAN, GERMAN ECHEVERRY, AND SUZANNE RUSSO

Introduction

There have been rapid and substantial advances in cancer treatment with improved systemic therapies, including chemotherapy, hormone therapy, targeted therapy, and immunotherapy, as well as recent technologic advances in radiation therapy. This has led to new combinations and sequences of cancer treatment, including the use of neoadjuvant and adjuvant therapies in surgical patients. Therapeutic advances in cancer treatments have significantly improved outcomes for many malignancies and have led to an increase in the number of patients undergoing surgery. Many of these patients are experiencing extended survival and sometimes long-term remission; hence the adverse effects of their oncologic treatments may impact subsequent oncologic and noncancer surgery for an increasing number of cancer survivors. The preoperative evaluation of a cancer patient may be challenging because of the physiologic deconditioning that this disease and its treatments can impose. It is important to identify individual patient risk factors and consider age-related comorbid conditions and cancer symptoms. It is also important to recognize the potential sequelae of various types of cancer therapies and their clinical implications on a patient's baseline functional status. A comprehensive history and physical examination can help guide targeted preoperative testing for the potential effects of specific cancer therapies and aid in medical optimization prior to surgery. Care may be further complicated by disruption of normal anatomy as a result of prior surgery and radiation, as well as vital organ dysfunction from systemic treatments leading to cardiopulmonary instability under general anesthesia. Postoperative management must meticulously account for the above maintaining great vigilance for complications related to surgery, thromboembolic events, wound healing, infection, and further deterioration of previously affected organ systems. This chapter provides an overview of the potential adverse effects of newer systemic chemotherapies, targeted therapies, and radiation therapy; describes recent advancements in cancer treatments; and reviews the impact of these newer cancer treatments and potential implications for the perioperative care of the cancer patient.

Surgical Considerations

Approximately 90% of patients with solid tumors will undergo a surgical resection for either cure or palliation.[1] There have been major advances in surgical techniques, including minimally invasive approaches such as laparoscopic surgery,[2] video-assisted thoracic surgery,[3,4] robotic surgery,[5] and improved intraoperative image guidance techniques[6] such as Brainlab navigation.[7] Additionally, indications for image-guided interventions, including endovascular embolization and ablations, continue to expand. These improvements can potentially result in improved safety and lower incidence of perioperative complications, but also mean that an increasing number of patients with advanced disease and likely multiple rounds of prior systemic treatments or local therapies are becoming candidates for surgical and image-guided interventions. Almost all cancer patients in the United States receive more than one treatment modality. The increasing use of preoperative therapies, including radiation therapy, interventional therapies, chemotherapy, targeted therapies, and immunotherapies, influences how cancer patients are surgically managed and require attention to planning with other oncology colleagues regarding the timing of surgery. Developments in effective systemic therapies have resulted in many cancers becoming chronic diseases, which require special considerations to reduce treatment-related toxicities in order to optimize survivorship. With the rapid development of new cancer therapies, cancer surgeons and anesthesiologists must understand the importance of relevant cancer-specific, considerations in the perioperative period, and undergo continuing education and training throughout their career.

It is also important for oncologic surgeons to understand the principles of the cancer in managing complex patients, work closely with other oncology disciplines, and know which patients need to be referred to high-volume specialty centers for optimal management, especially if they are at high risk of toxicity or complications.[8] The development of cancer centers that incorporate multidisciplinary teams of specialists which participate in comprehensive treatment planning for patients with specific oncologic conditions has improved outcome for many patients over recent years.[8] As such, there is increasing demand for cancer care to be delivered by specialists in multidisciplinary cancer centers. It has been demonstrated that surgeons who perform technically demanding procedures at centers with higher volumes achieve better outcomes with complex disease.[9] In addition, operative mortality has been shown to be significantly higher for patients treated at hospitals with lower annual caseloads for these procedures.[10] This does not mean that all cancer patients require treatment at high-volume centers. If patients are diagnosed early, many initial treatments are relatively protocolized and can be adequately provided in the community setting. For relatively more complex cases, increased utilization of telemedicine has facilitated cancer patient care at local hospitals by providing input from surgical oncology specialists.[9] These specialists assist by providing educational leadership within the general surgical community and have a central role in defining standards for treating surgical patients with cancer to achieve optimal care.

Chemotherapy and Targeted Therapy

The toxicity of cancer chemotherapy drugs and targeted agents and their relevance to perioperative management relates to the specific agents used. The most common toxicities encountered include cardiovascular, pulmonary, and hematologic toxicities, although gastrointestinal, hepatic, renal, endocrine, nutritional, and metabolic effects should also be considered.[11] Awareness of the common side effects associated with these various chemotherapeutic and targeted agents can direct preoperative clinical testing and subsequent patient management to ensure a well-prepared surgical patient. As with any preoperative evaluation, the considerations for the patient with cancer who is undergoing surgery can be grouped by organ system. Systemic therapies have been associated with cardiovascular toxicities (including ischemia, cardiomyopathy, conduction system abnormalities, and hypertension), pulmonary toxicity, hematologic toxicities (including cytopenias and coagulopathies), gastrointestinal toxicities (colitis), hepatotoxicity, nephrotoxicity, and endocrinopathies, all of which can complicate perioperative care of the cancer patient. These complications are described in greater detail earlier in this book. A quick review of systemic agents and their associated toxicities in cancer patients undergoing surgery is provided in Tables 5.1–5.5.

Newer Systemic Treatments: Immunotherapy

Systemic treatment of cancer has changed dramatically over the past two decades. Antineoplastic chemotherapy classically targets cell proliferation by delivering drugs intravenously in a cyclic schedule resulting in systemic toxicities.

TABLE 5.1 Chemotherapeutic and Targeted Agents Associated With Myocardial Ischemia

Drug	Incidence
Bevacizumab[53–55]	0.6%–1.5%
Capecitabine[56–59]	3%–9%
Docetaxel[60]	1.7%
Epirubicin[61]	0.9%–3.3%
Erlotinib[18]	2.3%
5-Fluorouracil[56,62]	1%–68%
Gemcitabine[63,64]	Rare
Paclitaxel[65]	<1%–5%
Sorafinib[66]	2.7%–3%
Vinblastine[67]	Rare
Vincristine[67]	Rare
Vinorelbine[68]	1.19%

A newer era of anticancer therapy emerged with targeted agents such as monoclonal antibodies that target more specific tumor cell antigens such as the CD20 protein in lymphoma, vascular endothelial growth factor (VEGF), and epidermal growth factor receptor (EGFR) in colon cancer. In addition to targeted antibodies, numerous oral tyrosine kinase inhibitors with different targets and indications have been developed for various hematological and solid tumors

TABLE 5.2 Chemotherapeutic and Targeted Agents Associated With Left Ventricular Dysfunction and Cardiomyopathy

Drug	Prevalence or Incidence
Bevacizumab[69,70]	1.7–3
Bortezomib[71]	2–5
Clofarabine[72]	27
Cyclophosphamide[73]	7–28
Dasatinib[74]	4
Docetaxel[75]	2.3–8
Doxorubicin[76]	3–26
Epirubicin[77]	5%
Idarubicin[78]	5–18
Imatinib mesylate[79]	0.5–1.7
Ifosfamide [78]	17
Lapatinib[80]	1.5–2.2
Mitoxantrone[81]	36%
Sunitinib[82,83]	2.7–11
Trastuzumab[84–86]	2–28

TABLE 5.3 Chemotherapeutic and Targeted Agents Associated With Pulmonary Toxicity

Drug	Pulmonary Toxicity	Incidence
Bevacizumab[87]	Hemoptysis	Up to 20%
Bleomycin[88]	Pulmonary fibrosis Bronchiolitis obliterans organizing pneumonia Pulmonary veno-occlusive disease	Up to 20%
Busulfan[89]	Pulmonary fibrosis Pulmonary alveolar lipoproteinosis	4%–10%
Carmustine[90]	Interstitial lung disease/pneumonitis Pulmonary fibrosis	Up to 35%
Cyclophosphamide[91]	Interstitial lung disease/pneumonitis Pulmonary fibrosis	<1%
Cytosine arabinoside[92]	Noncardiogenic pulmonary edema Pleural effusion	12.5%
Dasatinib[93]	Pleural effusion	7%–35%
Docetaxel[94]	Noncardiogenic pulmonary edema Pleural effusion	Up to 23%
Gefitinib[95]	Interstitial lung disease/pneumonitis	1%–2%
Gemcitabine[96]	Interstitial lung disease/pneumonitis Noncardiogenic pulmonary edema	5%–8%
Imatinib mesylate[93]	Pleural effusion	7%–35%
Methotrexate[97]	Noncardiogenic pulmonary edema Pulmonary fibrosis	1%–7%
Mitomycin[98]	Interstitial lung disease/pneumonitis Pulmonary fibrosis	<10%
Nilotinib[93]	Pleural effusion	7%–35%
Paclitaxel[99]	Pleural effusion	1%
Rituxumab[100]	Interstitial lung disease/pneumonitis	1%
Temsirolimus[101]	Interstitial lung disease/pneumonitis	30%
Trastuzumab[102]	Interstitial lung disease/pneumonitis Pulmonary hypertension	Rare

based on the principle of killing tumor cells by interrupting intracellular signals essential for cell proliferation and survival. Side effects associated with targeted agents are generally more specific to the treatment target than cytotoxic chemotherapies.

Over the last decade, immunotherapy has emerged as one of the most promising new cancer therapies and has become a component of standard treatment regimens for almost all solid tumors. **Chimeric antigen receptor (CAR) T cells and checkpoint inhibitors activate immune effectors decreasing their tolerance and allowing them to attack cancer cells. While cytotoxic cancer drugs cause adverse events by compromising defense mechanisms, the new classes of immune therapeutics often induce enhanced inflammatory responses and autoimmunity.** As such, the potential adverse effects of immunotherapy have introduced new challenges for perioperative management of these cancer patients. In addition, immunotherapy is most commonly used in combination therapy with chemotherapies, targeted therapies, or other immunotherapy agents. Hence the toxicities associated with immunotherapy often compound the side effects of systemic cancer therapies.

Immune checkpoint inhibitors (ICI) represent a promising emerging therapeutic modality by which the ability of tumor cells to evade immune cell activation via expression of inhibitory receptors at the cell surface is blocked. Monoclonal antibodies have been developed to target receptors and ligands involved in inhibitory signaling, including CTLA-4, PD-1, and PD-1L. Toxicities related to ICI can affect a variety of organ systems of great relevance in the perioperative period. Most commonly, gastrointestinal toxicities are seen, including nausea, vomiting, hepatitis, and enterocolitis.[12] Hypophysitis is common, leading to various endocrinopathies, including primary adrenal and thyroid hormone insufficiency.[13] This can cause cardiovascular compromise presenting as refractory vasoplegia, and signs and symptoms

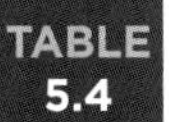

TABLE 5.4 Chemotherapeutic and Targeted Agents Associated With Hepatotoxicity

Drugs[103]	Hepatic Toxicity[103]
Methotrexate, sunitinib, pazopanib, regorafenib, brentuximab	Acute hepatic necrosis
Asparaginase, carmustine, floxuridine, lapatinib, imatinib, idelalisib, other tyrosine kinase inhibitors, interferon	Acute hepatitis
Estrogens, chlorambucil, cyclophosphamide, temozolomide, lenalidomide, azathioprine, mercaptopurine, erlotinib, floxuridine	Cholestasis
Azathioprine, flutamide, trabectedin	Hepatocellular-cholestatic hepatitis
Cytarabine, floxuridine	Biliary stricture
Tamoxifen, methotrexate, corticosteroids, L-asparaginase, 5-fluorouracil, trabectedin	Nonalcoholic fatty liver
Imatinib	Reactivation of chronic hepatitis B
High doses of alkylating agents (busulfan, melphalan, cyclophosphamide, etc.), high doses of mitomycin C and carboplatin, chronic administration of thiopurines (azathioprine, mercaptopurine, and 6-thioguanine), dacarbazine, oxaliplatin	Veno-occlusive disease
Azathioprine, thioguanine, mercaptopurine, methotrexate	Nodular regenerative hyperplasia
Estrogen, androgens	Hepatic adenoma
Methotrexate	Fibrosis or cirrhosis
Sunitinib and pazopanib	Ischemia

of hypothyroidism that can be severe and in rare cases, proceed to myxedema coma. Pituitary enlargement is noted on brain MRI, and confirmatory testing is performed based on laboratory results.[14] Treatment involves discontinuation of the agent for mild cases, thyroid hormone supplementation, and corticosteroids along with supportive measures when indicated. Long-term hormone supplementation is needed in some cases.[15] Pulmonary toxicity presenting as pneumonitis can occur especially when treating lung carcinoma and can lead to respiratory insufficiency requiring increasing levels of respiratory support.[16] Cardiovascular toxicities are rare, occurring in <1% of patients treated with ICI and include

TABLE 5.5 Chemotherapeutic and Targeted Agents Associated with Nephrotoxicity

Drugs[104]	Renal Toxicity[104]
Cisplatin, azacitidine	Salt wasting
Cisplatin, carboplatin, cetuximab, panitumumab	Magnesium wasting
Ifosfamide	Proximal tubular dysfunction
Sorafenib, sunitinib	Acute interstitial nephritis
IL-2, denileukin diftitox	Hemodynamic acute kidney injury (capillary leak syndrome)
Bevacizumab, tyrosine kinase inhibitors, gemcitabine, cisplatin, mitomycin C, interferon	Thrombotic microangiopathy
Interferon, pamidronate	Focal segmental glomerulosclerosis, minimal change disease
Platinums, zoledronate, ifosfamide, mithramycin, pentostatin, imatinib, diaziquone, pemetrexed	Acute tubular necrosis
Methotrexate	Crystal nephropathy
Cisplatin, ifosfamide, azacitidine, diaziquone, imatinib, pemetrexed	Fanconi sydrome
Cisplatin, ifosfamide, pemetrexed	Nephrogenic diabetes insipidus
Cyclophosamide[a], vincristine	Syndrome of inappropriate antidiuresis

[a]Cyclophosamide is also associated with hemorrhagic cystitis.

TABLE 5.6 Toxicities Associated With Immunotherapy and Potential Impact on Perioperative Course of the Cancer Patient

Drug	Class	Toxicity	Potential Impact on Perioperative Course
Ipilimumab Nivolumab Pembrolizumab Atezolizumab	ICI (anti-CTLA-4) ICI (anti-PD-1) ICI (anti-PD-1) ICI (anti-PD-1L)	Hypophysitis, adrenal insufficiency, hypothyroidism, gastroenteritis, pulmonary toxicity, dysrhythmias, cardiomyopathy	Patients may develop refractory hypotension due to primary adrenal insufficiency requiring stress dose hydrocortisone, may require thyroid hormone supplementation, aspiration risk due to protracted nausea and vomiting, at risk for hypoxemia including post-operative respiratory insufficiency/failure due to pulmonary toxicity, dysrhythmias in the perioperative period.[15]
Tisagenlecleucel Axicabtagene ciloleucel	CAR T cell (anti-CD19)	Cytokine release syndrome (CRS), neurotoxicity	Acute postinfusion side effects occur days to weeks following administration. Patients are usually pancytopenic as a result of conditioning chemotherapy. CRS presents as a hyperinflammatory state resulting in vasoplegia, pulmonary edema, cardiac dysrhythmias, and coagulopathy. Neurotoxicity may present with altered level of consciousness, increased ICP, epileptiform activity, and risk of cerebral herniation.[20]

Anti-CD19, B-lymphocyte antigen CD19, also known as CD19 molecule (Cluster of Differentiation 19); *anti-PD-1*, programmed cell death protein 1; *anti-PD-1L*, programmed cell death-1 ligand 1; *CAR T*, chimeric antigen receptor T cells; *CTLA*, cytotoxic T-lymphocyte-associated antigen; *ICI*, immune checkpoint inhibitors; *ICP*, intracranial pressure.

perimyocarditis, dysrhythmias, and heart failure. Though rare, cardiovascular complications carry a grave prognosis; treatment involves discontinuation of the offending agent, administration of pulse dose corticosteroids, and supportive care in a cardiac care unit if indicated.[15,17,18]

CAR T cells are another emerging form of immunotherapy demonstrating remarkable success at treating some hematologic malignancies, including B-ALL and non-Hodgkin's lymphoma. CAR T cells are patient's own T lymphocytes that are transfected ex vivo to express special chimeric receptors containing sufficient built-in costimulation to fully activate an immune response upon recognition of tumor-associated antigens.[19] Unfortunately, cost and their toxicity profile hinder widespread use. This therapy is currently only possible at tertiary care centers that are capable of managing associated side effects that could be life-threatening. The main side effects are cytokine release syndrome (CRS) and neurotoxicity. CRS results from an exaggerated inflammatory response that leads to shock and multiorgan dysfunction. It presents typically within days of CAR T-cell administration and ranges in severity from mild tachycardia, tachypnea, and electrolyte abnormalities to refractory vasoplegic shock, respiratory compromise, coagulopathy, multiorgan failure, and death.[20] Mild cases can be closely monitored; however, more severe cases may require additional interventions, including fluid resuscitation; respiratory support, including mechanical ventilation; and vasopressors and ionotropic agents for hemodynamic support.[20]

Neurotoxicity is a separate entity that usually presents days after CRS and is characterized by an expressive aphasia with focal neurologic deficits.[21] It can range in severity from mild word-finding difficulties to refractory status

TABLE 5.7 Potential Toxicities Resulting From Newer Cancer Therapies and Corresponding Perioperative Care Measures to Enhance Outcomes

Immune checkpoint inhibitors	Should include: • Complete history and physical examination inclusive of absence of cardiac, pulmonary, gastrointestinal side effects. • Imaging as needed including CXR or CT, PFTs, EKG. • Thyroid function tests, cortisol levels. • Aspiration precautions, thyroid hormone supplementation, and stress dose corticosteroids should be considered if needed based on findings.[15]
CAR T cells	• Must be aware of these patients. • Corticosteroids should be avoided as they could affect yield by suppressing T-cell populations. • Patients who have recently received CAR T cells should be evaluated for potential toxicity including any evidence of cytokine release syndrome and neurotoxicity. • An EKG should be obtained to rule out dysrhythmias and conduction or repolarization abnormalities. Tocilizumab should be considered for the treatment of any patient exhibiting signs of severe CRS. Patients should also be assessed for any evidence of neurotoxicity and any signs or symptoms of increased ICP and routine precautions should be undertaken accordingly. Patients experiencing severe neurotoxicity can be treated with pulse dose corticosteroids and antiepileptic agents when clinically indicated based on presentation.[20]

CAR T, Chimeric antigen receptor T cells; *CRS*, cytokine release syndrome; *CT*, computed tomography; *CXR*, chest x-ray; *EKG*, electrocardiogram; *ICP*, intracranial pressure; *PFTs*, pulmonary function tests.

epilepticus, cerebral edema, and brain herniation leading to death.[21] The exact etiologies of CRS and neurotoxicity are not well understood. The only FDA-approved agent to treat these toxicities is the IL-6 binder tocilizumab. Corticosteroids are also helpful in the management of severe cases in addition to supportive therapies.[20]

Table 5.6 describes the toxicities associated with immunotherapy and potential impact on the perioperative course of the cancer patient.

Table 5.7 reviews potential toxicities resulting from newer cancer therapies and corresponding perioperative care measures that enhance outcome for the cancer patient.

Radiation Therapy and Newer Techniques

Many cancer patients receive locoregional radiation therapy as a component of their cancer regimen preoperatively, alone or in combination with systemic treatments, which may have significant effects on the perioperative course and subsequent outcome. These effects can result from direct effects of the tumor or from effects of radiation therapy. The exact effects encountered are highly dependent on the location of the tumor, especially in relation to nearby normal tissue, and location, volume, and dose of radiation delivered. As with systemic therapies, potential adverse effects of radiation are also influenced by the toxicities encountered with concomitant treatments and the overall condition of the cancer patient. Tumors that cause anatomic effects of importance to perioperative management include head and neck tumors, especially those at risk for airway obstruction or poor dentition that may complicate intubation; mediastinal masses, especially those at risk for respiratory or cardiovascular compromise; or in patients with severe chronic obstructive pulmonary disease. Lung masses associated with large pleural effusions, pericardial effusion, cardiac tamponade, or superior vena cava syndrome are also at high risk for perioperative complications. In addition, esophageal cancers and other gastrointestinal tumors can cause baseline nutritional deficiencies from both tumor location and treatment. It is important to consider the anatomic effects of radiation therapy and consider potential toxicities related to radiation treatment location. This information provides a framework for discussing the effects of tumors and their therapy on the perioperative management of the cancer patient, and demonstrates the importance of close cooperation among surgeon, anesthesiologist, and cancer physician(s) to assure maximal safety of surgical procedures to provide the best outcome. Table 5.8 outlines potential radiation toxicities that should be considered in the perioperative care of the cancer patient.

Radiation therapy is typically divided into three forms: external beam or x-ray therapy, brachytherapy, and radionuclide radiation therapy. External beam radiation therapy (EBRT) or x-ray therapy is delivered by linear accelerators and the beams are modulated in order to focus the dose of radiation to the tumor while sparing adjacent normal tissues. Improvements in radiation technology have also been designed to reduce the dose to normal tissue during radiation therapy. For example, three-dimensional conformal radiation treatment (3DCRT) was historically used to treat esophageal cancer using an anterior posterior (AP)/posterior anterior (PA) field arrangement followed by a cone-down volume with oblique fields to minimize dose to the spinal cord. However, using 3DCRT to treat esophageal cancer results in a substantial radiation dose to the heart and lungs. Newer radiation techniques such as intensity-modulated radiation therapy (IMRT) and proton beam therapy (PBT) delivered under daily image guidance (IGRT) are providing more conformal and precisely delivered radiation treatment, which reduces the risk of radiation-induced side effects from normal tissue toxicity.

TABLE 5.8 Radiation Therapy Effects That May Complicate Perioperative Care

Radiation Treatment Location	Potential Toxicity
Head and neck	Dry mouth
	Dental caries
	Compromised nutritional status
	Osteoradionecrosis of the jaw
	Mandibular hypomobility
	Neck fibrosis/lymphedema
	Accelerated carotid artery disease
	Hypothyroidism
Thoracic	Acute pericarditis/pericardial effusion
	Constrictive pericarditis
	Coronary atherosclerosis
	Restrictive cardiomyopathy
	Conduction abnormalities
	Valvular stenosis/regurgitation
	Radiation pneumonitis
	Pulmonary fibrosis
	Esophageal stenosis/aspiration
	Compromised nutritional status
Abdomen	Malabsorption
	Compromised nutritional status
	Coagulopathy from vitamin deficiency
	Neutropenic or necrotizing enterocolitis
	Gastrointestinal bleeding
	Bowel strictures/fistulae/obstruction/perforation
Pelvic	Radiation cystitis
	Radiation proctitis
	Fistulae
Miscellaneous	Delayed wound healing

Intraoperative Radiation Therapy

Intraoperative radiation therapy (IORT or IOERT) is not considered a new technique but is often utilized at the time of surgery to deliver radiation directly to a small area of the body in the cavity where the tumor has just been removed at the area with biggest risk of cancer recurrence. It can be delivered externally with x-rays, electrons, or brachytherapy (see later). Both forms of IORT are delivered in a single dose. This is different from the usual method of delivering radiation, in which a larger part of the body (such as an entire organ) receives radiation for a longer period of time. IORT has been historically used in the abdomen and pelvis, especially in the setting of recurrent tumors in areas that have received prior radiation. More recently, there has been a renewed interest in this technology for delivering IORT as a radiation boost for breast cancer[22] or for low-risk breast cancer patients who meet criteria for partial breast radiation.[23] Similarly, IORT has been used for locally advanced or recurrent rectal cancer to reduce risk of local cancer recurrence and pancreas cancer to slow local progression. Perioperative complications associated with IORT have been studied in patients with rectal and pancreas cancer. Although operative time was significantly longer for rectal cancer patients receiving IORT than those who did not, no significant differences were found concerning anastomotic leakage rate, hospital stay, or wound infection rate.[24]

Brachytherapy

Although brachytherapy is also not considered a new technology, it is commonly used in the treatment of various malignancies. Brachytherapy is considered to be a direct radiation therapy because it is inserted into tumors or placed adjacent to the tumor or area at risk in order to deliver high doses of radiation over a short period of time. Brachytherapy can be delivered using a high dose rate (applicator is at the end of a wire that is passed by the cancer or areas at risk via hollow catheters implanted into the patient or hollow intracavitary applicators), or a low dose rate where the radioactive sources are placed directly into patient tissue (prostate seeds), into hollow catheters, or intracavitary applicators (gynecologic brachytherapy). With high-dose brachytherapy, treatment is delivered for shorter intervals (<1 h) over 3–5 days, and the patient is only exposed to radiation while treatments are being delivered. With low-dose brachytherapy, the radioactive sources remain in the patient for the duration of treatment and patients are isolated and monitored for several days. If these patients have acute surgical needs, the perioperative team must be aware of the risk of radiation exposure, and radiation precautions must be used.

Radionuclide Therapy

Targeted radionuclide therapy (also called molecular radiotherapy) involves a radioactive drug called a radiopharmaceutical that targets cancer cells. Radiopharmaceuticals typically consist of a radioactive atom (also known as a radionuclide) combined with a cell-targeting molecule that seeks and destroys cancer cells. Similarly, radionuclide therapy is not considered a new radiation treatment, albeit there have been recent improvements in technologies and delivery, and resurgence in use of radionuclides in the treatment of various cancers. Radionuclides may be administered intravenously for bone metastases (^{153}samarium-ethylenediamine tetramethylene phosphonate (EDTMP)[25] and ^{89}strontium[25]), thyroid cancer (^{131}I[26]), hematologic malignancies (Zevalin, ^{90}Y-ibritumomab tiuxetan[27]; Bexxar, ^{131}I-tositumomab[27]), metastatic castration-resistant prostate cancer (Xofigo, ^{223}Ra dichloride[28]), metastatic neuroendocrine cancers (peptide receptor Lutathera, ^{177}Lu-DOTA-Tyr^3-octreotate[29]), and neuroblastoma (^{131}I-MIBG[30]). Radionuclide therapy may also be delivered intraarterially to a segment or whole liver as targeted radioembolization via a minimally invasive procedure that combines embolization and radiation therapy. Selective internal radiation therapy (SIRT), otherwise known as radio embolization, is now becoming a common procedure performed for those patients with primary hepatocellular carcinoma, and liver-dominant metastatic disease.[31] Tiny glass or resin beads filled with the radioactive isotope yttrium Y-90 are placed directly inside the blood vessels that feed a tumor via catheterization by an interventional radiologist. This can block the supply of blood to the cancer cells and delivers a high dose of radiation to the tumor while sparing normal tissue.[31] Similar to the use of low-dose brachytherapy, patients who received radionuclide therapy who have acute surgical needs must be identified, so the perioperative team can be aware of the risk of radiation exposure and radiation precautions can be used.

Newer Radiation Techniques

Radiation therapy can affect all normal tissues, often resulting in irreversible late sequelae resulting from parenchymal, vascular, and connective tissue changes within the volume of irradiated tissue. The degree of damage to adjacent normal tissues (to the tumor) often correlates with the volume and dose of radiation that tissues receive. Improvements in radiation therapy delivery techniques have continued to reduce the area of collateral radiation to surrounding normal radiosensitive tissues. Modern, highly conformal treatment techniques with relatively low and inhomogeneous doses in the organs at risk (OARs) have enabled the characterization of the probability of specific radiation-induced normal tissue adverse effects as a function of individual dose-volume relationships.[32,33] Investigators continue to study these relations in order to improve outcomes for patients receiving radiation therapy by minimizing treatment-related toxicity. This concept is especially important for patients who are to receive surgery following radiation as part of a curative treatment regimen. For example, Wang et al. evaluated esophageal cancer patients treated with preoperative concurrent chemoradiation cisplatin, 5-FU, and thoracic radiation followed by surgical resection. The study reported on a primary endpoint of pulmonary complications that included pneumonia or acute respiratory distress syndrome (ARDS) within 30 days after surgery. Multivariate analysis showed that the volume of lung receiving ≥5 Gy (V5) was a significant independent factor for postoperative pulmonary complications (P = 0.005).[34] This suggests that ensuring an adequate volume of lung unexposed to radiation might reduce the incidence of postoperative pulmonary complications. Another study indicated that a V10 >40% is associated with a 35% risk of pneumonia or ARDS.[35] Similarly, the risk of pericarditis is approximately 27% for patients undergoing chemoradiation for esophageal carcinoma, with increased risk in patients who received lung V30 >46% and mean dose >26.1 Gy (73%) compared with patients who received lung V30 <46% and mean dose <26.1 Gy (13%).[36] In addition to defining dosevolume relationships for normal tissue toxicity risk assessments and incorporating these parameters as constraints in dosimetric radiation treatment planning, guidelines for normal tissue delineation and contouring have been published to reduce significant variability among practitioners.[37]

Reducing Toxicity

There have been considerable research efforts evaluating whether modern radiation technologies can spare critical organs, and whether improved radiation dose distributions are clinically meaningful. Most of the data are retrospective but suggest is large and significant benefit of IMRT over 3DCRT. Using esophageal cancer as an example, an analysis of seven dosimetric studies demonstrated significantly lower average irradiated volumes of the heart and lung using IMRT compared to 3DCRT in patients with esophageal cancer.[38] Furthermore, the ability of IMRT to minimize dose outside of the target volume appears to be clinically meaningful. Another study performing a dose-volume histogram (DVH) analysis demonstrated significant sparing of the heart and lung V30 and V45, and there was an overall survival benefit to patients receiving IMRT compared with 3DCRT.[39] In a meta-analysis comparing IMRT and 3DCRT for the treatment of esophageal carcinoma, IMRT was associated with overall improvement compared with 3DCRT.[38] The SCOPE1 (Study of Chemoradiotherapy in OesoPhageal cancer with Erbitux) trial found that higher conformality index was strongly associated with improved overall survival and that dosimetric plan quality was strongly related to receiving IMRT compared to 3DCRT.[40] Finally, a large cancer center registry study that included approximately 2500 elderly patients with esophageal cancer found that use of IMRT was associated with less all-cause, other-cause, and cardiovascular mortality compared with 3DCRT.[41]

This chapter specifically addresses the reduction in cardiopulmonary toxicity resulting from use of modern radiation techniques, as radiation-induced cardiopulmonary toxicity is known to contribute substantially to perioperative complications in a cancer patient undergoing surgery. It should be noted that similar reductions in normal tissue radiation exposures and associated radiation-induced adverse effects are similarly observed when using newer technologies to deliver radiation to other parts of the body. However, the impact of these reductions on perioperative complications is not as well studied.

Proton Beam Therapy

PBT has been shown to further reduce lung and heart radiation exposure compared to IMRT (Fig. 5.1).[42] PBT provides superior dose distributions and has a dosimetric advantage over photon beam therapy. The advantage of PBT is the physical characteristics of its depth-dose curve, with a dose peak (Bragg peak) at a well-defined depth in tissue. This Bragg peak allows for rapid fall-off of the radiation dose at the end of the range and a sharp lateral dose fall-off with the maximum energy deposition for each proton beam in the target region and almost no energy outside of the beam, as opposed to photons where there will be scatter. Comparison of passive scattering PBT with fixed-field IMRT plans for treatment of esophageal cancer patients demonstrated that PBT plans had improved lung sparing at low-to-moderate doses, as well as mean lung dose. PBT reduced the volume of lung receiving low-dose radiation (5 Gy) relatively by 36% to 70%, depending on the beam arrangements. Heart V40 was also reduced by up to 22% using PBT.[43] Intensity-modulated pencil-beam scanning PBT further increases dose conformality compared with passive scattering PBT.[44,45]

Others have investigated whether dosimetric superiority using PBT translates into improved clinical outcome. The MD Anderson Cancer Center (MDACC) first reported their experience using concurrent chemotherapy and passive scatter PBT in 62 patients with esophageal cancer. The complete pathologic response rate was 28%, and the near complete response rate was 50% at the time of surgical resection.[42] Wang et al. compared outcomes for 444 esophageal cancer patients treated with preoperative PBT, IMRT, or 3DCRT and concurrent chemotherapy and found that pretreatment pulmonary function and treatment modality were independent predictors of pulmonary complications. PBT was associated with the lowest rate of postoperative pulmonary complications (14%) compared with IMRT (24%) and 3DCRT (30%); however, no differences in cardiac complications were observed.[46] A Japanese study reported similar reductions in pulmonary toxicity in patients receiving PBT compared with IMRT, in addition to reduced cardiac toxicity.[47] Finally, a large study, including pooled data from three academic institutions, analyzed clinical outcomes for 580 patients with lower esophageal cancers treated with PBT (n = 111), IMRT (n = 255), or 3DCRT (n = 214). Patients treated with PBT were found to have significantly less pulmonary toxicity compared with 3DCRT patients (16% vs. 40%), but there was no statistically significant difference compared to IMRT patients (24%). In this study, fewer cardiac complications were experienced by PBT patients when compared with 3DCRT

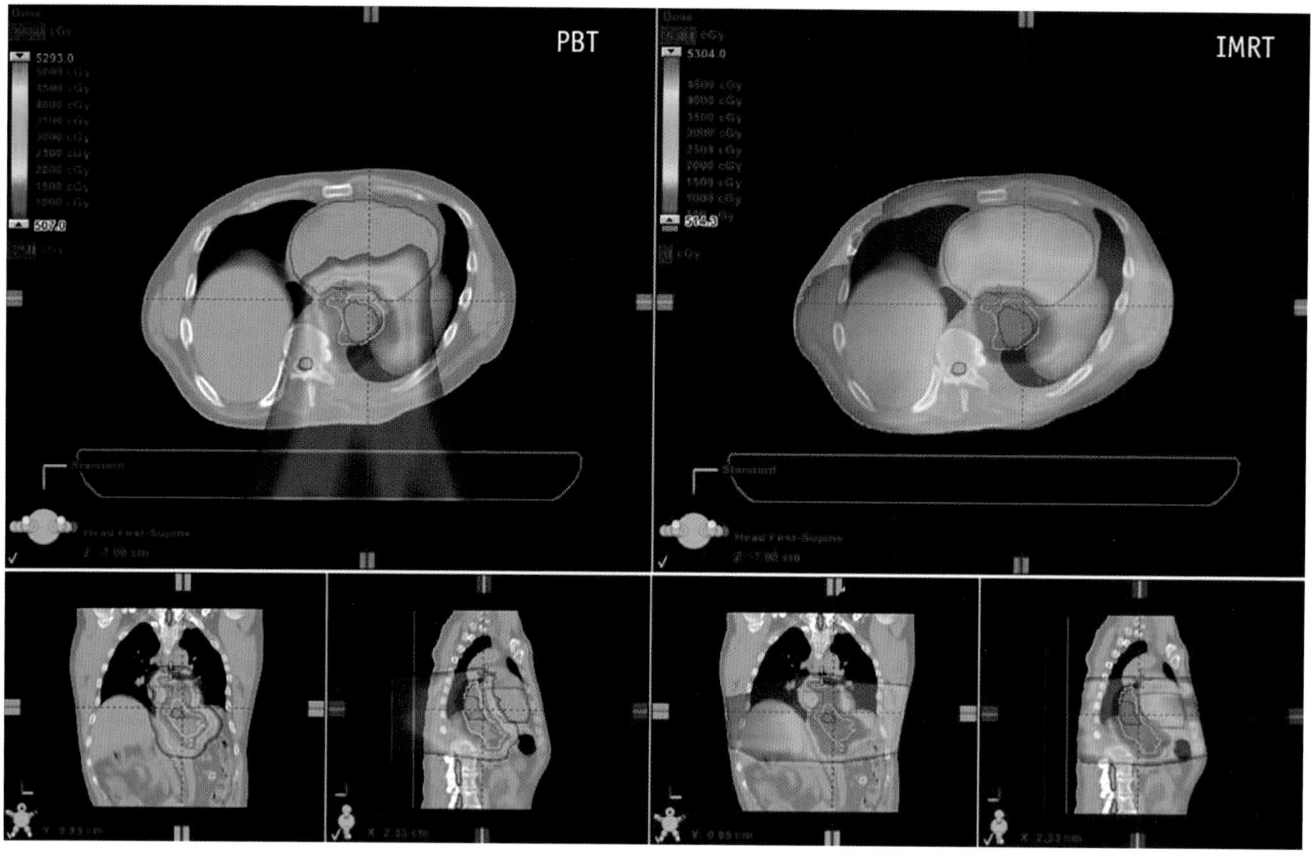

• **Fig. 5.1** Cardiac and lung sparing with proton beam therapy (*PBT*), with intensity modulated radiation therapy (*IMRT*) for distal esophageal cancer.

patients (12% vs. 27%), but there was no difference when compared with IMRT patients (12%).[48]

Stereotactic Body Radiotherapy

With conventional therapy, radiation is delivered in relatively small doses over the course of several weeks, with patients receiving daily treatments during that time. Various improvements in modulation allow millimeter accuracies of this radiation to be delivered over 1–5 days. This form is called stereotactic body radiation therapy (SBRT) or stereotactic radiosurgery (SRS) and may be used to treat carefully selected small, localized tumors utilizing delivery of a few image-guided, precisely localized, fractionated high-dose radiation treatments. Techniques to minimize motion (immobilization), breathing motion (breath-hold or gating), while improve targeting (use of markers or fiducials) and visualization (image guidance), allow for dose escalation while limiting the dose to normal tissues thus improving the therapeutic ratio. In addition, motion management should be used in conjunction with IGRT to ensure accurate target localization and delivery of treatment. Despite the fact that SBRT delivers higher biological dosage of radiation, carefully selected patients experience fewer side effects because SBRT utilizes multiple intersecting radiation beam arcs resulting in sharp dose gradient outside the tumor that minimizes dose to surrounding normal tissue (Fig. 5.2). SBRT has shown dramatically better local tumor control compared with conventional radiation therapy, especially for small lung tumors when adequate dose fractionation regimens are used.[49] However, due to the

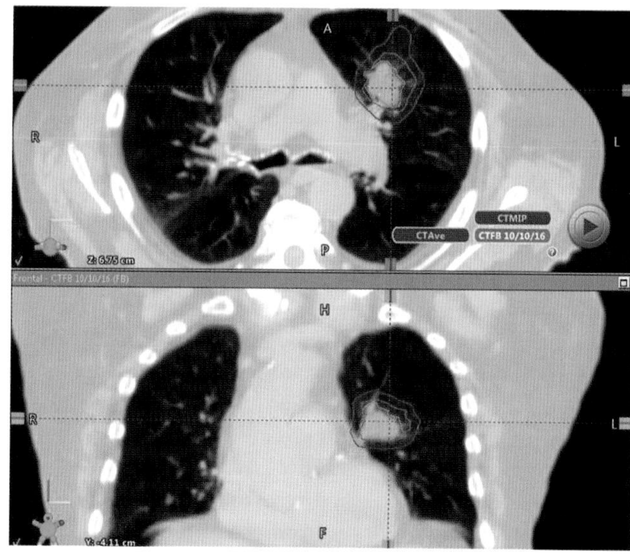

• **Fig. 5.2** Stereotactic body radiation therapy, for Stage 1 lung cancer with highly conformal radiation dose distribution around the treatment target volume and sparing of lung and heart.

TABLE 5.9 **Summary of Radiation Treatment Modalities**

Modality	Mechanism of Delivery	Level of Conformality	DeliveryTime/ Duration	Unique Characteristics for Perioperative Team
EBRT (conformal)	3DCRTIMRT	+	10–30 min, 5–6 weeks	Often given with chemo, more acute toxicity (1–3 months).
SBRT/SRS	Image-guided, usually with motion management	++	20–120 min, 1–5 days	Given with immunotherapy, more late toxicities (3–6 months).
IORT/IOERT	Intraoperative-focused radiation	++++	High dose, several minutes during surgery in addition to planning time	Prolonged operative time. Fibrosis of adjacent structures (vessels, ureters). Infection. Decreased healing.
Brachytherapy	High doseLow dose	++++	High dose: 30–60 min, 1–5 days Low dose: 1–3 days	Invasive, bleeding, infection. Fibrosis of adjacent structures (vessels, ureters). Decreased healing.
Radionuclide	Intravenous or targeted intraarterial	Targeted: ++ or segmental/whole liver (SIRT): +	~1–2 h/min for delivery	Acute toxicity, infection cytopenias.
Proton beam therapy	Passive scattering Pencil-beam scanning	+++	10–30 min, 5–6 weeks	Often given with chemo, more acute toxicity (1–3 months)

3DCRT, 3D conformal radiotherapy; *EBRT*, external beam radiotherapy; *IOERT*, intraoperative electron radiotherapy; *IORT*, intraoperative radiotherapy; *IMRT*, intensity-modulated radiotherapy; *SBRT*, stereotactic body radiotherapy; *SIRT*, selective internal radiotherapy; *SRS*, stereotactic radiosurgery.

potential damage to nearby normal tissues from delivery of high doses of radiation using SBRT, patients should be carefully selected, and more stringent dose-volume normal tissue constraints must be used for dosimetric planning. Acute toxicities during SBRT and within 3 months following completion are rare. However, late toxicity especially around 2–4 months after SBRT can be severe and can lead to bleeding, ulceration, or fibrosis (obstruction); therefore it is important for them to be aware of the timing from RT. It should be noted that patients who receive immunotherapy and SBRT are more likely to have a higher risk of these toxicities.[50]

SBRT is currently used to treat a variety of malignancies with limited tumor volume, including non–small cell lung cancer, primary and small volume secondary liver tumors, early stage prostate cancer, small volume pancreatic cancer, certain spine tumors, and selected oligometastases. SBRT is sometimes used in the neoadjuvant setting such as for pancreatic cancer. Perioperative complications associated with SBRT are mostly reported from small, single-institution experiences. Direct comparison with IMRT demonstrates that neoadjuvant SBRT and IMRT appear to have similar rates of resection and perioperative outcomes.[51]

Table 5.9 reviews the properties of various radiation modalities, both the classic and newer technologies.

Adaptive Radiation Therapy

The use of modern radiation therapy techniques, such as IMRT, PBT, and SBRT, can potentially improve target coverage with a much steeper dose gradient and minimize irradiated normal tissue volumes. Anatomic changes during radiotherapy may introduce discrepancies between planned and delivered doses, not only to tumor but also to surrounding normal tissues. The precision of radiation therapy may be limited by tumor shrinkage and other anatomic changes during treatment, as well as limitations in accuracy of daily image guidance. Adaptive radiation therapy (ART) is a radiation therapy process where treatment is adapted to account for internal anatomic changes. Adaptive treatment replanning can account for anatomic changes during the course of radiation and provide better normal tissue sparing, while allowing improved treatment targeting that may translate into improved local control. Evolving radiotherapy technologies, such as four-dimensional (4D) image-based motion management, daily on-board imaging, and ART based on volumetric images over the course of radiotherapy, facilitate delivery of higher doses to the target while minimizing normal tissue toxicities.

ART requires development of an initial treatment plan for the first few radiation fractions by evaluating treatment response using CT, CBCT, MR, or PET images; updating treatment target volumes based on the measured treatment response; revising the original prescription on the target volume according to an established adaptive protocol; and developing an adaptive plan through recontouring using deformable image registration, dose accumulation, and plan reoptimization (Fig. 5.3). ART holds promise for improved delivery of radiation to the clinical target while reducing normal tissue complications and remains an active area of clinical investigation.[52]

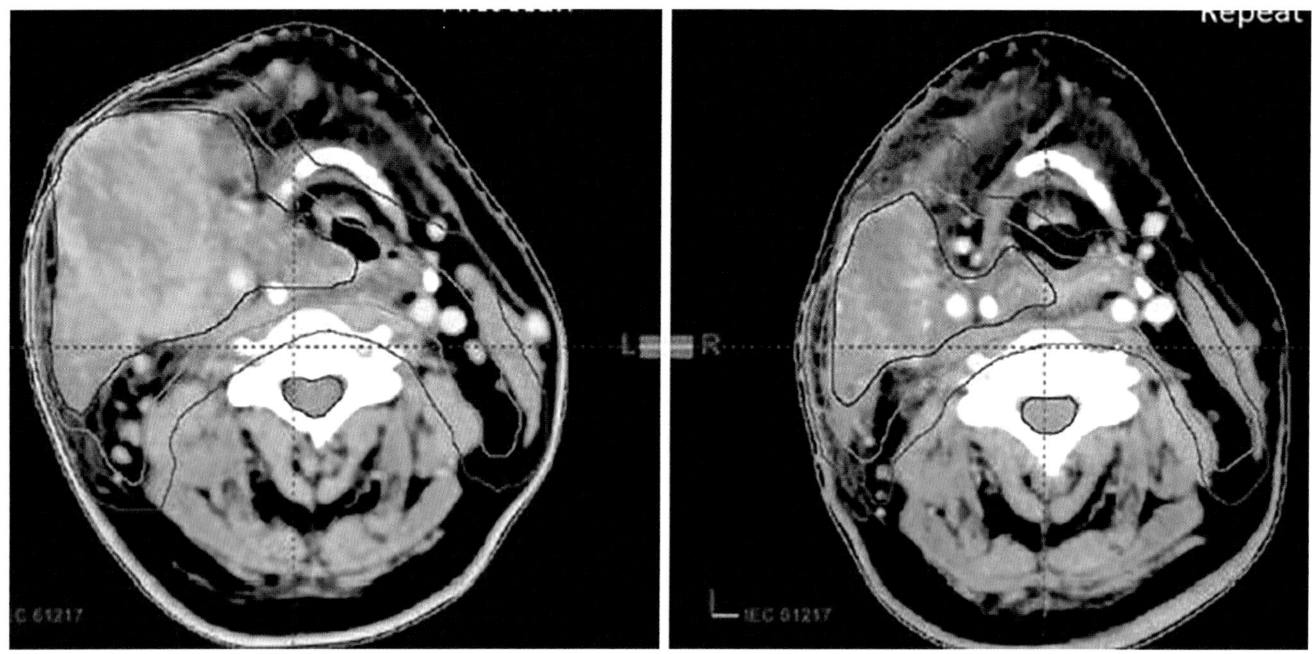

• **Fig. 5.3** Adaptive radiation therapy and the impact of reimaging and intensity-modulated radiation therapy replanning on radiation dose distributions in a head and neck cancer patient with good clinical response to initial treatment. Note the adjustments made in treatment planning after tumor shrinkage due to initial response to therapy *(outlined in blue)*.

Conclusion

Cancer therapies continue to rapidly evolve, resulting in a greater number of patients undergoing surgical and image-guided interventions. The multimodal approach to cancer therapy means most of these patients have either previously been exposed to systemic chemotherapies, radiation therapy, and immunotherapies, or will have a combination of these when they present for surgical or image-guided interventions. Physicians caring for patients in the perioperative period must understand advances in newer therapeutic modalities and their relevance in the care of the cancer patient undergoing surgery.

References

1. Wilson RF. Surgery in the patient with cancer. In: Goldman DR, Brown FH, Guarnieri DM, eds. *Perioperative Medicine: Medical Care of the Surgical Patient*: McGraw-Hill; 1994:283–293.
2. Kong SH, Haouchine N, Soares R, et al. Robust augmented reality registration method for localization of solid organs' tumors using CT-derived virtual biomechanical model and fluorescent fiducials. *Surg Endosc*. 2017;31(7):2863–2871.
3. Alam NZ, Flores RM. Extended video-assisted thoracic surgery (VATS) lobectomy. *Minerva Chir*. 2016;71(1):67–71.
4. Dmitrii S, Pavel K. Uniportal video-assisted thoracic surgery esophagectomy. *Thorac Surg Clin*. 2017;27(4):407–415.
5. Peters BS, Armijo PR, Krause C, Choudhury SA, Oleynikov D. Review of emerging surgical robotic technology. *Surg Endosc*. 2018;32(4):1636–1655.
6. Vasefi F, MacKinnon N, Farkas DL, Kateb B. Review of the potential of optical technologies for cancer diagnosis in neurosurgery: a step toward intraoperative neurophotonics. *Neurophotonics*. 2017;4(1):011010.
7. Metzger MC, Bittermann G, Dannenberg L, et al. Design and development of a virtual anatomic atlas of the human skull for automatic segmentation in computer-assisted surgery, preoperative planning, and navigation. *Int J Comput Assist Radiol Surg*. 2013;8(5):691–702.
8. Bilimoria KY, Bentrem DJ, Talamonti MS, Stewart AK, Winchester DP, Ko CY. Risk-based selective referral for cancer surgery: a potential strategy to improve perioperative outcomes. *Ann Surg*. 2010;251(4):708–716.
9. Birkmeyer JD, Stukel TA, Siewers AE, Goodney PP, Wennberg DE, Lucas FL. Surgeon volume and operative mortality in the United States. *N Engl J Med*. 2003;349(22):2117–2127.
10. Birkmeyer JD, Siewers AE, Finlayson EV, et al. Hospital volume and surgical mortality in the United States. *N Engl J Med*. 2002;346(15):1128–1137.
11. Sahai S, Ismail H. Perioperative implications of neoadjuvant therapies and optimization strategies for cancer surgery. *Curr Anesthesiol Rep*. 2015;5(3):305–317.
12. Stucci S, Palmirotta R, Passarelli A, et al. Immune-related adverse events during anticancer immunotherapy: pathogenesis and management. *Oncol Lett*. 2017;14(5):5671–5680.
13. Mahzari M, Liu D, Arnaout A, Lochnan H. Immune checkpoint inhibitor therapy associated hypophysitis. *Clin Med Insights Endocrinol Diabetes*. 2015;8:21–28.
14. Faje A. Immunotherapy and hypophysitis: clinical presentation, treatment, and biologic insights. *Pituitary*. 2016;19(1):82–92.
15. Brahmer JR, Lacchetti C, Schneider BJ, et al. Management of immune-related adverse events in patients treated with immune checkpoint inhibitor therapy: American Society of Clinical Oncology clinical practice guideline. *J Clin Oncol*. 2018;36(17):1714–1768.
16. Khunger M, Rakshit S, Pasupuleti V, et al. Incidence of pneumonitis with use of programmed death 1 and programmed

death-ligand 1 inhibitors in non-small cell lung cancer: a systematic review and meta-analysis of trials. *Chest*. 2017;152(2):271–281.

17. Johnson DB, Balko JM, Compton ML, et al. Fulminant myocarditis with combination immune checkpoint blockade. *N Engl J Med*. 2016;375(18):1749–1755.
18. Neelapu SS, Tummala S, Kebriaei P, et al. Chimeric antigen receptor T-cell therapy - assessment and management of toxicities. *Nat Rev Clin Oncol*. 2018;15(1):47–62.
19. Sadelain M, Riviere I, Brentjens R. Targeting tumours with genetically enhanced T lymphocytes. *Nat Rev Cancer*. 2003;3(1):35–45.
20. Lee DW, Santomasso BD, Locke FL, et al. ASTCT consensus grading for cytokine release syndrome and neurologic toxicity associated with immune effector cells. *Biol Blood Marrow Transplant*. 2019;25(4):625–638.
21. Santomasso BD, Park JH, Salloum D, et al. Clinical and biological correlates of neurotoxicity associated with CAR T-cell therapy in patients with B-cell acute lymphoblastic leukemia. *Cancer Discov*. 2018;8(8):958–971.
22. Malter W, Kirn V, Richters L, et al. Intraoperative boost radiotherapy during targeted oncoplastic breast surgery: overview and single center experiences. *Int J Breast Cancer*. 2014;2014:637898.
23. Kaiser J, Reitsamer R, Kopp P, et al. Intraoperative electron radiotherapy (IOERT) in the treatment of primary breast cancer. *Breast Care (Basel)*. 2018;13(3):162–167.
24. Klink CD, Binnebosel M, Holy R, Neumann UP, Junge K. Influence of intraoperative radiotherapy (IORT) on perioperative outcome after surgical resection of rectal cancer. *World J Surg*. 2014;38(4):992–996.
25. Guerra Liberal FDC, Tavares AAS, Tavares J. Palliative treatment of metastatic bone pain with radiopharmaceuticals: a perspective beyond strontium-89 and samarium-153. *Appl Radiat Isot*. 2016;110:87–99.
26. Hindie E, Taieb D, Avram AM, Giovanella L. Radioactive iodine ablation in low-risk thyroid cancer. *Lancet Diabetes Endocrinol*. 2018;6(9):686.
27. Sachpekidis C, Jackson DB, Soldatos TG. Radioimmunotherapy in non-Hodgkin's lymphoma: retrospective adverse event profiling of Zevalin and Bexxar. *Pharmaceuticals (Basel)*. 2019;12(4):141. doi:10.3390/ph12040141.
28. Parker C, Heidenreich A, Nilsson S, Shore N. Current approaches to incorporation of radium-223 in clinical practice. *Prostate Cancer Prostatic Dis*. 2018;21(1):37–47.
29. Severi S, Grassi I, Nicolini S, Sansovini M, Bongiovanni A, Paganelli G. Peptide receptor radionuclide therapy in the management of gastrointestinal neuroendocrine tumors: efficacy profile, safety, and quality of life. *Onco Targets Ther*. 2017;10:551–557.
30. Alexander N, Vali R, Ahmadzadehfar H, Shammas A, Baruchel S. Review: the role of radiolabeled DOTA-conjugated peptides for imaging and treatment of childhood neuroblastoma. *Curr Radiopharm*. 2018;11(1):14–21.
31. Wang EA, Stein JP, Bellavia RJ, Broadwell SR. Treatment options for unresectable HCC with a focus on SIRT with yttrium-90 resin microspheres. *Int J Clin Pract*. 2017;71(11):e12972. doi:10.1111/ijcp.12972.
32. Bentzen SM, Constine LS, Deasy JO, et al. Quantitative analyses of normal tissue effects in the clinic (QUANTEC): an introduction to the scientific issues. *Int J Radiat Oncol Biol Phys*. 2010;76(3 Suppl):S3–S9.
33. Emami B, Lyman J, Brown A, et al. Tolerance of normal tissue to therapeutic irradiation. *Int J Radiat Oncol Biol Phys*. 1991;21(1):109–122.
34. Wang SL, Liao Z, Vaporciyan AA, et al. Investigation of clinical and dosimetric factors associated with postoperative pulmonary complications in esophageal cancer patients treated with concurrent chemoradiotherapy followed by surgery. *Int J Radiat Oncol Biol Phys*. 2006;64(3):692–699.
35. Lee HK, Vaporciyan AA, Cox JD, et al. Postoperative pulmonary complications after preoperative chemoradiation for esophageal carcinoma: correlation with pulmonary dose-volume histogram parameters. *Int J Radiat Oncol Biol Phys*. 2003;57(5):1317–1322.
36. Wei X, Liu HH, Tucker SL, et al. Risk factors for pericardial effusion in inoperable esophageal cancer patients treated with definitive chemoradiation therapy. *Int J Radiat Oncol Biol Phys*. 2008;70(3):707–714.
37. Marks LB, Yorke ED, Jackson A, et al. Use of normal tissue complication probability models in the clinic. *Int J Radiat Oncol Biol Phys*. 2010;76(3 Suppl):S10–S19.
38. Xu D, Li G, Li H, Jia F. Comparison of IMRT versus 3D-CRT in the treatment of esophagus cancer: A systematic review and meta-analysis. *Medicine (Baltimore)*. 2017;96(31):e7685.
39. Lin SH, Wang L, Myles B, et al. Propensity score-based comparison of long-term outcomes with 3-dimensional conformal radiotherapy vs intensity-modulated radiotherapy for esophageal cancer. *Int J Radiat Oncol Biol Phys*. 2012;84(5):1078–1085.
40. Carrington R, Spezi E, Gwynne S, et al. The influence of dose distribution on treatment outcome in the SCOPE 1 oesophageal cancer trial. *Radiat Oncol*. 2016;11:19.
41. Lin SH, Zhang N, Godby J, et al. Radiation modality use and cardiopulmonary mortality risk in elderly patients with esophageal cancer. *Cancer*. 2016;122(6):917–928.
42. Lin SH, Komaki R, Liao Z, et al. Proton beam therapy and concurrent chemotherapy for esophageal cancer. *Int J Radiat Oncol Biol Phys*. 2012;83(3):e345–e351.
43. Zhang X, Zhao KL, Guerrero TM, et al. Four-dimensional computed tomography-based treatment planning for intensity-modulated radiation therapy and proton therapy for distal esophageal cancer. *Int J Radiat Oncol Biol Phys*. 2008;72(1):278–287.
44. Welsh J, Gomez D, Palmer MB, et al. Intensity-modulated proton therapy further reduces normal tissue exposure during definitive therapy for locally advanced distal esophageal tumors: a dosimetric study. *Int J Radiat Oncol Biol Phys*. 2011;81(5):1336–1342.
45. Zeng YC, Vyas S, Dang Q, et al. Proton therapy posterior beam approach with pencil beam scanning for esophageal cancer: clinical outcome, dosimetry, and feasibility. *Strahlenther Onkol*. 2016;192(12):913–921.
46. Wang J, Wei C, Tucker SL, et al. Predictors of postoperative complications after trimodality therapy for esophageal cancer. *Int J Radiat Oncol Biol Phys*. 2013;86(5):885–891.
47. Makishima H, Ishikawa H, Terunuma T, et al. Comparison of adverse effects of proton and X-ray chemoradiotherapy for esophageal cancer using an adaptive dose-volume histogram analysis. *J Radiat Res*. 2015;56(3):568–576.
48. Lin SH, Merrell KW, Shen J, et al. Multi-institutional analysis of radiation modality use and postoperative outcomes of neoadjuvant chemoradiation for esophageal cancer. *Radiother Oncol*. 2017;123(3):376–381.
49. Guckenberger M, Klement RJ, Allgauer M, et al. Local tumor control probability modeling of primary and secondary lung tumors in stereotactic body radiotherapy. *Radiother Oncol*. 2016;118(3):485–491.

50. Lin AJ, Roach M, Bradley J, Robinson C. Combining stereotactic body radiation therapy with immunotherapy: current data and future directions. *Transl Lung Cancer Res.* 2019;8(1):107–115.
51. Chapman BC, Gleisner A, Rigg D, et al. Perioperative outcomes and survival following neoadjuvant stereotactic body radiation therapy (SBRT) versus intensity-modulated radiation therapy (IMRT) in pancreatic adenocarcinoma. *J Surg Oncol.* 2018;117(5):1073–1083.
52. Sonke JJ, Aznar M, Rasch C. Adaptive radiotherapy for anatomical changes. *Semin Radiat Oncol.* 2019;29(3):245–257.
53. Kozloff M, Yood MU, Berlin J, et al. Clinical outcomes associated with bevacizumab-containing treatment of metastatic colorectal cancer: the BRiTE observational cohort study. *Oncologist.* 2009;14(9):862–870.
54. Scappaticci FA, Skillings JR, Holden SN, et al. Arterial thromboembolic events in patients with metastatic carcinoma treated with chemotherapy and bevacizumab. *J Natl Cancer Inst.* 2007;99(16):1232–1239.
55. Touyz RM, Herrmann J. Cardiotoxicity with vascular endothelial growth factor inhibitor therapy. *NPJ Precis Oncol.* 2018;2:13.
56. Kosmas C, Kallistratos MS, Kopterides P, et al. Cardiotoxicity of fluoropyrimidines in different schedules of administration: a prospective study. *J Cancer Res Clin Oncol.* 2008;134(1):75–82.
57. Ng M, Cunningham D, Norman AR. The frequency and pattern of cardiotoxicity observed with capecitabine used in conjunction with oxaliplatin in patients treated for advanced colorectal cancer (CRC). *Eur J Cancer.* 2005;41(11):1542–1546.
58. Saif MW, Tomita M, Ledbetter L, Diasio RB. Capecitabine-related cardiotoxicity: recognition and management. *J Support Oncol.* 2008;6(1):41–48.
59. Van Cutsem E, Hoff PM, Blum JL, Abt M, Osterwalder B. Incidence of cardiotoxicity with the oral fluoropyrimidine capecitabine is typical of that reported with 5-fluorouracil. *Ann Oncol.* 2002;13(3):484–485.
60. Vermorken JB, Remenar E, van Herpen C, et al. Cisplatin, fluorouracil, and docetaxel in unresectable head and neck cancer. *N Engl J Med.* 2007;357(17):1695–1704.
61. Fogarassy G, Vathy-Fogarassy A, Kenessey I, Kasler M, Forster T. Risk prediction model for long-term heart failure incidence after epirubicin chemotherapy for breast cancer - A real-world data-based, nationwide classification analysis. *Int J Cardiol.* 2019;285:47–52.
62. Jensen SA, Sorensen JB. Risk factors and prevention of cardiotoxicity induced by 5-fluorouracil or capecitabine. *Cancer Chemother Pharmacol.* 2006;58(4):487–493.
63. Bdair FM, Graham SP, Smith PF, Javle MM. Gemcitabine and acute myocardial infarction–a case report. *Angiology.* 2006;57(3):367–371.
64. Ozturk B, Tacoy G, Coskun U, et al. Gemcitabine-induced acute coronary syndrome: a case report. *Med Princ Pract.* 2009;18(1):76–80.
65. Arbuck SG, Strauss H, Rowinsky E, et al. A reassessment of cardiac toxicity associated with Taxol. *J Natl Cancer Inst Monogr.* 1993(15):117–130.
66. Escudier B, Eisen T, Stadler WM, et al. Sorafenib in advanced clear-cell renal-cell carcinoma. *N Engl J Med.* 2007;356(2):125–134.
67. Webster DR. Microtubules in cardiac toxicity and disease. *Cardiovasc Toxicol.* 2002;2(2):75–89.
68. Lapeyre-Mestre M, Gregoire N, Bugat R, Montastruc JL. Vinorelbine-related cardiac events: a meta-analysis of randomized clinical trials. *Fundam Clin Pharmacol.* 2004;18(1):97–105.
69. Miller K, Wang M, Gralow J, et al. Paclitaxel plus bevacizumab versus paclitaxel alone for metastatic breast cancer. *N Engl J Med.* 2007;357(26):2666–2676.
70. Miller KD, Chap LI, Holmes FA, et al. Randomized phase III trial of capecitabine compared with bevacizumab plus capecitabine in patients with previously treated metastatic breast cancer. *J Clin Oncol.* 2005;23(4):792–799.
71. Richardson PG, Sonneveld P, Schuster MW, et al. Bortezomib or high-dose dexamethasone for relapsed multiple myeloma. *N Engl J Med.* 2005;352(24):2487–2498.
72. Kremer LC, van der Pal HJ, Offringa M, van Dalen EC, Voute PA. Frequency and risk factors of subclinical cardiotoxicity after anthracycline therapy in children: a systematic review. *Ann Oncol.* 2002;13(6):819–829.
73. Braverman AC, Antin JH, Plappert MT, Cook EF, Lee RT. Cyclophosphamide cardiotoxicity in bone marrow transplantation: a prospective evaluation of new dosing regimens. *J Clin Oncol.* 1991;9(7):1215–1223.
74. Chaar M, Kamta J. Ait-Oudhia S. Mechanisms, monitoring, and management of tyrosine kinase inhibitors-associated cardiovascular toxicities. *Onco Targets Ther.* 2018;11:6227–6237.
75. Martin M, Pienkowski T, Mackey J, et al. Adjuvant docetaxel for node-positive breast cancer. *N Engl J Med.* 2005;352(22):2302–2313.
76. Swain SM, Whaley FS, Ewer MS. Congestive heart failure in patients treated with doxorubicin: a retrospective analysis of three trials. *Cancer.* 2003;97(11):2869–2879.
77. Ryberg M, Nielsen D, Cortese G, Nielsen G, Skovsgaard T, Andersen PK. New insight into epirubicin cardiac toxicity: competing risks analysis of 1097 breast cancer patients. *J Natl Cancer Inst.* 2008;100(15):1058–1067.
78. Pai VB, Nahata MC. Cardiotoxicity of chemotherapeutic agents: incidence, treatment and prevention. *Drug Saf.* 2000;22(4):263–302.
79. Atallah E, Durand JB, Kantarjian H, Cortes J. Congestive heart failure is a rare event in patients receiving imatinib therapy. *Blood.* 2007;110(4):1233–1237.
80. Perez EA, Koehler M, Byrne J, Preston AJ, Rappold E, Ewer MS. Cardiac safety of lapatinib: pooled analysis of 3689 patients enrolled in clinical trials. *Mayo Clin Proc.* 2008;83(6):679–686.
81. Shaikh AY, Suryadevara S, Tripathi A, et al. Mitoxantrone-induced cardiotoxicity in acute myeloid leukemia-a velocity vector imaging analysis. *Echocardiography.* 2016;33(8):1166–1177.
82. Chu TF, Rupnick MA, Kerkela R, et al. Cardiotoxicity associated with tyrosine kinase inhibitor sunitinib. *Lancet.* 2007;370(9604):2011–2019.
83. Khakoo AY, Kassiotis CM, Tannir N, et al. Heart failure associated with sunitinib malate: a multitargeted receptor tyrosine kinase inhibitor. *Cancer.* 2008;112(11):2500–2508.
84. Ewer MS, O'Shaughnessy JA. Cardiac toxicity of trastuzumab-related regimens in HER2-overexpressing breast cancer. *Clin Breast Cancer.* 2007;7(8):600–607.
85. Perez EA, Suman VJ, Davidson NE, et al. Cardiac safety analysis of doxorubicin and cyclophosphamide followed by paclitaxel with or without trastuzumab in the North Central Cancer Treatment Group N9831 adjuvant breast cancer trial. *J Clin Oncol.* 2008;26(8):1231–1238.

86. Suter TM, Procter M, van Veldhuisen DJ, et al. Trastuzumab-associated cardiac adverse effects in the herceptin adjuvant trial. *J Clin Oncol.* 2007;25(25):3859–3865.
87. Johnson DH, Fehrenbacher L, Novotny WF, et al. Randomized phase II trial comparing bevacizumab plus carboplatin and paclitaxel with carboplatin and paclitaxel alone in previously untreated locally advanced or metastatic non-small-cell lung cancer. *J Clin Oncol.* 2004;22(11):2184–2191.
88. Waid-Jones MI, Coursin DB. Perioperative considerations for patients treated with bleomycin. *Chest.* 1991;99(4):993–999.
89. Fernandez HF, Tran HT, Albrecht F, Lennon S, Caldera H, Goodman MS. Evaluation of safety and pharmacokinetics of administering intravenous busulfan in a twice-daily or daily schedule to patients with advanced hematologic malignant disease undergoing stem cell transplantation. *Biol Blood Marrow Transplant.* 2002;8(9):486–492.
90. O'Driscoll BR, Kalra S, Gattamaneni HR, Woodcock AA. Late carmustine lung fibrosis. Age at treatment may influence severity and survival. *Chest.* 1995;107(5):1355–1357.
91. Malik SW, Myers JL, DeRemee RA, Specks U. Lung toxicity associated with cyclophosphamide use. Two distinct patterns. *Am J Respir Crit Care Med.* 1996;154(6 Pt 1):1851–1856.
92. Andersson BS, Cogan BM, Keating MJ, Estey EH, McCredie KB, Freireich EJ. Subacute pulmonary failure complicating therapy with high-dose Ara-C in acute leukemia. *Cancer.* 1985;56(9):2181–2184.
93. Kelly K, Swords R, Mahalingam D, Padmanabhan S, Giles FJ. Serosal inflammation (pleural and pericardial effusions) related to tyrosine kinase inhibitors. *Target Oncol.* 2009;4(2):99–105.
94. Merad M, Le Cesne A, Baldeyrou P, Mesurolle B, Le Chevalier T. Docetaxel and interstitial pulmonary injury. *Ann Oncol.* 1997;8(2):191–194.
95. Cohen MH, Williams GA, Sridhara R, Chen G, Pazdur R. FDA drug approval summary: gefitinib (ZD1839) (Iressa) tablets. *Oncologist.* 2003;8(4):303–306.
96. Aapro MS, Martin C, Hatty S. Gemcitabine–a safety review. *Anticancer Drugs.* 1998;9(3):191–201.
97. Kremer JM, Alarcon GS, Weinblatt ME, et al. Clinical, laboratory, radiographic, and histopathologic features of methotrexate-associated lung injury in patients with rheumatoid arthritis: a multicenter study with literature review. *Arthritis Rheum.* 1997;40(10):1829–1837.
98. Verweij J, van Zanten T, Souren T, Golding R, Pinedo HM. Prospective study on the dose relationship of mitomycin C-induced interstitial pneumonitis. *Cancer.* 1987;60(4):756–761.
99. Khan A, McNally D, Tutschka PJ, Bilgrami S. Paclitaxel-induced acute bilateral pneumonitis. *Ann Pharmacother.* 1997;31(12):1471–1474.
100. Wagner SA, Mehta AC, Laber DA. Rituximab-induced interstitial lung disease. *Am J Hematol.* 2007;82(10):916–919.
101. Dabydeen DA, Jagannathan JP, Ramaiya N, et al. Pneumonitis associated with mTOR inhibitors therapy in patients with metastatic renal cell carcinoma: incidence, radiographic findings and correlation with clinical outcome. *Eur J Cancer.* 2012;48(10):1519–1524.
102. Romond EH, Perez EA, Bryant J, et al. Trastuzumab plus adjuvant chemotherapy for operable HER2-positive breast cancer. *N Engl J Med.* 2005;353(16):1673–1684.
103. Grigorian A, O'Brien CB. Hepatotoxicity secondary to chemotherapy. *J Clin Transl Hepatol.* 2014;2(2):95–102.
104. Perazella MA. Onco-nephrology: renal toxicities of chemotherapeutic agents. *Clin J Am Soc Nephrol.* 2012;7(10):1713–1721.

6

Cancer and Heart Disease

JOSE BANCHS AND SYED WAMIQUE YUSUF

Introduction

At the intersection of oncology and cardiology, the field of cardio-oncology is growing primarily with the aim of recognizing, monitoring, and treating cardiovascular complications resulting from cancer-related treatments. With advances in cardiac imaging technologies, we now have a much better understanding of the cardiac effects of cancer and cancer therapies; and are refining therapies in the subspecialty of heart failure (HF).

Although a number of different measures are recognized as capable of evaluating systolic function, the left ventricular ejection fraction (LVEF) continues to be the most widely utilized. In the clinical setting and in multiple research protocols, cardiotoxicity has been defined as a decline of LVEF ≥5% to final ejection fraction (EF) <55% with symptoms of congestive HF, or an asymptomatic decline of LVEF ≥10% to a final EF <55%. As controversial and arbitrary as this definition might be considered,[1] special attention is given to LVEF quantification in cardio-oncology oriented practices.

Quantification of Systolic Function in Cardio-oncology

In clinical practice, the most commonly accepted definition of cardiac toxicity comes from the independent Cardiac Review and Evaluation Committee's (CREC) retrospective review of patients enrolled onto a variety of trastuzumab clinical trials.[2] Echocardiography is the most used test for sequential measurement of LVEF in the assessment of potential cardiotoxicity from chemotherapy or immune therapy in patients with malignancies. In most oncology practices, the LVEF is followed closely, and the EF value is given significant clinical importance.

In practice, given the use of singular numbers for any particular cardiotoxicity definition used, it has been common for echocardiography clinicians in this field to report single numbers and avoid range EF reporting. It is understandable that it would be confusing for our oncology colleagues who make critical clinical decisions based on a 5% or 10% EF change, or a drop to under 50% or 55%, when, for example, the value reported from one study to the next is 55%–60% followed by 50%–55%.

The decisions that oncologists are faced with include the possibility of cessation of further anticancer therapy, which could have significant clinical consequences.[3] We also need to understand the history of single digit measure from the historic perspective in oncology. In this field, cardiac imaging was established in the late 70s and early 80s when a number of publications[4–8] supported the different available modalities, and over a short period, measurement of LVEF by nuclear methods (multiple-gated acquisition scan [MUGA]) became the established practice and was considered the gold standard for left ventricular function assessment during chemotherapy. LVEF by radionuclide imaging proved to be sensitive, specific, and reproducible and was reported as a single measure. Clearly, measurement of LVEF as a sole indicator of cardiotoxicity has significant limitations. These include image quality, the technical realities of the measurement that may include the single beat selection, operator experience, and volume drawing styles. In addition, the EF—the relative volume ejected in systole—can be load dependent.

It is important that our EF measurements are accurate with the lowest variability possible. The most commonly used LVEF methods in routine practice are the two-dimensional (2D) methods. Among the 2D options, the most commonly used method for volume calculations is the biplane method of disks summation (modified Simpson's rule). This is the recommended 2D echocardiographic method according to consensus and current published left ventricular quantification guidelines.[9] The literature is clear that among the 2D methods, using biplane volumes with the use of microbubble enhancement offers the best results in terms of intra- and interobserver variability; and contrast agents are recommended when there is a need to improve endocardial border delineation, particularly when two or more contiguous LV endocardial segments are poorly visualized in apical views. It is important to remember that microbubble-enhanced images provide larger volumes than unenhanced images. Volumes obtained in this fashion are closer to those obtained with cardiac magnetic resonance (CMR).[10]

Three-dimensional echocardiography (3DE) has been shown to be more accurate than 2D for both ventricular volume and EF measurements when compared with CMR imaging, and therefore it is an attractive modality in this field and should be used when available.[11,12] This method, while not routinely available in most centers, has been shown to offer the lowest temporal variability for EF and ventricular volumes on the basis of multiple echocardiograms performed over 1 year in women with breast cancer receiving chemotherapy.[13]

Diastolic Function and Detection of Cardiotoxicity

Measurements of diastolic function by Doppler echocardiography could represent a marker for the early detection of toxicity. One study found that the isovolumetric relaxation time was significantly prolonged after a cumulative doxorubicin dose of 100 to 120 mg/m^2. Any increase of more than 37% in volumetric relaxation time was 78% (7 of 9) sensitive and 88% (15 of 17) specific for predicting the ultimate development of doxorubicin-induced systolic dysfunction.[14] The myocardial performance (Tei) index is another important Doppler-derived tool.[15] This index expresses the ratio of the sum of the isovolumetric contraction time and the isovolumetric relaxation time divided by the ejection time. This formula combines systolic and diastolic myocardial performance without geometrical assumptions and correlates well with the results of invasive measurements. The value is appealing for use with cancer patients because it appears to be independent of heart rate, mean arterial pressure, and degree of mitral regurgitation. It has also been found to be sensitive and accurate in detecting subclinical cardiotoxicity associated with anthracycline therapy.[16]

Studies using the Tei index show that this index is better than the EF in detecting anthracycline-induced deterioration in LV function among adults; it detects this deterioration earlier in the course of treatment and is more likely to detect statistically significant differences.[17] However, the results regarding the value of diastolic dysfunction as an indicator of this diagnosis have been inconsistent. Because of the influence of hypertension and other risk factors on diastolic function, this signal appears to be nonspecific.

Cardiac Mechanics in Cardio-oncology

Earlier detection of cardiotoxicity allows for a time advantage in risk stratification. New techniques are aimed at detecting cardiotoxicity before the onset of a measurable decrease in LVEF or symptoms. These methods include echocardiographic assessment for strain using speckle-tracking imaging, as well as testing for elevations in cardiac biomarkers, including troponin. Speckle tracking takes full advantage of a new capacity for image acquisition at higher frame rates. Several reports regarding cancer populations receiving cardiotoxic agents and the use of this particular technology in the realm of cancer therapeutics–related cardiac dysfunction have been very exciting, particularly regarding the use of longitudinal deformation measures and the global longitudinal strain (GLS) value.

It was first reported in 2009 that changes in tissue deformation, assessed by myocardial strain and strain rate, were able to identify left ventricular dysfunction earlier than LVEF in women undergoing treatment with trastuzumab for breast cancer.[18] Following this, two reports resulted in comparable findings.[19,20] A multicenter collaboration[20] reported on the use of troponin and longitudinal strain measures to predict the development of cardiotoxicity in patients treated with anthracyclines and trastuzumab. Patients who demonstrated decreases in longitudinal strain measures or elevations in hypersensitive troponin had a ninefold increase in risk for cardiotoxicity at 6 months compared with those with no changes in either of these markers. Furthermore, diastolic function parameters and LVEF alone did not help predict cardiotoxicity.

In a review including over 30 studies, it was reported that although the best GLS value to predict cardiotoxicity is not clear, an early relative change between 10% and 15% appears to have the best specificity.[21] Similar studies, however, have found a stronger correlation with ventricular-arterial coupling and circumferential strain than longitudinal measures.[22] A consensus statement on the evaluation of adult patients during and after cancer therapy published by the American Society of Echocardiography and the European Association of Cardiovascular Imaging also reports that a relative percentage reduction in GLS of >15% is very likely to be abnormal, whereas a change of <8% appears to be of no clinical significance.[23]

Cardiac Dysfunction and the Heart Failure Spectrum

Cancer therapy–related cardiac dysfunction (CTRCD) is one of the most feared and undesirable side effects of chemotherapy despite occurring only in a small minority of cases.

Despite widespread screening recommendations, a clear universal definition of cardiotoxicity is lacking in the current literature. While there are different definitions of CTRCD presented by clinical trials and guideline statements, there is no universal consensus at this time. The first publication defining mild cardiotoxicity as a decline in EF by >10% and moderate cardiotoxicity as EF decline by >15% to a value less than 45% was by Alexander and colleagues in 1979.[24] In 1987 a large clinical trial defined CTRCD as a decline in EF by >10% to a final value <50%.[25] Both of these studies used MUGA scans as the method of screening and only included patients who had been treated with anthracycline. In 2002, after review of the trastuzumab trials, the CREC defined CTRCD as asymptomatic decline of LVEF ≥10%

to a final EF <55%.[2] Over a decade later (in 2014), the American Society of Echocardiography and European Association of Cardiovascular Imaging (ASE/EACI) chose a cutoff value of <53%.[23]

Controversy still persists regarding the definitions of cardiac toxicity, the true incidence, detection, monitoring, and treatment of the late effects in survivors of cancer of all ages. There are multiple explanations for the lack of consensus regarding clinical guidelines in CTRCD. Most importantly, there is a lack of large-scale randomized clinical trial data to support any evidence-proven, effective long-term treatment and/or surveillance strategies. Furthermore, there has been minimal success at showing the cost-effectiveness of aggressive cardiac surveillance and treatment to providers.

In this chapter, discussion of CTRCD will be limited to the proper management of the cardiac effects of anthracycline therapy in cancer survivors. The antitumor actions include inhibition of topoisomerase II, an enzyme that regulates the uncoiling of DNA strands and in doing so induces breaks in DNA and ultimately cell death. Anthracycline therapy results in the formation of toxic reactive oxygen species (ROS) and interferes with macromolecule synthesis with a subsequent increase in cardiac oxidative stress-associated apoptosis. In addition, a relationship between topoisomerase IIβ activity in the heart and cardiac toxicity was reported,[26] potentially opening a new avenue for future therapies.

Clinical presentations of toxicity can include arrhythmias, heart block, HF, pericarditis-myocarditis syndrome, and cardiac ischemia. Late toxicity is almost universally limited to myocardial systolic dysfunction. There are several known clinical risk factors associated with toxicity such as pre-existing cardiovascular disease (CVD), hypertension, the use of other cardiotoxic nonanthracycline agents (trastuzumab, taxanes), and exposure to mediastinal radiotherapy. It is also important to recognize that children are at particular risk for development of anthracycline-induced cardiomyopathy, but there is also increased incidence of systolic dysfunction with age, particularly in the elderly population. Although there is an accepted direct relationship between cardiotoxicity and cumulative anthracycline dose, cardiotoxicity has been reported in patients who have received doses under 100 mg/m^2 of doxorubicin, and there are patients who have received doses >550 mg/m^2 and never developed cardiotoxicity.

Biomarkers have been an exciting area of investigation in this arena, and there is increasing evidence that using a biomarker or a panel of them could significantly contribute to the clinical monitoring and surveillance of these patients in the future. The traditional tests have been troponin T/I, B-type natriuretic peptide (BNP), or N-terminal pro-BNP (NT-proBNP). However, new markers in the mRNA category such as miR-208b, miR-34a, and miR-150 have been recently reported, particularly for breast cancer patients receiving anthracyclines and/or trastuzumab.[27]

There is no specific therapy for systolic dysfunction in CTRCD. If a reduction in LVEF is detected, patients should be treated in accordance with established guidelines for the management of HF.[28] Drug antiremodeling therapy should include agents approved with appropriate indications such as angiotensin-converting enzyme (ACE) inhibitors or angiotensin receptor blockers (ARBs), and beta blockers as tolerated. There are no quality or long-term outcome data to guide treatment of CTRCD.

It is critical to consider alternate causes of LV dysfunction beyond chemotherapy, particularly in patients who present after low levels of anthracycline exposure or non-anthracycline regimens. It is always clinically mandatory to consider common causes such as coronary disease, hypertension, infiltrative conditions, and alcohol excess depending on the individual clinical picture.

Among patients who are still candidates for active cancer therapy, a multidisciplinary discussion, including the cardiologists and oncology providers, is usually beneficial. The risks and benefits of further chemotherapy should be carefully considered in planning subsequent treatments. It should be noted that there is some evidence that LVEF by echocardiography could be used to improve patient selection for enrollment in clinical trial–based regimens. One study suggests that it is safe to treat patients with LVEF between 35% and 50%.[29] However, in general, it is recommended to avoid further exposure to regimens containing known toxic agents in the presence of ongoing LV dysfunction. See Figs. 6.1 and 6.2.

Considerations in Radiation-Induced Heart Disease

Radiation-induced cardiac changes include a spectrum of pericardial disease, valvular disease, coronary/microvascular disease or dysfunction, and restrictive cardiomyopathy. Most commonly, these are pathologic processes that are late manifestations, becoming clinically significant years after radiation. Pericardial thickening appears as increased echogenicity of the pericardium on 2D echocardiography or M-mode imaging. Correct distinction between normal to thickened pericardium is challenging. Characteristic echocardiographic findings of constrictive pericarditis include a thickened pericardium, prominent respiratory phasic diastolic motion of the interventricular septum, restrictive diastolic filling pattern, and significant inspiratory variation of the mitral E-wave velocity (>25%). Other secondary findings include inferior vena cava dilatation and expiratory diastolic flow reversal in the hepatic veins. Typically, tissue Doppler interrogation of the medial mitral annulus reveals a normal or increased velocity that can be higher than the lateral annulus velocity.[30] Another important consideration is effusive-constrictive pericarditis. This clinical syndrome is characterized by concurrent pericardial effusion and pericardial constriction, with constrictive hemodynamics that persists after the drainage of the pericardial effusion. In effusive-constrictive pericarditis, the visceral layer of the pericardium, rather than the parietal layer, constricts

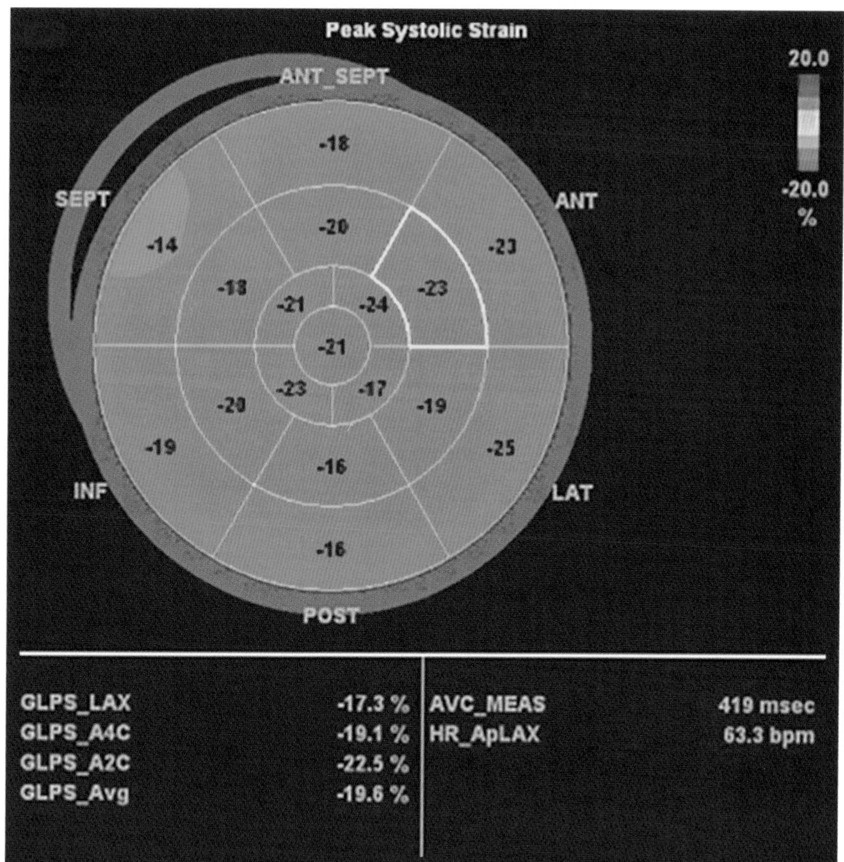

• **Fig. 6.1** A female with breast cancer treated with Herceptin has a GLS value of −19.6% at baseline. *GLS*, Global longitudinal strain.

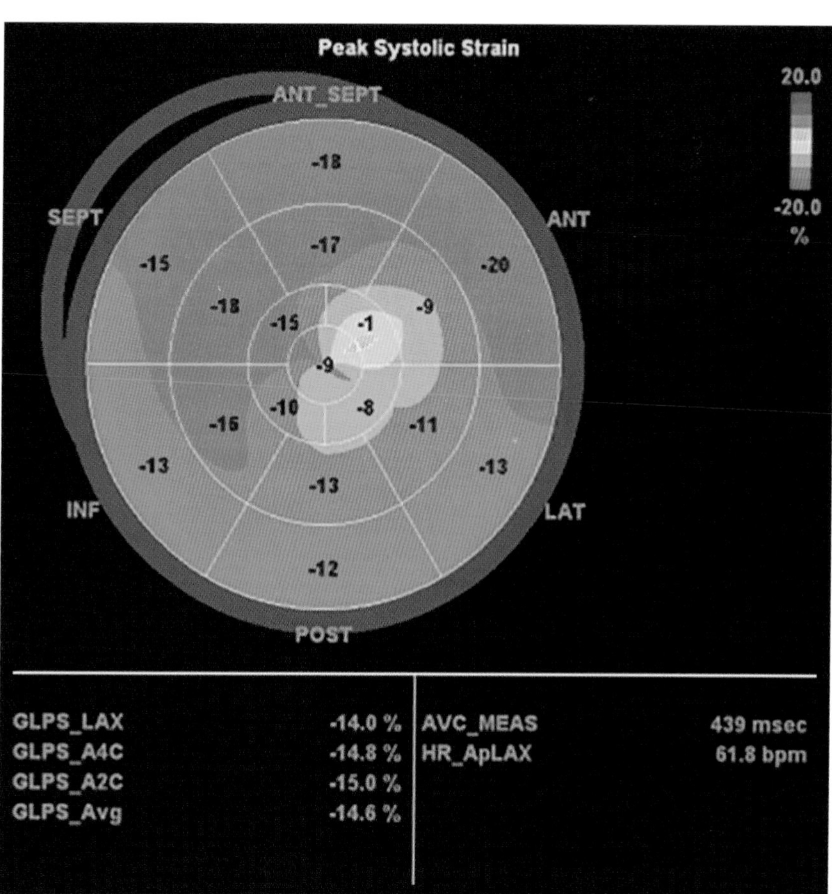

• **Fig. 6.2** The same patient with a GLS of −14.6, 3 months later. This preceded a 14% decrease in LVEF that was noted in her 6-month follow-up echocardiogram. *GLS*, Global longitudinal strain; *LVEF*, left ventricular ejection fraction.

the heart. This is a rare condition; however, effective recognition is important because pericardiectomy is sometimes indicated for management.

In the particular case of valvular disease, manifestations of radiation-induced heart disease (RIHD) include fibrosis and patchy calcification of structures, such as the aortic root, annulus, leaflets, the aorto-mitral intervalvular fibrosa, mitral annulus, and the base and mid-portions of the mitral valve leaflets usually sparing the tips and commissures (a key difference from rheumatic heart disease). Grading the severity of valvular disease should be based on published guidelines. Valve regurgitation is more commonly encountered than stenosis. Stenotic lesions more commonly involve the aortic valve. Reported incidence of clinically significant valve disease is 1% at 10 years, 5% at 15 years, and 6% at 20 years after radiation exposure. Incidence of valve disease increases significantly after >20 years following chest radiation (mild aortic regurgitation [AR] up to 45%, moderate AR up to 15%, aortic stenosis up to 16%, mild mitral regurgitation up to 48%, mild pulmonary regurgitation up to 12%).[31,32]

Cardiac Tumors

Cardiac tumors are rare, and are generally categorized as primary or secondary. Primary cardiac tumors are the rarest, with an autopsy incidence of 0.002%–0.3%.[33,34] Primary cardiac tumors include both benign and malignant neoplasms that originate from cardiac tissue. Secondary or metastatic cardiac tumors are around 30 times more common than primary malignancy, with a reported autopsy incidence of 1.7%–14%.[35]

Other possible categories of tumors could include those from the lower body that reach the cardiac cavities by extension through the inferior vena cava, and tumors that extend from the mediastinal space directly invading the pericardial layers. The infradiaphragmatic tumors can occur with almost any cell type, but the large majority of these have been attributed to renal cell carcinoma (RCC) where as much as 10% of patients will have tumor extension into the inferior vena cava.[35] In patients with RCC, involvement of the right atrium (RA) is encountered in up to 5% of cases, and pulmonary artery tumor emboli is rarely observed.[36] Other sources for this route of invasion include uterine malignancies[37] and hepatocellular carcinoma.[38,39] Tumors with direct extension in the mediastinal space again can occur with almost any cell type. Thymoma compromises 20%–25% of all mediastinal tumors and is the most commonly described anterior mediastinal tumor[40]; however, most case reports of direct mediastinal invasion are not from thymic origin.[41,42]

The clinical manifestation of cardiac tumor is variable and not unlikely to be found on routine surveillance echocardiogram examination or other chest imaging modality. In terms of clinical presentation, tumors cause signs and symptoms, depending on location, size, and etiology.[43–49] Presence of a growing mass inside a contractile and moving cavity can eventually cause hemodynamic compromise of blood flow in the affected or receiving chamber and even disrupt valve coaptation. In this setting, syndromes of congestive failure can be present. This can be further accelerated in the case of myocardial involvement and secondary limitations to contractility. See Table 6.1.

Careful evaluation of segmental ventricular dysfunction is pertinent, as direct occlusive pressure or extension of the tumor into the lumen of the coronary arteries (including the possible embolization of tumor fragments) has also been described.[50,51] Repolarization changes in patients with cardiac metastases are believed to occur by myocardial ischemia caused by the tumor's direct myocardial injury and invasion, as this presentation has been found in subjects without obstructive coronary lesion on angiography.[52]

Due to its noninvasive nature, availability, relative portability, and affordability (when compared with other modalities), echocardiography is the most widely used diagnostic modality for the evaluation of cardiac tumors. As indicated earlier, this technology has advanced to include mechanical function analysis, which may increase our sensitivity to recognize subtler wall motion defects.

A great complement to transthoracic echocardiogram (TTE) is the use of transesophageal echocardiography, which provides a significant upgrade in spatial resolution and overall image clarity compared to transthoracic imaging. This technique has also demonstrated impressive and rapidly improving quality of three-dimensional images. The use of echo contrast has also added a significant degree of confidence and accuracy to transthoracic echo; and is also frequently used for mass characterization.[53] See Fig. 6.3.

TABLE 6.1 Leading Reported Clinical Signs and Symptoms on Presentation for Cardiac Tumors

Dyspnea
Chest pain, common with malignant and pericardial tumors
Hypotension
Syncope
Edema (secondary to blood flow obstruction)
Cough or hemoptysis
Cardiac tamponade
Pericardial friction rubs
Auscultation: gallop or murmur
Systemic embolization of tumor fragments, stroke
Peripheral arterial occlusion associated with left sided tumors
Right heart failure/pulmonary hypertension as a complication of right-sided tumors

[a]Systemic emboli from left heart lesions are more frequently seen than pulmonary tumor emboli from right heart lesions

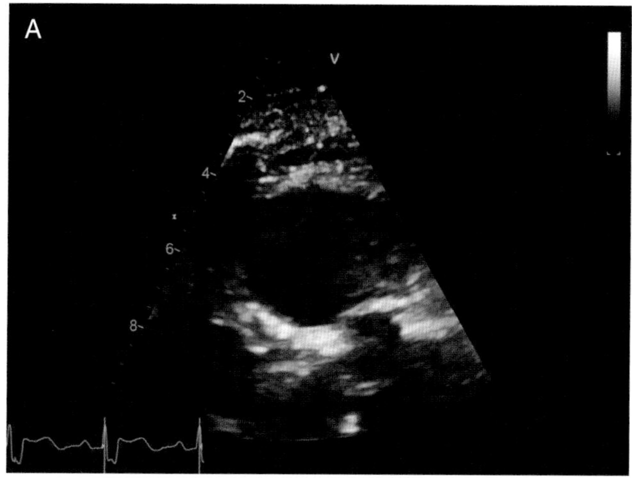

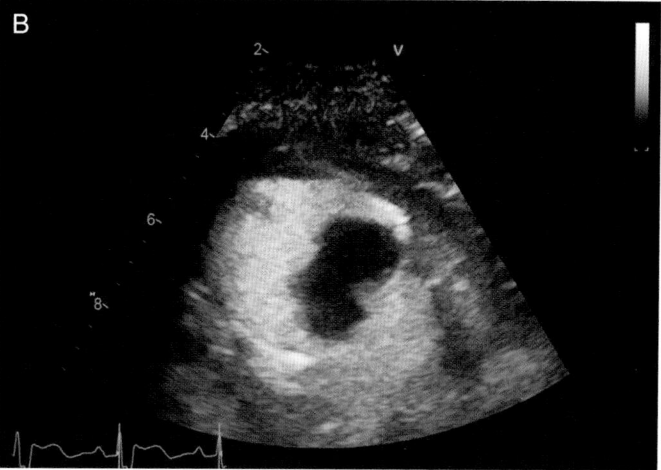

• **Fig. 6.3** A young woman with sarcoma. On echocardiogram, we see a mass at the base of the right ventricle. The mass is easily visible in the echo-contrast enhanced image (A), which the unenhanced image at the same angle fails to demonstrate clearly (B).

However, when it comes to more detailed characterization of a malignant lesion infiltrating the myocardium, CMR and cardiac computerized tomography (CCT) can give a more complete view of the mediastinum, extra cardiac structures, and the possible attachments of a mass outside of the cardiac cavities. This is considered critical information for the surgeon when planning resection. These modalities also have well-known advantages when it comes to tissue characterization. They do not suffer from the acoustic "window" limitations that often make transthoracic echocardiographic examination technically difficult, particularly in obese patients, subjects with history of previous chest surgery, and those with chronic lung disease.

Cardiac interventional procedures described in the diagnosis of cardiac tumors, both primary and secondary, include endomyocardial biopsy[54–57] and pericardiocentesis. The latter has been frequently used to confirm malignant cells within the fluid or as a palliative tool for patients with increased intrapericardial pressures secondary to progressive disease. Echocardiography (TEE) is often helpful for imaging guidance during these procedures.

Tumor Types, Physiology, and Treatment Considerations

There are limited detailed reports of large series of cardiac tumors in the existing literature. One of the largest reports comes from our institution, a 12-year experience, where we describe that roughly a quarter of cardiac tumors as primary and nearly three-quarters as secondary. We found that dyspnea is the most common symptom described by patients diagnosed with this condition.[58] The large majority (>80%) of primary cardiac tumors are benign; myxoma being the most common[59,60]; the remaining 20% are malignant primary cardiac tumors. The most common malignant primary tumor to be described unanimously in every large series is sarcoma. In our series, this was followed by paraganglioma and myxoma. Most sarcomas in our series were angiosarcomas. The most common location was the RA. This closely resembles the findings of other reported series.[61] From an echocardiography, perspective angiosarcomas are predominantly found on the right side, while osteosarcomas and unclassified sarcomas are predominantly found on the left side of the heart.[62,63] Pericardial angiosarcomas are rare. It is important to know that about 29% of cardiac sarcomas have metastatic disease at the time of presentation.[64]

Secondary cardiac tumors were, in large majority, metastases from renal cell carcinoma. These patients were generally older than those diagnosed with sarcoma. Again, the RA was the most frequent location affecting patients. The most common presenting symptom was, as expected, dyspnea. In our series, the majority of all secondary cardiac tumors were metastases from renal cell carcinoma, whereas in most other series metastasis from lung carcinoma appears to the commonest cause.[58] For secondary tumors in our experience, the second most common site was the left atrium, followed by right ventricle, right atria and right ventricle combined, left atria, mitral valve, an instance of left atria/right atria/mitral valve involvement, and an intrapericardial case. Almost half of the subjects (44%) died within 12 months of diagnosis; hence early recognition with imaging is considered critical.

Despite melanoma being described in a few reports as a neoplasm with a propensity to metastasize to the heart,[65–67] this represented a minority of cases in our series.[58] Recognition of cardiac lesions in these cases can yield a significant change in prognosis since once metastasized to other organs; melanoma is by definition stage IV, and associated with poor survival rates. The reported 5-year survival in these cases is 15% to 20%.[68] Of note, sarcomas that metastasize to the myocardium are frequently high grade and progress quickly. Myocardial infiltration, outflow obstruction, and distant metastasis result in death within a few weeks to 2 years of onset of symptoms, with median survival ranging from 6 to 12 months. Different series have documented the metastatic rate to be 26%–43% at presentation and 75% at the time of death.[62,64,69–77] In comparison to older series, there is a significant increase in the incidence of cardiac metastases in cancer patients after 1970.[60] This is possibly in an era of improved and more available cardiac imaging modalities.

The pericardium is most often involved due to direct invasion by the thoracic malignancies. The myocardium or epicardium is believed to be most involved through lymphatic spread and endocardial metastases through hematogenous spread.

Review of previous reports shows that lung cancer is the most common cause of cardiac metastasis followed by hematologic malignancy. Only a couple of reports show a different trend.[36,78–90]

Last, in contrast, in the pediatric population, rhabdomyosarcoma is the most common form of cardiac sarcoma. Leiomyosarcoma, synovial sarcoma, osteosarcoma, fibrosarcoma, myxoidsarcoma, liposarcoma, mesenchymal sarcoma, neurofibrosarcoma, and malignant fibrous histocytoma are the other cardiac sarcomas observed.[63,64] A recent systematic review of the literature reported a cumulative 30-day mortality rate of 6.7%.[91]

Cardiac Tumor Therapies

For treatment purposes, cardiac sarcomas are divided into three groups: right heart sarcomas, left heart sarcomas, and pulmonary artery sarcomas.[92] The treatment for right heart and left heart sarcomas is chemotherapy and surgical resection. Direct cardiac radiotherapy is avoided in patients, as it may cause myocardial injury. In brief, the history of cardiac tumor surgery dates back to the late 1550s when a case of primary cardiac neoplasm was first described.[93] The first series of cases was published in 1845[94] with six arterial tumors consistent with myxoma. A further 86 years later in 1931, Yater reported a postmortem series of nine cases of cardiac tumors, and a classification system that is still in use today.[95]

The surgical treatment of cardiac tumors began in the late 1930s with the removal of an intrapericardial cystic teratoma that extended to the right ventricle.[96] Surgery radically changed and progressed after the introduction of cardiopulmonary bypass in 1953.[97] This allowed controlled access to the interior chambers of the heart and led to multiple reports of successful cardiac mass excisions, mostly myxomas.[98,99] Cardiac tumor resection, however, has continued against challenges related to inherent technical difficulties of any major cardiac resection and the aggressive biology of these tumors. Against the challenges, survival has been shown to improve with surgical resection.[100] In addition, a major catalyst for the surgical treatment of cardiac tumors was the growth in cardiac imaging, specifically echocardiography. This allowed noninvasive, easy visualization of the interior and exterior of the heart. Over time, innovation has flourished in this field and novel approaches allowing a more complete tumor resection, such as cardiac autotransplantation, have been successful.[101,102]

Unlike other sarcomas, cardiac sarcomas have a very poor prognosis with a median survival rate of 6–25 months after diagnosis.[62,63] Presence of tumor necrosis and metastases is associated with a poor prognosis.[62,64] A recent study showed that 14.8% of the resected tumors were low grade and all the patients were alive at follow-up.[103] This underlies the importance of tumor grade in survival of postoperative patients. Sarcomas other than angiosarcomas, sarcomas on the left heart, and completely resected sarcomas have a better prognosis.[62,64] Angiosarcomas grow faster, infiltrate widely, and metastasize early; they therefore have a poor prognosis.

Treatment of metastatic cardiac tumors is usually palliative. Different series have shown that the median survival is 17–24 months for patients who can undergo complete resection, and 6–10 months for patients unable to undergo complete resection.[64,104] Surgery with postoperative chemotherapy and/or radiotherapy to prevent local recurrence is indicated in patients with better prognosis and when they only have cardiac metastasis without disseminated disease. Orthotopic heart transplantation is an option in selected patients, with improved survival.[105,106] In patients with disseminated disease, limited life expectancy, and poor performance status, radiotherapy might still represent a choice. Chemotherapy is recommended for tumors that are chemosensitive. In these patients, end-of-life care should be discussed, and all efforts should be made to improve patient quality of life.

Acute Coronary Syndromes

Rudolf Virchow postulated that three features predispose to thrombus formation, namely abnormalities in vessel wall, blood constituent, and blood flow. Although originally Virchow was referring to venous thrombosis, the concept also relates to arterial thrombosis. A number of patients with cancer show abnormalities in each component of Virchow's triad leading to a prothrombotic or hypercoagulable state.[107] Exposure to radiation and various chemotherapy agents predisposes to the development of cardiovascular disease.[108] Radiation damages the endothelium, predisposing to vascular disease and ischemic heart disease in a relatively younger patient population.[109,110] Of all chemotherapeutic agents, 5-flurouracil (and its analogue capecitabine) is particularly known to cause ischemic heart disease.[111,112] In addition to 5-fluorouracil, other medications, such as paclitaxel, docetaxel, bevacizumab, erlotinib, and sorafenib, are also implicated in the development of ischemic heart disease.[112]

In patients with cancer, in addition to underlying coronary atherosclerosis, there are multiple other etiologies and predisposing factors for cardiovascular abnormalities, including cardiac metastasis/coronary compression, tumor-related coagulation disorder (especially in patients with leukemia), coronary embolization from tumor or endocarditis, radiation, and chemotherapy, for example, 5-fluorouracil.[113] In terms of incidence and overall prognosis, there are limited reports available in the literature. However, a recent report from a national US database with more than 6 million patients showed a prevalence of acute myocardial infarction (AMI) of 9% in patients with cancer in the decade after 2004.[114] A very recent analysis on a large AMI population revealed that patients with active cancer have a 50% increased risk of major in-hospital adverse cardiac events than those without cancer.[115] In a 2017 study of more than 48,000 patients admitted with ST segment elevation myocardial infarctions, those with cancer had a significantly higher in-hospital and 1-year mortality than those without.[116] In summary, we have few observational, mainly retrospective studies comparing the clinical outcomes of patients with and without cancer and acute coronary syndromes. These analyses consistently report that patients with cancer are at higher risk of both in-hospital and long-term morbidity and mortality than those without.

Clinical Presentation and Diagnosis

Most patients with cancer and AMI usually have chest pain and dyspnea. Clinically a myocardial infarction denotes the presence of acute myocardial injury detected by abnormal cardiac biomarkers in the setting of evidence of acute myocardial ischemia. The diagnosis of myocardial infarction in cancer patients is based on the universal definition of myocardial infarction.[117] Myocardial infarction is further subclassified into various types.

Type 1 myocardial infarction is caused by atherothrombotic coronary artery disease and usually precipitated by atherosclerotic plaque disruption (rupture or erosion), whereas type 2 myocardial infarction is due to any condition causing a mismatch between oxygen supply and demand, leading to ischemic myocardial injury.[118] Majority of the cases in the intensive care unit setting are due to type 2 myocardial infarction, as some common conditions causing mismatch between oxygen supply and demand and resultant troponin are frequently seen in this setting, for example, tachycardia/arrhythmias, hypotension/shock, respiratory failure, severe hypertension, and HF/cardiomyopathy.

Treatment

Treatment of myocardial infarction in the cancer population is similar to the general population, which includes primary percutaneous intervention (in appropriate patients) antiplatelets, statin, and beta blockers.

Due to a lack of well-controlled trials, substantial data on cancer population are lacking. Nevertheless, current available evidence suggests that aspirin and beta blockers reduce mortality in these patients.[119] Primary percutaneous interventions should be considered as method of reperfusion, as a 1-year survival rate of 83% has been shown with this approach in the cancer population with ST elevation myocardial infarctions.[120]

The presence of thrombocytopenia poses special problems for management, but even in these patients aspirin should not be withheld, as one study amongst this subset of population showed that aspirin reduces mortality with no significant increase in bleeding.[121] The management of myocardial infarction in the cancer population, including those with thrombocytopenia, is outlined in an expert consensus statement.[122]

Acute Pericarditis

Acute pericarditis is acute inflammation of the pericardium resulting in a clinical syndrome consisting of pleuritic/positional chest pain, electrocardiogram changes, and a pericardial frictional rub. A pericardial effusion may or may not develop.[123,124] Malignancy is a common cause of pericardial disease in cancer, and in one study of 100 consecutive patients hospitalized with acute pericarditis, malignancy was found in 7% of the patients, with lung carcinoma being the commonest primary tumor.[125]

Acute pericarditis presents with retrosternal chest pain, which is typically worse on inspiration and in supine position and improves with sitting and on leaning forward. In some cases, it may radiate to the shoulder due to irritation of the phrenic nerve. On physical examination, the classic finding is a pericardial friction rub. The rub is best heard in end expiration with the patient leaning forward. It is a high-pitched scratchy sound that can have one, two, or all three components. A pericardial friction rub is present in approximately 34% of cases.[126]

Clinical criteria for diagnosis of acute pericarditis include typical chest pain, presence of audible pericardial friction rub, widespread ST-segment elevation on the electrocardiograms, and new or worsening pericardial effusion.[123,127] A diagnosis of acute pericarditis is made if at least two of the four criteria are present.[123,127]

Evidence of pericardial inflammation gained through the use of imaging techniques such as computerized tomographic scan or cardiac magnetic resonance, elevation of inflammatory markers, for example, C-reactive protein, white cell count, and erythrocyte sedimentation rate are additional supporting findings.[123] A 12-lead electrocardiogram is the most useful diagnostic test. The classic electrocardiogram finding is concave ST elevation and PR-segment depression in all leads, except AvR, which shows PR-segment elevation, and ST depression.[128] The electrocardiogram changes evolve in stages. In stage 1 the electrocardiogram shows ST-segment elevation and PR-segment depression. In stage 2 the normalization of PR and ST segments occurs. In stage 3 there are widespread T wave inversions and in stage 4 normalization of these T waves occurs.[128]

A chest x-ray is recommended in all patients with pericardial disease.[123] It is usually normal but may show other concomitant pathology such as pneumonia or enlarged cardiac silhouette in patients with associated pericardial effusion. Echocardiography is usually obtained to exclude a large pericardial effusion and tamponade.[123] Small pericardial effusion is present in about 60% of the cases and is responsive to medical therapy.[126] Computed tomography scan and CMR imaging can be used when the first level of investigations are not sufficient for diagnostic purposes or when there are complications related to pericarditis.[123,129]

Treatment

The mainstay of treatment are oral nonsteroidal anti-inflammatory drugs (NSAIDs), aspirin, and colchicine.[123,128] Steroids should not be used as a primary therapy in uncomplicated acute idiopathic pericarditis due to the high rate of relapse when the steroid is tapered or stopped.[130,131] Hence steroids should only be used in patients who are refractory and intolerant to aspirin/NSAIDs and colchicine combination or have an underlying condition for which steroids are indicated. For a first episode, aspirin should be given in a dose of 750–1000 mg three times a day, NSAIDs (e.g., ibuprofen) 600 mg three times a day for 1 to 2 weeks, and colchicine 0.5 mg twice daily or 0.5 mg daily in those weighing <70 kg or intolerant to high dose for 3 months.[128] If steroids are used, prednisone in a dose of 0.25–0.5 mg/kg/day is given for 1–2 weeks.[128] For recurrent cases, aspirin and NSAIDs are given for 2–4 weeks, colchicine for 6–12 months, and steroids for 2–4 weeks.[128]

Pericardial Effusion and Cardiac Tamponade

Generally, the pericardial space contains <50 mL of fluid. Accumulation of larger amounts of fluid is usually due to the disease process in the pericardium, which may or may not be related to cancer or a systemic disease. It may range from minimal to moderate and large, with symptoms and signs not only related to the size of effusion but also to the rapidity of fluid collection. In the general population, malignancy is the commonest cause of large pericardial effusion.[132]

The clinical symptoms and signs of pericardial effusion depend on the size, cause, and rate of accumulation of the pericardial fluid. A large but slowly growing effusion, for example, in a patient with malignancy, may lead to fewer symptoms and less-acute presentation, whereas a rapidly accumulating smaller pericardial fluid, for example, a complication of a radiofrequency ablation or cardiac biopsy, may cause acute tamponade. Common symptoms of pericardial effusion include dyspnea on exertion with orthopnea, palpations, chest pain, or tightness. Other nonspecific symptoms include weakness, fatigue, and anorexia. The classic clinical findings in tamponade consist of low blood pressure, distended neck veins, and muffled heart sounds, which is known as Beck's triad. Claude S. Beck described this in 1935 as two cardiac compression triads: acute cardiac compression (low arterial pressure, high venous pressure, quiet heart) and chronic cardiac compression (ascites, high venous pressure, quiet heart).[133]

A 2D echocardiogram is the most common noninvasive test utilized for the diagnosis of pericardial effusion. It not only provides information on the size but also on the features of increased intrapericardial pressure. As for the general population, in patients with cancer the effusion is categorized into small (≤1 cm), moderate (1–2 cm), and large (>2 cm).[134] Signs of hemodynamic compromise and tamponade include the presence of right atrial and right ventricular collapse/compression, respiratory variation in tricuspid and mitral valve inflow velocities, and usually associated with inferior vena cava plethora.[134] See Fig. 6.4.

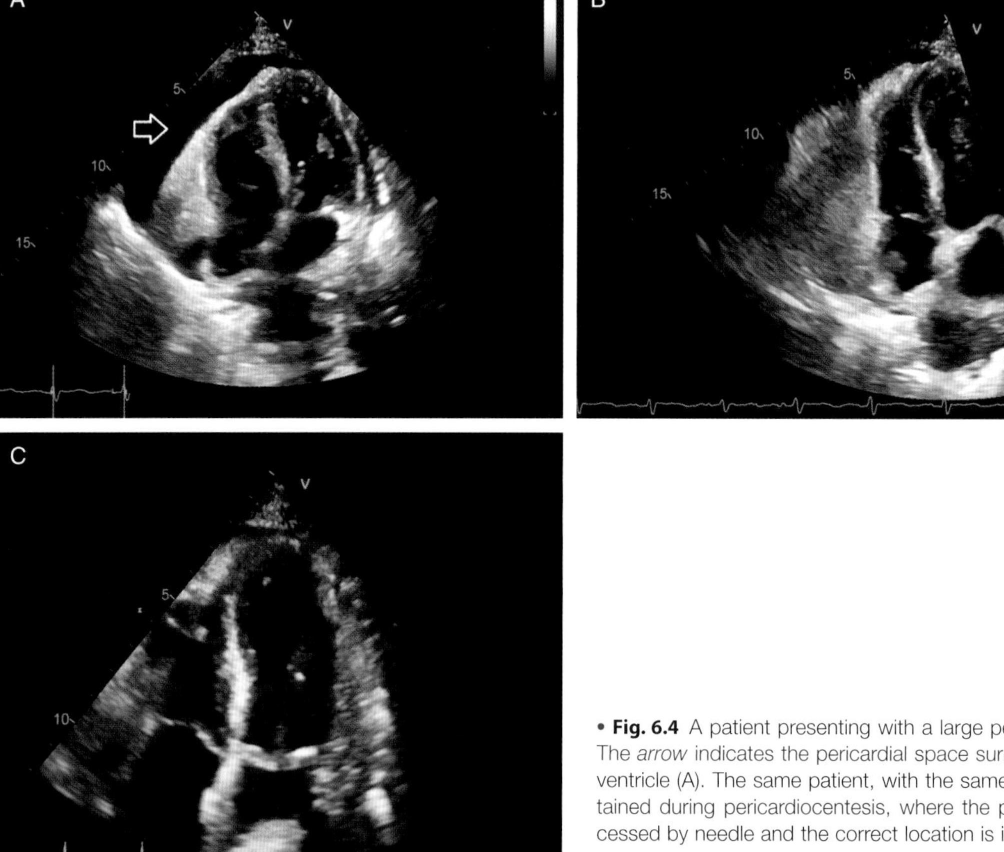

• **Fig. 6.4** A patient presenting with a large pericardial effusion. The *arrow* indicates the pericardial space surrounding the right ventricle (A). The same patient, with the same angle image obtained during pericardiocentesis, where the pericardium is accessed by needle and the correct location is identified by injection of agitated saline; therefore the space appears "white" (B). (C) The same patient when the effusion was fully drained.

The electrocardiogram findings in tamponade classically include low-voltage QRS complexes, electrical alternans, and sinus tachycardia. The combination of sinus tachycardia, low-voltage QRS, and electrical alternans has a high specificity and positive predictive value for the diagnosis of cardiac tamponade in patients with malignant pericardial effusion.[134]

Treatment

In cases with hemodynamic compromise, urgent pericardiocentesis under imaging guidance should be performed. Until pericardial drainage is set up, a patient should be started on intravenous hydration. Vasodilators and diuretics should be avoided. In cancer patients, a percutaneous approach is considered as the first-line therapy. Pericardiectomy is reserved for recurrent pericardial effusions. In the cancer population, percutaneous pericardiocentesis has been shown to be successful in 99% of cases with no procedure-related deaths and is even safe in patients with thrombocytopenia.[135] In one study, the median overall survival was 143 days; older age (i.e., >65 years), lung cancer, platelet count <20,000/mL, and malignant pericardial fluid were independently associated with poor prognosis.[135]

Conclusion

Patients with cancer are at increased risk of cardiovascular disease. Patients with cancer and heart disease are a growing population that deserves continued clinical study at present. They present with significant complexities, and further clinical studies regarding treatment strategies and outcomes are required. Close collaboration between oncologists, cardiologists, pharmacists, and ancillary staff is needed to provide an individualized approach for improving care and outcomes for every patient.

References

1. Lambert JT, Thavendiranathan P. Controversies in the Definition of Cardiotoxicity: Do We Care? Available at https://www.acc.org/latest-in-cardiology/articles/2016/07/07/14/59/controversies-in-the-definition-of-cardiotoxicity; 2016.
2. Seidman A, Hudis C, Pierri MK, et al. Cardiac dysfunction in the trastuzumab clinical trials experience. *J Clin Oncol.* 2002;20:1215–1221.
3. Moja L, Tagliabue L, Balduzzi S, et al. Trastuzumab containing regimens for early breast cancer. *Cochrane Database Syst Revs.* 2012;2012(4):CD006243.
4. Alcan KE, Robeson W, Graham MC, Palestro C, Oliver FH, Benua RS. Early detection of anthracycline-induced cardiotoxicity by stress radionuclide cineangiography in conjunction with Fourier amplitude and phase analysis. *Clin Nucl Med.* 1985;10:160–166.
5. Lenzhofer R, Dudczak R, Gumhold G, Graninger W, Moser K, Spitzy KH. Noninvasive methods for the early detection of doxorubicin-induced cardiomyopathy. *J Cancer Res Clin Oncol.* 1983;106:136–142.
6. McKillop JH, Bristow MR, Goris ML, Billingham ME, Bockemuehl K. Sensitivity and specificity of radionuclide ejection fractions in doxorubicin cardiotoxicity. *Am Heart J.* 1983;106:1048–1056.
7. Pauwels EK, Horning SJ, Goris ML. Sequential equilibrium gated radionuclide angiocardiography for the detection of doxorubicin cardiotoxicity. *Radiother Oncol.* 1983;1:83–87.
8. Ramos A, Meyer RA, Korfhagen J, Wong KY, Kaplan S. Echocardiographic evaluation of adriamycin cardiotoxicity in children. *Cancer Treat Rep.* 1976;60:1281–1284.
9. Lang RM, Badano LP, Mor-Avi V, et al. Recommendations for cardiac chamber quantification by echocardiography in adults: an update from the American Society of Echocardiography and the European Association of Cardiovascular Imaging. *J Am Soc Echocardiogr.* 2015;28:1–39.
10. Hoffmann R, von Bardeleben S, Kasprzak JD, et al. Analysis of regional left ventricular function by cineventriculography, cardiac magnetic resonance imaging, and unenhanced and contrast-enhanced echocardiography: a multicenter comparison of methods. *J Am Coll Cardiol.* 2006;47:121–128.
11. Jenkins C, Chan J, Hanekom L, Marwick TH. Accuracy and feasibility of online 3-dimensional echocardiography for measurement of left ventricular parameters. *J Am Soc Echocardiogr.* 2006;19:1119–1128.
12. Jenkins C, Moir S, Chan J, Rakhit D, Haluska B, Marwick TH. Left ventricular volume measurement with echocardiography: a comparison of left ventricular opacification, three-dimensional echocardiography, or both with magnetic resonance imaging. *Eur Heart J.* 2009;30:98–106.
13. Thavendiranathan P, Grant AD, Negishi T, Plana JC, Popovic ZB, Marwick TH. Reproducibility of echocardiographic techniques for sequential assessment of left ventricular ejection fraction and volumes: application to patients undergoing cancer chemotherapy. *J Am Coll Cardiol.* 2013;61:77–84.
14. McCall R, Stoodley PW, Richards DA, Thomas L. Restrictive cardiomyopathy versus constrictive pericarditis: making the distinction using tissue Doppler imaging. *Eur J Echocardiogr.* 2008;9:591–594.
15. Tei C, Ling LH, Hodge DO, et al. New index of combined systolic and diastolic myocardial performance: a simple and reproducible measure of cardiac function–a study in normals and dilated cardiomyopathy. *J Cardiol.* 1995;26:357–366.
16. Ishii M, Tsutsumi T, Himeno W, et al. Sequential evaluation of left ventricular myocardial performance in children after anthracycline therapy. *Am J Cardiol.* 2000;86:1279–1281.
17. Belham M, Kruger A, Mepham S, Faganello G, Pritchard C. Monitoring left ventricular function in adults receiving anthracycline-containing chemotherapy. *Eur J Heart Fail.* 2007;9:409–414.
18. Hare JL, Brown JK, Leano R, Jenkins C, Woodward N, Marwick TH. Use of myocardial deformation imaging to detect preclinical myocardial dysfunction before conventional measures in patients undergoing breast cancer treatment with trastuzumab. *Am Heart J.* 2009;158:294–301.
19. Fallah-Rad N, Walker JR, Wassef A, et al. The utility of cardiac biomarkers, tissue velocity and strain imaging, and cardiac magnetic resonance imaging in predicting early left ventricular dysfunction in patients with human epidermal growth factor receptor II-positive breast cancer treated with adjuvant trastuzumab therapy. *J Am Coll Cardiol.* 2011;57:2263–2270.
20. Sawaya H, Sebag IA, Plana JC, et al. Early detection and prediction of cardiotoxicity in chemotherapy-treated patients. *Am J Cardiol.* 2011;107:1375–1380.

21. Thavendiranathan P, Poulin F, Lim KD, Plana JC, Woo A, Marwick TH. Use of myocardial strain imaging by echocardiography for the early detection of cardiotoxicity in patients during and after cancer chemotherapy: a systematic review. *J Am Coll Cardiol.* 2014;63:2751–2768.
22. Narayan HK, French B, Khan AM, et al. Noninvasive measures of ventricular-arterial coupling and circumferential strain predict cancer therapeutics-related cardiac dysfunction. *JACC Cardiovasc Imaging.* 2016;9:1131–1141.
23. Plana JC, Galderisi M, Barac A, et al. Expert consensus for multimodality imaging evaluation of adult patients during and after cancer therapy: a report from the American Society of Echocardiography and the European Association of Cardiovascular Imaging. *J Am Soc Echocardiogr.* 2014;27:911–939.
24. Alexander J, Dainiak N, Berger HJ, et al. Serial assessment of doxorubicin cardiotoxicity with quantitative radionuclide angiocardiography. *N Engl J Med.* 1979;300:278–283.
25. Schwartz RG, McKenzie WB, Alexander J, et al. Congestive heart failure and left ventricular dysfunction complicating doxorubicin therapy. Seven-year experience using serial radionuclide angiocardiography. *Am J Med.* 1987;82:1109–1118.
26. Zhang S, Liu X, Bawa-Khalfe T, et al. Identification of the molecular basis of doxorubicin-induced cardiotoxicity. *Nat Med.* 2012;18:1639–1642.
27. Srikanthan K, Klug R, Tirona M, et al. Creating a biomarker panel for early detection of chemotherapy related cardiac dysfunction in breast cancer patients. *J Clin Exp Cardiol.* 2017;8:507.
28. Yancy CW, Jessup M, Bozkurt B, et al. 2013 ACCF/AHA guideline for the management of heart failure. *Circulation.* 2013;128:e240–e327.
29. Said R, Banchs J, Wheler J, et al. The prognostic significance of left ventricular ejection fraction in patients with advanced cancer treated in phase I clinical trials. *Ann Oncol.* 2014;25:276–282.
30. Reuss CS, Wilansky SM, Lester SJ, et al. Using mitral 'annulus reversus' to diagnose constrictive pericarditis. *Eur J Echocardiogr.* 2009;10:372–375.
31. Heidenreich PA, Hancock SL, Lee BK, Mariscal CS, Schnittger I. Asymptomatic cardiac disease following mediastinal irradiation. *J Am Coll Cardiol.* 2003;42:743–749.
32. Lund MB, Ihlen H, Voss BM, et al. Increased risk of heart valve regurgitation after mediastinal radiation for Hodgkin's disease: an echocardiographic study. *Heart.* 1996;75:591–595.
33. Al-Mamgani A, Baartman L, Baaijens M, de Pree I, Incrocci L, Levendag PC. Cardiac metastases. *Int J Clin Oncol.* 2008;13:369–372.
34. Eisenhauer EA, Therasse P, Bogaerts J, et al. New response evaluation criteria in solid tumours: revised RECIST guideline (version 1.1). *Eur J Cancer.* 2009;45:228–247.
35. Marshall VF, Middleton RG, Holswade GR, Goldsmith EI. Surgery for renal cell carcinoma in the vena cava. *J Urol.* 1970;103:414–420.
36. Hanfling SM. Metastatic cancer to the heart. Review of the literature and report of 127 cases. *Circulation.* 1960;22:474–483.
37. Xu ZF, Yong F, Chen YY, Pan AZ. Uterine intravenous leiomyomatosis with cardiac extension: imaging characteristics and literature review. *World J Clin Oncol.* 2013;4:25–28.
38. Jun CH, Sim da W, Kim SH, et al. Risk factors for patients with stage IVB hepatocellular carcinoma and extension into the heart: prognostic and therapeutic implications. *Yonsei Med J.* 2014;55:379–386.
39. Steinberg C, Boudreau S, Leveille F, Lamothe M, Chagnon P, Boulais I. Advanced hepatocellular carcinoma with subtotal occlusion of the inferior vena cava and a right atrial mass. *Case Rep Vasc Med.* 2013;2013:489373.
40. Detterbeck FC, Parsons AM. Thymic tumors. *Ann Thorac Surg.* 2004;77:1860–1869.
41. El Banna M, Geraldes L, Grapsa J, et al. Large mediastinal neoplasm penetrating the myocardium. *Perfusion.* 2019;34:170–172.
42. Ban-Hoefen M, Zeglin MA, Bisognano JD. Diffuse large B cell lymphoma presenting as a cardiac mass and odynophagia. *Cardiol J.* 2008;15:471–474.
43. Fuzellier JF, Torossian PF, Rubin S, Baehrel B. [Fibroelastoma of the tricuspid valve presenting with syncope]. *Arch Mal Coeur Vaiss.* 2004;97:67–69.
44. Aoyagi S, Tayama E, Yokokura Y, Yokokura H. Right atrial myxoma in a patient presenting with syncope. *Kurume Med J.* 2004;51:91–93.
45. Kubota H, Takamoto S, Kotsuka Y, et al. Surgical treatment of malignant tumors of the right heart. *Jpn Heart J.* 2002;43:263–271.
46. Alzeerah MA, Singh R, Jarrous A. Large B-cell lymphoma of the atria. *Tex Heart Inst J.* 2003;30:74–75.
47. Rettmar K, Stierle U, Sheikhzadeh A, Diederich KW. Primary angiosarcoma of the heart. Report of a case and review of the literature. *Jpn Heart J.* 1993;34:667–683.
48. Marti G, Galve E, Huguet J, Soler Soler J. [Cardiac metastases of malignant melanoma mimicking sick sinus syndrome]. *Rev Esp Cardiol.* 2004;57:589–591.
49. Schrepfer S, Deuse T, Detter C, et al. Successful resection of a symptomatic right ventricular lipoma. *Ann Thorac Surg.* 2003;76:1305–1307.
50. Reddy G, Ahmed MI, Lloyd SG, Brott BC, Bittner V. Left anterior descending coronary artery occlusion secondary to metastatic squamous cell carcinoma presenting as ST-segment-elevation myocardial infarction. *Circulation.* 2014;129:e652–e653.
51. Weinberg BA, Pinkerton CA, Waller BF. External compression by metastatic squamous cell carcinoma: a rare cause of left main coronary artery narrowing. *Clin Cardiol.* 1990;13:360–366.
52. Leeies M, Weldon E. STEMI stymie: metastatic cancer and cardiac tamponade presenting as inferior STEMI. *Ann Emerg Med.* 2011;57:221–224.
53. Kirkpatrick JN, Wong T, Bednarz JE, et al. Differential diagnosis of cardiac masses using contrast echocardiographic perfusion imaging. *J Am Coll Cardiol.* 2004;43:1412–1419.
54. Flipse TR, Tazelaar HD, Holmes Jr DR. Diagnosis of malignant cardiac disease by endomyocardial biopsy. *Mayo Clin Proc.* 1990;65:1415–1422.
55. Veinot JP. Endomyocardial biopsy of cardiac neoplastic involvement. *Ann Thorac Surg.* 2003;75:1363–1364.
56. Hosokawa Y, Kodani E, Kusama Y, et al. Cardiac angiosarcoma diagnosed by transvenous endomyocardial biopsy with the aid of transesophageal echocardiography and intra-procedural consultation. *Int Heart J.* 2010;51:367–369.
57. Kamiya K, Sakakibara M, Yamada S, et al. Diffuse large B-cell lymphoma diagnosed by intracardiac echocardiography-guided cardiac tumor biopsy. *Intern Med.* 2012;51:1043–1047.
58. Yusuf SW, Bathina JD, Qureshi S, et al. Cardiac tumors in a tertiary care cancer hospital: clinical features, echocardiographic findings, treatment and outcomes. *Heart Int.* 2012;7:e4.
59. Centofanti P, Di Rosa E, Deorsola L, et al. Primary cardiac tumors: early and late results of surgical treatment in 91 patients. *Ann Thorac Surg.* 1999;68:1236–1241.

60. Perchinsky MJ, Lichtenstein SV, Tyers GF. Primary cardiac tumors: forty years' experience with 71 patients. *Cancer.* 1997;79:1809–1815.
61. Bear PA, Moodie DS. Malignant primary cardiac tumors. The Cleveland Clinic experience, 1956 to 1986. *Chest.* 1987;92:860–862.
62. Burke AP, Cowan D, Virmani R. Primary sarcomas of the heart. *Cancer.* 1992;69:387–395.
63. Kim CH, Dancer JY, Coffey D, et al. Clinicopathologic study of 24 patients with primary cardiac sarcomas: a 10-year single institution experience. *Hum Pathol.* 2008;39:933–938.
64. Simpson L, Kumar SK, Okuno SH, et al. Malignant primary cardiac tumors: review of a single institution experience. *Cancer.* 2008;112:2440–2446.
65. Ambrosio GB. [Frequency of cardiac metastasis: review of 2222 autopsies and critical assessment]. *Arch Sci Med.* 1980;137:29–32.
66. Allen BC, Mohammed TL, Tan CD, Miller DV, Williamson EE, Kirsch JS. Metastatic melanoma to the heart. *Curr Probl Diagn Radiol.* 2012;41:159–164.
67. Glancy DL, Roberts WC. The heart in malignant melanoma. A study of 70 autopsy cases. *Am J Cardiol.* 1968;21:555–571.
68. Aerts BR, Kock MC, Kofflard MJ, Plaisier PW. Cardiac metastasis of malignant melanoma: a case report. *Neth Heart J.* 2014;22:39–41.
69. Silverman NA. Primary cardiac tumors. *Ann Surg.* 1980; 191:127–138.
70. Burke APTH, Butany J, Tazelaar H, et al. *Cardiac Sarcoma*: IARC Press; 2004.
71. Mayer F, Aebert H, Rudert M, et al. Primary malignant sarcomas of the heart and great vessels in adult patients–a single-center experience. *Oncologist.* 2007;12:1134–1142.
72. Llombart-Cussac A, Pivot X, Contesso G, et al. Adjuvant chemotherapy for primary cardiac sarcomas: the IGR experience. *Br J Cancer.* 1998;78:1624–1628.
73. Burgert SJ, Strickman NE, Carrol CL, Falcone M. Cardiac Kaposi's sarcoma following heart transplantation. *Catheter Cardiovasc Interv.* 2000;49:208–212.
74. Raaf HN, Raaf JH. Sarcomas related to the heart and vasculature. *Semin Surg Oncol.* 1994;10:374–382.
75. Knobel B, Rosman P, Kishon Y, Husar M. Intracardiac primary fibrosarcoma. Case report and literature review. *J Thorac Cardiovasc Surg.* 1992;40:227–230.
76. Laya MB, Mailliard JA, Bewtra C, Levin HS. Malignant fibrous histiocytoma of the heart. A case report and review of the literature. *Cancer.* 1987;59:1026–1031.
77. Donsbeck AV, Ranchere D, Coindre JM, et al. Primary cardiac sarcomas: an immunohistochemical and grading study with long-term follow-up of 24 cases. *Histopathology.* 1999;34:295–304.
78. Bussani R, De-Giorgio F, Abbate A, Silvestri F. Cardiac metastases. *J Clin Pathol.* 2007;60:27–34.
79. Cates CU, Virmani R, Vaughn WK, Robertson RM. Electrocardiographic markers of cardiac metastasis. *Am Heart J.* 1986;112:1297–1303.
80. Butany J, Leong SW, Carmichael K, Komeda M. A 30-year analysis of cardiac neoplasms at autopsy. *Can J Cardiol.* 2005; 21:675–680.
81. Rafajlovski S, Tatic V, Ilic S, Kanjuh V. [Frequency of metastatic tumors in the heart]. *Vojnosanit Pregl.* 2005;62:915–920.
82. Abraham KP, Reddy V, Gattuso P. Neoplasms metastatic to the heart: review of 3314 consecutive autopsies. *Am J Cardiovasc Pathol.* 1990;3:195–198.
83. Karwinski B, Svendsen E. Trends in cardiac metastasis. *APMIS.* 1989;97:1018–1024.
84. Goudie RB. Secondary tumours of the heart and pericardium. *Br Heart J.* 1955;17:183–188.
85. Lockwood WB, Broghamer, WL. Jr. The changing prevalence of secondary cardiac neoplasms as related to cancer therapy. *Cancer.* 1980;45:2659–2662.
86. Silvestri F, Bussani R, Pavletic N, Mannone T. Metastases of the heart and pericardium. *G Ital Cardiol (Rome).* 1997;27: 1252–1255.
87. Abioye AA, Maolomo IM. Prevalence of cardiac tumours at autopsy in Ibadan. *Trop Geogr Med.* 1975;27:25–30.
88. Deloach JF, Haynes JW. Secondary tumors of heart and pericardium; review of the subject and report of one hundred thirty-seven cases. *Arch Intern Med.* 1953;91:224–249.
89. MacGee W. Metastatic and invasive tumours involving the heart in a geriatric population: a necropsy study. *Virchows Archiv.* 1991;419:183–189.
90. Manojlovic S. Metastatic carcinomas involving the heart. Review of postmortem examination. *Zentralbl Allg Pathol.* 1990;136:657–661.
91. Tzani A, Doulamis IP, Mylonas KS, Avgerinos DV, Nasioudis D. Cardiac tumors in pediatric patients: a systematic review. *World J Pediatr Congenit Heart Surg.* 2017;8:624–632.
92. Reardon MJ, Walkes JC, Benjamin R. Therapy insight: malignant primary cardiac tumors. *Nat Clin Pract Cardiovasc Med.* 2006;3:548–553.
93. Burns A. *Observations on Some of the Most Frequent and Important Diseases of the Heart, etc.; on the Aneurism of the thoracic aorta; ... Illustrated by Cases.* Thomas Bryce and Co.; 1809.
94. Yater WM. Tumors of the heart and pericardium: pathology, symptomatology, and report of nine cases. *JAMA Intern Med.* 1931;48:627–666.
95. Barnes AR, Beaver DC, Snell AM. Primary sarcoma of the heart: report of a case with electrocardiographic and pathological studies. *Am Heart J.* 1934;9:480.
96. Mauer E. Successful removal of tumor of the heart. *J Thorac Surg.* 1952;3:479.
97. Craaford C. Panel discussion of late results of mitral commissurotomy. In: Lam CR, ed. *Henry Ford Hospital International Symposium on Cardiovascular Surgery.* W. B. Saunders Company; 1955:202–203.
98. Kay JH, Anderson RM, Meihaus J, et al. Surgical removal of an intracavitary left ventricular myxoma. *Circulation.* 1959;20:881–886.
99. Gerbode F, Kerth WJ, Hill JD. Surgical management of tumors of the heart. *Surgery.* 1967;61:94–101.
100. Cooley DA, Reardon MJ, Frazier OH, Angelini P. Human cardiac explantation and autotransplantation: application in a patient with a large cardiac pheochromocytoma. *Tex Heart Inst J.* 1985;12:171–176.
101. Hoffmeier A, Scheld HH, Tjan TD, et al. Ex situ resection of primary cardiac tumors. *Thorac Cardiovasc Surg.* 2003;51: 99–101.
102. Ewer MS, Benjamin RS. *Doxorubicin cardiotoxicity: clinical apect, recognition, monitoring, treatment, and prevention. Cancer and the Heart.* BC Decker; 2006.
103. Zhang PJ, Brooks JS, Goldblum JR, et al. Primary cardiac sarcomas: a clinicopathologic analysis of a series with follow-up information in 17 patients and emphasis on long-term survival. *Hum Pathol.* 2008;39:1385–1395.

104. Gross BH, Glazer GM, Francis IR. CT of intracardiac and intrapericardial masses. *Am J Roentgenol.* 1983;140:903–907.
105. Winther C, Timmermans-Wielenga V, Daugaard S, Mortensen SA, Sander K, Andersen CB. Primary cardiac tumors: a clinicopathologic evaluation of four cases. *Cardiovasc Pathol.* 2011;20:63–67.
106. Putnam JB, Jr, Sweeney MS, Colon R, Lanza LA, Frazier OH, Cooley DA. Primary cardiac sarcomas. *Ann Thorac Surg.* 1991;51:906–910.
107. Lip GY, Chin BS, Blann AD. Cancer and the prothrombotic state. *Lancet Oncol.* 2002;3:27–34.
108. Yusuf SW, Razeghi P, Yeh ET. The diagnosis and management of cardiovascular disease in cancer patients. *Curr Probl Cardiol.* 2008;33:163–196.
109. Venkatesulu BP, Mahadevan LS, Aliru ML, et al. Radiation-induced endothelial vascular injury: a review of possible mechanisms. *JACC Basic Transl Sci.* 2018;3:563–572.
110. Yusuf SW, Howell RM, Gomez D, Pinnix CC, Iliescu CA, Banchs J. Radiation-related heart and vascular disease. *Future Oncol.* 2015;11:2067–2076.
111. Bathina JD, Yusuf SW. 5-Fluorouracil-induced coronary vasospasm. *J Cardiovasc Med.* 2010;11:281–284.
112. Yeh ET, Bickford CL. Cardiovascular complications of cancer therapy: incidence, pathogenesis, diagnosis, and management. *J Am Coll Cardiol.* 2009;53:2231–2247.
113. Yusuf SW, Yeh E.T.H. *Acute coronary syndrome in cancer patients. Acute Care of the Cancer Patient.* Taylor & Francis; 2005:567–578.
114. Oren O, Herrmann J. Arterial events in cancer patients-the case of acute coronary thrombosis. *J Thorac Dis.* 2018;10:S4367–S4385.
115. Bharadwaj A, Potts J, Mohamed MO, et al. Acute myocardial infarction treatments and outcomes in 6.5 million patients with a current or historical diagnosis of cancer in the USA. *Eur Heart J.* 2020;41:2183–2193.
116. Pothineni NV, Shah NN, Rochlani Y, et al. Temporal trends and outcomes of acute myocardial infarction in patients with cancer. *Ann Transl Med.* 2017;5:482.
117. Thygesen K, Alpert JS, Jaffe AS, et al. Fourth universal definition of myocardial infarction. *J Am Coll Cardiol.* 2018;72:2231–2264.
118. Thygesen K, Alpert JS, Jaffe AS, et al. Fourth universal definition of myocardial infarction (2018). *Global Heart.* 2018;13:305–338.
119. Yusuf SW, Daraban N, Abbasi N, Lei X, Durand JB, Daher IN. Treatment and outcomes of acute coronary syndrome in the cancer population. *Clin Cardiol.* 2012;35:443–450.
120. Velders MA, Boden H, Hofma SH, et al. Outcome after ST elevation myocardial infarction in patients with cancer treated with primary percutaneous coronary intervention. *Am J Cardiol.* 2013;112:1867–1872.
121. Sarkiss MG, Yusuf SW, Warneke CL, et al. Impact of aspirin therapy in cancer patients with thrombocytopenia and acute coronary syndromes. *Cancer.* 2007;109:621–627.
122. Iliescu C, Grines CL, Herrmann J, et al. SCAI expert consensus statement: evaluation, management, and special considerations of cardio-oncology patients in the cardiac catheterization laboratory (Endorsed by the Cardiological Society of India, and Sociedad Latino Americana de Cardiologia Intervencionista). *Catheter Cardiovasc Interv.* 2016;87:895–899.
123. Adler Y, Charron P, Imazio M, et al. 2015 ESC Guidelines for the diagnosis and management of pericardial diseases: the task force for the diagnosis and management of Pericardial Diseases of the European Society of Cardiology (ESC) Endorsed by: The European Association for Cardio-Thoracic Surgery (EACTS). *Eur Heart J.* 2015;36:2921–2964.
124. Imazio M, Spodick DH, Brucato A, Trinchero R, Adler Y. Controversial issues in the management of pericardial diseases. *Circulation.* 2010;121:916–928.
125. Zayas R, Anguita M, Torres F, et al. Incidence of specific etiology and role of methods for specific etiologic diagnosis of primary acute pericarditis. *Am J Cardiol.* 1995;75:378–382.
126. Imazio M, Demichelis B, Cecchi E, et al. Cardiac troponin I in acute pericarditis. *J Am Coll Cardiol.* 2003;42:2144–2148.
127. Permanyer-Miralda G, Sagrista-Sauleda J, Soler-Soler J. Primary acute pericardial disease: a prospective series of 231 consecutive patients. *Am J Cardiol.* 1985;56:623–630.
128. Yusuf SW, Hassan SA, Mouhayar E, Negi SI, Banchs J, O'Gara PT. Pericardial disease: a clinical review. *Expert Rev Cardiovasc Ther.* 2016;14:525–539.
129. Klein AL, Abbara S, Agler DA, et al. American Society of Echocardiography clinical recommendations for multimodality cardiovascular imaging of patients with pericardial disease: endorsed by the Society for Cardiovascular Magnetic Resonance and Society of Cardiovascular Computed Tomography. *J Am Soc Echocardiogr.* 2013;26:965–1012.
130. Imazio M, Bobbio M, Cecchi E, et al. Colchicine in addition to conventional therapy for acute pericarditis: results of the COlchicine for acute PEricarditis (COPE) trial. *Circulation.* 2005;112:2012–2016.
131. Lotrionte M, Biondi-Zoccai G, Imazio M, et al. International collaborative systematic review of controlled clinical trials on pharmacologic treatments for acute pericarditis and its recurrences. *Am Heart J.* 2010;160:662–670.
132. Corey GR, Campbell PT, Van Trigt P, et al. Etiology of large pericardial effusions. *Am J Med.* 1993;95:209–213.
133. Beck CS. Two cardiac compression triads. *JAMA.* 1935;104:714–716.
134. Argula RG, Negi SI, Banchs J, Yusuf SW. Role of a 12-lead electrocardiogram in the diagnosis of cardiac tamponade as diagnosed by transthoracic echocardiography in patients with malignant pericardial effusion. *Clin Cardiol.* 2015;38:139–144.
135. El Haddad D, Iliescu C, Yusuf SW, et al. Outcomes of cancer patients undergoing percutaneous pericardiocentesis for pericardial effusion. *J Am Coll Cardiol.* 2015;66:1119–1128.

7

Personalized Cancer Care

ALEXANDER G. HERIOT

Introduction

The management of cancer patients has evolved exponentially over time. At the start of the 19th century surgery was the only available modality to treat cancer, and surgery itself was limited to superficial tumors such as breast and skin cancer due to the lack of anesthesia and the risk of sepsis. This resulted in surgery being a hazardous undertaking and the speed of surgery being the primary goal. The increasing availability of general anesthesia in the early 19th century, along with the introduction of aseptic techniques by Lister, opened the door to more invasive surgery and a number of surgeons across Europe and the United States, including Billroth, Kocher, Mayo, and Crile, developed new operations to treat malignancies. There was a progressive extension of both precision and radicality in approach, perhaps best personified by the work of William Halsted, who could perhaps be considered the "father" of cancer surgery. The development of the Halsted radical mastectomy, with the aim of removing all the areas of potential spread of breast cancer, led this mutilating surgery to become the standard of care for the next 75 years, even though the improvement in survival from breast cancer at that time had plateaued earlier with less radical surgery.

While surgery has remained the mainstay of cancer care, the introduction and development of other therapeutic pillars of cancer management have modified cancer care. The discovery of x-rays and radium by Roentgen and Curie led to the uptake of radiotherapy from the start of the 20th century, with varying efficacy across different tumors. The use of poisonous gas in the First World War led to the development of therapeutic drugs to treat cancer, initially "liquid" tumors such as leukemias and lymphomas, and then subsequently solid tumors. This has accelerated over the last 30 years as a result of the expansion of molecular biology and the increasing understanding of the molecular drivers of cancer, resulting in the development of targeted drug therapies aimed at specific molecular targets in a tumor type. More recently, the fourth pillar of cancer care has been the development of immunotherapy over the last decade. Immunotherapy, with drugs targeting CTLA-4 or PD-1 receptors, reducing immune suppression induced by the tumor has demonstrated dramatic results, predominantly in tumors with higher immunogenicity, such as melanomas, renal cell cancers, and microsatellite unstable tumors. The impact on other tumor types such as microsatellite stable bowel cancer has been far more limited, and research is in progress to explore how these drugs interact with standard chemotherapy, radiotherapy, and surgery.

The multiple available modalities of care pose challenges when determining the specific management of individual patients. The principle of utilizing all relevant modalities to deliver the best care and outcome for cancer patients is fundamental to modern cancer care and has been delivered through multidisciplinary care. The other principle has been the increased "tailoring" of care to the individual patient, rather than broad brushstroke care for particular tumor types. This "personalization" of cancer care has perhaps been the most significant change in management over the last 20 years. This chapter explores how this personalization has evolved and how it is delivered.

Multidisciplinary Care

The coordination of care across different modalities to deliver true multidisciplinary care poses several challenges. In the past this was undertaken through referral of patients from one clinician to another at varying stages of their treatment, without an integrated approach. This approach varied across different centers, with centers focused on cancer specifically having a more integrated approach; however, this was very specific to institutions and often the lack of integration led to inefficiencies in care and patient dissatisfaction. In the UK, the concept of multidisciplinary care first became more mainstream following the release of the Calman-Heine report in 1995.[1] This report recommended that cancer care should specifically involve nonsurgical oncologic input into services and that a lead clinician with a specific interest in cancer care should organize and coordinate the entire range of cancer services provided within a cancer unit. The report also recommended the instigation of multidisciplinary team (MDT) meetings to facilitate the delivery of multidisciplinary care, which will be discussed later. Although for a number of cancer units, this was business as usual, for others this was a radical change, and this report led to a broad adoption of this approach across the UK. This broad uptake perhaps happened later in the United States and was driven by other factors. For example, the adoption of tumor boards for rectal cancer management in the United States has more recently been driven by the Optimizing Surgical Treatment of Rectal Cancer (OSTRiCh) group, a consortium of 18 health care institutions whose purpose is to transform the delivery of rectal cancer care in the United States.[2] This is now supported by the American College of Surgeons, which has led to a significant uptake in a multidisciplinary approach to rectal cancer care in the United States.

The Multidisciplinary Team

The MDT is the collection of health care professionals across different disciplines, each providing specific services to ensure that the patient receives optimum care and management. While MDTs are now commonplace across a range of clinical areas, formal multidisciplinary meetings (MDMs) were initially instituted in a more general manner following the Calman-Heine report discussed earlier. The management of individual patients is discussed with representatives from all required specialties. Table 7.1 provides a summary of potential MDT members for a colorectal cancer MDT.

Coordination of care within an MDM has the potential to raise the quality of care for patients. For example, a study assessed the initiation of a colorectal cancer MDM in a hospital in the UK. Of the 310 patients, 176 were managed prior to the establishment of the MDT and 134 after establishment.[3] There was a significant increase in the administration of adjuvant chemotherapy to node-positive patients following the initiation of the MDT, with a subsequent increase in the 3-year survival of these patients from 58% to 66%. Multidisciplinary management is also cost-effective. Fader et al. reported on the cost-effectiveness of multidisciplinary management of 104 patients with melanoma in Michigan as compared to a consecutive sample of 104 patients treated in the Michigan community, with a saving of $1600 per patient with multidisciplinary management.[4]

The nature of a MDM is the focus on each individual patient. This facilitates the potential to shift from a protocolized management plan for a broad number of patients to a more tailored management plan for individual patients. Advances in imaging modalities have been the initial catalyst that has driven the individualization of care.

TABLE 7.1 Members of the Multidisciplinary Team for Colorectal Cancer

The multidisciplinary team may include the following members:
Care coordinator (as determined by multidisciplinary team members)[a]
Gastroenterologist with colorectal expertise[a]
General and/or colorectal surgeon[a]
Medical oncologist[a]
Nurse (with appropriate expertise)[a]
Pathologist[a]
Radiation oncologist[a]
Radiologist with expertise in MRI[a]
Stomal therapy nurse
Clinical psychologist
Clinical trials coordinator
Dietitian
Exercise physiologist
Fertility specialist
General practitioner
Geneticist or genetic counselor
Hepato-pancreatobiliary surgeon
Interventional radiologist
Nuclear medicine physician with PET expertise
Occupational therapist
Palliative care specialist
Pharmacist
Physiotherapist
Psychiatrist
Social worker
Spiritual/pastoral care
Thoracic surgeon.

[a]Denotes core members. The core members of the multidisciplinary team are expected to attend most multidisciplinary team meetings, either in person or remotely. *MRI*, Magnetic resonance imaging; *PET*, positron emission tomography.

Imaging

The development of imaging techniques is an essential driver for the development of cancer care. The management of solid tumors is determined primarily by the stage of the tumor, both local extent and distant metastases. Detailed staging classifications are available for each tumor type through the Union for International Cancer Control (UICC), with tumor stage divided into T (tumor), N (nodal), and M (metastases). The specific imaging required for each tumor type will vary; however, determination of the tumor stage prior to any therapeutic intervention is essential.

Computed Tomography

Computed tomography (CT) scanning was invented in 1967 by Sir Geoffrey Hounsfield at the EMI laboratories in the UK, with the first CT scanners installed in the United States in 1973.[5] By 1980, 3 million CT scans had been performed, and by 2005 that number had grown to 68 million CT scans performed annually. Shortened scan times and increased matrix size have been major developments allowing much greater resolution from the scanners. Hounsfield and McCormack were awarded the Nobel Prize for Medicine in 1979 for the development of computer-assisted tomography.

Cross-sectional imaging with a CT scan is the mainstay of cancer staging and is integral to cancer management. Cross-sectional imaging can be used to assess tumor response using the Response Evaluation Criteria in Solid Tumors (RECIST) criteria. This provides a simple and pragmatic methodology to evaluate the activity and efficacy of new cancer therapeutics in solid tumors, using validated and consistent criteria to assess changes in tumor burden.

Magnetic Resonance Imaging

The first magnetic resonance imaging (MRI) was performed in a patient in 1977 by Damadian in Nottingham. Utilizing a magnetic field, rather than radiation, it detects energy release by protons in the various tissues that have been aligned by the generated magnetic field, with the release of energy determined by the different tissue types. It can provide detailed cross-sectional imaging with greater resolution of soft tissues when compared to CT scans. Lauterber and Mansfield were subsequently awarded the Nobel Prize for Medicine in 2003 for their work on MRI.

Positron Emission Tomography

While CT and MRI provide anatomic cross-sectional imaging, positron emission tomography (PET) scans provide functional imaging and measure the metabolic activity of tissues. Utilization of radionucleotide tracers and measurement of positron emission from the breakdown of the tracers allows metabolic activity in tissues to be assessed. Most commonly, fluorodeoxyglucose (FDG) is utilized as the tracer with more glucose taken up by metabolically more active tissues. The use of different tracers allows specific tissues to be targeted, such as neuroendocrine tumors (NETs) in the case of a Gatate tracer. PET scans are usually combined with a CT scan to allow the anatomic resolution of the PET scan. In addition to staging tumors, PET scans can be used in follow up to assess the response to treatment, such as radiation or chemotherapy, by measuring changes in metabolic activity. Quantitative measurement is made using PET Response Criteria in Solid Tumors (PERCIST).

Molecular Aspects and Personalized Therapy

There has been a revolution in cancer management over the last 20 years, and this has continued to accelerate. Management decisions have previously been determined by clinical parameters and variables, the specifics of which have been improved by the developments in imaging described earlier. Although this has led to treatment becoming more individualized, this remains a fairly unidimensional approach, driven by tumor stage and taking no account of the biological variables between individual tumors. Information on the biology of individual tumors is now becoming available and is beginning to influence and direct aspects of cancer management. This led to the term "personalized medicine" to be applied to this approach. It was first applied in 1999 in an article in the *Wall Street Journal* entitled "New Era of Personalized Medicine – Targeting Drugs for each unique Genetic Profile." The article described the use of single-nucleotide polymorphism analysis for cancer drug development and generated significant excitement. Further advances in molecular biology and understanding of the hallmarks of cancer over the last 20 years have started to permeate and influence management across all modalities of treatment and even facilitated a new pillar of cancer management over the last decade in immunotherapy. It is a long way from the position where the biological and molecular tumor factors predominate over clinical factors such as tumor stage; however, the former definitely have an increasing impact on management. The "omic" information available for an individual tumor includes genomic, transcriptomic, and proteomic data that can now be obtained rapidly with readily available high throughput sequencers, allowing the molecular signature to be used in both a predictive and prognostic manner. The former allows identification of potential therapeutic targets and determining what therapy can be used, and the latter provides prognostic biomarkers that can provide information on the patients overall cancer outcome. The development of personalized or "precision" therapy is ongoing, and the degree of research and interest is reflected by the increasing number of publications on the subject. The degree and nature of personalization vary across different tumor types and treatment modalities. Some potential examples and the impact on therapies are considered in Fig. 7.1.

Treatment Modalities

Surgery

Surgery was the original cancer therapy and was inevitably anatomically based. The principle of personalization of care is also delivered through surgery. In 1996 Dr. Blake Cady in his Presidential Address to the New England Surgical Society commented that "the art of surgical oncology is to apply basic principles flexibly to the individual patient."[6] An example of this has been the refinement of lymphadenectomy across different tumors. The broad principle of removing all draining lymphatic tissue of a tumor such as a breast cancer or melanoma has been modified with the use of sentinel node sampling, allowing identification and excision of the primary draining lymph node alone, facilitating selective lymphadenectomy only if the sentinel lymph node is involved, thereby individualizing the surgical procedure and reducing morbidity.

The impact of "omic" data can also be used to directly influence whether a patient undergoes a surgical procedure.[7]

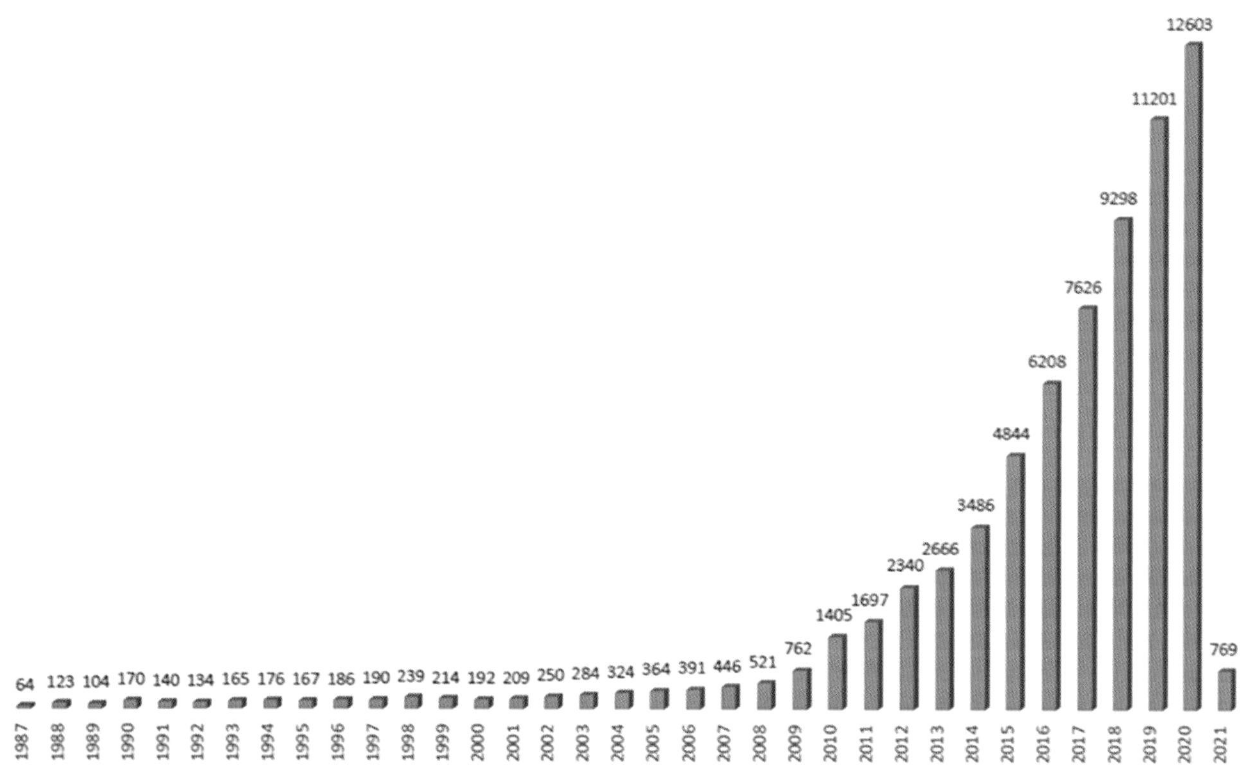

• **Fig. 7.1** Personalized medicine publications 1987–2021.

Percutaneous biopsies of thyroid nodules can be nondiagnostic in up to 30% of cases, necessitating surgical resection to make a diagnosis. The application of commercially available gene expression data obtained from biopsies using *Afirma* (Veracyte, San Francisco, CA, USA) testing can confirm a benign nodule with 92% sensitivity and a negative predictive value of 93%, allowing surgery to be avoided in these cases.[8]

An area where there has been a paradigm shift in management with personalized therapy, facilitated through both multidisciplinary management and molecular developments, has been gastrointestinal stromal tumors (GISTs), with dramatic changes to the management algorithms for these tumors. Historically, the only treatment option was surgical resection, with a significant number of patients having irresectable tumors or developing recurrent disease. Identification of c-KIT as a molecular driver for GIST tumors allowed the development of a small-molecule inhibitor against the KIT protein-tyrosine kinase. This molecule, imatinib mesylate, was one of the first “targeted” chemotherapies, and induced dramatic responses in many GIST tumors with significant reduction in size and growth stabilization. This has led to targeted therapy being used as first-line therapy in disease that is considered borderline resectability, with subsequent surgical resection being undertaken. Targeted therapy can also be applied to metastatic GISTs and generate an almost complete response of the tumor to treatment with stabilization and prevention of tumor growth. If subsequently any focal tumor area beings to grow, presumably as a result of a tumor “clone” escaping suppression, selective surgical resection can be applied to any focal tumor growth.[9]

Radiotherapy

Radiotherapy is a core component of multidisciplinary management of a number of tumors, and for selective tumors, such as anal cancer, it is the primary treatment modality. Clinical and technical factors have been major facilitators for the personalization of radiotherapy, with molecular factors starting to impact more recently. Advances in cross-sectional imaging and resolution have helped refine radiotherapy planning, reducing the amount of normal tissue to be irradiated while maximizing the dose to the body of the tumor and the margins. This anatomic and planning refinement has progressed to the application of stereotactic ablative body radiotherapy (SABR), which is a cutting-edge technique used to deliver highly focused doses of radiation to a very small area of the body, allowing delivery of a much higher dose to a small area in comparison with conventional radiotherapy. This can deliver local control for small areas of disease, such as small lung metastases, and is being trialed as an alternative to surgical resection.

NETs are a heterogeneous collection of tumors that can occur at multiple sites and are often categorized based on their site of origin such as the lung, pancreas, or small bowel. They develop from neuroendocrine cells of origin and as such, may express a spectrum of neuroendocrine secretory ability. This may manifest clinically as carcinoid syndrome, for example, in the case of secretory NET liver metastases. However, this capability may also be utilized therapeutically and treatment personalized to this capability. Somatostatin analogs (SSAs) such as octreotide may be administered to reduce endocrine symptoms and may also be administered prior to surgical resection to reduce the risk of a carcinoid crisis. In somatostatin receptor-positive tumors this can be targeted therapeutically. SSAs can be cross-linked to radioisotopes such as ^{177}Lu-Dotatate and deliver radioactivity specifically to the tumor site by directly binding to the somatostatin receptors. This approach, peptide receptor radionuclide therapy (PRRT), has demonstrated a survival improvement compared to systemic octreotide alone for metastatic NET tumors and was approved by the FDA in 2018.[10]

Chemotherapy

Chemotherapy is an area where the evolution of personalized therapy has been very significant and the changes are ongoing. Traditional cytotoxic chemotherapy is based on the principle of the direct effect of chemotherapy on cell division and the differential effect of this action on rapidly dividing malignant cells and their limitations in cellular repair as compared to normal tissue. Normal tissue may still be affected, albeit to a lesser degree, resulting in toxicity. The concept of targeted therapy was proposed over a 100 years earlier by Paul Erlich with the concept of a "magic bullet"; however, the reality has only started to be realized in more recent times with the advances in the molecular biology of cancer. There are three classes of targeted cancer agents: small-molecule therapies, mononuclear antibodies, and cancer vaccines.

Small molecule therapies have been a major growth area for chemotherapy and provide the opportunity to tailor the therapy to specific cancers. This area is expanding rapidly as new targets are identified in tumors, and active agents have subsequently developed. GIST tumors and the impact of imatinib have already been discussed earlier; however, tyrosine kinase inhibitors, including sunitinib, have been developed. As patients with metastatic GIST develop resistance to first-line tyrosine kinase inhibitors with failure of response to increased doses, they can be switched to second-line inhibitors such as sunitinib. Isolated clones of disease that demonstrate resistance to therapy, such as indicated by persistent metabolic uptake on a PET scan, can be surgically resected, thereby personalizing the therapy significantly.

The application of genomic profiling to routine management of specific tumors, which is essential information to be available at MDMs, is becoming much more mainstream. For melanoma, B-raf and MEK are recognized targets for which there are available active drugs such as vemurafenib, which is a B-raf inhibitor that has demonstrated effectiveness against metastatic disease. There is a multiplicity of agents with a range of targets. Dabrafenib is a B-raf inhibitor, and trametinib is an MEK inhibitor. In 2014, the FDA approved the combination of these two drugs for metastatic melanoma following a phase III trial comparing the combination to single agent vemurafenib. The application of this drug combination is not only a therapeutic strategy for metastatic melanoma. It has also been applied as neoadjuvant therapy in patients with resectable stage IIIB or IIIC B-rafV600 mutation-positive melanoma in the Neo-Combi trial, which was a single-arm, open-label, single-center, phase II trial. A high proportion of patients achieved a complete response on the Response Evaluation Criteria in Solid Tumors (RECIST) criteria, and around half of the 40 patients achieved a pathologic complete response, which improves prognosis, although a number of these later relapsed. The conclusion was that surgery was easier in over half of the patients.[11]

Monoclonal Antibodies

Monoclonal antibodies target tumor-associated antigens present on tumor cells by utilizing a form of passive immunotherapy. The initial challenges were a short half-life, limited tissue penetration, and failure to induce an adequate immune effector response in humans. Many of these issues have been resolved through the development of humanized antibodies. They are well tolerated because they are highly specific to their antigen-binding sites. An example is ErbB2, which is a cell surface receptor that is produced at high levels in approximately 30% of breast cancers, and is usually described as human epidermal growth factor receptor positive (HER-2) tumors. Trastuzumab (Herceptin) is a genetically engineered monoclonal antibody that inhibits tumor progression. It is used in HER2 breast cancers both as adjuvant therapy and treatment of metastatic disease, and is one of the first monoclonal antibodies used for solid tumors. HER2 receptors have been discovered in a number of other tumor types, including gastric cancer.

A more generic approach is the use of monoclonal antibodies that target the tumor microenvironment. Bevacizumab is an antivascular endothelial growth factor (VEGF) antibody that targets the VEGF receptor, which is a key mediator of tumor angiogenesis. Although it was first approved for metastatic colorectal cancer, it is also used for metastatic non–small cell lung cancer, advanced renal cell cancer, and glioblastoma[12].

Personalization of therapy can also be applied to decide whether to administer chemotherapy, rather than to identify novel therapeutic agents. Circulating tumor DNA or cDNA has been shown to be released by a number of tumors and has demonstrated a potential role as an "omic" biomarker. One study measured the sequential measurement of cDNA in a group of 250 stage II colorectal cancer patients who had undergone curative surgery.[13] A single specific mutation in each of the tumors was identified and measured regularly in the blood of the patient using cDNA. Patients with higher levels of cDNA were at a greater risk of recurrent disease, and the presence of cDNA after treatment with adjuvant chemotherapy was a predictor of worse survival. Elevation of cDNA was also present earlier than radiologically detectable recurrence in patients who developed recurrence. This biological feedback with respect to the use of cDNA as a biomarker for cancer care is likely to be the beginning of the application of cDNA to the tailoring of patient management. There may even be a potential role for cDNA in the early detection of resectable solid tumours.[14]

Immunotherapy

Immunotherapy is the fourth "pillar" of cancer management, along with surgery, radiotherapy, and chemotherapy, and has rapidly become an integral component of personalized cancer care. The relatively recent understanding of the ability to reinitiate innate tumor surveillance and killing by the innate immune system through removal of tumor-initiated immune suppression, enacted through the CTLA-4 and the PD-1 and PDL-1 receptors, combined with the ability to generate targeted therapies for these receptors has revolutionized cancer care. There are an increasing number of available immunotherapy drugs, predominantly monoclonal antibodies such as ipilimumab targeting CTLA-4 or pembrolizumab targeting PD-1. The selection of therapy, however, is relatively focused. There are a significant number of tumor types that currently receive no benefit from immunotherapy, including the majority of colorectal cancers. Highly immunogenic tumors, such as melanoma and some lung cancers, have demonstrated the greatest response to immunotherapy and utilization beyond the treatment of metastatic disease, such as in a neoadjuvant setting prior to surgery, is beginning to be explored. Assessment of PD-1 receptor levels in tumors may provide some indication of potential efficacy. On the other end of the spectrum, the use of immunotherapy in all microsatellite unstable tumors, regardless of the tissue of origin, has been approved as the drugs appear to be highly efficacious in these tumor types.

Conclusion

Cancer care is in a state of evolution and has been accelerating over the last 40 years. The advent of multidisciplinary care and meetings has streamlined cancer care with the inclusion of all treating clinicians and incorporating the different treatment modalities available. Treatment plans designed through MDMs play an essential role in staging patients, facilitating stratification of patients, and personalization of cancer care. Developments in imaging such as MRI and PET have been core facilitators of this development, as tumor staging remains the most important factor when stratifying cases. The ability to stratify individual cases has allowed for personalized care, with specific management plans tailored to the individual patient, rather than broad brush-stroke application of established treatment protocols. The other major catalyst beyond imaging that has driven the development and application of personalized care is the increasing availability of genetic and molecular data on individual tumors. This provides predictive and prognostic information on tumor behavior and has led to the development of a range of new treatment options, including targeted chemotherapy and immunotherapy. The advent of cDNA is also likely to play an increasing role in the selection of patients for treatment and monitoring.

The era of personalization of cancer care is here and this tailored approach is likely to only increase going forward.

Advances in molecular biology and availability of "omics" information have also significantly impacted the management of cancer, both influencing the type of treatment and timing of treatment, as well as generating novel therapies. This is resulting in increased tailoring of management for specific patients and personalization of care.

References

1. The Expert Advisory Group on Cancer to the Chief Medical Officers of England and Wales. A Policy Framework for Commissioning Cancer Services: A Report by the Expert Advisory Group on Cancer to the Chief Medical Officers of England and Wales. Department of Health; 1995.
2. Dietz DW, Consortium for Optimizing Surgical Treatment of Rectal Cancer (OSTRiCh). Consortium for Optimizing Surgical Treatment of Rectal Cancer. Multidisciplinary management of rectal cancer: the OSTRICH. *J Gastrointest Surg.* 2013;17(10):1863–1868.
3. MacDermid E, Hooton G, MacDonald M, et al. Improving patient survival with the colorectal cancer multi-disciplinary team. *Colorectal Dis.* 2009;11(3):291–295.
4. Fader DJ, Wise CG, Normolle DP, Johnson TM. The multidisciplinary melanoma clinic: a cost outcomes analysis of specialty care. *J Am Acad Dermatol.* 1998;38(5 Pt 1):742–751.
5. Hounsfield GN. Computerized transverse axial scanning (tomography). 1. Description of system. *Br J Radiol.* 1973;46(552):1016–1022.
6. Cady B. Basic principles in surgical oncology. *Arch Surg.* 1997;132(4):338–346.
7. Lidsky ME, D'Angelica MI. An outlook on precision surgery. *Eur J Surg Oncol.* 2017;43(5):853–855.
8. Alexander EK, Kennedy GC, Baloch ZW, et al. Preoperative diagnosis of benign thyroid nodules with indeterminate cytology. *N Engl J Med.* 2012;367(8):705–715.
9. Druker BJ. STI571 (Gleevec) as a paradigm for cancer therapy. *Trends Mol Med.* 2002;8(4)Supplement:S14–S18.
10. Strosberg J, El-Haddad G, Wolin E, et al. Phase 3 trial of 177Lu-Dotatate for midgut neuroendocrine tumors. *N Engl J Med.* 2017;376(2):125–135.

11. Long GV, Saw RPM, Lo S, et al. Neoadjuvant dabrafenib combined with trametinib for resectable, stage IIIB–C, BRAF^{V600} mutation-positive melanoma (NeoCombi): a single-arm, open-label, single-centre, phase 2 trial. *Lancet Oncol.* 2019;20(7):961–971.
12. Hurwitz H, Fehrenbacher L, Novotny W, et al. Bevacizumab plus irinotecan, fluorouracil, and leucovorin for metastatic colorectal cancer. *N Engl J Med.* 2004;350(23):2335–2342.
13. Tie J, Wang Y, Tomasetti C, et al. Circulating tumor DNA analysis detects minimal residual disease and predicts recurrence in patients with stage II colon cancer. *Sci Transl Med.* 2016;8(346):346ra92.
14. Cohen JD, Li L, Wang Y, et al. Detection and localization of surgically resectable cancers with a multi-analyte blood test. *Science.* 2018;359(6378):926–930.

SECTION 2

Inflammatory-Immune Responses, Perioperative Period, and Cancer Outcomes

8

Anemia, Thrombosis, Transfusion Therapy, and Cancer Outcomes

LACHLAN F. MILES, JUAN P. CATA, AND KATE L. BURBURY

Introduction

As surgical and anesthetic techniques have evolved, perioperative mortality in complex cancer surgical interventions has decreased significantly. However, complications and associated morbidity remain a challenge not only for surgical recovery, but also for functional restoration, completion of care for the patient, and long-term cancer outcomes. As such, optimization and preparation for major cancer surgery (prehabilitation) should be a high priority safety initiative and a fundamental strategy in perioperative medicine. Appropriate preparative management or optimization of functional capacity prior to an anticipated stressor can mitigate adverse outcomes, which carry substantial clinical and economic implications. Pivotal strategies with substantial impact include hematological optimization (including the correction of iron deficiency and anemia), appropriate use of blood products, and prevention of thromboembolic complications.

Blood loss is an inherent risk with more complicated cancer surgeries. Moreover, even prior to surgery, anemia and iron deficiency are common findings and remain important contributors to adverse postoperative outcomes and mortality. Equally, perioperative allogeneic red cell transfusions, which remain the most common strategy to correct anemia, are an independent predictor of postoperative complications and have been linked with an increased risk of cancer recurrence and reduced overall survival (OS).

Prevention of thromboembolism (TE) has been a high priority safety initiative for over a decade. TE is a common complication among patients with cancer, particularly in the postoperative period, and a leading cause of preventable morbidity and mortality. Yet systematic real-time approaches to TE prevention, particularly postsurgery, remain suboptimal.

Here we review the burden of these important contributors to outcomes in patients with cancer in association with the perioperative period. In addition, we propose pragmatic, expert, and evidence-based strategies that can be easily implemented and scaled in real-time to patient care.

Anemia

Anemia is a symptom of erythropoietic failure, reflecting inadequate substrate (particularly iron) or red cell production that is exceeded by loss. These processes frequently coexist in cancer patients and represent a continuum; even in the nonanemic patient, iron deficiency may still be present, impacting on skeletal muscle and respiratory chain function. Patients with cancer about to undergo major surgery require assessment of both hemoglobin and iron status and consideration of appropriate preoperative optimization prior to proceeding.

Burden of Anemia and Iron Deficiency in Cancer Patients

Iron deficiency and anemia contribute to cancer-associated morbidity. These reflect blood loss (particularly in tumors of the gastrointestinal tract) and the inflammatory response to the tumor and neoadjuvant therapy. The European Cancer Survey highlighted the prevalence of anemia in different cancer types; 39% of patients were anemic at time of diagnosis, with 68% becoming anemic within 6 months of starting treatment, a reflection of the additive effects of multiple rounds of chemotherapy and/or surgery.[1]

Emerging evidence suggests that iron deficiency, even in the absence of anemia, should be considered an actionable pathology in its own right. Data on the prevalence of iron deficiency as an independent laboratory abnormality in the oncological population are highest in the colorectal cancer population, ranging from 50%–60% in some series, as a reflection of chronic blood loss.[2,3] However, even in patients where ongoing bleeding is not a hallmark of the malignancy, iron deficiency is also found in up to 46% of cases.[4]

Pathophysiology of Anemia in Cancer

Causes of anemia can be divided into three categories:

1. Blood loss;
2. Increased red cell destruction;
3. Decreased red cell production.

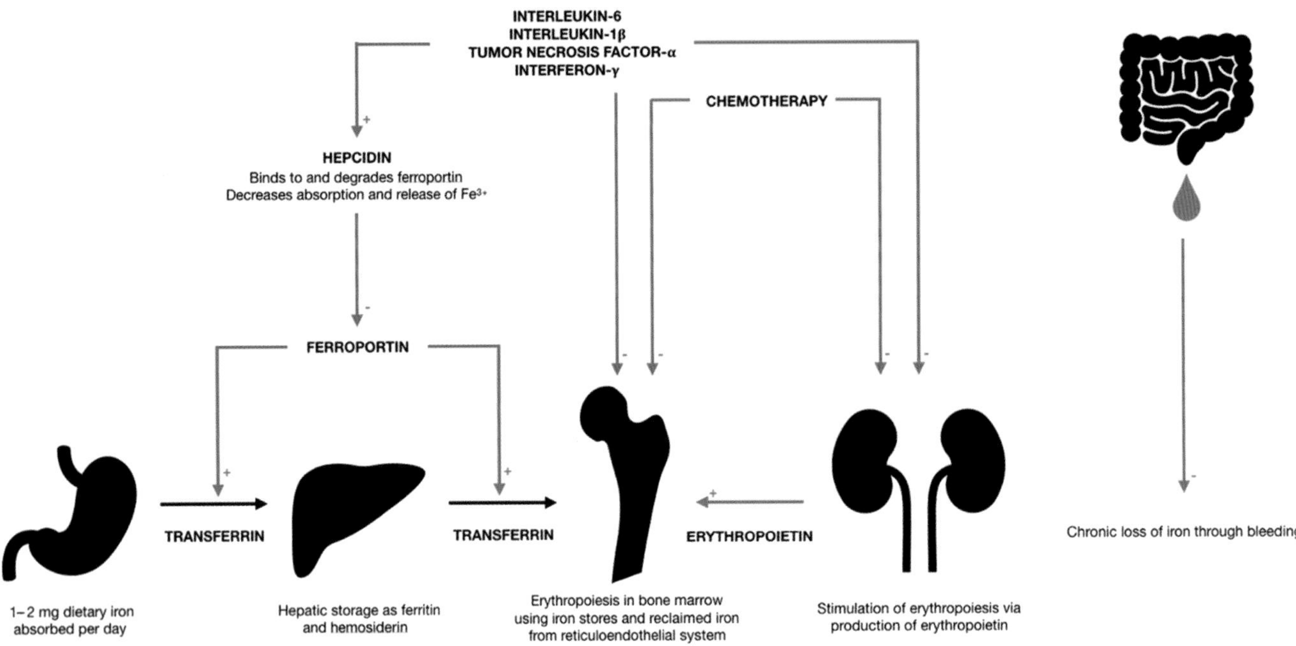

• **Fig. 8.1** Pathophysiology of anemia in the oncology patient. Various processes, some as a consequence of the malignancy itself, others as a consequence of treatment, contribute to this, although iron restricted erythropoiesis due to absolute or functional iron deficiency is frequently present.

Although certain tumors enable chronic, ongoing blood loss, most cancer-associated anemia is caused by diminished red cell production and is often due to iron deficiency (Fig. 8.1). Broadly speaking, iron deficiency can be defined as:

- a lack of stored iron due to chronic losses (absolute iron deficiency), and
- inability to access stored iron (functional iron deficiency).

Functional iron deficiency is a consequence of the inflammatory response.[5] A key contributor to the associated "anemia of inflammation" is dysregulation of the cytokine interleukin-6 (IL-6). Overexpression of IL-6 has been found in almost all types of tumor, promoting tumorigenesis, suppressing erythropoietin, and increasing expression of the iron regulatory hormone hepcidin. Hepcidin downregulates ferroportin-1, a transmembrane protein that enables iron to be transported across cell membranes. Consequently, iron cannot be absorbed from the gut, and stored iron cannot be accessed by bone marrow. This restricts erythropoiesis and limits the efficacy of oral iron supplementation. Additionally, overexpression of tumor necrosis factor-α (TNF-α) suppresses the hemoglobinization of erythroid progenitor cells, cytotoxic therapies impair hematopoiesis, and nephrotoxic therapeutics impact the production of erythropoietin. Consequently, perioperative risk is increased in patients who have undergone neoadjuvant treatment.[6]

Influence of Anemia and Iron Deficiency on Outcome in Cancer Patients

Separate to the perioperative period, anemia is associated with poor outcome in cancer patients,[7] both due to worsening of local tumor control[8] and increased requirement for allogeneic blood transfusion.[9] While some authors maintain that anemia is a marker of increased concomitant comorbidity, rather than an independent risk factor in its own right,[10] major randomized controlled trial data are lacking. Most guidelines promote hemoglobin concentration as a therapeutic target prior to proceeding to major surgery.[11]

Iron deficiency, independent of anemia, is gaining attention in the perioperative sphere. While clinicians often consider the two to be synonymous, physiological effects of iron deficiency (particularly fatigue and exercise intolerance) may be noted before hemoglobin drops below the anemic threshold. This is because iron is a key contributor to basic cellular function, with roles in energy metabolism, cell signaling, gene expression, and regulation of cell growth.[12] Most iron is inserted into protoporphyrin IX as the final step in the production of heme to allow oxygen binding to hemoglobin.[13] Additionally, iron serves as a prosthetic group for other oxygen-carrying molecules, notably myoglobin, cytochromes, and nitric oxide synthase,[14] and is integral to the function of enzyme systems responsible for DNA synthesis and repair, energy metabolism via the function of the respiratory chain, and production of ADP.[15] Hence iron deficiency can impact respiratory chain and skeletal muscle function adversely, affecting fatigability and recovery from exercise.[16] Early retrospective data from colorectal cancer populations have highlighted a possible association between iron deficiency and poor postoperative outcomes independent of anemia.[2,17] Consequently, some consensus statements recommend correction of iron deficiency in patients presenting to major surgery regardless of the starting hemoglobin concentration.[18] Prospective evidence for this practice is limited.

TABLE 8.1 **Metrics of Iron Status Obtained in Standard Iron Studies**

Test	Normal Values	Comment
Serum iron	>14 µmol/L	Little use for diagnosing iron deficiency Specificity lost in inflammation
Serum ferritin	10–300 µg/L	Allows safe storage of iron in Fe^{3+} form Appears in serum due to ICF leakage Acute phase reactant—cannot be used in isolation to determine iron status
Transferrin	2.0–3.5 g/L	Rarely used in isolation, but commonly combined with serum iron to determine transferrin saturation (TSAT)
Transferrin saturation	≥20%	Measure of binding capacity for iron Obtained by dividing serum transferrin by serum iron

*Other tests that are directly reflective of iron status include percentage of hypochromic red cells (normal, <5%) and reticulocyte hemoglobin concentration (>28 pg). Mean corpuscular hemoglobin (*MCH*) can also be used and is often routinely reported by standard hematology laboratory analyzers. However, due to the circulatory lifespan of red blood cells (120 days), this may not reflect recent onset iron deficiency.

Diagnosing Iron Deficiency in the Preoperative Cancer Patient

Differentiation and identification of iron deficiency as part of a program of preoperative optimization can be challenging, as ferritin (an acute phase reactant) may be elevated for a variety of reasons, possibly reflecting cellular damage and leakage of ferritin from storage sites into the bloodstream.[19] Indeed, serum ferritin in the normal reference range in the setting of a C-reactive protein greater than 5 mg/L will only be 39% sensitive for iron deficiency.[20] An alternative metric is transferrin saturation (TSAT). Taken as the quotient of serum iron divided by transferrin concentration and expressed as a percentage, TSAT is a more direct measure of the physiological demand for iron (although it may still be affected by inflammation independent of iron status). A value of less than 20% is interpreted as being reflective of iron deficiency (Table 8.1). Therefore a patient presenting for surgery with serum ferritin less than 100 µg/L regardless of TSAT, or a TSAT of less than 20% in the setting of serum ferritin at 100–300 µg/L, should be considered iron depleted.

More sensitive markers of iron deficiency have been described. These include soluble transferrin receptor, serum hepcidin, reticulocyte hemoglobin concentration, and percentage hypochromic red cells. Although these are increasingly being cited in best practice guidelines, they have not yet entered widespread use.[21,22]

Management of Iron Deficiency and Anemia in the Perioperative Period

All patients undergoing cancer treatment should be managed for reversible causes of anemia. While the most recent iteration of some medical oncology guidelines advocates for treating a hemoglobin concentration of less than 110 g/L,[21] guidelines pertaining to major surgery frequently target a hemoglobin concentration of greater than 120 g/L for women and greater than 130 g/L for men.[23] Indeed, emerging evidence and opinion suggest that 130 g/L be targeted in all patients, regardless of sex.[24–26]

Initial management of patients with preoperative anemia should involve a determination of iron status. Some sources recommend assessment of vitamin B_{12} and folate, but the incidence of actual deficiency of these substrates in the preoperative patient is rare. Formal testing should not be undertaken without clinical suspicion (elevated mean corpuscular volume, megaloblastic changes on blood film, or evidence of malnutrition).

If an iron deficient state has been identified (TSAT of less than 20%), or the patient is felt to have inadequate iron stores to facilitate postoperative erythropoiesis (serum ferritin of less than 100 µg/L), treatment with iron should be pursued. It is important to note that for the reasons outlined previously, patients with an active malignancy may not be able to absorb iron across the bowel wall. Intravenous iron supplementation is preferred, especially as the newer iron preparations are extremely stable, with a low rate of adverse reaction.[27] In order to facilitate incrementation of hemoglobin prior to surgery, current consensus opinion suggests that 3 weeks is required to see a meaningful increase in hemoglobin concentration,[28] although evidence from orthopedic and cardiac surgical populations suggests intervention as little as 24 hours prior to surgery can yield some benefit.[29,30] The PREVENTT trial called into practice the routine administration of intravenous iron to patients with preoperative anaemia undergoing major abdominal surgery.[138] In this randomized trial, no short-term (within 30 days postoperatively) benefit was observed in patients who received intravenous iron at a median of 14 days prior to operation, relative to those who received placebo. While a statistically significant reduction in late readmission was seen at 8-month follow up, together with an increase in hemoglobin concentration, this was a secondary outcome that the study was not powered to examine, and that occured in the setting of a negative primary outcome. At the time of writing, the results of this trial have not yet been translated

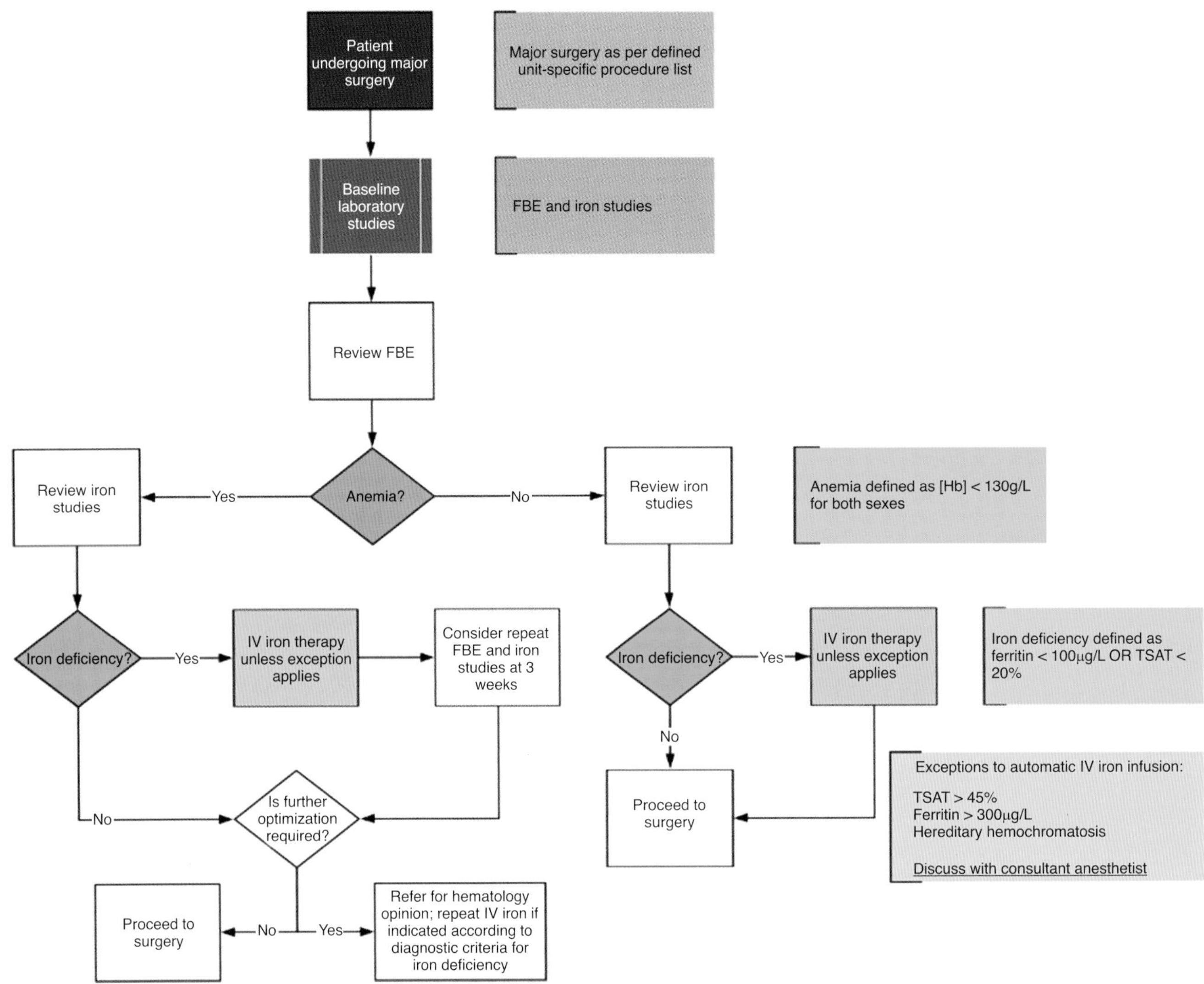

• **Fig. 8.2** Example practice nomogram to guide the use of iron therapy preoperatively. Note that the lack of consensus around erythropoiesis stimulating agents (ESAs), particularly duration and regimen, precludes their inclusion in this algorithm despite multiple studies and trials having described their use in the oncological context. *TSAT*, Transferrin saturation.

to best practice guidelines, and routine administration of intravenous iron in patients with iron deficiency anemia prior to major surgery remains standard of care. An example nomogram for preoperative iron therapy is shown in Fig. 8.2.

Exogenous erythropoietin and other erythropoiesis stimulating agents (ESAs) were historically avoided in patients with an active malignancy, as it was thought that erythropoietin promotes tumorigenesis. However, subsequent registry studies have not replicated this signal and recent clinical guidelines, particularly in North America, are beginning to recommend the use of ESAs in patients with chemotherapy-associated anemia and an apparently adequate iron status.[21,31] Perioperative guidelines, particularly those from Europe, have been more reluctant to recommend the routine use of these agents to improve preoperative hemoglobin concentration. Although systematic reviews have suggested that there is benefit to combining ESAs with iron therapy relative to iron therapy alone,[32] there is undoubtedly an increased risk of venous TE that may be magnified in the presence of malignancy. Current FDA recommendations advocate for concomitant anticoagulation in patients receiving ESAs in a perioperative context, particularly where the hemoglobin concentration exceeds 120 g/L. A further important caveat in the use of these agents is the time required for effect, and a course of treatment of up to 4 months is frequently required to realize maximum benefit. Finally, there is considerable heterogeneity in the literature regarding the correct dose of ESAs, which has contributed to the uncertainty surrounding their use.

Transfusion- and Cancer-Related Outcomes

Clinical Evidence

Perioperative red blood cell transfusion (RBCT) remains a common strategy to manage acute anemia in patients with cancer. In this population, the rate of perioperative RBCT ranges from 9.4% to 90% depending on the type surgery, patient risk factors, and the lack of clear definitions on when transfusions should be applied perioperatively.[33–37] Transfusion triggers in patients with cancer remain ill-defined and controversial.[38] Hemoglobin concentrations of 70–100 g/L have been used; however, these do not necessarily reflect the delivery of oxygen to tissues. Therefore perioperative physicians still transfuse using poorly defined hemoglobin thresholds, or demonstrative hemodynamic instability and/or signs of organ hypoperfusion. A recent trial by de Almeida et al. found a negative impact on short-term outcomes when hemoglobin at 70 g/L was used to trigger RBCT, compared with a liberal transfusion (90 g/L) strategy in critically ill cancer patients.[38,39] In these patients, a trigger of 80 g/L could therefore be considered to initiate RBCT with a modified threshold in those with objective signs of organ hypoperfusion.[40]

Transfusion-Related Immunomodulation and Cancer Outcomes

Blood products contain high concentrations of interleukins (IL-1β, IL-6, IL-8), chemokines, prostaglandin E, thromboxanes, histamine, leukocytes (particularly in non-leukoreduced units), growth factors, nonpolar lipids, pro-inflammatory lysophosphatidylcholines, CD40 ligand, and microparticles.[41] The administration of blood products can therefore have particular profound effects on transfusion-related immunomodulation (TRIM) defined as:

1. donor-specific transfusion-related immune suppression,
2. "generalized" transfusion-related immune suppression.

The former primarily suppresses adaptive immunity; in contrast, the generalized form appears to be mediated by macrophages and neutrophils and has a significant suppressive impact on the innate immunity. TRIM alters the function of natural killer cells, reduces proliferation of T and B lymphocytes, increases activity of T regulatory cells, and impairs the maturation and antigen-presenting activity of dendritic cells.[42] It has been proposed that infections and cancer recurrence would be a consequence of the "generalized" transfusion-related immune suppression, rather than the donor-specific form.[43] The timing of transfusion may also have different effects on the inflammatory and immune response. Thus when blood products are administered during or immediately after surgery, the so-called systemic inflammatory response syndrome can be further exaggerated by transfusions delaying inflammatory resolution, which can also participate in the pathogenesis of transfusion-related adverse outcomes.[44]

Age of Stored Blood and Cancer Recurrence

It has been theorized that the age of the blood may influence perioperative outcomes.[45] Although biological impact theoretically exists, studies that have investigated the impact of blood storage duration on the survival of patients with cancer are limited. Cata et al. reported that neither the use of "new" allogeneic nor autologous RBCs had a beneficial effect on recurrence-free survival or OS in patients with non-metastatic prostate cancer.[46] In large cohort study of 27,591 patients with mixed malignancies, the administration of "old" blood defined as 28 days of storage or older also did not influence OS or cancer recurrence.[46]

Impact of Blood Transfusions on Outcomes of Patients With Cancers

Perioperative RBCT remains common in patients undergoing head and neck cancer surgeries. Azmy et al. reported a transfusion rate of 11.2% in a cohort of 3090 patients undergoing neck dissection; however, this number can be doubled in those undergoing free-flap surgery.[47] Two retrospective studies indicated that RBCT given perioperatively in patients with head and neck cancers were linked to reduced OS and increased tumor recurrence.[48,49] However, this negative association was recently disputed by Goubran et al. who studied 354 patients.[50]

The rate of perioperative RBCT among patients with lung cancer is approximately 10% and an independent predictor of short-term postoperative complications.[51] Luan et al. conducted a meta-analysis of retrospective studies that included 3588 patients undergoing surgery for primary lung malignancies. They assessed the impact on cancer-related outcomes and reported a negative association between RBCT, recurrence-free survival, and OS.[33] A more recent observational study included 5709 patients and demonstrated a dose-dependent relationship between the number of units transfused and a negative effect on cancer progression and OS.[52]

Current evidence on whether the administration of RBCs is an independent risk factor for esophageal and gastric cancer recurrence is also controversial.[53–57] Boshier et al. conducted a meta-analysis and concluded that the administration of autologous RBCs, and a low transfusion volume (<1–2 RBC units), is associated with better survival rates than with allogeneic transfusion or >3 RBC units transfused.[55] However, a more recent retrospective study has demonstrated (after using propensity score matching) that perioperative blood transfusions are not an independent risk factor of reduced OS.[58]

Evidence from two meta-analyses by Amato et al. that included randomized controlled trials and observational studies demonstrates that RBCT in patients with colorectal cancers had a negative impact on survival regardless of timing (pre-, intra-, or postoperative), type (allogeneic or autologous), leukodepletion status, and number of RBCT units.[37,59–65] In patients with pancreatic and hepatocellular carcinoma, RBCT is also associated with negative perioperative outcomes, including increased risk of death, recurrence, and perioperative complications.[66–69] Tai et al. reported a rate of RBCT after liver resections for hepatocellular carcinomas of 42%, and the risk of dying from any cause, including cancer, was almost doubled compared to nontransfused subjects.[70] Shiba et al. reported the impact of the transfusion of fresh frozen plasma (FFP) after surgery for pancreatic ductal adenocarcinoma. Patients receiving FFP had a significantly shorter OS.[71]

A negative impact of autologous blood transfusions on cancer progression was not observed after colorectal metastatic liver resections[72]; however, this was observed with FFP. Nakaseko et al. reviewed the outcomes of 127 patients who had colorectal metastatic liver resections; those who received FFP (24%) had a twofold higher risk of dying of cancer or any cause than those who were not transfused.[73]

Regarding cholangiocarcinoma, a meta-analysis by Wang et al. reported that the administration of RBCTs negatively affected the OS, while a more recent retrospective study using a propensity score matching method did not demonstrate negative survival outcomes.[74–76]

Multiple studies have assessed perioperative RBCTs in patients with urological malignancies and demonstrated increased cancer recurrence and decreased survival. In patients with bladder cancer who underwent radical cystectomy, two meta-analyses suggested an association.[77–84] Furrer et al. investigated the effect of RBCTs alone or in combination with FFP on oncological outcomes in a cohort of 885 patients who underwent radical cystectomy. While the risk of dying from any cause was similar between patients who received RBCTs alone or in combination with FFP, the odds of dying from cancer were higher in those receiving the combination therapy.[85] The findings in patients with renal cancers are mixed,[86–90] although it appears that RBCT had a negative impact in prostate cancer patients and those with adrenocortical carcinomas.[36,91]

There is no definitive evidence of the impact of RBCT in cancer recurrence or survival in patients undergoing radical hysterectomy for cervical or ovarian cancer.[92–94] Although De Oliveira et al. found an increased risk of recurrence in patients with advanced ovarian cancer, subsequent investigations by Altman et al., Warner et al., and Manning-Geist et al. showed no association.[95–98] More recently, Hunsicker et al. also reviewed the impact of allogeneic blood transfusions in 529 women with stage I–IV ovarian cancer. After adequate propensity score matching, the authors did not find any association between blood transfusion and shorter progression-free and OS.[99]

Consequently, evidence of a deleterious effect of perioperative blood transfusion on cancer progression remains controversial for most malignancies. Although the association with RBCT and poor oncological outcomes has been demonstrated for colorectal cancer, there is low level of evidence to recommend or contraindicate perioperative RBCT in other malignancies. Nevertheless, the presence of anemia and the requirement for RBCT are associated with more adverse surgical outcomes in patients with cancer.

Thrombosis

Hemostatic Dysfunction and Cancer

Patients with cancer are at high risk of both thromboembolic and hemorrhagic events during the course of their disease.[100] The interplay between cancer and the hemostatic system is well recognized, but complex, and involves a diverse range of factors and pathophysiological mechanisms related to the cancer itself, patient factors, and "anticancer therapies," including surgical stressors. There is a wide spectrum of clinical manifestations from macrovascular complications such as pulmonary embolus (PE), deep vein thrombosis (DVT), and arterial thrombotic events, through to microvascular pathology such as disseminated intravascular coagulopathy and thrombotic thrombocytopenic purpura. All of these are relevant throughout the perioperative period and confer significant clinical consequences for patients and their surgical outcomes.

The hemostatic system is pivotal to maintain vascular integrity and the surrounding tissue microenvironment during surgery, and incorporates the most fundamental immediate responses to vascular injury and termination of blood loss through to the complex maintenance of the vascular microenvironment and biological continuum of cell–cell interaction, inflammatory responses, stromal cell recruitment, and cellular repair.[101]

The key physiological events required during surgery—when the vasculature and tissue microenvironment are breached—include:

- vasoconstriction of blood vessels,
- platelet aggregation and adhesion,
- generation of the thrombin burst to accelerate conversion of soluble fibrinogen to fibrin polymers to stabilize the platelet plug to the endothelium,
- activation of protease inhibitors to contain coagulation and clot formation only to sites of damage, and
- activation of fibrinolysis to remove excess blood clot once the structural integrity of the vasculature has been restored.

Many of these processes are perpetually disturbed in patients with cancer and during anticancer therapy, even prior to the event of major cancer surgery.[101,102] Importantly, the coagulation system appears to be a systematic target of oncogenic dysregulation and cellular signaling, as a consequence of both the tumor cells and the applied therapies.[101,103] Moreover, the surgical stress as a systemic response involving cytokine release, ischemia reperfusion, sympathetic activation, inflammatory response, and hemodynamic changes may further exaggerate hemostatic dysregulation, as well as tumor growth and metastases.[104] Efforts to understand this pathophysiology may have the capacity to prevent important TE and bleeding events, but also impact perisurgical "wound" restoration, patient recovery, and overall cancer outcomes.[101,104]

Importance of Prevention of Thromboembolism in Patients Undergoing Cancer Surgery

The hemostatic system is particularly challenged during the perioperative period, with potential for adverse clinical and economic consequences.[105–110] Postoperative TE among patients with cancer accounts for more than a third of TE-associated deaths. Nonfatal events remain common (up to 40% in some cohorts) with attributable morbidity, impaired quality of life, increased length of hospital stay, increased rates of recurrent events (2-3 fold), increased rates of bleeding complications on anticoagulant therapy, and negative predictors of OS.[105–107] Importantly, an index TE event represents a significant clinical hurdle for patients following cancer surgery, not only related to the morbidity and mortality of the TE and the requirement for high-dose anticoagulant therapy, but also the impact on both the recovery and potential interruption to ongoing requirement for therapy. Moreover, TE rates remain high despite the availability of safe, efficacious, and cost-effective thromboprophylaxis (TP) strategies, and more than a third of the events occur postdischarge (within 30 days postoperatively) when routine TP is not universally applied.[111–114]

Furthermore, in terms of clinical impact this burden is significantly underestimated, with the focus on clinically apparent macrovascular events such as DVT and PE, overlooking the hemostatic and endothelial dysfunction at a microvascular, surgical bed, and tumor biology level, which contributes to morbidity, postsurgical recovery, cancer progression, metastatic potential, and mortality. This interplay between hemostatic dysfunction and tumor cell survival, proliferation, and metastatic spread,[115] as well as the antiangiogenic and antitumor properties of anticoagulants,[116,117] highlights additional opportunity for therapeutic impact. The key is identifying for whom and when this impact is maximal.

Risk-Directed Approach to Prevention Thromboembolism Associated With Cancer Surgery

While all patients with cancer, particularly in the perioperative period, should be considered at risk of TE, the risk is heterogeneous and dynamic, with the absolute magnitude and duration not equal for all patient cohorts, or within cohorts. The net risk varies according to patient factors (e.g., age, body mass index, comorbid disease), cancer type and stage, and treatment-related factors (e.g., chemoradiotherapy, biological therapy, hospitalization, presence of vascular access devices). This risk heterogeneity—for both TE and bleeding—is exaggerated during the course of the disease and different intervention phases, most notably the perioperative period, emphasizing the importance of some degree of risk stratification, rather than broad application of preventative strategies.

In retrospective and prospective studies, the TE risk for patients with cancer undergoing surgery increases over the age of 40 years, with a 2–3-fold increased risk for those aged 60 years or older. Moreover, irrespective of cancer, increasing age is associated with other risk factors, such as comorbidities, decreased exercise and functional status, and greater immobility, which all play a role in the TE risk post-procedurally.[110,118]

Cancer-related factors are important, including histological subtype, grade, site, stage, and therapy. The highest TE rates occur in mucin-producing adenocarcinomas and the primary site tumors of the pancreas, gastrointestinal system, lung, brain, uterus, and kidney. However, the frequency of cancer and surgical requirements equally dictate this landscape, with TE-related complications reported in breast, gynecological, and lung cancers in women and prostate, colorectal, and lung cancers in men. Patients with more advanced stage are at substantially greater TE risk with both regional and distant metastases compared with local disease undergoing resection. The highest risk period is immediately following the diagnosis or at relapse, during the first 3–6 months, and particularly during chemotherapy/chemoradiotherapy, which is a common strategy prior to surgical resection.[119] The awareness of this escalated TE risk prior to surgical resection is imperative, given that surgery alone confers a 2–3-fold TE risk compared with similar procedures in patients without cancer.[108,120]

Efforts to apply risk stratification have focused largely on primary tumor site, stage, and comorbid disease, with some consideration to anesthetic and surgical techniques. Such factors lack potency, and real-time clinical application of risk stratification strategies has been challenging. Nevertheless, a systematic approach via prehabilitation programs allows preemptive assessment and identification of TE risk, with integration and the ultimate decision regarding application of pharmacologic prophylaxis (P-TP) in conjunction with neuroaxial blockade, real-time intraoperative assessment of hemostasis, and bleeding risk.

Application of Prophylaxis in Cancer Surgery

P-TP is a proven preventative and safe strategy, with up to 80% reduction in TE in cancer cohorts.[121–126] However, the heterogeneity in TE risk and concerns regarding cumulative bleeding risk has restricted "routine" P-TP utilization and caused uncertainty regarding real-time clinical application. Meta-analysis demonstrated a 14-fold variation in surgical TE risk in a broad population of patients who did not receive postoperative P-TP using the Caprini risk assessment model. Moreover, Pannucci et al. demonstrated that although P-TP significantly reduced postoperative TE (odds ratio [OR], 0.66; 95% confidence interval [CI], 0.52–0.85; $P = 0.001$), this was associated with an increased incidence of clinically significant bleeding (OR, 1.69; 95% CI, 1.16–2.45; $P = 0.006$).[127] Importantly the maximal benefit of P-TP was identified in patients determined to be at high surgical TE risk (Caprini score ≥7), without an increased risk of bleeding.

All major expert clinical guidelines highlight the clinical and economic importance of postoperative TE and as a consequence are largely explicit that all patients undergoing major surgical intervention should be offered P-TP (generally recommending low-molecular-weight heparin), unless contraindicated. It should either commence preoperation or 6 hours postoperation and continue for 7–10 days, with consideration of extension (28 days) for major abdominopelvic surgery.[100] Mechanical methods for TP can be added to, but not replace, P-TP as a single strategy except if P-TP is contraindicated, with the focus being on active or high risk of bleeding. A combined strategy may be considered in high TE risk patients, targeting the potential for improved efficacy.[100]

Despite consensus on the effectiveness of primary TE prevention strategies and presence of international clinical practice guidelines, surgical (and medical) patients with identifiable risk factors continue to be admitted to acute care hospitals without receiving appropriate TP.[128,129] The reasons are multifactorial, but largely reflect poor (or highly variable) implementation into clinical practice due to the complexity and relevance of the feasibility of real-time risk assessment of patients and the decision-making provision of appropriate prophylaxis in accordance with that assessment.[109,130,131] Guidelines often do not allow for flexibility and adaptability to acknowledge the patient and procedural factors that alter risk or the real-time nuances of surgical clinical interaction. Equally there is a perception that TE is less problematic due to improved surgical and anesthetic techniques and earlier discharge. It is therefore not surprising that reported rates of compliance with TE preventative guidelines are as low as 6% at baseline and 36% postintervention. This suggests that the availability of evidence-based recommendations is insufficient to ensure consistent adoption.

Appropriate, but simple and practical, TE risk stratification is essential to guide appropriate TP for maximal clinical benefit. This precision medicine approach, while widely advocated, has found little practical application in TE prevention, and to date there have been few prospective studies supporting its use. Decision-support tools that allow real-time surgical application incorporating competing thrombotic and bleeding risks are increasingly being explored. One such application, the Surgical Thromboembolism Prevention protocol (STEP), is a smartphone application that uses a risk assessment model that considers both procedural and patient risk to generate an overall TE risk. It also integrates surgical hemostasis at the time of surgical "time out" to generate a decision-making algorithm for the appropriate application of TP strategies, including application of both P-TP (choice of agent, time to commence, duration, dose, cautions, and contraindications) and M-TP (strategy, duration, and cautions). Implementation of this protocol has demonstrated sustained, routine TE prevention postsurgery (99% adherence across 24,953 surgical admissions) with a substantial reduction in both TE (relative risk reduction [RRR], 79%; 95% CI, 39%–93%; $P = 0.02$) and bleeding events (RRR, 37%; 95% CI, 6.2%–57.5%; $P = 0.02$—which included major bleeding RRR of 31% and nonmajor bleeding RRR of 50%). This program was led by anesthetic perioperative physicians at Peter MacCallum Cancer Centre and is scalable across health institutions and all cancer surgery. This strategy has the capacity to overcome the most important lingering challenge in this clinical area: appropriate, real-time utilization of TP strategies among all patients with cancer undergoing surgical interventions.

Conclusion

The clinical and economic value of systematic identification and management of anemia and the appropriate use (even avoidance) of blood products and TE risk in all patients undergoing surgery for cancer are profound. Despite advances in surgical and anesthetic techniques, these pathologies remain major, potentially preventable, contributors to morbidity and mortality postsurgery. Consequently, routine patient blood management and TP are rightly considered to be the standard of care for the cancer patient.

Among patients with cancer, both anemia and the delivery of blood products in the perioperative period are associated with reduced postoperative survival. Anemia remains the most common hematological abnormality among cancer populations, with prevalence and severity varying by cancer type, stage, and therapy. Retrospective and prospective studies have reported anemia in 30%–90% of oncological patients at diagnosis.[132–135] Importantly, anemia is a consequence of potentially avoidable and/or reversible drivers.[136,137] Early identification can allow optimization and reduction in, or avoidance of, unnecessary allogeneic transfusion in the perioperative period.

Hemostatic dysfunction, in particular the hypercoagulable state, with macro- and microvascular events, remains an important phenomenon, further exaggerated in the postoperative setting. Simplistically, TE is a common and preventable complication of major cancer surgery, with negative implications for survival. Predictive models and decision-making algorithms can identify high TE risk patients, drive systematic preventative strategies, and positively impact postsurgical recovery, morbidity, and mortality among patients with cancer.

References

1. Ludwig H, Müldür E, Endler G, Hübl W. Prevalence of iron deficiency across different tumors and its association with poor performance status, disease status and anemia. *Ann Oncol.* 2013;24(7):1886–1892.
2. Wilson MJ, Dekker JWT, Harlaar JJ, Jeekel J, Schipperus M, Zwaginga JJ. The role of preoperative iron deficiency in colorectal cancer patients: prevalence and treatment. *Int J Colorectal Dis.* 2017:1617–1624.
3. Beale AL, Penney MD, Allison MC. The prevalence of iron deficiency among patients presenting with colorectal cancer. *Colorectal Dis.* 2005;7(4):398–402.
4. Aapro M, Österborg A, Gascón P, Ludwig H, Beguin Y. Prevalence and management of cancer-related anaemia, iron deficiency and the specific role of I.V. iron. *Ann Oncol.* 2012;23(8):1954–1962.
5. Ganz T. Anemia of inflammation. *N Engl J Med.* 2019;381:1148–1157.
6. Musallam KM, Tamim HM, Richards T, et al. Preoperative anaemia and postoperative outcomes in non-cardiac surgery: a retrospective cohort study. *Lancet.* 2011;378(9800):1396–1407.
7. Caro JJ, Salas M, Ward A, Goss G. Anemia as an independent prognostic factor for survival in patients with cancer. *Cancer.* 2002;94(10):2793–2796.

8. Knight K, Wade S, Balducci L. Prevalence and outcomes of anemia in cancer: a systematic review of the literature. *Am J Med.* 2004;116(7):11–26.
9. Baron DM, Hochrieser H, Posch M, et al. Preoperative anaemia is associated with poor clinical outcome in non-cardiac surgery patients. *Br J Anaesth.* 2014;113(3):416–423.
10. Saager L, Turan A, Reynolds LF, Dalton JE, Mascha EJ, Kurz A. The association between preoperative anemia and 30-day mortality and morbidity in noncardiac surgical patients. *Anesth Analg.* 2013;117(4):909–915.
11. Muñoz M, Gómez-Ramírez S, Martín-Montañez E, Auerbach M. Perioperative anemia management in colorectal cancer patients: a pragmatic approach. *World J Gastroenterol.* 2014; 20(8):1972–1985.
12. Musallam KM, Taher AT. Iron deficiency beyond erythropoiesis: should we be concerned? *Curr Med Res Opin.* 2018;34:81–93.
13. Ajioka RS, Phillips JD, Kushner JP. Biosynthesis of heme in mammals. *Biochim Biophys Acta.* 2006;1793:723–736.
14. B. H-CU, Flögel U, Kelm M, Rassaf T. Unmasking the Janus face of myoglobin in health and disease. *J Exp Biol.* 2010; 213:2734–2740.
15. Paul BT, Manz DH, Torti FM, Torti SV. Mitochondria and iron: current questions. *Expert Rev Hematol.* 2017;10:65–79.
16. Charles-Edwards G, Amaral N, Sleigh A, et al. Effect of iron isomaltoside on skeletal muscle energetics in patients with chronic heart failure and iron deficiency: FERRIC-HF II randomized mechanistic trial. *Circulation.* 2019;139:2386–2398.
17. Miles LF, Sandhu RN, Grobler A, et al. Associations between non-anaemic iron deficiency and outcomes following surgery for colorectal cancer: an exploratory study of outcomes relevant to prospective observational studies. *Anaesth Intensive Care.* 2018;46(6):52–159.
18. Muñoz M, Acheson AG, Auerbach M, et al. International consensus statement on the peri-operative management of anaemia and iron deficiency. *Anaesthesia.* 2017;72(2):233–247.
19. Kell DB, Pretorius E. Serum ferritin is an important inflammatory disease marker, as it is mainly a leakage product from damaged cells. *Metallomics.* 2014;6(4):748–773.
20. Thomas C, Thomas L. Biochemical markers and hematologic indices in the diagnosis of functional iron deficiency. *Clin Chem.* 2002;48(7):1066–1076.
21. Aapro M, Beguin Y, Bokemeyer C, et al. Management of anaemia and iron deficiency in patients with cancer: ESMO clinical practice guidelines. *Ann Oncol.* 2018;29:iv271.
22. Thomas DW, Hinchliffe RF, Briggs C, Macdougall IC, Littlewood T, Cavill I. Guideline for the laboratory diagnosis of functional iron deficiency. *Br J Haematol.* 2013;161(5):639–648.
23. National Blood Authority. *Perioperative Patient Blood Management Guidelines: Module 2*: National Blood Authority; 2012:177.
24. Butcher A, Richards T, Stanworth SJ, Klein AA. Diagnostic criteria for pre-operative anaemia–time to end sex discrimination. *Anaesthesia.* 2017;72(7):811–814.
25. Miles LF, Larsen T, Bailey MJ, Burbury KL, Story DA, Bellomo R. Borderline anaemia and postoperative outcome in women undergoing major abdominal surgery: a retrospective cohort study. *Anaesthesia.* 2020;75(2):210–217.
26. Blaudszun G, Munting KE, Butchart A, Gerrard C, Klein AA. The association between borderline pre-operative anaemia in women and outcomes after cardiac surgery: a cohort study. *Anaesthesia.* 2018;73(5):572–578.
27. Avni T, Bieber A, Grossman A, Green H, Leibovici L, Gafter-Gvili A. The safety of intravenous iron preparations: systematic review and meta-analysis. *Mayo Clin Proc.* 2015;90(1):12–23.
28. Low MSY, Grigoriadis G. Iron deficiency and new insights into therapy. *Med J Aust.* 2017;207(2):81–87.
29. Spahn DR, Schoenrath F, Spahn GH, et al. Effect of ultra-short-term treatment of patients with iron deficiency or anaemia undergoing cardiac surgery: a prospective randomized trial. *Lancet.* 2019;393(10187):2201–2212.
30. Muñoz M, Gómez-Ramírez S, Cuenca J, et al. Very-short-term perioperative intravenous iron administration and postoperative outcome in major orthopedic surgery: a pooled analysis of observational data from 2547 patients. *Transfusion.* 2014;54(2):289–299.
31. Bohlius J, Bohlke K, Castelli R, et al. Management of cancer-associated anemia with erythropoiesis-stimulating agents: ASCO/ASH clinical practice guideline update. *Blood Adv.* 2019;3(8):1197–1210.
32. Kei T, Mistry N, Curley G, et al. Efficacy and safety of erythropoietin and iron therapy to reduce red blood cell transfusion in surgical patients: a systematic review and meta-analysis. *Can J Anesth.* 2019;66(6):716–731.
33. Luan H, Ye F, Wu L, Zhou Y, Jiang J. Perioperative blood transfusion adversely affects prognosis after resection of lung cancer: a systematic review and a meta-analysis. *BMC Surg.* 2014;14:34.
34. Rinker BD, Bowling JT, Vasconez HC. Blood transfusion and risk of metastatic disease or recurrence in patients undergoing immediate TRAM flap breast reconstruction: a clinical study and meta-analysis. *Plast Reconstruct Surg.* 2007;119(7):2001–2007.
35. Soubra A, Zabell JR, Adejoro O, Konety BR. Effect of perioperative blood transfusion on mortality for major urologic malignancies. *Clin Genitourin Cancer.* 2015;13(3):e173–e181.
36. Li SL, Ye Y, Yuan XH. Association between allogeneic or autologous blood transfusion and survival in patients after radical prostatectomy: a systematic review and meta-analysis. *PLoS One.* 2017;12(1):e0171081.
37. Acheson AG, Brookes MJ, Spahn DR. Effects of allogeneic red blood cell transfusions on clinical outcomes in patients undergoing colorectal cancer surgery: a systematic review and meta-analysis. *Ann Surg.* 2012;256(2):235–244.
38. American Society of Anesthesiologists Task Force on Perioperative Blood Management. Practice guidelines for perioperative blood management: an updated report by the American Society of Anesthesiologists Task Force on perioperative blood management*. *Anesthesiology.* 2015;122(2):241–275.
39. de Almeida JP, Vincent JL, Galas FR, et al. Transfusion requirements in surgical oncology patients: a prospective, randomized controlled trial. *Anesthesiology.* 2015;122(1):29–38.
40. Cata JP. Perioperative anemia and blood transfusions in patients with cancer: when the problem, the solution, and their combination are each associated with poor outcomes. *Anesthesiology.* 2015;122(1):3–4.
41. Durante C, Agostini F, Abbruzzese L, et al. Growth factor release from platelet concentrates: analytic quantification and characterization for clinical applications. *Vox Sang.* 2013;105(2):129–136.
42. Long K, Meier C, Ward M, Williams D, Woodward J, Bernard A. Immunologic profiles of red blood cells using in vitro models of transfusion. *J Surg Res.* 2013;184(1):567–571.
43. Dzik WH, Mincheff M, Puppo F. An alternative mechanism for the immunosuppressive effect of transfusion. *Vox Sang.* 2002;83(Suppl 1):417–419.

44. Bilgin YM, Brand A. Transfusion-related immunomodulation: a second hit in an inflammatory cascade? *Vox Sang.* 2008;95(4): 261–271.
45. Garcia-Roa M, Del Carmen Vicente-Ayuso M, Bobes AM, et al. Red blood cell storage time and transfusion: current practice, concerns and future perspectives. *Blood Transfus.* 2017;15(3):222–231.
46. Kekre N, Mallick R, Allan D, Tinmouth A, Tay J. The impact of prolonged storage of red blood cells on cancer survival. *PLoS One.* 2013;8(7):e68820.
47. Azmy MC, Pinto J, Patel NM, Govindan A, Kalyoussef E. Risk factors for blood transfusion with neck dissection. *Otolaryngol Head Neck Surg.* 2019;161(6):922–928.
48. Woolley AL, Hogikyan ND, Gates GA, Haughey BH, Schechtman KB, Goldenberg JL. Effect of blood transfusion on recurrence of head and neck carcinoma. Retrospective review and meta-analysis. *Ann Otol Rhinol Laryngol.* 1992;101(9):724–730.
49. Chau JK, Harris JR, Seikaly HR. Transfusion as a predictor of recurrence and survival in head and neck cancer surgery patients. *Otolaryngol Head Neck Surg.* 2010;39(5):516–522.
50. Goubran H, Baumeister P, Canis M, Reiter M. Preoperative anemia and perioperative blood transfusion in head and neck squamous cell carcinoma. *PLoS One.* 2018;13(10):e0205712.
51. Shewale JB, Correa AM, Brown EL, et al. Time trends of perioperative outcomes in early stage non-small cell lung cancer resection patients. *Ann Thorac Surg.* 2020;109(2):404–411.
52. Latif MJ, Tan KS, Molena D, et al. Perioperative blood transfusion has a dose-dependent relationship with disease recurrence and survival in patients with non–small cell lung cancer. *J Thorac Cardiovasc Surg.* 2019;157(6):2469–2477.e10.
53. Li L, Zhu D, Chen X, Huang Y, Ouyang M, Zhang W. Perioperative allogenenic blood transfusion is associated with worse clinical outcome for patients undergoing gastric carcinoma surgery: a meta-analysis. *Medicine.* 2015;94(39):e1574.
54. Agnes A, Lirosi MC, Panunzi S, Santocchi P, Persiani R, D'Ugo D. The prognostic role of perioperative allogeneic blood transfusions in gastric cancer patients undergoing curative resection: a systematic review and meta-analysis of non-randomized, adjusted studies. *Eur J Surg Oncol.* 2018;44(4):404–419.
55. Boshier PR, Ziff C, Adam ME, Fehervari M, Markar SR, Hanna GB. Effect of perioperative blood transfusion on the long-term survival of patients undergoing esophagectomy for esophageal cancer: a systematic review and meta-analysis. *Dis Esophagus.* 2018;31(4). doi:10.1093/dote/dox134.
56. Reeh M, Ghadban T, Dedow J, et al. Allogenic blood transfusion is associated with poor perioperative and long-term outcome in esophageal cancer. *World J Surg.* 2017;41(1):208–215.
57. Lee J, Chin JH, Kim JI, Lee EH, Choi IC. Association between red blood cell transfusion and long-term mortality in patients with cancer of the esophagus after esophagectomy. *Dis Esophagus.* 2018;31(2). doi:10.1093/dote/dox123.
58. Liu J, Chen S, Chen Y, Wang N, Ye X. Perioperative blood transfusion has no effect on overall survival after esophageal resection for esophageal squamous cell carcinoma: a retrospective cohort study. *Int J Surg.* 2018;55:24–30.
59. Amato AC, Pescatori M. Effect of perioperative blood transfusions on recurrence of colorectal cancer: meta-analysis stratified on risk factors. *Dis Colon Rectum.* 1998;41(5):570–585.
60. Amato A, Pescatori M. Perioperative blood transfusions for the recurrence of colorectal cancer. *Cochrane Database Syst Rev.* 2006(1):CD005033.
61. Lyu X, Qiao W, Li D, Leng Y. Impact of perioperative blood transfusion on clinical outcomes in patients with colorectal liver metastasis after hepatectomy: a meta-analysis. *Oncotarget.* 2017;8(25):41740–41748.
62. Saxena A, Valle SJ, Liauw W, Morris DL. Allogenic blood transfusion is an independent predictor of poorer peri-operative outcomes and reduced long-term survival after cytoreductive surgery and hyperthermic intraperitoneal chemotherapy: a review of 936 cases. *J Gastrointest Surg.* 2017;21(8):1318–1327.
63. Aquina CT, Blumberg N, Becerra AZ, et al. Association among blood transfusion, sepsis, and decreased long-term survival after colon cancer resection. *Ann Surg.* 2017;266(2):311–317.
64. Patel SV, Brennan KE, Nanji S, Karim S, Merchant S, Booth CM. Peri-operative blood transfusion for resected colon cancer: practice patterns and outcomes in a population-based study. *Cancer Epidemiol.* 2017;51:35–40.
65. Deeb A-P, Aquina CT, Monson JRT, Blumberg N, Becerra AZ, Fleming FJ. Allogeneic leukocyte-leduced red blood cell transfusion is associated with postoperative infectious complications and cancer recurrence after colon cancer resection. *Dig Surg.* 2020;37(2):163–170.
66. Liu L, Wang Z, Jiang S, et al. Perioperative allogenenic blood transfusion is associated with worse clinical outcomes for hepatocellular carcinoma: a meta-analysis. *PLoS One.* 2013; 8(5):e64261.
67. Mavros MN, Xu L, Maqsood H, et al. Perioperative blood transfusion and the prognosis of pancreatic cancer surgery: systematic review and meta-analysis. *Ann Surg Oncol.* 2015; 22(13):4382–4391.
68. Abe T, Amano H, Hanada K, et al. Perioperative red blood cell transfusion is associated with poor long-term survival in pancreatic adenocarcinoma. *Anticancer Res.* 2017;37(10):5863–5870.
69. Hwang HK, Jung MJ, Lee SH, Kang CM, Lee WJ. Adverse oncologic effects of intraoperative transfusion during pancreatectomy for left-sided pancreatic cancer: the need for strict transfusion policy. *J Hepatobiliary Pancreat Sci.* 2016;23(8):497–507.
70. Tai YH, Wu HL, Mandell MS, Tsou MY, Chang KY. The association of allogeneic blood transfusion and the recurrence of hepatic cancer after surgical resection. *Anaesthesia.* 2020; 75(4):464–471.
71. Shiba H, Misawa T, Fujiwara Y, et al. Negative impact of fresh-frozen plasma transfusion on prognosis of pancreatic ductal adenocarcinoma after pancreatic resection. *Anticancer Res.* 2013;33(9):4041–4047.
72. Kang R, Seath BE, Huang V, Barth RJ. Impact of autologous blood transfusion on survival and recurrence among patients undergoing partial hepatectomy for colorectal cancer liver metastases. *J Am Coll Surg.* 2019;228(6):902–908.
73. Nakaseko Y, Haruki K, Shiba H, et al. Impact of fresh frozen plasma transfusion on postoperative inflammation and prognosis of colorectal liver metastases. *J Surg Res.* 2018;226:157–165.
74. Wang Q, Du T, Lu C. Perioperative blood transfusion and the clinical outcomes of patients undergoing cholangiocarcinoma surgery: a systematic review and meta-analysis. *J Eur Gastroenterol Hepatol.* 2016;28(11):1233–1240.
75. Zhou PY, Tang Z, Liu WR, et al. Perioperative blood transfusion does not affect recurrence-free and overall survivals after curative resection for intrahepatic cholangiocarcinoma: a propensity score matching analysis. *BMC Cancer.* 2017;17(1):762.
76. Gomez-Gavara C, Doussot A, Lim C, et al. Impact of intraoperative blood transfusion on short and long term outcomes after

curative hepatectomy for intrahepatic cholangiocarcinoma: a propensity score matching analysis by the AFC-IHCC study group. *HPB (Oxford)*. 2017;19(5):411–420.

77. Wang YL, Jiang B, Yin FF, et al. Perioperative blood transfusion promotes worse outcomes of bladder cancer after radical cystectomy: a systematic review and meta-analysis. *PLoS One*. 2015;10(6):e0130122.
78. Cata JP, Lasala J, Pratt G, Feng L, Shah JB. Association between perioperative blood transfusions and clinical outcomes in patients undergoing bladder cancer surgery: a systematic review and meta-analysis study. *J Blood Transfus*. 2016;2016:9876394.
79. Chalfin HJ, Liu JJ, Gandhi N, et al. Blood transfusion is associated with increased perioperative morbidity and adverse oncologic outcomes in bladder cancer patients receiving neoadjuvant chemotherapy and radical cystectomy. *Ann Surg Oncol*. 2016;23(8):2715–2722.
80. Moschini M, Bianchi M, Gandaglia G, et al. The impact of perioperative blood transfusion on survival of bladder cancer patients submitted to radical cystectomy: role of anemia status. *Eur Urol Focus*. 2016;2(1):86–91.
81. Siemens DR, Jaeger MT, Wei X, Vera-Badillo F, Booth CM. Peri-operative allogeneic blood transfusion and outcomes after radical cystectomy: a population-based study. *World J Urol*. 2017;35(9):1435–1442.
82. Moschini M, Soria F, Abufaraj M, et al. Impact of intra- and postoperative blood transfusion on the incidence, timing, and pattern of disease recurrence after radical cystectomy. *Clin Genitourin Cancer*. 2017;15(4):e681–e688.
83. Buchner A, Grimm T, Schneevoigt BS, et al. Dramatic impact of blood transfusion on cancer-specific survival after radical cystectomy irrespective of tumor stage. *Scand J Urol*. 2017;51(2):130–136.
84. Vetterlein MW, Gild P, Kluth LA, et al. Peri-operative allogeneic blood transfusion does not adversely affect oncological outcomes after radical cystectomy for urinary bladder cancer: a propensity score-weighted European multicentre study. *BJU Int*. 2018;121(1):101–110.
85. Furrer MA, Fellmann A, Schneider MP, Thalmann GN, Burkhard FC, Wuethrich PY. Impact of packed red blood cells and fresh frozen plasma given during radical cystectomy and urinary diversion on cancer-related outcome and survival: an observational cohort study. *Eur Urol Focus*. 2018;4(6):916–923.
86. Linder BJ, Thompson RH, Leibovich BC, et al. The impact of perioperative blood transfusion on survival after nephrectomy for non-metastatic renal cell carcinoma (RCC). *BJU Int*. 2014;114(3):368–374.
87. Park YH, Kim YJ, Kang SH, et al. Association between perioperative blood transfusion and oncologic outcomes after curative surgery for renal cell carcinoma. *J Cancer*. 2016;7(8):965–972.
88. Soria F, de Martino M, Leitner CV, Moschini M, Shariat SF, Klatte T. Perioperative allogenic blood transfusion in renal cell carcinoma: risk factors and effect on long-term outcomes. *Clin Genitourin Cancer*. 2017;15(3):e421–e427.
89. Tsivian M, Abern MR, Tsivian E, et al. Effect of blood transfusions on oncological outcomes of surgically treated localized renal cell carcinoma. *Urol Oncol*. 2018;36(8):362.e1–362.e7.
90. Abu-Ghanem Y, Zilberman DE, Dotan Z, Kaver I, Ramon J. Perioperative blood transfusion adversely affects prognosis after nephrectomy for renal cell carcinoma. *Urol Oncol*. 2018;36(1):12 e5–12.e20.
91. Poorman CE, Postlewait LM, Ethun CG, et al. Blood transfusion and survival for resected adrenocortical carcinoma: a study from the United States Adrenocortical Carcinoma Group. *Am Surg*. 2017;83(7):761–768.
92. Monk BJ, Tewari K, Gamboa-Vujicic G, Burger RA, Manetta A, Berman ML. Does perioperative blood transfusion affect survival in patients with cervical cancer treated with radical hysterectomy? *Obstet Gynecol*. 1995;85(3):343–348.
93. Spirtos NM, Westby CM, Averette HE, Soper JT. Blood transfusion and the risk of recurrence in squamous cell carcinoma of the cervix: a gynecologic oncology group study. *Am J Clin Oncol*. 2002;25(4):398–403.
94. Bogani G, Ditto A, Martinelli F, et al. Impact of blood transfusions on survival of locally advanced cervical cancer patients undergoing neoadjuvant chemotherapy plus radical surgery. *Int J Gynecol Cancer*. 2017;27(3):514–522.
95. De Oliveira GS, Jr., Schink JC, Buoy C, Ahmad S, Fitzgerald PC, McCarthy RJ. The association between allogeneic perioperative blood transfusion on tumor recurrence and survival in patients with advanced ovarian cancer. *Transfus Med*. 2012;22(2):97–103.
96. Altman AD, Liu XQ, Nelson G, Chu P, Nation J, Ghatage P. The effects of anemia and blood transfusion on patients with stage III-IV ovarian cancer. *Int J Gynecol Cancer*. 2013;23(9):1569–1576.
97. Warner LL, Dowdy SC, Martin JR, et al. The impact of perioperative packed red blood cell transfusion on survival in epithelial ovarian cancer. *Int J Gynecol Cancer*. 2013;23(9):1612–1619.
98. Manning-Geist BL, Alimena S, del Carmen MG, et al. Infection, thrombosis, and oncologic outcome after interval debulking surgery: does perioperative blood transfusion matter? *Gynecol Oncol*. 2019;153(1):63–67.
99. Hunsicker O, Gericke S, Graw JA, et al. Transfusion of red blood cells does not impact progression-free and overall survival after surgery for ovarian cancer. *Transfusion*. 2019;59(12):3589–3600.
100. Key NS, Khorana AA, Kuderer NM, et al. Venous thromboembolism prophylaxis and treatment in patients with cancer: ASCO clinical practice guideline update. *J Clin Oncol*. 2020;38(5):496–520.
101. Burbury K, MacManus MP. The coagulome and the oncomir: impact of cancer-associated hemostatic dysregulation on the risk of metastasis. *Clin Exp Metastasis*. 2018;35(4):237–246.
102. Falanga A, Schieppati F, Russo L. Pathophysiology 1. Mechanisms of thrombosis in cancer patients. *Cancer Treat Res*. 2019;179:11–36.
103. Falanga A, Marchetti M. Hemostatic biomarkers in cancer progression. *Thromb Res*. 2018;164(Suppl 1):S54–S61.
104. Chen Z, Zhang P, Xu Y, et al. Surgical stress and cancer progression: the twisted tango. *Mol Cancer*. 2019;18(1):132.
105. Agnelli G, Verso M, Ageno W, et al. The MASTER registry on venous thromboembolism: description of the study cohort. *Thromb Res*. 2008;121(5):605–610.
106. Khorana AA, Francis CW, Culakova E, Kuderer NM, Lyman GH. Frequency, risk factors, and trends for venous thromboembolism among hospitalized cancer patients. *Cancer*. 2007;110(10):2339–2346.
107. Otten HM, Prins MH, Smorenburg SM, Hutten BA. Risk assessment and prophylaxis of venous thromboembolism in non-surgical patients: cancer as a risk factor. *Haemostasis*. 2000;30(Suppl 2):72–76, discussion 63.

108. Spyropoulos AC, Brotman DJ, Amin AN, Deitelzweig SB, Jaffer AK, McKean SC. Prevention of venous thromboembolism in the cancer surgery patient. *Cleve Clin J Med.* 2008;75(Suppl 3):S17–S26.
109. Gordon RJ, Lombard FW. Perioperative venous thromboembolism: a review. *Anesth Analg.* 2017;125(2):403–412.
110. Agnelli G, Bolis G, Capussotti L, et al. A clinical outcome-based prospective study on venous thromboembolism after cancer surgery: the @RISTOS project. *Ann Surg.* 2006;243(1):89–95.
111. Ma L, Wen Z. Risk factors and prognosis of pulmonary embolism in patients with lung cancer. *Medicine.* 2017;96(16):e6638.
112. Khorana AA, Dalal MR, Lin J, Connolly GC. Health care costs associated with venous thromboembolism in selected high-risk ambulatory patients with solid tumors undergoing chemotherapy in the United States. *Clinicoecon Outcomes Res.* 2013;5:101–108.
113. Trujillo-Santos J, Nieto JA, Tiberio G, et al. Predicting recurrences or major bleeding in cancer patients with venous thromboembolism. Findings from the RIETE Registry. *Thromb Haemost.* 2008;100(3):435–439.
114. Schulman S, Lindmarker P, Holmstrom M, et al. Post-thrombotic syndrome, recurrence, and death 10 years after the first episode of venous thromboembolism treated with warfarin for 6 weeks or 6 months. *J Thromb Haemost.* 2006;4(4):734–742.
115. Burbury K, MacManus M. The coagulome and the oncomir: impact of cancer-associated hemostatic dysregulation on the risk of metastasis. *Clin Exp Metastasis.* 2018;35(4):237–246.
116. Amirkhosravi A, Mousa SA, Amaya M, Francis JL. Antimetastatic effect of tinzaparin, a low-molecular-weight heparin. *J Thromb Haemost.* 2003;1(9):1972–1976.
117. Mousa SA, Linhardt R, Francis JL, Amirkhosravi A. Anti-metastatic effect of a non-anticoagulant low-molecular-weight heparin versus the standard low-molecular-weight heparin, enoxaparin. *Thromb Haemost.* 2006;96(6):816–821.
118. Becattini C, Rondelli F, Vedovati MC, et al. Incidence and risk factors for venous thromboembolism after laparoscopic surgery for colorectal cancer. *Haematologica.* 2015;100(1):e35–e38.
119. Alexander M, Ball D, Solomon B, et al. Dynamic thromboembolic risk modelling to target appropriate preventative strategies for patients with non-small cell lung cancer. *Cancers (Basel).* 2019;11(1):50.
120. Kakkar AK, Haas S, Wolf H, Encke A. Evaluation of perioperative fatal pulmonary embolism and death in cancer surgical patients: the MC-4 cancer substudy. *Thromb Haemost.* 2005;94(4):867–871.
121. Di Nisio M, Porreca E, Candeloro M, De Tursi M, Russi I, Rutjes AW. Primary prophylaxis for venous thromboembolism in ambulatory cancer patients receiving chemotherapy. *Cochrane Database Syst Rev.* 2016;12:CD008500.
122. Fuentes HE, Oramas DM, Paz LH, Casanegra AI, Mansfield AS, Tafur AJ. Meta-analysis on anticoagulation and prevention of thrombosis and mortality among patients with lung cancer. *Thromb Res.* 2017;154:28–34.
123. Bergqvist D, Agnelli G, Cohen AT, et al. Duration of prophylaxis against venous thromboembolism with enoxaparin after surgery for cancer. *N Engl J Med.* 2002;346(13):975–980.
124. Vedovati MC, Becattini C, Rondelli F, et al. A randomized study on 1-week versus 4-week prophylaxis for venous thromboembolism after laparoscopic surgery for colorectal cancer. *Ann Surg.* 2014;259(4):665–669.
125. Carrier M, Altman AD, Blais N, et al. Extended thromboprophylaxis with low-molecular weight heparin (LMWH) following abdominopelvic cancer surgery. *Am J Surg.* 2019;218(3):537–550.
126. Htun KT, Lee AYY. Thromboprophylaxis in cancer patients undergoing surgery. *Semin Thromb Hemost.* 2017;43(7):672–681.
127. Pannucci CJ, Swistun L, MacDonald JK, Henke PK, Brooke BS. Individualized venous thromboembolism risk stratification using the 2005 Caprini score to identify the benefits and harms of chemoprophylaxis in surgical patients: a meta-analysis. *Ann Surg.* 2017;265(6):1094–1103.
128. Krell RW, Scally CP, Wong SL, et al. Variation in hospital thromboprophylaxis practices for abdominal cancer surgery. *Ann Surg Oncol.* 2016;23(5):1431–1439.
129. Cohen AT, Tapson VF, Bergmann JF, et al. Venous thromboembolism risk and prophylaxis in the acute hospital care setting (ENDORSE study): a multinational cross-sectional study. *Lancet.* 2008;371(9610):387–394.
130. Kotaska A. Venous thromboembolism prophylaxis may cause more harm than benefit: an evidence-based analysis of Canadian and international guidelines. *Thromb J.* 2018;16:25.
131. Pannucci CJ, Fleming KI. Comparison of face-to-face interaction and the electronic medical record for venous thromboembolism risk stratification using the 2005 Caprini score. *J Vasc Surg Venous Lymphat Disord.* 2018;6(3):304–311.
132. Knight K, Wade S, Balducci L. Prevalence and outcomes of anemia in cancer: a systematic review of the literature. *Am J Med.* 2004;116(Suppl 7A):11S–26S.
133. Tas F, Eralp Y, Basaran M, et al. Anemia in oncology practice: relation to diseases and their therapies. *Am J Clin Oncol.* 2002;25(4):371–379.
134. Liu L, Liu L, Liang LC, et al. Impact of preoperative anemia on perioperative outcomes in patients undergoing elective colorectal surgery. *Gastroenterol Res Pract.* 2018;2018:2417028.
135. Liu X, Qiu H, Huang Y, et al. Impact of preoperative anemia on outcomes in patients undergoing curative resection for gastric cancer: a single-institution retrospective analysis of 2163 Chinese patients. *Cancer Med.* 2018;7(2):360–369.
136. Aapro M, Osterborg A, Gascon P, Ludwig H, Beguin Y. Prevalence and management of cancer-related anaemia, iron deficiency and the specific role of i.v. iron. *Ann Oncol.* 2012;23(8):1954–1962.
137. Aapro M, Van Erps J, MacDonald K, et al. Managing cancer-related anaemia in congruence with the EORTC guidelines is an independent predictor of haemoglobin outcome: initial evidence from the RESPOND study. *Eur J Cancer.* 2009;45(1):8–11.
138. Richards T., Baikady R.R., Clevenger B., et al. Preoperative intravenous iron to treat anaemia before major abdominal surgery (PREVENTT): a randomised, double-blind, controlled trial. *Lancet.* 2020;396(10259):1353–1361. doi:10.1016/S0140-6736(20)31539-7.

9

Improving Cancer Survival Through Perioperative Attenuation of Adrenergic-Inflammatory Signaling

ITAY RICON-BECKER, JONATHAN G. HILLER, AND SHAMGAR BEN-ELIYAHU

The Perioperative Period—An Underutilized "Window-of-Opportunity" to Prevent Metastatic Disease

The occurrence of metastatic disease is the leading cause of death in most patients with cancer. Accumulating evidence suggests that the perioperative period, days to weeks before and after surgery, is a critical time frame in which multiple factors profoundly affect initiation, progression, and/or elimination of metastases, providing a critical window of opportunity to prevent metastatic disease.[1–5] Surgery is the primary life-saving therapeutic approach for many patients with cancer. However, even after successful surgery, minimal residual disease (MRD) in the form of scattered single tumor cells and/or micrometastases are evident in a substantial portion of patients.[6] Additionally, several aspects of oncological surgery have been shown or suggested to promote metastasis,[2] including: (i) increased secretion of stress hormones[7,8]; (ii) local and systemic inflammation[9,10]; (iii) shedding of tumor cells into the circulation[11,12]; (iv) blood transfusions[13,14]; (v) hypothermia[15]; and (vi) use of specific anesthetic/analgesic agents[5,16,17] (e.g., intravenous lidocaine and propofol-TIVA are potentially preferred approaches in colorectal and lung cancers).[18–21] Specifically, these processes act directly on tumor cells and promote their capacity to survive, extravasate, migrate, seed, and release proangiogenic factors and additional progrowth/prometastatic factors while inhibiting a patient's antimetastatic immune response.[1–3] These processes are hypothesized to act synergistically on preexisting micrometastases and on isolated tumor cells scattered at the time of surgery, and thereby catalyze cancer recurrence that may not become evident for months or years following surgery when metastases reach a detectable size. For the patient receiving cancer resection surgery, the perioperative period thereby represents a vulnerability to cancer recurrence, which also provides an opportunity for effective intervention.

Clinical examples indicate that the inhibition of prometastatic perioperative processes can improve long-term cancer outcomes, indicating the nonproportional high impact of this short timeframe, specifically: (i) adherence to Enhanced Recovery After Surgery (ERAS) protocols in colorectal cancer (CRC) surgery[22,23]; (ii) enhancing perioperative immunity through use of short preoperative interleukin-2 (IL-2) treatment in colorectal and pancreatic cancer[24,25]; and (iii) perioperative hormone (progesterone) therapy in patients with breast cancer (BC),[26] have all been shown to improve long-term cancer outcomes. Such clinical trials suggest that brief, targeted perioperative therapies could offset perioperative prometastatic processes, ultimately improving cancer survival. Additional therapies under investigation include inhibition of neutrophil extracellular trap (NET) formation[27] and the use of neuroaxial anesthesia to reduce surgical stress.[5,28] Taken together, current evidence suggests that short-perioperative interventions (some already part of best practice guidelines[22,23]) may improve patients' long-term survival following cancer surgery.

As elaborated later, driving many of the prometastatic effects of the perioperative period is the abundant release of inflammatory and stress-related hormones that accompanies surgery.[29] Prominent among these are prostaglandins (PGs) and catecholamines (CAs; epinephrine, EPI; norepinephrine, NE).[1–3] Both PGs and CAs have been consistently shown in animal models and clinical trials to promote metastasis through their perioperative impact on tumor cells and immunity.[2] The effects of inflammation, a hallmark of cancer,[30] on cancer progression were noted over a hundred years ago,[31] and the deleterious effects of CAs on cancer progression have also been thoroughly documented during the last two decades.[32,33] More recently, perioperative care has been dominated by ERAS programs designed to maximize short-term clinical recovery and have been utilized with great success.[34] However, for the patient with cancer, a focus must also be placed on limiting the adrenergic-inflammatory response to reduce perioperative vulnerability to cancer metastasis, thereby improving long-term survival.

In this chapter, we (i) provide evidence for the importance of synergistically addressing inflammatory and adrenergic stress responses to surgery in order to reduce the risk for post-surgical metastatic disease and (ii) discuss how this may be achieved with simple and readily available clinical therapies.

Perioperative Stress-Inflammatory Responses: the Prometastatic Edge of the Sword

During the last three decades, translational[9,7,35–39] and clinical research[2,3,40–43] has shown that the perioperative secretion of PGs and CAs induced by anxiety, tissue damage, pain, and a variety of surgery-related procedures[3] affects cancer cells directly[44–46] and further promotes metastasis through their impact on immunity and the cancer microenvironment[36,37,47,48] (reviewed in Horowitz et al., 2015[1]). Importantly, PGs and CAs (i) copotentiate each other's synthesis and secretion and (ii) their impact eventually converges on the same intracellular molecular pathways (e.g., cAMP-PKA), establishing a synergistic inflammatory-stress response (ISR) to surgery.[1] ISRs drive cancer cells' epithelial-to-mesenchymal transition (EMT), migration, motility, survival, invasiveness, and angiogenesis, as well as suppress anti metastatic immune activities.[1,2] The effects of these ISRs, mediated also through PGs and CAs, could transform a life-saving operation into a double-edged sword, excising the malignant tissue but increasing the risk of recurrence.

ISRs Are Initiated Before Surgery

ISRs are known to be induced while anticipating threatening events (e.g., skydiving, public speaking, and surgery).[32,49–51] Specifically, expecting such events was shown to be accompanied by elevated levels of NE, EPI, cortisol, and proinflammatory cytokines such as CRP and IL-6.[50,51] Similarly, elevated levels of stress and inflammatory agents are evident a day before surgery.[52,53] Thus, the preoperative period is one in which ISRs are already elevated and facilitate prometastatic processes and immune inhibition, suggesting the need to therapeutically address ISRs even before surgery.

Inflammatory and Stress Responses Mutually Potentiate Each Other

Although stress responses and inflammatory responses are triggered separately, they also potentiate each other, creating an integrated ISR. CAs are secreted systemically (EPI) and locally released (NE) in response to sympathetic nervous system (SNS) activation due to stress and/or tissue damage.[32,33] Tissue damage also leads to the release of arachidonic acid, which is eventually metabolized by COX enzymes to synthesize PGs. SNS activation, through adrenergic signaling, promotes the metabolism of arachidonic acid and facilitates the synthesis of PGs.[33] In vivo exposure to chronic stress and in vitro exposure to EPI leads to upregulation of COX2 expression in cancer cell lines and in macrophages,[39,54] and to increased production of PG-E2[39] (the most abundant PG) and proinflammatory cytokines such as IL-6.[55] Importantly, adrenergic signaling can also lead to changes in lymphatic structure[39] and flow,[39,56] and to recruitment of immune cells from the spleen and bone marrow into the circulation, modulating their activity[57] in a manner that may potentiate proinflammatory responses. Peripheral inflammatory processes initiated by PG synthesis and mediated by cytokines crossing the blood–brain barrier can induce central nervous system (CNS) neuroinflammation and is known to increase and sustain adrenergic signaling.[57] In addition, proinflammatory cytokines (e.g., IL-6) can activate nociceptors, leading to local secretion of NE, and sustained pain can induce anxiety and systemic release of EPI.[58] Taken together, inflammatory and adrenergic signaling copotentiate each other in a manner that can lead to a self-perpetuating cycle of increasing inflammatory-adrenergic signaling (see Fig. 9.1).

Converging Intracellular Molecular Pathways of PGs and CAs

Although PGs and CAs act on different extracellular receptor systems, they often activate the same intracellular molecular pathways, leading to similar prometastatic consequences. EPI and NE bind to α and β receptors, of which binding to β2 receptors was repeatedly shown to promote many of the prometastatic effects of adrenergic signaling,[32,33] but other adrenergic receptors (e.g., β3) were also reported to deleteriously affect metastasis.[33] PGs are synthesized by epithelial, cancer, and immune cells (e.g., macrophages) through the metabolism of arachidonic acid by the constitutively active COX1 and tissue-damage (e.g., surgery)-induced COX2 enzymes. PG and CA receptors are expressed by most immunocytes and epithelial cells and are overly expressed by many tumors.[59,60] Both PGs and CAs elevate intracellular cAMP levels and subsequently lead to activation of various prometastatic signaling pathways (e.g., cAMP-PKA, cAMP-EPAC).[42,59] Notably, activation of both adrenergic and prostanoid receptors affects similar transcription pathways (e.g., NF-κB, STAT-3, CREB, AP1, GATA1, ETS) through which they exert potent prometastatic effects on cancer and immune cells.[32,33,55,59]

Overall, during the perioperative period, both PGs and CAs (i) are induced independently and through multiple mechanisms, starting even before surgery; (ii) potentiate the synthesis and release of each other; and (iii) activate similar intracellular prometastatic pathways. Thus combined

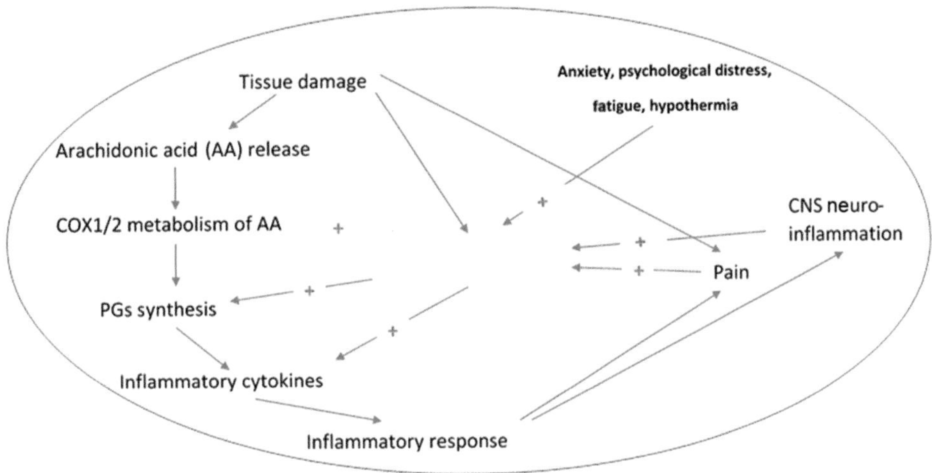

• **Fig. 9.1** Copotentiation of inflammatory-stress responses. The inflammatory stress response copotentiation cycle. Tissue damage leads to both arachidonic acid (*AA*) release and to local activation of adrenergic signaling. AA metabolism by COX enzymes is enhanced by adrenergic signaling, thus increasing prostaglandin (*PG*) synthesis. The secretion of inflammatory cytokines is induced by PGs and enhanced by adrenergic signaling, leading to an increased inflammatory response that enhances local and systemic adrenergic signaling through activation of nociceptors, and through induction of CNS neuroinflammation leading to increased systemic adrenergic signaling. Additionally, anxiety, psychological distress, fatigue, and hypothermia also induce adrenergic signaling throughout the perioperative period. Thus inflammation leads to an increased adrenergic response that leads to an increased inflammatory response.

beta-adrenergic and COX inhibition initiated before surgery could be optimal.

Herein, we will discuss the specific cancer-promoting mechanisms of PGs and CAs and the pharmacological agents currently available to block their effects perioperatively.

Direct Effects of PGs and CAs on Cancer Cells

The activation of the cAMP pathway by PGs and CAs induces prometastatic transcription activity. Specifically, NF-κB stimulation of the Snail, Slug, and TWIST1 transcription factors induces the tumor prometastatic processes necessary for the survival and dissemination of cancer cells. This includes the initiation of EMT and upregulation of HIF-1α, which enhances hypoxic conditioning and facilitates survival of circulating tumor cells with the potential to establish metastasis.[61] Additionally, cAMP-PKA-NF-κB activation leads to tumor secretion of (i) prometastatic and proinflammatory cytokines, such as IL-6, IL-1, IL-8, and TNFα; (ii) proangiogenic VEGF; and (iii) extracellular matrix degrading MMP2 and MMP9.[32,33,61]

Importantly, proinflammatory cytokines, such as TNF secreted by tumor cells, lead to activation of NF-κB, thus creating an autocrine positive feedback loop sustaining inflammatory conditions in the tumor microenvironment.

NF-κB is a prominent pathway by which many of the prometastatic effects of CAs and PGs are manifested. It was recently suggested that NF-κB regulation by NE is cell and context specific, such that elevated systemic levels of NE and EPI could potentially suppress inflammation in one context while elevating it in another.[55] Thus the blockade of beta-adrenoceptors may not always suppress inflammation and/or prometastatic processes. A recent review of clinical studies also suggested that the impact of beta blockers is cancer and context specific.[41] This and the fact that both CAs and PGs are simultaneously elevated[29,62] during the perioperative period may explain why in some animal models only the combined treatment of nonsteroidal antiinflammatory drugs (NSAIDs) and beta blockers has been effective in reducing postsurgical metastatic burden.[9,35,36]

ISRs and Immunity

Both animal and human studies demonstrate that PGs and CAs suppress immunity.[1,2] Specifically, CAs recruit immunocytes into the circulation,[32,52] and in parallel CAs and PGs induce tumor cell secretion of chemokines[61,63,64] that attract monocytes into the malignant tissue. Additionally, CAs and PGs directly facilitate polarization of tumor-associated macrophages (TAMs) into the M2 prometastatic phenotype.[65] Importantly, M2-like TAMs were shown to promote extravasation and metastasis and inhibit cell-mediated immunity.[65–67] Furthermore, TAMs express COX2 and produce PGs,[68] and this can be enhanced by beta-adrenergic signaling.[39] Additionally, macrophages are known to secrete NE in response to LPS stimulation[69] (in vitro) or in hypothermic animals.[70] Hence, adrenergic and prostanoid signaling leads to the recruitment of TAMs into the tumor environment, and TAMs in turn facilitate a proinflammatory prometastatic environment and can potentially secrete PGs and NE in a non-SNS dependent manner. Clinically, this suggests that even patients who do not exhibit anxiety and/or a systemic adrenergic response pre- or perioperatively may still benefit from pharmacological inhibition of CAs and PGs signaling.

ISRs exert extensive immune suppression as most immune cells express receptors for PGs and CAs.[33,55,71] Binding of PGs and CAs to these receptors was shown to (i) suppress NK cytotoxicity in vitro and in vivo[7,47] and reduce the cytotoxicity of T cells,[54,72] (ii) shift the Th2/Th1 balance toward Th2 dominance[73] (regarded as prometastatic), (iii) reduce lymphocyte number in critical compartments where circulating cancer cells might be retained (e.g., lung marinating pool),[35] and (iv) inhibit lymphocyte infiltration into tumor tissue.[32] Thus the combined effects of CAs and PGs can lead to immune suppression and can change the systemic and tumor immunocyte milieu in a manner that supports cancer progression.[10,36]

ISRs and the Cancer Microenvironment

CAs and PGs can facilitate prometastatic changes in the tumor microenvironment through a number of mechanisms. Both CAs and PGs can cause immune cells (e.g., macrophages, lymphocytes) to secrete MMP2 and MMP9, leading to extracellular matrix degradation that promotes tumor cell intravasation.[55,64] Notably, NE was shown to induce inhibin b A (INHBA) secretion by cancer cells, promoting a cancer-associated fibroblast (CAF) phenotype that can substantially potentiate tumor growth, invasion, and migration.[74] Inflammatory processes through COX signaling can induce platelet activation and aggregation, which provides protection and cloaking to circulating tumor cells, thus promoting their migration capacity.[75] Notably, EPI can also promote platelet activation and aggregation and is routinely used in in vitro studies for experimental activation of platelets.[76,77] Further assisting the migration of tumor cells, adrenergic signaling can increase the density of lymphatic vessels and lymphatic flow, as was shown in both animal models and recently in humans.[39,56] Such changes in the lymphatic vasculature were shown to be correlated with increased lymphatic presence of tumor cells, increased lymph-node involvement, and increased lung metastases.[39]

Given the abundant release of both CAs and PGs in the perioperative period, preventing the multiple prometastatic effects of ISRs may be especially important during this critical period. The "double-edged sword" of the perioperative period is such that while surgery represents a mainstay of solid tumor cure, the potential exists for perioperative ISRs to promote cancer recurrence and for their blockade to prevent it.

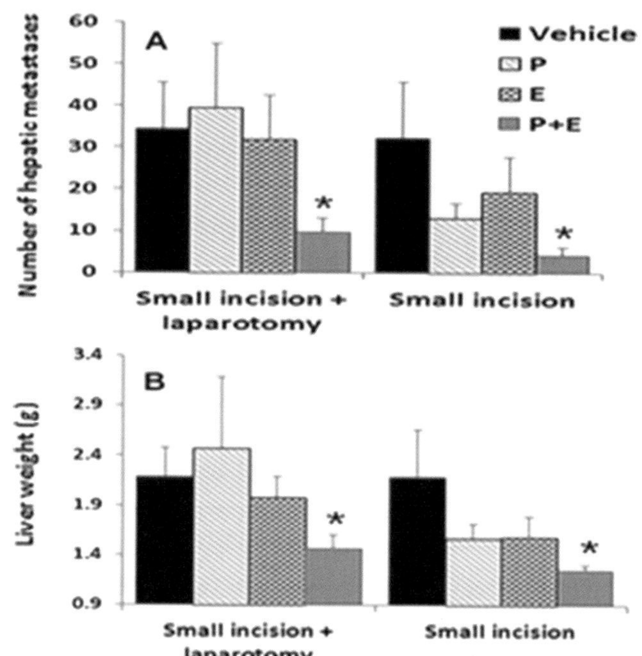

• **Fig. 9.2** Colon cancer (CT26). The beneficial effects of propranolol, etodolac, and their combined administration on the number of surface hepatic metastases and on liver weight (A and B). All animals underwent surgery for the injection of tumor cells through the spleen. A total of 57 mice (32 males and 25 females) were injected with propranolol (n = 13), etodolac (n = 16), both drugs (n = 14), or vehicles (n = 14), and 30 min later underwent one of two surgical procedures (small incision with or without laparotomy, approximately half from each drug treatment) for the injection of CT26 tumor cells into the spleen. Twenty-one days later, surface hepatic metastases were counted and livers were weighted. (A) Only the combined drug treatment, but not each drug alone, significantly reduced the number of surface-hepatic metastases compared to no drug treatment (vehicle), as indicated by an *, in both surgical procedures (PLSD $P < 0.05$ in all comparisons). (B) Liver weight showed the exact same pattern of results, and livers without tumors weighed ~1 g. Data are presented as mean + SEM.
From Sorski, L. et al. Reducing liver metastases of colon cancer in the context of extensive and minor surgeries through beta-adrenoceptors blockade and COX2 inhibition. *Brain Behav Immun*. 2016;58:91–98, doi:10.1016/j.bbi.2016.05.017

Addressing Perioperative Inflammation and Adrenergic Stress Responses

Based on preclinical studies, preventing the prometastatic effects of prostanoid and adrenergic signaling was suggested by us and others to be most effective in the initial stages of metastatic development.[3,4,28,36,46] The perioperative period is characterized by high levels of CAs and PGs, and in most patients also by MRD in the form of scattered tumor cells and micrometastases.[2] Several animal translational studies indicated that in the context of stress and/or surgery, the inhibition of inflammatory and/or adrenergic signaling can significantly reduce metastatic burden (e.g., number/weight of metastases) and increase survival rates[9,7,35–37,47] (see Figs. 9.2 and 9.3 for examples). As PGs and CAs converge to the same molecular pathways, in many animal models their combined blockade has been found to be particularly effective and in some models was the only effective approach using etodolac (semi-selective COX inhibitor) and propranolol (nonselective beta blocker).[9,35–37]

Clinical studies regarding beta blockade and/or COX inhibition and their effects on cancer outcomes are mostly retrospective cohort studies and meta-analyses[41,42,78–81] that have produced encouraging yet inconsistent evidence.[41,42] These studies, however, have only addressed the use of one family of drugs (i.e., beta-adrenergic blockers or COX inhibitors)

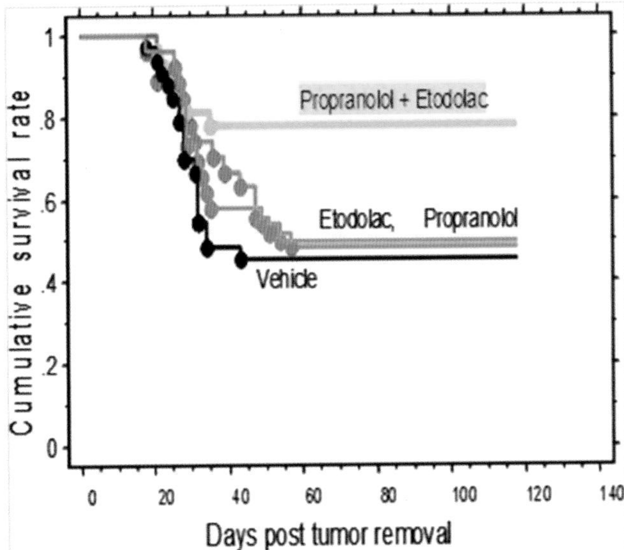

• **Fig. 9.3** Spontaneous metastasis and long-term survival following excision of a primary melanoma (B16F10.9). The beneficial effect of propranolol, etodolac, and their combined administration on long-term survival. All animals underwent surgery for the removal of a primary tumor (n = 234). Only the combined treatment of propranolol and etodolac significantly increased survival rates (but not either drug alone). Methods: mice were injected with B16F10.9 melanoma cells into the footpad subcutaneous space. Once a developing tumor reached 100–150 µL in volume, mice received drug/vehicle treatment, the tumor was completely excised, and long-term survival rates were assessed.
From Glasner, A. et al. Improving survival rates in two models of spontaneous postoperative metastasis in mice by combined administration of a beta-adrenergic antagonist and a cyclooxygenase-2 inhibitor. *J Immunol*. 2010;184:2449–2457. doi:10.4049/jimmunol.0903301

used acutely or chronically, but not the combined effects of both agents. Drawing conclusions based on these studies is challenging as they are highly heterogeneous with respect to the type of medication, timing of treatment and treatment duration, cancer characteristics, heterogeneity of co morbid diseases, and selection bias of the chosen populations. Overall, the strongest retrospective evidence for perioperative or chronic use of COX inhibitors or beta-adrenergic blockers is reported in CRC and melanoma.[41,42] Importantly, NSAIDs are now recommended by government advisory boards as a first-line CRC prevention strategy, indicating their anticancer properties, as reflected in a recent recommendation by the "US preventive services task force" to men between the ages of 50–59 years.[82] Furthermore, retrospective studies that have indicated beneficial effects of attenuating adrenergic or prostanoid signaling suggest that the use of a nonselective beta blocker (e.g., propranolol) may be more effective than selective blockers,[83–85] and that the blockade of both COX1 and COX2 enzymes (e.g., using aspirin or etodolac) could be more advantageous than the blockade of each enzyme separately.[86,87] Taken together, robust evidence from animal studies and mixed results from retrospective human studies indicate potential benefits from blocking inflammation and/or adrenergic stress responses (ISRs) in the perioperative oncological context. As discussed later, recent small randomized controlled trials (RCTs) are now showing promising findings for the separate and/or combined perioperative use of beta blockers and NSAIDs.

Perioperative Beta-adrenergic Blockade in RCTs

Recent clinical trials provide evidence for the potential short- and possible long-term benefits of perioperative beta blockade. For example, in patients with ovarian cancer, three different RCTs have provided promising results. In one study, 5 days of perioperative oral propranolol (a nonselective beta blocker) treatment, initiated 2 days before surgery, reduced serum levels of CA-125 (a biomarker indicating cancer burden) for up to 3 weeks following surgery (n = 22).[88] Another RCT studied the effects of low-dose (10–20 mg twice daily) propranolol, initiated 2 days prior to ovarian cancer surgery or as neoadjuvant therapy, and found decreased anxiety, depression, and increased quality of life (n = 32).[89] A third RCT studying the effects of propranolol treatment (40 mg b.i.d.) initiated 3 days before surgery and continued until completion of chemotherapy treatment demonstrated significant reductions in VEGF, IL-6, MCP-1, and IL-8 serum levels at several time points along the treatment course (n = 84).[90] These findings demonstrate the effectiveness of propranolol in reducing (i) markers of tumor burden, (ii) perioperative inflammation, and (iii) anxiety and distress.

A recent study assessing the effects of intraoperative intravenous landiolol hydrochloride (an ultra-short acting b1 blocker) administration to patients with lung cancer showed a trend toward increased 2-year relapse-free survival, with 89% (95% confidence interval [CI], 0.78–1.01) in landiolol-treated patients compared with 76% (95% CI, 0.6–0.91) in the placebo group, although this was not statistically significant (P = 0.1828, n = 57).[91] A recently concluded triple-blinded RCT study (n = 60) assessed the effects of an escalating dose of preoperative propranolol for 7 days prior to BC resection surgery. The trial focused on changes in prometastatic and proinflammatory gene expression between biopsy (prior to drug treatment) and tumor resection. Propranolol reduced mesenchymal gene expression (P = 0.002), down-regulated intratumoral inflammatory transcription factors (Snail/Slug, NF-κB/Rel, AP-1), and promoted tumor infiltration of $CD68^+$ macrophages and $CD8^+$ T cells.[92]

Taken together, clinical evidence from RCTs indicates the potential efficacy of perioperative beta blockade in reducing the metastatic potential of different cancers.

Perioperative RCTs of NSAIDs During Cancer Surgery

Evidence regarding the effects of perioperative NSAID use on cancer outcomes is also emerging. In a clinical trial of patients with thyroid cancer (n = 57), preoperative analgesia using intravenous parecoxib sodium (a highly selective COX2 inhibitor) reduced plasma levels of NE, cortisol, and blood glucose, indicating a reduced stress response to surgery through blockade of PG synthesis.[93] Interestingly, this clinical evidence suggests that inhibition of COX2 may itself reduce local adrenergic (NE) signaling. In separate trials the use of perioperative parecoxib[94] and flurbiprofen[95] (nonselective COX inhibitor) enhanced antitumor immunity among patients with cervical and gastric cancer, restored Th1/Th2/Treg balance,[94] and reduced postoperative suppression of CTLs and NK cell activity.[95] In patients with CRC (n = 28), 3 days of preoperative NSAID treatment (the nonselective COX inhibitor indomethacin or the COX2 selective celecoxib) increased CTL infiltration into tumor stroma.[96] Among patients with prostate cancer (n = 45), 4 weeks of presurgical treatment with celecoxib, initiated following biopsy, suggested that treatment decreased histological markers of proliferation and angiogenesis, and enhanced tumor apoptosis.[97] Notably, standard dosing of celecoxib during cancer surgery only weakly reduced perioperative PG production,[98] and post hoc analysis found that neo-CTX impaired celecoxib's ability to reduce PGs. Thus it may be hypothesized that semi-selective COX inhibitors may be advantageous in some circumstances. In addition, effective reduction of perioperative inflammation may be assisted by beta blockade, either through intraoperative intravenous administration or oral administration initiated prior to surgery.

Perioperative Combined Blockade of Inflammatory Stress Responses

The rationale for clinical trials assessing the combined perioperative blockade of CA and PG signaling relies on the (i) copotentiating and synergistic pathways by which CAs and PGs affect cancer progression, (ii) simultaneous perioperative increase in both CAs and PGs, and (iii) preclinical studies indicating the superior impact of their combined blockade.

A recent retrospective study, published as an abstract,[99] assessed the impact of perioperative separate and combined use of NSAIDs and/or beta blockers in patients with ovarian cancer, and found that their use was correlated with improved overall survival. Importantly, the combined use of propranolol and etodolac was correlated with a lower number of tumor nodules to a greater extent than each drug family used alone, suggesting that combined treatment increases inhibition of metastatic processes.

In two recently concluded RCTs, we treated BC[10,52] (n = 38) and CRC[100] (n = 34) patients with a combination (see Tables 9.1 and 9.2) of etodolac and slow-release (SR) propranolol (vs. placebo). Treatment was initiated 5 days before surgery and continued for 5 (BC) or 14 days (CRC) following surgery. Etodolac was given at a dose of 400 mg b.i.d. throughout the entire intervention. SR propranolol was initiated at a dose of 20 mg b.i.d., increased to 80 mg b.i.d. on the day of surgery, and then down-titrated to 40 (only in CRC) and 20 mg postoperatively. Impor-

TABLE 9.1 Drug/Placebo Schedule in the Breast Cancer Study

	Days −5 to −1	Day of Surgery	Days 1 to 7
Propranolol slow release oral, b.i.d.	20 mg	80 mg	20 mg
Etodolac oral, b.i.d.	400 mg	400 mg	400 mg

This table describes the perioperative combined treatment used in the study of Shaashua et al. (2017).[52] The treatment regimen of oral slow-release propranolol was scheduled as follows: (i) 20 mg b.i.d. for 5 days prior to surgery, (ii) 80 mg b.i.d. on the day of surgery, and (iii) 20 mg b.i.d. for 7 days following surgery. Four hundred milligram pills of the semi-selective COX2 inhibitor etodolac were scheduled twice a day throughout the intervention period. b.i.d., bis-in-die (twice a day). Data from Shaashua, L. et al. Perioperative COX-2 and beta-Adrenergic Blockade Improves Metastatic Biomarkers in Breast Cancer Patients in a Phase-II Randomized Trial. *Clin Cancer Res* 23, 4651–4661, doi:10.1158/1078-0432.CCR-17-0152 (2017).

TABLE 9.2 Drug/Placebo Schedule in the Colorectal Cancer Study

	Days −5 to −1	Day of Surgery	Days 1 to 7	Days 8 to 14
Propranolol slow release oral, b.i.d.	20 mg	80 mg	40 mg	20 mg
Etodolac oral, b.i.d.	400 mg	400 mg	400 mg	400 mg

This table describes a perioperative combined treatment given to patients with colorectal cancer as described by Haldar et al. (2017).[100] The treatment regimen of oral slow-release propranolol was scheduled as follows: (i) 20 mg b.i.d. for 5 days prior to surgery, (ii) 80 mg b.i.d. on the day of surgery, and (iii) 20 mg b.i.d. for 7 days following surgery. Four hundred milligram pills of the semi-selective COX2 inhibitor etodolac were scheduled twice a day throughout the intervention period. b.i.d., bis-in-die (twice a day).

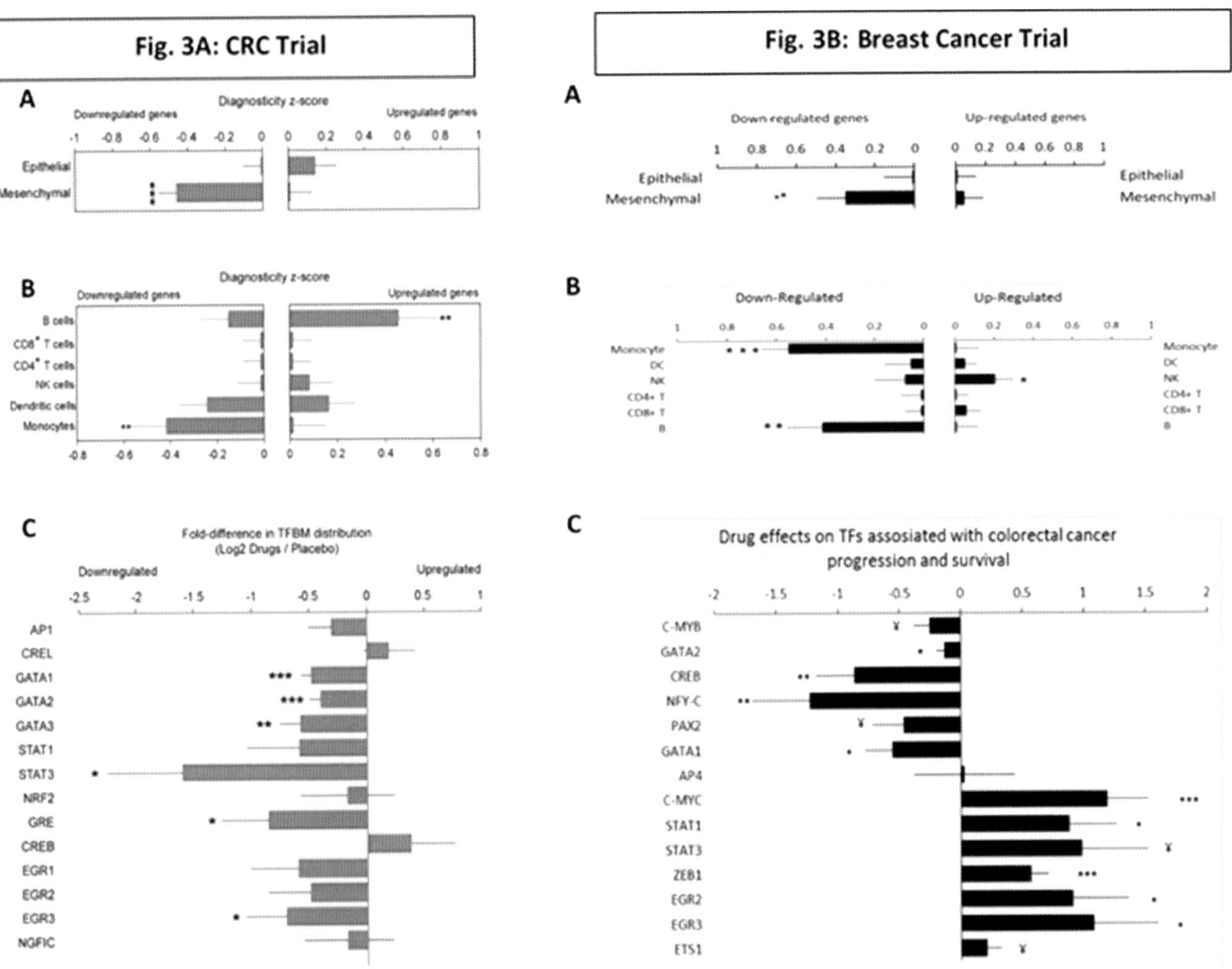

• **Fig. 9.4** Combined perioperative blockade effect on transcription activity within CRC and BC tumors. The effects of 5 days of presurgical treatment with the nonselective beta blocker propranolol and the semi-selective COX2 inhibitor etodolac on transcription activity within CRC[100] and BC[10,52] tumors. Tumor samples (from FFPE blocks) were subjected to whole-genome mRNA profiling. In both cancer types: (A) reduced EMT, (B) reduced monocytes infiltration, (C) activity of prometastatic/proinflammatory transcription factors. In BC tumor samples an increase in NK cells infiltration was also evident. $^{*}P < 0.05$, $^{**}P < 0.001$, $^{***}P < 0.0001$, γ borderline significant. *BC*, Breast cancer; *CRC*, colorectal cancer; *EMT*, epithelial-to-mesenchymal transition; *FFPE*, formalin-fixed paraffin-embedded.

tantly, no drug-related adverse events were noted. In both CRC and BC tumor tissue samples extracted at surgery, 5 preoperative days of combined treatment led to decreased EMT and downregulation of proinflammatory and pro-malignant transcription pathways in the malignant tissue, including NF-κB, STAT-3, CREB, and the GATA family (see Fig. 9.4). The treatment also reduced monocyte presence in the tumor tissue; in BC patients the tumor proliferation marker Ki67 was reduced, and in CRC tumors NK cell infiltration was increased. Analyses of blood samples, which were collected only in the BC study, indicated that the perioperative treatment reduced serum IL-6 and CRP, improved markers of NK cell cytotoxicity, and enhanced IL-12- and IFN-γ-induced production, but did not affect antiinflammatory IL-10 and cortisol serum levels. Finally, the increase in circulating monocyte number on postoperative day 1 was completely abolished by the treatment. Notably, in the CRC study, the 3 years following surgery recurrence rates were 1/15 in treated patients, and 5/19 in the placebo group (see Fig. 9.5) ($P = 0.23$) in intent to treat analysis, and 0/11 vs. 5/17 in protocol compliant patients ($P = 0.054$). Taken together, recent studies in the clinical setting indicate that the combined approach improves perioperative immune function and reduces prometastatic processes. Efforts to examine the long-term significance of these results are now underway in two RCTs in CRC (NCT03919461) and pancreatic (NCT03838029) cancer patients.

Safety Concerns

Perioperative use of either NSAIDs or beta blockers has been extensively studied. Beta blockers were initially recommended for the reduction of postsurgical cardiac events.[101] This recommendation was reversed following the POISE1 study,[102] which assessed the effects of administering the

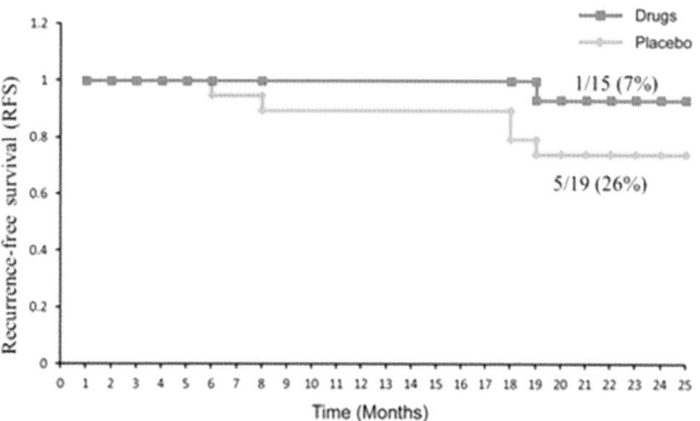

• **Fig. 9.5** Intent-to-treat. Disease-free survival (DFS) following combined perioperative inflammatory-adrenergic blockade: 3-year follow up after the combined perioperative treatment of propranolol and etodolac indicated that 1 of 15 (7%) patients in the medication treatment experienced recurrence, and 5 of 19 (26%) in the placebo group experienced recurrence. *P* = 0.23. Data are presented as DFS curves.

selective β1 blocker metoprolol, initiated on the day of surgery until 30 days following it. The treatment with this β1 blocker not only reduced postsurgical myocardial infraction (hazard ratio [HR], 0.73; 95% CI, 0.6–0.89; *P* = 0.0017), but also increased the number of postsurgical hypotension- and stroke-related deaths (HR, 1.33; 95% CI, 1.03–1.74; *P* = 0.0317). The researchers noted that the moderate-to-high dosage, lack of titration, and treatment initiation on the day of surgery contributed to the increase in treatment-related mortality. A subsequent cohort study assessed the impact of in-hospital beta blocker treatment on postsurgical stroke occurrences. Of 44,092 consecutive patients, 10,756 patients received beta blockers, of which 0.2% (88) suffered a stroke within 7 days of surgery.[103] Notably, the study concluded that the observation of increased stroke was specific to metoprolol, in contrast to other drugs of the beta blocker class.[103] Importantly, propranolol, a nonselective beta blocker, was not included in the POISE trial or this follow up trial, and clinical studies in the context of oncological studies report favorable safety outcomes for propranolol (see earlier). Current guidelines recommend that the perioperative use of beta blockers be considered on an individual patient basis.[101] Given what has been learned from the POISE1 trial, patients with high risk of cerebrovascular events receiving intermediate-to-high risk cancer surgery are not good candidates to receive moderate-to-high dose beta blockers (in particular metoprolol), especially without preoperative dose escalation. The American Heart Association (AHA), the American College of Cardiology (ACC), and the European Society of Cardiology (ESC) recommend initiating perioperative beta blocker treatment, when indicated, prior to surgery.[104,105]

Chronic NSAID use is associated with several adverse side effects, including increased risk for gastrointestinal bleeding and thrombotic events. However, regarding the more acute perioperative contexts, current ERAS guidelines recommend NSAID use in order to reduce opioid and opioid-related side effects[106] in patients with low risk for cardiovascular events. In addition, a number of studies assessing the safety of COX2 inhibitors during the perioperative period did not find evidence for increased thrombotic, renal, or cardiac risk.[107–109] Importantly, in patients with elevated risk for cardiovascular complications, the administration of NSAIDs should be for short durations and at low doses.[110]

In our two concluded clinical trials[52,100] (see Tables 9.1 and 9.2), we used propranolol in titration and etodolac at a medium dosage for a short perioperative duration, initiated 5 days before surgery (see earlier). Treatment was well tolerated with equivalent adverse event rates between treatment and placebo groups, and few treated patients expectedly exhibited temporary asymptomatic bradycardia that was not sustained. In all of the studies described earlier, in which NSAIDs and beta blockers were administered separately, treatment was also well tolerated.

Conclusion

Evidence suggests that blocking ISRs could beneficially affect prometastatic processes to which patients may be extremely vulnerable during the perioperative period. Use of the COX2 inhibitor etodolac and the nonselective beta blocker propranolol provide a safe, accessible, prophylactic approach in a manner that also reduces pain and carries a low risk of side effects. Clinical trials have provided promising safety and efficacy results, and larger clinical trials assessing impacts on long-term cancer outcomes are underway. Furthermore, as many cancer therapies induce inflammation and stress responses (including adjuvant and neoadjuvant chemo-, radio-, and immunotherapies), combined beta blocker and COX2 therapy could be considered as adjuncts to such therapies.

Perioperative clinicians are responsible for progressing research into anti-PG and anti-CA therapies during cancer surgery, and the insight gained from perioperative research must be disseminated to medical oncologists. Both propranolol and COX inhibitors are widely available and are routinely and safely used in the perioperative context with patients without contraindications. Protocols for the use of a combined drug regimen and the contraindications list used in our two RCTs mentioned earlier are available upon request.

References

1. Horowitz M, Neeman E, Sharon E, Ben-Eliyahu S. Exploiting the critical perioperative period to improve long-term cancer outcomes. *Nat Rev Clin Oncol.* 2015;12:213–226. doi:10.1038/nrclinonc.2014.224.
2. Hiller JG, Perry NJ, Poulogiannis G, Riedel B, Sloan EK. Perioperative events influence cancer recurrence risk after surgery. *Nat Rev Clin Oncol.* 2018;15:205–218. doi:10.1038/nrclinonc.2017.194.
3. Forget P, Aguirre JA, Bencic I, et al. How anesthetic, analgesic and other non-surgical techniques during cancer surgery

might affect postoperative oncologic outcomes: a summary of current state of evidence. *Cancers*. 2019;11:592. doi:10.3390/cancers11050592.
4. Wall T, Sherwin A, Ma D, Buggy DJ. Influence of perioperative anaesthetic and analgesic interventions on oncological outcomes: a narrative review. *Br J Anaesth*. 2019;123:135–150. doi:10.1016/j.bja.2019.04.062.
5. Nagrath S, Sequist LV, Maheswaran S, et al. Isolation of rare circulating tumour cells in cancer patients by microchip technology. *Nature*. 2007;450:1235–1239. doi:10.1038/nature06385.
6. Rosenne E, Sorski L, Shaashua L, et al. In vivo suppression of NK cell cytotoxicity by stress and surgery: glucocorticoids have a minor role compared to catecholamines and prostaglandins. *Brain Behav Immun*. 2014;37:207–219. doi:10.1016/j.bbi.2013.12.007.
7. Inbar S, Neeman E, Avraham R, Benish M, Rosenne E, Ben-Eliyahu S. Do stress responses promote leukemia progression? An animal study suggesting a role for epinephrine and prostaglandin-E2 through reduced NK activity. *PLoS One*. 2011;6:e19246. doi:10.1371/journal.pone.0019246.
8. Sorski L, Melamed R, Matzner P, et al. Reducing liver metastases of colon cancer in the context of extensive and minor surgeries through beta-adrenoceptors blockade and COX2 inhibition. *Brain Behav Immun*. 2016;58:91–98. doi:10.1016/j.bbi.2016.05.017.
9. Ricon I, Hanalis-Miller T, Haldar R, Jacoby R, Ben-Eliyahu S. Perioperative biobehavioral interventions to prevent cancer recurrence through combined inhibition of beta-adrenergic and cyclooxygenase 2 signaling. *Cancer*. 2019;125:45–56. doi:10.1002/cncr.31594.
10. Haldar R, Shaashua L, Lavon H, et al. Perioperative inhibition of beta-adrenergic and COX2 signaling in a clinical trial in breast cancer patients improves tumor Ki-67 expression, serum cytokine levels, and PBMCs transcriptome. *Brain Behav Immun*. 2018;73:294–309. doi:10.1016/j.bbi.2018.05.014.
11. Hardingham JE, Grover P, Winter M, Hewett PJ, Price TJ, Thierry B. Detection and clinical significance of circulating tumor cells in colorectal cancer–20 years of progress. *Mol Med*. 2015;21(Suppl 1):S25–S31. doi:10.2119/molmed.2015.00149.
12. Rahbari NN, Aigner M, Thorlund K, et al. Meta-analysis shows that detection of circulating tumor cells indicates poor prognosis in patients with colorectal cancer. *Gastroenterology*. 2010;138:1714–1726. doi:10.1053/j.gastro.2010.01.008.
13. Atzil S, Arad M, Glasner A, et al. Blood transfusion promotes cancer progression: a critical role for aged erythrocytes. Anesthesiology. 2018;109:989–997. doi:10.1097/ALN.0b013e31818ddb72.
14. Cata JP, Gutierrez C, Mehran RJ, et al. Preoperative anemia, blood transfusion, and neutrophil-to-lymphocyte ratio in patients with stage I non-small cell lung cancer. *Cancer Cell Microenviron*. 2016;3:e1116. doi:10.14800/ccm.1116.
15. Ben-Eliyahu S, Shakhar G, Rosenne E, Levinson Y, Beilin B. Hypothermia in barbiturate-anesthetized rats suppresses natural killer cell activity and compromises resistance to tumor metastasis: a role for adrenergic mechanisms. *Anesthesiology*. 1999;91:732–740.
16. Cata JP, Keerty V, Keerty D, et al. A retrospective analysis of the effect of intraoperative opioid dose on cancer recurrence after non-small cell lung cancer resection. *Cancer Med*. 2014;3:900–908. doi:10.1002/cam4.236.
17. Oh TK, Jeon JH, Lee JM, et al. Association of high-dose postoperative opioids with recurrence risk in esophageal squamous cell carcinoma: reinterpreting ERAS protocols for long-term oncologic surgery outcomes. *Dis Esophagus*. 2017;30:1–8. doi:10.1093/dote/dox074.
18. Wigmore TJ, Mohammed K, Jhanji S. Long-term survival for patients undergoing volatile versus IV anesthesia for cancer surgery. *Anesthesiology*. 2016;124:69–79. doi:10.1097/Aln.0000000000000936.
19. Enlund M, Berglund A, Andreasson K, Cicek C, Enlund A, Bergkvist L, The choice of anaesthetic-sevoflurane or propofol-and outcome from cancer surgery: a retrospective analysis. *Upsala J Med Sci*. 2014;119:251–261. doi:10.3109/03009734.2014.922649.
20. Yap A, Lopez-Olivo MA, Dubowitz J, Hiller J, Riedel B Anesthetic technique and cancer outcomes: a meta-analysis of total intravenous versus volatile anesthesia. *Can J Anesth*. 2019;66:546–561. doi:10.1007/s12630-019-01330-x.
21. Wang HL, Yan HD, Liu YY, et al. Intraoperative intravenous lidocaine exerts a protective effect on cell-mediated immunity in patients undergoing radical hysterectomy. *Mol Med Rep*. 2015;12:7039–7044. doi:10.3892/mmr.2015.4235.
22. Gustafsson UO, Oppelstrup H, Thorell A, Nygren J, Ljungqvist O. Adherence to the ERAS protocol is associated with 5-year survival after colorectal cancer surgery: a retrospective cohort study. *World J Surg*. 2016;40:1741–1747. doi:10.1007/s00268-016-3460-y.
23. Pisarska M, Torbicz G, Gajewska N, et al. Compliance with the ERAS protocol and 3-year survival after laparoscopic surgery for non-metastatic colorectal cancer. *World J Surg*. 2019;43:2552–2560. doi:10.1007/s00268-019-05073-0.
24. Caprotti R, Brivio F, Fumagalli L, et al. Free-from-progression period and overall short preoperative immunotherapy with IL-2 increases the survival of pancreatic cancer patients treated with macroscopically radical surgery. *Anticancer Res*. 2008;28:1951–1954.
25. Brivio F, Fumagalli L, Lissoni P, et al. Pre-operative immunoprophylaxis with interleukin-2 may improve prognosis in radical surgery for colorectal cancer stage B-C. *Anticancer Res*. 2006;26:599–603.
26. Badwe R, Hawaldar R, Parmar V, et al. Single-injection depot progesterone before surgery and survival in women with operable breast cancer: a randomized controlled trial. *J Clin Oncol*. 2011;29:2845–2851. doi:10.1200/JCO.2010.33.0738JCO.2010.33.0738.
27. Tohme S, Yazdani HO, Al-Khafaji AB, et al. Neutrophil extracellular traps promote the development and progression of liver metastases after surgical stress. *Cancer Res*. 2016;76:1367–1380. doi:10.1158/0008-5472.Can-15-1591.
28. Dubowitz JA, Sloan EK, Riedel BJ. Implicating anaesthesia and the perioperative period in cancer recurrence and metastasis. *Clin Exp Metastasis*. 2018;35:347–358. doi:10.1007/s10585-017-9862-x.
29. Desborough JP. The stress response to trauma and surgery. *Brit J Anaesth*. 2000;85:109–117. doi:10.1093/bja/85.1.109.
30. Hanahan D, Weinberg RA. Hallmarks of cancer: the next generation. *Cell*. 2011;144:646–674. doi:10.1016/j.cell.2011.02.013.
31. Balkwill F, Mantovani A. Inflammation and cancer: back to Virchow? *Lancet*. 2001;357:539–545. doi:10.1016/S0140-6736(00)04046-0.

32. Cole SW, Nagaraja AS, Lutgendorf SK, Green PA, Sood AK. Sympathetic nervous system regulation of the tumour microenvironment. *Nat Rev Cancer*. 2015;15:563–572. doi:10.1038/nrc3978.
33. Cole SW, Sood AK. Molecular pathways: beta-adrenergic signaling in cancer. *Clin Cancer Res*. 2012;18:1201–1206. doi:10.1158/1078-0432.CCR-11-0641.
34. Kehlet H. ERAS implementation-time to move forward. *Ann Surg*. 2018;267:998–999. doi:10.1097/SLA.0000000000002720.
35. Benish M, Bartal I, Goldfarb Y, et al. Perioperative use of beta-blockers and COX-2 inhibitors may improve immune competence and reduce the risk of tumor metastasis. *Ann Surg Oncol*. 2008;15:2042–2052. doi:10.1245/s10434-008-9890-5.
36. Glasner A, Avraham R, Rosenne E, et al. Improving survival rates in two models of spontaneous postoperative metastasis in mice by combined administration of a beta-adrenergic antagonist and a cyclooxygenase-2 inhibitor. *J Immunol*. 2010;184:2449–2457. doi:10.4049/jimmunol.0903301.
37. Melamed R, Rosenne E, Shakhar K, Schwartz Y, Abudarham N, Ben-Eliyahu S. Marginating pulmonary-NK activity and resistance to experimental tumor metastasis: suppression by surgery and the prophylactic use of a beta-adrenergic antagonist and a prostaglandin synthesis inhibitor. *Brain Behav Immun*. 2005;19:114–126.
38. Lamkin DM, Sung HY, Yang GS, et al. alpha2-Adrenergic blockade mimics the enhancing effect of chronic stress on breast cancer progression. *Psychoneuroendocrinology*. 2015;51:262–270. doi:10.1016/j.psyneuen.2014.10.004.
39. Le CP, Nowell CJ, Kim-Fuchs C, et al. Chronic stress in mice remodels lymph vasculature to promote tumour cell dissemination. *Nat Commun*. 2016;7:1–14. doi: ARTN 1063410.1038/ncomms10634.
40. Neeman E, Ben-Eliyahu S. Surgery and stress promote cancer metastasis: new outlooks on perioperative mediating mechanisms and immune involvement. *Brain Behav Immun*. 2013;30(Suppl):S32–S40. doi:10.1016/j.bbi.2012.03.006S0889-1591(12)00097-9.
41. Yap A, Lopez-Olivo MA, Dubowitz J, et al. Effect of beta-blockers on cancer recurrence and survival: a meta-analysis of epidemiological and perioperative studies. *Br J Anaesth*. 2018;121:45–57. doi:10.1016/j.bja.2018.03.024.
42. Cata JP, Guerra CE, Chang GJ, Gottumukkala V, Joshi GP. Non-steroidal anti-inflammatory drugs in the oncological surgical population: beneficial or harmful? A systematic review of the literature. *Br J Anaesth*. 2017;119:750–764. doi:10.1093/bja/aex225.
43. Forget P, Aguirre JA, Bencic I, et al. How anesthetic, analgesic and other non-surgical techniques during cancer surgery might affect postoperative oncologic outcomes: a summary of current state of evidence. *Cancers*. 2019;11:592. doi:ARTN 59210.3390/cancers11050592.
44. Lutgendorf SK, Cole S, Costanzo E, et al. Stress-related mediators stimulate vascular endothelial growth factor secretion by two ovarian cancer cell lines. *Clin Cancer Res*. 2003;9:4514–4521.
45. Sood AK, Armaiz-Pena GN, Halder J, et al. Adrenergic modulation of focal adhesion kinase protects human ovarian cancer cells from anoikis. *J Clin Investig*. 2010;120:1515–1523. doi:10.1172/JCI40802.
46. Kim-Fuchs C, Le CP, Pimentel MA, et al. Chronic stress accelerates pancreatic cancer growth and invasion: a critical role for beta-adrenergic signaling in the pancreatic microenvironment. *Brain Behav Immun*. 2014;40:40–47. doi:10.1016/j.bbi.2014.02.019.
47. Yakar I, Melamed R, Shakhar G, et al. Prostaglandin e(2) suppresses NK activity in vivo and promotes postoperative tumor metastasis in rats. *Ann Surg Oncol*. 2003;10:469–479.
48. Ben-Eliyahu S, Shakhar G, Page GG, Stefanski V, Shakhar K. Suppression of NK cell activity and of resistance to metastasis by stress: a role for adrenal catecholamines and beta-adrenoceptors. *Neuroimmunomodulation*. 2000;8:154–164.
49. Hiller J, Schier R, Riedel B. *Perioperative Inflammation as Triggering Origin of Metastasis Development*. Springer; 2017:83–107.
50. Carroll JE, Low CA, Prather AA, et al. Negative affective responses to a speech task predict changes in interleukin (IL)-6. *Brain Behav Immun*. 2011;25:232–238. doi:10.1016/j.bbi.2010.09.024.
51. Breen MS, Beliakova-Bethell N, Mujica-Parodi LR, et al. Acute psychological stress induces short-term variable immune response. *Brain Behav Immun*. 2016;53:172–182. doi:10.1016/j.bbi.2015.10.008.
52. Shaashua L, Shabat-Simon M, Haldar R, et al. Perioperative COX-2 and beta-adrenergic blockade improves metastatic biomarkers in breast cancer patients in a phase-II randomized trial. *Clin Cancer Res*. 2017;23:4651–4661. doi:10.1158/1078-0432.CCR-17-0152.
53. Bartal I, Melamed R, Greenfeld K, et al. Immune perturbations in patients along the perioperative period: alterations in cell surface markers and leukocyte subtypes before and after surgery. *Brain Behav Immun*. 2010;24:376–386. doi:S0889-1591(09)00060-9 [pii]10.1016/j.bbi.2009.02.010 .
54. Muthuswamy R, Okada NJ, Jenkins FJ, et al. Epinephrine promotes COX-2-dependent immune suppression in myeloid cells and cancer tissues. *Brain Behav Immun*. 2017;62:78–86. doi:10.1016/j.bbi.2017.02.008.
55. Kolmus K, Tavernier J, Gerlo S. beta(2)-Adrenergic receptors in immunity and inflammation: stressing NF-kappa B. *Brain Behav Immun*. 2015;45:297–310. doi:10.1016/j.bbi.2014.10.007.
56. Hiller JG, Ismail HM, Hofman MS, Narayan K, Ramdave S, Riedel BJ. Neuraxial anesthesia reduces lymphatic flow: proof-of-concept in first in-human study. *Anesth Analg*. 2016;123:1325–1327. doi:10.1213/Ane.0000000000001562.
57. Carnagarin R, Matthews V, Zaldivia MTK, Peter K, Schlaich MP. The bidirectional interaction between the sympathetic nervous system and immune mechanisms in the pathogenesis of hypertension. *Br J Pharmacol*. 2019;176:1839–1852. doi:10.1111/bph.14481.
58. Schlereth T, Birklein F. The sympathetic nervous system and pain. *Neuromol Med*. 2008;10:141–147. doi:10.1007/s12017-007-8018-6.
59. Umar A, Steele VE, Menter DG, Hawk ET. Mechanisms of nonsteroidal anti-inflammatory drugs in cancer prevention. *Semin Oncol*. 2016;43:65–77. doi:10.1053/j.seminoncol.2015.09.010.
60. Regulski M, Regulska K, Prukała W, Piotrowska H, Stanisz B, Murias M. COX-2 inhibitors: a novel strategy in the management of breast cancer. *Drug Discov Today*. 2016;21:598–615. doi:10.1016/j.drudis.2015.12.003.
61. Taniguchi K, Karin M. NF-kappa B, inflammation, immunity and cancer: coming of age. *Nat Rev Immunol*. 2018;18:309–324. doi:10.1038/nri.2017.142.

62. Buvanendran A, Kroin JS, Berger RA, et al. Upregulation of prostaglandin E-2 and interleukins in the central nervous system and peripheral tissue during and after surgery in humans. *Anesthesiology.* 2006;104:403–410. doi:10.1097/00000542-200603000-00005.
63. Armaiz-Pena GN, Cole SW, Lutgendorf SK, Sood AK. Neuroendocrine influences on cancer progression. *Brain Behav Immun.* 2013;30(Suppl):S19–S25. doi:10.1016/j.bbi.2012.06.005.
64. Kim TH, Rowat AC, Sloan EK. Neural regulation of cancer: from mechanobiology to inflammation. *Clin Transl Immunol.* 2016;5(e78):1–9. doi:10.1038/cti.2016.18.
65. Lamkin DM, Ho HY, Ong TH, et al. beta-Adrenergic-stimulated macrophages: comprehensive localization in the M1-M2 spectrum. *Brain Behav Immun.* 2016;57:338–346. doi:10.1016/j.bbi.2016.07.162.
66. Heusinkveld M, van Steenwijk PJDV, Goedemans R, et al. M2 macrophages induced by prostaglandin E2 and IL-6 from cervical carcinoma are switched to activated M1 macrophages by CD4+ Th1 cells. *J Immunol.* 2011;187:1157–1165. doi:10.4049/jimmunol.1100889.
67. Wang Z, Brandt S, Medeiros A, et al. MicroRNA 21 is a homeostatic regulator of macrophage polarization and prevents prostaglandin E-2-mediated M2 generation. *PLos One.* 2015;10:1–13. doi:ARTN e011585510.1371/journal.pone.0115855.
68. Yao C, Narumiya S. Prostaglandin-cytokine crosstalk in chronic inflammation. *Br J Pharmacol.* 2019;176:337–354. doi:10.1111/bph.14530.
69. Flierl MA, Rittirsch D, Nadeau BA, et al. Phagocyte-derived catecholamines enhance acute inflammatory injury. *Nature.* 2007;449:721–U728. doi:10.1038/nature06185.
70. Nguyen KD, Qiu Y, Cui X, et al. Alternatively activated macrophages produce catecholamines to sustain adaptive thermogenesis. *Nature.* 2011;480:104–U272. doi:10.1038/nature10653 .
71. Sun XT, Li Q. Prostaglandin EP2 receptor: novel therapeutic target for human cancers (Review). *Int J Mol Med.* 2018;42:1203–1214. doi:10.3892/ijmm.2018.3744.
72. Zalli A, Riddell N, Goodyear O, et al. Targeting beta 2 adrenergic receptors regulate human T cell function directly and indirectly. *Brain Behav Immun.* 2015;45:211–218. doi:10.1016/j.bbi.2014.12.001.
73. Lubahn CL, Lorton D, Schaller JA, Sweeney SJ, Bellinger DL. Targeting alpha- and beta-adrenergic receptors differentially shifts Th1, Th2, and inflammatory cytokine profiles in immune organs to attenuate adjuvant arthritis. *Front Immunol.* 2014;5:346. doi:10.3389/fimmu.2014.00346.
74. Nagaraja AS, Dood RL, Armaiz-Pena G, et al. Adrenergic-mediated increases in INHBA drive CAF phenotype and collagens. *JCI Insight.* 2017;2:e93076. doi:10.1172/jci.insight.93076.
75. Sharma D, Brummel-Ziedins KE, Bouchard BA, Holmes CE. Platelets in tumor progression: a host factor that offers multiple potential targets in the treatment of cancer. *J Cell Physiol.* 2014;229:1005–1015. doi:10.1002/jcp.24539.
76. Martin A, Zlotnik D, Bonete GP, et al. Epinephrine rescues platelet functions inhibited by ticagrelor: a mechanistic approach. *Arch Cardiovasc Dis Suppl.* 2019;11:192.
77. Spiryova DV, Karmatskih OY, Vorob'ev AY, Moskalensky AE. Towards optical control of single blood platelet activation. *Proc Spie.* 2018;10717:1071722. doi:10.1117/12.2305477.
78. Musselman RP, Bennett S, Li W, et al. Association between perioperative beta blocker use and cancer survival following surgical resection. *Eur J Surg Onc.* 2018;44:1164–1169. doi:10.1016/j.ejso.2018.05.012.
79. Na ZJ, Qiao X, Hao X, et al. The effects of beta-blocker use on cancer prognosis: a meta-analysis based on 319,006 patients. *Oncotargets Ther.* 2018;11:4913–4944. doi:10.2147/Ott.S167422.
80. Schack A, Fransgaard T, Klein MF, Gogenur I. Perioperative use of nonsteroidal anti-inflammatory drugs decreases the risk of recurrence of cancer after colorectal resection: a cohort study based on prospective data. *Ann Surg Oncol.* 2019;26:3826–3837. doi:10.1245/s10434-019-07600-8.
81. Spini A, Roberto G, Gini R, et al. Evidence of beta-blockers drug repurposing for the treatment of triple negative breast cancer: a systematic review. *Neoplasma.* 2019;66(6):963–970. doi:10.4149/neo_2019_190110N34.
82. Bibbins-Domingo K. U.S. Preventive Services Task Force. Aspirin use for the primary prevention of cardiovascular disease and colorectal cancer: US Preventive Services Task Force Recommendation Statement. *Ann Intern Med.* 2016;164:836–U103. doi:10.7326/M16-0577.
83. Heitz F, Hengsbach A, Harter P, et al. Intake of selective beta blockers has no impact on survival in patients with epithelial ovarian cancer. *Gynecol Oncol.* 2017;144:181–186. doi:10.1016/j.ygyno.2016.11.012.
84. Renz BW, Graf S, Dantes Z, et al. Clinical impact of nonselective beta-blockers on survival in patients with pancreatic cancer-revival of well known drugs? *Pancreatology.* 2017;17:S32–S33.
85. Barron TI, Connolly RM, Sharp L, Bennett K, Visvanathan K. Beta blockers and breast cancer mortality: a population-based study. *J Clin Oncol.* 2011;29:2635–2644. doi:10.1200/Jco.2010.33.5422.
86. Patrignani P, Sacco A, Sostres C, et al. Low-dose aspirin acetylates cyclooxygenase-1 in human colorectal mucosa: implications for the chemoprevention of colorectal cancer. *Clin Pharmacol Ther.* 2017;102:52–61. doi:10.1002/cpt.639.
87. Forget P, Bentin C, Machiels JP, Berlière M, Coulie PG, De Kock M. Intraoperative use of ketorolac or diclofenac is associated with improved disease-free survival and overall survival in conservative breast cancer surgery. *Br J Anaesth.* 2014;113:82–87. doi:10.1093/bja/aet464.
88. Jang HI, Lim SH, Lee YY, et al. Perioperative administration of propranolol to women undergoing ovarian cancer surgery: a pilot study. *Obstet Gynecol Sci.* 2017;60:170–177. doi:10.5468/ogs.2017.60.2.170.
89. Ramondetta L, Hu W, Thaker PH, et al. No need to stress: prospective clinical trial of adrenergic blockade during primary treatment in women with epithelial ovarian cancer. *Gynecol Oncol.* 2017;145:33–34.
90. Thaker P, Kuroki LM, Hu W, et al. Overcoming stress effects: a prospective feasibility trial of beta-blockers with upfront ovarian cancer therapy. *Gynecol Oncol.* 2017;145:18.
91. Sakamoto A, Yagi K, Okamura T, Harada T, Usuda J. Perioperative administration of an intravenous beta-blocker landiolol hydrochloride in patients with lung cancer: a Japanese retrospective exploratory clinical study. *Sci Rep.* 2019;9:1–6. doi:10.1038/s41598-019-41520-7.
92. Hiller J, Cole SW, Crone EM, et al. Pre-operative β-blockade with propranolol reduces biomarkers of metastasis in breast cancer: a phase II randomized trial. *Clin Cancer Res.* 2020;26(8):1803–1811. doi:10.1158/1078-0432.CCR-19-2641
93. Wang LD, Gao X, Li JY, et al. Effects of preemptive analgesia with parecoxib sodium on haemodynamics and plasma

stress hormones in surgical patients with thyroid carcinoma. *Asian Pac J Cancer Prev.* 2015;16:3977–3980. doi:10.7314/apjcp.2015.16.9.3977.

94. Ma W, Wang K, Du J, Luan J, Lou G. Multi-dose parecoxib provides an immunoprotective effect by balancing T helper 1 (Th1), Th2, Th17 and regulatory T cytokines following laparoscopy in patients with cervical cancer. *Mol Med Rep.* 2015;11:2999–3008.
95. Shen J-C, Sun HL, Zhang MQ, Liu XY, Wang Z, Yang JJ. Flurbiprofen improves dysfunction of T-lymphocyte subsets and natural killer cells in cancer patients receiving post-operative morphine analgesia. *Int J Clin Pharmacol Ther.* 2014;52:669–675.
96. Lonnroth C, Andersson M, Arvidsson A, et al. Preoperative treatment with a non-steroidal anti-inflammatory drug (NSAID) increases tumor tissue infiltration of seemingly activated immune cells in colorectal cancer. *Cancer Immun.* 2008;8:5.
97. Sooriakumaran P, Coley HM, Fox SB, et al. A randomized controlled trial investigating the effects of celecoxib in patients with localized prostate cancer. *Anticancer Res.* 2009;29:1483–1488.
98. Hiller JG, Sampurno S, Millen R, et al. Impact of celecoxib on inflammation during cancer surgery: a randomized clinical trial. *Can J Anaesth.* 2017;64:497–505. doi:10.1007/s12630-017-0818-z.
99. Dood R, Nagaraja AS, Lyons YA, et al. Knocking out stress: a systems-based identification of optimal drug combinations to improve ovarian cancer outcomes. *Gynecol Oncol.* 2017;145:15.
100. Haldar R, Ricon I, Cole S, Zmora O, Ben-Eliyahu S. Perioperative beta-adrenergic blockade and COX2 inhibition in colorectal cancer patients improves pro-metastatic indices in the excised tumor: EMT, tumor infiltrating lymphocytes (TILs), and gene regulatory pathways. *Brain Beh Immun.* 2017;66:e9.
101. Priebe H-J. The controversy of peri-operative ß-blockade: what should I do? *Eur J Vasc Endovasc Surg.* 2014;47:119–123.
102. POISE Study Group. Effects of extended-release metoprolol succinate in patients undergoing non-cardiac surgery (POISE trial): a randomised controlled trial. *Lancet.* 2008;371:1839–1847. doi:10.1016/S0140-6736(08)60601-7.
103. Ashes C, Judelman S, Wijeysundera DN, et al. Selective β1-antagonism with bisoprolol is associated with fewer postoperative strokes than atenolol or metoprolol. A single-center cohort study of 44,092 consecutive patients. *Anesthesiology.* 2013;119:777–787.
104. Fleisher LA, Fleischmann KE, Auerbach AD, et al. 2014 ACC/AHA guideline on perioperative cardiovascular evaluation and management of patients undergoing noncardiac surgery: a report of the American College of Cardiology/American Heart Association Task Force on practice guidelines. *J Am Coll Cardiol.* 2014;64:e77–e137. doi:10.1016/j.jacc.2014.07.944.
105. Kristensen SD, Knuuti J. New ESC/ESA guidelines on non-cardiac surgery: cardiovascular assessment and management. *Eur Heart J.* 2014;35:2344–2345. doi:10.1093/eurheartj/ehu285.
106. Gustafsson UO, Scott MJ, Schwenk W, et al. Guidelines for perioperative care in elective colonic surgery: Enhanced Recovery After Surgery (ERAS®) Society recommendations. *World J Surg.* 2013;37:259–284. doi:10.1007/s00268-012-1772-0.
107. Wattchow D, De Fontgalland D, Bampton PA, Leach PL, McLaughlin K, Costa M. Clinical trial: the impact of cyclooxygenase inhibitors on gastrointestinal recovery after major surgery–a randomized double blind controlled trial of celecoxib or diclofenac vs. placebo. *Aliment Pharmacol Ther.* 2009;30:987–998.
108. Cheung R, Krishnaswami S, Kowalski K. Analgesic efficacy of celecoxib in postoperative oral surgery pain: a single-dose, two-center, randomized, double-blind, active-and placebo-controlled study. *Clin Ther.* 2007;29:2498–2510.
109. Huang MT, Chen ZX, Wei B, et al. Preoperative growth inhibition of human gastric adenocarcinoma treated with a combination of celecoxib and octreotide 1. *Acta Pharmacol Sin.* 2007;28:1842–1850.
110. FDA Drug Safety Communication. FDA strengthens warning that non-aspirin nonsteroidal anti-inflammatory drugs (NSAIDs) can cause heart attacks or strokes. July 9, 2015. Available at https://www.fda.gov/drugs/drug-safety-and-availability/fda-drug-safety-communication-fda-strengthens-warning-non-aspirin-nonsteroidal-anti-inflammatory.

10

Local Anesthetics and Cancer

TIM G. HALES AND DANIEL T. BAPTISTA-HON

The Perioperative Period Is Critical for Postsurgical Cancer Outcomes

Surgery is the primary and often the most effective treatment for many solid tumors. However, even otherwise successful surgeries may disrupt and disseminate tumor cells. Disseminated tumor cells increase the risk of recurrence and metastasis. Indeed, the number of postsurgical circulating cancer cells is a negative prognostic indicator of disease-free survival.[1]

A number of prometastatic events occur during the perioperative period as a direct consequence of surgery.[2] For instance, direct injury to tissue causes local inflammation and a wound-healing response characterized by increased proliferation and enhanced release of angiogenic factors. These events promote the viability of residual or disseminated cancer cells. Inflammation also leads to edema, which increases the pressure of local drainage (via the lymphatic system) and enhances the propulsion of disseminated tumor cells away from the surgical site. Surgical trauma also induces a more general surgical stress response, characterized by systemic increases in catecholamines and inflammatory mediators. This can lead to immunosuppression and a reduction in the cytotoxic activity of natural killer (NK) cells. These events may tip the balance enabling micrometastases, previously suppressed by the immune system, to thrive.[3,4]

Anesthetics and analgesics administered during the perioperative period have the potential to exacerbate prometastatic events, and there is considerable interest in the possibility that the type of anesthetic and/or analgesic agent may influence cancer recurrence. Indeed, a number of retrospective clinical studies suggest that regional anesthesia by local anesthetics increases disease-free survival following breast and prostate cancer surgery.[5] Here, we explore the potential benefits of using local anesthetics during the perioperative period of surgical tumor excision with regard to subsequent disease progression and/or recurrence and the mechanisms, which may underpin it.

Potential Detrimental Effects of Anesthetics and Opioid Analgesics

Opioid analgesics are effective for the management of severe pain but can cause opioid-induced respiratory depression, constipation, hyperalgesia, tolerance, and dependence.[6] Of particular concern in the context of the perioperative period is the possibility that some opioids may cause immunosuppression. For instance, fentanyl and morphine may activate mu-opioid receptors on NK cells, attenuating their cytotoxic activity.[7,8] Furthermore, fentanyl and morphine may also stimulate the hypothalamic-pituitary axis to raise glucocorticoid levels, causing indirect immunosuppression.[9] The presence of mu-opioid receptors on some tumor cells (particularly non–small cell lung cancer) suggests that opioids may directly influence cancer cell function. The impact of opioids on cancer is discussed in detail in Chapter 12.

Volatile general anesthetics such as sevoflurane may also suppress the immune response.[10] In mice, sevoflurane treatment reduced total leukocyte and lymphocyte cell counts in blood.[11] There is also less infiltration of NK and T-helper cells in breast cancer tissue biopsies from patients receiving sevoflurane.[12] Furthermore, serum from breast cancer patients receiving sevoflurane reduces the cytotoxicity of NK cells in vitro.[13] Volatile general anesthetics may also have direct procancer effects. For instance, serum taken from breast or colon cancer patients receiving sevoflurane impairs apoptosis of breast or colon cancer cells, respectively, in vitro.[14,15] Sevoflurane may also enhance migration and invasion in ovarian cancers and glioblastomas.[15–19] The impact of volatile anesthetics on cancer is discussed further in Chapter 11.

Indirect Benefits of Perioperative Local Anesthetics

Local anesthetics are often used to provide analgesia during the perioperative period as part of a balanced multimodal anesthesia. This diminishes the need for volatile anesthetics and opioid analgesics and may be beneficial for subsequent cancer outcomes.[20,21] Furthermore, local anesthetics may attenuate the stress response itself and mitigate the extent of perioperative immunosuppression.[22,23]

However, a recent large prospective multicenter trial comparing outcomes after breast cancer surgery with inhalational anesthesia with or without paravertebral analgesia by ropivacaine or levobupivacaine revealed no difference in disease-free survival.[24] The findings suggest that opioid and volatile anesthetic sparing effects of paravertebral analgesia do not account for any potential beneficial effects of local anesthetics on cancer outcomes in patients undergoing surgery for breast cancer. There are several other ongoing clinical trials exploring the impact of anesthetic technique on cancer outcomes; most predicated on the idea that the potential benefit of local anesthetics is conferred indirectly through their anesthetic sparing effects (Table 10.1).

However, there is mounting evidence that local anesthetics may have direct beneficial effects during the perioperative period. They may be antiinflammatory.[25–27] This may be significant because there is a possibility that antiinflammatory drugs administered perioperatively increase disease-free survival after breast cancer excision.[28,29] Furthermore, some cancers express membrane protein targets of local anesthetics, including voltage-activated sodium ion channels (VASCs), not seen in their nonmalignant cellular counterparts. It is therefore possible that local anesthetics such as lidocaine, ropivacaine, and levobupivacaine might provide a direct beneficial effect by inhibiting the function of these proteins.

Direct Effects of Local Anesthetics on Cancer Cells

VASCs are the canonical target for local anesthetics. However, in vitro evidence also implicates the muscarinic acetylcholine receptor (mAChR) and Src kinase as targets for local anesthetic inhibition.[30,31] These proteins may play important roles in cancer cell oncophysiology, and their presence raises the possibility of additional beneficial effects of local anesthetics beyond general anesthetic and opioid analgesic sparing. Furthermore, emerging evidence suggests that lidocaine can stimulate the function of NK cells,[32] inhibit tumor angiogenesis,[33] as well as sensitize resistant cancer cells to the actions of several cytotoxic agents, such as cisplatin, pirarubicin, and 5-fluorouracil.[34]

If this is the case, then a more beneficial approach for the use of local anesthetics might be to administer them directly into the tumor, or systemically (e.g., intravenously or intraperitoneally). Indeed lidocaine, a class 1b antiarrhythmic agent, can be safely administered intravenously and is also used as a circulating analgesic,[35] and may be more beneficial in terms of pain control than epidural anesthesia.[36] A number of ongoing clinical trials will test whether local anesthetics delivered directly onto breast tumors prior to excision, intravenously or intraperitoneally during the perioperative period for breast, colon, and ovarian cancer surgery, will prolong postoperative disease-free survival (NCT01916317, NCT02786329, and NCT04065009; Table 10.1).

Voltage-Activated Sodium Channel Oncochannelopathy

VASCs are ion channels most noted for their role in generating the action potential in excitable cells. Diseases involving VASCs in excitable cells are called Na^+ channelopathies.[37] Notable examples are the congenital long QT3 (Romano-Ward) and Brugada syndromes involving $Na_V1.5$ (cardiac VASC), febrile seizures ($Na_V1.1$ and $Na_V1.2$), and painful inherited neuropathy ($Na_V1.7$). These classic channelopathies involve VASC dysfunction caused by mutations. In cancer, however, a number of hallmarks characterize oncogenic transformation.[38] The term "oncochannelopathy" is

TABLE 10.1 Clinical Trials Investigating the Influence of Local Anesthetic Use in the Perioperative Period

ClinicalTrials.gov ID	Study Start Date	Resection Site	LA Delivery	GA Alone Versus GA + LA	Direct LA Benefit
NCT00418457	Jan-07	Breast	NB	✓	
NCT00938171	Jun-08	Breast	NB	✓	
NCT01204242	Aug-09	Breast	IV	✓	
NCT01916317	Dec-11	Breast	IT		✓
NCT02089178	Feb-14	Breast	IV	✓	
NCT02786329	Jun-16	Colorectal	IV	✓	✓
NCT02839668	Aug-16	Breast	IV	✓	
NCT04065009	Jan-20	Ovary	IP		✓

The studies either compare general anesthesia (GA) alone with GA combined with local anesthetic (LA) regional block or examine the potential direct beneficial effects of local anesthetics delivered intravenously (IV), intraperitoneally (IP), local nerve block (NB), or into the tumor (IT).

used to describe the aberrant expression or function of a particular ion channel, leading to one or multiple cancer hallmarks.[39] No underlying mutation is implied in oncochannelopathies, although mutations in VASC genes have been observed in breast and colon cancer cells.[40]

VASC oncochannelopathies have been implicated in many different types of cancers.[41–43] We focus on $Na_V1.5$, which is one of the most studied in metastatic tumors such as colon cancer[44,45] and breast cancer.[46–48] $Na_V1.5$ is also found in prostate, lung (small and non–small cell), and ovarian cancers.[41] $Na_V1.5$ expressed in breast and colon cancer cells is functional, and $Na_V1.5$-mediated ionic currents can be recorded using the patch-clamp technique from colon and breast cancer cells.[44,47–49] Metastatic SW620 colon cancer cells exhibit greater $Na_V1.5$-mediated currents compared to their SW480 adenocarcinoma cell counterparts.[44] Inhibition of $Na_V1.5$ by tetrodotoxin or local anesthetics in colon and breast cancer cells reduces proliferation, migration, and invasive behavior, as does reduction in $Na_V1.5$ expression.[44,45,47,48,50–52] Conversely, increasing Na^+ flux via $Na_V1.5$ in colon cancer cells using veratridine enhances invasive activity.[45,49] This highlights the importance of $Na_V1.5$ function in the signal transduction cascades necessary to initiate invasive behavior in cancer cells. It also raises the possibility of directly targeting $Na_V1.5$ using local anesthetics during the perioperative period and highlights the importance of the few clinical trials looking at the direct effects of local anesthetics (Table 10.1).

Research into the role played by VASCs in oncophysiology is also beginning to unravel a unique and complex system of intracellular signaling and ionic homeostasis, which could be targeted by local anesthetics (Fig. 10.1). $Na_V1.5$ activity in colon cancer cells can influence the expression of a number of invasion-related genes in a mitogen-activated protein kinase (MAPK)-dependent manner.[49] This may be mediated via $Na_V1.5$ activity raising $[Na^+]_i$. The Na^+ gradient is often utilized by cells to drive the transport of other molecules such as Ca^{2+}, a key second messenger. It is possible that some of the changes in gene expression attributed to $Na_V1.5$ activity are mediated by altered $[Ca^{2+}]_i$.

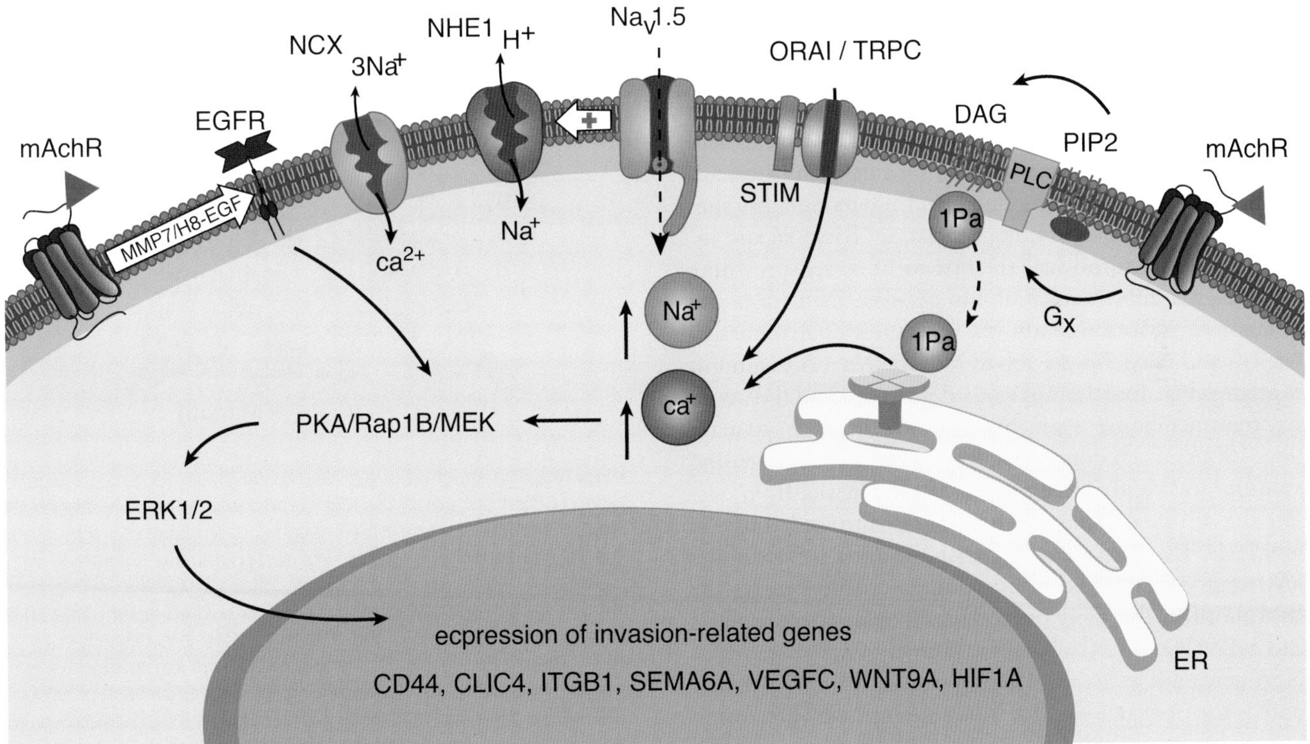

• **Fig. 10.1** The roles of $Na_V1.5$ and muscarinic acetylcholine receptors *(mAChR)* in cancer metastasis A diagram summarizing the results of studies investigating $Na_V1.5$ and mAChR signaling in cancer cells. Persistent Na^+ entry via $Na_V1.5$ may increase $[Na^+]_i$ and enhance Ca^{2+} entry via reverse mode Na^+/Ca^{2+} exchanger *(NCX)* activity. Activation of mAChRs by ambient acetylcholine also increases $[Ca^{2+}]_i$ via the production of inositol triphosphate (IP3) and activation of IP3 receptors. Depletion of endoplasmic reticulum *(ER)* Ca^{2+} activates store-operated Ca^{2+} entry mechanisms via ORAI/TRPC ion channels, further raising $[Ca^{2+}]_i$. Ca^{2+} is a second messenger which can cause the transcription of genes involved in the metastatic cascade. This could be mediated via a MEK/PKA/ERK pathway known to be enhanced by persistent $Na_V1.5$ activity.[49] The MEK/PKA/ERK pathway can also be activated by signaling through epidermal growth factor receptors *(EGFRs)*. mAChR activation can lead to the cleavage of inactive pro-HB-EGF to its active form via metalloproteinase 7 (MMP7) and activate EGFRs.[84] Finally $Na_V1.5$ may directly transactivate the sodium-proton exchanger *(NHE1)*, leading to extracellular acidification, which is required for the degradation of the extracellular matrix by matrix metalloproteinases.[53]

Other targets of local anesthetics (such as mAChRs) may also exert their effects by regulating $[Ca^{2+}]_i$. The presence of Na_V1.5 protein may also have direct effects on the function of other transporters, for example, by directly transactivating the sodium-proton exchanger (NHE1).[53,54] NHE1 mediates extracellular acidification which is required for the degradation of the extracellular matrix by matrix metalloproteinases. This puts Na_V1.5 in the center of a complex signaling pathway of cancer oncophysiology contributing to proliferation and invasion. It also highlights the potential of targeting Na_V1.5 function in cancer cells. In the following sections we will discuss recent advances in our understanding of the structure and function of Na_V1.5 VASCs, which provides new insights into the mechanism of their block by local anesthetics in the context of cancer.

Na_V1.5 Structure and Function

Na_V1.5 is encoded by the SCN5A gene located on chromosome 3p21. The α-subunit encoded by SCN5A is sufficient to form functional ion channels. Four auxiliary β-subunits are encoded by additional genes (SCN1B to SCN4B) and augment the function of some VASCs. VASC β-subunits may also play a role in breast cancers in which Na_V1.5 is found.[55]

The pore-forming α-subunit of Na_V1.5 is a large protein (>200 kDa in size) with more than 2000 amino acids and contains binding sites for various drugs (including local anesthetics), β-subunits, calmodulin, and also modulatory sites for phosphorylation and ubiquitinylation. Bacterial and insect VASC structures were the first to be solved providing new insights into the relationship between their form and function.[56,57] More recently, the structures of mammalian Na_V1.5 and Na_V1.7 were solved.[58,59] The Na_V1.5 α-subunit is arranged in four homologous domains (DI–DIV) with six transmembrane segments (S1–S6) in each domain (Fig. 10.2A). Each domain is divided into a voltage-sensing module (VM) and a pore module (PM). Viewed from outside the cell membrane, the ion pore is surrounded by the four PMs. The VMs are arranged on the outer surface of the PMs (Fig. 10.2B). The inactivation gate is formed by the IFM motif in the short intracellular loop connecting DIII and DIV (Fig. 10.2C). Alternative mRNA splicing of SCN5A generates at least 13 Na_V1.5 variants.[60] Of particular note is the neonatal Na_V1.5e splice variant, which is found in both breast and colon cancer cells.[45,48] The neonatal splice variant arises from alternative usage of exon 6, which codes for part of the VM.

The gating of Na_V1.5 and other VASCs involves three key steps: voltage-dependent activation, the rapid opening of an Na^+ selective ion channel pore, and voltage-dependent inactivation. Structurally, these involve transitions into discrete conformations: closed, active, and inactive. These are illustrated in Fig. 10.3. Activation is caused by a voltage-dependent movement of S4 along its long axis and outward perpendicular to the membrane.[61,62] This movement opens the Na^+ selective pore lined by the PMs. Na^+ selectivity is governed by a conserved quartet of amino acids (DEKA) (Fig. 10.2A). VASCs, including Na_V1.5, inactivate within 1–2 ms following activation. This is caused by the

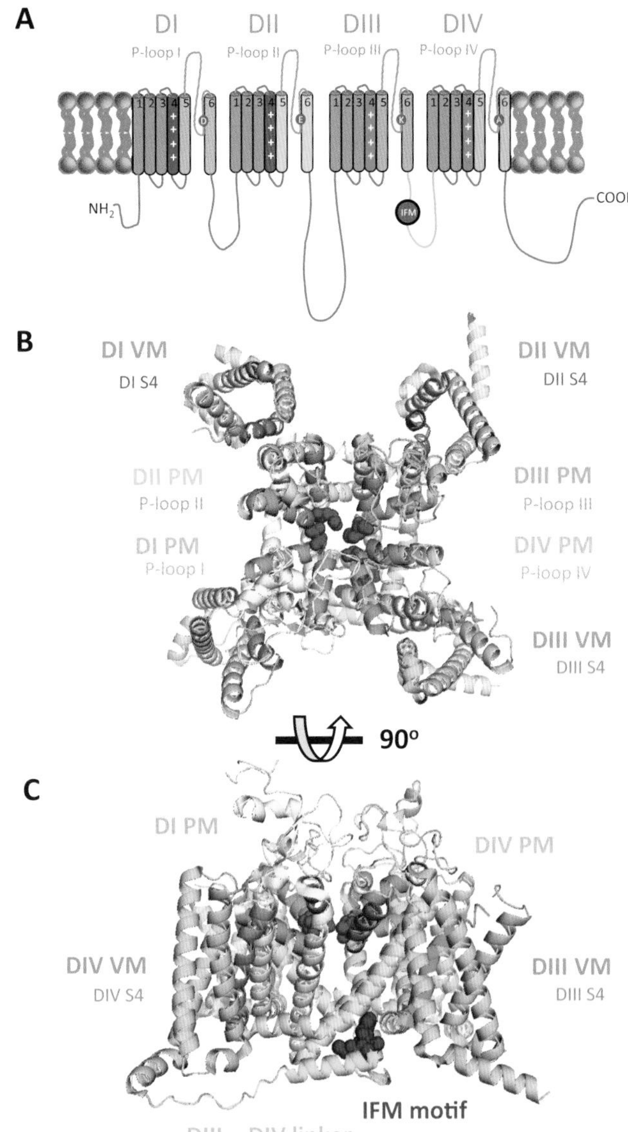

• **Fig. 10.2** The structure of the Na_V1.5 VASC. (A) Topological organization of Na_V1.5. Each of the four homologous domains is labeled DI through DIV. The transmembrane segments are labeled 1 through 6. The voltage sensor in segment 4 of each domain is highlighted with a series of "+". Together with the residues comprising segments 1 through 3 each voltage-sensing module is colored in *light blue*. The pore module (segments 5 and 6) is highlighted in a different color in each domain. Each pore loop is in *grey* and the key residues, which form the selectivity filter (DEKA), are depicted in *red* on each pore loop. The loop connecting DIII and DIV, which contains the inactivation gate, is highlighted in *yellow*, and the key IFM motif, which is required for the stabilization of the inactive state, is in *purple*. (B) Top down (from the extracellular aspect) view of the Na_V1.5 channel structure (protein data bank entry 6UZ3). The structure is rendered in ribbon format to highlight the location of the membrane spanning α-helices. The key structures are color coded and labeled according to the topological figure in (A). (C) Side view (from DI and DIV) highlighting the inactivation gate, with DIII VM, DIV VM, D1 PM, and DIV PM facing forward. The DIII–DIV linker is in *yellow* and the IFM motif is in *purple*, corresponding to the topological diagram in (A).

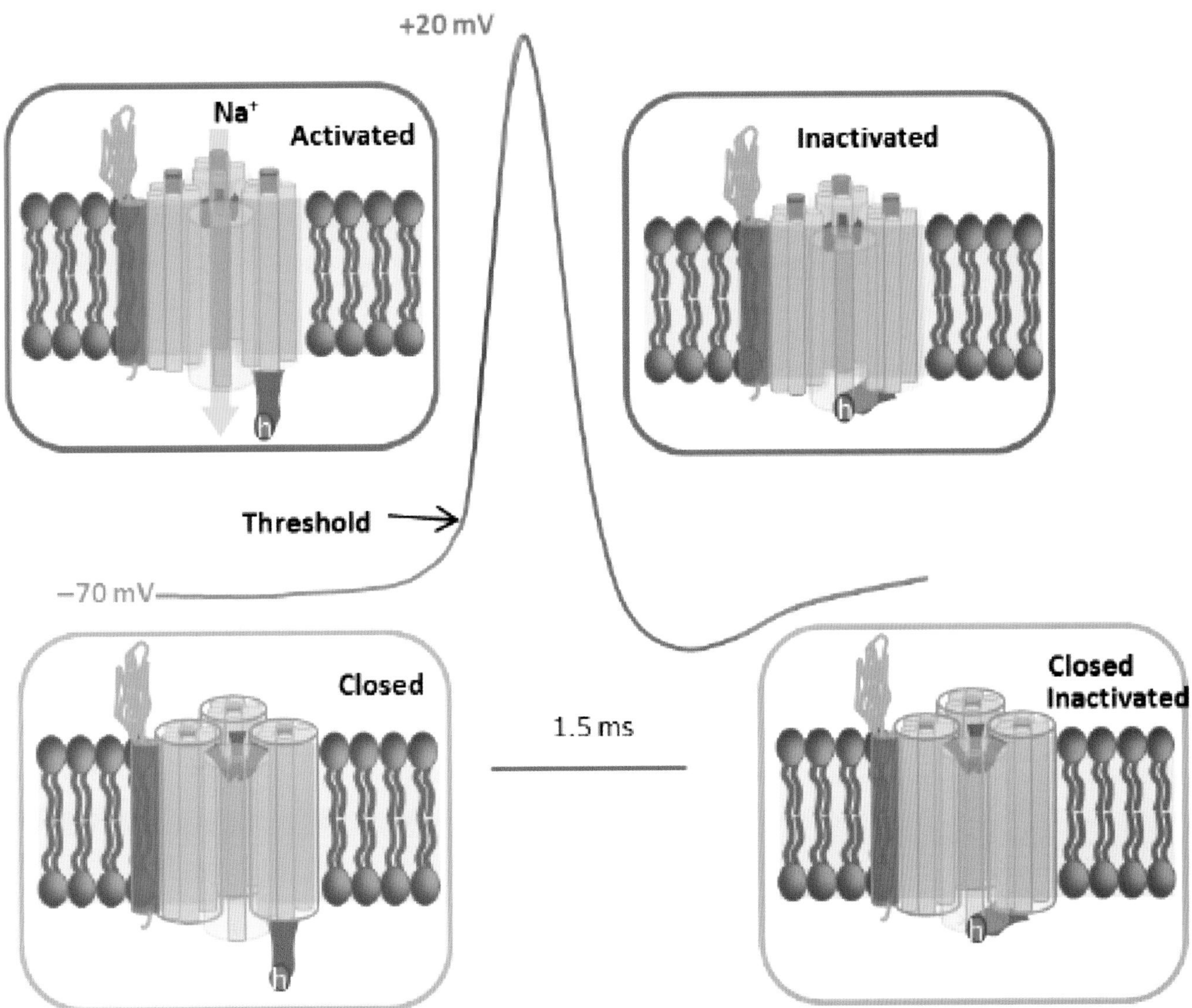

• **Fig. 10.3** State-dependent voltage-activated sodium ion channel (VASC) function. A schematic diagram illustrating the key states of VASC activity. VASC function can be broadly divided into conducting (activated) and nonconducting states (closed and inactivated). In excitable cells, cycling between these conducting and nonconducting states is associated with the different phases of the action potential. In cancer cells, where the resting membrane potential is more depolarized, such cyclic activity is not possible, and most of the VASCs are likely to be found in the inactive state (note the position of the h-gate). The large proportion of VASCs in this state at equilibrium allows the possibility for state-dependent inhibition by local anesthetics.

inactivation gate (also sometimes referred to as the h-gate) containing the IFM motif folding into the intracellular opening of the pore blocking ion permeation.[63,64]

$Na_V1.5$ channels (and other VASCs) are found primarily in excitable cells, such as cardiomyocytes and neurons, where they mediate rapid depolarization of the membrane during the action potential (Fig. 10.4). The expression of VASCs in these cells, together with the ability to maintain a hyperpolarized resting membrane potential (RMP) (more negative than -60 mV), is key to the generation of action potentials.[65] While $Na_V1.5$ are functional in cancer cells, they do not confer the ability to fire action potentials because of the relatively depolarized RMP of approximately -40 mV[45] (Fig. 10.4).

$Na_V1.5$ function can be characterized by their voltage dependence of activation and inactivation. This is illustrated in Fig. 10.5A (left panel). The relationship between the extent of activation and the voltage is sigmoidal and can be fitted with a mathematical function enabling determination of the voltage at which 50% activation or inactivation (V_{50}) occurs. The V_{50} of activation and inactivation are important parameters in the investigation of $Na_V1.5$ not least because the block by local anesthetics of $Na_V1.5$ is highly state-dependent and shifts the V_{50} parameter.[45,66] Experimentally, state-dependent inhibition of $Na_V1.5$ by local anesthetics manifests as (1) a reduction in the absolute amount of available current evoked by depolarization, and (2) a leftward shift in the voltage dependence of inactivation (Fig. 10.5B).

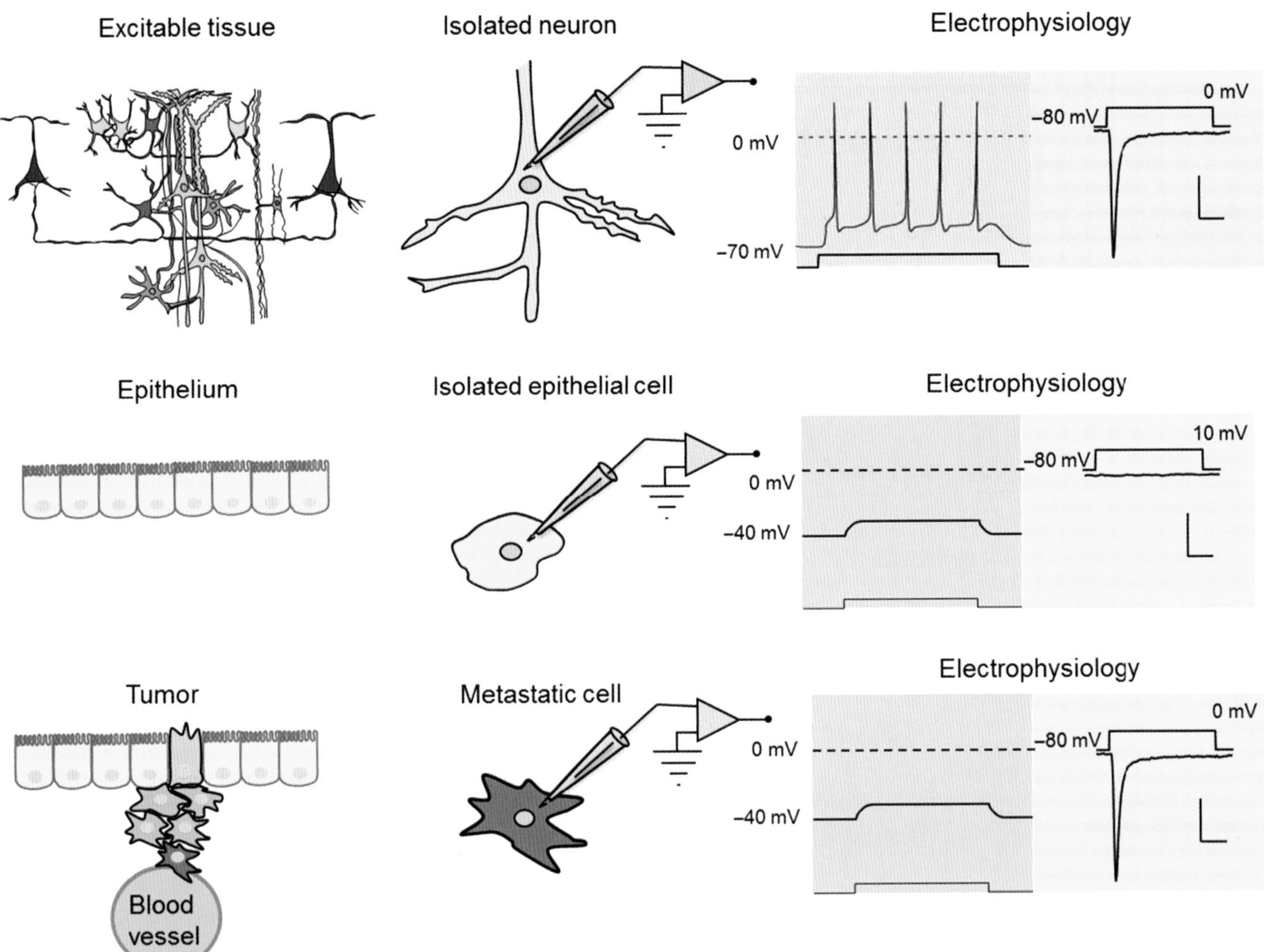

• **Fig. 10.4** Voltage-activated sodium ion channels (VASCs) play different roles in excitable tissues and tumor cells *(Top)*. Electrical activity recorded from cells in excitable tissues, such as central nervous system structures and heart tissues, can be determined directly by patch-clamp recordings. The diagram illustrates how the injection of current, while recording membrane potential, can evoke action potentials. Robust VASC (and Ca^{2+}, K^{+}) currents can be evoked using step depolarization pulses while recording under voltage clamp. *(Middle)* Epithelial cells do not express many voltage-activated ion channels. The diagram illustrates how depolarization fails to activate action potentials. *(Bottom)* Cancer cells of an epithelial origin often exhibit upregulated expression of VASCs. In the case of colon and breast cancers, there is evidence that the upregulation of $Na_V1.5$ is correlated with cancer stage, with metastatic cells expressing higher levels of $Na_V1.5$. These cells, like the epithelial cells from which they originated, have a depolarized resting membrane potential. The diagram illustrates that despite expressing VASCs cancer cells of epithelial origin are unable to fire action potentials. However, when voltage is clamped at −80 mV, depolarization evokes robust VASC-mediated currents.

It is apparent from Fig. 10.5A (middle panel) that at the RMP of colon cancer cells (approximately -40 mV), most $Na_V1.5$ are unavailable for activation, that is, they are in the inactivated state. Nevertheless, at equilibrium a minor proportion of channels are still active at −40 mV, resulting in a small tonic current. The voltages at which there is tonic (or persistent) Na^+ current (referred to as the window current) are represented by the area bounded by the activation and inactivation curves (Fig. 10.5A, right panel). It is this component of persistent Na^+ entry which is likely to account for the proinvasion effects of $Na_V1.5$ activity.[45,49]

VASCs are blocked by a variety of drugs, including local anesthetics, antiarrhythmics, and antiepileptics (Table 10.2).[45,66] Local anesthetics show a strong preference for the inactivated state of the $Na_V1.5$ channel, and this may provide a strategy for targeting cancer cells and avoiding cardiac effects.[66–71] Local anesthetic concentrations in the low-to-mid micromolar range are safely achievable in the blood.[72,73] At these concentrations, local anesthetics have negligible effects on the activity of $Na_V1.5$ channels at membrane potentials more negative than −80 mV. The RMP of human cardiac myocytes is approximately −90 mV,[74] which require millimolar concentrations of local anesthetics to inhibit $Na_V1.5$ channels.[66] By contrast, inactivation is prevalent in colon cancer cells due to their depolarized RMP.[45] Persistent Na^+ entry therefore likely underlies the function of $Na_V1.5$, manifesting as the window current. Indeed, local anesthetics reduce the size of this window current and hence the amount of persistent Na^+ entry.[45]

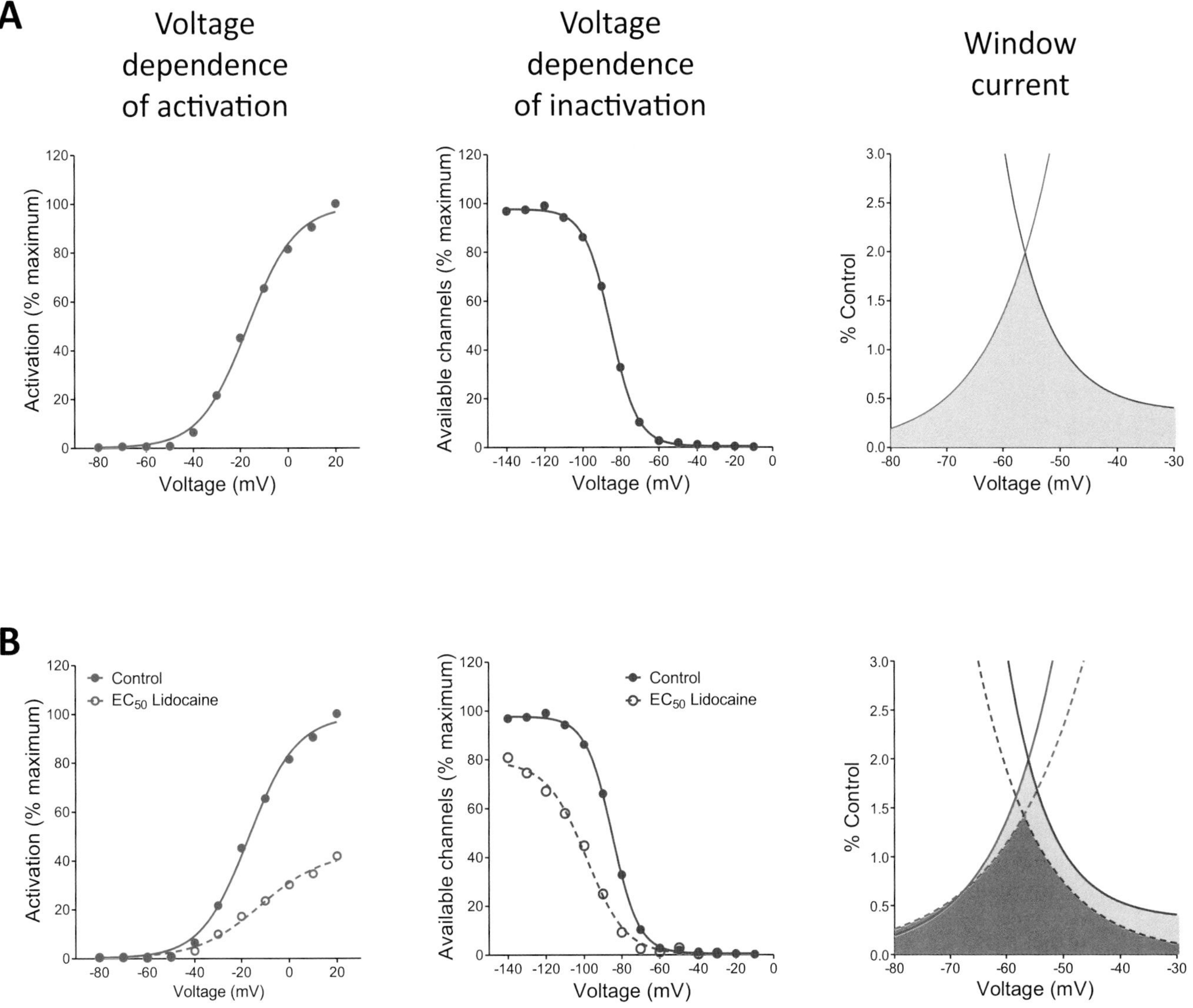

• **Fig. 10.5** Electrophysiological properties of $Na_V1.5$ in cancer cells. (A) Representative examples of $Na_V1.5$ voltage dependence of activation *(red)* and voltage dependence of inactivation *(blue)*. A sigmoidal Boltzmann relationship was fitted to the data, from which the V_{50} of activation and inactivation can be derived. In this example, the V_{50} of activation is −17 mV and that of inactivation is −85 mV. These examples are obtained from voltage-clamp recordings from SW620 colon cancer cells. The third figure shows the window current formed by the area under the curve of the voltage dependence of activation and inactivation. This is shaded in *grey*. (B) The effect of lidocaine on the electrophysiological properties of $Na_V1.5$. Shown in *open circles* and the *dotted lines* are representative examples of $Na_V1.5$ voltage dependence of activation and inactivation in the presence of an EC_{50} concentration of lidocaine and their associated Boltzmann relationship. In this example, the V_{50} values of activation and inactivation in the presence of lidocaine are −12 mV and −99 mV, respectively. Note the large hyperpolarizing (more negative) shift in the V_{50} of inactivation, characteristic of lidocaine stabilizing/favoring the inactivated state. The influence of lidocaine on the window current is shown in the third panel, where there is a reduction in the size of the window current. This will likely manifest as a reduction in the persistent Na^+ entry in these metastatic colon cancer cells.

The prevalence of inactivation, highlighted in Fig. 10.5B (right panel), raises the possibility of state-dependent targeting of $Na_V1.5$ channels on cancer cells, while sparing cardiac tissue. The strong state dependence of local anesthetics and many of the other VASC-inhibiting drugs in Table 10.2 is a major contributing factor to their relatively high therapeutic indexes and particularly in the case of lidocaine, enabling its safe systemic administration.[35]

The class 1C antiarrhythmic agent flecainide has a structure similar to that of lidocaine and shares common molecular determinants for its block of $Na_V1.5$ channels.[75] A recent structural model sheds light on the molecular mechanism of $Na_V1.5$ inhibition by flecainide,[59] which binds to the intracellular aspect of the selectivity filter, lined by Phe1420, Lys1421, and Phe1461 from the PM of DIII, and Phe1762 from the PM of DIV (Fig. 10.6A). Phe1762 is a known residue for lo-

TABLE 10.2 VASC Inhibitors With Potential for Repurposing as Anticancer Agents

Drugs	Primary Action
Antidepressants	
Fluoxetine, sertraline, paroxetine	Selective serotonin reuptake inhibitors
Amitriptyline, nortriptyline, clomipramine, imipramine, desipramine	Tricyclic antidepressants
Maprotiline, nisoxetine, reboxetine	Norepinephrine reuptake inhibitors
Mianserin, mirtazapine	Noradrenergic and specific serotonergic antidepressants
Bupropion, venlafaxine	Norepinephrine-dopamine reuptake inhibitor
Nefazodone	Serotonin-norepinephrine reuptake inhibitor
Trazodone	Serotonin antagonist and reuptake inhibitor
Antipsychotics	
Haloperidol, chlorpromazine, chlorprothixene, clozapine	D2 antagonist
Antiepileptics	
Carbamazepine, lamotrigine, phenytoin, topiramate, valproate	VASC inhibitors
Antiarrhythmics	
Mexiletine, flecainide, procainamide, propafenone, ranolazine	VASC inhibitors
Verapamil	VASC inhibitor
Other Drugs	
Memantine	NMDA receptor antagonist
Diclofenac	Nonsteroidal antiinflammatory drug
Ritanserin	5-HT2A antagonist
Ambroxol, lifarizine, riluzole, tolperisone	VASC inhibitor
Flunarizine	VASC inhibitor

cal anesthetic interaction with VASCs.[76] The movement of this residue in DIV-S6 during inactivation may enhance the interaction with flecainide and local anesthetics, providing a plausible mechanism for state-dependent inhibition.[57] Access to the binding site by some VASC inhibitors from the cytoplasm will require the activation gate to open.[77] This is consistent with use-dependent block that is characteristic of many local anesthetics and antiarrhythmic inhibitors of VASCs. However, the wall of the central cavity of the $Na_V1.5$ channel is penetrated by four fenestrations, one on each surface, formed between adjacent PMs.[59] These fenestrations are large enough for hydrophobic inhibitors such as lidocaine to penetrate and access the binding pocket via the lipid bilayer[78] (Fig. 10.6B). This provides a plausible mechanism of inhibition of $Na_V1.5$ channels in cancer cells where the vast majority will be in the inactive state and very few will be open due to the depolarized RMP in cancer cells.

Muscarinic Acetylcholine Receptors

Local anesthetics are not entirely selective for their canonical target. For example, local anesthetics inhibit M1 and M3 mAChR.[79,80] While this promiscuity may be a disadvantage in the usual therapeutic setting, it may be advantageous for the cancer patient in whom aberrant upregulation of many different proteins underlies complex pathology. Indeed, mAChR overexpression has been linked with a number of cancers, such as brain, breast, pancreatic, ovarian, gastric, and colon cancers.[81] mAChRs are G-protein-coupled receptors widely expressed in central and peripheral tissues where they mediate biological functions such as glandular secretion, blood vessel dilation, and smooth muscle contraction.[82] Lidocaine modulates M3 mAChR signaling via inhibition of G_q proteins, rather than by a direct action on the receptor.[83] Activation of mAChRs can directly activate epidermal growth factor receptors (EGFRs) on the cell membrane.[84] In addition, G_q-protein-mediated activation of phospholipase C (PLC) raises intracellular inositol triphosphate (IP3), leading to increased $[Ca^{2+}]_i$. This, together with EGFR signaling, mediates gene transcription relevant to proliferation and invasion via MAPK signaling, such as those described earlier (Fig. 10.1).

M3 mAChR-deficient mice exhibit reduced cell proliferation and tumor size following chemically induced colon

A

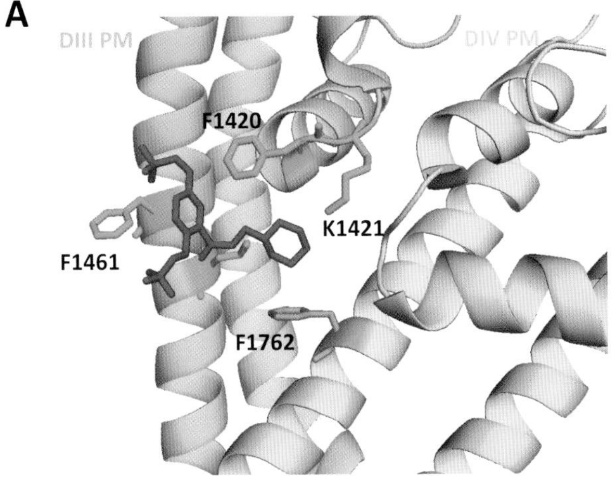

B

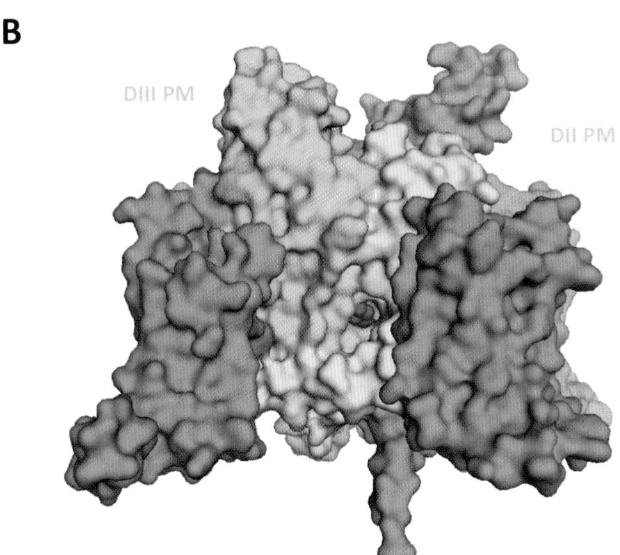

• **Fig. 10.6** Interaction of $Na_V1.5$ with flecainide. (A) Ribbon rendering of DIII *(green)* and DIV *(brown)* with flecainide rendered in stick format in *red* (protein data bank entry 6UZ0). The residues contributing to the binding of flecainide are labeled in *green* for those in DIII and *orange* in DIV. (B) Space fill rendering of $Na_V1.5$ viewed from the side highlighting the fenestration formed between the pore domain of DII *(pink)* and DIII *(green)*. It is possible to see flecainide *(red space fill)* in its binding pocket through the fenestration.

cancer.[85] Consistent with a role for the activity of mAChRs in cancer, their direct stimulation using muscarinic agonists increases proliferation.[86] In gastric cancers, pharmacologic blockade of M3 mAChRs inhibits tumorigenesis.[87,88] Furthermore, denervation via surgical vagotomy attenuated tumorigenesis in mouse models of gastric cancers, highlighting the importance of acetylcholine signaling in tumorigenesis.[87,89] In breast cancer, stimulation of M3 mAChR activity increases breast cancer cell proliferation.[90–92] The influence of lidocaine on the prooncogenic effects of M3 mAChRs remains to be elucidated.

Conclusion

The inhibition by local anesthetics of a number of key targets relevant to oncophysiology highlights their potential value in the treatment of cancer. The perioperative period may be an opportune time to deploy local anesthetics when the cancer patient is most vulnerable to seeding micrometastases. Basic research into the role played by VASCs and mAChRs (plus other proteins) in oncophysiology is beginning to unravel a unique and complex system of intracellular signaling and ionic homeostasis, which could be targeted by local anesthetics. There is also a need to investigate the expression of these proteins in patients, which may provide an opportunity for disease stratification, enabling a personalized treatment regimen.

References

1. Yu JJ, Xiao W, Dong SL, et al. Effect of surgical liver resection on circulating tumor cells in patients with hepatocellular carcinoma. *BMC Cancer*. 2018;18:835.
2. Hiller JG, Perry NJ, Poulogiannis G, Riedel B, Sloan EK. Perioperative events influence cancer recurrence risk after surgery. *Nat Rev Clin Oncol*. 2018;15:205–218.
3. Ogawa K, et al. Suppression of cellular immunity by surgical stress. *Surgery*. 2000;127:329–336.
4. Kvarnström AL, Sarbinowski RT, Bengtson JP, Jacobsson LM, Bengtsson AL. Complement activation and interleukin response in major abdominal surgery. *Scand J Immunol*. 2012;75:510–516.
5. Forget P, et al. How anesthetic, analgesic and other non-surgical techniques during cancer surgery might affect postoperative oncologic outcomes: a summary of current state of evidence. *Cancers*. 2019;11.
6. Colvin LA, Bull F, Hales TG. Perioperative opioid analgesia—when is enough too much? A review of opioid-induced tolerance and hyperalgesia. *Lancet*. 2019;393:1558–1568.
7. Xie N, et al. Activation of μ-opioid receptor and Toll-like receptor 4 by plasma from morphine-treated mice. *Brain Behav Immun*. 2017;61:244–258.
8. Boland JW, Pockley AG. Influence of opioids on immune function in patients with cancer pain: from bench to bedside. *Br J Pharmacol*. 2018;175:2726–2736.
9. Franchi S, Panerai AE, Sacerdote P. Buprenorphine ameliorates the effect of surgery on hypothalamus-pituitary-adrenal axis, natural killer cell activity and metastatic colonization in rats in comparison with morphine or fentanyl treatment. *Brain Behav Immun*. 2007;21:767–774.
10. Stollings LM, et al. Immune modulation by volatile anesthetics. *Anesthesiology*. 2016;125:399–411.
11. Elena G, et al. Effects of repetitive sevoflurane anaesthesia on immune response, select biochemical parameters and organ histology in mice. *Lab Anim*. 2003;37:193–203.
12. Desmond F, McCormack J, Mulligan N, Stokes M, Buggy DJ. Effect of anaesthetic technique on immune cell infiltration in breast cancer: a follow-up pilot analysis of a prospective, randomised, investigator-masked study. *Anticancer Res*. 2015;35:1311–1320.

13. Buckley A, McQuaid S, Johnson P, Buggy DJ. Effect of anaesthetic technique on the natural killer cell anti-tumour activity of serum from women undergoing breast cancer surgery: a pilot study. *Br J Anaesth*. 2014;113(Suppl 1):i56–i62.
14. Jaura AI, Flood G, Gallagher HC, Buggy DJ. Differential effects of serum from patients administered distinct anaesthetic techniques on apoptosis in breast cancer cells in vitro: A pilot study. *Br J Anaesth*. 2014;113(Suppl 1):i63–i67.
15. Xu YJ, et al. Effects of anaesthesia on proliferation, invasion and apoptosis of LoVo colon cancer cells in vitro. *Anaesthesia*. 2016;71:147–154.
16. Zhu M, et al. Isoflurane enhances the malignant potential of glioblastoma stem cells by promoting their viability, mobility in vitro and migratory capacity in vivo. *Br J Anaesth*. 2016;116:870–877.
17. Ecimovic P, Mchugh B, Murray D, Doran P, Buggy DJ. Effects of sevoflurane on breast cancer cell function in vitro. *Anticancer Res*. 2013;33:4255–4260.
18. Iwasaki M, et al. Volatile anaesthetics enhance the metastasis related cellular signalling including CXCR2 of ovarian cancer cells. *Oncotarget*. 2016;7:26042–26056.
19. Luo X, et al. Impact of isoflurane on malignant capability of ovarian cancer in vitro. *Br J Anaesth*. 2015;114:831–839.
20. Sessler DI, Ben-Eliyahu S, Mascha EJ, Parat M-O, Buggy DJ. Can regional analgesia reduce the risk of recurrence after breast cancer? Methodology of a multicenter randomized trial. *Contemp Clin Trials*. 2008;29:517–526.
21. Wigmore TJ, Mohammed K, Jhanji S. Long-term survival for patients undergoing volatile versus IV anesthesia for cancer surgery: a retrospective analysis. *Anesthesiology*. 2016;124:69–79.
22. Fant F, et al. Thoracic epidural analgesia inhibits the neuro-hormonal but not the acute inflammatory stress response after radical retropubic prostatectomy. *Br J Anaesth*. 2013;110:747–757.
23. Siekmann W, et al. Surgical and not analgesic technique affects postoperative inflammation following colorectal cancer surgery: A prospective, randomized study. *Color Dis*. 2017;19:O186–O195.
24. Sessler DI, et al. Recurrence of breast cancer after regional or general anaesthesia: a randomised controlled trial. *Lancet*. 2019;394:1807–1815.
25. Hollmann MW, Durieux ME, Fisher DM. Local anesthetics and the inflammatory response: a new therapeutic indication? *Anesthesiology*. 2000;93:858–875.
26. Beaussier M, Delbos A, Maurice-Szamburski A, Ecoffey C, Mercadal L. Perioperative use of intravenous lidocaine. *Drugs*. 2018;78:1229–1246.
27. Caracas HCPM, Maciel JVB, Martins PMRES, deSouza MMG, Maia LC. The use of lidocaine as an anti-inflammatory substance: a systematic review. *J Dent*. 2009;37:93–97.
28. Forget P, et al. Intraoperative ketorolac in high-risk breast cancer patients. A prospective, randomized, placebo-controlled clinical trial. *PLoS One*. 2019;14.
29. Forget P, et al. Intraoperative use of ketorolac or diclofenac is associated with improved disease-free survival and overall survival in conservative breast cancer surgery. *Br J Anaesth*. 2014;113(Suppl 1):i82–i87.
30. Piegeler T, et al. Antimetastatic potential of amide-linked local anesthetics: Inhibition of lung adenocarcinoma cell migration and inflammatory Src signaling independent of sodium channel blockade. *Anesthesiology*. 2012;117:548–559.
31. Wall TP, Crowley PD, Sherwin A, Foley AG, Buggy DJ. Effects of lidocaine and src inhibition on metastasis in a murine model of breast cancer surgery. *Cancers (Basel)*. 2019;11.
32. Cata JP, et al. Lidocaine stimulates the function of natural killer cells in different experimental settings. *Anticancer Res*. 2017;37:4727–4732.
33. Gao J, Hu H, Wang X. Clinically relevant concentrations of lidocaine inhibit tumor angiogenesis through suppressing VEGF/VEGFR2 signaling. *Cancer Chemother Pharmacol*. 2009;83:1007–1015.
34. Zhou D, et al. Repositioning lidocaine as an anticancer drug: the role beyond anesthesia. *Front Cell Dev Biol*. 2020;8:565.
35. Vigneault L, et al. Perioperative intravenous lidocaine infusion for postoperative pain control: a meta-analysis of randomized controlled trials. *Can J Anesth*. 2011;58:22–23.
36. Yardeni IZ, Beilin B, Mayburd E, Levinson Y, Bessler H. The effect of perioperative intravenous lidocaine on postoperative pain and immune function. *Anesth Analg*. 2009;109:1464–1469.
37. George AL. Inherited disorders of voltage-gated sodium channels. *J Clin Investig*. 2005;11:1990–1999.
38. Hanahan D, Weinberg RA. Hallmarks of cancer: The next generation. *Cell*. 2011;14:646–674.
39. Prevarskaya N, Skryma R, Shuba Y. Ion channels in cancer: are cancer hallmarks oncochannelopathies? *Physiol Rev*. 2018;98:559–621.
40. Wood LD, et al. The genomic landscapes of human breast and colorectal cancers. *Science*. 2007;318(80):1108–1113.
41. Roger S, Gillet L, LeGuennec JY, Besson P. Voltage-gated sodium channels and cancer: is excitability their primary role? *Front Pharmacol*. 2015;6 2015.
42. Mao W Zhang J, Körner H, Jiang Y, Ying S. The emerging role of voltage-gated sodium channels in tumor biology. *Front Oncol*. 2019;9:124.
43. Djamgoz MBA, Fraser SP, Brackenbury WJ. In vivo evidence for voltage-gated sodium channel expression in carcinomas and potentiation of metastasis. *Cancers*. 2019;11(11):1675.
44. House CD, et al. Voltage-gated Na+ channel SCN5A is a key regulator of a gene transcriptional network that controls colon cancer invasion. *Cancer Res*. 2010;70:6957–6967.
45. Baptista-Hon DT, et al. Potent inhibition by ropivacaine of metastatic colon cancer SW620 cell invasion and Na V 1.5 channel function. *Br J Anaesth*. 2014;113:i39–i48.
46. Yildirim S, Altun S, Gumushan H, Patel A, Djamgoz MBA. Voltage-gated sodium channel activity promotes prostate cancer metastasis in vivo. *Cancer Lett*. 2012;323:58–61.
47. Fraser SP, et al. Voltage-gated sodium channel expression and potentiation of human breast cancer metastasis. *Clin Cancer Res*. 2005;11:5381–5389.
48. Brackenbury WJ, Chioni AM, Diss JKJ, Djamgoz MBA. The neonatal splice variant of Nav1.5 potentiates in vitro invasive behaviour of MDA-MB-231 human breast cancer cells. *Breast Cancer Res Treat*. 2007;101:149–160.
49. House CD, et al. Voltage-gated Na+ channel activity increases colon cancer transcriptional activity and invasion via persistent MAPK signaling. *Sci Rep*. 2015;5:11541.
50. Nelson M, Yang M, Dowle AA, Thomas JR, Brackenbury WJ. The sodium channel-blocking antiepileptic drug phenytoin inhibits breast tumour growth and metastasis. *Mol Cancer*. 2015;14:13.
51. Siekmann W, Tina E, Koskela von Sydow A, Gupta A. Effect of lidocaine and ropivacaine on primary (SW480) and metastatic (SW620) colon cancer cell lines. *Oncol Lett*. 2019;18(1):395–401. doi:10.3892/ol.2019.10332.
52. D'Agostino G, et al. Lidocaine inhibits cytoskeletal remodelling and human breast cancer cell migration. *Br J Anaesth*. 2018;121:962–968.

53. Brisson L, et al. NaV1.5 Na+ channels allosterically regulate the NHE-1 exchanger and promote the activity of breast cancer cell invadopodia. *J Cell Sci*. 2013;126:4835–4842.
54. Brisson L, et al. Na v 1.5 enhances breast cancer cell invasiveness by increasing NHE1-dependent H efflux in caveolae. *Oncogene*. 2011;30:2070–2076.
55. Bon E, et al. SCN4B acts as a metastasis-suppressor gene preventing hyperactivation of cell migration in breast cancer. *Nat Commun*. 2016;7:13648.
56. Shen H, et al. Structure of a eukaryotic voltage-gated sodium channel at near-atomic resolution. *Science*. 2017; 355(80):eaal4326.
57. Payandeh J, Scheuer T, Zheng N, Catterall WA. The crystal structure of a voltage-gated sodium channel. *Nature*. 2011; 475:353–359.
58. Shen H, Liu D, Wu K, Lei J, Yan N. Structures of human Na v 1.7 channel in complex with auxiliary subunits and animal toxins. *Science*. 2019;363(80):1303–1308.
59. Jiang D, et al. Structure of the cardiac sodium channel. *Cell*. 2020;180:122–134.
60. Schroeter A, et al. Structure and function of splice variants of the cardiac voltage-gated sodium channel Nav1.5. *J Molecular Cellular Cardiol*. 2010;49:16–24.
61. Yarov-Yarovoy V, et al. Structural basis for gating charge movement in the voltage sensor of a sodium channel. *Proc Natl Acad Sci USA*. 2012;109:E93–E102.
62. Vargas E, et al. An emerging consensus on voltage-dependent gating from computational modeling and molecular dynamics simulations. *J Gen Physiol*. 2012;140:587–594.
63. Vassilev PM, Scheuer T, Catterall WA. Identification of an intracellular peptide segment involved in sodium channel inactivation. *Science*. 1988;241(80):1658–1661.
64. West JW, et al. A cluster of hydrophobic amino acid residues required for fast Na+-channel inactivation. *Proc Natl Acad Sci USA*. 1992;89:10910–10914.
65. Hille B. *Ion Channels of Excitable Membranes*: Sinauer Associates, Inc.; 2001.
66. Elajnaf T, Baptista-Hon DT, Hales TG. Potent inactivation-dependent inhibition of adult and neonatal NaV1.5 channels by lidocaine and levobupivacaine. *Anesth Analg*. 2018;127: 650–660.
67. Schwoerer AP, Scheel H. Friederich PA Comparative analysis of bupivacaine and ropivacaine effects on human cardiac SCN5A channels. *Anesth Analg*. 2015;120:1226–1234.
68. Nadrowitz F, et al. The distinct effects of lipid emulsions used for 'lipid resuscitation' on gating and bupivacaine-induced inhibition of the cardiac sodium channel nav 1.5. *Anesth Analg*. 2013;117:1101–1108.
69. Song W, et al. The human Nav 1.5 F1486 deletion associated with long QT syndrome leads to impaired sodium channel inactivation and reduced lidocaine sensitivity. *J Physiol*. 2012;590:5123–5139.
70. Balser JR, Nuss HB, Romashko DN, Marban E, Tomaselli GF. Functional consequences of lidocaine binding to slow-inactivated sodium channels. *J Gen Physiol*. 1996;107:643–658.
71. Bean BP, Cohen CJ, Tsien RW. Lidocaine block of cardiac sodium channels. *J Gen Physiol*. 1983;81:613–642.
72. Litonius E, Tarkkila P, Neuvonen PJ, Rosenberg PH. Effect of intravenous lipid emulsion on bupivacaine plasma concentration in humans. *Anaesthesia*. 2012;67:600–605.
73. Prieto-Álvarez P, et al. Comparison of mepivacaine and lidocaine for intravenous regional anaesthesia: pharmacokinetic study and clinical correlation. *Br J Anaesth*. 2002;88:516–519.
74. Trautwein W, Kassebaum D, Nelson R, Hecht H. Electrophysiological study of human heart muscle. *Circ Res*. 1962;10: 306–312.
75. Liu H, Atkins J, Kass RS. Common molecular determinants of flecainide and lidocaine block of heart Na+ channels: evidence from experiments with neutral and quaternary flecainide analogues. *J Gen Physiol*. 2003;121:199–214.
76. Ragsdale DS, McPhee JC, Scheuer T, Catterall WA. Molecular determinants of state-dependent block of Na+ channels by local anesthetics. *Science*. 1994;265(80):1724–1728.
77. Hille B. Local anesthetics: hydrophilic and hydrophobic pathways for the drug-receptor reaction. *J Gen Physiol*. 1977; 69:497–515.
78. Gamal El-Din TM, Lenaeus MJ, Zheng N, Catterall WA. Fenestrations control resting-state block of a voltage-gated sodium channel. *Proc Natl Acad Sci USA*. 2018;115:13111–13116.
79. Hollmann MW, et al. Inhibition of m3 muscarinic acetylcholine receptors by local anaesthetics. *Br J Pharmacol*. 2001;133: 207–216.
80. Hollmann MW, Fischer LG, Byford AM, Durieux ME. Local anesthetic inhibition of m1 muscarinic acetylcholine signaling. *Anesthesiology*. 2000;93:497–509.
81. Shah N, Khurana S, Cheng K, Raufman JP. Muscarinic receptors and ligands in cancer. *Am J Physiol Cell Physiol*. 2009;296:C221–C232.
82. Kruse AC, Li J, Hu J, Kobilka BK, Wess J. Novel insights into M3 muscarinic acetylcholine receptor physiology and structure. *J Mol Neurosci*. 2014;53:316–323.
83. Hollmann MW, McIntire WE, Garrison JC, Durieux ME. Inhibition of mammalian Gq protein function by local anesthetics. *Anesthesiology*. 2002;97:1451–1457.
84. Cheng K, Xie G, Raufman J-P. Matrix metalloproteinase-7-catalyzed release of HB-EGF mediates deoxycholyltaurine-induced proliferation of a human colon cancer cell line. *Biochem Pharmacol*. 2007;73:1001–1012.
85. Raufman J-P, et al. Genetic ablation of M3 muscarinic receptors attenuates murine colon epithelial cell proliferation and neoplasia. *Cancer Res*. 2008;68:3573–3578.
86. Peng Z, Heath J, Drachenberg C, Raufman J-P, Xie G. Cholinergic muscarinic receptor activation augments murine intestinal epithelial cell proliferation and tumorigenesis. *BMC Cancer*. 2013;13:204.
87. Zhao CM, et al. Denervation suppresses gastric tumorigenesis. *Sci Transl Med*. 2014;6:115–250 250ra115.
88. Yu H, et al. Acetylcholine acts through M3 muscarinic receptor to activate the EGFR signaling and promotes gastric cancer cell proliferation. *Sci Rep*. 2017;7:40802.
89. Rabben H-L, Zhao C-M, Hayakawa YC, Wang T, Chen D. Vagotomy and gastric tumorigenesis. *Curr Neuropharmacol*. 2016;14:967–972.
90. Fiszman GL, et al. Activation of muscarinic cholinergic receptors induces MCF-7 cells proliferation and angiogenesis by stimulating nitric oxide synthase activity. *Cancer Biol. Ther*. 2007;6:1106–1113.
91. Negroni MP, et al. Immunoglobulin G from breast cancer patients in stage i stimulates muscarinic acetylcholine receptors in MCF7 cells and induces proliferation. Participation of nitric oxide synthase-derived nitric oxide. *J Clin Immunol*. 2010;30:474–484.
92. Jiménez E, Montiel M. Activation of MAP kinase by muscarinic cholinergic receptors induces cell proliferation and protein synthesis in human breast cancer cells. *J Cell Physiol*. 2005;204:678–686.

11

Volatile and Intravenous Anesthetics and Cancer

JULIA A. DUBOWITZ, SANKETH RAMPES, MATS ENLUND, AND DAQING MA

General Introduction: Anesthesia and Cancer Progression

Surgery remains a central treatment modality for patients with solid cancers, with more than 60% of cancer patients presenting for surgical resection, and more than 80% of cancer patients exposed to a surgical procedure during their treatment journey.[1,2] Together with a rapidly growing and aging population, it is estimated that in 2030 17.3 million cancer patients will need surgery as part of their oncologic treatment.[3]

Accompanying surgical intervention is a perioperative stress response characterized by systemic release of inflammatory mediators, activation of cells of the innate and adaptive immune system, and prothrombotic responses.[4] While evolutionarily appropriate to aid healing after surgical tissue damage, excessive and prolonged upregulation of these responses results in a period of prolonged postoperative immunosuppression and has the potential to alter the biological environment of tumor cells. The perioperative surgical response has thus been implicated in the progression of malignant disease.

Surgical intervention requires anesthesia and the role of anesthetic agents in modulating this perioperative stress response, cancer cell biology, and even long-term cancer outcomes is emerging. This chapter aims to provide a comprehensive overview of the current evidence supporting the impact of anesthetic agents on cancer progression.

Mechanisms of Cancer Development and Progression

Tumor cells have the ability to grow, proliferate, and spread within their host.[5] In order to facilitate the tumor's development, tumor angiogenesis is also established. This occurs when tumors are just 1 mm in size; therefore tumors have developed the potential to metastasize well before they are amenable to surgical resection. In addition, with surgical manipulation of tumors, cancer cells are released into circulation and can deposit in distant sites where they can develop into overt metastatic disease.[6] However, not all patients who undergo surgery ultimately die from overwhelming metastatic disease, suggesting that not all tumor cells have the same propensity to spread into the blood stream or to establish themselves at distant sites as metastases.

The concept of immunoediting describes the role of the immune system in suppression and proliferation of oncologic disease.[7] It recognizes the complex interplay between tumor cells and their environment, which is responsible for the removal of malignant cells (elimination) and control of disease (equilibrium), but also the unwanted progression of malignant disease (escape).[8,9] With this understanding, the importance of supporting an antitumorigenic immune state, particularly at times of physiologic perturbation such as during surgery, becomes increasingly significant.[10] Macrophages, natural killer cells, and T cells play an important role in the survival, proliferation, and invasion of tumor cells within their host[9] and are known to be suppressed in number and function after major surgical insult.[4] It is- therefore- plausible that the immunosuppressive environment induced after major surgery has the potential to promote the growth and spread of potentially fatal disease.

Molecular Actions of Anesthetics and Cancers

While the complete mechanism of action of general anesthetic agents remains unclear, both volatile anesthetics and propofol exert their hypnotic and amnesic effects by positive modulation of the inhibitory neurotransmitter gamma-aminobutyric acid (GABA), primarily through $GABA_A$ receptor activity[11,12] in the brain and spinal cord. Activity of anesthetic agents at other receptors has been identified, including potassium (K^+) channels and *N*-methyl-D-aspartate (NMDA) receptors, and may be responsible for the secondary effects of anesthetic agents such as their effect on tumor and immune cells.

TABLE 11.1 Effect of Anesthetic Agents on Cancer Cell Biology

Mechanism	Effect of Anesthetic Agent	Cancer Type (Reference)
Proliferation	↓ Propofol	Breast[17] Endometrial[29] Prostate[30] Osteosarcoma[31] Esophageal SCC[32] Ovarian[28]
	↑ Volatile	Hepatocellular[22]
Apoptosis	↑ Propofol	Nonsmall cell lung[33] Endometrial[29] Osteosarcoma[31] Lung[34] Esophageal SCC[32] Glioblastoma[35] Breast[36]
NK-mediated cell apoptosis	↑ Propofol-paravertebral treated patient serum	Breast[110]
	↓ Volatile anesthesia treated patient serum	Breast[110]
Cell viability	↓ Propofol	Cervical[37] Endometrial[29] Lung[40] Glioma[38] Lung[34] Gastric[39]
Metabolism	↓ Propofol	Colorectal[44] Glioma[38]
EMT	↓ Propofol	Prostate[47]
Invasion and migration	↓ Propofol	Endometrial[29] Lung[40] Glioma[38] Breast[36] Osteosarcoma[31] Lung[41]
	↑ Propofol (in esophageal SCC)	Esophageal SCC[32]
	↑ Volatile	Ovarian[28]

EMT, Epithelial-mesenchymal transition; *SCC*, squamous cell carcinoma.

While these receptor interactions may explain the non-anesthetic (cardiovascular, respiratory, hepatic, and renal) side effects of commonly used anesthetic agents, it has been interestingly observed that affinity for these receptors explains the potential direct effect of anesthetic agents on cells of the immune system and tumor cells alike.[13,14]

Preclinical In Vitro and In Vivo Studies of Cancer and Anesthetics

Studies have examined the effect of different anesthetic agents on tumor cell biology in vitro and in vivo, across a number of different tumor cell lines (Tables 11.1 and 11.2). In addition to volatile anesthetics and propofol, studies of the most common intravenous agents studied have investigated the effect of other analgesic and hypnotic agents, including the NMDA-receptor antagonist ketamine, the alpha-2 adrenoreceptor agonist dexmedetomidine, and the benzodiazepine midazolam (Table 11.3).

Inhalational Anesthetics

Volatile anesthetics are the mainstay of anesthesia worldwide and are the most commonly used agents for maintenance of anesthesia.[15,16] Preclinical data have identified direct protumorigenic effects of volatile anesthetics across multiple cell lines.[17–19]

In addition, volatile anesthetic agents have been shown to activate receptors on immune cells and have been shown in vitro to modulate the function of immune cells.[13,14] Impaired neutrophil, macrophage, and NK cell recruitment and activity has been shown in vitro in response to direct exposure to volatile anesthetics.[13,14] Conversely, exposure to propofol has been shown to preserve the function of immune cells.[20,21] Exploratory research is beginning to interrogate the clinical implications of these findings, in particular, to determine if the type of anesthesia used for surgery is indeed responsible for postoperative immune modulation and to assess the impact

TABLE 11.2 Mechanistic Pathways Involved in Anesthetic Modulation of Tumor Cell Growth

Mechanism	Effect of Anesthetic Agent	Reference
PD-L1	↓ Propofol	Breast[17]
ERK1/2	↓ Propofol	Non–small cell lung[33] Colorectal[44]
PUMA	↑ Propofol	Non–small cell lung[33]
AMPK/mTOR	↑ Propofol	Cervical[37]
HIF-1α	↓ Propofol	Colorectal[44] Prostate[47] Prostate[27] Squamous cell carcinoma[49]
	↑ Volatile	Prostate[27] Renal cell[25]
N-cadherin, vimentin and Snail expression (EMT)	↓ Propofol	Lung[40]
Akt/mTOR	↓ Propofol	Chronic myeloid leukemia[43]
NF-κB signaling	↓ Propofol	Gliosarcoma[19]
Inflammatory cytokine production	↓ Propofol	Gliosarcoma[19]
CPAR-system-xc	↓ Propofol	Glioma[38]
Receptor target genes	↓ Propofol	Prostate[30]
Caspase-3	↑ Propofol	Lung[34]
mIR-486 mIR-218 mIR-21	↑ Propofol	Gliosarcoma[19] Lung[34] Pancreas[111]
Slug-dependent PUMA and e-cadherin	↓ Propofol	Pancreas[111]
VEGF	↑ Volatile	Ovarian[24] Renal[25] Ovarian[28]
MMP-11	↑ Volatile	Ovarian[24]
MMP-13	↓Propofol	Osteosarcoma[45]
MMP-2, 7, 9[113]	↓Propofol	Glioblastoma[46] Lung[41]
MMP-2, 9	↑ Volatile	Ovarian[28]
Repair-associated genes	↓Propofol	Leukemia[112]
mTOR	↓Propofol	Cervical[51]

Akt-mTOR, Protein kinase B-mammalian target of rapamycin; *AMPK/mTOR*, adenosine monophosphate-activated protein kinase; *EMT*, epithelial-mesenchymal transition; *ERK 1/2*, extracellular signal-related kinase 1/2; *HIF 1α*, hypoxia-inducible factor 1α; *MMP*, matrix metalloproteinase; *PD-L1*, programmed death ligand-1; *VEGF*, vascular endothelial growth factor.

on postoperative outcomes. These data are presented elsewhere in this chapter.

Sevoflurane

Sevoflurane is a widely used fluorinated methyl isopropyl ether anesthetic agent. Its effects on in vitro tumor cell mechanics have been investigated in hepatocellular carcinoma, breast, renal cell carcinoma, and ovarian cancer cell lines with consistent results.

Hepatocellular carcinoma cells treated with sevoflurane displayed increased proliferation compared to control,[22] and the sera of patients who underwent surgical resection of breast cancer under propofol-paravertebral anesthesia showed increased apoptosis in HCC1500 breast cancer cells[23] compared with sera from patients treated with sevoflurane-general anesthesia.

Exposure of ovarian cancer cells to the volatile anesthetics agents sevoflurane, isoflurane, and desflurane increased expression of vascular endothelial growth factor (VEGF) and matrix metalloproteinases (MMPs),[24,25] factors known to support angiogenesis and epithelial-mesenchymal transformation, processes vital to the growth and spread of malignant cells.[26]

TABLE 11.3 Effect of Hypnotic Anesthetic Agents

Mechanism	Effect of Anesthetic Agent	Cancer Type (Reference)
Proliferation	↑ Dexmedetomidine	Breast[57, 61, 62] Colorectal[57] Lung[57]
	↓ Midazolam	Head and neck[67, 68] Leukemia[69] Colorectal[69]
	↓ Ketamine	Pancreas[80]
	↑ Ketamine	Breast[84]
Apoptosis	↓ Dexmedetomidine	Lung[33, 56]
	↑ Dexmedetomidine	Neuroglioma[56] Bone[63]
	↑ Midazolam	Lung[56] Neuroglioma[56] Leukemia[69] Colorectal[69] Testicular[70]
	↑ Ketamine	Lung[81] Pancreas[80] Brain[82]
Necrosis	↑ Midazolam	Oral squamous cell carcinoma[71] Lymphoma[72] Neuroblastoma[72]
Invasion and migration	↑ Dexmedetomidine	Breast[58]
	↓ Dexmedetomidine	Lung[56] Neuroglioma[56] Osteosarcoma[63]
	↓ Ketamine	Breast[84]

Isoflurane

Induction of hypoxia-inducible factors (HIF-1α) is associated with increased tumor cell proliferation. Upregulation of HIF-1α via upregulation of PI-3K-Akt[27] has been shown in prostate[27] and renal cell carcinoma[25] cells exposed to isoflurane. Increased invasion and expression of VEGF-A and MMP-11 was seen in ovarian cancer cells upon exposure to isoflurane.[28]

Desflurane

Only one study in ovarian cancer has examined the effect of exposure to desflurane on tumor cell dynamics. Desflurane exposure led to the greatest expression of vascular endothelial growth factor-a (VEGF-A), matrix metalloproteinase-11 (MMP-11), C-X-C motif chemokine receptor-2 (CXCR2), and tumor growth factor-beta (TGF-β) expression compared with sevoflurane and isoflurane.[24]

Intravenous Anesthetics

Consistently, propofol has been shown to reduce proliferation,[17,28-32] increase cancer cell apoptosis,[29,31-36] reduce cancer cell viability,[29,34,37-39] and inhibit cancer cell migration and invasion,[29,31,32,36,38,40,41] in breast, endometrial, prostate, osteosarcoma, squamous cell carcinoma (SCC), lung, and glioblastoma cells. Interestingly, only one study found contradictory results with propofol increasing the velocity and migration of breast cancer cells.[42]

To further understand the mechanism driving anesthetic agent modulation of tumor cell biology, in vitro data have implicated key target pathways. Propofol has been shown to increase apoptosis and inhibit tumor cell viability, epithelial-mesenchymal transition (EMT), invasion and migration via inhibition of the extracellular signal-related kinase 1/2 (ERK 1/2),[17] protein kinase B-mammalian target of rapamycin (Akt-mTOR)[43] and adenosine monophosphate-activated protein kinase (AMPK)/mTOR[44] pathways, and programmed death ligand-1 (PD-L1).[17] Expression of proteins required for EMT and invasion, MMPs,[45,46] VEGF,[24,25,28] e-cadherin, vimentin, and Snail[40] has been shown to be reduced in cells treated with propofol. Similarly, induction of HIF-1α, crucial for angiogenesis in tumor cells, has been reduced with exposure to propofol in vitro in colorectal cancer[44] and prostate cancer[47,48] and in ex vivo studies in head and neck SCC.[49]

A small number of in vivo studies have examined the effects of anesthetic agents on tumor growth and metastasis, using varying experimental models (Table 11.4). Treatment

TABLE 11.4 In Vivo Studies

Mechanism	Effect of Anesthetic Agent	Cancer Type (Reference)
Pulmonary metastasis count	↓ Propofol	Breast[50]
		Osteosarcoma[113]
	↑ Volatile	Melanoma[114]
		Breast[50]
Tumor size	↓ Propofol	Cervical[51]
		CML[43]
		Gliosarcoma[19]
Tumor growth	↓ Propofol (treated cells)	Colorectal[44]
Survival time	↑ Propofol	Gliosarcoma[19]
Lung tumor retention	↓ Propofol	Breast[18]
	↑ Volatile	Breast[18]

CML, Chronic myeloid leukemia.

with volatile anesthesia increased pulmonary metastasis in a murine model of breast cancer,[50] while treatment with propofol consistently reduced primary tumor growth, pulmonary metastasis, improved response to chemotherapy and improved overall survival in models of breast,[50] chronic myeloid leukemia (CML),[43] cervical,[51] glioblastoma,[19] and colorectal[44] cancer.

Dexmedetomidine

Dexmedetomidine is a relatively new drug available to anesthetists and intensivists. Dexmedetomidine is a highly selective alpha-2-adrenoreceptor agonist with sedative, analgesic, and anxiolytic properties.[52] It exerts its sedative effect through stimulation of the alpha-2-adrenoreceptor in the locus coeruleus, which blunts excitation of the central nervous system.[52] The purported benefits of dexmedetomidine include a reduction in the surgical stress response,[53] concurrent need for analgesia,[54] and need for volatile anesthesia.

Laboratory evidence suggests that dexmedetomidine stimulates metastasis through stimulation of proliferation[55-58] and invasion[56,58] of cancer cells. However, large retrospective studies have demonstrated no effect on cancer recurrence.[59,60] Dexmedetomidine has been shown to stimulate proliferation in human breast cancer cell lines through stimulation of alpha-2-adrenoreceptors.[61] An in vivo study in mice has confirmed this finding.[62] The alpha-2-adrenoreceptorextracellular receptor kinase (ERK) signaling pathway has been shown to promote proliferation, migration, and invasion of human breast cancer cells both in vitro and in vivo.[58] Autocrine/paracrine prolactin signaling has also been shown to contribute to alpha-2-adrenoreceptor stimulation of breast cancer cell proliferation.[55] Dexmedetomidine has also been shown to stimulate the upregulation of the antiapoptotic proteins Bcl-2 and Bcl-xL.[56] A study involving the human osteosarcoma cell line MG63 found that dexmedetomidine inhibited cell proliferation and migration, and promoted apoptosis through upregulation of the miR-520a-3p, which directly targets AKT1 and represses the Akt/ERK pathway.[63] These conflicting results might be explained due to the different tumor types studied; however, further research is needed to elucidate the reason for this difference. In vivo rodent models of breast, lung, and colon cancers have shown that short-term use of clinically relevant doses of dexmedetomidine promotes metastasis.[57]

Dexmedetomidine may also affect tumorigenesis through immunomodulation. Dexmedetomidine has been shown in vivo in metastatic mouse models to expand monocytic myeloid-derived suppressor cells (M-MDSCs) in the postoperative period.[64] These M-MDSCs were able to promote metastasis through increasing the production of the proangiogenic factor VEGF.[64] These findings have been confirmed in lung cancer patients who were administered dexmedetomidine postthoracotomy.[64] Subhypnotic doses of dexmedetomidine may downregulate antitumor immunity through decreasing the production of interleukin-12 (IL-12) from antigen-presenting cells, resulting in Th2 shift and increased cytotoxic T lymphocyte activity.[65]

Midazolam

Midazolam is a benzodiazepine sedative drug that is used intraoperatively due to its rapid onset and short duration of action relative to other benzodiazepines. It also has significant anticonvulsant, amnesic, anxiolytic, and hypnotic properties that occur through modulation of $GABA_A$ receptors in the central nervous system.[66] Several studies have demonstrated the antitumor properties of midazolam; however, clinical trials establishing the effect of midazolam on cancer recurrence are yet to be conducted.

In vitro and in vivo evidence has demonstrated that midazolam inhibits cell proliferation[67-69] and induces both apoptosis[63,69,70] and necrosis[71,72] in cancer cells. Midazolam's antitumorigenic properties are partially mediated through the peripheral $GABA_A$ receptor.[73] Midazolam is thought to inhibit cell proliferation in FaDu human hypopharyngeal SCC cells partially through downregulating the expression of the EP300 gene, which controls the expression of numerous genes throughout the body and prevents tumor growth.[67,74,75] Midazolam has also been shown to exert its antiproliferative effect in FaDu cells through inhibition of transient receptor potential melastatin 7 (TRPM7).[68] Similar results were also demonstrated in T-98-MG malignant glioblastoma cells.[76]

Midazolam induces apoptosis in human lymphoma and neuroblastoma cell lines, and lung carcinoma cell lines in a concentration-dependent manner.[56,72] The activation of caspase-3, caspase-9, and PARP by midazolam indicates the induction of the intrinsic mitochondrial apoptosis pathway.[69] Midazolam also inhibited pERK1/2 signaling causing activation of the pro-apoptotic protein Bid and downregulation of antiapoptotic proteins Bcl-XL and XIAP. Midazolam did not induce generation of apoptotic markers in oral squamous cell carcinoma (OSCC) cells but did induce mitochondrial swelling, vacuoles, and plasma membrane rupture.[77] Another study demonstrated a switch from apoptotic cell death to necrotic cell death at high concentrations of midazolam.[72]

Ketamine

Ketamine is a drug used for induction and maintenance of general anesthesia and for the treatment of pain. The main mechanism of action is through antagonism of NMDA receptors, which are associated with central sensitization.[78] Ketamine also decreases presynaptic release of glutamate and interacts with opioid receptors.[79] Ketamine has been shown to exert antitumor effects in vitro and in vivo through the suppression of cell proliferation[80] and induction of apoptosis.[80-82]

Ketamine has been shown to induce apoptosis in a lung adenocarcinoma cell line in a concentration-dependent manner through upregulation of CD69 expression.[81] Downregulation of CD69 blocked the function of ketamine on inducing apoptosis.[81] Another in vitro study of human embryonic stem cells revealed that ketamine induced neuronal apoptosis via a mitochondrial pathway as revealed through the activation of caspase 3 activity, loss of the mitochondrial membrane potential, and release of cytochrome c.[82] Ketamine induced apoptosis in human hepatoma HepG2 cells through activation of a Bax-mitochondria-caspase protease pathway. Administration of Z-VEID-FMK, a caspase 6 inhibitor, prevented the ketamine-induced cellular apoptosis.[83] Interestingly, one study found that ketamine facilitates breast cancer cell line MDA-MB-231 proliferation and invasion through increasing the expression of the antiapoptotic protein Bcl-2.[84] Ketamine has been shown to inhibit the malignant potential of colorectal cancer cells via blockade of the NMDA receptor. NMDA blockade resulted in decreased phosphorylation of AKT, ERK, and Ca^{2+}/calmodulin-dependent protein kinase II (CaMK II), decreased expression of HIF-1α, and a decrease in the intracellular Ca^{2+} level.[85] This resulted in decreased VEGF expression and migration of colorectal cancer cells.[85]

Ketamine has been suggested to additionally affect tumor development through immunomodulation. Ketamine suppresses NK cell activity.[86] Ketamine induces human lymphocyte apoptosis via the mitochondrial pathway and inhibits dendritic cell maturation.[87,88] Ketamine also decreases the production of proinflammatory cytokines, including tumor necrosis factor kappa B (NF-κB) and IL-6. Animal models have shown that ketamine increases lung and liver metastases with one study in a rat model showing that ketamine increased lung metastases via NK cell suppression.[18,89]

Clinical Studies

Volatile and Total Intravenous Anesthesia Anesthetics

A large body of literature has emerged investigating the association between choice of anesthetic agent and cancer outcomes in different populations (Table 11.5). However, the studies are predominantly small and retrospective in nature, limiting the ability to delineate a clear association. The largest of the retrospective studies[90,91] have both shown a 5–10 percent-unit improvement in overall survival across multiple cancers with propofol compared with volatile anesthesia. Of note, Wigmore et al.[91] found that the survival benefit of total intravenous anesthesia (TIVA) was predominantly due to its effect in gastrointestinal and urological cancers, and Enlund et al.[90] attributed most of the reported survival benefit to the colorectal cancer cohort, suggesting a differential effect dependent on the biology of the cancer. Smaller retrospective studies have shown an improved recurrence-free survival with the use of TIVA in breast cancer[92] and improved overall survival in oesophageal,[93] glioma,[94] gastric,[95] and colorectal[96] cancers.

Only two small prospective randomized control trials have been undertaken in 120 non–small cell lung cancer[97] and 80 breast cancer[98] patients, respectively, and both found no difference in survival between propofol TIVA and volatile anesthesia. It is important to note, however, that both of these studies were significantly underpowered to detect a difference, and the lack of significant findings does not preclude the possibility of a true clinical effect. A recently published prospective trial (NCT00418457) investigating the impact of regional anesthesia-analgesia (paravertebral blocks and propofol) and general anesthesia (sevoflurane and opioid analgesia) on breast cancer recurrence found no statistically significant difference in a post hoc analysis of patients who received sevoflurane ($n = 1203$) or not ($n = 901$) (log rank $P = 0.78$), although the trial was not powered to detect a difference between these two groups.[99]

There are a number of other studies which have not shown a difference in cancer outcomes as a result of choice of anesthetic agents in glioblastoma,[100] breast cancer,[101,102] non–small cell lung cancer,[103] gastric cancer,[104] and appendiceal carcinoma[105] (Table 11.4). The retrospective nature of these

TABLE 11.5 Clinical Studies Investigating the Impact of Anesthetic Technique on Cancer Outcomes

Study	Cancer Type	Study Type	No. VOLA	No. TIVA	Median Follow up (Months)	Outcome	Reported Outcome	HR of Reported Outcome/Event Rate	95% CI
Enlund et al.[115], 2014 Sweden	Breast, colon, colorectal	Retrospective	1935	903	60	Overall survival	TIVA superior	5% difference favoring TIVA	0.03–0.06
Wigmore et al. [91], 2016 UK	Mixed	Retrospective	3316	3714	32	Overall survival	Volatile inferior	1.46	1.29–1.66
Lee et al.[92], 2016 South Korea	Breast	Retrospective	173	152	60	Recurrence-free survival	TIVA superior	0.55	0.311–0.973
Xu et al.[97], 2017 China	NSCLC	Prospective	60	60	36	Tumor-free survival Cumulative survival	No difference No difference	26.78 months (TIVA) 27.12 months (volatile) 78.33 months (TIVA), 80.00 months (volatile)	*P* = 0.877 *P* > 0.05
Cata et al.[115], 2017 United States	Glioblastoma	Retrospective	170	208	N/A	Overall survival Progression-free survival	No difference No difference	1.13 1.07	0.86–1.48 0.85–1.37
Jun et al.[93], 2017	Esophageal	Retrospective	731	191	37.9	Overall survival	Volatile inferior	1.58	1.24–2.01
Kim et al.[101], 2017	Breast	Retrospective	2589	56	70.1	Recurrence-free survival	No difference	1.14	0.49–2.60
Zheng et al. [95], 2018	Gastric	Retrospective	897	897	39.7	Overall survival	TIVA superior	0.65	0.64–1.26
Oh et al.[103], 2018 Korea	NSCLC	Retrospective	181	181	60	Recurrence-free survival Overall survival	No difference No difference	0.9 1.31	0.64–1.26 0.84–2.04
Wu et al.[96], 2018 China	Colon	Retrospective	579	579	44.4 (TIVA) 38.4 (volatile)	Overall survival	TIVA superior	0.27	0.22–0.35
Yan et al.[98], 2018 China	Breast	Prospective	40	40	28	Recurrence-free survival	No difference	Event rate: 78% (volatile) 95% (TIVA)	*P* = 0.221
Dong et al.[94], 2019 China	Glioma	Retrospective	140	154	12	Overall mortality	Volatile inferior	1.66	1.08–2.57
Yoo et al.[102], 2019 Korea	Breast	Retrospective	1776	1776	67 (TIVA) 53 (volatile)	Recurrence-free survival Overall survival	No difference No difference	0.96 0.96	0.69–1.32 0.69–1.33
Oh et al.[104], 2019 Korea	Gastric	Retrospective	769	769	12	Overall mortality Cancer-related mortality	No difference No difference	0.92 0.91	0.50–1.67 0.50–1.67
Cata et al.[105], 2019 United States	Appendiceal carcinoma	Retrospective	263	110	N/A	Progression-free survival Overall survival	No difference No difference	1.45 1.66	0.94–2.22 0.86–3.20

CI, Confidence interval; *HR*, hazard ratio; *NSCLC*, non–small cell lung cancer; *TIVA*, total intravenous anesthesia; *VOLA*, volatile anesthesia.

studies limits their ability to draw conclusions on the causative effect of anesthesia and cancer outcomes due to significant heterogeneity amongst the cancer patient populations and confounding from other perioperative interventions.

In summary of the current available data, a recent meta-analysis by Yap et al.[106] found volatile anesthesia to be associated with a worse disease-free survival (pooled hazard ratio [HR], 0.79; 95% confidence interval [CI], 0.62–1.0; P = 0.05) and overall survival (pooled HR, 0.76; 95% CI, 0.63–0.92; $P < 0.01$) across breast, esophageal, colorectal, lung, and mixed cancer types. Significant heterogeneity and bias exist in the available literature, which means that the results of this meta-analysis need to be interpreted with caution.

The conduct of high-quality, large prospective clinical trials is needed to directly address this question. Several studies are registered at ClinicalTrials.gov (NCT03034096, NCT02786329, NCT03447691, NCT02660411), of which the largest is NCT01975064 with another international randomized control trial to commence in 2020 (VAPOR-C trial). One trial comparing sevoflurane and propofol on postoperative long-term outcome after cancer surgery has completed the recruitment of patients,[107] but the results are not yet published.

Dexmedetomidine, Ketamine, and Midazolam

Despite accumulating laboratory evidence suggesting a detrimental impact of dexmedetomidine on cancer surgery, the limited clinical evidence available suggests negligible impact on cancer outcomes and recurrence. A retrospective single-center study of 93 pediatric patients who underwent cytoreductive surgery with hyperthermic intraperitoneal chemotherapy for peritoneal carcinomatosis found that the intraoperative or early postoperative administration of dexmedetomidine was not associated with altered progression-free or overall survival.[59] Another retrospective single-center study of 250 patients who underwent surgery for nonsmall cell lung cancer found no association between intraoperative use of dexmedetomidine and altered recurrence-free survival; however, they found a significant association between intraoperative use of dexmedetomidine and decreased overall survival. Clonidine is another alpha-2-adrenoreceptor agonist widely used during surgery. A retrospective study of 657 patients who underwent surgery for lung or breast cancer found no association between low-dose clonidine and recurrence-free or overall survival.[108] There is currently one ongoing randomized controlled trial, NCT03109990, of 460 patients investigating the effect of dexmedetomidine on breast cancer recurrence following surgery. The estimated primary completion date is April 2021, and these results will be eagerly awaited. Further prospective trials should be conducted to definitively determine the impact of dexmedetomidine in postoperative cancer recurrence.

Thus far, one single-center retrospective trial on 90 patients treated for hepatic malignancies with percutaneous microwave ablation found that midazolam was associated with lower local tumor progression-free survival (LTPFS) compared with propofol and general anesthesia.[109] Further retrospective studies and prospective studies should be conducted to definitively test the role of midazolam in cancer recurrence following surgery.

There have been no retrospective or prospective studies analyzing the impact of ketamine on cancer recurrence. In vivo models have associated intrinsic weaknesses but are useful for hypothesis development. Prospective studies are required to definitively test the influence of ketamine on postoperative cancer recurrence.

Ongoing Clinical Trials

To definitively answer the question of whether choice of anesthetic agent for cancer surgery impacts long-term cancer outcomes requires high-quality evidence. As mentioned, a number of prospective randomized control trials are currently underway. The results of these trials are expected to help delineate the causative effect, if any, of anesthetic agents on cancer outcome in patients presenting for surgical resection of cancers. It is important to note, however, that anesthetic agents are not administered in isolation, and it is likely the magnitude of surgery itself; other concomitant immunomodulatory interventions, including the administration of steroids, opioids and other analgesics, nonsteroidal antiinflammatory drugs, beta blockers, blood transfusions, temperature regulation; and the incidence and severity of postoperative complications (which themselves can generate a significant inflammatory-immune response) all have the potential to impact long-term cancer outcomes. This renders the task of characterizing the isolated effect of anesthetic agents a difficult and daunting one, but it also helps us to remember that the perioperative period as a whole is a major iatrogenic intervention that causes significant physiological perturbation and has the potential to dramatically impact the tumor microenvironment and, in turn, the progression of cancer in its host.

Implication and Conclusions

Emerging preclinical and clinical evidence support the theory that different anesthetic agents have differential effects on cancer cell biology and long-term cancer outcomes in patients presenting for surgical resection (Fig. 11.1). Currently, however, limitations in the available literature mean that they are not sufficient to support a change in clinical practice. A number of mechanisms have been implicated, namely in the protumorigenic effects of volatile anesthesia and the potentially antitumorigenic effects of TIVA anesthesia. It is plausible that any beneficial effect of TIVA with propofol, if any, may be in major surgery. Sufficient data are lacking to delineate the impact of other hypnotic agents in the modulation of cancer biology and long-term cancer outcomes. Limitations in the currently available data are due to the retrospective nature of the majority of evidence, with limited power and significant confounders for which the analyses cannot adjust, as well as conflictin biological

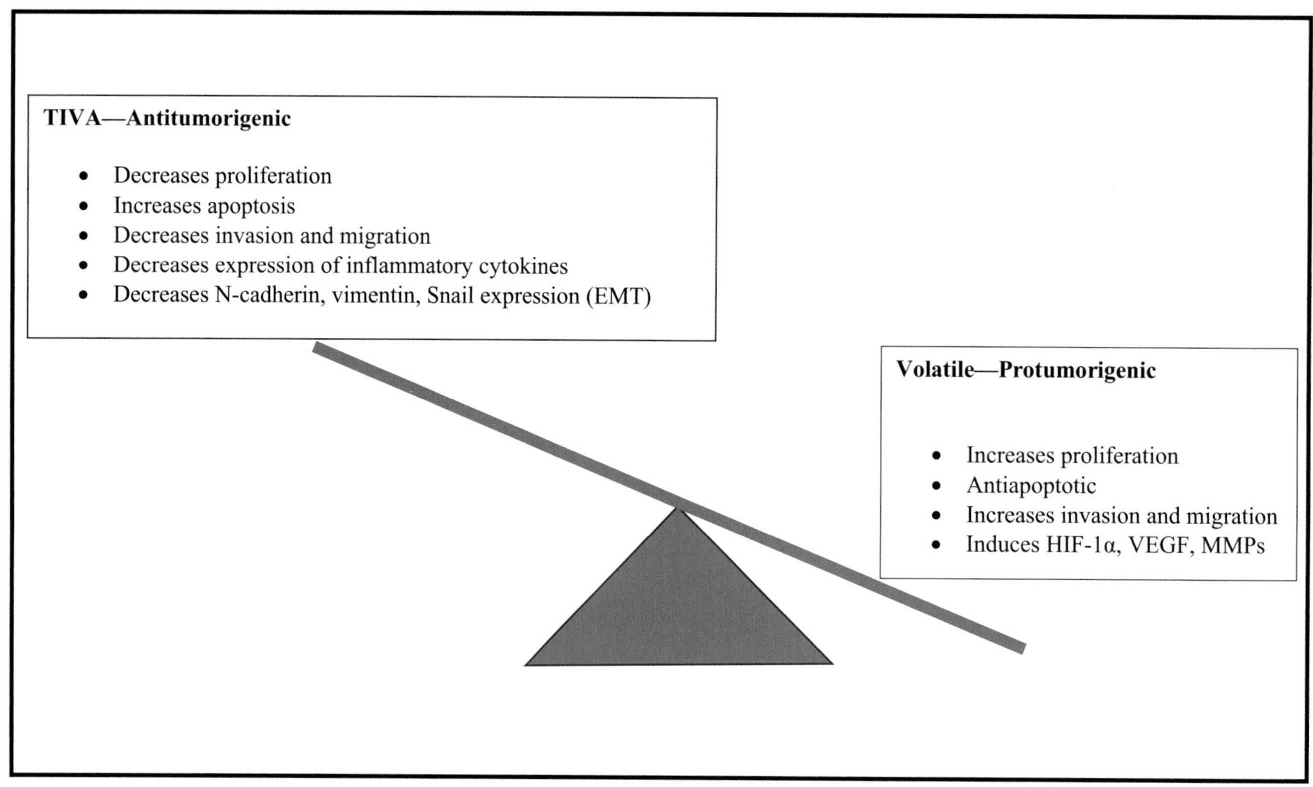

TIVA—Antitumorigenic
Decreases proliferation
Increases apoptosis
Decreases invasion and migration
Decreases expression of inflammatory cytokines
Decreases N-cadherin, vimentin, Snail expression (EMT)
Volatile—Protumorigenic
Increases proliferation
Antiapoptotic
Increases invasion and migration
Induces HIF-1α, VEGF, MMPs

• **Fig. 11.1** Mechanistic overview: anesthetic agents and cancer progression. *EMT*, Epithelial-mesenchymal transition; *HIF-1α*, hypoxia-inducible factors-1α; *MMP*, matrix metalloproteinase; *VEGF*, vascular endothelial growth factor.

mechanisms being implicated in both in vitro and in vivo studies. As such, the exact role anesthetic agents play in modulating cancer progression and the exact mechanisms involved remains unclear.

Given the plausible connection between anesthetic technique and long-term cancer outcomes, and the lack of definitive answers from the currently available literature, prospective clinical trials are needed to further understand the role of anesthesia and the potential ways of changing clinical practice to improve patient outcomes. If identified, simple, cheap, and easy to implement changes to clinical practice should rapidly be implemented to improve the care of the perioperative cancer patient and improve long-term cancer outcomes. Given that more than 60% of cancers are amenable to surgical resection, and the anticipated 21.6 million new cancer diagnoses anticipated worldwide in 2030,[3] herein lies the potential to significantly impact the prognosis of millions of cancer patients worldwide.

References

1. Sullivan R, Peppercorn J, Sikora K, et al. Delivering affordable cancer care in high-income countries. *Lancet Oncol.* 2011;12(10):933–980.
2. Alkire B, Raykar N, Shrime M. et al. Global access to surgical care: a modelling study. *Lancet Glob Health.* 2015;3(6):e316–e323.
3. Sullivan R, Alatise O, Anderson B. et al. Global cancer surgery: delivering safe, affordable, and timely cancer surgery. *Lancet Oncol.* 2015;16(11):1193–1224.
4. Desborough J. The stress response to trauma and surgery. *Br J Anaesth.* 2000;85(1):109–117.
5. Bielenberg DR, Zetter BR. The contribution of angiogenesis to the process of metastasis. *Cancer J (Sudbury, Mass.).* 2015;21(4):267–273.
6. Martin OA, Anderson R, Narayan K. et al. Does the mobilization of circulating tumour cells during cancer therapy cause metastasis? *Nat Rev Clin Oncol.* 2017;14(1):32–44.
7. Dunn G, Old L, Schreiber R. The immunobiology of cancer immunosurveillance and immunoediting. *Immunity.* 2004;21(2):137–148.
8. Mittal D, Gubin M, Schreiber R. et al. New insights into cancer immunoediting and its three component phases–elimination, equilibrium and escape. *Curr Opin Immunol.* 2014;27:16–25.
9. Hanahan D, Weinberg R. Hallmarks of cancer: the next generation. *Cell.* 2011;144(5):646–674.
10. Demicheli R, Retsky M, Hrushesky W, et al. The effects of surgery on tumor growth: a century of investigations. *Ann Oncol.* 2008;19(11):1821–1828.
11. Trapani G, Altomare C, Liso G, et al. Propofol in anesthesia. Mechanism of action, structure-activity relationships, and drug delivery. *Curr Med Chem.* 2000;7(2):249–271.
12. Khan KS, Hayes I, Buggy DJ. Pharmacology of anaesthetic agents II: inhalation anaesthetic agents. *BJA Educ.* 2013;14(3):106–111.
13. Stollings L, Jia L, Tang P, et al. Immune modulation by volatile anesthetics. *Anesthesiology.* 2016;125(2):399–411.
14. Yuki K, Eckenhoff R. Mechanisms of the immunological effects of volatile anesthetics: a review. *Anesth Analg.* 2016;123(2):326–335.
15. Pandit JJ, Andrade J, Bogod D, et al. 5th National Audit Project (NAP5) on accidental awareness during general anaesthesia:

protocol, methods, and analysis of data. *Br J Anaesth*. 2014; 113(4):540–548.

16. Lim A, Braat S, Hiller J, et al. Inhalational versus propofol-based total intravenous anaesthesia: practice patterns and perspectives among Australasian anaesthetists. *Anaesth Intensive Care*. 2018;46(5):480–487.
17. Zhang X, Li F, Zheng Y, et al. Propofol reduced mammosphere formation of breast cancer stem cells via PD-L1/Nanog in vitro. *Oxid Med Cell Longev*. 2019;2019:9078209.
18. Melamed R, Bar-Yosef S, Shakhar G, et al. Suppression of natural killer cell activity and promotion of tumor metastasis by ketamine, thiopental, and halothane, but not by propofol: mediating mechanisms and prophylactic measures. *Anesth Analg*. 2003;97(5):1331–1339.
19. Zheng Y, Liu H, Liang Y. Genistein exerts potent antitumour effects alongside anaesthetic, propofol, by suppressing cell proliferation and nuclear factor-kappaB-mediated signalling and through upregulating microRNA-218 expression in an intracranial rat brain tumour model. *J Pharm Pharmacol*. 2017;69(11):1565–1577.
20. Tazawa K, Koutsogiannaki S, Chamberlain M, et al. The effect of different anesthetics on tumor cytotoxicity by natural killer cells. *Toxicol Lett*. 2017;266:23–31.
21. Zhou M, Dai J, Zhou Y, et al. Propofol improves the function of natural killer cells from the peripheral blood of patients with esophageal squamous cell carcinoma. *Exp Ther Med*. 2018;16(1):83–92.
22. Nishiwada T, Kawaraguchi Y, Uemura K, et al. Effect of sevoflurane on human hepatocellular carcinoma HepG2 cells under conditions of high glucose and insulin. *J Anesth*. 2015;29(5):805–808.
23. Ni Eochagain A, Burns D, Riedel B, et al. The effect of anaesthetic technique during primary breast cancer surgery on neutrophil-lymphocyte ratio, platelet-lymphocyte ratio and return to intended oncological therapy. *Anaesthesia*. 2018;73(5):603–611.
24. Iwasaki M, Zhao H, Jaffer T, et al. Volatile anaesthetics enhance the metastasis related cellular signalling including CXCR2 of ovarian cancer cells. *Oncotarget*. 2016;7(18):26042–26056.
25. Benzonana LL, Perry N, Watts H, et al. Isoflurane, a commonly used volatile anesthetic, enhances renal cancer growth and malignant potential via the hypoxia-inducible factor cellular signaling pathway in vitro. *Anesthesiology*. 2013;119(3):593–605.
26. Rundhaug JE. Matrix metalloproteinases, angiogenesis, and cancer. Commentary re: A. C. Lockhart et al., Reduction of wound angiogenesis in patients treated with BMS-275291, a broad spectrum matrix metalloproteinase inhibitor. *Clin Cancer Res*. 2003;9(2):551–554 9:00–00, 2003.
27. Huang H, Benzonana L, Zhao H, et al. Prostate cancer cell malignancy via modulation of HIF-1alpha pathway with isoflurane and propofol alone and in combination. *Br J Cancer*. 2014;111(7):1338–1349.
28. Luo X, Zhao H, Hennah L. et al. Impact of isoflurane on malignant capability of ovarian cancer in vitro. *Br J Anaesth*. 2015;114(5):831–839.
29. Du Q, Liu J, Zhang X, et al. Propofol inhibits proliferation, migration, and invasion but promotes apoptosis by regulation of Sox4 in endometrial cancer cells. *Braz J Med Biol Res*. 2018;51(4):e6803.
30. Tatsumi K, Hirotsu A, Daijo H, et al. Effect of propofol on androgen receptor activity in prostate cancer cells. *Eur J Pharmacol*. 2017;809:242–252.
31. Xu YB, Jiang W, Zhao F, et al. Propofol suppresses invasion and induces apoptosis of osteosarcoma cell in vitro via downregulation of TGF-beta1 expression. *Eur Rev Med Pharmacol Sci*. 2016;20(7):1430–1435.
32. Guo XG, Wang S, Xu Y, et al. Propofol suppresses invasion, angiogenesis and survival of EC-1 cells in vitro by regulation of S100A4 expression. *Eur Rev Med Pharmacol Sci*. 2015;19(24):4858–4865.
33. Xing SG, Zhang K, Qu J, et al. Propofol induces apoptosis of non-small cell lung cancer cells via ERK1/2-dependent upregulation of PUMA. *Eur Rev Med Pharmacol Sci*. 2018; 22(13):4341–4349.
34. Yang N, Liang Y, Yang P, et al. Propofol inhibits lung cancer cell viability and induces cell apoptosis by upregulating microRNA-486 expression. *Braz J Med Biol Res*. 2017;50(1):e5794.
35. Liang WZ, Jan CR, Lu CH. Investigation of 2,6-diisopropylphenol (propofol)-evoked Ca2+ movement and cell death in human glioblastoma cells. *Toxicol In Vitro*. 2012;26(6):862–871.
36. Siddiqui RA, Zerouga M, Wu M, et al. Anticancer properties of propofol-docosahexaenoate and propofol-eicosapentaenoate on breast cancer cells. *Breast Cancer Res*. 2005;7(5):R645–R654.
37. Chen X, Li K, Zhao G. Propofol inhibits HeLa cells by impairing autophagic flux via AMP-activated protein kinase (AMPK) activation and endoplasmic reticulum stress regulated by calcium. *Med Sci Monit*. 2018;24:2339–2349.
38. Wang XY, Li Y, Wang H, et al. Propofol inhibits invasion and proliferation of C6 glioma cells by regulating the Ca(2+) permeable AMPA receptor-system xc(-) pathway. *Toxicol In Vitro*. 2017;44:57–65.
39. Yang C, Gao J, Yan N, et al. Propofol inhibits the growth and survival of gastric cancer cells in vitro through the upregulation of ING3. *Oncol Rep*. 2017;37(1):587–593.
40. Liu WZ, Liu N. Propofol inhibits lung cancer A549 cell growth and epithelial-mesenchymal transition process by upregulation of microRNA-1284. *Oncol Res*. 2018;27(1):1–8.
41. Wu KC, Yang S, Hsia T, et al. Suppression of cell invasion and migration by propofol are involved in down-regulating matrix metalloproteinase-2 and p38 MAPK signaling in A549 human lung adenocarcinoma epithelial cells. *Anticancer Res*. 2012;32(11):4833–4842.
42. Garib V, Niggemann B, Zanker K, et al. Influence of non-volatile anesthetics on the migration behavior of the human breast cancer cell line MDA-MB-468. *Acta Anaesthesiol Scand*. 2002;46(7):836–844.
43. Tan Z, Peng A, Xu J, et al. Propofol enhances BCR-ABL TKIs' inhibitory effects in chronic myeloid leukemia through Akt/mTOR suppression. *BMC Anesthesiol*. 2017;17(1):132.
44. Chen X, Wu Q, Sun P, et al. Propofol disrupts aerobic glycolysis in colorectal cancer cells via inactivation of the NMDAR-CAMKII-ERK pathway. *Cell Physiol Biochem*. 2018;46(2):492–504.
45. Ye Z, Jingzhong L, Yangbo L, et al. Propofol inhibits proliferation and invasion of osteosarcoma cells by regulation of microRNA-143 expression. *Oncol Res*. 2013;21(4):201–207.
46. Xu J, Xu W, Zhu J. Propofol suppresses proliferation and invasion of glioma cells by upregulating microRNA-218 expression. *Mol Med Rep*. 2015;12(4):4815–4820.
47. Qian J, Shen S, Chen W, et al. Propofol reversed hypoxia-induced docetaxel resistance in prostate cancer cells by preventing epithelial-mesenchymal transition by inhibiting hypoxia-inducible factor 1alpha. *Biomed Res Int*. 2018;2018:4174232.

48. Huang H, Benzonana L, Zhao H, et al. Prostate cancer cell malignancy via modulation of HIF-1α pathway with isoflurane and propofol alone and in combination. *Br J Cancer.* 2014;111(7):1338–1349.
49. Ferrell JK, Cattano D, Brown R, et al. The effects of anesthesia on the morphoproteomic expression of head and neck squamous cell carcinoma: a pilot study. *Transl Res.* 2015;166(6):674–682.
50. Freeman J, Crowley P, Foley A, et al. Effect of perioperative lidocaine, propofol and steroids on pulmonary metastasis in a murine model of breast cancer surgery. *Cancers (Basel).* 2019;11(5)613.
51. Zhang D, Zhou X, Zhang J, et al. Propofol promotes cell apoptosis via inhibiting HOTAIR mediated mTOR pathway in cervical cancer. *Biochem Biophys Res Commun.* 2015;468(4):561–567.
52. Scott-Warren V, Sebastian J. Dexmedetomidine: its use in intensive care medicine and anaesthesia. *BJA Education.* 2015;16(7):242–246.
53. Bulow NM, Colpo E, Pereira R, et al. Dexmedetomidine decreases the inflammatory response to myocardial surgery under mini-cardiopulmonary bypass. *Braz J Med Biol Res.* 2016;49(4):e4646.
54. Grosu I, Lavand'homme P. Use of dexmedetomidine for pain control. *F1000 Med Rep.* 2010;2:90.
55. Castillo LF, Rivero E, Goffin V, et al. Alpha2-adrenoceptor agonists trigger prolactin signaling in breast cancer cells. *Cell Signal.* 2017;34:76–85.
56. Wang C, Datoo T, Zhao H, et al. Midazolam and dexmedetomidine affect neuroglioma and lung carcinoma cell biology in vitro and in vivo. *Anesthesiology.* 2018;129(5):1000–1014.
57. Lavon H, Matzner P, Benbenishty A, et al. Dexmedetomidine promotes metastasis in rodent models of breast, lung, and colon cancers. *Br J Anaesth.* 2018;120(1):188–196.
58. Xia M, M, Ji N, Duan M, et al. Dexmedetomidine regulate the malignancy of breast cancer cells by activating alpha2-adrenoceptor/ERK signaling pathway. *Eur Rev Med Pharmacol Sci.* 2016;20(16):3500–3506.
59. Owusu-Agyemang P, Cata J, Kapoor R, et al. An analysis of the survival impact of dexmedetomidine in children undergoing cytoreductive surgery with hyperthermic intraperitoneal chemotherapy. *Int J Hyperth.* 2018;35(1):435–440.
60. Cata JP, Singh V, Lee B, et al. Intraoperative use of dexmedetomidine is associated with decreased overall survival after lung cancer surgery. *J Anaesthesiol Clin Pharmacol.* 2017;33(3):317–323.
61. Vazquez SM, Mladovan A, Perez C, et al. Human breast cell lines exhibit functional alpha2-adrenoceptors. *Cancer Chemother Pharmacol.* 2006;58(1):50–61.
62. Bruzzone A, Pinero C, Castillo L, et al. Alpha2-adrenoceptor action on cell proliferation and mammary tumour growth in mice. *Br J Pharmacol.* 2008;155(4):494–504.
63. Wang X, Xu Y, Chen X, et al. Dexmedetomidine inhibits osteosarcoma cell proliferation and migration, and promotes apoptosis by regulating miR-520a-3p. *Oncol Res.* 2018;26(3):495–502.
64. Su X, Fan Y, Yang L, et al. Dexmedetomidine expands monocytic myeloid-derived suppressor cells and promotes tumour metastasis after lung cancer surgery. *J Transl Med.* 2018; 16(1):347.
65. Inada T, Shirane A, Hamano N, et al. Effect of subhypnotic doses of dexmedetomidine on antitumor immunity in mice. *Immunopharmacol Immunotoxicol.* 2005;27(3):357–369.
66. Alvaro-Bartolome M, Garcia-Sevilla JA. The neuroplastic index p-FADD/FADD and phosphoprotein PEA-15, interacting at GABAA receptor, are upregulated in brain cortex during midazolam-induced hypnosis in mice. *Eur Neuropsychopharmacol.* 2015;25(11):2131–2144.
67. Dou YL, Lin J, Liu F, et al. Midazolam inhibits the proliferation of human head and neck squamous carcinoma cells by downregulating p300 expression. *Tumour Biol.* 2014;35(8):7499–7504.
68. Dou Y, Li Y, Chen J, et al. Inhibition of cancer cell proliferation by midazolam by targeting transient receptor potential melastatin 7. *Oncol Lett.* 2013;5(3):1010–1016.
69. Mishra SK, Kang J, Lee C, et al. Midazolam induces cellular apoptosis in human cancer cells and inhibits tumor growth in xenograft mice. *Mol Cells.* 2013;36(3):219–226.
70. So EC, Lin Y, Tseng C, et al. Midazolam induces apoptosis in MA-10 mouse Leydig tumor cells through caspase activation and the involvement of MAPK signaling pathway. *Onco Targets Ther.* 2014;7:211–221.
71. Ohno S, Kobayashi K, Uchida S, et al. Cytotoxicity and type of cell death induced by midazolam in human oral normal and tumor cells. *Anticancer Res.* 2012;32(11):4737–4747.
72. Stevens MF, Werdehausen R, Gaza N, et al. Midazolam activates the intrinsic pathway of apoptosis independent of benzodiazepine and death receptor signaling. *Reg Anesth Pain Med.* 2011;36(4):343–349.
73. Wang D-S, Kaneshwaran K, Lei G, et al. Dexmedetomidine prevents excessive γ-aminobutyric acid type A receptor function after anesthesia. *Anesthesiology.* 2018;129(3):477–489.
74. Selvi RB, Swaminathan A, Chatterjee S, et al. Inhibition of p300 lysine acetyltransferase activity by luteolin reduces tumor growth in head and neck squamous cell carcinoma (HNSCC) xenograft mouse model. *Oncotarget.* 2015;6(41):43806–43818.
75. Bedford DC, Kasper L, Fukuyama T, et al. Target gene context influences the transcriptional requirement for the KAT3 family of CBP and p300 histone acetyltransferases. *Epigenetics.* 2010;5(1):9–15.
76. Chen J, Dou Y, Zheng X, et al. TRPM7 channel inhibition mediates midazolam-induced proliferation loss in human malignant glioma. *Tumour Biol.* 2016;37(11):14721–14731.
77. Braun S, Bauer I, Pannen B, et al. Pretreatment but not subsequent coincubation with midazolam reduces the cytotoxicity of temozolomide in neuroblastoma cells. *BMC Anesthesiol.* 2015;15:151.
78. Zgaia AO, Irimie A, Sandesc D, et al. The role of ketamine in the treatment of chronic cancer pain. *Clujul Med.* 2015;88(4):457–461.
79. Pai A, Heining M. Ketamine. *BJA Education.* 2007;7(2):59–63.
80. Malsy M, Gebhardt K, Gruber M, et al. Effects of ketamine, s-ketamine, and MK 801 on proliferation, apoptosis, and necrosis in pancreatic cancer cells. *BMC Anesthesiol.* 2015;15(1):111.
81. Zhou X, Zhang P, Luo W, et al. Ketamine induces apoptosis in lung adenocarcinoma cells by regulating the expression of CD69. *Cancer Med.* 2018;7(3):788–795.
82. Bai X, Yan Y, Canfield S, et al. Ketamine enhances human neural stem cell proliferation and induces neuronal apoptosis via reactive oxygen species-mediated mitochondrial pathway. *Anesth Analg.* 2013;116(4):869–880.
83. Lee ST, Wu T, Yu P, et al. Apoptotic insults to human HepG2 cells induced by S-(+)-ketamine occurs through activation of a Bax-mitochondria-caspase protease pathway. *Br J Anaesth.* 2009;102(1):80–89.

84. He H, Chen J, Xie W, et al. Ketamine used as an acesodyne in human breast cancer therapy causes an undesirable side effect, upregulating anti-apoptosis protein Bcl-2 expression. *Genet Mol Res*. 2013;12(2):1907–1915.
85. Duan W, Hu J, Liu Y. Ketamine inhibits colorectal cancer cells malignant potential via blockage of NMDA receptor. *Exp Mol Pathol*. 2019;107:171–178.
86. Forget P, Collet V, Lavand'homme P, et al. Does analgesia and condition influence immunity after surgery? Effects of fentanyl, ketamine and clonidine on natural killer activity at different ages. *Eur J Anaesthesiol*. 2010;27(3):233–240.
87. Ohta N, Ohashi Y, Fujino Y. Ketamine inhibits maturation of bone marrow-derived dendritic cells and priming of the Th1-type immune response. *Anesth Analg*. 2009;109(3):793–800.
88. Braun S, Gaza N, Werdehausen R, et al. Ketamine induces apoptosis via the mitochondrial pathway in human lymphocytes and neuronal cells. *Br J Anaesth*. 2010;105(3):347–354.
89. Shapiro J, Jersky J, Katzav S, et al. Anesthetic drugs accelerate the progression of postoperative metastases of mouse tumors. *J Clin Invest*. 1981;68(3):678–685.
90. Enlund M, Berglund A, Andreasson K, et al. The choice of anaesthetic—sevoflurane or propofol—and outcome from cancer surgery: a retrospective analysis. *Ups J Med Sci*. 2014;119(3):251–261.
91. Wigmore T, Mohammed K, Jhanji S. Long-term survival for patients undergoing volatile versus IV anesthesia for cancer surgery. A retrospective analysis. *Anesthesiology*. 2016;124(1):69–79.
92. Lee JH, Kang S, Kim Y, et al. Effects of propofol-based total intravenous anesthesia on recurrence and overall survival in patients after modified radical mastectomy: a retrospective study. *Korean J Anesthesiol*. 2016;69(2):126–132.
93. Jun IJ, Jo JY, Kim JI, et al. Impact of anesthetic agents on overall and recurrence-free survival in patients undergoing esophageal cancer surgery: a retrospective observational study. *Sci Rep*. 2017;7(1):14020.
94. Dong J, Zeng M, Ji N, et al. Impact of anesthesia on long-term outcomes in patients with supratentorial high-grade glioma undergoing tumor resection: a retrospective cohort study. *J Neurosurg Anesthesiol*. 2019;32(3):227–233.
95. Zheng X, Wang Y, Dong L, et al. Effects of propofol-based total intravenous anesthesia on gastric cancer: a retrospective study. *Onco Targets Ther*. 2018;11:1141–1148.
96. Wu ZF, Lee MS, Wong CS, et al. Propofol-based total intravenous anesthesia is associated with better survival than desflurane anesthesia in colon cancer surgery. *Anesthesiology*. 2018;129(5):932–941.
97. Xu Q, Shi N, Zhang H, et al. Effects of combined general-epidural anesthesia and total intravenous anesthesia on cellular immunity and prognosis in patients with nonsmall cell lung cancer: a comparative study. *Mol Med Rep*. 2017;16(4):4445–4454.
98. Yan T, Zhang GH, Wang BN, et al. Effects of propofol/remifentanil-based total intravenous anesthesia versus sevoflurane-based inhalational anesthesia on the release of VEGF-C and TGF-beta and prognosis after breast cancer surgery: a prospective, randomized and controlled study. *BMC Anesthesiol*. 2018;18(1):131.
99. Sessler DI, Pei L, Huang Y, et al. Recurrence of breast cancer after regional or general anaesthesia: a randomised controlled trial. *Lancet*. 2019;394(10211):1807–1815.
100. Cata J, Hagan K, Bhavsar S, et al. The use of isoflurane and desflurane as inhalational agents for glioblastoma surgery. A survival analysis. *J Clin Neurosci*. 2017;35:82–87.
101. Kim MH, Kim DW, Kim JH, et al. Does the type of anesthesia really affect the recurrence-free survival after breast cancer surgery? *Oncotarget*. 2017;8(52):90477–90487.
102. Yoo S, Lee HB, Noh DY, et al. Total intravenous anesthesia versus inhalation anesthesia for breast cancer surgery: a retrospective cohort study. *Anesthesiology*. 2019;130(1):31–40.
103. Oh TK, Kim K, Jheon S, et al. Long-term oncologic outcomes for patients undergoing volatile versus intravenous anesthesia for non-small cell lung cancer surgery: a retrospective propensity matching analysis. *Cancer Control*. 2018;25(1):1073274818775360.
104. Oh TK, Kim HH, Jeon YT. Retrospective analysis of 1-year mortality after gastric cancer surgery: total intravenous anesthesia versus volatile anesthesia. *Acta Anaesthesiol Scand*. 2019;63(9):1169–1177.
105. Cata JP, Nguyen L, Ifeanyi-Pillette I, et al. An assessment of the survival impact of multimodal anesthesia/analgesia technique in adults undergoing cytoreductive surgery with hyperthermic intraperitoneal chemotherapy: a propensity score matched analysis. *Int J Hyperthermia*. 2019;36(1):369–375.
106. Yap A, Lopez-Olivo M, Dubowitz J, et al. Anesthetic technique and cancer outcomes: a meta-analysis of total intravenous versus volatile anesthesia. *Can J Anaesth*. 2019;66(5):546–561.
107. Zhang Y, Li HJ, Wang DX, et al. Impact of inhalational versus intravenous anaesthesia on early delirium and long-term survival in elderly patients after cancer surgery: study protocol of a multicentre, open-label, and randomised controlled trial. *BMJ Open*. 2017;7(11):e018607.
108. Forget P, Berliere M, Poncelet A, et al. Effect of clonidine on oncological outcomes after breast and lung cancer surgery. *Br J Anaesth*. 2018;121(1):103–104.
109. Puijk RS, Ziedses des Plantes V, Nieuwenhuizen S, et al. Propofol compared to midazolam sedation and to general anesthesia for percutaneous microwave ablation in patients with hepatic malignancies: a single-center comparative analysis of three historical cohorts. *Cardiovasc Intervent Radiol*. 2019;42(11):1597–1608.
110. Buckley A, McQuaid S, Johnson P, et al. Effect of anaesthetic technique on the natural killer cell anti-tumour activity of serum from women undergoing breast cancer surgery: a pilot study. *Br J Anaesth*. 2014;113(Suppl 1):i56–i62.
111. Liu Z, Zhang J, Hong G, et al. Propofol inhibits growth and invasion of pancreatic cancer cells through regulation of the miR-21/Slug signaling pathway. *Am J Transl Res*. 2016;8(10):4120–4133.
112. Wu KC, Yang ST, Hsu SC, et al. Propofol induces DNA damage in mouse leukemic monocyte macrophage RAW264.7 cells. *Oncol Rep*. 2013;30(5):2304–2310.
113. Mammoto T, Mukai M, Mammoto A, et al. Intravenous anesthetic, propofol inhibits invasion of cancer cells. *Cancer Lett*. 2002;184(2):165–170.
114. Moudgil G, Singal D. Halothane and isoflurane enhance melanoma tumour metastasis in mice. *Can J Anaesth*. 1997;44(1):90–94.
115. Cata JP, Hagan KB, Bhavsar S, et al. The use of isoflurane and desflurane as inhalational agents for glioblastoma surgery. A survival analysis. *J Clin Neurosci*. 2017;35:82–87.

12

Opioids and Cancer

IQIRA SAEED, ADAM LA CAZE, PAUL N. SHAW, AND MARIE-ODILE PARAT

Introduction

Cancer is the second leading cause of death globally, accounting for approximately 9.6 million deaths in 2018.[1] The impact of cancer morbidity is significant and continues to rise, with an annual cost of approximately US$1.16 trillion in 2010.[2] There has been significant research in cancer therapeutics and identification of the causes of cancer. Despite the availability of more than 500 drugs[3] to treat various cancers, surgery continues to remain an important part of cancer therapy.

The risk of recurrence after solid tumor removal is a well-established phenomenon. A number of factors have been identified to influence the risk of cancer progression in the perioperative period, including (1) the potential release of tumor cells into the systemic circulation; (2) the influence of the surgical process on cancer cell proliferation, invasiveness, adhesion, apoptosis, and angiogenesis; (3) the invasiveness of the surgical technique (laparotomy vs. laparoscopy); (4) the choice of anesthetic and perioperative analgesia; and (5) the extent of the surgical stress and resulting pain.[4]

It is known that pain-induced immunosuppression plays a key role in promoting tumor recurrence.[5] Painful stimuli such as surgery induce a neuroendocrine response and centrally activate the hypothalamic pituitary adrenal (HPA) axis, which stimulates the release of immunosuppressive glucocorticosteroids, thereby decreasing anticancer immunity.[6] Consequently, the administration of adequate pain relief in the perioperative period is essential for more than one reason.

Opioids are widely used for the management of both malignant and surgical pain. However, there is growing evidence to suggest that opioids may alter the course of cancer, especially when administered in the perioperative period. Opioids have been shown to modulate the tumor microenvironment via direct effects on tumor cell growth and apoptosis, and an indirect effect on immunity, inflammation, and angiogenesis. While evidence on the overall *direction* of the effects of opioids on cancer outcomes is still unclear, the focus of current research has shifted toward the use of opioid-sparing techniques such as regional analgesia/anesthesia (RAA), nonsteroid antiinflammatory drugs (NSAIDs), local anesthetics (LA), and propofol, and elucidating whether this influences perioperative outcomes.

In this chapter the link between opioids and cancer is reviewed, including the mechanisms by which opioids influence the tumor microenvironment, the influence of opioid-sparing techniques on cancer outcomes, the effect of opioids in clinically diverse patient groups, and the complexities of assessing opioid use and cancer risk at the cellular, animal, and human levels. While certain topics within this chapter have been extensively reviewed, we will focus on the most current literature.

Mechanisms

Tumor Proliferation and Apoptosis

The ability of opioids to modulate tumor growth in both perioperative and nonsurgical settings has been of great interest to scientists and clinicians. The mechanisms underlying the role of opioids in regulating tumor cell growth are complex. In practice, cancer patients often receive high opioid doses; therefore the relationship between opioid dose and tumor proliferation has significant clinical ramifications. The literature reports a range of plasma concentrations of opioids commonly consumed for cancer pain in the surgical setting (Table 12.1).

Opioids exert their effects on both malignant and nonmalignant cells, with the ability to influence proliferation and apoptotic pathways, thereby modulating tumor growth.[15] The effects of morphine on tumor growth in vitro and in vivo have been extensively reviewed,[15–17] and these reviews highlight that the results are inconsistent. These discrepancies can be partially explained by the differences in cell types and the concentrations of opioids used.

It is known that opioids have both pro-[18,19] and antiproliferative[20,21] effects on tumor cells. In vitro studies testing the effect of various opioids on cancer cell survival and/or proliferation have been reviewed previously.[22] It has been proposed that at higher opioid concentrations, tumor cell growth is inhibited, whereas at lower concentrations the inverse is true.[23] The literature further suggests the potential involvement of various opioid receptors in tumor cell

TABLE 12.1 Examples of Opioid Concentrations in the Circulation of Cancer Patients

Opioid	Plasma Concentration Range (μM)
Morphine[7,8]	0.035–0.9
Oxycodone[7,9]	0.06–0.9
Fentanyl[10]	2.97×10^{-4}–0.03
Methadone[11]	0.1–0.37
Tramadol[12]	0.05–6
Remifentanil[13,14]	5×10^{-3}–1.3×10^{-2}

growth (Table 12.2). It has been reported that stimulation of the κ-opioid receptor induces apoptosis of CNE2 human epithelial cancer cells via a phospholipase C-mediated pathway.[24] Over the years, several studies have shown the presence of μ-opioid receptors (MORs) in various cancer types and have investigated their roles in promoting cell proliferation, adhesion, migration, and tumorigenesis.[25–28] A recent study found that MOR expression is positively associated with hepatocarcinoma (HCC) progression, and MOR silencing decreased HCC tumorigenesis in vitro and in vivo, significantly extending the survival of tumor-bearing mice.[29] A triple-negative breast cancer mouse model treated with morphine and naloxone showed that over 30 days, naloxone was able to prevent the morphine-induced increase in tumor volume.[30]

It has been proposed that instead of MOR involvement, opioid growth factor receptors (OGFR) may be involved in control of tumor proliferation. Research has shown that exogenous morphine reduced the growth of H1975 human adenocarcinoma cells that overexpressed OGFR but not MOR.[37] This antiproliferative effect of morphine was attenuated upon OGFR knockdown, suggesting a potential underlying morphine-OGFR binding mechanism.[37] Current research in the field has found that methionine enkephalin upregulated OGFR expression and significantly inhibited the growth of human gastric cancer cell lines (SG7901 and HGC27).[38] This induced G0/G1 cell cycle arrest and caspase-dependent apoptosis, suggesting the application of methionine enkephalin as a potential anticancer drug for the treatment of gastric cancers.[38]

Tumor Cell Invasion, Migration, and Metastasis

The spread of a tumor from its primary site to a distant organ accounts for approximately 90% of all cancer-related deaths.[39] During the metastatic process, disruptions in the cell matrix and cell-cell adhesion are of upmost importance.[40] Epithelial-mesenchymal transition (EMT) is a key step in converting cancer cells into a migratory population that is capable of systemic metastasis.[40] A number of factors are involved in cancer cell metastasis, including invasion/extravasation through the basement membrane and extracellular matrix via the secretion of urokinase-type plasminogen activator (uPA), matrix metalloproteinase (MMP) production, and increased vascular basement membrane permeability.

Various studies have shown that morphine can both increase[25,26] and decrease[41,42] the invasion of cancer cells through the vascular basement membrane. Morphine also increases vascular permeability (i.e., decreases endothelial barrier function).[43–45] A more recent study has found that morphine promoted, whereas naloxone and nalmefene (MOR antagonists) suppressed migration and invasion in various hepatocellular carcinoma cell lines and in mouse models.[28] Morphine has also been reported to increase[46,47] or decrease[48] uPA secretion by cancer cells.

Earlier studies showed that morphine inhibits adhesion and migration of colon 26-L5 carcinoma cells to the extracellular matrix and invasion into basement membrane matrigel, inhibiting the production of both MMP-2 and MMP-9.[49] Naloxone did not attenuate the inhibitory effects of morphine on MMP production from tumor cells, suggesting that morphine may inhibit cell adhesion and enzymatic degradation of the extracellular matrix via nonopioid receptor mechanisms.[49]

Several mechanisms have been proposed to explain the inhibitory effects of morphine on MMP production. The

TABLE 12.2 Receptor Types Currently Proposed to Be Involved in Modulation of Tumor Cell Proliferation

Receptors	Type	Ligands (Endogenous or Synthetic)	Cells
Classical opioid receptors (GPCR)[28,31,32]	Mu, kappa, delta	Enkephalin Endomorphins β-endorphin Alkaloids Semisynthetic and synthetic opioid agonists and antagonists	Immune and cancer cells
Nonclassical opioid receptors (GPCR)[33–36]	Nociceptin orphanin FQ peptide receptor (ORL-1, NOP)	Nociceptin/orphanin FQ (N/OFQ)	Lymphocytes, monocytes, PBMC, astrocytes, T cells, B cells, and cancer cells

involvement of a MOR-independent, nitric oxide synthase-dependent mechanism has been suggested[50]; morphine has been shown to decrease both endothelial oxide synthase (NOS) mRNA and nitric oxide secretion in MCF-7 cells.[51] In a coculture of breast cancer cells and macrophages or endothelial cells, morphine reduced the levels of MMP-9, while increasing the levels of its endogenous inhibitor, TIMP-1; this was not observed in cells grown individually.[48] It has been suggested that morphine may exert its antitumor effects via modulation of paracrine communication between cancer and nonmalignant cells.[48] Morphine prevented the increase in IL-4-induced MMP-9 by inhibiting the conversion of macrophages to an M2 phenotype via an opioid receptor-mediated mechanism.[42] A more recent study found that when compared with serum from saline-treated controls, serum from morphine-treated mice (10 mg/kg for 3 days) reduced the chemotaxis of breast cancer and endothelial cells and reduced cancer cell invasion.[52] This was also associated with a decrease in MMP-9 and an increase in TIMP-1 and TIMP3/4 levels. Inhibition of MMP-9 abolished the reduction in chemotactic attraction, indicating that MMP9 reduction in the serum of morphine-treated mice may mediate the decrease in chemoattraction.[52]

The effect of opioids on migration can further be seen in noncancer models where remifentanil was shown to increase the migration of C2C12 cells (mouse pluripotent mesenchymal cell line), significantly increasing osteoblast differentiation.[53] It has previously been shown that morphine can induce microglial migration via an interaction between the MOR and ionotropic P2 × 4 purinergic receptors, dependent on PI3K/Akt pathway activation.[54] This occurred in vitro at a low (100 nM) concentration of morphine and is proposed to have implications in morphine-induced side effects such as tolerance or hyperalgesia.[54]

Immunosuppression

The immune system plays a vital role in the defense against cancer. However, exogenous opioids have been reported to influence key aspects of the immune system, including lymphocyte proliferation, natural killer cell and phagocytic activity, expression of important cytokines, and antibody production.[4] The inhibitory effect of opioids on the immune system has attracted great interest from researchers and clinicians especially because of its potential consequences for postsurgical outcomes. The surgical process is often accompanied by pain and surgical stress, known triggers for the release of mast cells, neutrophils, macrophages, eosinophils, monocytes, and most importantly, natural killer cells. Opioids have been identified to influence this cascade via two main mechanisms: (1) peripheral and (2) central.[6] Opioids can directly act on immune cells (e.g., B and T lymphocytes) through the MOR, which can inhibit NK cell migration, or indirectly via nonopioid receptors such as Toll-like receptor 4.[6] Centrally, acute morphine administration activates periaqueductal gray (PAG), which in turn activates the CNS to induce lymphoid organs, i.e., the spleen, to trigger the release of biological amines, suppressing NK cell activity and lymphocyte proliferation in the spleen.[6] Following surgery, some patients take opioids long-term, which stimulates the HPA axis to produce glucocorticoids, thereby decreasing NK cell activity.[6]

Opioids can act directly on immune cells and have been reported to exert a number of effects on macrophages. Morphine reduces the proliferation of macrophage progenitor cells, their recruitment, Fc gamma receptor (Fcg R)-mediated phagocytosis, and the release of nitric oxide.[17] Recent literature suggests that morphine may exert its antitumor effect in the tumor microenvironment by modulating the paracrine communication between nonmalignant and cancer cells[48] and modulates tumor aggressiveness by influencing M2 polarization and the production of macrophage proteases within the tumor environment.[42] Results from the same laboratory have further shown that morphine can prevent proangiogenic interactions between macrophages and breast cancer cells in the tumor microenvironment.[55]

To place these mechanisms in the context of cancer surgery, it is important to acknowledge that: (1) in the context of pain, which itself is immunosuppressive, opioids are protective due to the analgesia they provide, (2) in response to surgical stress the body itself can trigger the release of endogenous opioids, and (3) the level of immunosuppression may vary greatly between opioids (Table 12.3).

Remifentanil, an opioid analgesic used intraoperatively, has been shown to significantly reduce neutrophil migration and cell adhesion molecule expression in vitro when compared to fentanyl.[62] Remifentanil inhibited lipopolysaccharide (LPS)-induced activation of human neutrophils and decreased the expression of various proinflammatory factors. No effect, however, was seen with the structurally related opioids, including sufentanil, alfentanil, fentanyl, delta, or kappa receptor antagonists.[63] A more recent study conducted in 40 gynecological laparotomy patients found that at 2 h postincision when compared with oxycodone or nonopioid analgesia, morphine significantly downregulated

TABLE 12.3 Opioids and their Proposed Level of Immune Modulation

Level of Proposed Immune Modulation in the Current Literature	Opioids
Highly immunosuppressive	Morphine[56] Fentanyl[57] Remifentanil[58] Methadone[59] Diamorphine (heroin)
Weakly immunosuppressive	Codeine[56,57]
Nonimmunosuppressive	Buprenorphine[56] Oxycodone[57] Hydromorphone[59]
Immunoprotective	Tramadol[59,60,61]

the expression of various genes in CD4+, CD8+, and NK cells; increased IL-6 concentration; and suppressed NK cell activity.[64] A number of studies have found that following incubation of blood from gastric or blood cancer patients with opioids ex vivo, fentanyl increased the number of regulatory T cells.[65,66]

In contrast, the administration of tramadol (20 and 40 mg/kg) before and after laparotomy prevented surgery-induced NK cell suppression in rat models.[61] Oxycodone has been shown to increase the generation of reactive oxygen intermediates and nitric oxide by macrophages in mice, while also increasing the release of IL-6, TNF-α, and TNF-β.[67] In this study oxycodone did not influence the humoral immune response, whereas morphine suppressed and buprenorphine enhanced B-cell activation.[67] Buprenorphine has been shown to reduce corticosterone levels, with no effect on immune parameters such as CD4+ and CD8+[68] or NK cell activity.[69] In the context of surgery-induced immunosuppression, it was found that when compared to fentanyl or morphine, buprenorphine ameliorated the effects of surgery on the HPA axis, NK cell activity, and metastatic colonization in rats.[70]

Opioids are commonly administered in the perioperative period; hence their immunosuppressive profile and ability to influence cancer outcomes are of clinical importance. While opioids such as morphine, remifentanil, fentanyl, and methadone are proposed to be highly immunosuppressive, the literature suggests nonimmunosuppressive and immunoprotective roles for buprenorphine and tramadol, respectively.

Inflammation

The inflammatory response plays a key role in various stages of tumor development, including initiation, tumor growth, invasion, and metastasis.[71] Opioids have been shown to modulate the inflammatory response via regulating the expression of key inflammatory cytokines and their receptors[72] and mediating the release of endogenous opioids (i.e., β-endorphin) from immune cells at the site of inflammation.[73] Morphine significantly enhanced the release of neuropeptide substance P (SP) from mast cells in a transgenic sickle mouse model.[74] Similarly, morphine was shown to promote mast cell activation and degranulation in a murine breast cancer model[75] while also increasing the expression of inflammatory cytokines and neuropeptide SP release.[76] A more recent study showed that morphine increased CD11b+ cells and microglia at the site of injury in vivo, exacerbating the inflammatory response; pretreatment with minocycline (an antibiotic with antiinflammatory properties), however, reduced this effect, aiding functional recovery.[77]

In contrast, several studies have suggested an inhibitory effect of opioids on the production of key inflammatory markers. Morphine decreases inflammation-induced angiogenesis and inhibits the early recruitment of phagocytes to an inflammatory signal, with a significant reduction in monocyte chemoattractant protein-1 (MCP-1).[78] Morphine also attenuated peripheral inflammation in a rat model of chronic antigen-induced arthritis (AIA).[79] Interestingly, opposing roles of opioid receptors have been reported, whereby the activation of the kappa (κ) opioid receptor (KOR) induces an antiinflammatory response, while MOR activation favors a proinflammatory response.[42,72]

Angiogenesis

The formation of new blood vessels plays an integral role in tumor development and progression. Angiogenesis is required for primary tumors or metastases to grow beyond a critical size. Localized tumor growth is often characterized by hypoxia, which upregulates the expression of hypoxia inducible factor (HIF) and stimulates the secretion of vascular endothelial growth factor (VEGF), a key player in the formation of new blood vessels that promotes tumor growth. The current literature suggests that morphine can have both stimulatory[19,80–82] and inhibitory[83,85] effects on angiogenesis.

At clinically relevant (analgesic) concentrations, morphine significantly reduced angiogenesis and tumor growth in a Lewis lung carcinoma mouse model.[83] This inhibitory effect was mediated through a hypoxia-induced p38 MAPK pathway.[83] A simple chorioallantoic membrane model, evaluating the effects of codeine, morphine, and tramadol on angiogenesis at three different concentrations, concluded that morphine had an antiangiogenic effect at 1 and 10 μM, whereas tramadol and codeine only inhibited angiogenesis at high concentrations.[84] In the context of opioids and angiogenesis, morphine significantly inhibited hypoxia-induced VEGF expression in rat cardiac myocytes, and coculture induced VEGF production by macrophages and cancer cells, which was significantly reversed by naloxone, suggesting potential opioid receptor involvement.[55,85]

In contrast, morphine increased tumor neovascularization in MCF-7 human breast cancer *cells* in vivo, induced the in vitro proliferation of human endothelial cells, and stimulated angiogenesis.[80] The results of this study must be clinically translated with care, since mice and humans metabolize morphine differently, and hence mg/kg dosing in humans cannot necessarily be applied to a mouse model. Chronic morphine treatment not only stimulated angiogenesis but also increased prostaglandin E2 (PGE2) and cyclooxygenase (COX)-2 in a breast cancer mouse model, but this was successfully prevented by coadministration of celecoxib (a selective COX-2 inhibitor).[81] A more recent study showed that δ-opioid receptor stimulation in breast cancer cells may lead to COX-2 expression and the PI3K/Akt-dependent activation of HIF-1α, which stimulates endothelial cell sprouting via paracrine activation of PGE2 receptors.[86] While discrepancies exist in the literature, it is apparent that opioids may influence the angiogenic process in the perioperative period.

Opioids Versus Opioid-Sparing Analgesia/Anesthesia for Cancer Surgery

Surgical excision of primary tumors is an essential component of cancer therapy; however, the surgical process itself can trigger the metastatic process. The presence of circulating tumor cells following cancer surgery has been shown to be independently associated with an elevated risk of tumor recurrence and reduced disease-free survival in various cancer types.[87–89] Most importantly, the current literature suggests that there are three perioperative-associated factors that impair cellular immunity: (1) surgical stress and tissue injury as a result of tumor resection, which may influence the risk of tumor metastasis through the release of angiogenic factors and suppression of NK cells[90]; (2) general anesthesia (GA), which has been shown to impair various immune functions; and (3) opioid analgesia, which has been shown to impair both cellular and humoral immunity in humans.[91]

In the context of surgery, the focus of current research has shifted toward the use of opioid-sparing techniques such as RAA, NSAIDs, LA, and propofol, and elucidating whether this influences perioperative outcomes. Current prospective clinical studies predominantly compare regimens where opioids are present to different extents but are primarily not designed to study the effects of opioids on cancer outcomes. A number of publications have reviewed the influence of opioid-sparing techniques on oncological outcomes in which opioids are part of both interventions,[15,92,93] but there are only few ex vivo, in vivo, and clinical studies (in which opioids are only part of one regimen) (Table 12.4) that have compared the influence of opioid-sparing techniques versus opioid analgesia on cancer outcomes.

Regional Anesthesia and Analgesia

Regional anesthesia and analgesia attenuate the immunosuppressive and potentially tumor-promoting effects of both opioids and GA by preventing the neuroendocrine stress response that results from surgical excision.[106] The combination of RAA and GA decreases the amount of GA utilized during surgery as well as the need for subsequent postoperative opioid analgesia, obviating subsequent immune-related effects while providing adequate pain relief.[107] Studies have shown that epidural anesthesia (EA) attenuates the stress response but not the inflammatory response.[108,109]

Several retrospective studies comparing the effect of PVA/EA + GA with GA + opioid analgesia have shown a reduced risk of cancer recurrence[110] or increased overall survival (OS)[111] following cancer surgery. However, it was unclear whether this beneficial effect was due to the reduced perioperative opioid requirements. While it is known that in the context of pain RAA is protective, the results from systematic reviews and meta-analyses in assessing the influence of perioperative RAA versus GA + opioid analgesia on cancer outcomes have reported a benefit on OS but not recurrence-free survival (RFS).[112,113] A recent article by the American Society of Regional Anesthesia and Pain Medicine (ASRA) and the European Society of Regional Anesthesia and Pain Therapy (ESRA) concluded that there is currently weak evidence to suggest that the use of regional anesthesia and analgesia may reduce metastasis or cancer recurrence.[114] Findings from a Cochrane review further concluded that there is currently inadequate evidence supporting the benefits of regional anesthesia techniques on tumor recurrence.[115] Results from a recently completed large randomized controlled trial comparing the use of opioids (morphine) + GA versus propofol + thoracic epidural or PVA/A for breast cancer surgery found no difference between the groups in terms of cancer-specific survival or overall quality of life despite the RAA group receiving half the amount of opioids compared with the GA group.[116] This study was the first prospective randomized multicenter trial specifically designed to assess whether anesthesia and analgesia techniques could affect the long-term outcome of breast cancer surgery.[107] It is important to acknowledge that in this study RAA was not compared to opioids alone; therefore, the study was not designed to determine the role of opioids.

NSAIDs

Inflammation plays a key role in tumor development. An in vivo study found that prostaglandin (PGE2) promotes the formation of liver metastases in mice via various mechanisms.[117] The influence of NSAIDs on cancer has been proposed to be through the decreased synthesis of PGE2 as a result of COX inhibition. In a murine breast cancer model the COX-2 inhibitor celecoxib has been shown to prevent morphine-induced stimulation of tumor cell growth, angiogenesis, metastasis, PGE2, and COX-2.[81] Several studies have reported that the combination of NSAIDs and opioids better preserves immune function[36] in vitro and increases survival[81] in vivo when compared with opioids alone. In the clinical setting a number of studies have associated NSAID use with improved RFS postcancer surgery.[118,119]

Local Anesthetics

Intravenous LA such as lidocaine, bupivacaine, and ropivacaine are commonly used as part of multimodal analgesia and are known to possess antiinflammatory properties.[120] LA have been reported to exert a number of antitumor effects on various cancer cells in vitro such as the inhibition of epidermal growth factor receptor (EGFR) and EGF-induced proliferation of human tongue cancer cells,[121] reduced metastatic progression,[122] and demethylation of DNA in breast cancer cells[123] while also reducing tumor cell proliferation, viability, and migration of prostate, ovarian,[124] and breast cancer cells.[125] Intraperitoneally injected lidocaine was further shown to suppress human hepatocellular carcinoma HepG2 xenograft tumor growth in vivo.[124] Results from an ASRA/ESRA special article reported that there is strong evidence, arising from in vitro data, suggesting a protective effect of LA on cancer recurrence; however, there is a lack of preclinical and clinical studies to suggest a beneficial role in cancer surgery. In the context of pain, LA are likely to

TABLE 12.4 Specific Studies Comparing the Effects of Opioid Sparing Techniques Versus Opioid + GA in Which the Use of Opioids Is Restricted to One Group, on Oncological Outcomes

Study Type	Surgical Procedure	Intervention	Influence on Cancer
Ex vivo	Mastectomy (breast cancer)	PVA + GA (n = 15) Opioids + GA (n = 15)	Lower stress response to surgery from PVA, but no effect on PGE_2 or VEGF levels.[94]
Retrospective	Radical prostatectomy	EA + GA (n = 102) Opioids + GA (n = 123)	Reduced risk of BCR with EA.[95]
Retrospective	Resection of colon cancer	EA + GA (n = 85) IV opioids + GA (n = 92)	Improved survival with EA in the first 1.46 years prior to metastases. No effect on postmetastasis.[96]
Secondary analysis of subjects undergoing radical prostatectomy	Radical prostatectomy	EA + GA (n = 49) IV morphine + GA (n = 50)	No difference in disease-free survival observed at 4.5 years postsurgery.[97]
Retrospective	Radical prostatectomy	EA + GA (n = 105) IV opioids/NSAID + GA (n = 158)	Improved RFS with EA; however, no difference in OS, CSS, or BCR.[98]
Prospective RCT	Major abdominal surgery	EA + GA (n = 230) IV opioids + GA (n = 216)	No difference in cancer recurrence, RFS, or mortality.[99]
Retrospective	Open radical prostatectomy	EA + GA (n = 67) IV opioids/NSAID + GA (n = 81)	No difference in OS, RFS, or BCR.[100]
In vitro (derived from randomized prospective study)	Primary breast cancer surgery	PVA + propofol (n = 5) opioids + sevoflurane GA (n = 5)	Elevated serum NK cell cytotoxicity in vitro with PVA.[101]
In vitro	Breast cancer surgery	PVA/propofol (n = 11) Opioids + sevoflurane GA (n = 11)	Greater inhibition of proliferation in breast cancer cells with PVA/propofol but no effect on migration.[102]
In vitro	Breast cancer surgery	PVA/propofol (n = 15) Opioids + GA (n = 17)	PVA/propofol altered cytokines, influencing perioperative cancer immunity.[103]
In vitro	Breast cancer surgery	PVA/propofol (n = 20) Morphine + GA (n = 20)	GA enhanced serum VEGF C levels and reduced serum concentration of TGF-β in breast cancer patients.[104]
In vivo	Invasive SCK breast cancer model	Equal groups: Normal saline + methylcellulose SC morphine + methylcellulose Celecoxib + methylcellulose Morphine + celecoxib (via gavage)	Coadministration of morphine + celecoxib increased survival when compared with morphine alone, significantly influences key component of the tumor microenvironment.[81]
In vitro	Pancreatic and colon cancer	Ropivacaine or bupivacaine or sufentanil alone Ropivacaine + sufentanil	Antiproliferative effects only visible at high concentrations; however, no influence on cell cycle or apoptosis.[105]

BCR, Biochemical recurrence; *CSS*, cancer-specific survival; *EA*, epidural analgesia; *GA*, general anesthesia; *IV*, intravenous; *NSAID*, nonsteroidal antiinflammatory; *OS*,overall survival; *PGE2*, prostaglandin E2; *PVA*, paravertebral anesthesia; *RCT*, randomised controlled trial; *RFS*, recurrence-free survival; *SC*, subcutaneous; *TGF*, transforming growth factor; *VEGF*, vascular endothelial growth factor.

be protective; this requires validation by prospective clinical studies designed to compare the long-term oncological effects of opioids and LA on cancer surgery.

Propofol

Propofol, an intravenous anesthetic, is commonly used during cancer surgery and has been shown to affect malignant cancer cells via multiple mechanisms.[126–128] A number of studies suggest that propofol exerts a stimulatory[101,129] effect on immune parameters and possesses antiinflammatory properties in vitro.[130] In an ex vivo study, when compared with opioids + GA, PVA + propofol administered to breast cancer surgery patients altered the circulating cytokine profile, which may indicate an influence on perioperative cancer immunity.[103] Several retrospective clinical studies have shown improved OS[41,131] with propofol-based anesthesia following colon and gastric cancer surgery, while reduced cancer recurrence[132,133] has been shown following breast and esophageal cancer surgery in other retrospective clinical studies. The long-term oncological effects of propofol have not been well established.

Clinical Trials Involving Opioids Versus Alternative Technique

As of 2019, there is one ongoing prospective randomized controlled trial (RCT) (listed at clinicaltrials.gov) studying the influence of an opioid-sparing technique versus opioid + GA on cancer recurrence and survival (Table 12.5).

Based on the evidence mentioned earlier, it is apparent that there is still no consensus on whether opioid-sparing techniques positively influence cancer outcomes in humans in the context of surgery. The issue is the lack of prospective trials primarily designed to determine the effect of opioids on long-term cancer outcomes. Opioid-sparing techniques all have protective effects independent of their opioid sparing, and there has never been a group that entirely lacks opioids as part of their analgesic regime. However, due to ethical concerns, it is difficult to deprive humans of opioids, which are widely used for perioperative pain control during and after cancer surgery.

Effect of Opioids in Clinically Diverse Patient Groups

Opioid Use in Noncancer Patients

Chronic opioid abuse and dependence has been significantly associated with morbidity and mortality, including cancer-related outcomes; however, this is most likely attributed to factors other than direct opioid effects.

A retrospective cohort study conducted by Australian researchers showed that opioid use was associated with a particular risk of mortality from certain site-specific cancers.[134] The standard mor tality ratio (SMR) was significantly elevated in the liver (6.9; 95% confidence interval [CI], 4.3–10.5), lung (3.6; 95% CI, 2.8–4.6), and anogenital cancers (2.8, 95% CI, 1.3–5.3), while it was significantly reduced for breast cancer (0.4; 95% CI, 0.1–0.9).[134] In this study, however, the likely cause of this altered risk of cancer is thought to be associated with the indirect effects of opioids or confounders, rather than opioid use itself. Overall, opioid-dependent individuals were reported to be at a 1.7 times higher risk of death from cancer than the general Australian population (SMR 95% CI, 1.4–1.9).[134] The authors of this study proposed that elevated cancer mortality may reflect a higher cancer incidence among opioid users.[134] A similar retrospective longitudinal follow up study showed no difference in the rates of cancer among methadone, buprenorphine, and implant naltrexone groups.[135] Opioid users had a lower survival rate (hazard ratio [HR], 2.68; CI, 1.03–6.97; $P = 0.04$) when compared with nonopioid using controls.[135] Mortality rates were significantly higher among methadone patients, but naltrexone and buprenorphine did not significantly differ from the controls.[135] While this study also found an increased rate of respiratory and female genital cancers, it was concluded that the lower survival rate among opioid-dependent patients may be due to a higher rate of cancer-related mortality in this cohort.[135]

In a cohort of opioid-dependent individuals, it was found that the standard incidence ratio (SIR) for various cancer types did not differ from the general population.[136] Similarly, an elevated risk for liver (6.8; 95% CI, 1.76–11.83), larynx (3.62; 95% CI, 1.11–6.13), lung (1.97; 95%

TABLE 12.5 Ongoing Prospective Clinical Trial Investigating the Influence of an Opioid-Sparing Technique Versus Opioids + GA on Cancer Recurrence and Survival

Trial ID	Title	Design and Intervention	Primary Outcome
NCT02840227	The Effect of Combined General/Regional Anesthesia on Cancer Recurrence in Patients Having Lung Cancer Resections	RCT (n = 2000) GA + EA vs. GA + postoperative patient controlled opioid analgesia	Disease-free survival (cancer)

GA, in which the use of opioids is restricted to one group, on oncological outcomes.

EA, Epidural analgesia/anesthesia; *GA*, general anesthesia; *PVA/A*, paravertebral anesthesia/analgesia; *RCT*, randomzed controlled trial.

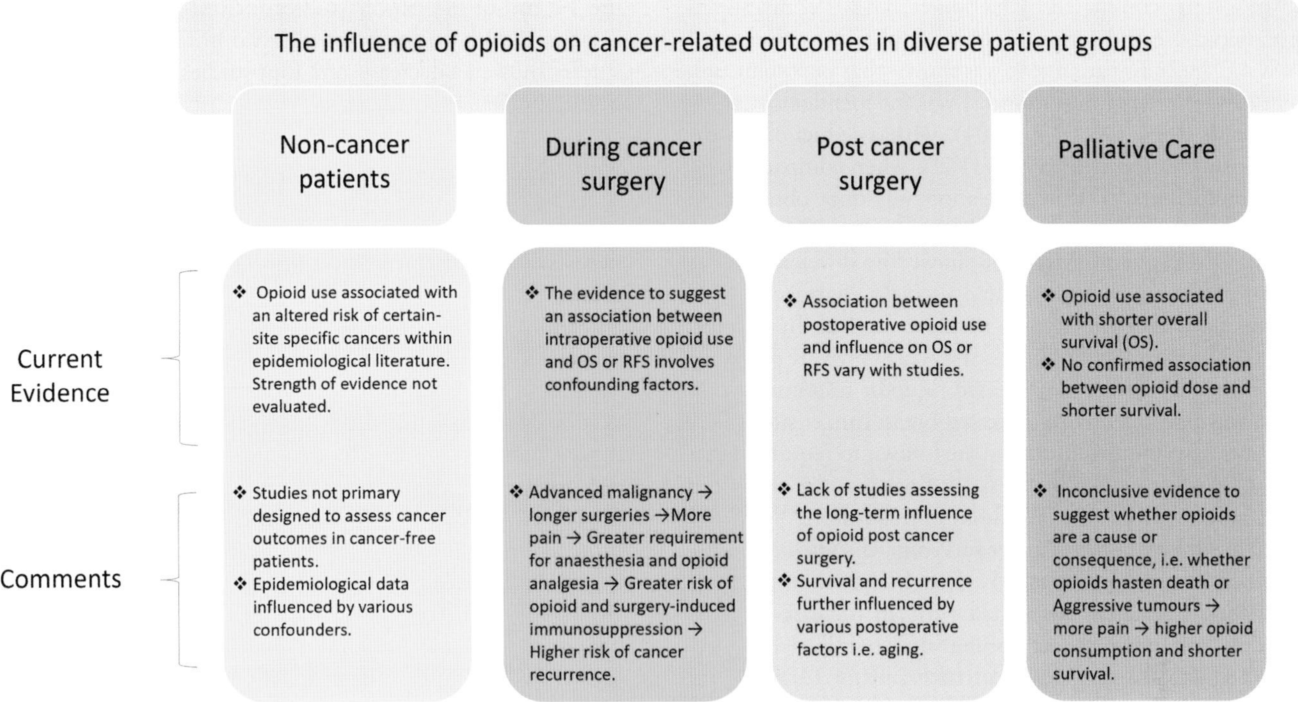

The influence of opioids on cancer-related outcomes in diverse patient groups
Non-cancer patients
During cancer surgery
Post cancer surgery
Palliative Care
Current Evidence
❖ Opioid use associated with an altered risk of certain-site specific cancers within epidemiological literature. Strength of evidence not evaluated.
❖ The evidence to suggest an association between intraoperative opioid use and OS or RFS involves confounding factors.
❖ Association between postoperative opioid use and influence on OS or RFS vary with studies.
❖ Opioid use associated with shorter overall survival (OS).
❖ No confirmed association between opioid dose and shorter survival.
Comments
❖ Studies not primary designed to assess cancer outcomes in cancer-free patients.
❖ Epidemiological data influenced by various confounders.
❖ Advanced malignancy → longer surgeries →More pain → Greater requirement for anaesthesia and opioid analgesia → Greater risk of opioid and surgery-induced immunosuppression → Higher risk of cancer recurrence.
❖ Lack of studies assessing the long-term influence of opioid post cancer surgery.
❖ Survival and recurrence further influenced by various postoperative factors i.e. aging.
❖ Inconclusive evidence to suggest whether opioids are a cause or consequence, i.e. whether opioids hasten death or Aggressive tumours → more pain → higher opioid consumption and shorter survival.

• **Fig. 12.1** The influence of opioids on cancer-related outcomes in diverse patient groups.

CI, 1.13–2.82), and uterine cervical cancer (2.41; 95% CI, 0.99–3.84) was found, while finding a reduction in the incidence of breast cancer (0.36; 95% CI, 0.00–0.71).[134–136] It was concluded that this elevated cancer mortality may indicate that opioid-dependent patients may be more likely to be diagnosed with tumor types that have a lower rate of survival (e.g., lung cancer) or late-stage tumors.[136]

The current literature on the influence of opioids on noncancer patients suggests an altered risk of cancer for certain site-specific cancers; however, most studies are not powered to assess cancer risk as a primary endpoint and may be influenced by the presence of additional confounding variables (Fig. 12.1).

Opioid Use During Cancer Surgery

A study investigating intraoperative opioid use and survival following oral cancer surgery in 268 patients showed that patients who received a median fentanyl dose of 1081.63 μg had a 77% and 27% reduction in OS and RFS, respectively.[137] It was apparent in the study design that 86% of the cohort had advanced malignancy (ASA physical status III or IV), and patients with more severe cancer were given higher doses of opioids when compared to early stage cancer (1.5 vs. 0.8 mg).[137] Hence the reduction observed in OS may be due to the underlying differences in the cohorts.

A recent retrospective study that investigated intraoperative fentanyl use, and its impact on survival or recurrence following curative colorectal tumor resection in 1679 patients with stage I–III colorectal cancer, showed no dose-dependent association between the amount of fentanyl and RFS or OS.[138] Findings from a recent systematic review assessing perioperative opioid use and colorectal cancer recurrence showed that 7/13 included studies assessed OS as a primary endpoint, of which 4/7 studies reported a decrease in OS, whereas the results from 3/7 studies were not statistically significant.[139] The review found no conclusive evidence to terminate the perioperative use of opioids in colorectal cancer patients.[139]

Findings from a retrospective analysis indicated a significant association between intraoperative fentanyl doses of >710 μg and longer OS and RFS in patients with esophageal squamous cell carcinoma; no association was found in adenocarcinoma patients.[140] Another retrospective study comprising 901 patients who underwent surgery for non–small cell lung cancer (NSCLC) found that intraoperative opioid use (median fentanyl dose of 10.15 μg/kg) was only associated with a reduced OS and RFS in stage I NSCLC patients and not stages II and III.[141] Overall, the current literature indicates that the association between intraoperative opioid use and altered OS or RFS is influenced by various factors including surgical duration, the use of additional anesthetic or analgesic agents, and surgery-induced stress and immunosuppression.

Opioid Use Following Cancer Surgery

Studies investigating the effects of postoperative opioid use on patient survival and cancer recurrence have shown no effect of opioids on OS or RFS, a modest effect on OS but no effect on RFS or rarely, an effect on both overall and RFS in cancer patients.

In a study conducted by Nelson et al. (2019) investigating opioid use and survival following lobectomy for stage I NSCLC in 2884 patients, it was shown that persistent opioid use (for at least 3–6 months) was independently associated with worse OS ($P < 0.001$), with a reduction in the 5-year survival postsurgery by 11.2% when compared with nonopioid users.[142] This association was only observed in patients taking high oral morphine equivalent (OME) doses (≥300 OME) as an OME ≤300 showed no difference in OS when compared with nonopioid users.[142] Pharmacogenetic factors have also been shown to affect survival. In a cohort of 2039 breast cancer patients, the A118G MOR polymorphism, which results in decreased receptor response to opioids, was associated with increased breast cancer survival.[143] Patients carrying this mutation are known to require higher opioid doses to reach analgesia[144]; however, the study did not analyze opioid administration in this cohort.[143]

In a cohort of breast cancer survivors, chronic opioid use (defined as opioid use for 75+ days in a 90-day window) was not significantly associated with an increased risk of a secondary breast cancer event (SBCE) (HR, 1.20; 95% CI, 0.85–1.70) or cancer recurrence (HR, 1.14; 95% CI, 0.76–2.70) when compared with nonchronic users.[17] In a similar retrospective cohort study, assessing opioid use for 8 days postoperatively and postoperative complications in 121 esophageal cancer surgery patients, there was no significant association between opioid use and OS ($P = 0.520$) and RFS ($P = 0.818$).[145] A prospective cohort study comprising 34,188 primary breast cancer patients found no association between opioid use and breast cancer recurrence (crude HR, 0.98; 95% CI, 0.90–1.1) irrespective of cumulative dose, type of opioid consumed, strength, or chronicity of use (>6 months).[146]

A similar study comprising 99 patients with stage I or II NSCLC who underwent video-assisted thoracoscopic surgery with lobectomy showed that 26% of the patients had recurrence within 5 years.[147] The results showed that the total opioid dose in cancer-free groups was 124 mg OME versus 232 mg OME in the recurrence group ($P = 0.02$), suggesting an association between increased total opioid dose in the first 96 h postsurgery and reduced RFS within 5 years.[147] No association between age and risk of cancer recurrence in stage 1 NSCLC patients was found; OS, however, was reduced in the elderly. This may be a result of aging and thus be related to other postoperative complications.[148]

Based on the current literature, there is insufficient evidence to suggest a causal association between postoperative opioid use and OS or RFS, and a lack of studies assessing postoperative opioid use and long-term oncological outcomes.

Opioid Use in the Palliative Care Setting

Opioids are widely used in palliative care settings to reduce pain as a result of advanced malignant disease. Recent literature has investigated whether opioid use in palliative care may impact survival and hasten death. A systematic review evaluating opioid use in palliative care found that out of the 11 end-of-life cancer studies included, opioid use was associated with an increased survival in four studies, three studies showed a decrease, and four studies found no change in the survival of cancer patients.[58]

A prospective cohort study showed that in 150 patients with advanced NSCLC, opioid use was associated with a shorter OS compared to no opioids (median OS 627 vs. 242 days), and there was no difference in OS between patients who received low or high opioid doses (less than or greater than 60 mg OME).[149] Results from a similar study also showed that the opioid dose was not associated with a shortened survival.[150] On the contrary, in newly diagnosed stage IV nonhematologic malignancies, patients with high opioid doses (>5 mg OME/day) had a shorted median survival time (12.4 months) when compared to low opioid doses (<5 mg OME/day) (5.5 months).[151] An important consideration in these studies is that tumors that are more aggressive are likely to cause more pain and therefore be associated with a higher morphine intake. A retrospective cohort study including 566 patients with unresectable pancreatic cancer, of which 75% were stage IV, showed that both initial opioid dose and rate of dose increase were negatively correlated with survival time in terminally ill cancer patients.[145]

Complexities of Linking Opioid Use and Cancer Risk

Estimating the effects of opioids on cancer outcomes is complex. Some of the factors that contribute to this complexity include variations in study design (in vitro, ex vivo, in vivo, and human), experimental models used, dosing regimens, cancer type(s), tumor grade/organ affected, and the circulating concentrations of opioids. The effect of opioids on cancer is further influenced by the presence of pain or surgical stress, genetic polymorphisms influencing opioid function, central versus peripheral effects of opioids (tolerance, hyperalgesia), and the release of endogenous opioids by immune cells at the sites of inflammation. In the context of surgery, where opioid intake is not the only factor that differs between patient groups, variations exist because of the inability to control for various perioperative factors. More importantly, however, the variability in the conclusions of published data arises from the complexities of the underlying biological mechanisms and our abilities to integrate mechanisms across various streams of evidence (in vitro, in vivo, and human) (Fig. 12.2).

Cellular Level (In Vitro)

At the cellular level, while cells grown in vitro cannot mimic the complexities of the tumor microenvironment, discrepancies may exist due to the involvement of various receptors (opioid and nonopioid) and signaling pathways engaged, the type and clinical relevance of the concentrations of opioid used, the concentration responses, the chronicity of

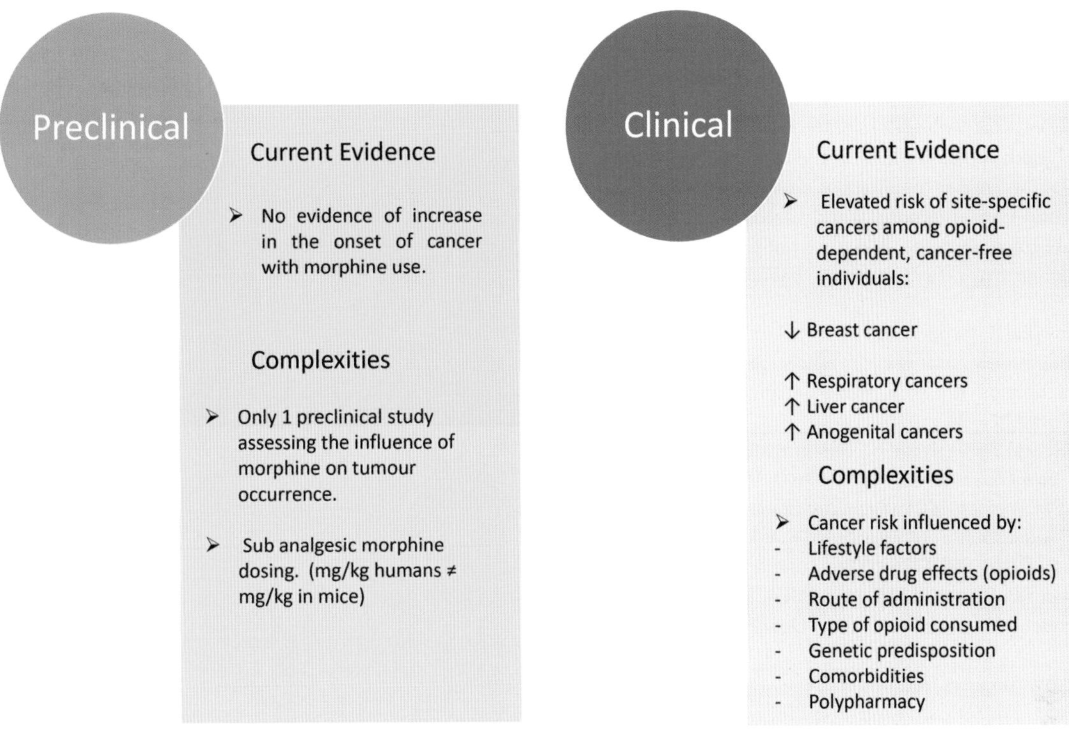

• **Fig. 12.2** Factors influencing opioid use and cancer risk in preclinical and clinical studies.

exposure, the type of cells involved (e.g., cancer, immune or endothelial), the subsequent release of cytokines, and the influence of these cytokines on the tumor microenvironment.

Animal Level (In Vivo)

The number of animal studies evaluating whether opioid administration affects the onset of tumor development is limited. Using transgenic mice spontaneously developing metastatic breast cancer, a study showed that morphine administration starting prior to the onset of tumor growth did not have a significant effect on the weight or number of tumors when compared with controls (buffer treatment).[75]

Human Level

The complexity of assessing the effects of opioids on the risk of developing cancer in humans arises from a number of factors. The current epidemiological literature attempting to assess opioid use and cancer risk is mostly retrospective, often focusing on specific population types (e.g., opioid-dependent individuals). The primary outcomes of epidemiological studies are mostly limited to opioid-related mortality and cause-specific morbidity or mortality, and such studies are often not designed to investigate cancer-related outcomes (i.e., cancer incidence). Multiple mechanisms/factors can influence the incidence or severity of cancer independent of opioid use. Some of these factors may include adverse drug effects inherent to opioid use (constipation, urinary retention, gastroesophageal reflux disease, immunosuppression, and hypogonadism), the lifestyle of the cohort (smoking, alcohol consumption, age of first pregnancy, BMI, and immune-related infections), comorbidities that increase the risk of developing cancer, genetic predisposition, and the use of concurrent illicit substances. Epidemiological studies further suggest that opium use may be an emerging risk factor for cancer. However, it is unclear whether the risk of cancer stems from the alkaloid component of opium, for example, morphine, nonalkaloid-based additional constituents, or is due to the route of administration, namely the inhalation/smoking of carcinogenic compounds arising through opium pyrolysis.[152,153]

Future Outlook and Conclusion

Opioids are an important component of cancer patient analgesia, especially during the perioperative period. The current literature investigating the influence of opioids on tumor growth remains disputed, showing both pro- and antitumor effects on cell proliferation, apoptosis, invasion, migration, inflammation, and angiogenesis. It is apparent that the ability to assess opioid use and cancer outcomes, especially in humans, is further complicated by the presence of various confounders. Future prospective clinical studies may be able to assess the long-term impact of opioid use on OS and RFS, especially when compared to alternate modes of anesthesia and analgesia.

References

1. World Health Organization. *Cancer*. 2018. Available at https://www.who.int/health-topics/cancer#tab=tab_1.
2. World Health Organization. World Cancer Report. 2014. Available at https://publications.iarc.fr/Non-Series-Publications/World-Cancer-Reports/World-Cancer-Report-2014.
3. National Cancer Institute. A to Z List of Cancer Drugs. 2019. Available at https://www.cancer.gov/about-cancer/treatment/drugs.
4. Zajączkowska R, Leppert W, Mika J, et al. Perioperative immunosuppression and risk of cancer progression: the impact of opioids on pain management. *Pain Res Manag*. 2018;2018:9293704.
5. Page GG, and Ben-Eliyahu S. The immune-suppressive nature of pain. *Sem Oncol Nursing*. 1997;13:10–15.
6. Boland JW, Pockley AG. Influence of opioids on immune function in patients with cancer pain: from bench to bedside. *Br J Pharmacol*. 2018;175:2726–2736.
7. Heiskanen TE, Ruismäki PM, Seppälä TA, Kalso EA. Morphine or oxycodone in cancer pain? *Acta Oncologica*. 2000;39:941–947.
8. Oosten AW, Abrantes JA, Jönsson S, et al. A prospective population pharmacokinetic study on morphine metabolism in cancer patients. *Clin Pharmacokinet*. 2017;56:733–746.
9. Sato H, Naito T, Ishida T, Kawakami J. Relationships between oxycodone pharmacokinetics, central symptoms, and serum interleukin-6 in cachectic cancer patients. *Eur J Clin Pharmacol*. 2016;72:1463–1470.
10. Kuip EJM, Oldenmenger WH, Thijs-Visser MF, et al. Effects of smoking and body mass index on the exposure of fentanyl in patients with cancer. *PLoS One*. 2018;13:1932–6203.
11. George R, Haywood A, Good P, et al. Can saliva and plasma methadone concentrations be used for enantioselective pharmacokinetic and pharmacodynamic studies in patients with advanced cancer? *Clin Therapeut*. 2017;39:1840–1848.
12. Tanaka H, Naito T, Sato H, Hiraide T, Yamada Y, Kawakami J. Impact of CYP genotype and inflammatory markers on the plasma concentrations of tramadol and its demethylated metabolites and drug tolerability in cancer patients. *Eur J Clin Pharmacol*. 2018;74:1461–1469.
13. Zhao X, Jin YW, Li HB, Wang ZG, Feng H, Feng C. Effects of maintaining intravenous infusion of remifentanil or propofol on anesthesia and palinesthesia during anesthesia and analepsia. *Genet Mol Res*. 2014;13:2865–2872.
14. Wu G, Fu G, Zhang L, Zhang Z, Wang X. EEffects of neoadjuvant chemotherapy on the depth of total intravenous anesthesia in patients with breast cancer undergoing unilateral modified radical mastectomy: A prospective observational study. *Medicine*. 2018;97:e13776.
15. Afsharimani B, Cabot PJ, Parat MO. Morphine use in cancer surgery. *Front Pharmacol*. 2011;2:46.
16. Brinkman D, Wang JH, Redmond HP. Morphine as a treatment of cancer-induced pain – is it safe? A review of in vivo studies and mechanisms. *Naunyn Schmiedebergs Arch Pharmacol*. 2018;391:1169–1178.
17. Tuerxun H, Cui J. The dual effect of morphine on tumor development. *Clin Transl Oncol*. 2019;21:695–701.
18. Sergeeva MG, Grishina ZV, Varfolomeyev SD. Morphine effect on proliferation of normal and tumor cells of immune origin. *Immunology Letters*. 1993;36:215–218.
19. Leo S, Nuydens R, Meert TF. Opioid-induced proliferation of vascular endothelial cells. *J Pain Res*. 2009;2:59–66.
20. Hatzoglou A, Bakogeorgou E, Castanas E. The antiproliferative effect of opioid receptor agonists on the T47D human breast cancer cell line, is partially mediated through opioid receptors. *Eur J Pharmacol*. 1996;296:199–207.
21. Chen Y, Qin Y, Li L, Chen J, Zhang X, Xie Y. Morphine can inhibit the growth of breast cancer MCF-7 cells by arresting the cell cycle and inducing apoptosis. *Biol Pharm Bull*. 2017;40:1686–1692.
22. Xie N, Parat M-O. Opioid analgesic agents and cancer cell biology. *Curr Anesthesiol Rep*. 2015;5:278–284.
23. Gonzalez-Nunez V, Noriega-Prieto JA, Rodríguez RE. Morphine modulates cell proliferation through mir133b & mir128 in the neuroblastoma SH-SY5Y cell line. *Biochim Biophys Acta*. 2014;1842:566–572.
24. Diao CT, Li L, Lau SY, Wong TM, Wong NS. kappa-Opioid receptor potentiates apoptosis via a phospholipase C pathway in the CNE2 human epithelial tumor cell line. *Biochim Biophys Acta*. 2000;1499:49–62.
25. Mathew B, Lennon FE, Siegler J, et al. The novel role of the mu opioid receptor in lung cancer progression: a laboratory investigation. *Anesth Analg*. 2011;112:558–567.
26. Lennon FE, Mirzapoiazova T, Mambetsariev B, Salgia R, Moss J, Singleton PA. Overexpression of the μ-opioid receptor in human non-small cell lung cancer promotes Akt and mTOR activation, tumor growth, and metastasis. *Anesthesiology*. 2012;116:857–867.
27. Singleton PA, Mirzapoiazova T, Hasina R, Salgia R, Moss J. Increased μ-opioid receptor expression in metastatic lung cancer. *Br J Anaesth*. 2014;113(Suppl 1):i103–i108.
28. Chen DT, Pan JH, Chen YH, et al. The mu-opioid receptor is a molecular marker for poor prognosis in hepatocellular carcinoma and represents a potential therapeutic target. *Br J Anaesth*. 2019;122:e157–e167.
29. Li Y, Li G, Tao T, et al. The μ-opioid receptor (MOR) promotes tumor initiation in hepatocellular carcinoma. *Cancer Lett*. 2019;453:1–9.
30. Bimonte S, Barbieri A, Cascella M, et al. Naloxone counteracts the promoting tumor growth effects induced by morphine in an animal model of triple-negative breast cancer. *In Vivo*. 2019;33:821–825.
31. Börner C, Kraus J, Bedini A, Schraven B, Höllt V. T-cell receptor/CD28-mediated activation of human T lymphocytes induces expression of functional μ-opioid receptors. *Mol Pharmacol*. 2008;74:496–504.
32. Pasternak GW, Pan YX. Mu opioids and their receptors: evolution of a concept. *Pharmacol Rev*. 2013;65:1257–1317.
33. Williams J. Basic opioid pharmacology. *Rev Pain*. 2008;1:2–5.
34. Donica CL, Awwad HO, Thakker DR, Standifer KM. Cellular mechanisms of nociceptin/orphanin FQ (N/OFQ) peptide (NOP) receptor regulation and heterologous regulation by N/OFQ. *Mol Pharmacol*. 2013;83:907–918.
35. Meyer LC, Paisley CE, Mohamed E, et al. Novel role of the nociceptin system as a regulator of glutamate transporter expression in developing astrocytes. *Glia*. 2017;65:2003–2023.
36. Wang K, Zheng Y, Yang Y, et al. Nociceptin receptor is overexpressed in non-small cell lung cancer and predicts poor prognosis. *Front Oncol*. 2019;9:235.
37. Kim JY, Ahn HJ, Kim JK, Kim J, Lee SH, Chae HB. Morphine suppresses lung cancer cell proliferation through the interaction

with opioid growth factor receptor: an in vitro and human lung tissue study. *Anesth Analg*. 2016;123:1429–1436.
38. Wang X, Tian J, Jiao X, et al. The novel mechanism of anticancer effect on gastric cancer through inducing G0/G1 cell cycle arrest and caspase-dependent apoptosis in vitro and in vivo by methionine enkephalin. *Cancer Manag Res*. 2018;10:4773–4787.
39. Siegel R, Ward E, Brawley O, Jemal A. Cancer statistics, 2011: the impact of eliminating socioeconomic and racial disparities on premature cancer deaths. *CA Cancer J Clin*. 2011;61:212–236.
40. Bravo-Cordero JJ, Hodgson L, Condeelis J. Directed cell invasion and migration during metastasis. *Curr Opin Cell Biol*. 2012;24:277–283.
41. Koodie L, Yuan H, Pumper JA, et al. Morphine inhibits migration of tumor-infiltrating leukocytes and suppresses angiogenesis associated with tumor growth in mice. *Am J Pathol*. 2014;184:1073–1084.
42. Khabbazi S, Goumon Y, Parat MO. Morphine modulates interleukin-4- or breast cancer cell-induced pro-metastatic activation of macrophages. *Sci Rep*. 2015;5:11389.
43. Liu HC, Anday JK, House SD, Chang SL. Dual effects of morphine on permeability and apoptosis of vascular endothelial cells: morphine potentiates lipopolysaccharide-induced permeability and apoptosis of vascular endothelial cells. *J Neuroimmunol*. 2004;146:13–21.
44. Singleton PA, Moreno-Vinasco L, Sammani S, Wanderling SL, Moss J, Garcia JG. Attenuation of vascular permeability by methylnaltrexone: Role of mOP-R and S1P3 transactivation. *CA Cancer J Clin*. 2007;37:222–231.
45. Moss J, Rosow CE. Development of peripheral opioid antagonists: new insights into opioid effects. *Mayo Clin Proc*. 2008;83:1116–1130.
46. Nylund G, Pettersson A, Bengtsson C, Khorram-Manesh A, Nordgren S, Delbro DS. Functional expression of μ-opioid receptors in the human colon cancer cell line, HT-29, and their localization in human colon. *Dig Dis Sci*. 2008;53:461–466.
47. Gach K, Szemraj J, Fichna J, Piestrzeniewicz M, Delbro DS, Janecka A. The influence of opioids on urokinase plasminogen activator on protein and mRNA level in MCF-7 breast cancer cell line. *Chem Biol Drug Des*. 2009;74:390–396.
48. Afsharimani B, Baran J, Watanabe S, Lindner D, Cabot PJ, Parat MO. Morphine and breast tumor metastasis: the role of matrix-degrading enzymes. *Clin Exp Metastasis*. 2014;31: 149–158.
49. Harimaya Y, Koizumi K, Andoh T, Nojima H, Kuraishi Y, Saiki I. Potential ability of morphine to inhibit the adhesion, invasion and metastasis of metastatic colon 26-L5 carcinoma cells. *Cancer Lett*. 2002;187:121–127.
50. Shariftabrizi A, Nifli AP, Ansari M, et al. Matrix metalloproteinase 2 secretion in WEHI 164 fibrosarcoma cells is nitric oxide-related and modified by morphine. *Eur J Pharmacol*. 2006;530:33–39.
51. Gach K, Szemraj J, Wyrębska A, Janecka A. The influence of opioids on matrix metalloproteinase-2 and -9 secretion and mRNA levels in MCF-7 breast cancer cell line. *Mol Biol Rep*. 2011;38:1231–1236.
52. Xie N, Khabbazi S, Nassar ZD, et al. Morphine alters the circulating proteolytic profile in mice: functional consequences on cellular migration and invasion. *FASEB J*. 2017;31:5208–5216.
53. Yoon JY, Kim TS, Ahn JH, Yoon JU, Kim HJ, Kim EJ. Remifentanil promotes osteoblastogenesis by upregulating Runx2/osterix expression in preosteoblastic C2C12 cells. *J Dent Anesth Pain Med*. 2019;19:91–99.
54. Horvath RJ, Deleo JA. Morphine enhances microglial migration through modulation of P2X4 receptor signaling. *J Neurosci*. 2009;29:998–1005.
55. Khabbazi S, Nassar ZD, Goumon Y, Parat MO. Morphine decreases the pro-angiogenic interaction between breast cancer cells and macrophages in vitro. *Sci Rep*. 2016;6:31572.
56. Sacerdote P. Opioids and the immune system. *Palliat Med*. 2006;20(Suppl 1):s9–s15.
57. Al-Hashimi M, Scott SWM, Thompson JP, Lambert DG. Opioids and immune modulation: more questions than answers. *Br J Anaesth*. 2013;111:80–88.
58. Boland JW, Ziegler L, Boland EG, McDermid K, Bennett MI. Is regular systemic opioid analgesia associated with shorter survival in adult patients with cancer? A systematic literature review. *Pain*. 2015;156:2152–2163.
59. Wiese AD, Griffin MR, Schaffner W, et al. Long-acting opioid use and the risk of serious infections: a retrospective cohort study. *Clin Infecs Dis*. 2019;68:1862–1869.
60. Beilin B, Grinevich G, Yardeni IZ, Bessler H. Tramadol does not impair the phagocytic capacity of human peripheral blood cells. *Can J Anaesth*. 2005;52:1035–1039.
61. Gaspani L, Bianchi M, Limiroli E, Panerai AE, Sacerdote P. The analgesic drug tramadol prevents the effect of surgery on natural killer cell activity and metastatic colonization in rats. *J Neuroimmunol*. 2002;129:18–24.
62. Hofbauer R, Frass M, Gmeiner B, et al. Effects of remifentanil on neutrophil adhesion, transmigration, and intercellular adhesion molecule expression. *Acta Anaesthesiol Scand*. 2000;44:1232–1237.
63. Hyejin J, Mei L, Seongheon L, et al. Remifentanil attenuates human neutrophils activation induced by lipopolysaccharide. *Immunopharmacol Immunotoxicol*. 2013;35:264–271.
64. Wodehouse T, Demopoulos M, Petty R, et al. A randomized pilot study to investigate the effect of opioids on immunomarkers using gene expression profiling during surgery. *Pain*. 2019;160:2691–2698.
65. Gong L, Qin Q, Zhou L, et al. Effects of fentanyl anesthesia and sufentanil anesthesia on regulatory T cells frequencies. *Int J Clin Exp Pathol*. 2014;7:7708–7716.
66. Hou M, Zhou N-B, Li H, et al. Morphine and ketamine inhibit immune function of gastric cancer patients by increasing percentage of CD4+ CD25+ Foxp3+ regulatory T cells in vitro. *J Orthop Res*. 2016;203:306–312.
67. Filipczak-Bryniarska I, Nazimek K, Nowak B, Kozlowski M, Wąsik M, Bryniarski K. In contrast to morphine, buprenorphine enhances macrophage-induced humoral immunity and, as oxycodone, slightly suppresses the effector phase of cell-mediated immune response in mice. *Int Immunopharmacol*. 2018;54:344–353.
68. D'Elia M, Patenaude J, Hamelin C, Garrel DR, Bernier J. No detrimental effect from chronic exposure to buprenorphine on corticosteroid-binding globulin and corticosensitive immune parameters. *Clin Immunol*. 2003;109:179–187.
69. Martucci C, Panerai AE, Sacerdote P. Chronic fentanyl or buprenorphine infusion in the mouse: similar analgesic profile but different effects on immune responses. *Pain*. 2004;110:385–392.
70. Franchi S, Panerai AE, Sacerdote P. Buprenorphine ameliorates the effect of surgery on hypothalamus–pituitary–adrenal axis, natural killer cell activity and metastatic colonization in rats in comparison with morphine or fentanyl treatment. *Brain Behav Immun*. 2007;21:767–774.

71. Fernandes JV, Cobucci RN, Jatobá CA, Fernandes TA, de Azevedo JW, de Araújo JM. The role of the mediators of inflammation in cancer development. *Pathol Oncol Res*. 2015;21:527–534.
72. Finley MJ, Happel CM, Kaminsky DE, Rogers TJ. Opioid and nociceptin receptors regulate cytokine and cytokine receptor expression. *Cellular Immunol*. 2008;252:146–154.
73. Cabot PJ, Carter L, Gaiddon C, et al. Immune cell-derived beta-endorphin. Production, release, and control of inflammatory pain in rats. *J Clinical Invest*. 1997;100:142–148.
74. Vincent L, Vang D, Nguyen J, et al. Mast cell activation contributes to sickle cell pathobiology and pain in mice. *Blood*. 2013;122:1853–1862.
75. Nguyen J, Luk K, Vang D, et al. Morphine stimulates cancer progression and mast cell activation and impairs survival in transgenic mice with breast cancer. *Br J Anaesth*. 2014;113(Suppl 1): i4–i13.
76. Aich A, Afrin LB, Gupta K. Mast cell-mediated mechanisms of nociception. *Intl J Mol Sci*. 2015;16:29069–29092.
77. Aceves M, Terminel MN, Okoreeh A, et al. Morphine increases macrophages at the lesion site following spinal cord injury: protective effects of minocycline. *Brain Behav Immun*. 2019;79:125–138.
78. Martin JL, Charboneau R, Barke RA, Roy S. Chronic morphine treatment inhibits LPS-induced angiogenesis: implications in wound healing. *Cell Immunol*. 2010;265:139–145.
79. Boettger MK, Weber K, Gajda M, Bräuer R, Schaible HG. Spinally applied ketamine or morphine attenuate peripheral inflammation and hyperalgesia in acute and chronic phases of experimental arthritis. *Brain Behav Immun*. 2010;24:474–485.
80. Gupta K, Kshirsagar S, Chang L, et al. Morphine stimulates angiogenesis by activating proangiogenic and survival-promoting signaling and promotes breast tumor growth. *Cancer Res*. 2002;62:4491–4498.
81. Farooqui M, Li Y, Rogers T, et al. COX-2 inhibitor celecoxib prevents chronic morphine-induced promotion of angiogenesis, tumour growth, metastasis and mortality, without compromising analgesia. *Br J Cancer*. 2007;97:1523–1531.
82. Bimonte S, Barbieri A, Rea D, et al. Morphine promotes tumor angiogenesis and increases breast cancer progression. *Biomed Res Int*. 2015;2015:161508.
83. Koodie L, Ramakrishnan S, Roy S. Morphine suppresses tumor angiogenesis through a HIF-1α/p38MAPK pathway. *Am J Pathol*. 2010;177:984–997.
84. Karaman H, Tufek A, Karaman E, Tokgoz O. Opioids inhibit angiogenesis in a chorioallantoic membrane model. *Pain Physician*. 2017;20:SE11–SE21.
85. Balasubramanian S, Ramakrishnan S, Charboneau R, Wang J, Barke RA, Roy S. Morphine sulfate inhibits hypoxia-induced vascular endothelial growth factor expression in endothelial cells and cardiac myocytes. *J Mol Cell Cardiol*. 2001;33:2179–2187.
86. Schoos A, Gabriel C, Knab VM, Fux DA. Activation of HIF-1α by δ-opioid receptors induces COX-2 expression in breast cancer cells and leads to paracrine activation of vascular endothelial cells. *J Pharmacol Exp Ther*. 2019;370:480–489.
87. Peach G, Kim C, Zacharakis E, Purkayastha S, Ziprin P. Prognostic significance of circulating tumour cells following surgical resection of colorectal cancers: a systematic review. *Br J Cancer*. 2010;102:1327–1334.
88. Park Y, Kitahara T, Urita T, Yoshida Y, Kato R. Expected clinical applications of circulating tumor cells in breast cancer. *World J Clin Oncol*. 2011;2:303–310.
89. Iinuma H, Watanabe T, Mimori K, et al. Clinical significance of circulating tumor cells, including cancer stem-like cells, in peripheral blood for recurrence and prognosis in patients with Dukes' stage B and C colorectal cancer. *J Clin Oncol*. 2011;29:1547–1555.
90. Bar-Yosef S, Melamed R, Page GG, Shakhar GG, Shakhar K, Ben-Eliyahu S. Attenuation of the tumor-promoting effect of surgery by spinal blockade in rats. *Anesthesiology*. 2001;94:1066–1073.
91. Sacerdote P, Bianchi M, Gaspani L, et al. The effects of tramadol and morphine on immune responses and pain after surgery in cancer patients. *Anesth Analgesia*. 2000;90:1411–1414.
92. Connolly C, Buggy DJ. Opioids and tumour metastasis: does the choice of the anesthetic-analgesic technique influence outcome after cancer surgery? *Current Opin Anaesthesiol*. 2016;29:468–474.
93. Wall T, Sherwin A, Ma D, Buggy DJ. Influence of perioperative anaesthetic and analgesic interventions on oncological outcomes: a narrative review. *Br J Anaesth*. 2019;123:135–150.
94. O'Riain SC, Buggy DJ, Kerin MJ, Watson RW, Moriarty DC. Inhibition of the stress response to breast cancer surgery by regional anesthesia and analgesia does not affect vascular endothelial growth factor and prostaglandin E2. *Anesth Analg*. 2005;100:244–249.
95. Biki B, Mascha E, Moriarty DC, Fitzpatrick JM, Sessler DI, Buggy DJ. Anesthetic technique for radical prostatectomy surgery affects cancer recurrence: a retrospective analysis. *Anesthesiology*. 2008;109:180–187.
96. Christopherson R, James KE, Tableman M, Marshall P, Johnson FE. Long-term survival after colon cancer surgery: a variation associated with choice of anesthesia. *Anesth Analg*. 2008;107:325–332.
97. Tsui BC, Rashiq S, Schopflocher D, et al. Epidural anesthesia and cancer recurrence rates after radical prostatectomy. *Can J Anaesth*. 2010;57:107–112.
98. Wuethrich PY, Hsu Schmitz SF, Kessler TM, et al. Potential influence of the anesthetic technique used during open radical prostatectomy on prostate cancer-related outcome: a retrospective study. *Anesthesiology*. 2010;113:570–576.
99. Myles PS, Peyton P, Silbert B, et al. Perioperative epidural analgesia for major abdominal surgery for cancer and recurrence-free survival: randomised trial. *Br Med J*. 2011;342:d1491.
100. Wuethrich PY, Thalmann GN, Studer UE, Burkhard FC. Epidural analgesia during open radical prostatectomy does not improve long-term cancer-related outcome: a retrospective study in patients with advanced prostate cancer. *PLoS One*. 2013;8:e72873.
101. Buckley A, McQuaid S, Johnson P, Buggy DJ. Effect of anaesthetic technique on the natural killer cell anti-tumour activity of serum from women undergoing breast cancer surgery: a pilot study. *Br J Anaesth*. 2014;113(Suppl 1):i56–i62.
102. Deegan CA, Murray D, Doran P, Ecimovic P, Moriarty DC, Buggy DJ. Effect of anaesthetic technique on oestrogen receptor-negative breast cancer cell function in vitro. *Br J Anaesth*. 2009;103:685–690.
103. Deegan CA, Murray D, Doran P, et al. Anesthetic technique and the cytokine and matrix metalloproteinase response to primary breast cancer surgery. *Region Anesth Pain Med*. 2010;35:490–495.
104. Looney M, Doran P, Buggy DJ. Effect of anesthetic technique on serum vascular endothelial growth factor C and transforming growth factor beta in women undergoing anesthesia and surgery for breast cancer. *Anesthesiology*. 2010;113:1118–1125.

105. Bundscherer A, Malsy M, Gebhardt K, et al. Effects of ropivacaine, bupivacaine and sufentanil in colon and pancreatic cancer cells in vitro. *Pharmacol Res.* 2015;95–96:126–131.
106. Buggy DJ, Smith G. Epidural anaesthesia and analgesia: better outcome after major surgery? Growing evidence suggests so. *Br Med J.* 1999;319:530–531.
107. Sessler DI, Ben-Eliyahu S, Mascha EJ, Parat MO, Buggy DJ. Can regional analgesia reduce the risk of recurrence after breast cancer? Methodology of a multicenter randomized trial. *Contemp Clin Trials.* 2008;29:517–526.
108. Fant F, Tina E, Sandblom D, et al. Thoracic epidural analgesia inhibits the neuro-hormonal but not the acute inflammatory stress response after radical retropubic prostatectomy. *Br J Anaestha.* 2013;110:747–757.
109. Siekmann W, Eintrei C, Magnuson A, et al. Surgical and not analgesic technique affects postoperative inflammation following colorectal cancer surgery: a prospective, randomized study. *Colorectal Dis.* 2017;19:O186–O195.
110. Exadaktylos AK, Buggy DJ, Moriarty DC, Mascha E, Sessler DI. Can anesthetic technique for primary breast cancer surgery affect recurrence or metastasis? *Anesthesiology.* 2006;105:660–664.
111. Lin L, Liu C, Tan H, Ouyang H, Zhang Y, Zeng W. Anaesthetic technique may affect prognosis for ovarian serous adenocarcinoma: a retrospective analysis. *Br J Anaesth.* 2011;106:814–822.
112. Lee BM, Singh Ghotra V, Karam JA, Hernandez M, Pratt G, Cata JP. Regional anesthesia/analgesia and the risk of cancer recurrence and mortality after prostatectomy: a meta-analysis. (Report). *Pain Manag.* 2015;5:387.
113. Sun Y, Li T, Gan TJ. The effects of perioperative regional anesthesia and analgesia on cancer recurrence and survival after oncology surgery: a systematic review and meta-analysis. *Reg Anesth Pain Med.* 2015;40:589–598.
114. Missair A, Cata JP, Votta-Velis G, et al. Impact of perioperative pain management on cancer recurrence: an ASRA/ESRA special article. *Reg Anesth Pain Med.* 2019;44:13–28.
115. Cakmakkaya OS, Kolodzie K, Apfel CC, Pace NL. Anaesthetic techniques for risk of malignant tumour recurrence. *Cochrane Database Syst Rev.* 2014(11):CD008877.
116. Sessler DI, Pei L, Huang Y, et al. Recurrence of breast cancer after regional or general anaesthesia: a randomised controlled trial. *Lancet.* 2019;394:1807–1815.
117. Wang FL, Sun H, Guo L, DuBois RN. Prostaglandin E2 promotes colorectal cancer stem cell expansion and metastasis in mice. *Gastroenterology.* 2015;149:1884–1895.
118. Ng K, Meyerhardt JA, Chan AT, et al. Aspirin and COX-2 inhibitor use in patients with stage III colon cancer. *J Natl Cancer Inst.* 2015;107:345.
119. Huang X, Gao P, Sun J, et al. Aspirin and nonsteroidal anti-inflammatory drugs after but not before diagnosis are associated with improved breast cancer survival: a meta-analysis. *Cancer Causes Control.* 2015;26:589–600.
120. Cassuto J, Sinclair R, Bonderovic M. Anti-inflammatory properties of local anesthetics and their present and potential clinical implications. *Acta Anaesthesiol Scand.* 2006;50:265–282.
121. Sakaguchi M, Kuroda Y, Hirose M. The antiproliferative effect of lidocaine on human tongue cancer cells with inhibition of the activity of epidermal growth factor receptor. *Anesth Analg.* 2006;102:1103–1107.
122. Yoon JR, Whipple RA, Balzer EM, et al. Local anesthetics inhibit kinesin motility and microtentacle protrusions in human epithelial and breast tumor cells. *Breast Cancer Res Treat.* 2011;129:691–701.
123. Lirk P, Berger R, Hollmann MW, Fiegl H. Lidocaine time- and dose-dependently demethylates deoxyribonucleic acid in breast cancer cell lines in vitro. *Br J Anaesth.* 2012;109:200–207.
124. Wei X, Hailin Z, James H, Lin C, Shanglong Y, Daqing M. Local anesthetic bupivacaine induced ovarian and prostate cancer apoptotic cell death and underlying mechanisms in vitro. *Sci Rep.* 2016;6:26277.
125. Li R, Xiao C, Liu H, Huang Y, Dilger JP, Lin J. Effects of local anesthetics on breast cancer cell viability and migration (Report). *BMC Cancer.* 2018;18:666.
126. Huang H, Benzonana LL, Zhao H, et al. Prostate cancer cell malignancy *via* modulation of HIF-1alpha pathway with isoflurane and propofol alone and in combination. *Br J Cancer.* 2014;111:1338–1349.
127. Zhou CL, Li JJ, Ji P. Propofol suppresses esophageal squamous cell carcinoma cell migration and invasion by down-regulation of sex-determining region Y-box 4 (SOX4). *Med Sci Mon Int Med J Exp Clin Res.* 2017;23:419–427.
128. Tatsumi K, Hirotsu A, Daijo H, Matsuyama T, Terada N, Tanaka T. Effect of propofol on androgen receptor activity in prostate cancer cells. *Eur J Pharmacol.* 2017;809:242–252.
129. Jaura AI, Flood G, Gallagher HC, Buggy DJ. Differential effects of serum from patients administered distinct anaesthetic techniques on apoptosis in breast cancer cells in vitro: a pilot study. *Br J Anaesth.* 2014;113(Suppl 1):i63–i67.
130. Jiang S, Liu Y, Huang L, Zang F, Kang R. Effects of propofol on cancer development and chemotherapy: potential mechanisms. *Eur J Pharmacol.* 2018;831:46–51.
131. Zheng X, Wang Y, Dong L, et al. Effects of propofol-based total intravenous anesthesia on gastric cancer: a retrospective study (Report). *Onco Targets Ther.* 2018;11:1141–1148.
132. Lee JH, Kang SH, Kim Y, Kim HA, Kim BS. Effects of propofol-based total intravenous anesthesia on recurrence and overall survival in patients after modified radical mastectomy: a retrospective study. *Korean J Anesthesiol.* 2016;69:126–132.
133. Jun IJ, Jo JY, Kim JI, et al. Impact of anesthetic agents on overall and recurrence-free survival in patients undergoing esophageal cancer surgery: a retrospective observational study. *Scic Rep.* 2017;7:14020.
134. Randall D, Degenhardt L, Vajdic CM, et al. Increasing cancer mortality among opioid-dependent persons in Australia: a new public health challenge for a disadvantaged population. *Aust N Z J Public Health.* 2011;35:220–225.
135. Kelty E, Dobbins T, Hulse G. Incidence of cancer and cancer related mortality in opiate dependent patients treated with methadone, buprenorphine or implant naltrexone as compared with non-opiate using controls. *Heroin Addict Relat Clin Probl.* 2017:19.
136. Grinshpoon A, Barchana M, Lipshitz I, Rosca P, Weizman A, Ponizovsky AM. Methadone maintenance and cancer risk: an Israeli case registry study. *Drug Alcohol Depend.* 2011;119:88–92.
137. Patino MA, Ramirez RE, Perez CA, et al. The impact of intraoperative opioid use on survival after oral cancer surgery. *Oral Oncol.* 2017;74:1–7.
138. Tai YH, Wu HL, Chang WK, Tsou MY, Chen HH, Chang KY. Intraoperative fentanyl consumption does not impact cancer recurrence or overall survival after curative colorectal cancer resection. *Sci Rep.* 2017;7:10816.
139. Diaz-Cambronero O, Mazzinari G, Cata JP. Perioperative opioids and colorectal cancer recurrence: a systematic review of the literature. *Pain Manag.* 2018;8:353–361.

140. Du KN, Feng L, Newhouse A, et al. Effects of intraoperative opioid use on recurrence-free and overall survival in patients with esophageal adenocarcinoma and squamous cell carcinoma. *Anesth Analg.* 2018;127:210–216.
141. Cata JP, Keerty V, Keerty D, et al. A retrospective analysis of the effect of intraoperative opioid dose on cancer recurrence after non-small cell lung cancer resection. *Cancer Med.* 2014;3: 900–908.
142. Nelson DB, Cata JP, Niu J, et al. Persistent opioid use is associated with worse survival after lobectomy for stage I non-small cell lung cancer. *Pain.* 2019;160:2365–2373.
143. Bortsov AV, Millikan RC, Belfer I, Boortz-Marx RL, Arora H, McLean SA. mu-Opioid receptor gene A118G polymorphism predicts survival in patients with breast cancer. *Anesthesiology.* 2012;116:896–902.
144. Hwang IC, Park JY, Myung SK, Ahn HY, Fukuda K, Liao Q. OPRM1 A118G gene variant and postoperative opioid requirement: a systematic review and meta-analysis. *Anesthesiology.* 2014;121:825–834.
145. Oh TK, Kim K, Jheon SH, et al. Long-term oncologic outcomes, opioid use, and complications after esophageal cancer surgery. *J Clin Med.* 2018;7(2):33.
146. Cronin-Fenton DP, Heide-Jørgensen U, Ahern TP, et al. Opioids and breast cancer recurrence: a Danish population-based cohort study. *Cancer.* 2015;121:3507–3514.
147. Maher DP, Wong W, White PF, et al. Association of increased postoperative opioid administration with non-small-cell lung cancer recurrence: a retrospective analysis. *Br J Anaesth.* 2014;113(Suppl 1):i88–i94.
148. Goodgame B, Viswanathan A, Zoole J, et al. Risk of recurrence of resected stage I non-small cell lung cancer in elderly patients as compared with younger patients. *J Thorac Oncol.* 2009;4:1370–1374.
149. Hasegawa T, Oguri T, Osawa T, et al. pioid dose and survival of patients with incurable nonsmall cell lung cancer: a prospective cohort study. *J Palliat Med.* 2018;21:1436–1441.
150. Sathornviriyapong A, Nagaviroj K, Anothaisintawee T. The association between different opioid doses and the survival of advanced cancer patients receiving palliative care. *BMC Palliative Care.* 2016;15:95.
151. Zylla D, Steele G, Shapiro A, Richter S, Gupta P. Impact of opioid use on health care utilization and survival in patients with newly diagnosed stage IV malignancies. *Support Care Cancer.* 2018;26:2259–2266.
152. Kamangar F, Shakeri R, Malekzadeh R, Islami F. Opium use: an emerging risk factor for cancer? *Lancet Oncol.* 2014;15:e69–e77.
153. Hosseini SY, Safarinejad MR, Amini E, Hooshyar H. Opium consumption and risk of bladder cancer: a case-control analysis. *Urol Oncol.* 2010;28:610–616.

13

Can Regional Anesthesia and Analgesia Influence the Risk of Cancer Recurrence?

DYLAN FINNERTY AND DONAL J. BUGGY

What Is Regional Anesthesia?

Regional anesthesia may be defined as the administration of local anesthetic drugs around a nerve or plexus of nerves, or anatomical plane through which nerves pass, in order to render a distal site anesthetized. It can be used in conjunction with general anesthesia (GA), or it can be the sole means of anesthesia, thereby sometimes allowing the patient to be fully awake during surgery without feeling any pain.

General Benefits of Regional Anesthesia

The potential established benefits of regional anesthesia to surgical cancer patients may be summarized as:

- A reduction in intraoperative and postoperative systemic analgesia requirements[1]
- Shorter lengths of hospital stay[2]
- Inhibition of the surgical stress response[3]
- Reduction in postoperative nausea and vomiting[4]
- Fewer postoperative pulmonary complications[5]

How Regional Anesthesia Might Influence Cancer

In 2006, a retrospective analysis of women undergoing mastectomy for breast cancer with paravertebral anesthesia and analgesia found an association between the use of this technique and improved disease-free survival time, compared with women who received volatile anesthesia and opioid analgesia.[6] This study, although limited by its retrospective design, sparked a global interest in the question of whether regional anesthesia or analgesia during surgery of curative intent might reduce the risk of later recurrence or metastasis.

There are biologically plausible mechanisms to explain why regional anesthesia may have a role to play in reducing cancer recurrence (Table 13.1) including the following.

Regional anesthesia can inhibit the stress response that is associated with surgery.[7] The stress response to surgery has been shown to have a negative effect on natural killer cells (NK cells) and T cells, which play a key role in eliminating minimal residual cancer disease or circulating tumor cells (CTC) at the time of surgery.[8] Simultaneously, the surgical stress response stimulates immune cells which have a protumor effect such as regulatory T cells (Tregs) and type 2 helper T cells (Th2):

1. This surgical stress response also leads to activation of the hypothalamic-pituitary-adrenal (HPA) axis, which results in secretion of cortisol and catecholamines. Many cancer cells contain adrenoreceptors that when activated by catecholamines, secrete substances such as interleukin 6 (IL-6), vascular endothelial growth factor (VEG-F), and matrix metalloproteinase (MMP) enzymes, which all increase the propensity for tumor cells to invade and proliferate.[9]
2. The superior pain relief that regional anesthesia provides means that opioids can be used sparingly or not at all. While controversial, some experimental and retrospective studies suggest that perioperative use of opioids may be associated with cancer recurrence.[3,10] Morphine appears to have immunosuppressant effects by reducing the activity of NK cells, which play a crucial role in suppressing tumor growth.[10] It may act directly to suppress NK cells via opioid receptors or nonopioid receptors present on immune cells, e.g., Toll-like receptor 4 (TLR-4).[11] Morphine also acts indirectly on the periaqueductal grey area in the brain stem and sympathetic nervous system that release chemical messengers that suppress NK cytotoxicity.[12] Cancer cells can also express opioid receptors that, when activated, can trigger a tumorigenic cascade that can result in metastasis.[13] This has also been observed clinically with retrospective studies showing that tumors that overexpress opioid receptors are associated with poorer outcomes in prostate and squamous cell carcinoma of the esophagus.[14,15] Poorly

TABLE 13.1 Summary of Mechanisms by Which Regional Anesthesia May Reduce Cancer Recurrence

Proposed Mechanism	Subsequent Effects
Attenuation of surgical stress response	↑ NK and CD 8 – T cells ↓ Tregs and Th2 cells ↓ Cortisol and catecholamine secretion ↓ MMPs, VEGF, IL6
Opiate-sparing effect means possible negative effects of opiates are reduced	Less suppression of NK cells Cancer cells with opiate receptors are not stimulated to replicate
Avoidance or dose reduction of volatile anesthetic gasses	↓ Expression of HIFs, which can promote angiogenesis
Improved pain relief postoperatively	↓ Stimulation of sympathetic system and HPA axis ↓ Beta endorphin ↓ Suppression of NK activity
Action of local anesthetic drugs	↑ Apoptosis of tumor cells Inhibition of metastatic pathways via VGSCs ↓ Src activation ↓ EGFR Demethylation of DNA in cancer cells
Reduction in intraoperative blood loss	Reduced requirement for blood transfusion, which in itself has been associated with cancer recurrence

EGFR, Epidermal growth factor receptor; *HIF*, hypoxia inducible factor; *HPA*, hypothalamic pituitary adrenal; *IL-6*, interleukin 6; *MMP*, matrix metalloproteinase; *NK*, natural killer cells; *Th2*, Type 2 helper T cells; *Treg*, regulatory T cells; *VEGF*, vascular endothelial growth factor; *VGCS*, voltage-gated sodium channel.

controlled pain *per se* postoperatively has been shown to be a driving force for cancer recurrence in an animal model.[16] Effective regional anesthesia can improve pain scores postoperatively[4] and offer superior analgesia when compared with parenteral opioids in patients undergoing cancer operations.[17] Pain itself is thought to have an immunosuppressive effect via stimulation of the sympathetic system and the hypothalamic pituitary adrenal axis, hence reducing the body's defense systems against invading malignant cells. Painful stimuli can also increase circulating levels of β-endorphin which has immunosuppressant effects specifically by reducing the cytotoxic effects of NK cells.[18] An experimental cancer model showed that effective analgesia can reduce the incidence and number of metastases.[19]

3. Similarly, volatile anesthetics have been implicated in cancer recurrence.[20] Effective regional anesthesia can provide a dose reduction in the amount of volatile required[21] or in some cases negate its usage entirely by allowing the operation to be performed completely under regional anesthesia with the patient awake or lightly sedated. Volatile anesthetics have been shown to upregulate the expression of hypoxia inducible factor (HIF), which can promote angiogenesis and have been implicated in facilitating cancer recurrence.[22] However, studies have not been consistent in their findings with some suggesting that sevoflurane (a commonly used volatile anesthetic gas) may have antiproliferative effects on non–small cell lung carcinoma (NSCLC) cells.[23] While uncertainty continues regarding the pros and cons of volatile anesthetic use during cancer surgery, regional anesthesia may, if it is the sole anesthetic technique, circumnavigate this issue entirely or perhaps reduce volatile anesthesia requirements if used in combination with general anesthesia.
4. Emerging evidence suggests that amide local anesthetics may reduce the metastatic burden in both in vitro and animal models.[24] A number of potential mechanisms exist that may explain this antitumor effect. The primary use of amide local anesthetics in anesthesia is to block sensory nerve transmission and hence provide pain relief. This is achieved by blockade of voltage-gated sodium channels (VGSCs). These channels also exist in the membrane of many cancer cells and they tend to be constitutively active. Inhibition of the alpha subunit of these channels can halt the metastatic potential of cancerous cells.[25] While evidence to support this theory is weak, other medications that work on VGSCs such as phenytoin have been found to suppress the metastatic potential of breast cancer cells.[26]

Non-VGSC-dependent mechanisms of tumor suppression have also been identified. Lidocaine has been shown to reduce the tyrosine kinase activity of the epidermal growth factor receptor (EGFR) and hence suppress replication in human tongue squamous cell carcinoma cells. This was seen at concentrations that occur in clinical practice.[27] The same study also demonstrated a direct cytotoxic effect on cancer cells with lidocaine but this was seen at concentrations much higher than could safely be achieved in vivo.

The amide local anesthetics (lidocaine and ropivacaine) have been shown to have a direct inhibitory effect on the Src oncogene.[28] The Src pathway is involved in promoting the epithelial to mesenchymal transition which allows invasion of cancerous cells to occur.[29] In recent years the Src tyrosine protein kinase has been viewed as an important research focus and specific "targeted therapies" (e.g., Dasatinib, Bristol-Myers Squibb, New York, NY)[30] have been developed to inhibit its actions. Interestingly, while the amide local anesthetics were seen to have an inhibitory effect on the pathway the same was not seen for the ester class of local anesthetics (chloroprocaine).[28]

As well as possibly enhancing the efficacy of conventional chemotherapeutic drugs,[31] local anesthetics have also been shown to demethylate DNA in breast cancer cells in vitro[32]; this action can decrease tumor progression through the upregulation of tumor suppressor genes.[33] These effects were seen at concentrations of local anesthetic typically achieved during epidural infusions. All of these antitumor effects of local anesthetic drugs may in some part explain the beneficial effects on tumor recurrence when melanoma excision is performed under local anesthetic as opposed to general anesthesia.[34,35] Lignocaine and bupivacaine have been shown to trigger apoptosis in human breast cancer cells.[36] The authors of this study suggested that it might be beneficial to infiltrate tissues with these drugs during breast cancer resections. In vivo evidence suggests that lidocaine may also exert antimetastatic effects when given intravenously.[37]

Some evidence exists that regional anesthesia may reduce intraoperative blood loss in comparison with general anesthesia[2] (however, this was in observational trials and the quality of this evidence was rated as low). This may be an indirect benefit of regional anesthesia in terms of reducing cancer recurrence as perioperative blood transfusion may also be associated with cancer recurrence.[38]

Evidence for a Benefit of Regional Anesthesia in Cancer Surgery

In Vivo Data

In a rat model of mammary adenocarcinoma, rats that received spinal anesthesia as opposed to GA (with isoflurane) had lower rates of postoperative tumor burden.[39] The potential rationale for this is that spinal anesthesia reduces the neuroendocrine stress response that occurs during surgery. This stress response has been shown to have an immunosuppressant effect, reducing the activity of NK cells in particular. These lymphocytes are an integral part of the body's immune response to fighting tumor cells. The aforementioned study showed that regional anesthesia appeared to preserve the numbers and activity of NK cells. In the group without regional anesthesia, NK cell activity was inhibited, and this may explain the greater rate of tumor recurrence and metastasis seen in this group.

A 2007 study in mice also showed a similar benefit to spinal anesthesia, when combined with GA, in reducing the amount of liver metastasis postsurgery.[40] Again, spinal blockade appeared to preserve the ability of NK cells to perform its defensive role against invading cancerous cells.

These animal studies provide modest evidence for the potential beneficial role of regional anesthesia in patients undergoing cancer surgery. Unfortunately, promising results from animal studies frequently do not show the same effect in human studies. In fact, only in approximately one-third of studies are results of animal trials in accordance with those of human randomized control trials and the vast majority of animal studies (approximately 90%) are not repeated using human subjects.[41] There should be caution in extrapolating results of these experiments to our clinical practice. There remain unanswered questions as to how well the animal model replicates human physiology, particularly in the intricate arena of cancer recurrence.

Translational Studies

Translational studies may be defined as studies that bridge the gap between laboratory research and clinical research, sometimes referred to as "bedside to bench" studies. A number of recent translational studies have demonstrated a potential benefit to regional anesthesia in the cancer setting. In a pilot study, 32 women undergoing breast cancer surgery were randomized to one of either two anesthetic techniques, propofol GA combined with paravertebral regional anesthesia or GA with sevoflurane and opioid analgesia.[42] Of the 14 cytokines associated with cancer biology that were measured in this study, 10 showed no difference between the groups; however, MMP 3 and MMP 9 were decreased postoperatively in the propofol/paravertebral group. MMPs are enzymes capable of degrading proteins of the extracellular matrix and hence play an essential role in tumor cell invasion, angiogenesis, and metastasis.[43] MMPs are upregulated in many cancers and are associated with advanced disease and higher mortality.[44] This study showed that regional anesthesia (with propofol) reduces MMPs and hence may have a protective role in cancer recurrence at the time of surgery.

In another translational study, 40 women undergoing breast cancer surgery were randomized to receive either paravertebral anesthesia and analgesia combined with GA or volatile anesthesia and opioid analgesia alone. The authors found that vascular endothelial growth factor C (VEGF-C) levels were elevated in the GA-alone group while they remained virtually unchanged in the patients who received paravertebral anesthesia. VEGF-C stimulates angiogenesis, which is the process by which cancerous cells generate a blood supply from the host. Angiogenesis is an essential step in tumor development and metastasis, as the tumor mass increases in size. It has been demonstrated that tumor tissue greater than 2 mm in diameter cannot survive without its own blood supply.[45] This process of developing new blood and lymph vessels also facilitates the dissemination of cancerous cells into the systemic circulation and hence the development of metastasis. The observation that patients who received a paravertebral block had lower levels of VEGF-C postoperatively compared with those without suggests that perhaps the paravertebral block creates a microenvironment less conducive to tumor growth and metastatic spread.

Evidence from translational studies would also suggest that regional anesthesia may preserve the antitumor effect of NK cells. The effect of serum from women undergoing cancer surgery on healthy human donor NK function and cytotoxicity was evaluated.[46] Preservation of NK function and cytotoxicity was noted in patients who had received regional anesthesia. As mentioned previously, the main function of NK cells is the recognition and destruction of virus-infected cells and tumor cells, making it one of the front-line defenses against cancerous cells. A reduction in NK cell activity is mediated via beta-adrenoreceptors located on the surface of these cells, which, when activated, trigger an increase in cAMP and protein kinase A. Regional anesthesia may ameliorate this catecholamine-driven suppression of NK cells via its ability to attenuate the stress response associated with surgery.

Cancer cells can express μ-opioid receptors (MORs). Increased expression of this receptor is associated with a higher incidence of metastasis in gastric,[47] prostate,[14] and non-small cell lung cancer.[48] Another study demonstrated that anesthetic technique can influence MOR expression.[49] In a group of 20 breast cancer patients, those who had volatile GA with opioid analgesia had higher levels of MOR expression on intraoperative biopsy specimens compared with those who had a propofol-paravertebral-based anesthetic technique. Again, this study suggests a potential benefit to regional anesthesia in cancer surgeries.

Retrospective Analysis

The initial hypothesis suggesting a benefit from regional anesthesia in cancer patients came from retrospective studies (Table 13.2). Patients undergoing radical prostatectomy who received epidural analgesia combined with GA were associated with a 57% lower risk of cancer recurrence (95% confidence interval [CI], 17%–78%) compared with those who had GA and opioids.[50] Cancer recurrence in this study was defined as increase in postoperative prostate-specific antigen (PSA) compared with its postoperative nadir that prompted adjunctive therapy. However, subsequent retrospective studies showed no significant benefit in terms of disease-free survival[51] or biochemical recurrence[52] in patients given neuraxial anesthesia undergoing a radical prostatectomy.

Similarly, in patients undergoing breast cancer surgery, retrospective analysis seemed to suggest a benefit of regional anesthesia; in this case, paravertebral analgesia was used. Metastasis and recurrence-free survival was 94% (95% CI, 87%–100%) and 77% (95% CI, 68%–87%) in the paravertebral and GA patients, respectively ($P = 0.012$).[6] However, similar to what was seen in the prostate cancer trials, more recent retrospective analysis in breast cancer patients suggests that paravertebral anesthesia may not be associated with longer survival after surgery.[53]

In laryngeal and hypopharyngeal cancer surgery a survival benefit has been seen with the use of cervical epidurals. In a single-center, retrospective study of more than 100 patients with a 4.5-year follow up, the cervical epidural and GA group had a significantly increased cancer-free survival compared with the GA group alone.[54]

Other retrospective analysis looking at the role of regional anesthesia and potential beneficial cancer outcomes in bladder,[55,56] colon,[57,58] and ovarian[59,60] cancers have also shown mixed results.

Certain studies have even demonstrated worse oncologic outcomes for patients receiving regional anesthesia. In a propensity-matched cohort of 430 patients of patients undergoing radical cystectomy those who received epidural and GA as opposed to GA had a higher risk of recurrence at 2 years. Epidural usage was a significant predictor of worse recurrence-free survival (adjusted hazard ratio [HR], 1.67; 95% CI, 1.14–2.45; $P = 0.009$) and cancer-specific survival (HR, 1.53; 95% CI, 1.04–2.25; $P = 0.030$) on multivariable analyses. Interestingly, the regional group received sufentanil via the epidural and also received higher median total intravenous morphine equivalents (ivMEQ) versus those in the GA group (75 ivMEQ [11–235] vs. 50 ivMEQ [7–277], $P < 0.0001$).[61]

All retrospective studies examining a potential link between regional anesthesia and cancer recurrence suffer similar limitations. Patients with major comorbidities may be more likely to receive regional anesthesia, hence introducing a selection bias into the cohort. While multivariate analysis attempts to control for confounders, other risk factors that were not recorded at the time, or simply not accounted for, are quite often present. This design is often prone to recall bias, and temporal relationships can be difficult to assess. Ultimately, the greatest limitation of this study design is that it can demonstrate an association but not causative effect between regional anesthesia and cancer recurrence. However, these early retrospective studies were certainly hypothesis generating (which is the intent) and paved the way for future investigation in the area.

Another study looked at the effects of epidural anesthesia on patients undergoing surgery for colorectal malignancy.[62] This study looked at two groups, epidural and GA, and GA alone. At 24 h the epidural group had lower levels of markers that are associated with tumor recurrence and metastatic progression (namely VEGF-C and IL-6), and higher level levels of IL-10, which inhibits proinflammatory cytokines and can enhance the ability of NK cells to eliminate tumor cells. However, this study had relatively small numbers with 20 in each group and data were only collected 24 h after surgery. Immunosuppressive effects of surgery have been observed up to 30 days after surgery.[63,64]

To date, the bulk of evidence pertaining to regional anesthesia and cancer recurrence has come from retrospective studies. A number of RCTs designed to look at different outcomes have used post hoc analyses to examine a potential link between regional anesthesia and cancer recurrence. Tsui and colleagues showed no difference in disease-free survival among patients undergoing a radical prostatectomy under general anesthetic[51]; similarly, Myles et al. showed a survival benefit with epidural analgesia in patients undergoing abdominal surgery for a variety of cancers.[65] Of note, this trial was adequately powered to detect an approximately 30% treatment effect but was underpowered to detect any smaller effects that could still have considerable clinical relevance.

TABLE 13.2 Selected Studies of Regional Anesthesia and Cancer-Related Outcomes

Study Authors	Year	Trial Design	Surgery Type	Techniques Compared	Significant Results
Exadaktylos et al.	2006	RETR	Breast cancer requiring mastectomy +/− axillary clearance	GA + PVB (n = 50) vs. GA + opioid (n = 79)	Increased recurrence-free survival in PVB group at 3 years (88% vs. 77%; $P = 0.012$)
Bar-Yosef et al.	2001	Animal model of breast cancer metastasis	Laparotomy and inoculation with syngeneic MADB106 adenocarcinoma cells	Spinal anesthesia IV morphine	Spinal anesthesia reduced the number of pulmonary metastasis 37.2 ± 24.4 to 10.5 ± 4.7 ($P = 0.0043$)
Wada et al.	2007	Mouse model of liver metastasis	Inoculation with EL4 tumor cells	Spinal + GA GA alone	Spinal group had a reduced number of liver metastasis 33.7 ± 8.9 to 19.8 ± 9.1 ($P < 0.05$) and preserved NK cell activity
Deegan et al.	2010	Pilot RCT	Breast cancer surgery	Propofol/PVB (n = 15) Sevoflurane/opioid (n = 17)	Significant attenuation of elevated MMP-3 and MMP-9 in propofol/PVB group
Looney et al.	2010	RCT	Breast cancer	Propofol/PVB (n = 20) GA (n = 20)	PVB group had a decreased rise in VEGF-C postoperatively
Buckley et al.	2014	In vitro translational study	Breast cancer	Propofol/PVB (n = 5) vs. sevoflurane/opioid (n = 5)	Greater NK cell cytotoxicity seen in PVB group
Biki et al.	2008	RETR	Prostate cancer	GA + epidural vs. GA + opioid	57% lower incidence of cancer recurrence in epidural group (95% CI, 17%–78%)
Tsui et al.	2010	RCT–PHA	Prostate cancer	GA + epidural (n = 49) GA (n = 50)	No difference in disease-free survival
Tseng et al.	2014	RETR	Prostate cancer	Spinal + sedation (n = 1166) GA (n = 798)	No difference in biochemical recurrence
Cata et al.	2016	RETR	Breast cancer	PVB (n = 198); Opioid-based analgesia (n = 594)	Use of PVB not associated with a significant change in recurrence-free survival or overall survival
Merquiol et al.	2013	RETR	Laryngeal and hypopharyngeal cancer	GA + cervical epidural (n = 111) GA + opioid (n = 160)	↑ 5-year cancer-free survival in epidural group
Doiron et al.	2016	RETR	Cystectomy for bladder cancer	Thoracic epidural + GA (n = 887); GA (n = 741)	Thoracic epidural not associated with cancer-specific survival
Koumpan et al.	2018	RETR	TURBT for bladder cancer	Spinal (n = 135) GA (n = 96)	Lower incidence of cancer recurrence in spinal group
Holler et al.	2013	RETR	Colorectal cancer	Epidural + GA (n = 442) GA (n = 307)	↑ 5-year survival rate with epidural (62% vs. 54%, $P < 0.02$)

Continued

TABLE 13.2 Selected Studies of Regional Anesthesia and Cancer Related Outcomes—cont'd

Study Authors	Year	Trial Design	Surgery Type	Techniques Compared	Significant Results
Day et al.	2012	RETR	Laparoscopic colorectal resection for colorectal cancer	GA + epidural (n = 107) GA + spinal (n = 144) GA + opiate (n = 173)	No difference in overall survival or 5-year disease-free survival
Oliveira et al.	2011	RETR	Ovarian cancer debulking	GA + epidural (n = 55) GA (n = 127)	Intraoperative epidural use associated with reduced recurrence risk (HR, 0.37)
Capmas et al.	2012	RETR	Ovarian cancer	GA + epidural (n = 47) GA (n = 47)	Epidural had no clear impact on cancer recurrence
Chipollini et al.	2018	RETR	Bladder cancer	GA + epidural (n = 215) GA (n = 215)	↓ Recurrence-free survival (HR, 1.67) and cancer-specific survival (HR, 1.53) in epidural group, interestingly epidural group received higher doses of morphine equivalents
Xu et al.	2014	Randomized trial	Colon cancer	Propofol + epidural (n = 20); GA (n = 20)	Epidural group had decreases in VEGF-C and IL-6 compared to GA group at 24 h post surgery
Myles et al.	2011	RCT–PHA	Abdominal cancer surgery	GA + epidural (n = 230) GA (n = 16)	No difference in overall survival or recurrence-free survival between groups
Cata et al.	2018	RETR	Craniotomies for malignant brain tumors	Scalp block + GA GA	Scalp block not associated with longer progression-free survival or longer overall survival
Lee et al.	2015	Meta-analysis	Prostate cancer surgery	Epidural/spinal GA	Improved overall survival with regional anesthesia (HR, 0.81; 95% CI, 0.68–0.96; *P* = 0.016)
Weng et al.	2016	Meta-analysis	21 studies including breast, prostate, colorectal, laryngeal, hepatocellular, cervical, and ovarian cancer	Neuraxial anesthesia GA	Improved overall survival in regional group (HR, 0.853; 95% CI, 0.741–0.981; *P* = 0.026)
Grandhi et al.	2017	Meta- analysis	Variety of cancer surgeries 67,577 patients 28 studies	RA GA	No significant benefit to RA in cancer surgery
Sessler, et al.	2019	Prospective multicenter RCT	Primary breast cancer surgery	PVB + propofol vs. sevoflurane + opioid	PVB and propofol does not improve cancer recurrence (median follow up, 36 months)

GA, General anesthesia; *HR*, hazard ratio; *IL-6*, interleukin 6; *IV*, intravenous; *MMP*, matrix metalloproteinase; *NK*, natural killer cells; *PVB*, paravertebral block; *RA*, regional anesthesia; *RCT*, randomized controlled trial; *RCT–PHA*, randomized control trial–post hoc analysis; *RETR*, retrospective; *VEG-F*, vascular endothelial growth factor.

Prospective Evidence

A recent review on the potential effect of anesthesia, analgesic, and perioperative interventions during primary cancer surgery on long-term oncologic outcomes[3] anticipated the future publication of ongoing prospective RCTs, which would definitively address whether a causal relationship exists between anesthetic technique and oncologic outcome.

The first and largest such RCT (NCT00418457) evaluated the effect of paravertebral regional anesthesia, combined with propofol total intravenous general anesthesia versus sevoflurane volatile anesthesia with opioid analgesia, among more than 2100 women undergoing primary breast cancer surgery in nine globally distributed centers. The primary outcome was local or metastatic breast cancer recurrence. Secondary outcomes included chronic persistent incisional pain at 6 and 12 months. Primary analyses were on an intent-to-treat basis.

The study was halted after crossing a preplanned futility boundary with 213 cancer recurrence events (61% of the maximum required number of recurrences). Median (25%–75%) follow up was 36 (24–49) months. There were 102 (9.8%) recurrences among 1043 women assigned to paravertebral anesthesia versus 111 (10.4%) among 1065 women who received sevoflurane anesthesia. HR for cancer recurrence in paravertebral versus GA was an estimated 0.97 (95% CI, 0.74–1.3; $P = 0.84$). The incidence of chronic neuropathic breast pain was 10% at 6 months and 7% at 12 months in each group, which did not differ according to anesthetic technique.

It was concluded that paravertebral-propofol anesthesia improves neither breast cancer recurrence nor the incidence and severity of persistent incisional breast pain after potentially curative surgery compared with sevoflurane-opioid anesthesia.[66]

However, this should not put an end to research in the field. Since undertaking this trial, new data have emerged showing multiple mechanisms by which systemically administered amide local anesthetics inhibit cancer cell biology, raising the hypothesis that systemic lidocaine during tumor removal surgery could plausibly attenuate cancer cell progression.[67] Systemically administered lidocaine enables significantly higher plasma levels compared with absorption from a regional anesthetic technique. Further, different types of tumor may respond differently to anesthetic technique. Therefore although the data indicate that regional anesthesia is unlikely to affect breast cancer outcome, we await ongoing and emerging RCT results evaluating other anesthetic techniques and in different tumors.

Peripheral Nerve Blocks and Cancer Recurrence

Many orthopedic cancer operations are amenable to regional anesthesia.[68] In the case of upper-limb resections, the brachial plexus can be infiltrated with local anesthetic at different sites, which can give very effective anesthesia and analgesia throughout the operation and into the postoperative period. It is worth remembering that the surgeon can also place an infusion catheter intraoperatively in the location of the nerve plexus, which can provide excellent postoperative analgesia. By the time cancer patients present for surgery, they may be quite opioid tolerant and regional anesthesia can therefore provide very effective pain relief.

Similarly in lower-limb surgery, apart from neuraxial anesthesia (epidural and spinal), a range of blocks, such as the sciatic, femoral, lumbar plexus, or popliteal block, can be employed. Unfortunately, evidence that regional anesthesia influences oncologic outcomes in orthopedic oncology cases is currently lacking. A systematic review of the literature on this topic found no eligible studies.[69] Adequately powered RCTs designed to investigate the relationship between regional anesthesia and orthopedic oncology surgery will likely be very difficult to perform given that the overall incidence of bone tumors in the general population is quite low (osteosarcoma, the most common bone sarcoma, has an incidence of 4.6 per million people).[68]

Postoperative pain is a significant problem for patients undergoing musculoskeletal resections. Orthopedic patients have the highest incidence of pain in the ambulatory setting.[70] Any reduction in opioid usage due to peripheral nerve block might theoretically benefit cancer recurrence. The peripheral opioid antagonist methylnaltrexone is associated with increased survival in patients with advanced cancer[71,72] in retrospective analysis of patients randomized to receive methylnaltrexone or not for constipation associated with opioid use for cancer pain.

Scalp blocks have also been investigated during neurosurgery for brain tumor resections. Evidence exists that scalp blocks have an opiate-sparing effect and reduce the stress response in patients undergoing craniotomy.[73,74] These observations led investigators to postulate that scalp blocks might have a benefit in patients undergoing resections of malignant gliomas. A retrospective review of 808 patients undergoing craniotomies for malignant brain tumors showed no difference in progression-free survival and overall survival in those that had the block and those that did not.[73]

Systematic Reviews and Meta-Analysis

With such differing outcomes from conducted retrospective research, it comes as no surprise that the published systematic reviews on the topic of regional anesthesia and cancer recurrence equally show varying results. In prostate cancer surgery a systematic review of available retrospective studies demonstrated that regional anesthesia was not associated with longer biochemical recurrence-free survival but was associated with improved overall survival (HR, 0.81; 95% CI, 0.68–0.96; $P = 0.016$).[75]

A meta-analysis of 21 retrospective studies of different cancer types (including prostate, ovarian, colorectal, and breast cancer) found a positive association with neuraxial anesthesia and improved overall survival HR of 0.853 with a 95% CI of 0.741–0.981 ($P = 0.026$) (in particular in colorectal cancer surgery: HR, 0.653; 95% CI, 0.430–0.991, $P = 0.045$).[76] However, a more recent meta-analysis consisting of 28 retrospective studies concluded that regional anesthesia is not associated with improved overall survival or recurrence-free survival.[77]

A 2014 Cochrane review[78] concluded that there was insufficient evidence to support the theory that regional anesthesia could positively affect outcomes for patients undergoing cancer surgery. The review consisted of four studies with 746 patients in total undergoing abdominal operations for cancer surgery with or without epidural anesthesia. The four studies were post hoc analyses of previously conducted RCTs, meaning that none of these studies were originally designed to look at the incidence of cancer recurrence in relation to regional anesthesia. All participants were followed up for at least 7.8 years after the initial surgery.

Conclusion

The stress response to surgery elicits an inflammatory milieu in which cancer cells could flourish. The immune system is transiently undermined by both the stress response to surgery and potentially some of the anesthetic techniques that we use. Surgical resection is likely to remain the primary modality for the treatment of solid organ tumors for the foreseeable future. Therefore anesthesia will remain a prerequisite for these patients. As surgery aspires to deliver better patient outcomes, so must anesthesiologists investigate how their techniques and medications can impact recurrence of cancer in the postoperative setting. Many of the RCTs that have been performed in this area were not initially designed to investigate cancer outcomes and so any conclusions drawn are made with the inherent limitations of post hoc analyses.

The first prospective RCT published on this topic concluded that regional anesthesia in the form of paravertebral analgesia does not appear to influence tumor recurrence in primary breast cancer surgery.[66] However, this by no means closes the chapter on this important research question. Emerging evidence from translational studies would suggest that systemically administered lidocaine may have a positive impact on tumor recurrence after cancer surgery.[24] Further studies in the field of oncoanesthesia are needed to evaluate how choice of anesthetic technique could influence outcomes for cancer surgery patients.

Therefore the choice of whether to use regional anesthesia and analgesia techniques in cancer patients should be focused on other patient-centered outcomes, such as improved quality of recovery, rather than to specifically reduce the incidence of cancer recurrence. While a biologically plausible theory exists, no conclusive evidence has been published to date to recommend or dissuade use of a particular anesthetic technique in patients presenting for cancer surgery in terms of reducing the likelihood of cancer recurrence.

References

1. Schug SA, Palmer GM, Scott DA, et al. *Acute Pain Management: Scientific Evidence*: ANZCA and FPM; 2015.
2. Smith LM, Cozowicz C, Uda Y, et al. Neuraxial and combined neuraxial/general anesthesia compared to general anesthesia for major truncal and lower limb surgery: a systematic review and meta-analysis. *Anesth Analg*. 2017;125(6):1931–1945. doi:10.1213/ane.0000000000002069.
3. Wall T, Sherwin A, Ma D, et al. Influence of perioperative anesthetic and analgesic interventions on oncological outcomes: a narrative review. *Br J Anaesth*. 2019;123:135–150.
4. Liu SS, Strodtbeck WM, Richman JM, et al. A comparison of regional versus general anesthesia for ambulatory anesthesia: a meta-analysis of randomized controlled trials. *Anesth Analg*. 2005;101(6):1634–1642.
5. van Lier F, van der Geest PJ, Hoeks SE, et al. Epidural analgesia is associated with improved health outcomes of surgical patients with chronic obstructive pulmonary disease. *Anesthesiology*. 2011;115(2):315–321.
6. Exadaktylos AK, Buggy DJ, Moriarty DC, et al. Can anesthetic technique for primary breast cancer surgery affect recurrence or metastasis? *Anesthesiology*. 2006;105(4):660–664.
7. Fant F, Tina E, Sandblom D, et al. Thoracic epidural analgesia inhibits the neuro-hormonal but not the acute inflammatory stress response after radical retropubic prostatectomy. *Br J Anaesth*. 2013;110(5):747–757. doi:10.1093/bja/aes491.
8. Alazawi W, Pirmadjid N, Lahiri R, et al. Inflammatory and immune responses to surgery and their clinical impact. *Ann Surg*. 2016;264(1):73–80.
9. Neeman E, Ben-Eliyahu S. Surgery and stress promote cancer metastasis: new outlooks on perioperative mediating mechanisms and immune involvement. *Brain Behav Immun*. 2013;30:S32–S40.
10. Boland JW, Pockley AG. Influence of opioids on immune function in patients with cancer pain: from bench to bedside. *Br J Pharmacol*. 2018;175(14):2726–2736.
11. Xie N, Gomes FP, Deora V, et al. Activation of μ-opioid receptor and Toll-like receptor 4 by plasma from morphine-treated mice. *Brain Behav Immun*. 2017;61:244–258.
12. Gomez-Flores R, Weber RJ. Differential effects of buprenorphine and morphine on immune and neuroendocrine functions following acute administration in the rat mesencephalon periaqueductal gray. *Immunopharmacology*. 2000;48(2):145–156.
13. Wigmore T, Farquhar-Smith P. Opioids and cancer: friend or foe? *Palliat Support Care*. 2016;10(2):109–118.
14. Zylla D, Gourley BL, Vang D, et al. Opioid requirement, opioid receptor expression, and clinical outcomes in patients with advanced prostate cancer. *Cancer*. 2013;119(23):4103–4110.
15. Zhang Y-F, Xu Q-X, Liao L-D, et al. Association of mu-opioid receptor expression with lymph node metastasis in esophageal squamous cell carcinoma. *Dis Esophagus*. 2015;28(2):196–203.
16. Page GG, Blakely WP, Ben-Eliyahu S. Evidence that postoperative pain is a mediator of the tumor-promoting effects of surgery in rats. *Pain*. 2001;90(1–2):191–199.
17. Weinbroum AA. Superiority of postoperative epidural over intravenous patient-controlled analgesia in orthopedic oncologic patients. *Surgery*. 2005;138(5):869–876.
18. Sacerdote P, Manfredi B, Bianchi M, et al. Intermittent but not continuous inescapable footshock stress affects immune responses and immunocyte beta-endorphin concentrations

in the rat. *Brain Behav Immun*. 1994;8(3):2512–2560. doi:10.1006/brbi.1994.1023.

19. Hooijmans CR, Geessink FJ, Ritskes-Hoitinga M, et al. A systematic review and meta-analysis of the ability of analgesic drugs to reduce metastasis in experimental cancer models. *Pain*. 2015;156(10):1835–1844. doi:10.1097/j.pain. 0000000000000296.
20. Luo X, Zhao H, Hennah L, et al. Impact of isoflurane on malignant capability of ovarian cancer in vitro. *Br J Anaesth*. 2014;114(5):831–839.
21. Hodgson PS, Liu SS. Epidural lidocaine decreases sevoflurane requirement for adequate depth of anesthesia as measured by the Bispectral Index® monitor. *Anesthesiology*. 2001;94(5):799–803.
22. Benzonana LL, Perry NJ, Watts HR, et al. Isoflurane, a commonly used volatile anesthetic, enhances renal cancer growth and malignant potential via the hypoxia-inducible factor cellular signaling pathway in vitro. *Anesthesiology*. 2013;119(3):593–605.
23. Ciechanowicz S, Zhao H, Chen Q, et al. Differential effects of sevoflurane on the metastatic potential and chemosensitivity of non-small-cell lung adenocarcinoma and renal cell carcinoma in vitro. *Br J Anaesth*. 2018;120(2):368–375.
24. Johnson MZ, Crowley PD, Foley AG, et al. Effect of perioperative lidocaine on metastasis after sevoflurane or ketamine-xylazine anesthesia for breast tumor resection in a murine model. *Br J Anaesth*. 2018;121(1):76–85. doi:10.1016/j.bja.2017.12.043.
25. Mao L, Lin S, Lin J. The effects of anesthetics on tumor progression. *Int J Physiol Pathophysiol Pharmacol*. 2013;5(1):1.
26. Yang M, Kozminski DJ, Wold LA, et al. Therapeutic potential for phenytoin: targeting Na v 1.5 sodium channels to reduce migration and invasion in metastatic breast cancer. *Breast Cancer Res Treat*. 2012;134(2):603–615.
27. Sakaguchi M, Kuroda Y, Hirose M. The antiproliferative effect of lidocaine on human tongue cancer cells with inhibition of the activity of epidermal growth factor receptor. *Anesth Analg*. 2006;102(4):1103–1107.
28. Piegeler T, Votta-Velis EG, Liu G, et al. Antimetastatic potential of amide-linked local anesthetics inhibition of lung adenocarcinoma cell migration and inflammatory Src signaling independent of sodium channel blockade. *Anesthesiology*. 2012;117(3):548–559.
29. Thiery JP. Epithelial–mesenchymal transitions in tumor progression. *Nat Rev Cancer*. 2002;2(6):442.
30. Das J, Chen P, Norris D, et al. 2-Aminothiazole as a novel kinase inhibitor template. Structure–activity relationship studies toward the discovery of N-(2-chloro-6-methylphenyl)-2-[[6-[4-(2-hydroxyethyl)-1-piperazinyl)]-2-methyl-4-pyrimidinyl] amino)]-1, 3-thiazole-5-carboxamide (dasatinib, BMS-354825) as a potent pan-Src kinase inhibitor. *J Med Chem*. 2006;49(23):6819–6832.
31. Esposito M, Fulco RA, Collecchi P, et al. Improved therapeutic index of cisplatin by procaine hydrochloride. *J Natl Cancer Inst*. 1990;82(8):677–684.
32. Lirk P, Hollmann M, Fleischer M, et al. Lidocaine and ropivacaine, but not bupivacaine, demethylate deoxyribonucleic acid in breast cancer cells in vitro. *Br J Anaesth*. 2014;113(Suppl 1):i32–i38.
33. Navada SC, Steinmann J, Lübbert M, et al. Clinical development of demethylating agents in hematology. *J Clin Invest*. 2014;124(1):40–46.
34. Schlagenhauff B, Ellwanger U, Breuninger H, et al. Prognostic impact of the type of anesthesia used during the excision of primary cutaneous melanoma. *Melanoma Res*. 2000;10(2):165–169.
35. Sekandarzad MW, van Zundert AA, Lirk PB, et al. Perioperative anesthesia care and tumor progression. *Anesth Analg*. 2017;124(5):1697–1708.
36. Chang Y-C, Liu C-L, Chen M-J, et al. Local anesthetics induce apoptosis in human breast tumor cells. *Anesth Analg*. 2014;118(1):116–124.
37. Johnson M, Crowley P, Foley A, et al. Does perioperative iv lidocaine infusion during tumor resection surgery reduce metastatic disease in the 4T1 mouse model of breast cancer? *Br J Anaesth*. 2018;120(1):e1–e2.
38. Amato A, Pescatori M. Perioperative blood transfusions and recurrence of colorectal cancer. *Cochrane Database Syst Rev*. 2006;2006(1):CD005033. doi:10.1002/14651858.CD005033.pub2.
39. Bar-Yosef S, Melamed R, Page GG, et al. Attenuation of the tumor-promoting effect of surgery by spinal blockade in rats. *Anesthesiology*. 2001;94(6):1066–1073.
40. Wada H, Seki S, Takahashi T, et al. Combined spinal and general anesthesia attenuates liver metastasis by preserving TH1/TH2 cytokine balance. *Anesthesiology*. 2007;106(3):499–506.
41. Van der Worp HB, Howells DW, Sena ES, et al. Can animal models of disease reliably inform human studies? *PLoS Med*. 2010;7(3):e1000245.
42. Deegan CA, Murray D, Doran P, et al. Anesthetic technique and the cytokine and matrix metalloproteinase response to primary breast cancer surgery. *Reg Anesth Pain Med*. 2010;35(6):490–495. doi:10.1097/AAP.0b013e3181ef4d05.
43. Duffy MJ, Maguire TM, Hill A, et al. Metalloproteinases: role in breast carcinogenesis, invasion and metastasis. *Breast Cancer Res*. 2000;2(4):252.
44. Sier C, Kubben F, Ganesh S, et al. Tissue levels of matrix metalloproteinases MMP-2 and MMP-9 are related to the overall survival of patients with gastric carcinoma. *Br J Cancer*. 1996;74(3):413.
45. Wittekind C, Neid M. Cancer invasion and metastasis. *Oncology*. 2005;69(Suppl. 1):14–16.
46. Buckley A, McQuaid S, Johnson P, et al. Effect of anesthetic technique on the natural killer cell anti-tumor activity of serum from women undergoing breast cancer surgery: a pilot study. *Br J Anaesth*. 2014;113(Suppl 1):i56–i62.
47. Yao Y, Yao R, Zhuang L, et al. MOR1 expression in gastric cancer: a biomarker associated with poor outcome. *Clin Transl Sci*. 2015;8(2):137–142.
48. Singleton P, Mirzapoiazova T, Hasina R, et al. Increased µ-opioid receptor expression in metastatic lung cancer. *Br J Anaesth*. 2014;113(Suppl 1):i103–i108.
49. Levins KJ, Prendeville S, Conlon S, et al. The effect of anesthetic technique on µ-opioid receptor expression and immune cell infiltration in breast cancer. *J Anesth*. 2018;32(6):792–796.
50. Biki B, Mascha E, Moriarty DC, et al. Anesthetic technique for radical prostatectomy surgery affects cancer recurrence: a retrospective analysis. *Anesthesiology*. 2008;109(2):180–187. doi:10.1097/ALN.0b013e31817f5b73.
51. Tsui BCH, Rashiq S, Schopflocher D, et al. Epidural anesthesia and cancer recurrence rates after radical prostatectomy. *Can J Anaesth*. 2010;57(2):107–112. doi:10.1007/s12630-009-9214-7.
52. Tseng KS, Kulkarni S, Humphreys EB, et al. Spinal anesthesia does not impact prostate cancer recurrence in a cohort of men undergoing radical prostatectomy: an observational study. *Reg Anesth Pain Med*. 2014;39(4):284–288. doi:10.1097/aap.0000000000000108.

53. Cata JP, Chavez-MacGregor M, Valero V, et al. The impact of paravertebral block analgesia on breast cancer survival after surgery. *Reg Anesth Pain Med.* 2016;41(6):696. doi:10.1097/AAP.0000000000000479.
54. Merquiol F, Montelimard A-S, Nourissat A, et al. Cervical epidural anesthesia is associated with increased cancer-free survival in laryngeal and hypopharyngeal cancer surgery: a retrospective propensity-matched analysis. *Reg Anesth Pain Med.* 2013;38(5):398. doi:10.1097/AAP.0b013e31829cc3fb.
55. Doiron RC, Jaeger M, Booth CM, et al. Is there a measurable association of epidural use at cystectomy and postoperative outcomes? A population-based study. *Can Urol Assoc J.* 2016;10(9–10):321.
56. Koumpan Y, Jaeger M, Mizubuti GB, et al. Spinal anesthesia is associated with lower recurrence rates after resection of non-muscle invasive bladder cancer. *J Urol.* 2018;199(4):940–946.
57. Holler JP, Ahlbrandt J, Burkhardt E, et al. Peridural analgesia may affect long-term survival in patients with colorectal cancer after surgery (PACO-RAS-Study): an analysis of a cancer registry. *Ann Surg.* 2013;258(6):989–993.
58. Day A, Smith R, Jourdan I, et al. Retrospective analysis of the effect of postoperative analgesia on survival in patients after laparoscopic resection of colorectal cancer. *Br J Anaesth.* 2012;109(2):185–190.
59. de Oliveira GS, Ahmad S, Schink JC, et al. Intraoperative neuraxial anesthesia but not postoperative neuraxial analgesia is associated with increased relapse-free survival in ovarian cancer patients after primary cytoreductive surgery. *Reg Anesth Pain Med.* 2011;36(3):271–277. doi:10.1097/AAP.0b013e318217aada.
60. Capmas P, Billard V, Gouy S, et al. Impact of epidural analgesia on survival in patients undergoing complete cytoreductive surgery for ovarian cancer. *Anticancer Res.* 2012;32(4):1537–1542.
61. Chipollini J, Alford B, Boulware DC, et al. Epidural anesthesia and cancer outcomes in bladder cancer patients: is it the technique or the medication? A matched-cohort analysis from a tertiary referral center. *BMC Anesthesiol.* 2018;18(1):157.
62. Xu Y, Chen W, Zhu Y, et al. Effect of thoracic epidural anesthesia on serum vascular endothelial growth factor C and cytokines in patients undergoing anesthesia and surgery for colon cancer. *Br J Anaesth.* 2014;113(Suppl 1):i49–i55.
63. Crane CA, Han SJ, Barry JJ, et al. TGF-β downregulates the activating receptor NKG2D on NK cells and CD8+ T cells in glioma patients. *Neuro-Oncol.* 2009;12(1):7–13. doi:10.1093/neuonc/nop009.
64. Baxevanis CN, Papilas K, Dedoussis GV, et al. Abnormal cytokine serum levels correlate with impaired cellular immune responses after surgery. *Clin Immunol Immunopathol.* 1994;71(1):82–88.
65. Myles PS, Peyton P, Silbert B, et al. Perioperative epidural analgesia for major abdominal surgery for cancer and recurrence-free survival: randomized trial. *Br Med J.* 2011;342:d1491.
66. Sessler DI, Pei L, Huang Y, Buggy DJ. Recurrence of breast cancer after regional or general anesthesia: a randomized controlled trial. *Lancet.* 2019;394(10211):1807–1815. doi:10.1016/S0140-6736(19)32313-X.
67. Hermanns H, Hollmann MW, Stevens MF, et al. Molecular mechanisms of action of systemic lidocaine in acute and chronic pain. *Br J Anaesth.* 2019;123(3):335–349.
68. Anderson MR, Jeng CL, Wittig JC, et al. Anesthesia for patients undergoing orthopedic oncologic surgeries. *J Clin Anesth.* 2010;22(7):565–572.
69. Cata JP, Hernandez M, Lewis VO, Kurz A. Can regional anesthesia and analgesia prolong cancer survival after orthopedic oncologic surgery? *Clin Orthop Relat Res.* 2014;472(5):1434–1441.
70. Chung F, Ritchie E, Su J. Postoperative pain in ambulatory surgery. *Anesth Analg.* 1997;85(4):808–816.
71. Singleton PA, Moss J. Effect of perioperative opioids on cancer recurrence: a hypothesis. *Future Oncol.* 2010;6(8):1237–1242.
72. Janku F, Johnson L, Karp DD, et al. Treatment with methylnaltrexone is associated with increased survival in patients with advanced cancer. *Ann Oncol.* 2016;27(11):2032–2038.
73. Cata JP, Bhavsar S, Hagan KB, et al. Scalp blocks for brain tumor craniotomies: a retrospective survival analysis of a propensity match cohort of patients. *J Clin Neurosci.* 2018;51:46–51.
74. Geze S, Yilmaz AA, Tuzuner F. The effect of scalp block and local infiltration on the haemodynamic and stress response to skull-pin placement for craniotomy. *Eur J Anaesthesiol.* 2009;26(4):298–303.
75. Lee BM, Singh Ghotra V, Karam JA, et al. Regional anesthesia/analgesia and the risk of cancer recurrence and mortality after prostatectomy: a meta-analysis. *Pain Manag.* 2015;5(5):387–395.
76. Weng M, Chen W, Hou W, et al. The effect of neuraxial anesthesia on cancer recurrence and survival after cancer surgery: an updated meta-analysis. *Oncotarget.* 2016;7(12):15262.
77. Grandhi RK, Lee S, Abd-Elsayed A. The relationship between regional anesthesia and cancer: a metaanalysis. *Ochsner J.* 2017;17(4):345–361.
78. Cakmakkaya OS, Kolodzie K, Apfel CC, et al. Anaesthetic techniques for risk of malignant tumor recurrence. *Cochrane Database Syst Rev.* 2014;(11):CD008877. doi:10.1002/14651858.CD008877.pub2.

SECTION 3

Perioperative/Periprocedural Care in the Cancer Patient

14

Preoperative Evaluation and Medical Optimization of the Cancer Patient

KIMBERLY D. CRAVEN AND SUNIL K. SAHAI

Introduction

Although many of the goals of preoperative evaluation and optimization are the same for patients with and without cancer, cancer patients present a unique set of challenges that perioperative physicians must be familiar with. The overall goals of preoperative evaluation are to understand the whole patient, identify undiagnosed or undertreated conditions, and acknowledge patient- and procedure-related risk factors in order to prepare the patient optimally for surgery. A comprehensive preoperative evaluation lays the groundwork for high-quality care of the surgical patient. Additionally, a comprehensive preoperative evaluation of the cancer patient lends insight into potential risks and complications that may occur in the postoperative period.

History and Physical Examination

For all patients, the preoperative evaluation should involve information gathering through history taking, review of medical records, diagnostic testing, and a focused physical examination. All medications must be reviewed and confirmed with the patient. The history of each medical condition should be reviewed in detail to develop an understanding of the level of control of each and to determine if additional treatment or optimization is needed. The physical examination should be focused as to add insight into findings from the review of the history.

For cancer patients, it is especially important to take a detailed history that includes initial presenting symptoms and how the diagnosis of cancer was made. A thorough review for any history of cancer and prior cancer treatments should be conducted. As treatment of cancer is, more often than not, multi-disciplinary, it is of particular importance to note current treatment in the neoadjuvant period. Recent cancer treatment, including chemotherapy and radiation therapy, must also be reviewed as these may have systemic effects relevant to perioperative management (addressed elsewhere). It is important to note that recent imaging should be reviewed in order to understand the nature of any solid tumors and other organ involvement that may impact perioperative care (e.g., head or neck tumor compromising the airway). Care should be taken to ensure that the physical examination includes findings related to the area of tumor involvement, and these findings should be documented carefully (for example, hepatomegaly in liver cancer).

Preoperative Testing

In general, routine preoperative testing should not be performed.[1] Institutional policies that mandate blanket testing for all patients should be avoided. Laboratory tests and other diagnostic testing should be performed only if indicated based on patient factors and if results are anticipated to affect or improve management.[2] This should generally also apply to cancer patients. Given the systemic effects of cancer and cancer treatments, it is likely that many cancer patients will warrant some preoperative testing based on focused history and physical examination findings if it has not been done already. It would be prudent to check laboratory markers for nutrition in the patient who presents with a gastrointestinal malignancy and weight loss. Likewise, patients with a history of radiation therapy to the neck may need testing of thyroid function and possibly vascular studies if carotid bruits are present.[3,4] Additionally, if a patient has experienced a side effect or complication due to recent treatment, it is prudent to check for laboratory studies that may be abnormal. For example, a patient who has experienced nausea and vomiting after chemotherapy and just prior to surgery might have electrolyte derangements that need correcting.

Preoperative evaluation may take many different forms. Some institutions may rely on the patient's usual primary care physician to provide a preoperative evaluation, while many large academic institutions have highly developed

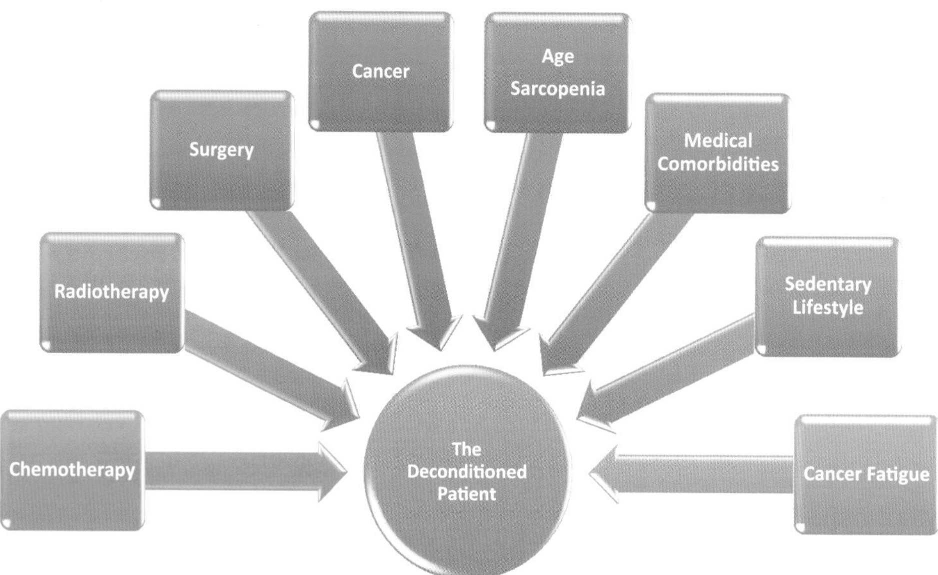

• **Fig. 14.1** Multiple hit hypothesis for cancer deconditioning. (Reprinted with permission from Sahai SK, Ismail H. Perioperative implications of neoadjuvant therapies and optimization strategies for cancer surgery. *Curr Anesthesiol Rep.* 2015;5(3):305–317.)

preoperative evaluation clinics staffed by practitioners with training and experience in perioperative medicine.[5–7] These clinics are often a key component in facilitating coordinated perioperative care and enrollment of patients in preoperative pathways (addressed elsewhere). There are numerous reports of potential benefits of a dedicated preoperative clinic and interdisciplinary coordinated care, with some studies citing improvement in patient satisfaction, decrease in unnecessary testing and consultations, reduction in surgical delays and cancelations, shorter length of stay, fewer postoperative complications, and even reduced in-patient mortality.[5,8–10] Although a preoperative evaluation is a requisite for surgery, there is no consensus on a superior method for accomplishing this, and it ultimately depends on the resources and priorities of the institution where the surgery will be performed.

One of the major principles that must be kept in mind for cancer patients is that cancer surgery is not usually truly elective. The time-sensitive nature of cancer surgery means that careful attention must be paid to avoid preoperative management plans that would unnecessarily delay surgical treatment. The benefit of performing additional tests or delaying surgery for better control of a medical condition must be weighed against the risk of cancer progression and a potentially worse prognosis that may develop in the interim.[11] Collaboration between the oncologist, surgeon, anesthesiologist, primary care physician, and other specialists is especially important in this case to determine the optimal time to proceed with surgery. A useful concept in evaluating patients facing cancer is the multihit hypothesis for cancer deconditioning (Fig. 14.1).[12] Perioperative physicians should identify potential concerns along the domains of prior treatment, age and sarcopenia, medical comorbidities, sedentary lifestyle, and cancer fatigue.

Cardiovascular Risk Assessment

As in preoperative evaluation of all surgical patients, assessment of risk for cardiovascular events should be performed for all cancer patients planning for surgery. In general, the stepwise approach provided in the 2014 ACC/AHA Guideline on Perioperative Cardiovascular Evaluation and Management of Patients Undergoing Noncardiac Surgery can be applied.[13] The first step of the approach for cancer patients planning for nonemergent surgery will be to estimate the risk of major adverse cardiac events (MACE) for the combined clinical/surgical risk. The 2014 ACC/AHA guidelines recommend the use of the Revised Cardiac Risk Index (RCRI) or the American College of Surgeons National Surgical Quality Improvement Program (NSQIP) calculator to determine if the risk is low (<1%) or elevated. If the risk is low then no further testing is indicated. If the risk is elevated then functional capacity should be assessed. If it is determined that a patient can achieve four metabolic equivalents (METs) or more, then no further testing is indicated. If the patient cannot achieve four METs or if functional capacity is unknown, then additional cardiac testing is considered only if the results of testing will change the management (i.e., delay surgery for revascularization, choose alternative management strategy, or decide not to proceed with surgery).

Studies have previously suggested that subjective assessment with self-reported exercise tolerance is predictive of cardiovascular complications,[14] and this has been a commonly used method of determining whether the patient requires further cardiac workup prior to surgery. With the publication of the results of the multicenter, international, prospective cohort METS study, the reliability of subjective assessment of exercise tolerance is now being questioned. When compared with subjective assessment of exercise tolerance, only the Duke Activity Status Index (DASI) was found to be predictive of death or myocardial infarction within 90 days of surgery.[15] Based on the results of the study the authors recommend that given the lack of predictive ability found, subjective assessment of exercise tolerance no longer be used. How this finding will be applied in future recommendations is not yet known.

Pulmonary Risk Assessment

In regard to perioperative evaluation of the patient presenting with dyspnea and/or chest pain, it is especially important to obtain a history that includes details of recent treatment. Numerous treatments can affect the cardiopulmonary system, and it is important to determine if symptoms existed prior to treatment or developed during treatment.[12] Patients with preexisting symptoms may have known or undiagnosed cardiovascular conditions, and targeted testing should be performed. For patients who develop dyspnea and/or fatigue during neoadjuvant treatment, it is important to discern if the treatment itself has cardiotoxic or pulmotoxic side effects. If a previously healthy and active patient has developed these symptoms and has not received treatment that may affect the cardiopulmonary system, it is reasonable to assume that cancer treatment–associated fatigue is the etiology behind the deconditioning and the patient may proceed to surgery.

The Older Patient

In 2012 the American College of Surgeons and the American Geriatrics Society released best practices guidelines for preoperative assessment of the geriatric patient, which recommends screening for frailty, cognitive impairment, and nutrition.[16] All cancer patients considering surgery should be screened for nutritional status. Older cancer patients planning for major surgery should also be screened for frailty and cognitive impairment. Frailty is a better predictor of mortality, complications, and prolonged length of stay in older surgical patients than chronological age.[17] Although screening for these risk factors is clearly recommended, interventions for management once the patient has been screened are emerging and many hospitals are not yet equipped to provide additional resources that might be of benefit. Patients who have been identified as frail and planning major surgery should undergo a comprehensive geriatric assessment with a specialist in geriatrics. Additional benefit may be gained for frail patients with early involvement of a multidisciplinary comanagement team involving social workers and geriatrics specialists.[10,17–19] A multimodal prehabilitation program may benefit patients with these risk factors as well (addressed elsewhere).

Certain types of cancer and cancer treatments will require that special attention be paid to specific features preoperatively in order to facilitate carefully coordinated intra- and postoperative management (cancer therapies and perioperative implications addressed elsewhere). This is especially important for cancers that have the potential to cause airway compromise or hemodynamic disturbance intraoperatively.

Cancer-Specific Concerns

Patients with head and neck cancer warrant a detailed airway examination ideally by a practitioner experienced in airway management. A careful history should be performed to elicit symptoms that may suggest airway involvement, such as dyspnea, stridor, and voice change. Imaging should also be carefully reviewed preoperatively. Normal anatomic landmarks may be obscured, and a preoperative examination should be performed to document any abnormalities that might suggest difficult airway management[20] (addressed in detail elsewhere).

Similarly, a patient with solid tumor with involvement of major cardiovascular or airway structures must be carefully assessed preoperatively with a review of imaging. Especially in the case of anterior mediastinal and other large intrathoracic masses, careful communication and coordination between the surgeon and anesthesiologist preoperatively is imperative in order to ensure plans for intraoperative management, should severe hemodynamic or airway disturbances occur.[21]

Presence of malignant ascites or pleural effusions may have significant hemodynamic and respiratory significance during anesthetic management. Especially if drainage of ascites is planned intraoperatively, fluid needs to be carefully managed intraoperatively. Patients may benefit from preoperative drainage of fluid to prevent large fluid shifts or difficulty with ventilation intraoperatively.

Anemia is frequently seen preoperatively in cancer patients. It is usually multifactorial, as it can be related to blood loss, hemolysis, underlying hereditary disease, renal insufficiency, nutritional deficiency, chronic disease, cancer treatment, or a combination of these. Cancer patients should be screened for anemia early and treatment started as soon as possible to avoid transfusion of blood products whenever possible [22] (addressed elsewhere).

Conclusion

As previously stated, medical comorbidities, including cancer treatment–related side effects, should be carefully noted and commented on for perioperative management concerns. The preoperative visit should also be viewed as a chance to impact those lifestyle behaviors that correlate with poorer outcomes, such as smoking and sedentary lifestyle.[23] The perioperative consultation should also highlight immediate medical management concerns such as anticoagulation and management of devices, including, but not limited to, pacemakers, defibrillators, and insulin pumps. In summary, a thoughtful and concise perioperative evaluation of the cancer patient should anticipate potential complications from the cancer itself, previous cancer treatment, and medical comorbidities for the patient undergoing surgery.

References

1. National Institute for Health and Care Excellence. Routine Preoperative Tests for Elective Surgery. NICE Guideline [NG45]. 2016. Available at https://www.nice.org.uk/guidance/ng45.
2. Edwards AF, Forest DJ. Preoperative laboratory testing. *Anesthesiol Clin*. 2018;36(4):493–507.
3. Sinard RJ, Tobin EJ, Mazzaferri EL, et al. Hypothyroidism after treatment for nonthyroid head and neck cancer. *Arch Otolaryngol Head Neck Surg*. 2000;126(5):652–657.
4. Xu J, Cao Y. Radiation-induced carotid artery stenosis: a comprehensive review of the literature. *Interv Neurol*. 2014;2(4): 183–192.
5. Blitz JD, Kendale SM, Jain SK, Cuff GE, Kim JT, Rosenberg AD. Preoperative evaluation clinic visit is associated with decreased risk of in-hospital postoperative mortality. *Anesthesiology*. 2016;125(2):280–294.
6. Blitz JD, Mabry C. Designing and running a preoperative clinic. *Anesthesiol Clin*. 2018;36(4):479–491.
7. Sahai S. Abstracts of the 2008 international MASCC/ISOO symposium. *Support Care Cancer*. 2008;16(6):619–756.
8. Epstein RH, Dexter F, Schwenk ES, Witkowski TA. Bypass of an anesthesiologist-directed preoperative evaluation clinic results in greater first-case tardiness and turnover times. *J Clin Anesth*. 2017;41:112–119.
9. Nelson SE, Li G, Shi H, Terekhov M, Ehrenfeld JM, Wanderer JP. The impact of reduction of testing at a preoperative evaluation clinic for elective cases: value added without adverse outcomes. *J Clin Anesth*. 2019;55:92–99.
10. McDonald SR, Heflin MT, Whitson HE, et al. Association of integrated care coordination with postsurgical outcomes in high-risk older adults: the perioperative optimization of senior health (POSH) initiative. *JAMA Surg*. 2018;153(5):454–462.
11. Sahai SK, Zalpour A, Rozner MA. Preoperative evaluation of the oncology patient. *Anesthesiol Clin*. 2009;27(4):805–822.
12. Sahai SK, Ismail H. Perioperative implications of neoadjuvant therapies and optimization strategies for cancer surgery. *Curr Anesthesiol Rep*. 2015;5(3):305–317.
13. Fleisher LA, Fleischmann KE, Auerbach AD, et al. 2014 ACC/AHA guideline on perioperative cardiovascular evaluation and management of patients undergoing noncardiac surgery: executive summary: a report of the American College of Cardiology/American Heart Association Task Force on Practice Guidelines. *Circulation*. 2014;130(24):2215–2245.
14. Reilly DF, McNeely MJ, Doerner D, et al. Self-reported exercise tolerance and the risk of serious perioperative complications. *Arch Intern Med*. 1999;159(18):2185–2192.
15. Wijeysundera DN, Pearse RM, Shulman MA, et al. Assessment of functional capacity before major non-cardiac surgery: an international, prospective cohort study. *Lancet*. 2018;391(10140):2631–2640.
16. Chow WB, Rosenthal RA, Merkow RP, et al. Optimal preoperative assessment of the geriatric surgical patient: a best practices guideline from the American College of Surgeons National Surgical Quality Improvement Program and the American Geriatrics Society. *J Am Coll Surg*. 2012;215(4):453–466.
17. Lin HS, Watts NM, Peel JN, Hubbard RE. Frailty and postoperative outcomes in older surgical patients: a systematic review. *BMC Geriatr*. 2016;16(1):157.
18. Goldstein DP, Sklar MC, de Almeida JR, et al. Frailty as a predictor of outcomes in patients undergoing head and neck cancer surgery. *Laryngoscope*. 2019;130(5):E340–E345.
19. Alvarez-Nebreda ML, Bentov N, Urman RD, et al. Recommendations for preoperative management of frailty from the society for perioperative assessment and quality improvement (SPAQI). *J Clin Anesth*. 2018;47:33–42.
20. Artime CA, Roy S, Hagberg CA. The difficult airway. *Otolaryngol Clin North Am*. 2019;52(6):1115–1125.
21. Rath L, Gullahorn G, Connolly N, Pratt T, Boswell G, Cornelissen C. Anterior mediastinal mass biopsy and resection: anesthetic techniques and perioperative concerns. *Semin Cardiothorac Vasc Anesth*. 2012;16(4):235–242.
22. Rodgers GM. A perspective on the evolution of management of cancer- and chemotherapy-induced anemia. *J Natl Compr Canc Netw*. 2012;10(4):434–437.
23. van Rooijen SJ, Molenaar CJL, Schep G, et al. Making patients fit for surgery: introducing a four pillar multimodal prehabilitation program in colorectal cancer. *Am J Phys Med Rehabil*. 2019;98(10):888–896.

15

Functional Assessment and Prehabilitation

HILMY ISMAIL, GABRIELE BALDINI, CELENA SCHEEDE BERGDAHL, AND FRANCO CARLI

The Physiologic Impact of Cancer and Surgery on Patient Function

As the volume and complexity of surgical procedures will increase in the next decades, the age and number of associated comorbid conditions of patients presenting for these procedures is also projected to rise.[1] In this context, preventative strategies aimed at reducing postoperative complications by mitigating the stress response to cancer and surgery before it occurs is an area of increasing clinical activity and research.

The physical, metabolic, emotional, and systemic impacts of cancer on patient function while waiting for surgery are compounded by the effects of age, frailty, comorbidities, and cancer treatment. Frailty is a syndrome associated with decline across multiple organ systems with effects on cognitive, psychologic, and social well being, resulting in impaired homeostatic reserve and physical activity. [2–4] The presence of cancer exacerbates the influence of disability and chronic disease on frailty. Over half of older patients with cancer have frailty or prefrailty, and this results in a progressive decrease in resiliency and adaptive capacity to stressors such as surgery and related neoadjuvant treatments such as chemotherapy and radiotherapy. This makes frail patients extremely vulnerable to postoperative complications.[5]

Patients with cancer diagnoses awaiting surgery frequently lose lean body mass (LBM) due to age-related factors and immobility, while fat mass remains constant or increases. This combination of decreased LBM and increased body mass index (BMI), defined as sarcopenic obesity (SO), represents an extreme state of vulnerability to adverse postoperative outcomes. Cancer-related cachexia is also another multifactorial syndrome characterized by an ongoing loss of skeletal muscle mass (with or without loss of fat mass) and leads to progressive functional impairment. Notwithstanding the fact that there remains considerable variation in definitions of these terms, methods of assessment, and cutoff values for these entities, underpinning many of these overlapping concepts is the common thread of reduction in functional capacity and activity.[6]

In patients presenting for cancer surgery, the effects of frailty, multiple comorbidities, sedentary lifestyle, and neoadjuvant treatments have been described as "multiple hits" to the oxygen cascade[7] and cardiovascular reserve capacity (CVRC).[8] These "multiple hits" result in progressive reduction in patients' functional capacity.

The impact of a cancer diagnosis requiring surgery has been shown to adversely affect all modalities of quality-of-life measures, especially affecting the domains of vitality and mental health.[9] Among the common emotional responses to a cancer diagnosis, fear, anxiety, and worry appear to have the most relevance to patients' abilities to cope with the diagnosis and make choices related to their treatments. These emotions can both facilitate decision-making and at the same time serve as barriers for making choices available to them, such as prehabilitation.[10]

The Surgical Insult and the Importance of Preparing Patients for Stress

Similar to increased activity and intense exercise, the stress of surgery and the postoperative period are associated with an increase in oxygen consumption ($\dot{V}O_2$) especially in states of acute inflammation[11] or sepsis.[12] The inability to match oxygen delivery to increased oxygen demand is associated with anaerobic metabolism, and this is not sustainable, neither during exercise nor in the postoperative period.[13] This inability to reduce oxygen debt at times of "stress" has been putatively proposed as the underlying mechanism for developing postoperative complications.[14,15] In a meta-analysis of more than 3632 patients with adult onset cancer, exercise was found to be safe and effective in increasing $\dot{V}O_{2peak}$ compared with no exercise.[16]

Multiple clinical studies, including the recent Measurement of Exercise Tolerance before Surgery (METS) study[17] and a study by Barberan-Garcia et al.,[18] have demonstrated the significance of oxygen carrying mechanisms in terms of prognosticating and optimizing patients for postoperative complications and long-term disease-free survival after major cancer surgery.

The Enhanced Recovery After Surgery (ERAS) program has identified some determinants of the surgical stress response, which lead to hyperglycemia and protein catabolism. With the understanding of the pathophysiology of the stress response and insulin resistance, ERAS elements, such as minimally invasive surgery, multimodal analgesia, oral carbohydrate drink, early mobilization, and early nutrition, have shown an impact on postoperative recovery.[19]

More recent trials that have combined multimodal prehabilitation with ERAS programs appear to result in increased postoperative functional capacity and improved disease-free survival.[20–22]

Changes brought about at various points in the oxygen cascade, such as optimization of cardiac output, improved ventilatory capacity, matching of lung ventilation to perfusion, increased oxygen carrying capacity, improved antiinflammatory effects, and increased end-organ capillary and mitochondrial density, may explain the possible impact of perioperative optimization.

Functional Assessment and Risk Stratification

Preoperative risk assessment is commonly based on the presence of medical comorbidities and on the invasiveness or clinical setting of the surgical procedure (elective vs. emergency). As a result, physicians commonly utilize general or organ-specific scoring systems that include a variety of medical conditions and/or surgical factors to stratify preoperative risk.[23]

Despite extensive evidence demonstrating that poor preoperative functional capacity is associated with prolonged hospital stay, increased morbidity and mortality, decreased quality of life, and level of independence,[17,24–26] the importance of measuring preoperative functional capacity is frequently underestimated and inconsistently or inadequately measured. Recently, the American College of Surgeons National Surgical Quality Improvement Program (ACS NSQIP) Surgical Risk Calculator incorporated the level of functional dependency and basic geriatric assessment measures to predict not only complications, but also functional decline, postoperative delirium, the use of a mobility aid, and the probability to be discharged to a nursing or rehabilitation facility (https://riskcalculator.facs.org/RiskCalculator/).

Aging, comorbidities, physical fitness, and nutritional and psychologic status are the main pillars of functional capacity. Preoperative functional capacity of oncologic patients can be weakened by several factors: some related to their underlying diseases, such as malnutrition, cachexia, sarcopenia, frailty, depression, anxiety, and anemia; others related to the oncologic treatment, such as chemotherapy, radiotherapy, and/or surgery.

As preoperative functional capacity is complex in nature, its assessment cannot rely on a single preoperative test. Moreover, measuring functional capacity with multiple tools could be particularly useful when patients have physical limitations that prevent daily activities (e.g., musculoskeletal or neurologic disorders, obesity or pain) and therefore the use of certain tests. Today, several tests can be used in the preoperative period to estimate patients' functional capacity (Table 15.1).[27]

(a) The Cardiopulmonary Exercise Test (CPET) is considered the gold standard for measuring cardiorespiratory capacity. It is a noninvasive stress test that measures patient's functional reserve, providing objective information on the integrated cardiopulmonary and musculoskeletal function. It allows for the determination of the oxygen consumption at the anaerobic threshold ($\dot{V}O_{2AT}$) and the peak oxygen consumption ($\dot{V}O_{2peak}$) through the analysis of breath-by-breath ventilation volumes, oxygen consumption, and carbon dioxide

TABLE 15.1 Utility of Preoperative Cardiopulmonary Exercise Testing (CPET)

	Grade of the Recommendation
To estimate the likelihood of perioperative morbidity and mortality and contribute to preoperative risk assessment	B
To inform the processes of multidisciplinary shared decision-making and consent	C
To guide clinical decisions about the most appropriate level of perioperative care (ward vs. critical care)	C
To direct preoperative referrals/interventions to optimize comorbidities	C
To identify previously unsuspected pathology	B
To evaluate the effects of neoadjuvant cancer therapies including chemotherapy and radiotherapy.	B
To guide prehabilitation and rehabilitation training programs	B
To guide intraoperative anesthetic practice	D

production.[28] These variables inform the perioperative physician about the patient's ability to withstand the increased metabolic demand induced by surgical stress. Several studies conducted in different surgical populations have demonstrated that poor functional capacity as measured by different CPET-derived variables, such as $\dot{V}O_{2AT}$, $\dot{V}O_{2peak}$, or ventilatory equivalent for CO_2 at the AT ($\dot{V}E/\dot{V}CO_2$ at AT), are associated with adverse outcomes.[17,24–26] In general, a $\dot{V}O_{2AT}$ <10–11 mL/kg/min and a $\dot{V}O_{2peak}$ <15 mL/kg/h may identify high-risk patients. $\dot{V}O_{2AT}$ and $\dot{V}O_{2peak}$ should always be expressed as a percentage of the age-predicted $\dot{V}O_{2max}$, because $\dot{V}O_2$ physiologically declines with age. These variables not only inform about surgical risk, but also guide physicians to plan the appropriate intensity of perioperative care (e.g., advanced monitoring, intensive care admission vs. high-dependency unit vs. surgical wards), and develop tailored preoperative interventions aiming at improving functional capacity and thus attenuating surgical risk.[18,28] However, performing CPET is not always feasible, and it is resource-intensive and costly. Moreover, interpretation of its results requires appropriate training, as $\dot{V}O_{2AT}$ can be influenced by several factors and produce misleading results. These could consequently lead to an inappropriate clinical management.[29]

It is common practice to measure preoperatively functional capacity by estimating metabolic equivalents (METs). This is also recommended by several international guidelines on preoperative risk assessment.[30,31] In fact, estimation of METs is a key element in deciding whether patients will require further preoperative evaluation and if patients are "fit" for surgery. Traditionally METs equivalent less than 4 (i.e., the ability of a patient to climb 1–2 flights of stairs in the absence of symptoms) has been associated with an increase in complications.[30] However, recent evidence strongly discourages from continuing to subjectively assess preoperative functional capacity. In fact, the results of a recent international prospective cohort study, including 1401 patients (METS trial), have clearly demonstrated that preoperative subjective assessment of functional capacity (estimating METs by asking patients questions about common daily activities) is inadequate for predicting 30-day death or complications after major elective noncardiac surgery.[17] Most importantly, the authors demonstrated that a subjective assessment of poor functional capacity (<4 METs) had a sensitivity of 19.2% (95% confidence interval [CI], 14.2–25.0) and a specificity of 94.7% (95% CI, 93.2–95.9) for identifying patients with peak oxygen consumption of <14 mL/kg/min (equivalent to <4 METs). These important findings demonstrate that preoperative physicians should correctly identify patients reporting poor fitness (positive likelihood ratio, 3.8). However, among those physicians rating adequate exercise tolerance, poor cardiopulmonary fitness is missed 84% of the time (negative likelihood ratio, 0.85).[17] This implies that several high-risk patients with poor functional capacity, and that could be potentially optimized, are improperly "cleared" for surgery when objective and more sensitive measures of physical fitness are not utilized in the preoperative period. These findings have also been confirmed by the results of the recent National Health and Nutrition Examination Survey conducted in 522 nonsurgical patients.[32]

(b) Dynamic tests, such as the 6- and 2-min walking tests, shuttle walking test, timed up and go (TUG), and gait speed, have also been used to measure preoperative functional capacity and predict surgical risk and postoperative recovery.[27] The 6- and 2-min walking tests evaluate the ability to maintain a moderate level of physical activity by measuring the distance covered over 2 or 6 min. These tests are easy to apply and can be used as screening tools to identify high-risk patients with reduced functional capacity who deserve a more thorough and accurate evaluation (e.g., CPET). Moreover, in high-risk patients, 6-minute walk test (6MWT) distance weakly correlates with both 12-month disability-free survival (Spearman's correlation coefficient [ρ] = –0.23; $P < 0.0005$) and 30-day 15-item quality of recovery ($\rho = 0.14$; $P < 0.001$).[33] Its sensitivity and specificity improve when patients walk short distances (<370 m).[33]

(c) The Duke Activity Status Index (DASI) is a self-administered questionnaire that was originally developed and validated as a measure of functional capacity and to predict $\dot{V}O_{2peak}$ in nonsurgical cardiovascular patients.[34] In fact, this score moderately correlates with $\dot{V}O_{2peak}$ ($\rho = 0.58$, $P < 0.001$).[34] In contrast to the 6MWT or the CPET, where the assessment of functional capacity depends on the patient's performance during the test, the DASI includes measures of physical and emotional fitness covering a period of time, thus better reflecting overall patient functional capacity. Not surprisingly, the DASI has been recently shown to predict 30-day death or myocardial infarction after major elective noncardiac surgery (adjusted odds ratio [AOR], 0.91; 95% CI, 0.83–0.99; $P = 0.03$), while $\dot{V}O_{2peak}$ or N-terminal pro-B-type natriuretic peptide (NT-pro BNP) have not.[17] In the same study, the DASI also predicted 30-day death or myocardial injury (AOR, 0.96; 95% CI, 0.92–0.99; $P = 0.05$).[17] Interestingly, in a secondary analysis of the METS trial, the DASI predicts 12-month disability-free survival (AOR, 1.06; $P < 0.0005$), better than the 6MWT (area under the curve [AUC], 0.63; 95% CI 0.57–0.70) and the $\dot{V}O_{2peak}$ (AUC, 0.60; 95% CI, 0.53–0.67),[33] further confirming the clinical utility of this multidimensional assessment tool.

In an observational study of 50 elderly patients undergoing major abdominal surgery and in whom functional capacity was measured with different tests, a DASI score ≥46 has been proposed as a threshold to identify high-risk patients ($\dot{V}O_{2AT}$ ≤11 mL/kg/min and $\dot{V}O_{2peak}$ ≤15 mL/kg/min; positive predictive value, 1.00).[35] However, it underestimated functional capacity in almost two-thirds of low-risk patients (negative predictive value, 0.40).[35] These results suggest that a DASI score <46 should not be used as a single test to identify high-risk patients. Moreover, larger validation studies are needed to confirm this threshold and its association with clinical outcomes.

(d) Most recently, plasma brain natriuretic peptides such as the brain natriuretic peptide (BNP) or the NT-pro BNP have been proposed as biomarkers to estimate cardiovascular risk[36] and functional capacity.[17] BNPs are mainly produced by cardiomyocytes in response to ventricular and atrial stretching (mechanical strain), but other causes such as inflammation and hypoxia can trigger its release. High plasma BNP and NT-proBNP concentrations are frequently measured in patients with a variety of chronic and acute cardiac conditions, such as ventricular hypertrophy, diastolic dysfunction, and congestive heart failure.[37] In this clinical context, the prognostic value of plasma BNPs has been well established. Similarly, the prognostic value of plasma BNP/NT-pro BNP has also been demonstrated in surgical patients undergoing major noncardiac surgery.[38] Patients with high preoperative BNP/NT-pro BNP concentrations were more likely to develop postoperative 30-day cardiac complications, including death, cardiovascular death, and myocardial infarction (odds ratio [OR], 44.2; 95% CI, 7.6–257).[38] Recently, the ability of the NT-pro BNP to estimate functional capacity has been evaluated.[17] The results of the METS trial demonstrate that NT-pro BNP negatively correlates with $\dot{V}o_{2peak}$ (Spearman $\rho = -0.21$, $P < 0.0001$), and positively with the DASI (Spearman $\rho = 0.43$, $P < 0.0001$). However, it predicts 30-day death or myocardial injury (AOR, 1.78; 95% CI, 1.21–2.62; $P = 0.003$), 1-year death (AOR, 2.91; 95% CI, 1.54–5.49; $P = 0.001$), but not disability-free survival (AUC, 0.56; 95% CI, 0.49–0.63, $P = 0.08$) or in hospital moderate or severe complications (AUC, 1.10; 95% CI, 0.77–1.57; $P = 0.61$).[17,33] Estimating preoperative functional capacity by measuring preoperative BNPs may be useful in patients with physical impairments or in the preoperative setting with limited personnel or resources. However, further research is needed to understand the causes of high plasma BNP levels and to validate these biomarkers as accurate measures of functional capacity.

Prehabilitation

Prehabilitation can be defined as the process that initiates before surgery and enables patients to enhance their functional capacity in anticipation of surgical stressors. The term, as proposed by Topp, is opposed to rehabilitation where the intervention occurs after surgery.[39]

Another definition of prehabilitation for oncology was proposed by Silver and is more comprehensive: "A process on the cancer continuum of care that occurs between the time of cancer diagnosis and the beginning of acute treatment and includes physical and psychological assessments that establish a baseline functional level, identify impairments, and provide interventions that promote physical and psychological health to reduce the incidence and/or severity of future impairments."[40]

The explanation of the term prehabilitation is based on understanding that by applying an interventional program aiming at improving functional ability before the stress of surgery, patients would retain a higher level of functional reserve over their entire surgical admission. It would then mean that postoperative recovery would occur more rapidly compared to patients who remain inactive throughout the whole surgical admission (Fig. 15.1).[41]

While the prehabilitation cancer literature in the first instance focused on exercise as a single modality intervention, recent studies have highlighted the importance of other modalities such as nutrition, either together with exercise or alone.[41] The addition of psychologic strategies to the other two elements, as part of the prehabilitation program, in cancer patients with depression demonstrates how important the trimodal approach is in the enhancement of functional capacity.[42] This model represents a much more holistic approach and is based on the understanding that physical

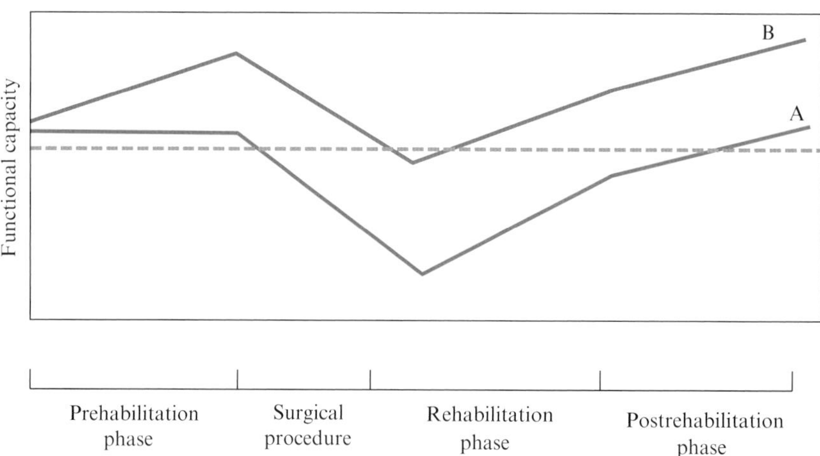

• **Fig. 15.1** (A) Functional capacity throughout the surgical process (B) Perioperative trajectory of multimodal prehabilitation, rehabilitation, and control groups Ref. 42.

fitness, optimal nutrition, and emotional well being are closely interrelated and complement each other.

Furthermore, the more general scope of prehabilitation recognizes that nonexercise interventions, as mentioned above, may also be beneficial to a specific population, as well as prescribing exercise as a single modality. This supports the concept that prehabilitation is not a "one size fits all" program but rather involves specific, individualized assessments and structured interventions delivered by a team of experts.

Successful surgery is dependent upon many factors—anesthesia, surgery, surgical care, and most importantly on how well the patient is able to return to a physically and psychologically healthy state. While fast track and ERAS protocols have been shown to shorten the length of hospitalization, it is important to consider how well, physically, nutritionally, and emotionally, patients need to be before surgery in order to facilitate their recovery process once discharged from the hospital. In view of this, there is strong published evidence that low cardiorespiratory fitness not only limits access to surgery and other therapies, but also that when patients are operated on, the risk of postoperative complications, and mortality is high.[43] The question is whether surgeons wish to operate on deconditioned frail elderly patients or run the risk of the cancer spreading due to delays to surgery. A commonly accepted position would be to accept a delay of 4 to 6 weeks of prehabilitation in patients presenting for high-risk surgical procedures.

Recent studies have shown that prolonging the time interval between diagnosis and surgery does not impact the immediate- and long-term outcome in patients scheduled for elective colorectal cancer resection. This would imply that optimization of patients' health status can be justified in those who are at high risk of postoperative complications.[44,45]

Prehabilitation not only prepares the cancer patient in anticipation of the surgery, but also plays an important role in continuing the best comprehensive care and subsequent cancer treatment, as chemotherapy, radiotherapy, and hormonal treatment are all known to have a negative impact on functional capacity. This can also be said for those patients who undergo neoadjuvant therapy followed by surgery. In fact, poor physical and nutritional statuses have been identified as important reasons for low adherence and responsiveness to neoadjuvant therapy. In addition, delays in the commencement of adjuvant treatment due to poor physical status are associated with higher mortality rates.

In light of these important concerns, there is a growing interest in prehabilitation as a part of a cancer care continuum for the prevention and/or attenuation of treatment-driven disorders, improvement in access, and adherence to treatment.

While in principle all patients anticipating cancer surgery can be enrolled in a prehabilitation program, there is a need to assess individual patients and determine whether some conditions can be modified during the time interval between diagnosis and surgery. This is particularly true for different types of cancer, the age of the patient, comorbidities, and the site where the prehabilitation can be conducted. While some comorbidities and patient factors cannot be modified, others, such as smoking cessation, sedentary activity, poor nutrition, and high anxiety, can be amenable to modification. This requires a concerted action by an interdisciplinary group working on a common platform. Patients who are frail with low fitness and low functional reserve can improve their functional capacity over a minimum period of 4 weeks before colorectal cancer surgery when multimodal prehabilitation is administered.[46] In the case of malnutrition, which is very common in cancer patients, a minimum of 7–10 days of either enteral or parenteral nutrition is recommended.[47]

The initial assessment of patient fitness from the physical, nutritional, and mental point of view would determine the necessity to plan an intervention that includes various elements with the intention to create a synergy between them. This of course needs to consider patient comorbidities and access to care. All these elements represent the potential risk factors (sedentary activity, malnutrition, anxiety, depression) that feature in the pathogenesis of cancer. Therefore it becomes necessary to determine how to modulate these elements to counteract the negative impact of these factors on outcome. The concept of the multimodal, synergistic effect of these elements needs to be integrated with other interventions, such as the optimization of medical morbidities, smoking and alcohol cessation, and modification of surgical care within the (ERAS) pathway programs.

Exercise and Physical Activity for the Surgical Cancer Patient

It is becoming increasing clear that a paradigm shift must occur, moving from the traditional belief that a patient must rest in preparation for surgery to a more proactive approach with the goal of optimizing patient functional status in the preoperative time frame. Physical inactivity and bed rest are associated with insulin and protein resistance, which together contribute to increased systemic inflammation and loss of muscle mass.[48] This may, in addition, further exacerbate preexisting age-related comorbidities, such as low cardiovascular fitness, sarcopenia, and insulin resistance/diabetes. All of these factors not only hinder the cancer patient's ability to cope with acute treatment, such as surgery, chemotherapy, or radiation therapy, but can also impact the patient's recovery and potentially, postpone subsequent intervention.[49]

A conventional approach to improving patient physical status focuses on rehabilitating the patient after treatment. Although there are clear benefits from posttreatment intervention, it may be more challenging to initiate and adhere to major behavioral changes such as commencing an exercise program when the patient is both mentally and physically stressed and in the early stages of recovery.[49] This may be especially challenging when the individual is already facing a diminished functional status resulting from sedentarism in the pretreatment phase, as depicted in Fig. 15.1. Recent advances in the area of prehabilitation support the notion that the pretreatment phase is an important opportunity to both physically

TABLE 15.2 Goals, Guidelines, Specifics, and Strategies for Exercise, Physical Activity, and Nutrition in the Presurgical Period

Goal	Guideline	Specifics	Strategies
Improve cardiovascular fitness	*Accumulate 150 min of moderate to vigorous activity per week.*	*150 min can be divided into multiple sessions per week (i.e., 30 min per session, 5 times per week). Intensity should be between 5–8/10 on Borg scale.*	*Swimming, jogging, brisk walk, aerobics class, or other continuous activity that the patient can perform safely and enjoy.*
Improve skeletal muscle fitness	*Exercise all major muscle groups, for at least one set of 8 to 12 repetitions. Patient should find last repetition challenging.*	*Strength exercises should happen every second day to allow for adequate recovery. If patient finds it easy to complete 12 repetitions, resistance should be increased. Ensure that motion is controlled and both concentric and eccentric phases are equal in velocity.*	*Resistance bands, hand weights, barbells, gym equipment. Pay attention to strain at joints.*
Increase amount of weekly physical activity	*Accumulate a minimum of 30 min of physical activity per day.*	*Light intensity activity, between 3 and 4/10 on Borg scale, can be broken up over days.*	*Patient should perform physical activities that may include gardening, walking, bicycle rides, dancing, housekeeping*
Improve balance	*Include balance exercises if necessary.*	*Perform exercises that involve balance on one leg or agility tests. Activities will be dependent on abilities of patient.*	*Patient can perform yoga, tai chi, and other exercises specific to needs.*
Improve flexibility	*Include flexibility exercises.*	*Hold stretches for at least 20 s to point of "tightness" but not to pain. Activities will be dependent on abilities of patient.*	*Patient can perform lunges, attempt to touch toes (standing or seated), attempt to "scratch back."*
Reduce sitting/sedentary time	*Provide strategies for breaking up sitting time.*	*Patient should not be immobile for more than 30 min without moving or standing.*	*Every 30 min, patient should use strategies to move or stand.*

Goal	Strategy
Establish whether a nutrition-based intervention is required in the presurgical period	*Perform a detailed analysis of patient dietary habits, along with relevant hospital tests at baseline.*
Intervene if patient is malnourished or at risk for malnourishment	*Provide nutritional counseling or supplementation and follow up to ensure patient improvement.*
Time protein ingestion throughout day	*Plan daily diet with patient to include protein (approximately 25–35 g) at each meal.*
Time protein ingestion postexercise to take advantage of "anabolic window"	*Ingest an easily digestible protein (i.e., whey protein) within 90 min postexercise.*

and mentally optimize the patient in order to mitigate the decline in functional status and enhance the recovery process.[42]

Physical activity has been defined as any bodily movement produced by skeletal muscles that results in energy expenditure. Exercise, however, encompasses a subset of physical activity that is planned, structured, and repetitive and aims to improve or maintain physical fitness. Physical fitness describes and quantifies a set of attributes that are either health- or skill-related and can be measured by specific tests or assessments.[50] These tests or assessments will not only provide insight into the patient's baseline but also how each individual responds to the exercise stimulus. In order to optimize patient functional status and encourage program adherence, a comprehensive prescription may include both a physical activity and exercise component. The exercise component, in particular, should also be accompanied by regular assessments in order to ensure that the patient is training effectively. This combination will not only serve as a backbone for presurgical intervention but can also provide important groundwork for the postoperative period and beyond.

A structured exercise program includes either some or all of the following training elements, depending on the specific needs and abilities of each patient: cardiovascular, resistance, flexibility, neuromotor (balance), and respiratory (Table 15.2). Each exercise session should also include a warm up and cool down, which allows for the patient to physiologically transition in and out of exercise.

Exercise prescription is based on the FITT principle, which specifies the frequency (how many times per week?), intensity (how hard should the patient be working?), time (how long should each exercise session be?), and type (what kind of exercise should they be doing?). This provides the structure, reproducibility, and overview that will not only

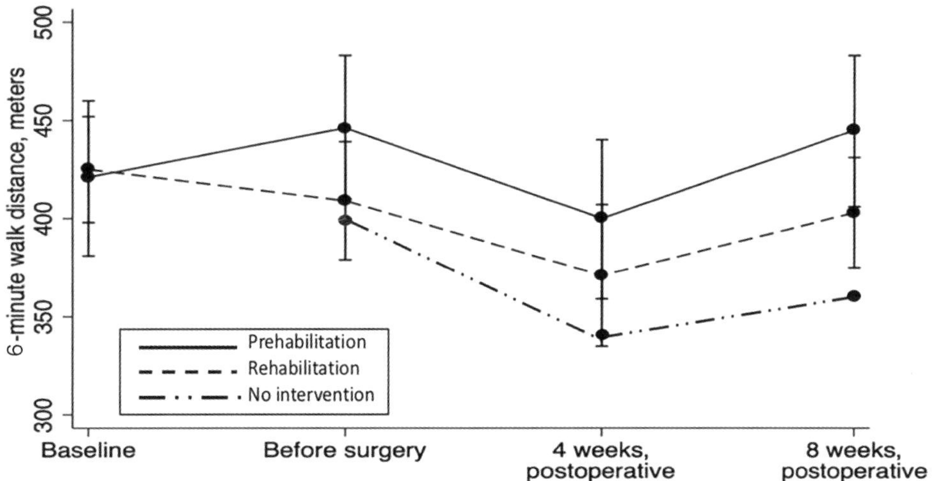

• **Fig. 15.2** Modified Borg scale. This scale allows for patients to monitor themselves throughout the training period and make self-adjustments in intensity to accommodate periods where they either improve due to training (higher intensity to maintain same target number on scale) or are fatigued due to illness or treatment (lower intensity to maintain same target number on scale). The patient or health professional may point or refer to a number (out of a scale of 20) to reflect intensity.

help with understanding what the patient is able to do but also when the program should be progressed and by how much.[49] The exercise prescription must be progressed or intensified as the body adapts to provide an ongoing physiologic stimulus. If the individual trains at an intensity that they are physically accustomed to or that is below their functional capacity, it will result in a training plateau (i.e., no further improvements) or detraining. A benefit of using a self-adjusting scale, such as the Borg scale (Fig. 15.2), not only allows for the patient to be able to easily monitor themselves through a variety of training modalities but also compensates for the effects of training; therefore as they adapt to the exercise, they will have to work harder to maintain the same intensity range.[51] Monitoring intensity by heart rate is also self-adjusting but cannot be relied upon if the patient is taking a chronotropic pharmacologic agent.

Adequate recovery between bouts of exercise must be also be considered in order to maximize the benefits of the training program, and prevent fatigue and physical maladaptation. Jones et al. provided a review suggesting a comprehensive approach to, and a rationale for, exercise prescription specific to the cancer population.[52] Rest between sets or repetitions, between bouts, and between sessions are important components of comprehensive exercise prescriptions.

Current recommendations for the general population include 150 min of moderate or 75 min of vigorous physical activity per week, which is well tolerated by cancer patients in the presurgical time frame.[53] For the purpose of prescription, these recommendations are typically broken down into bouts of aerobic training that should occur at least every second day, for approximately 30–45 minute, at a moderate level of intensity (e.g., 50%–75% of age-predicted maximum heart rate or 13–16 on the Borg scale). How this exercise is performed (i.e., cycling, walking, jogging, rowing machine, swimming, elliptical machine) is dependent on the availability of equipment, and patient preference and capability. More recently, to address both preferred modalities, as well as time restraints, high-intensity interval training has been introduced to patients during prehabilitation programs and shown to be an effective and well-tolerated means of exercise prescription.[54] Resistance exercises should be performed at least twice a week, targeting all major muscle groups, and performed at a weight where 8 to 12 repetitions are possible but difficult to achieve at the end of the set. Intensity can also be assessed by the Borg scale, as well as by a percentage of repetition maximum (either estimated or measured), elastic band color, percentage of body weight, or time (either holding weight or how many repetitions of a movement in a given period of time). Programs, as previously mentioned, may also include flexibility, neuromotor or balance, and respiratory muscle training as determined by the needs and preferences of the patient.[55,56]

Physical activity, as per the definition provided here, is also important to include in patient education, as it decreases overall sedentary behavior. These recommendations may include post dinner walks, activity for fun (such as sports, games, or dancing), hikes, bicycle rides, or gardening. Minimizing sitting time is also an important approach to preventing cardiovascular and metabolic complications, which are independent from the amount of exercise performed.[57]

When prescribing exercise as a component of prehabilitation, it is important to consider the patients' capabilities/capacities and their willingness to adhere to the program. If they do not exercise or perform any physical activity, either because they cannot or do not wish to, this will impact the prehabilitation program. In addition, both the level of supervision required and whether the program is home-based or to be performed in a clinical environment will impact the intensity and modality of the exercise, especially for the sake of patient safety. Concurrent medical conditions must be identified, especially those which may limit the ability of the patient to participate in a safe and effective manner. It is also important to identify clear program goals and determine whether they are consistent with the available resources. Last, to maximize adherence, there must be a dialogue with the patient in order for the program to be meaningful for them.[57] The successful implementation of a prehabilitation program in the critical presurgical period is strategic for changing behaviors and improving functional capacity.[58]

Nutrition and the Importance of Protein for the Colorectal Cancer Patient

Nutrition is a critical element of an effective multimodal approach to prehabilitation.[59] Cancer patients who are malnourished are in a suboptimal state for subsequent surgery, chemotherapy, or recovery. Malnutrition is related to adverse outcomes for treatment and independently predicts poor survival.[59] Approximately 50% of deaths worldwide are attributed to the cancer types most associated with malnutrition, such as pancreatic, esophageal, gastric, lung, hepatic, and colorectal. Clinically, it remains a challenge to determine which patients are malnourished because many who are overweight or obese do not fit into the "at risk" categories as defined by weight loss but require intervention nonetheless.[60] The development of standardized nutritional care pathways is complex and depends on the individual needs of each patient and the services available. In order to be effective, nutrition needs to be addressed in a multimodal context throughout the care continuum for cancer patients.[61]

Nutritional prehabilitation should focus on determining whether malnourishment or risk of malnourishment exists. A detailed analysis of patient dietary habits, along with any relevant hospital tests, should help to establish whether a nutrition-based intervention is required in the presurgical period.[62] Nutritional guidelines advise early screening (i.e., immediately after diagnosis), followed by a more complete assessment in the case that risk has been determined. A nutritionist or dietitian can provide the patient with individualized counseling, taking into consideration their estimated resting energy expenditure, lifestyle factors, habitual food intake, and preferences, along with disease state and symptoms. Effective dietary counseling involves patient education and motivation to initiate behavioral changes that reflect the altered nutritional requirements of their disease state.[63]

In conditions associated with stress and tissue injury, such as cancer and its treatment, additional protein is necessary to compensate for acute-phase reactants that respond to inflammation and the synthesis of proteins involved in immune function and wound healing.[63,64] In addition, protein is also important for the maintenance of lean muscle mass, which is required for the preservation or amelioration of functional capacity. Malnourishment negatively impacts functional capacity due to the lack of substrates necessary for metabolism and anabolic signaling.[42] Although the exact amount of protein required in this patient population has not been determined, The European Society for Clinical Nutrition and Metabolism (ESPEN) expert panels recommend a protein intake of a minimum of 1 g/kg/day and preferably 1.5 g/kg/day. These values are based on previously published values that range from a minimum protein supply of 1 g/kg/day and a target supply of 1.2–2 g/kg/day, with higher values being preferable under conditions of physical inactivity and systemic inflammation.[59]

The two most important determinants of lean muscle mass are food intake and contractile activity,[65] thus highlighting the important interactions between nutrition and exercise/physical activity.[59] After exercise, in particular resistance-based, the amino acid-mediated stimulation of muscle protein synthesis is enhanced, thus augmenting anabolic signaling.[66,67] Exercise-mediated increases in blood flow facilitate amino acid delivery to skeletal muscle.[68] These interactions are an important basis of prehabilitation programs[59] and for this reason should be coordinated for optimal benefits to the patient.

Psychologic Support

For patients undergoing major life-altering surgery, anxiety and depression are common and have a negative impact on postoperative pain control, hospital admission, readmissions, and functional limitations with poor compliance to exercise.[69,70] The prevalence of anxiety and depressive disorders in patients with a cancer diagnosis varies between 10% and 60%; this has been attributed to differences in populations, disease stage, study methodologies, cutoff values for depression, and point prevalence of depression in the different populations studied.[71,72] Many instruments with a varying degree of complexity exist to measure depressive symptoms. Among the commonly measured in prehabilitation literature is the Hospital Anxiety and Depression Scale (HADS),[73] the Edmonton Symptom Assessment System (ESAS),[74] and the NCCN Distress Thermometer.[75] A study of more than 800 patients prior to colorectal cancer surgery demonstrated that lower levels of self-efficacy and social support and higher levels of anxiety and depression adversely affect the quality of postoperative recovery. Interestingly, older age was significantly associated with higher levels of well being after surgery.[69] Other psychologic factors that have been associated with poor postoperative outcomes are trait anxiety, state anxiety, depression, intramarital hostility, state anger, and psychologic distress. In contrast, greater self-efficacy, low pain expectation, external locus of control, optimism, religiousness, and anger control have been related to improved postoperative outcomes.[70] These results allow future researchers to understand the burden of psychologic morbidity in patients who are on prehabilitation programs and to provide targeted interventional strategies.

Multiple studies using interventions, such as individual and group therapy with relaxation therapy, psychoeducation, behavioral and cognitive counseling, education, nonbehavioral counseling, social support, and music therapy, have been described in the oncology literature with varying results. The use of medications to treat depressive illness in patients with cancer has shown mixed results with improvements in depression scores observed after therapy with mianserin, paroxetine, and methyl prednisone.[71] A review of seven studies of psychologic interventions prior to cancer surgery did not show an effect on traditional surgical outcomes (e.g., length of hospital stay, complications, analgesia use, or mortality) but positively affected patients' immunologic function and appeared to have an impact on patient-reported outcome measures, including psychologic outcomes, quality of life, and somatic symptoms.[76] Psychologic interventions have also been used as a component of multimodal prehabilitation with significant positive results, including improvements in functional capacity, psychologic outcomes, and reduction in postoperative complications.[77] Behavioral change requires considerable motivation on the part of both clinicians and patients. Motivational strategies, including support from family or peer group combined with preoperative individual and group patient education through initiatives, such as preoperative surgery school[78] and preoperative respiratory education interviews[79] have been successfully shown to reduce postoperative complications. Psychologic interventions when delivered in the context of multimodal prehabilitation programs could potentially achieve the multiple aims of reducing anxiety and depression, facilitating behavioral change (exercise) and facilitating shared decision making (SDM).

Medical Optimization: Glycemic Control, Anemia

Preoperative identification of high-risk patients provides the important opportunity to optimize modifiable risk factors, and therefore potentially change the patient's surgical risk. Among several patient comorbidities and modifiable risk factors, poor glycemic control, anemia, and patient behaviors such as smoking have all been associated with adverse perioperative events. It is important to highlight that optimization of these conditions requires time. Therefore, prompt referral to the preoperative physician is essential to initiate the optimization process as soon as possible, especially considering that most of these problems are already known to the patient and/or to the treating physician or surgeon. This will avoid the preoperative dilemma, especially when evaluating oncologic patients, of whether to defer surgery or accepting to expose patients to preventable risks.

Poor perioperative glycemic control, identified by high blood glucose levels or elevated hemoglobin A1c (HbA1c) levels in diabetic and nondiabetic patients undergoing major cardiac and noncardiac surgery, has been associated with reduced survival and increased overall morbidity, especially surgical site infections and wound healing complications.[80–82] These data suggest that preoperative intervention aiming at reducing blood glucose levels and improving insulin sensitivity could be beneficial for avoiding postoperative complications. However, studies demonstrating that preoperative glycemic optimization improves outcomes are lacking. Moreover, authors suggest that the increased morbidity and mortality observed in patients with high HbA1c is linked more to the severity of the underlying disease—and therefore to a longstanding history of poor glycemic control—than to the perioperative hyperglycemia observed in these patients. Finally, the optimal preoperative HbA1c threshold triggering preoperative glycemic optimization remains controversial. Depending on the type of surgery, an HbA1c level ranging between 6% and 8% has been shown to be acceptable.[80,82]

Preoperative anemia is common,[83] especially in oncologic patients for whom its prevalence has been reported as high as 90%.[84] The pathogenesis of anemia is multifactorial (iron deficiency, anemia of chronic inflammatory diseases, renal dysfunction, myelosuppression) and multiple causes frequently coexist in the same patient. Both anemia and allogeneic blood transfusion have been associated with organ injury and increased morbidity and mortality after major surgery,[85–87] although several perioperative confounding factors raise questions regarding these relationships. However, a further secondary analysis of the METS trial recently confirmed this association demonstrating that hemoglobin concentration was strongly associated with moderate or severe complications, even after adjusting for measurements of physical fitness such as $\dot{V}O_{2peak}$ (OR per 10 g/L increase in hemoglobin concentration, 0.86; 95% CI, 0.77–0.96; $P = 0.007$) or $\dot{V}O_{2AT}$ (OR per 10 g/L increase in hemoglobin concentration, 0.86; 95% CI, 0.77–0.97, $P = 0.01$).[88] For a 10 g/L increase in hemoglobin concentration, $\dot{V}O_{2peak}$ and $\dot{V}O_{2AT}$ increased by 0.71 mL/kg/min and 0.32 mL/kg/min, respectively.[88] These results are important to consider when planning prehabilitation programs aiming at improving functional capacity in anemic patients. Preliminary evidence also suggests that allogeneic blood transfusion is associated with worse oncologic outcomes.[86] Considering that the risk of anemia is present throughout the surgical journey, interventions to optimize preoperative anemia should be part of a perioperative multimodal and multidisciplinary patient blood management program, including blood sparing technique and alternatives to transfusion.[89,90] The implementation of such programs has demonstrated reduction in allogeneic blood transfusion and postoperative complications such as acute renal failure.[91] Preoperative intravenous iron infusion is frequently utilized in the preoperative period, as the majority of anemic patients have either iron deficiency anemia and/or anemia of inflammatory chronic disease. Oral iron supplementation should be reserved when there is sufficient time to allow optimization before surgery (>6 weeks from the time of diagnosis to the time of surgery).[85] Nephrology consultation is advocated in patients with reduced glomerular filtration rate.[85,89]

Literature on Prehabilitation and Impact on Outcome

The current body of literature on prehabilitation represented in the seven systematic reviews with meta-analyses published to date, and numerous systematic and narrative reviews, includes over 40 randomized controlled trials (RCTs) (Fig. 15.3).

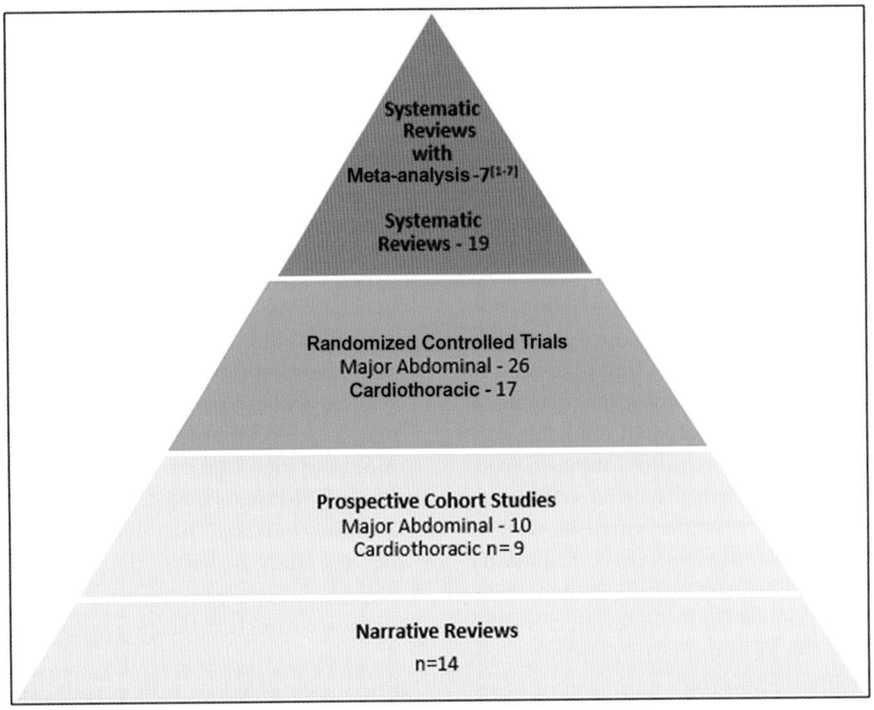

• **Fig. 15.3** The hierarchy of evidence in the current literature on prehabilitation prior to cancer surgery, illustrating the growing body of literature. The numbers indicate current publications (excluding conference abstracts) based on an EMBASE search (1974 to October 11, 2019).

This exponential increase in publications in the last decade is indicative of the interest in prehabilitation among a wide range of clinical craft groups. However, they include a number of low to moderate quality studies with often widely heterogeneous metrics of patient selection, study methodologies, measurements, and outcomes.

The evidence from RCTs and cohort studies for the majority of major cancer surgeries supports the notion that prehabilitation strategies (multi- and unimodal) are feasible and safe, and can improve mobility, functional capacity, and physical fitness. In most of these studies postoperative complications have only been explored as secondary outcomes.[92–99]

Two RCTs in cancer stand out, having explored the effects of prehabilitation on postoperative complications resulting in remarkably similar results. Barberan-Garcia et al.[100,101] assessed the impact of a personalized 6-week prehabilitation program on postoperative complications in high-risk patients undergoing elective major abdominal surgery using a blinded, RCT design. One hundred and twenty-four elderly (>70 years), high-risk (ASA 3 and 4) patients were randomized to multimodal prehabilitation consisting of a motivational interview, increased activity, and supervised, structured, responsive aerobic exercise training vs. standard care. This intervention enhanced aerobic capacity by 135% (Δ endurance time [ET], 135% (standard deviation [SD], 218); $P < 0.001$), reduced the number of patients with postoperative complications by 51% (relative risk [RR], 0.5; 95% CI, 0.3–0.8; $P = 0.001$), and reduced the rate of all complications by 64% (1.4% [SD, 1.6] and 0.5% [SD, 1.0] per patient; $P = 0.001$) compared with controls. The intervention also showed a lower mean number of cardiovascular complications per patient (RR, 0.1; 95% CI, 0.1–1.0; $P = 0.033$). There was a significant reduction in the number of days in intensive care in the group admitted to the intensive care unit comparing the intervention and control groups (n = 44; 3 [SD, 2] vs. 12 [SD, 20]; $P = 0.046$).

A subsequent cost analysis of this prehabilitation program by the same group showed a sustained clinical benefit at 6 months after surgery and reduced perioperative complications (RR, 0.5; 95% CI, 0.3–0.8) without increasing direct health care costs.[102]

LIPPSMAck-POP[79] was an RCT testing the hypothesis that preoperative respiratory physiotherapy education and training prevents postoperative pulmonary complications (POPC) following abdominal surgery. The intervention group was administered a 30-min educational and instructional educational interview on strategies to prevent postoperative pulmonary complications, while the control group received printed educational material. This intervention resulted in a reduction of postoperative pulmonary complications within 14 postoperative hospital days by 50%. The adjusted hazard ratio was 0.48 (95% CI, 0.30–0.75; $P = 0.001$), the absolute risk reduction was 15% (95% CI, 7%–22%), and the number needed to treat (NNT) was 7 (95% CI, 5–14). However, the contrast in results to a similar study[103] highlights the need for caution when applying such results to populations having different types of surgery and lower baseline incidence of pulmonary complications utilizing different definitions for the clinical outcomes concerned.

Future research needs to address the variability inherent in current study designs. More standardized methods of risk stratification, and defining prehabilitation strategies (dose, duration, and modality) and outcomes (clinical and operational) could improve the evidence base and facilitate implementation on larger scales.

We are currently awaiting the outcomes of several large studies to provide us with further evidence on the efficacy, effectiveness, and ability to implement prehabilitation interventions. These studies include:

1. The Implementation of Collaborative Self-Management Services to Promote Physical Activity[104] (NEXT-CARE-PA). This is a parallel assigned, nonrandomized study of implementation of prehabilitation involving 2300 participants looking at cost effectiveness of increasing physical activity in a range of cohorts, including high-risk patients, presenting for abdominal surgery. The study is scheduled to complete by June 2020.
2. The Wessex Fit-4-Cancer Surgery Trial. This is an efficacy trial looking at the effect of a Structured Responsive Exercise Training Program (SRETP) and psychologic intervention on postoperative outcomes in 1560 participants, due to complete in March 2022.[105]
3. PREPARE-ABC trial for patients undergoing curative colorectal cancer surgery. This multicenter trial will compare a home or hospital-based exercise program to standard care and intends to recruit 1146 patients by August 2020.[106]
4. International multicenter RCT, currently recruiting, based in the Netherlands for patients undergoing colorectal surgery for cancer. This study will include 714 patients randomized to a 4-week period of multimodal prehabilitation or control. This trial will be conducted within an ERAS program framework and will include a cost analysis. It will be the first trial of its kind to include a comprehensive multimodal intervention consisting of interval exercise training, nutritional intervention using whey protein, vitamins and micronutrient supplements, smoking cessation support, and psychologic support. The primary outcomes of this trial will be postoperative complications scored using a Compressive Complication Index and change in the 6MWT result between baseline and 4 weeks after surgery.[107]

The results of this study could strengthen the case for implementing multimodal prehabilitation into the perioperative pathways for patients undergoing cancer surgery. Incorporating prehabilitation into ERAS programs could add value by improving clinical and patient-reported outcomes with reduced health care expenditure.

Prehabilitation as a Compelling Strategy: Successes and Challenges Ahead

With the increasing number of oncology patients who are in need of surgery, we are presented with new challenges as patients tend to be older, frail, physically unfit, and sarcopenic, with multiple comorbidities, impacted by delays in treatments due to the COVID 19 epidemic, and undergoing oncologic neoadjuvant therapies. While ERAS has contributed immensely to addressing the importance of better surgical care through the identification of elements based on sound evidence within the intraoperative and postoperative phases, it is still necessary to address the preoperative component of the perioperative trajectory, and prehabilitation becomes the missing link.

To this extent, the optimization of medical conditions must be accompanied by better physical conditions and a more robust nutritional environment. Prehabilitation can in fact be a compelling strategy offered to our oncologic patients at the time of diagnosis. It is at this point that the patient can receive support in identifying the challenges ahead and overcome, step by step, all the obstacles associated with the organization of care.

The prehabilitation unit, where all the interdisciplinary team meets the patient, can be a place where the patient-physician partnership is established and where the patient becomes empowered and engaged in self-care, and guided through the various stages of cancer care. As surgery represents a large percentage of cancer therapy, it would make sense that patients are also prepared for the upcoming stress of surgery. The proposition offered to the patient to become stronger, physically, nutritionally, and mentally, reassures the patient that they can overcome the impairments associated with immediate and subsequent therapies.

The benefits of introducing prehabilitation programs on functional outcomes have been demonstrated consistently, particularly in colorectal cancer surgery and lung cancer, although with regard to the impact on other outcomes the immediate effect has been modest and deserves further research.[105] This is particularly true for clinical outcomes such as postoperative complications and hospital readmissions, which are important from the clinician and payer point of view.

It has to be said that the impact of ERAS on clinical outcomes has been consistent, and when prehabilitation is an added part of the perioperative strategy, it is plausible that the effect might not be evident. Nevertheless, the long-term effect of prehabilitation on oncologic outcome might be of interest to this population, as it might be a target for more therapies. This point has been shown recently by two studies demonstrating the positive impact of prehabilitation on tumor regression and 5-year disease-free survival.[20,22]

Although prehabilitation strategies have focused on optimizing short-term recovery, it is now evident that current elements of prehabilitation may need to be modified and expanded to take account of the growing literature that identifies other factors that may influence long-term oncologic outcomes. The challenge will be to design and conduct trials with sufficient sample sizes to prove the value of each and combined interventions.

References

1. Popat K, McQueen K, Feeley TW. The global burden of cancer. *Best Pract Res Clin Anaesthesiol.* 2013;27:399–408.
2. Clegg A, Young J, Iliffe S, Rikkert MO, Rockwood K. Frailty in elderly people. *Lancet.* 2013;381(9868):752–762. doi:10.1016/S0140-6736(12)62167-9.

3. Bauer JM, Wirth R, Volkert D, Werner H, Sieber CC. Malnutrition, sarcopenia and cachexia in the elderly: from pathophysiology to treatment. Conclusions of an international meeting of experts, sponsored by the BANSS Foundation Teilnehmer des BANSS-Symposiums 2006. *Dtsch Med Wochenschr.* 2008;133(7):305–310. doi:10.1055/s-2008-1046711.
4. Singh M, Stewart R, White H. Importance of frailty in patients with cardiovascular disease. *Eur Heart J.* 2014;35(26):1726–1731. doi:10.1093/eurheartj/ehu197.
5. Ethun CG, Bilen MA, Jani AB, Maithel SK, Ogan K, Master VA. Frailty and cancer: implications for oncology surgery, medical oncology, and radiation oncology. *CA Cancer J Clin.* 2017;67(5):362–377. doi:10.3322/caac.21406.
6. Mei KL, Batsis JA, Mills JB, Holubar SD. Sarcopenia and sarcopenic obesity: do they predict inferior oncologic outcomes after gastrointestinal cancer surgery? *Perioper Med (Lond).* 2016;26(5):30.
7. Jones LW, Haykowsky MJ, Swartz JJ, Douglas PS, Mackey JR. Early breast cancer therapy and cardiovascular injury. *J Am Coll Cardiol.* 2007;50(15):1435–1441.
8. Koelwyn GJ, Khouri M, Mackey JR, Douglas PS, Jones LW. Running on empty: cardiovascular reserve capacity and late effects of therapy in cancer survivorship. *J Clin Oncol.* 2012;30(36):4458–4461. doi:10.1200/JCO.2012.44.0891.
9. Visser MR, van Lanschot JJ, van der Velden J, Kloek JJ, Gouma DJ, Sprangers MA. Quality of life in newly diagnosed cancer patients waiting for surgery is seriously impaired. *J Surg Oncol.* 2006;93(7):571–577.
10. Mazzocco K, Masiero M, Carriero MC, Pravettoni G. The role of emotions in cancer patients' decision-making. *Ecancermedicalscience.* 2019;13:914. doi:10.3332/ecancer.2019.914.
11. Oudemans-van Straaten HM, Jansen PG, te Velthuis H, et al. Increased oxygen consumption after cardiac surgery is associated with the inflammatory response to endotoxemia. *Intensive Care Med.* 1996;22(4):294–300.
12. Dunn OC, Mythen MG. Physiology of oxygen transport. *BJA Educ.* 2016;16(10):341–348.
13. Older PO, Levett DZH. Cardiopulmonary exercise testing and surgery. *Ann Am Thorac Soc.* 2017;14:S74–S83.
14. Davies SJ, Wilson RJ. Preoperative optimization of the high-risk surgical patient. *Br J Anaesth.* 2004;93(1):121–128.
15. Moonesinghe SR, Mythen MG, Grocott MP. High-risk surgery: epidemiology and outcomes. *Anesth Analg.* 2011;112(4):891–901.
16. Scott JM, Zabor EC, Schwitzer E, et al. Efficacy of exercise therapy on cardiorespiratory fitness in patients with cancer: a systematic review and meta-analysis. *J Clin Oncol.* 2018;36(22):2297–2305. doi:10.1200/JCO.2017.77.5809.
17. Wijeysundera DN, Pearse RM, Shulman MA, et al. Assessment of functional capacity before major non-cardiac surgery: an international, prospective cohort study. *Lancet.* 2018;391(10140):2631–2640. doi:10.1016/S0140-6736(18)31131-0.
18. Barberan-Garcia A, Ubré M, Roca J, et al. Personalised prehabilitation in high-risk patients undergoing elective major abdominal surgery: a randomized blinded controlled trial. *Ann Surg.* 2018;267(1):50–56.
19. Ljungqvist O, Scott M, Fearon KC. Enhanced recovery after surgery: a review. *JAMA Surg.* 2017;152(3):292–298. doi:10.1001/jamasurg.2016.4952.
20. Minnella EM, Awasthi R, Loiselle SE, Agnihotram RV, Ferri LE, Carli F. Effect of exercise and nutrition prehabilitation on functional capacity in esophagogastric cancer surgery: a randomized clinical trial. *JAMA Surg.* 2018;153(12):1081–1089.
21. West MA, Astin R, Moyses HE, et al. Exercise prehabilitation may lead to augmented tumor regression following neoadjuvant chemoradiotherapy in locally advanced rectal cancer. *Acta Oncol.* 2019;58(5):588–595.
22. Trépanier M, Minnella EM, Paradis T, et al. Improved disease-free survival after prehabilitation for colorectal cancer surgery. *Ann Surg.* 2019;270(3):493–501.
23. Baldini G, Fawcett WJ. Anesthesia for colorectal surgery. *Anesthesiol Clin.* 2015;33(1):93–123.
24. Baldini G, Ferreira V, Carli F. Preoperative preparations for enhanced recovery after surgery programs: a role for prehabilitation. *Surg Clin North Am.* 2018;98(6):1149–1169.
25. Wilson RJ, Davies S, Yates D, Redman J, Stone M. Impaired functional capacity is associated with all-cause mortality after major elective intra-abdominal surgery. *Br J Anaesth.* 2010;105(3):297–303.
26. West MA, Asher R, Browning M, et al. Validation of preoperative cardiopulmonary exercise testing-derived variables to predict in-hospital morbidity after major colorectal surgery. *Br J Surg.* 2016;103(6):744–752.
27. Carli F, Minnella EM. Preoperative functional assessment and optimization in surgical patient: changing the paradigm. *Minerva Anestesiol.* 2017;83(2):214–218.
28. Levett DZH, Jack S, Swart M, et al. Perioperative cardiopulmonary exercise testing (CPET): consensus clinical guidelines on indications, organization, conduct, and physiological interpretation. *Br J Anaesth.* 2018;120(3):484–500.
29. Nyasavajjala SM, Low J. Anaerobic threshold: pitfalls and limitations. *Anaesthesia.* 2009;64(9):934–936.
30. Fleisher LA, Fleischmann KE, Auerbach AD, et al. 2014 ACC/AHA guideline on perioperative cardiovascular evaluation and management of patients undergoing noncardiac surgery: a report of the American College of Cardiology/American Heart Association Task Force on practice guidelines. *J Am Coll Cardiol.* 2014;64(22):e77–e137.
31. Kristensen SD, Knuuti J, Saraste A, et al. 2014 ESC/ESA Guidelines on non-cardiac surgery: cardiovascular assessment and management: The Joint Task Force on non-cardiac surgery: cardiovascular assessment and management of the European Society of Cardiology (ESC) and the European Society of Anaesthesiology (ESA). *Eur J Anaesthesiol.* 2014;31(10):517–573.
32. Rubin DS, Huisingh-Scheetz M, Hung A, et al. Accuracy of physical function questions to predict moderate-vigorous physical activity as measured by hip accelerometry. *Anesthesiology.* 2019;131(5):992–1003.
33. Shulman MA, Cuthbertson BH, Wijeysundera DN, et al. Using the 6-minute walk test to predict disability-free survival after major surgery. *Br J Anaesth.* 2019;122(1):111–119.
34. Hlatky MA, Boineau RE, Higginbotham MB, et al. A brief self-administered questionnaire to determine functional capacity (The Duke Activity Status Index). *Am J Cardiol.* 1989;64(10):651–654.
35. Struthers R, Erasmus P, Holmes K, Warman P, Collingwood A, Sneyd JR. Assessing fitness for surgery: a comparison of questionnaire, incremental shuttle walk, and cardiopulmonary exercise testing in general surgical patients. *Br J Anaesth.* 2008;101(6):774–780.
36. Duceppe E, Parlow J, MacDonald P, et al. Canadian cardiovascular society guidelines on perioperative cardiac risk assessment and management for patients who undergo noncardiac surgery. *Can J Cardiol.* 2017;33(1):17–32.
37. Levin ER, Gardner DG, Samson WK. Natriuretic peptides. *N Engl J Med.* 1998;339(5):321–328.

38. Karthikeyan G, Moncur RA, Levine O, et al. Is a pre-operative brain natriuretic peptide or N-terminal pro-B-type natriuretic peptide measurement an independent predictor of adverse cardiovascular outcomes within 30 days of noncardiac surgery? A systematic review and meta-analysis of observational studies. *J Am Coll Cardiol.* 2009;54(17):1599–1606.
39. Topp R, Ditmyer M, King K, Doherty K, Hornyak J. 3rd. The effect of bed rest and potential of prehabilitation on patients in the intensive care unit. *AACN Clin Issues.* 2002;13(2):263–276.
40. Silver JK, Baima J. Cancer prehabilitation: an opportunity to decrease treatment-related morbidity, increase cancer treatment options, and improve physical and psychological health outcomes. *Am J Phys Med Rehabil.* 2013;92(8):715–727.
41. Carli F, Zavorsky GS. Optimizing functional exercise capacity in the elderly surgical population. *Curr Opin Clin Nutr Metab Care.* 2005;8(1):23–32.
42. Carli F, Bousquet-Dion G, et al. Improving perioperative functional capacity: a case for prehabilitation in geriatric anesthesiology. In: Reves JG, Barnett SR, McSwain J et al, eds. *Geriatric Anaesthesiology.* 3rd ed.: Springer International Publishing AG; 2018.
43. Carli F, Scheede-Bergdahl C. Prehabilitation to enhance perioperative care. *Anesthesiol Clin.* 2015;33(1):17–33.
44. Snowden CP, Prentis J, Jacques B, et al. Cardiorespiratory fitness predicts mortality and hospital length of stay after major elective surgery in older people. *Ann Surg.* 2013;257(6):999–1004.
45. Strous MTA, Janssen-Heijnen MLG, Vogelaar FJ. Impact of therapeutic delay in colorectal cancer on overall survival and cancer recurrence – is there a safe timeframe for prehabilitation? *Eur J Surg Oncol.* 2019;45(12):2295–2301.
46. Curtis NJ, West MA, Salib E, et al. Time from colorectal cancer diagnosis to laparoscopic curative surgery—is there a safe window for prehabilitation? *Int J Colorectal Dis.* 2018;33(7):979–983.
47. Minnella EM, Awasthi R, Gillis C, et al. Patients with poor baseline walking capacity are most likely to improve their fuctional status with multimodal prehabilitation. *Surgery.* 2016;160:1070–1079.
48. Weimann A, Braga M, Carli F, et al. ESPEN guideline: clinical nutrition in surgery. *Clin Nutr.* 2017;36(3):623–650.
49. Crossland H, Skirrow S, Puthucheary ZA, Constantin-Teodosiu D, Greenhaff PL. The impact of immobilisation and inflammation on the regulation of muscle mass and insulin resistance: different routes to similar end-points. *J Physiol.* 2019;597(5):1259–1270.
50. Scheede-Bergdahl C, Minnella EM, Carli F. Multi-modal prehabilitation: addressing the why, when, what, how, who and where next? *Anaesthesia.* 2019;74(suppl 1):20–26.
51. Caspersen CJ, Powell KE, Christenson GM. Physical activity, exercise, and physical fitness: definitions and distinctions for health-related research. *Public Health Rep.* 1985;100(2):126–131.
52. Borg G. Psychophysical scaling with applications in physical work and the perception of exertion. *Scand J Work Environ Health.* 1990;16(suppl 1):55–58.
53. Cormie P, Atkinson M, Bucci L, et al. Clinical Oncology Society of Australia position statement on exercise in cancer care. *Med J Aust.* 2018;209(4):184–187. doi:10.5694/mja18.00199.
54. Jones LW, Eves ND, Scott JM. Bench-to-bedside approaches for personalized exercise therapy in cancer. *Am Soc Clin Oncol Educ Book.* 2017;37:684–694.
55. van Rooijen SJ, Molenaar CJL, Schep G, et al. Making patients fit for surgery: introducing a four pillar multimodal prehabilitation program in colorectal cancer. *Am J Phys Med Rehabil.* 2019;98(10):888–896.
56. Kushi LH, Doyle C, McCullough M, et al. American Cancer Society Guidelines on nutrition and physical activity for cancer prevention: reducing the risk of cancer with healthy food choices and physical activity. *CA Cancer J Clin.* 2012;62(1):30–67.
57. Wolin KY, Schwartz AL, Matthews CE, Courneya KS, Schmitz KH. Implementing the exercise guidelines for cancer survivors. *J Support Oncol.* 2012;10(5):171–177.
58. Ferreira V, Agnihotram RV, Bergdahl A, et al. Maximizing patient adherence to prehabilitation: what do the patients say? *Support Care Cancer.* 2018;26(8):2717–2723.
59. Chen BP, Awasthi R, Sweet SN, et al. Four-week prehabilitation program is sufficient to modify exercise behaviors and improve preoperative functional walking capacity in patients with colorectal cancer. *Support Care Cancer.* 2017;25(1):33–40.
60. Carli F, Gillis C, Scheede-Bergdahl C. Promoting a culture of prehabilitation for the surgical cancer patient. *Acta Oncol.* 2017;56(2):128–133.
61. Baracos VE. Cancer-associated malnutrition. *Eur J Clin Nutr.* 2018;72(9):1255–1259.
62. Cotogni P, Pedrazzoli P, De Waele E, et al. Nutritional therapy in cancer patients receiving chemoradiotherapy: should we need stronger recommendations to act for improving outcomes? *J Cancer.* 2019;10(18):4318–4325.
63. Gillis C, Carli F. Promoting perioperative metabolic and nutritional care. *Anesthesiology.* 2015;123(6):1455–1472.
64. Arends J, Bachmann P, Baracos V, et al. ESPEN guidelines on nutrition in cancer patients. *Clin Nutr.* 2017;36(1):11–48.
65. Wolfe RR. The underappreciated role of muscle in health and disease. *Am J Clin Nutr.* 2006;84(3):475–482.
66. Rennie MJ. Control of muscle protein synthesis as a result of contractile activity and amino acid availability: implications for protein requirements. *Int J Sport Nutr Exerc Metab.* 2001;11(suppl 1):S170–S176.
67. Moore DR, Tang JE, Burd NA, Rerecich T, Tarnopolsky MA, Phillips SM. Differential stimulation of myofibrillar and sarcoplasmic protein synthesis with protein ingestion at rest and after resistance exercise. *J Physiol.* 2009;587(Pt 4):897–904.
68. Phillips SM, Hartman JW, Wilkinson SB. Dietary protein to support anabolism with resistance exercise in young men. *J Am Coll Nutr.* 2005;24(2):134S–139S.
69. Timmerman KL, Dhanani S, Glynn EL, et al. A moderate acute increase in physical activity enhances nutritive flow and the muscle protein anabolic response to mixed nutrient intake in older adults. *Am J Clin Nutr.* 2012;95(6):1403–1412.
70. Foster C, Haviland J, Winter J, et al. Pre-surgery depression and confidence to manage problems predict recovery trajectories of health and wellbeing in the first two years following colorectal cancer: results from the CREW cohort study. *PLoS One.* 2016;11(5):e0155434.
71. Levett DZH, Grimmett C. Psychological factors, prehabilitation and surgical outcomes: evidence and future directions. *Anaesthesia.* 2019;74(suppl 1):36–42.
72. Pirl WF. Evidence report on the occurrence, assessment, and treatment of depression in cancer patients. *J Natl Cancer Inst Monogr.* 2004(32):32–39.
73. Jadoon NA, Munir W, Shahzad MA, Choudhry ZS. Assessment of depression and anxiety in adult cancer outpatients: a cross-sectional study. *BMC Cancer.* 2010;10:594.
74. Snaith RP. The hospital anxiety and depression scale. *Health Qual Life Outcomes.* 2003;1:29.

75. Hui D, Bruera E. The Edmonton symptom assessment system 25 years later: past, present, and future developments. *J Pain Symptom Manage*. 2017;53(3):630–643.
76. Cutillo A, O'Hea E, Person S, Lessard D, Harralson T, Boudreaux E. The distress thermometer: cutoff points and clinical use. *Oncol Nurs Forum*. 2017;44(3):329–336.
77. Tsimopoulou I, Pasquali S, Howard R, et al. Psychological prehabilitation before cancer surgery: a systematic review. *Ann Surg Oncol*. 2015;22(13):4117–4123.
78. Bousquet-Dion G, Awasthi R, Loiselle SE, et al. Evaluation of supervised multimodal prehabilitation programme in cancer patients undergoing colorectal resection: a randomized control trial. *Acta Oncol*. 2018;57(6):849–859.
79. Moore JA, Conway DH, Thomas N, Cummings D, Atkinson D. Impact of a peri-operative quality improvement programme on postoperative pulmonary complications. *Anaesthesia*. 2017;72(3):317–327.
80. Boden I, Skinner EH, Browning L, et al. Preoperative physiotherapy for the prevention of respiratory complications after upper abdominal surgery: pragmatic, double blinded, multicentre randomised controlled trial. *Br Med J*. 2018;360:j5916.
81. Duggan EW, Carlson K, Umpierrez GE. Perioperative hyperglycemia management: an update. *Anesthesiology*. 2017;126(3):547–560.
82. Sato H, Carvalho G, Sato T, Lattermann R, Matsukawa T, Schricker T. The association of preoperative glycemic control, intraoperative insulin sensitivity, and outcomes after cardiac surgery. *J Clin Endocrinol Metab*. 2010;95(9):4338–4344.
83. Levy N, Dhatariya K. Pre-operative optimisation of the surgical patient with diagnosed and undiagnosed diabetes: a practical review. *Anaesthesia*. 2019;74(suppl 1):58–66.
84. Musallam KM, Tamim HM, Richards T, et al. Preoperative anaemia and postoperative outcomes in non-cardiac surgery: a retrospective cohort study. *Lancet*. 2011;378(9800):1396–1407.
85. Knight K, Wade S, Balducci L. Prevalence and outcomes of anemia in cancer: a systematic review of the literature. *Am J Med*. 2004;116(suppl 7A):11S–26S.
86. Munting KE, Klein AA. Optimisation of pre-operative anaemia in patients before elective major surgery—why, who, when and how? *Anaesthesia*. 2019;74(suppl 1):49–57.
87. Cata JP. Perioperative anemia and blood transfusions in patients with cancer: when the problem, the solution, and their combination are each associated with poor outcomes. *Anesthesiology*. 2015;122(1):3–4.
88. Shander A, Javidroozi M, Ozawa S, Hare GM. What is really dangerous: anaemia or transfusion? *Br J Anaesth*. 2011;107(suppl 1):i41–i59.
89. Bartoszko J, Thorpe KE, Laupacis A, et al. Association of preoperative anaemia with cardiopulmonary exercise capacity and postoperative outcomes in noncardiac surgery: a substudy of the Measurement of Exercise Tolerance before Surgery (METS) Study. *Br J Anaesth*. 2019;123(2):161–169.
90. Goodnough LT, Shander A. Patient blood management. *Anesthesiology*. 2012;116(6):1367–1376.
91. Frank SM, Chaturvedi S, Goel R, Resar LMS. Approaches to bloodless surgery for oncology patients. *Hematol Oncol Clin North Am*. 2019;33(5):857–871.
92. Meybohm P, Herrmann E, Steinbicker AU, et al. Patient blood management is associated with a substantial reduction of red blood cell utilization and safe for patient's outcome: a prospective, multicenter cohort study with a noninferiority design. *Ann Surg*. 2016;264(2):203–211.
93. Moran J, Guinan E, McCormick P, et al. The ability of prehabilitation to influence postoperative outcome after intra-abdominal operation: a systematic review and meta-analysis. *Surgery*. 2016;160(5):1189–1201.
94. Jones LW, Liang Y, Pituskin EN, et al. Effect of exercise training on peak oxygen consumption in patients with cancer: a meta-analysis. *Oncologist*. 2011;16(1):112–120.
95. Sebio Garcia R, Yanez Brage MI, Gimenez Moolhuyzen E, Granger CL, Denehy L. Functional and postoperative outcomes after preoperative exercise training in patients with lung cancer: a systematic review and meta-analysis. *Interact Cardiovasc Thorac Surg*. 2016;23(3):486–497.
96. Lee CHA, Kong JC, Ismail H, Riedel B, Heriot A. Systematic review and meta-analysis of objective assessment of physical fitness in patients undergoing colorectal cancer surgery. *Dis Colon Rectum*. 2018;61(3):400–409.
97. Treanor C, Kyaw T, Donnelly M. An international review and meta-analysis of prehabilitation compared to usual care for cancer patients. *J Cancer Surviv*. 2018;12(1):64–73.
98. Steffens D, Beckenkamp PR, Hancock M, Solomon M, Young J. Preoperative exercise halves the postoperative complication rate in patients with lung cancer: a systematic review of the effect of exercise on complications, length of stay and quality of life in patients with cancer. *Br J Sports Med*. 2018;52(5):344.
99. Kamarajah S, Bundred J, Weblin J, Tan B. Critical appraisal on the impact of preoperative rehabilitation and outcomes after major abdominal and cardiothoracic surgery: A systematic review and meta-analysis. *Surgery*. 2020;167(3):540–549. doi:10.16/j.surg.2019.07.032.
100. Bolshinsky V, Li M H, Ismail H, Burbury K, Riedel B, Heriot A. Multimodal prehabilitation programs as a bundle of care in gastrointestinal cancer surgery: a systematic review. *Dis Colon Rectum*. 2018;61:124–138.
101. Barberan-Garcia A, Ubre M, Roca J, et al. Personalised prehabilitation in high-risk patients undergoing elective major abdominal surgery: a randomized blinded controlled trial. *Ann Surg*. 2018;267(1):50–56.
102. Barberan-Garcia A, Ubre M, Pascual-Argente N, et al. Post-discharge impact and cost-consequence analysis of prehabilitation in high-risk patients undergoing major abdominal surgery: secondary results from a randomised controlled trial. *Br J Anaesth*. 2019;123(4):450–456.
103. Brasher PA, McClelland KH, Denehy L, Story I. Does removal of deep breathing exercises from a physiotherapy program including pre-operative education and early mobilisation after cardiac surgery alter patient outcomes? *Aust J Physiother*. 2003;49(3):165–173.
104. Implementation of collaborative self-management services to promote physical activity (NEXTCARE-PA). ClinicalTrials.gov identifier: NCT02976064. https://clinicaltrials.gov/ct2/show/NCT02976064.
105. The Wessex fit-4-cancer surgery trial (WesFit). ClinicalTrials.gov identifier: NCT03509428. https://clinicaltrials.gov/ct2/show/NCT03509428.
106. Murdoch J, Varley A, McCulloch J, et al. Implementing supportive exercise interventions in the colorectal cancer care pathway: a process evaluation of the PREPARE-ABC randomised controlled trial. *BMC Cancer*. 2021;21:1137.
107. van Rooijen S, Carli F, Dalton S, et al. Multimodal prehabilitation in colorectal cancer patients to improve functional capacity and reduce postoperative complications: the first international randomized controlled trial for multimodal prehabilitation. *J Clin Oncol*. 2019;19(1):98. doi:10.1186/s12885-018-5232-6.

16

Redesign of Perioperative Care Pathways

MICHAEL P.W. GROCOTT AND DENNY Z.H. LEVETT

Introduction

Patients follow a journey through time when they progress from the first symptoms or screening tests, through investigations and receiving a new diagnosis of cancer, to the initiation of treatment and beyond. The notions of "survivorship" and "living with and beyond cancer"[1] encapsulate the changing face of this journey and emphasize the chronicity of experience that people with cancer now have. Increasingly effective cancer treatments are facilitating prolonged survival living with, or cure from, cancer.[2] With these changes come ever more complex clinical pathways, as each patient navigates their unique journey through the intricate landscape of treatments, tumor response, and personal resilience.

Surgery is the most common first intervention for solid tumors, but many patients will receive systematic anticancer treatments (e.g., chemotherapy targeted therapies or hormonal treatment) and/or radiotherapy during their treatment.[3] As survival following cancer continues to increase, so the likelihood of having multiple sequential different treatments rises. While these journeys may not feel like simple linear paths to the person with cancer, health care providers often focus on the idea of such a linear pathway in order to conceptualize the patient journey and to contrast this thinking with a "silo" focused approach, which has historically been associated with limited attention on how different components of each pathway interact together.

Pathway-based thinking has been driven by a number of factors, including policy, economics (funding mechanisms), and patient engagement in health care. Integrated care, meaning seamless integration of care between primary and secondary care settings, is increasingly seen as more efficient and effective than alternatives for both practical and financial reasons. Modifying underpinning funding mechanisms, which incentivize the way that care is delivered, may be the most economical approach to the challenge of managing relentlessly escalating health costs. The transition from fee-for-service through bundled payments to, in some cases, capitation payment mechanisms exemplifies this and contributes to the drive toward improved integration of care. Finally, better informed patients have less patience with constraints on care delivery that are driven by provider, rather than patient, convenience. Each of these factors serves as a driver toward a focus on pathways rather than silos of care.

This chapter will explore these drivers for pathway-based care, the processes through which pathway reorganization may be achieved, and the consequences for perioperative care in general and in relation to specific elements of that care.

Drivers for Pathway-Based Care

Patient Versus Provider Perspectives

Care providers often contextualize themselves according to their setting. Their thinking and actions are typically based on their immediate physical and organizational interactions. For example, surgeons and anesthetists/anesthesiologists typically focus primarily on the operating room environment and adjacent areas (preoperative ward and recovery). Moreover, operational budgets within hospitals are characteristically held at a department level, with surgery separate from anesthesiology or medicine. In fee-for-service settings, this division is magnified by the consequences of which particular individuals or departments receive fees. Such an environment has been described as "silo-based care,"[4] in which the boundaries between specialty silos are identified as obstacles to the efficient and effective delivery of care. These boundaries may be physical, for example the setting of care, or organizational, for example the way departments or budgets are arranged. These issues are of particular relevance to elective/scheduled secondary care pathways where the efficient integrated function of many components of the hospital, working in concert with primary/community care, is essential to facilitate the best preparation for and recovery from significant intervention such as major surgery.

Currently, it can be argued that the "timing, location and manner of interactions between patients and health care providers are frequently dictated by provider priorities rather than patient wishes." "Control of the pathway resides almost exclusively with the providers, not those being provided for."[5] Services are often arranged for the convenience of providers. Patients typically come to doctors, during normal working hours, and at a place of convenience for the doctor, not the patient.[5] To date, limited effort has been invested in remote consultation for most patients, and those developments that have taken place in this area have often been driven by financial efficiency considerations, rather than patient convenience.

A variety of approaches are available that can readily facilitate the delivery of more patient-focused care and overcome some of the challenges presented by health care delivery "silos." Technologic developments, including remote consultations and diagnostics, facilitated via telemedicine,[6] the use of wearable technologies[7] for screening diagnosis and monitoring of physiologic signals, and the use of mobile devices for collecting health data and disseminating health information (so-called m-health).[8] The requirement for the patient to attend a face-to-face interaction with a health care worker may diminish as these innovations are adopted more widely among secondary care providers. Such changes enable patients to interact with health care professionals at a time and in a setting of their choice, rather than at the convenience of others. Furthermore, it may allow them to have important communications, such as the diagnosis of cancer, to be delivered in a timelier manner than is possible with traditional face-to-face interactions. While not all patients may be attracted to such methods of communication, some may cherish the face-to-face clinical interaction; these approaches offer the potential for better and more efficient interactions for many.

Patients are increasingly involved in contributing to the development of health care services. Experienced-based co-design (EBCD)[9] is becoming more common and incorporates the "lived experience" of non-health care professionals (patients and public) in contributing to service design across primary[10] and secondary care.[11] Examples have included cancer care,[9] palliative, and end-of-life care pathways.[12]

Early evidence supports the notion that patients may engage better with such pathways.

Health Policy Developments

The "Triple Aim" proposed by the US Institute for Health care Improvement encapsulates improving individual patient experience of care (including quality and experience), health of the population, and value.[13,14] Two current areas of policy that are linked to this are personalized care and integrated care.

The concept of personalized care links two distinct concepts. First, the ever growing availability of data with which to make decisions about health care, for example, in relation to the various "omics" techniques (genomics, metabolomics, etc.) has the potential to provide information to guide care at an individual patient level.[15] Second, patients increasingly expect to take more control over their own health as the paternalistic model of health care becomes less common. One example of improving patient control is the idea of "personal health budgets" in which patients within a publicly funded health care system have control over some of the resources available to fund their care and allocate them according to best information and advice.[16] This is linked with initiatives around shared decision-making (SDM), such as the international "Choosing Wisely" movement,[17] as well as the provision of better and clearer data to inform choices, for example through the UK NHS Choices website in the UK.[18] Such developments are symptomatic of the evolution from traditional paternalistic approaches to health care, in which the physician made decisions about the patient care, to so-called "patient-centered care" in which decisions are made in partnership between health care provider and patient.[16] In some situations, patients may behave as independent consumers with little reference to health care providers, particularly in relation to diagnostic services such as "screening scans" and over-the-counter genetic information.[19]

Integrated Care Organizations (ICOs) deliver care across a defined geography by an alliance of relevant health care providers in primary, secondary, and social care.[20] The development of ICOs has, in part, been a response to the economic challenges outlined in the following section and the quest for value in modern health care. There is a perception that fundamental changes in methods of service provision (e.g., pathway redesign) are required to meet current funding challenges; incremental cost-saving and gradual refinement of services are unlikely to offer a solution. ICOs stand in contrast to the concept of market-driven local health economies and certainly in the UK, represent a response to the perceived failure of a local health care market embodying arrangements such as the "purchaser-provider" split.[21] An important aspect of ICOs is that funding is allocated at the level of geographically defined populations resulting in a so-called "capitation" mechanism (see later). Such capitation mechanisms may be a more efficient means of achieving value, defined as outcome per unit cost,[22] than traditional fee-for-service or more recent "bundled payment" mechanisms, which tend to incentivize activity, rather than improved outcome.

Health Economics

The fundamental challenge in relation to health economics in high-income countries is the relentlessly rising cost of health care as a consequence of apparently limitless demand. Achieving health care cost containment has become a political imperative as the proportion of gross domestic product that is allocated to health care approaches one-fifth in the United States and exceeds 10% in many high-income countries.[23]

The key drivers of cost escalation are health care innovation and demographic change. Health care innovation is probably the primary driver: interventions from knee replacements through complex cancer surgery and novel biological anticancer agents are new to our therapeutic repertoire and each innovation becomes a new drain on the limited available pool of health care resource. However, each of these innovations also contributes to improvements in the quantity and/or quality of life for patients for whom they provide benefit. This benefit is, in turn, at least partially responsible for the demographic change that is taking place in high-income countries, where life expectancy is rising in parallel with the duration of life living with comorbidities. As the population ages, life expectancy in good health rises more slowly, and consequently time lived with ill health is progressively increasing with the associated attendant health care costs.[24]

One way in which health care controls may be brought under control may be through modification of funding mechanisms within health care systems. Incentivization resulting from different funding mechanisms is recognized to be a key driver of behavior within health systems. For example, "fee for service" models incentivize physician activity through encouraging the conduct of tests and procedures that can be billed for and thereby increase the income of health care providers.[25] With this funding model, it may be argued that physician and patient interests are not aligned and perverse incentives may arise: physicians get more remuneration the longer and more complicated a patient's hospital stay. In such a setting, there is little financial incentive to make a decision against surgery as both the procedure and any adverse consequences will provide revenue to the provider. By contrast, so-called capitation involves the provision of funding to particular geographically or functionally defined groups of patients to provide for their entire health care needs.[26] In such a system, the incentives for health care providers are to maximize positive health outcomes and minimize burden on the health care system to provide the greatest benefit to the largest number of patients. So called "bundled payment" systems reside in the middle ground between these two approaches.[27] Bundled payments involve the provision of funding for all the care of a particular category of patients with a specific problem. For example, elective hip surgery may attract a certain monetary tariff that is fixed for all patients. Hospitals that deliver good efficient care with few adverse outcomes will be rewarded through the generation of an operating surplus within such a system. Less efficient and effective systems with worse outcomes will lose money and may therefore exit the market, invest in improving their processes, or focus more attention on decision-making with respect to which patients they operate on.

Each system favors a particular type of thinking in relation to organization of activity. Fee-for-service models will tend to drive organizations into provider silos with types of practitioners who receive payments (e.g., surgeons) being protective of this situation and tending to make choices that contribute to increasing activity, and therefore income. Bundled payments tend to drive behavior at an institutional level, which may for example encourage institutions to avoid higher-risk patients because of the institutional level-financial risk. Capitation systems tend to drive thinking across the whole health care system, in order to maximize positive outcomes while minimizing cost. Both bundled payments and capitation systems tend to encourage attention to pathways in contrast to silos. Saving money in one silo is of little benefit to an institution or health care system if the consequence is to drive up costs in another part of the system. Movement toward capitation funding mechanisms is an important element of the ICOs discussed above.

Pathway Reengineering

One approach to addressing the challenge of silo-based care and moving toward a pathway focus is encapsulated in the methods of business process reengineering (BPRE).[28,29] BPRE is an approach borrowed from the corporate management literature that is based on the analysis of workflows and process in order to facilitate fundamental redesign of a more efficient and effective health care system. The aims of BPRE are to improve "customer experience" and efficiency and thereby lower costs. In the context of health care, "customer experience" can be reframed as "patient outcomes and experience," and the effectiveness of the pathway in delivering patient outcomes becomes an important driver of value along with attention to cost containment. Self-evidently, these ambitions are consistent with the recognized aims of health care systems, including the IHI Triple Aim discussed earlier.[13,14]

In the health care setting, execution of BPRE requires careful mapping of the relevant clinical pathway(s), with attention to the timing and scale of flow of patients at different decision points followed by deconstruction/reconstruction according to the aims of patient focus, efficiency, and value. Experience with pathway remodeling in relation to the introduction of enhanced recovery pathways has taught us that achieving such reengineering is only likely to be successful in the context of a multi-disciplinary approach.[30]

In the perioperative context a critical element of such reengineering is moving the encounter between perioperative specialist and patient earlier in the pathway. As an example, preoperative assessment clinics typically take place a few days before surgery. The consequence of this timing is that opportunities for preoperative intervention and decision-making are substantially limited. The alternative approach involves restructuring the pathway to ensure that the encounter between specialist and patient occurs as soon as possible after the "moment of contemplation of surgery"—the first time that surgery becomes a significant likelihood. Such a change enables improved decision-making in relation to future treatments as well as providing the opportunity to improve patient resilience in the face of an imminent physiologically challenging treatment (e.g., surgery, chemotherapy). Examples of traditional and "reengineered" pathways are shown in Fig. 16.1.[29] However, such changes require close inter-disciplinary working with a focus on best patient outcomes, rather than on provider convenience.

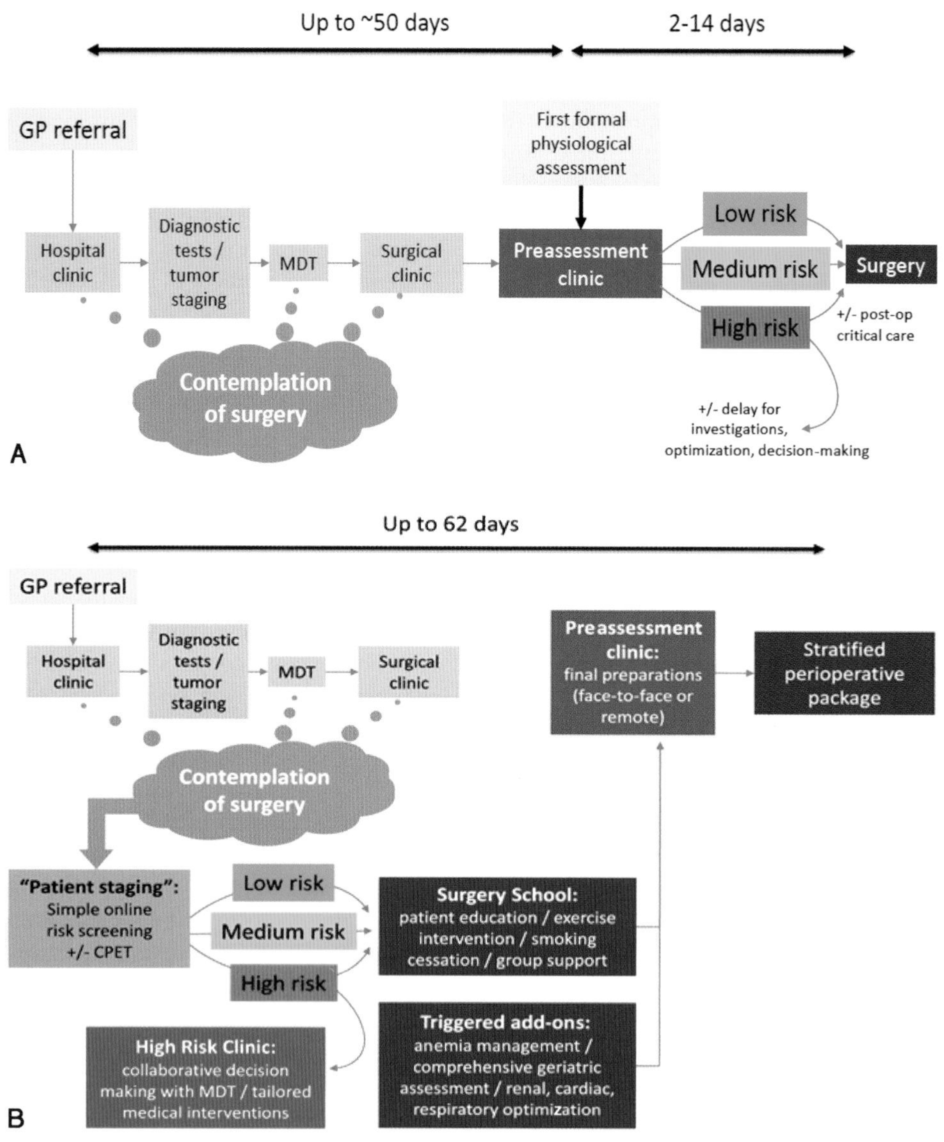

• **Fig. 16.1** Examples of traditional and "reengineered" pathways

Implications of Pathway-Focused Care

Before Surgery

Reengineering of patients pathways to surgery may facilitate improved decision-making with respect to treatment choice (SDM) and improving preparation for surgery through prehabilitation and comorbidity management.

Shared Decision-Making

The notion of SDM has become increasingly important as the patient-physician interaction has evolved from a traditional, paternalistic interaction to a more collaborative and balanced relationship.[31] For many patients, the idea that their physician will "make decisions for them" is not acceptable, and the concept of patient as consumer is increasingly prevalent, particularly in contexts where the patient is a direct purchaser of care. However, for many other patients the doctor is seen as the decision maker whose opinion they would not consider challenging. Clearly, a spectrum of interactions exists within which SDM may contribute.[32]

The shorthand for SDM has been "no decision about me, without me." As a movement, SDM has been embraced by patient groups, policy makers, and health care providers as well some, but not all, health care practitioners. For patients, the benefits in terms of autonomy and self-determination are obvious. Policy makers and providers embrace the health economic argument, which is based on the understanding that those patients at greatest risk of adverse outcome should, in general, be most likely to choose against a particular treatment and will also most likely present a financial burden to the system due to the likelihood of adverse outcomes (e.g., postoperative complications and increased length of stay).

While practitioners also recognize these arguments, there is evidence of variable enthusiasm for SDM among health care professionals.[33,34] It is also interesting that there may be discordance in patients' and physicians' views on goals of care[34] when presented with decisions about health care interventions; medical professionals' views about treatment that they would want for themselves may be different from what they would suggest for their patients (more or less conservative), including in the context of cancer diagnoses.[35,36] This striking observation suggests that physicians have a greater appreciation of the scope and magnitude of adverse consequences from major interventions, such as surgery or chemotherapy, and therefore tend to choose against them, all other things being equal.

While as first glance, SDM may not seem to be particularly relevant to patients having cancer, where many therapies are "life-saving," in fact in many cases the situation is much more nuanced. The nature of the natural history of the underlying cancer is clearly critical in this respect, with striking contrasts between fast-growing and aggressive tumors that are associated with poor short- and medium-term outcomes (e.g., pancreas) in contrast to more indolent tumors where many patients may die with, rather than of, their cancer (e.g., prostate).

As an example, it is now clear that for patients with prostate cancer, there is no meaningful survival difference between watchful waiting and treatment with surgery or radiotherapy.[37] There are, however, substantial qualitative differences in the likelihood of various complications. Decision-making between therapies are therefore much more about choice of different types of decrement in quality of life, rather than any quantitative differences in survival. In this context, SDM has a very obvious and valuable role. However, even with much more aggressive tumors, SDM may have substantial utility. SDM is considered in more detail in Chapter 55.

Prehabilitation

Prehabilitation involves enhancing the functional capacity of a person to enable them to withstand a stressful event, for example the physiologic challenge of most anticancer treatments, including surgery and chemotherapy.[38] To quote the recently published principles and guidance for prehabilitation within the management and support of people with cancer: "Prehabilitation enables people with cancer to prepare for treatment by promoting healthy behaviors in order to maximize resilience to treatment and improve long-term health. Prehabilitation empowers people with cancer to enhance their own physical and mental health and well-being and thereby supports them to live life as fully as they can."[39] Prehabilitation includes exercise, nutrition, and psychologic interventions, as well as alcohol and smoking cessation, often supported by specific behavioral change techniques.[39,40] Prehabilitation is something that patients do, supported by health care professionals, and is centered around changes in patient behavior. This is in contrast with the medical management of long-term conditions that typically involves pharmacologic or procedural interventions.[40] Practically, prehabilitation involves screening to identify needs based on assessment and prescription of relevant interventions. Trials in this area have shown high levels of adherence to hospital-based interventions before surgery and home-based interventions seem to have much lower adherence rates.[38] Randomized studies have also shown improved patient satisfaction, and early data suggest that substantial reductions in complication rates are achievable in some centers.[38] A number of major trials are currently evaluating prehabilitation before cancer surgery. Prehabilitation is discussed in more detail in Chapter 15.

Comorbidity Management

The prevalence of comorbidities increases with age: more than 50% of people over the age of 50 years have at least one comorbidity.[24] Consequently, multimorbidity—defined as the existence of multiple medical conditions in a single individual—is also becoming increasingly common.[41] Patients most commonly present with cancer over the age of 50 years, and many of the risk factors for cancer (inactivity, obesity, poor diet) are also predisposing factors for a variety of other long-term conditions that majorly impact the risk profile of many cancer interventions. Management of these long-term conditions or comorbidities (e.g., diabetes, heart disease) is an important element of preoperative preparation to maximize resilience to the physiologic challenges of the surgical episode. Once again, such management is most likely to be effective if more time is available for interventions to be scheduled and benefits to be realized. Pathway reengineering to enable early screening and referral for comorbidity management maximizes the likelihood that such comorbidities will be optimally managed.[29] Comorbidity-specific preoperative clinics are becoming integral to effective preoperative pathways. Anemia clinics are probably the most prevalent,[42] but diabetes, cardiac, respiratory, and other specialist areas are also being served. Although some clinics may be face to face, many are virtually configured with established standard operating procedures for most common problems and specialist involvement only required for complex or difficult cases. Comorbidity management is covered in more detail in Chapter 14.

During Surgery

Two fundamental concepts are of relevance to the intraoperative period in relation to pathway thinking: minimizing physiologic harm and standardizing delivery of care.

Minimizing Physiologic Harm

The first of these is the concept that a core element of intraoperative care for both surgeons and anesthesiologists is the minimization of physiologic harm. This is in keeping with the principals of enhanced recovery,[43] which has championed minimally invasive surgery and is also an essential complement to the principles of prehabilitation and comorbidity management. The conceptual framework of resilience, response, and recovery from injury (Fig. 16.2) is useful in this regard. Prehabilitation and comorbidity management serve to maximize resilience to the imminent

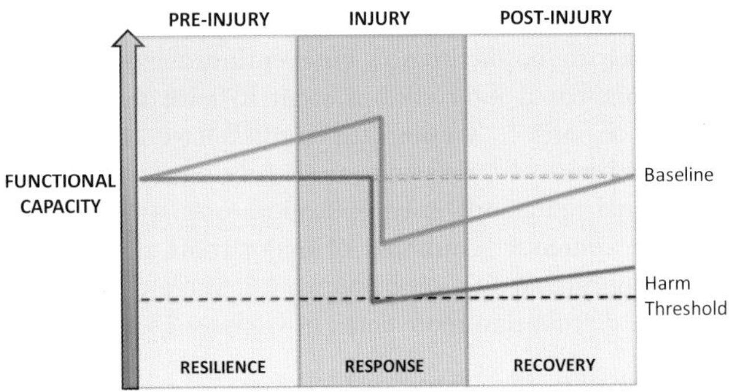

• **Fig. 16.2** Resilience-response-recovery injury model. The green trajectory indicates a prepared patient who undertakes prehabilitation and rehabilitation; by contrast, the red trajectory indicates an unprepared patient. In the green trajectory, functional capacity does not encroach upon the harm threshold. In the red trajectory, functional capacity encroaches on the harm threshold and may not recover above this level. Injury responses are heterogeneous and the unprepared patient is more vulnerable to long-term harm due to low resilience. Harm threshold indicates level at which patient may experience adverse outcome, for example death, complications, or new care dependency.

physiologic challenge of surgery. The degree of injury from surgery is dependent on both patient preoperative resilience and their individual response to the injurious stimulus. It is clear that the responses to surgical and nonsurgical trauma demonstrate substantial heterogeneity between individuals, and controlling this response is an important future therapeutic target. However, minimizing the injurious stimulus through optimizing surgical or anesthetic techniques that limit physiologic disturbance is an opportunity that is available to us now.

Standardizing Individualized Perioperative Care

The availability of "big data" to describe perioperative care on a large scale has revealed striking findings in relation to the determinants of some aspects of perioperative care. For example, in a 30,000 patient study of fluid therapy in two US institutions, the strongest determinant of fluid prescription was not any patient factor (e.g., duration of surgery, blood loss, operation type) but was the identity of the attending anesthetist (the second strongest determinant was the identity of the attending surgeon).[44] Clearly, not all these anesthesiologists can be administering the "optimal" amount of fluid and it seems implausible that most of such practice is evidence based. Such observations are repeated for other interventions (e.g., blood transfusion) and such unwarranted variation should be a cause for substantial reflection for all anesthetic practitioners.

After Surgery

The progress of patients through the recovery phase following surgery may also be helped by pathway-focused approaches. A variety of factors are relevant to patient pathways in the postoperative period, including effective implementation of enhanced recovery principles, minimization of adverse effects from medical interventions, particularly drug treatments, efficient and effective transitions from hospital to community, and rehabilitation interventions.

Arguably the most important element of enhanced recovery is the enabling of early eating, drinking, and mobilization after surgery. Not only does this so-called "DrEaMing" triad (drinking, eating, and mobilizing)[45] signify a rapid return to normal physiologic function for the patient, it also provides a useful measure of effectiveness of the care pathway and enables early discharge from hospital and thereby promotes effective use of limited resources.[45] Importantly, the effective management of postoperative pain, which has long been a core element of enhanced recovery, may facilitate early "DrEaMing." This is best achieved through balancing sufficient analgesia to control symptoms sufficiently to enable mobilization and return of normal gastrointestinal function while avoiding the harms associated with excessive analgesic treatment.[46] Concerns about the consequences for excess opioid prescription in the short (in-hospital adverse effects) and longer term (epidemic of opioid use in the community) are driving interest in opioid-free and opioid-minimizing analgesia.[47] More generally deprescribing, defined as the process of withdrawal or dose reduction of medications that are considered inappropriate in an individual[48] particularly around the time of hospital discharge, has an important role to play in minimizing long-term polypharmacy.

Early mobilization, early oral intake, and effective pain management facilitate early hospital discharge. Reliable and effective communication among hospitals and community health care and social care providers is a critical part of facilitating safe and efficient discharges.[49] Transitions of care into and out of hospital are a critical part of the patient journey around the time of surgery and failures of these processes may significantly impact patient recovery and satisfaction. Pathways designed to enable efficient return of patients to their normal living environment and, where relevant, their workplace, promote patient satisfaction and minimize resource use within health care systems. Integration of rehabilitation interventions into these pathways will promote recovery and accelerate this return to normal life.

Conclusion

People with cancer are experiencing increasingly complex medical journeys as options for treatment expand with the advent of novel therapies. The relative harms and benefits of each treatment are increasingly nuanced when the likely benefits, in terms of tumor regression, are considered alongside the possible harms of treatment, including known adverse effects and physical deconditioning. The preoperative period offers a particular opportunity to address these challenges through improved decision-making and/or interventions to reduce the risks of harm related to treatment.

Careful collaborative informed decision-making about treatments through an SDM process might contribute to improving the patient experience (greater satisfaction, reduced regret) as well as to the rational allocation of resources. Prehabilitation and comorbidity management offer the opportunity to prepare patients better for treatment (surgery, systemic anticancer therapy, radiotherapy) through improving physiologic resilience to treatments and thereby enabling more effective treatment of the underlying cancer.

Fundamental to the execution of these strategies is the reshaping of preoperative pathways to enable early SDM, prehabilitation, and comorbidity management. This may be achieved through processes such as "business process reengineering" that involve pathway mapping, deconstruction, and reconstruction to improve patient experience, clinical outcomes, and value.

References

1. Campbell S. Living with and beyond cancer: an evolving landscape. *Br J Nurs*. 2020;29(3):S3.
2. Quaresma M, Coleman MP, Rachet B. 40-year trends in an index of survival for all cancers combined and survival adjusted for age and sex for each cancer in England and Wales, 1971–2011: A population-based study. *Lancet*. 2015;385(14): 1206–1218.
3. National Cancer Registration & Analysis Service and Cancer Research UK. *Chemotherapy, Radiotherapy and Tumour Resections in England: 2013–2014 workbook*: NCRAS; 2017.
4. Hajek AM. Breaking down clinical silos in health care. *Front Health Serv Manage*. 2013;29(4):45.
5. Grocott MP. Pathway redesign: putting patients ahead of professionals. *Clin Med*. 2019;19(6):468–472.
6. Kahn JM. Virtual visits–confronting the challenges of telemedicine. *N Engl J Med*. 2015;372(18):1684–1685.
7. Bahadori S, Immins T, Wainwright TW. A review of wearable motion tracking systems used in rehabilitation following hip and knee replacement. *J Rehabil Assist Technol Eng*. 2018;5:2055668318771816.
8. Brørs G, Pettersen TR, Hansen TB, et al. Modes of e-Health delivery in secondary prevention programmes for patients with coronary artery disease: A systematic review. *BMC Health Serv Res*. 2019;19(1):36.
9. Tsianakas V, Robert G, Maben J, et al. Implementing patient-centred cancer care: Using experience-based co-design to improve patient experience in breast and lung cancer services. *Support Care Cancer*. 2012;20(11):2639–2647.
10. Litchfield I, Bentham L, Hill A, McManus RJ, Lilford R, Greenfield S. The impact of status and social context on health service co-design: An example from a collaborative improvement initiative in UK primary care. *BMC Med Res Methodol*. 2018;18(1):136.
11. Rawson TM, Moore LSP, Castro-Sanchez E, et al. Development of a patient-centred intervention to improve knowledge and understanding of antibiotic therapy in secondary care. *Antimicrob Resist Infect Control*. 2018;7:43.
12. Borgstrom E, Barclay S. Experience-based design, co-design and experience-based co-design in palliative and end-of-life care. *BMJ Support Palliat Care*. 2019;9(1):60–66.
13. Grocott MPW, Edwards M, Mythen MG, Aronson S. Perioperative care pathways: re-engineering care to achieve the 'triple aim'. *Anaesthesia*. 2019;74(Suppl 1):90–99.
14. Berwick DM, Nolan TW, Whittington J. The triple aim: Care, health, and cost. *Health Aff*. 2008;27(3):759–769.
15. Prodan Žitnik I, Černe D, Mancini I, et al. Personalized laboratory medicine: a patient-centered future approach. *Clin Chem Lab Med*. 2018;56(12):1981–1991.
16. Welch E, Jones K, Caiels J, Windle K, Bass R. Implementing personal health budgets in England: A user-led approach to substance misuse. *Health Soc Care Community*. 2017;25(5):1634–1643.
17. Santhirapala R, Fleisher LA, Grocott MPW. Choosing wisely: just because we can, does it mean we should? *Br J Anaesth*. 2019;122(3):306–310.
18. NHS website datasets. Available at https://www.nhs.uk/about-us/nhs-website-datasets/
19. Gustafson DH. Expanding on the role of patient as consumer. *QRB Qual Rev Bull*. 1991;17(10):324–325.
20. Asthana S, Gradinger F, Elston J, Martin S, Byng R. Capturing the role of context in complex system change: an application of the Canadian Context and Capabilities for Integrating Care (CCIC) Framework to an Integrated Care Organisation in the UK. *Int J Integr Care*. 2020;20(1):4.
21. Iacobucci G. STPs will end purchaser-provider split in parts of England, says NHS chief. *BMJ*. 2017;356:j1125.
22. Porter ME. What is value in health care? *N Engl J Med*. 2010;363:2477–2481.
23. Grocott MP, Mythen MG. Perioperative medicine: the value proposition for anesthesia? A UK perspective on delivering value from anesthesiology. *Anesthesiol Clin*. 2015;33:617–628.
24. Barnett K, Mercer SW, Norbury M, Watt G, Wyke S, Guthrie B. Epidemiology of multimorbidity and implications for health care, research, and medical education: A cross-sectional study. *Lancet*. 2012;380(9836):37–43.
25. McPherson E, Hedden L, Regier DA. Impact of oncologist payment method on health care outcomes, costs, quality: A rapid review. *Syst Rev*. 2016;5(1):160.
26. Goodson JD, Bierman AS, Fein O, Rask K, Rich EC, Selker HP. The future of capitation: The physician role in managing change in practice. *J Gen Intern Med*. 2001;16(4):250–256.
27. Porter ME, Kaplan RS. How to pay for health care. *Harv Bus Rev*. 2016;94(7–8):88–98.
28. Hammer M. Reengineering work: don't automate, obliterate. *Harv Bus Rev*. 1990:104–112.
29. Grocott MPW, Plumb JOM, Edwards M, Fecher-Jones I, Levett DZH. Re-designing the pathway to surgery: Better care and added value. *Perioper Med*. 2017;6:9.
30. Roulin D, Najjar P, Demartines N. Enhanced recovery after surgery implementation: from planning to success. *J Laparoendosc Adv Surg Tech A*. 2017;27(9):876–879.
31. Glance LG, Osler TM, Neuman MD. Redesigning surgical decision making for high-risk patients. *N Eng J Med*. 2014;370:1379–1381.
32. Chin JJ. Doctor-patient relationship: from medical paternalism to enhanced autonomy. *Singapore Med J*. 2002;43(3):152–155.
33. Bailoor K, Valley T, Perumalswami C, Shuman AG, DeVries R, Zahuranec DB. How acceptable is paternalism? A survey-based study of clinician and nonclinician opinions on paternalistic decision making. *AJOB Empir Bioeth*. 2018;9(2):91–98.
34. Zeuner R, Frosch DL, Kuzemchak MD, Politi MC. Physicians' perceptions of shared decision-making behaviours: A qualitative study demonstrating the continued chasm between aspirations and clinical practice. *Health Expect*. 2015;18(6):2465–2476.
35. Harrison M, Milbers K, Hudson M, Bansback N. Do patients and health care providers have discordant preferences about which aspects of treatments matter most? Evidence from a

systematic review of discrete choice experiments. *BMJ Open.* 2017;7(5):e014719.

36. Ubel PA, Angott AM, Zikmund-Fisher BJ. Physicians recommend different treatments for patients than they would choose for themselves. *Arch Intern Med.* 2011;171:630–634.
37. Donovan JL, Hamdy FC, Lane JA, et al. Patient-reported outcomes after monitoring, surgery, or radiotherapy for prostate cancer. *N Engl J Med.* 2016;375(15):1425–1437.
38. Richardson K, Levett DZH, Jack S, Grocott MPW. Fit for surgery? Perspectives on pre-operative exercise testing and training. *Br J Anaesth.* 2017;119(Suppl 1):i34–i43.
39. Macmillan Cancer Support, Royal College of Anaesthetists and NIHR Cancer and Nutrition Collaboration. Principles and guidance for prehabilitation within the management and support of people with cancer. 2019. Available at https://www.macmillan.org.uk/assets/prehabilitation-guidance-for-people-with-cancer.pdf
40. Levett DZ, Edwards M, Grocott M, Mythen M. Preparing the patient for surgery to improve outcomes. *Best Pract Res Clin Anaesthesiol.* 2016;30(2):145–157.
41. The Academy of Medical Sciences. Multimorbidity: a priority for global health research. 2018. Available at https://acmedsci.ac.uk/file-download/82222577.
42. Guinn NR, Guercio JR, Hopkins TJ, et al. How do we develop and implement a preoperative anemia clinic designed to improve perioperative outcomes and reduce cost? *Transfusion.* 2016;56(2):297–303.
43. Grocott MP, Martin DS, Mythen MG. Enhanced recovery pathways as a way to reduce surgical morbidity. *Curr Opin Crit Care.* 2012;18:385–392.
44. Lilot M, Ehrenfeld JM, Lee C, et al. Variability in practice and factors predictive of total crystalloid administration during abdominal surgery: retrospective two-centre analysis. *Br J Anaesth.* 2015;114:767–776.
45. Levy N, Mills P, Mythen M. Is the pursuit of DREAMing (drinking, eating and mobilising) the ultimate goal of anaesthesia? *Anaesthesia.* 2016;71:1008–1012.
46. McEvoy MD, Scott MJ, Gordon DB, et al. American Society for Enhanced Recovery (ASER) and Perioperative Quality Initiative (POQI) joint consensus statement on optimal analgesia within an enhanced recovery pathway for colorectal surgery: part 1-from the preoperative period to PACU. *Perioper Med.* 2017;6:8.
47. Wu CL, King AB, Geiger TM, et al. American Society for Enhanced Recovery and Perioperative Quality Initiative joint consensus statement on perioperative opioid minimization in opioid-naïve patients. *Anesth Analg.* 2019;129(2):567–577.
48. Kelly M. Faith in Subtraction: deprescribing in older patient facilitates needed surgery. *Am Fam Physician.* 2018;98(11):634.
49. Levy N, Grocott MPW, Lobo DN. Restoration of function: The holy grail of peri-operative care. *Anaesthesia.* 2020;75(Suppl 1):e14–e17.

17

Airway Management in Special Situations

GANG ZHENG

Special situations in cancer airway management, including unexpected difficult tracheal intubation, airway bleeding, and extubating a difficult airway, are major challenges in cancer airway management. Although the majority of airway events are managed uneventfully, failure of airway management occurs despite the application of various techniques and leads to fatal outcomes, emphasizing the importance of situation awareness, preparing for unexpected difficulties, appropriate working environment, and team collaboration.

Management of Unanticipated Difficult Airway

Due to rapid progress and local invasion of the cancerous disease in the upper aerodigestive tract, the complex changes in airway anatomy from previous surgery, the tissue changes resulting from head and neck radiotherapy, and so on, management of unexpected situations occurs more often in patients undergoing head and neck cancer resection than in those with gross normal anatomy in the airway. These cases often present unique challenges. However, the obstruction of airflow and/or the intubation path are primary issues in management of the cancer airway regardless of the underlying pathologic change; therefore the principle of airway management in these cases is not different from any other airway management. A systemic approach with appropriate strategies for various unexpected situations ahead of time and abundant clinical experiences plays key roles in these scenarios.

Cancer Airway Assessment

Understanding the baseline condition and underlying airway mechanism is essential for formulating a practical strategy. A comprehensive perioperative assessment of a patient undergoing head and neck cancer surgery should include a focused history related to respiratory symptoms, issues of intolerance of hypoxia, history of anticancer therapy, including surgery and radiotherapy, and records of previous airway management. Conventional airway assessment tools focus on the patients' characteristics to evaluate the potential issues of (1) patient cooperation or consent, (2) difficult mask ventilation, (3) difficult supraglottic airway placement, (4) difficult laryngoscopy, (5) difficult intubation, and (6) difficult surgical airway access.[1] In general, bedside airway assessment tools have low sensitivity and high variability.[2] For a cancer airway, the following information is also carefully inquired and assessed:

- **Primary versus recurring disease:** For a primary neoplasm, the mass effect and corresponding anatomic change due to the tumor growth are the primary assessing points. For a recurring disease, the impacts of tissue change to the airway management from previous cancer therapies, including surgery and radiotherapy, must also be included in the airway assessment.
- **Cancer stage and location:** The staging system (TNM) for cancer in the upper aerodigestive tract is the tumor (T), node (N), and metastasis (M). The stage and location of cancer pathology exert significant influence on airway management. The "T" is the primary consideration in managing the airway. Oral cavity or oropharyngeal cancer rarely causes significant obstruction of the intubation path, whereas a cancer located in the hypopharynx or larynx will be more likely to cause obstruction of not only the airflow, but also of the intubation path. Invasion of cancer into cartilage at an advanced cancer (stage 3–4) will markedly restrict the intubation pathway and curb the insertion of an endotracheal tube (ETT) through the tumor site. It is worth mentioning that forcing an ETT though a critical stenosis site may result in immediate airway obstruction and a fatal outcome.
- **Head and neck radiation:** Radiation toxicity induces significant tissue changes and organ dysfunction. The issues that affect the airway management include acute airway edema (early stage change), lymph edema and/or diffused tissue thickness, and tissue fibrosis (later stage change). Crucial laryngeal edema is rare but may require tracheostomy to maintain the airway. A study showed that more than 50% of patients who received a full dose

of head and neck radiotherapy develop acute laryngeal edema.[3] Tissue fibrosis, lymphedema, and/or diffused tissue thickening are common late issues. One study (n = 81) showed that 75% of patients developed lymphedema and 30% had edema only in the aerodigestive tract.[4] Therefore facial edema is not always correlated to the internal change in the airway and should not be used as a predictor of airway edema. Lymphedema lasts many years and imposes remarkable adverse impacts to airway management in these patients. Loss of tissue compliance after tissue fibrosis challenges the exposure of the glottis and increases the failure of laryngoscopy. Coexisting restriction in neck range of motion and trismus resulting from tissue fibrosis further curb the intubation efforts. One must understand that these problems cannot be solved by administration of a neuromuscular relaxant.

- **Anatomic changes from previous surgery:** Although previous surgery in the upper aerodigestive tract may raise the concern of local anatomic changes, clinical experiences have indicated that a well-healed surgical site rarely curbs face mask ventilation and the performance of tracheal intubation. One study of 472 oral cavity and oropharyngeal cancer airways showed that only 7.4% of these airways managed with an advanced technique were due to the concern of distorted airway anatomy from previous surgery, and failure of airway management in this population is low.[5]
- **Inability to support the airway immediately after surgery:** Inability to support the airway immediately after surgery is not uncommon in cases of free tissue transfer (free flap) reconstruction surgery. The airway manipulation and pressure added to the flap during rescue of the airway may result in severe flap damage or failure. The potential risks of extubating the airway in these cases must be carefully assessed ahead of time.

Limits of Diagnostic Imaging Studies for Cancer Airway Evaluation

The primary goal of various cancer imaging studies is to facilitate cancer evaluation, rather than airway assessment. The limits of imaging findings in airway assessment should be fully appreciated. The commonly used imaging studies for cancer evaluation include magnetic resonance imaging (MRI), contrast enhanced computed tomography (CECT), and ultrasound study. Diagnostic imaging studies depict the tumor margin and the anatomic location of the tumor. However, the caliber of the airway varies depending on the respiratory circle. Deep inspiration increases the caliber of the airway and expiration reduces it. MRI or CT scan cannot capture the dynamic changes of the airway space. Unless special techniques are applied, such as a second pass with breath holding during deep inspiration, the maximal airway space available at the tumor site, and therefore the appropriate tube size, cannot be determined (Fig. 17.1). The interpretation of imaging findings must therefore be combined with clinical evaluation. Although a high-resolution ultrasound study may be used to assess vocal fold mobility and the maximal airway caliber, inadequate spatial resolution remains an issue for accurately measuring the airway space.

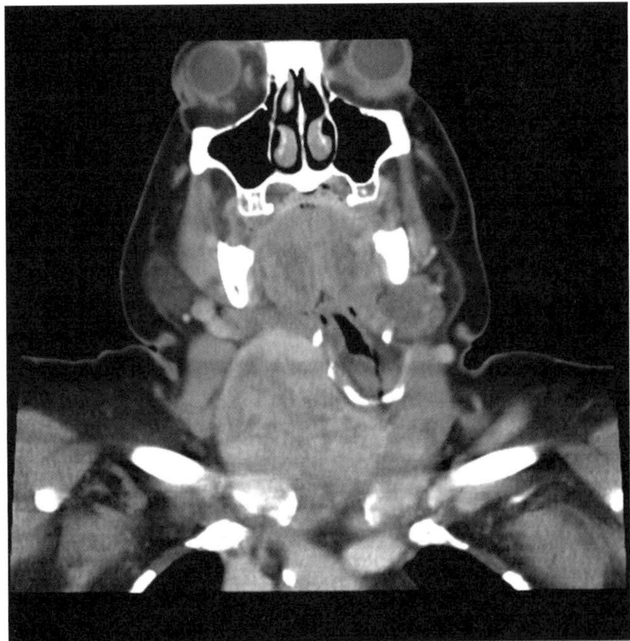

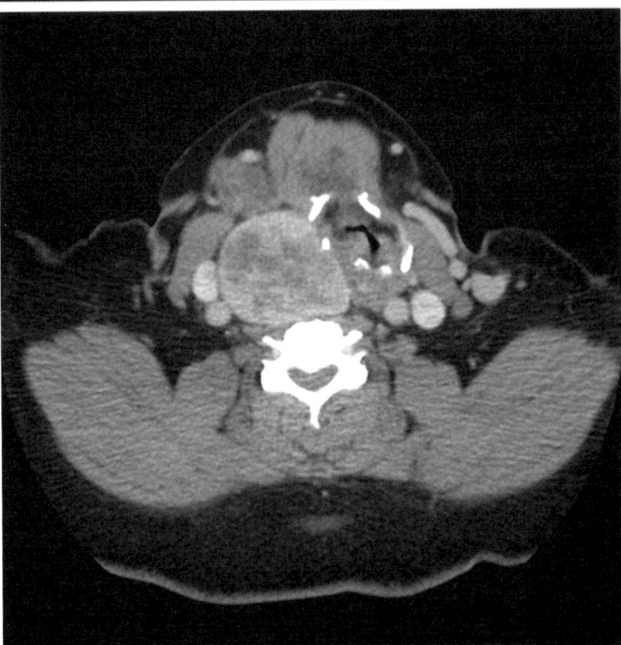

• **Fig. 17.1** Coronal *(upper)* and transverse *(lower)* planes of computed tomography (CT) images from a large thyroid mass. The CT images show significant left shift and compression of the larynx and trachea by the thyroid mass effect. However, the clinical evaluation indicated an asymptomatic patient with respect to respiratory status. The subsequent flexible scope intubation revealed insignificant airway compression suggesting a mismatch between CT findings and clinical presentation.

Guidelines and Cognitive Aids in Managing Difficult Airways

Globally, all the major societies of anesthesiology or airway management have published guidelines and algorithms for management of the airway in various situations.[1,6] These documents consist of fundamental elements in daily airway management and should be routinely applied to cancer airway management. Further, an appropriately designed cognitive aid is an important tool in the management of an unexpected airway event and should be routinely included in the cancer airway management strategy. A study showed that when appropriately implemented, a cognitive aid is effective for improving team communication and promoting situation awareness.[7] A meta-analysis of outcome measures showed that the surgical safety checklist improves the effect on teamwork and communication by 1.2-fold and enhances heterogeneity.[8] Effective implementation of a checklist requires that the entire team participate in the process, receive support from senior personnel, have appropriate education and training, and address the barriers to the implementation of the checklist. Implementing a safety checklist should consider the needs of the patient population, the procedures, and the practice environment.

Training and Education in Cancer Airway Management

Difficult or failed tracheal intubation due to inadequate skill in using advanced tools is not uncommon. Lack of skill curbs the efforts of managing an unexpected airway event. Training should emphasize the critical skills in managing cancer airway such as flexible scope intubation (awake or asleep) and lifesaving skills such as cricothyroidotomy (needle or scalp) that are not used as routine anesthesia practice. One survey from 147 directors of an anesthesiology residency program in the United States and Canada showed that approximately one-third of graduating residents were estimated to have performed 25 awake fiber optic intubations during their training.[9] The skill level for preforming an awake flexible bronchoscopy will rapidly decay if it is not used in routine practice after residency. Cricothyroidotomy is a lifesaving technique. Correct identification of the cricothyroid membrane (CTM) is not only the key to success but also to reducing the risk of major complications. Inability to identify the CTM is a common issue among anesthesiologists and surgeons. One study showed that less than 50% of anesthesia providers and trauma surgeons were able to identify the CTM in nonobese females with optimized neck extension. Prior experience of emergency surgical airway did not improve the success rate,[10] emphasizing the importance of training on a regular basis. Further, clinical data showed that in comparing elective cases, emergency airway management bears a significantly higher morbidity and mortality, suggesting that training should not be focused on clinical skills only but must be performed in different environments and situations.

Human Factor in Airway Management

The 4th National Audit Project (NAP4) studied the major complications of airway management in the UK and showed that the majority of the major complications of airway management in the emergency department would have been preventable through an improved system, better preparation, and good communication,[11] suggesting that human factors impose significant adverse impacts in patient outcomes. The NAP4 also revealed that we are unable to effectively manage the difficult situations with our existing knowledge, "...the vast majority of the reports concerned events that are already well known to the anesthetic community but it seems that we have not learned from the past..."[12] Acknowledging the human limits and inclusion of human factors in training and education curricula will enhance teamwork, communication, situation awareness, and the decision-making process.

Principles and Strategies of Managing an Unexpected Difficult Cancer Airway

Following the first airway management guidelines published in 1993 by the American Society of Anesthesiologists (ASA), all the major societies of anesthesiology or airway management have published their corresponding guidelines. These guidelines provide step-by-step approaches to managing the difficult airway in different clinical scenarios. The practice guideline for management of the difficult airway by the ASA (2013) proposed basic preparations for difficult airway management including:

- Availability of appropriate equipment with at least one portable storage unit containing specialized equipment for difficult airway management readily available,
- Informing the patient with a known or suspected difficult airway and procedures pertaining to managing a difficult airway,
- Ascertaining an assigned individual to provide assistance,
- Preanesthetic preoxygenation by mask before initiation of anesthetic induction, and
- Actively pursuing the chance to deliver supplemental oxygen throughout the process of managing the difficult airway.

The guidelines for management of unanticipated difficult intubation in adults by the Difficult Airway Society (DAS, 2015)[6] proposed a simplified, single algorithm, including a four-plan strategy consisting of:

- Face mask ventilation and tracheal intubation as an initial step (Plan A),
- Maintaining oxygenation by a supraglottic airway device (SAD) after an unsuccessful initial intubation attempt (Plan B),
- Final attempt at face mask ventilation as the last effort of noninvasive intervention (Plan C), and
- Performing emergency front of neck access (FONA, Plan D).

These recommendations and step-by-step approaches comprise the fundamental components in management of the difficult airway in different clinical situations.

Techniques and Tools for Management of the Difficult Cancer Airway

Ventilation and oxygenation of the lungs is the primary determinant of an urgent or emergency airway event. The tools that are commonly used to achieve effective lung ventilation and oxygenation include face mask and SAD. In recent years, application of heated, humidified high-flow oxygen devices such as Optiflow (Fisher & Paykel, Healthcare Ltd., Auckland, New Zealand) has increased in airway management and is reported to enhance oxygen delivery, counterbalance auto-PEEP (positive end-expiratory pressure), and increase ventilatory efficiency.[13] One early study in 25 patients showed that at an oxygen flow rate of 70 L/min, the patients maintained oxygen saturation above 90% with a median apneic time of 14 min (range, 5–65 min).[14] Another study on 21 healthy volunteers showed that Optiflow provided rapid oxygenation. With a flow rate of 70 L/min, patients achieved 72% end-tidal oxygen concentration (ETo_2) in 30 s and reached the ETo_2 peak level of 88% in 150 s.[15] Use of a nasal oxygen cannula as a machine-human interface increases patient tolerance and compliance during the course of preoxygenation, especially for patients with claustrophobia. Current studies favor its usage in airway management although the benefits for cancer airway management need to be further studied.

Due to significant risk of airway bleeding after failed airway intubation, the initial intubation technique should be carefully selected based on the anesthesiologist's previous experiences. In general, videolaryngoscope is a preferred tool for an unobstructed airway, and flexible scope remains the most popular tool to intubate a partially obstructed airway. Multiple randomized controlled trials (RCTs) have compared the outcomes of direct laryngoscopy and videolaryngoscopy intubation. Tracheal intubation by videolaryngoscopy had higher success rates on the first attempt in patients with predictors of difficult airway (C-MAC; Karl Storz, Tuttlingen, Germany)[16] in patients with restricted neck mobility (Pentax-AWS; Pentax Corporation, Tokyo Japan),[17] or in simulated difficult airway (GlideScope, Bothell, MA, USA).[18]

Comparing videolaryngoscopes, the flexible scope remains a nonreplaceable tool in managing various levels of obstructive airways. However, performing flexible scope intubation demands an experienced hand, a clean field, and is time-consuming. Further, the flexible scope is limited during a time-sensitive event. Inability to maintain adequate oxygenation during the procedure due to various causes is a common problem and curbs the success of flexible scope intubation. The tube impinging on laryngeal structure during the flexible scope intubation resulting in difficulty or impossibility in sliding the ETT into the trachea is also a common issue.[19] This may be especially true when intubating the trachea via a partially obstructed pathway at the tumor site. It is important to select an appropriate ETT for flexible scope intubation in cancer airway management. One RCT on 80 patients compared outcomes of flexible scope oral intubation using a Parker Flex-Tip tube (PFT) (Parker Medical, Highlands Ranch, CO, USA) (Fig. 17.2) and a standard-tip tube and found that use of the PFT resulted in a two-thirds reduction in the rate of resistance to passage of the tube into the trachea.[20] Another randomized study on 40 individuals during transnasal fiber optic intubation reported that PFT significantly reduced the incidence of traumatic nose bleeding when compared with using a standard-tip tube during nasal intubation.[21]

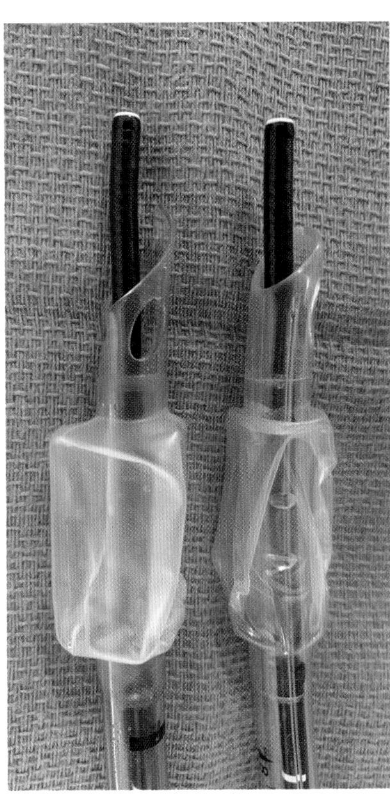

• **Fig. 17.2** The effect of a 7-mm ID Parker Flex-Tip ET tube *(left)* and a 7-mm ID regular endotracheal tube (ETT) *(right)* on a 3.8-mm flexible scope. The inward-pointed tip of the Parker Flex-Tip tube reduces the chance of tube impingement on the surrounding structure or hanging tissue along the intubation path. In comparison, the thick and noncompliant tip of the regular ETT is more likely to strike a hanging structure along its pathway.

Combined techniques may be used to improve the performance and success rate of tracheal intubation. One example is videolaryngoscopy-assisted flexible scope intubation for laryngeal or hypopharyngeal cancer airway, in which videolaryngoscopy facilitates the insertion of a flexible scope to bypass the base of tongue and improve the view of the scope, and guides the suction tip to clear airway secretions and blood. However, the requirement for two people to collaborate with each other increases the complexity of the operation. Trans-intubation laryngeal mask airway (iLMA) tracheal intubation has been used in routine practice or emergency situations. This technique not only provides the chance of uninterrupted oxygenation during the procedure but also guides the flexible scope to bypass the base of tongue and locate the glottic opening. The selection of technique and tool should be based on the findings from the preanesthetic assessment, underlying airway issues, and personal experiences.

Establishing a successful invasive airway is the last chance to save a life in the course of managing an emergency airway. In all the major airway guidelines, the final common pathway in managing the situation of CICO (can't intubate, can't oxygenate) is to establish an emergency invasive airway. However, delay in performing such a procedure remains a major issue. In the NAP4 report, three of six deaths out of a total of 58 anesthetic patients undergoing emergency surgical airway were the result of failed emergency airway. The report of "A closed claims analysis" by Peterson et al. (2005) revealed that the percentage of patients undergoing attempted surgical airway who died or sustained brain damage was 84%.[22] Clinical evidence suggests that reluctance to perform such a procedure and inadequate training are the major causes of delay and failure of the operation. In practice, among the three most commonly performed techniques in establishing an invasive airway via CTM, including narrow bore cannula, wide bore cannula, and surgical airway, cricothyroidotomy by scalpel-bougie tube technique to establish an emergency airway (FONA) is the preferred technique recommended by the DAS. Although no special cricothyroidotomy technique was recommended by ASA practice guidelines, the use of a familiar technique and an early decision are general principles for performing an invasive airway. In practice, inability of appropriate identification of CTM is also a recognized issue hindering the success of cricothyroidotomy. The study showed that the overall success rate by palpation to recognize the CTM was less than 50%. The performance was not different between anesthesia providers and trauma surgeons (95% confidence interval [CI], −23 to 3; $P = 0.15$). Further, no significant difference was found in the success rates for identifying the CTM by either clinical experience or the previous emergency surgical airway experience.[10]

Extubation of the Difficult Airway

In the NAP4 report, the major airway events occurring during anesthetic emergence or recovery generally fall into one of two categories: airway obstruction or pulmonary aspiration. Head and neck cases constituted a third of all the cases, and 70% of reported head and neck cases were associated with airway obstruction. The multiple issues identified in these cases included inappropriate assessment and planning, substandard working environment, technique and performance errors, and so on.[11] Human factors were also identified in the majority of these fatal events.

The overall outcome of extubation failure in cancer airway management is unclear. Multiple issues impact the airway extubation in these patients. Premature removal of the ETT due to fear of hematoma development, local edema after surgery in the upper aerodigestive tract, inability to support the airway immediately after tracheal extubation due to the sensitive surgical site, and bleeding in the airway due to failure of initial airway manipulation are not uncommon and markedly increase the difficulty of airway management. Multiple failures in technique often coexist with the aforementioned situations. Developing effective strategies for extubating a difficult airway is therefore essential in managing the cancer airway. Existing guidelines published by the major anesthesiology or airway management societies, including the ASA and DAS, provide systemic approaches for managing these challenging situations.

Current Guidelines for Managing Extubation Failure or At-Risk Extubation

The ASA Practice Guidelines for Management of the Difficult Airway (2013) stated that "an extubation strategy is considered to be a logical extension of the intubation strategy" and should include consideration of evaluating the advantages of awake versus deep extubation, assessing the risks and establishing management strategies when failing to maintain adequate ventilation after tracheal extubation, and the short-term use of devices for expedited reintubation when indicated.

The DAS extubation guidelines/algorithms (2015) delineated patient characteristics for extubation into the conditions of low risk and at risk. Compared with the ASA guidelines (2013), the DAS at-risk extubation guideline covers a wide range of situations. The condition of at-risk extubation was generally described as uncertainty of the patient to remain extubated for a prolonged duration, including the situations of expected difficult reintubation or presenting certain conditions such as inability to protect the airway and various severe systemic derangements. Four steps were described in the at-risk extubation algorithm, including planning extubation (step 1), preparing for extubation (step 2), performing extubation (step 3), and postextubation care (step 4). The key elements to be considered prior to tracheal extubation include ability to oxygenate, potential difficult reintubation, present general risk factors, and optimizing the patient's systemic derangement and environmental conditions for airway management.

Recognizing the Risk Factors Leading to Extubation Failure

Although multiple issues are responsible for extubation failure, airway obstruction is the most commonly reported cause,[11,23] and obesity or obstructive sleep apnea (OSA) were found to be common patient characteristics in these cases.[11,24]

The spectrum of head and neck cancer surgery is broad, and the risk of acquired difficult airway from surgery varies from case to case. Although there is a lack of study data, clinical observations have indicated that surgical technique and the location and duration of surgery significantly influence the outcomes of postoperative airway management. For instance, compared with laser ablation of an early-stage cancer in the oral cavity, the resection of a cancer in the hypopharynx, such as robotic resection of the base of the tongue, carries a high risk of developing airway obstruction after surgery. In general, cancer surgery in the hypopharynx and larynx renders a higher risk of airway obstruction and extubation failure after surgery than the corresponding risk of extubation failure after oral cavity or oropharyngeal surgery. Compared with a laser procedure, "cold knife" surgery has an increased risk of surgical bleeding. Airway edema is more common in prolonged surgery than in a short procedure.

General Strategies for Extubation of the Difficult Airway

Optimizing the patient's condition and physicians' working environment is essential for extubation of a difficult airway. Inappropriate preparation for managing a potential adverse airway event, poor working environment, and lack of team collaboration are the common issues hindering the efforts to manage a difficult airway. Multiple techniques may be used for extubation of a difficult airway, such as extubation over an assistant device, including a flexible scope, a gum-elastic bougie, a commercial tube exchanger, and so on. Depending on the clinical situation, deep tracheal extubation is also beneficial for selected cases.

Awake Versus Deep Extubation

Wakefulness and establishment of a regular respiratory pattern and adequate respiratory minute volume (5–7 L/min) comprise the essential components for awake tracheal extubation. The advantages of awake tracheal extubation include recovery of spontaneous respiration and airway protection, the capability to follow commands, and timely feedback of difficulty in breathing. The major challenge of awake extubation is the potential difficult emergence. Bucking and fighting with the ventilator leads to elevation of intrathoracic pressure and increases the risks of bleeding and/or hematoma at the surgical site. In extreme cases, the patient may become combative and uncontrollable. Difficult emergence may also lead to premature extubation before effective spontaneous respiration is established and therefore potentiates the risks of laryngospasm and postextubation respiratory insufficiency.

Contrary to awake extubation, deep extubation refers to the technique in which the trachea is extubated under deep anesthesia. When performing deep extubation, the patient must have regular respiratory rhythm and appropriate minute volume. The most common clinical indication for deep extubation in airway cases is to avoid difficult emergence as mentioned earlier. Successful deep extubation leads to smooth and uneventful anesthetic emergence. However, deep extubation requires experience to manage the airway. Unrecognized airway obstruction is the most dreaded situation after deep extubation. This is due to a decrease in muscular tone in the airway under deep anesthesia. With ceased or decreasing airflow due to airway obstruction, the inhalation anesthetic effect will remain constant resulting in prolonged emergence. It is well known that the airway muscular tone in both the upper (skeletal muscle) and lower airway (smooth muscle) is reduced during sleeping, leading to increased respiratory resistance.[25,26] Multiple studies have shown that tracheal extubation under deep anesthesia increases respiratory complications both in the operating room and during anesthetic recovery.[27,28] In cancer airway management, additional risks of airflow obstruction by mass effect or surgery render deep extubation a high-risk operation. The benefit over the risk of deep extubation must therefore be carefully evaluated prior to decision-making. Studies show that extreme age, oversedation, use of neuromuscular blockers, head and neck surgery, and the duration of surgery (>3 h) are risk factors of tracheal reintubation in early anesthetic recovery. In addition, patients with poor cardiac, respiratory, or renal function have increased risks for extubation failure. These risk factors must be carefully evaluated prior to extubating the airway.[29]

Strategies for Extubating the Difficult Airway

It is worth mentioning that not all difficult airways for intubation are difficult for extubation in cancer airway management. For instance, a difficult airway before the surgery may become easy after surgical resection of the airway pathology and vice versa. Bucking and fighting at anesthetic emergence promote hemorrhage at the surgical site and render the previous easy airway difficult. Continuously considering changes in airway mechanics is essential for the success of managing these cases. The principles and strategies of extubating the difficult airway are described in the airway management guidelines of many societies worldwide and should be followed in routine practice. For example, extubation of difficult airway over an airway exchange catheter (AEC) is described in the practice guidelines by the ASA and multiple clinical reports. Leaving an AEC in the airway after removal of the ETT from the trachea is thought to provide an extra safety measure when reintubation is indicated. One study of 51 intensive care unit patients showed that 92% of reintubation was successfully performed over an indwelling AEC, and 87% were achieved on the first attempt.[30] An indwelling AEC, depending on the type, may provide support for oxygen delivery by jet ventilation or insufflation and can be used as a guide for reintubation when indicated.[31,32] However, retaining an AEC in the airway after airway surgery is also risky. For those who are intolerant of an indwelling catheter, traumatic coughing and the corresponding movement of the AEC in the airway promote wound bleeding. The benefits versus the risks of performing AEC-assisted extubation must therefore be carefully balanced. The other significant risks of using AEC for airway management include barotrauma, perforation of the respiratory tract, and loss of the airway.[33,34] Replacing the ETT with a laryngeal mask airway to facilitate smooth anesthetic emergence is another technique in managing some of the challenging situations. When performed by an experienced practitioner, extubation of the airway over a SAD reduces the airway reaction during emergence. It is especially helpful in cases such as thyroidectomy, parathyroidectomy, and neck dissection.

Extubating the trachea in certain cases, such as free flap reconstruction surgery after major tumor resection in the anterior oral cavity or lower facial areas, is particularly challenging. These cases are lengthy and complex, with an average surgery duration of 8–12 h and a fluid load of 4–5 L. Due to the location of the flap in these cases, application of airway support increases the risk of flap damage. Carefully assessing the airway condition and respiratory status and ensuring smooth emergence and extubation of the airway in a fully conscious patient are essential.

Management of Upper Airway Bleeding

The mechanism of upper airway bleeding from cancer may be categorized as one of the three conditions including: (1) spontaneous bleeding from the tumor, (2) bleeding from traumatic intubation, and (3) bleeding from a surgical site. The strategy of managing a bleeding airway should be based on the underlying problem and the urgency of the condition. In general, blood in the airway and inability to maintain adequate oxygenation constitute the major challenges in these cases. An advanced intubation tool such as a videolaryngoscope or flexible bronchoscope attached to a large screen viewer should be the primary consideration. Combined techniques such as videolaryngoscopy-assisted flexible bronchoscopy or via iLMA flexible scope intubation may also be used. The person who performs the intubation should be experienced with the available tools.

Massive spontaneous bleeding from an airway tumor is a rare clinical entity. The occurrences of airway bleeding and the outcomes in these cases remain unclear. Massive upper airway bleeding usually causes suffocation and quickly results in a fatal outcome. Surgical airway should be rapidly established in those who survive the initial insult of airway bleeding. Attempts to intubate the airway should be avoided since the operation may further traumatize the bleeding site, resulting in a life-threatening condition. In contrast, intubation of the airway is often required to facilitate the surgical intervention. In these cases, awake intubation by a flexible bronchoscope is preferred in a patient with stable oxygenation and hemodynamic conditions. Videolaryngoscopy should be performed with great caution since insertion of a laryngoscope blade into the airway may further injure the bleeding site. Mild bleeding from a cancerous disease may present with bloody sputum or coughed-up blood. These cases are usually closely followed without immediate surgical intervention; therefore control of airway for these cases is not indicated.

Traumatic intubation is the most common cause of airway hemorrhage. Clinical observation indicates that the unsighted insertion of a laryngoscope blade into the tumor airway, especially a hyperangulated one such as the "D" blade of a C-MAC videolaryngoscope, can lead to laceration of the tumor and result in bleeding. Placing a blade into the airway should be performed under direct vision at all the times. In spite of the aforementioned problems, videolaryngoscopy is still the preferred primary technique in intubation of the cancer airway. Compared with the flexible scope technique, videolaryngoscopy has advantages including: (1) better field visualization, (2) ability to assess the bleeding condition, and (3) ability to guide a large suction device to clean the field, and therefore a higher first-pass success rate.

Airway bleeding at the surgical site is a surgical emergency. Spilling or coughing up copious amounts of blood after a procedure is the indication for surgical intervention. However, continuously swallowing the blood or confining it to soft tissue, especially in a suture-closed wound, often conceals the problem from early recognition. Intubation of these airways is challenging due to significant field contamination and a narrow intubation pathway by active bleeding and/or a large hematoma. Removal of the sutures may help to decompress the hematoma (Fig. 17.3). Except in a life-threatening emergency, airway management should be performed in the operation room with the surgeon standing by. Maintaining spontaneous respiration during intubation is preferred. Despite technique challenges due to field contamination, flexible scope intubation in a patient with effective spontaneous ventilation is a preferred technique due to its flexibility of operation in a narrow field. Clinical experience indicates that a patient with mild or moderate airway bleeding usually tolerates airway manipulation with application of a topical anesthetic. Use of a tranquilizer for intubation in these cases should be kept to a minimum. Meanwhile, great caution should be paid to possible massive vomiting of blood during airway manipulation.

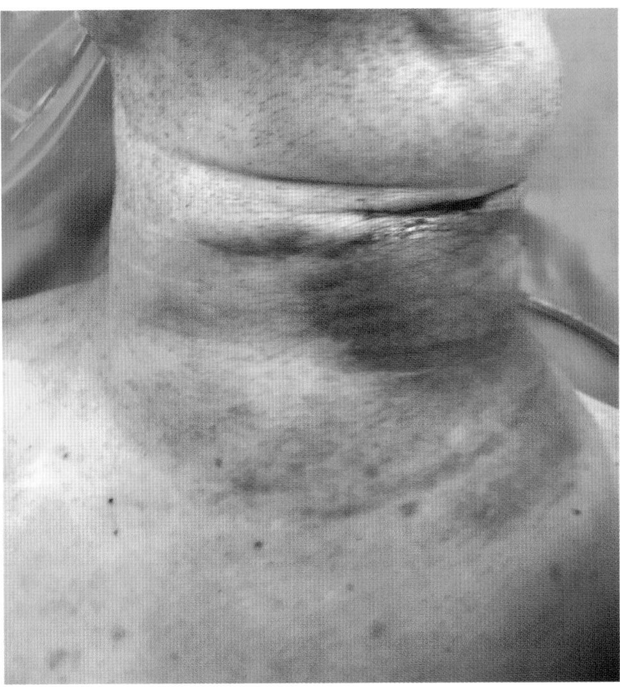

• **Fig. 17.3** Hemorrhage of multiple surgical sites, including the base of the tongue and neck dissection site, after surgery in a patient who underwent robotic partial glossectomy and unilateral neck dissection. The effects of the neck hematoma on the airway may include the airway shifting from the midline and reducing lymphatic drainage resulting in significant tissue edema.

Conclusion

Unexpected difficult cancer airway management during intubation and extubation and managing a bleeding airway comprise the major and emerging challenges in cancer airway management. Prediction of such situations is not always possible. With a high mortality rate in these cases, the urgency and emergency of the situation allows no room for erroneous decisions. There is no perfect solution for these challenging issues. Regardless of the technique used to support the airway, prioritizing the tasks, team collaboration, an adequate physician-working environment, and readiness for managing such an airway event are paramount to achieving success.

References

1. Apfelbaum JL, Hagberg CA, Caplan RA, et al. American Society of Anesthesiology task force on management of the difficult airway. Practice guidelines for management of the difficult airway: an updated report by the American Society of Anesthesiologists task force on management of the difficult airway. *Anesthesiology*. 2013;118:251–270.
2. Roth D, Pace NL, Lee A, et al. Airway physical examination tests for detection of difficult airway management in apparently normal patients. *Cochrane Database Syst Rev*. 2018;15(5):CD008874.
3. Bae JS, Roh JL, Lee SW, et al. Laryngeal edema after radiotherapy in patients with squamous cell carcinomas of the larynx and hypopharynx. *Oral Oncol*. 2012;48(9):853–858.
4. Deng J, Ridner SH, Dietrich MS, et al. Prevalence of secondary lymphedema in patients with head and neck cancer. *J Pain Symptom Manage*. 2012;43(2):244–252.
5. Zheng G, Feng L, Lewis CM. A data review of airway management in patients with oral cavity or oropharyngeal cancer: a single-institution experience. *BMC Anesthesiol*. 2019;19:92.
6. Frerk C, Mitchell VS, McNarry AF, et al. Difficult Airway Society 2015 guidelines for management of unanticipated difficult intubation in adults. *Br J Anaesth*. 2015;115(6):827–848.
7. Chrimes N. The Vortex: a universal 'high-acuity implementation tool' for emergency airway management. *Br J Anaesth*. 2016;117(S1):i20–i27.
8. Lyons VE, Popejoy LL. Meta-analysis of surgical safety checklist effects on teamwork, communication, morbidity, mortality, and safety. *West J Nurs Res*. 2014;36(2):245–261.
9. Pott LM, Randel GI, Straker T, et al. A survey of airway training among U.S. and Canadian Anesthesiology residency programs. *J Clin Anesth*. 2011;23:15–26.
10. Hiller KN, Karni RJ, Cai C, et al. Comparing success rates of anesthesia providers versus trauma surgeons in their use of palpation to identify the circothyroid membrane in female subjects: a prospective observational study. *Can J Anesth*. 2016;63(7):807–817.
11. Cook TM, Woodall N, Frerk C. 4th National Audit Project (NAP4): Major complications of airway management in the UK. 2011. Available at https://www.rcoa.ac.uk/nap4.
12. Frerk C, Pearce A. Induction and maintenance of anaesthesia. 4th National Audit Project (NAP4): Major complications of airway management in the UK. Available at https://www.rcoa.ac.uk/nap4.
13. Spoletini G, Alotaibi M, Blasi F, Hill NS. Heated humidified high flow nasal oxygen in adults: mechanisms of action and clinical implications. *Chest*. 2015;148(1):252–261.
14. Patel A, Nouraei SA. Transnasal humidified rapid insufflation ventilatory exchange (THRIVE): a physiological method of increasing apnoea time in patients with difficult airway. *Anaesthesia*. 2015;70(3):323–329.
15. Ang KS, Green A, Ramaswamy KK, Frerk C. Preoxygenation using the Optiflow™ system. *Br J Anaesth*. 2017;118(3):463–464.
16. Aziz MF, Dillman D, Fu R, Brambrink AM. Comparative effectiveness of the C-MAC video laryngoscope versus direct laryngoscopy in the setting of the predicted difficult airway. *Anesthesiology*. 2012;116(3):629–636.
17. Enomoto Y, Asai T, Kamishma K, Okuda Y. Pentax-AWS, a new videolaryngoscope, is more effective than the Macintosh laryngoscope for tracheal intubation in patients with restricted neck movements: a randomized comparative study. *Br J Anaesth*. 2008;100(4):544–548.
18. Lim Y, Yeo SW. A comparison of the GlideScope with the Macintosh laryngoscope for tracheal intubation in patients with simulated difficult airway. *Anaesth Intensive Care*. 2005;33(2):243–247.
19. Jones HE, Pearce AC, Moore P. Fiberoptic intubation: Influence of tracheal tube tip design. *Anaesthesia*. 1993;48:672–674.
20. Kristensen MS. The Parker Flex-Tip tube versus a standard tube for fiber optic orotracheal intubation. *Anesthesiology*. 2003;98(2):354–358.
21. Prior S, Heaton J, Jatana KR, Rashid RG. Parker Flex-Tip and standard-tip endotracheal tubes: A comparison during nasotracheal intubation. *Anesth Prog*. 2010;57(1):18–24.
22. Peterson GN, Domino KB, Caplan RA, et al. Management of the difficult airway: a closed claim analysis. *Anesthesiology*. 2005;103:33–39.
23. Mathew JP, Rosenbaum SH, O'Connor T, Barash PG. Emergency tracheal intubation in the postanesthesia care unit: Physician error or patient disease? *Anesth Analg*. 1990;71:691–697.
24. Benumof JL. Obesity, sleep apnea, the airway and anesthesia. *Curr Opin Anaesthesiol*. 2004;17:21–30.
25. Canning BJ. Reflex regulation of airway smooth muscle tone. *J Appl Physiol*. 2006;101:971–985.
26. Anttalainen U, Tenhunen M, Rimpila V, et al. Prolonged partial upper airway obstruction during sleep – an underdiagnosed phenotype of sleep disordered breathing. *Eur Clin Respir J*. 2016;3:31806.
27. Asai T, Koga K, Vaughan RS. Respiratory complication associated with tracheal intubation and extubation. *Br J Anaesth*. 1998;80:767–775.
28. Parr SM, Robinson BJ, Glover PW, Galletly DC. Level of consciousness on arrival in the recovery room and the development of early respiratory morbidity. *Anaesth Intensive Care Med*. 1991;19:369–372.
29. Rujirojindakul P, Geater AF, McNeil EB, et al. Risk factors for reintubation in the post-anesthetic care unit: a case-control study. *Br J Anaesth*. 2012;109:636–642.
30. Mort TC. Continuous airway access for the difficult extubation: the efficacy of the airway exchange catheter. *Anesth Analg*. 2007;105:1357–1362.
31. Benumof JL. Airway exchange catheters for safer extubation (Editorials). *Chest*. 1997;111:1483.
32. Baraka AS. Tension pneumothorax complicating jet ventilation via a Cook airway exchange catheter. *Anesthesiology*. 1990;91:557–558.
33. De Almeida JP, Hajjar LA, Fukushima JT, et al. Bronchial injury and pneumothorax after reintubation using an airway exchange catheter. *Rev Bras Anesthesiol*. 2013;63(1):107–112.
34. Cooper RM, Khan S. Extubation and reintubation of the difficult airway. In: Hagberg CA, ed. *Benumof and Hagberg's Airway Management*. Elsevier; 2017:844. 4th ed.

18

Procedural Care of the Adult Cancer Patient Outside of the Operating Room

ALAN KOTIN AND JENNIFER MASCARENHAS

Introduction

The cancer patient often requires complex diagnostic, therapeutic, and palliative care procedures in nonoperating room (non-OR) sites, which has created an increasing demand for anesthesia services in remote locations outside of the traditional operating room (OR). Remote areas requiring anesthesia continues to expand, and anesthesia services are now frequently requested for endoscopy, diagnostic radiology, interventional radiology (IR), radiation oncology, nuclear medicine, as well as for procedures such as bone marrow aspiration and biopsy. Technological advancement and movement toward minimally invasive approaches have moved procedures that were once performed in the OR to non-OR locations. Historically, patients in these remote locations were given conscious sedation by a certified nurse under the supervision of the proceduralist. The relationship between anesthesia services and proceduralists can be complex and challenging, requiring that the medical specialties gain familiarity with one another. The proceduralists and personnel in remote areas must be familiar with the anesthesia practice guidelines and standards of anesthesia to promote the highest level of safety possible for the patient. The anesthesiologist must be knowledgeable of the procedure, treatment or imaging technique, potential complications, and the anesthetic needs required for a successful procedure, treatment, or scan. The increased need for anesthesia in complex diagnostic, therapeutic, and palliative procedures performed in the cancer patient has created a demand for expertise in non-OR anesthesia (NORA). This chapter discusses the principles of sedation and analgesia as well as the role and challenges of the anesthesia team while providing services in the various NORA locations such as diagnostic radiology, IR, interventional gastroenterology and endoscopy (GI), and radiation therapy (RT).

Practice Guidelines

The American Society of Anesthesiologists (ASA) has long been an advocate for patient safety. Although anesthesiologists may not be directly involved in the care of all patients receiving sedation and analgesia for a procedure outside of the OR, there is a high likelihood that they are involved in creating, revising, and organizing sedation services throughout the hospital. Some medical subspecialties, such as the American College of Radiology (ACR), have practice parameters for the safe administration and monitoring of sedation and analgesia for NORA.[1] The key components of these guidelines and regulations are defining the continuum for sedation and anesthesia and the qualifications for those administering the sedatives and analgesia. This requirement states that qualified individuals must have competency-based education, training, and experience to evaluate patients appropriately prior to sedation; administer sedation safely; and have the ability to rescue patients from the next level of sedation. Because sedation is a continuum, it is not always possible to predict how an individual patient will respond, therefore the practitioners administering sedation must be qualified to recover or rescue the patient from the next level of sedation. This requirement states that qualified individuals must have competency-based education, training, and experience to evaluate patients appropriately prior to sedation; administer sedation safely; and have the ability to rescue patients from the next level of sedation. Practitioners intending to induce moderate sedation must be competent to manage a compromised airway and inadequate oxygenation and ventilation. Practitioners intending to induce deep sedation are competent to rescue a patient from general anesthesia (GA), being able to manage an unstable cardiovascular system as well as a compromised airway and inadequate oxygenation and ventilation.[2]

Screening

All patients requiring anesthesia services should be evaluated according to the ASA practice advisory for preanesthesia evaluation.[2–5] Each institution or department may decide what preprocedure tests are appropriate. Specifically, guidelines for moderate and deep sedation include:

- Presedation assessment
- Appropriate patient selection
- Immediate reevaluation prior to sedation
- Post Anesthesia Care Unit (PACU) admission and discharge assessment
- Sedation plan and communication among all patient providers
- Informed consent
- ASA monitors
- Outcome collections to improve patient care[2]

There is a wide spectrum of cancer patients who present for NORA. Some may have no other comorbidities, and some may have psychiatric or pain syndromes, rendering them unable to tolerate the required position for their diagnostic or therapeutic procedure. Some cancer patients have multiple comorbidities or may require a palliative procedure. Although the same types of patients may also come to the OR, there may be a different plan for patients who are critically ill because they may not be appropriate surgical candidates. Critically ill patients often undergo procedures that are considered minimal but urgent, such as drainage of an abscess, placement or exchange of a stent, central venous line placement, or ablation of a lesion that is not surgically treatable. Most of the procedures scheduled for NORA locations are planned and usually bloodless; however, timing is essential and may be uncertain based on patient acuity. These patients often have complex medical problems, are critically ill, and can be extremely challenging from an anesthetic and positioning standpoint.

There are several commonly used approaches to screening patients scheduled for NORA. These include one of the following formats: an anesthetic preoperative visit prior or medical proceduralist office visit prior to the day of the procedure, telephone interview with a review of a health survey, or preprocedure screening on the morning of surgery.[3–9] Each option has its own advantages and disadvantages. To satisfy the Joint Commission (TJC) requirements, the medical proceduralist will select one of these approaches.[10] Like surgeons, some proceduralists may choose to have a clinic for consultation prior to the actual day of the procedure. The preprocedure assessment reviews medical history, medications, allergies, and fasting guidelines, and determines the need for an anesthesiologist. In the traditional OR the anesthesia care provider is always present and will select the type of anesthesia based upon the patient's comorbidities and surgeon's request. NORA procedures differ in that the proceduralist or oncologist must recognize the need for an anesthesia care provider and request this service. For a procedure that mandates deep sedation or a general anesthetic, the consultation is clear; however, patient factors that determine the need for an anesthesia care provider for minimal or moderate sedation are not well defined.

The ASA Task Force on Sedation and Analgesia by Non-anesthesiologists has developed guidelines to assist medical proceduralists to identify higher risk patients, such as major comorbidities, abnormal or difficult airway, and increased tolerance to pain medications that may require the presence of an anesthesia care provider.[2] Other factors that may contribute to the need for anesthesia services are pediatric patients and patients with known or suspected difficult airways, morbid obesity, sleep apnea, prone position, claustrophobia, pain syndromes, family history of difficulty with anesthesia, or those who have had prior difficulties with nurse administered sedation. These guidelines should be transformed into an algorithm that is followed during the preprocedural assessment schedule, which can be used to determine the need for an anesthesiologist during the procedure.

Scheduling

Scheduling procedures between anesthesiology, oncologists, and proceduralists can be challenging. Most anesthesiology departments typically have clinical coordinators who are responsible for daily scheduling and staffing needs. The same is true for IR, GI, RT, and radiology, and is often referred to as the "traffic coordinator." Anesthesiology clinical coordinators responsible for staffing and scheduling prefer a consistent day of procedures, which allows for the most efficient use of personnel. If an entire day of anesthesia services is not required, it is preferred for procedures requiring anesthesia services to be performed as "first cases." Proceduralists typically prefer to schedule outpatient procedures prior to inpatient procedures. While the number of procedures requiring anesthesia services is increasing, there may not be a full day's worth of procedures to require a dedicated anesthesia team. Creating a schedule requires daily communication between the "traffic" coordinator and the anesthesiology coordinator. The two service coordinators share the responsibility to keep both services on schedule. In our institution each proceduralist has a NORA suite assigned to them. The need for anesthesia personnel in a suite is determined by whether at least one of the procedures requires anesthesia services. The anesthesia team will then care for all the patients scheduled for that NORA suite. This allows for efficient use of the anesthesia staff. It also allows the medical department performing procedures to effectively staff their other suites requiring minimal or moderate sedation without anesthesia services.[11]

Anesthesia Provider Evaluation

Although sometimes difficult to arrange, the preprocedural interview and evaluation by an anesthesiologist is beneficial. In addition to lessening anxiety about the treatment and anesthesia, the anesthesiologist will be able to identify potential medical problems, determine their etiology, and if indicated, initiate appropriate corrective measures, thereby minimizing any potential delays, cancellations as well as complications on the day of the procedure. For NORA, it is often the anesthesiologist who is most involved in the direct medical care of the patient. The anesthesiologist must ensure that the patient is appropriately screened, evaluated, and informed prior to the procedure. The anesthesiologist-patient relationship often takes on a primary care quality in NORA.

An important component of the preanesthesia evaluation is assigning ASA Physical Status to the patient (Table 18.1). The anesthetic risk attributed to a procedure depends on the preoperative status of the patient. The presence of comorbidities that may influence the incidence of postoperative morbidity and mortality needs to be recognized at the preoperative visit and then clinically optimized prior to the procedure. Detailed evaluation of these major organ systems with a focus on corrective measures is combined with selected pharmacologic agents, anesthetic technique, and monitoring to provide optimal care.

Extrapolating from the traditional and ambulatory surgery literature, geriatric and higher risk (ASA III and IV) patients may be considered acceptable candidates for NORA procedures if their systemic diseases are well controlled, and the patient's medical condition is optimized preoperatively.[3–6,11] Often it is the presence of comorbidities that makes the risk/benefit ratio of an image-guided procedure more acceptable than traditional surgery. The anesthesiologist must have an informed discussion with the patient or the health care proxy about the increased risk of morbidity and mortality. If necessary, the anesthesiologist may collaborate with other members of the patient's care team to determine whether any consultations or preprocedure therapies are indicated prior to the procedure to minimize the risk of anesthesia. The anesthesiologist may be asked to care for a patient whose illness is life threatening and the proceduralist's intention may be palliative. For procedures aimed at improving the patient's quality of life, the anesthesia care provider requires flexibility and complex case management skills. With few exceptions, the appropriateness of a case for NORA is determined by a combination of factors, including type of procedure, anesthetic technique, and risk/benefit ratio.

Non-operating Room Anesthesia

The anesthesiologist must adopt and adapt to a new mindset when providing services outside of the traditional OR. The health care providers from anesthesiology and the medical department performing the procedure are often unfamiliar with one another. The location, equipment, and room arrangement vary from the OR. In addition, the types of procedures are unfamiliar and the scheduling patterns differ. At our institution, proceduralists schedule and perform elective procedures, but they are often called upon to perform

TABLE 18.1 ASA Physical Status Classification System

ASA Physical Status Classification	Definition	Adult Examples, Including But Not Limited to:
ASA I	A normal healthy patient	Healthy, nonsmoking, no or minimal alcohol use
ASA II	A patient with mild systemic disease	Mild diseases only without substantive functional limitations. Current smoker, social alcohol drinker, pregnancy, obesity (30<BMI<40), well-controlled DM/HTN, mild lung disease
ASA III	A patient with severe systemic disease	Substantive functional limitations; One or more moderate to severe diseases. Poorly controlled DM or HTN, COPD, morbid obesity (BMI ≥40), active hepatitis, alcohol dependence or abuse, implanted pacemaker, moderate reduction of ejection fraction, ESRD undergoing regularly scheduled dialysis, history (>3 months) of MI, CVA, TIA, or CAD/stents
ASA IV	A patient with severe systemic disease that is a constant threat to life	Recent (<3 months) MI, CVA, TIA or CAD/stents, ongoing cardiac ischemia or severe valve dysfunction, severe reduction of ejection fraction, shock, sepsis, DIC, ARD or ESRD not undergoing regularly scheduled dialysis
ASA V	A moribund patient who is not expected to survive without the operation	Ruptured abdominal/thoracic aneurysm, massive trauma, intracranial bleed with mass effect, ischemic bowel in the face of significant cardiac pathology or multiple organ/system dysfunction
ASA VI	A declared brain-dead patient whose organs are being removed for donor purposes	

ARD, Acute renal disease; *ASA*, American Society of Anesthesiologists; *BMI*, body mass index (kg/m^2); *CAD*, coronary artery disease; *COPD*, chronic obstructive pulmonary disease; *CVA*, cerebrovascular accident; *DIC*, disseminated intravascular coagulation; *DM*, diabetes mellitus; *ESRD*, end-stage renal disease; *HTN*, hypertension; *MI*, myocardial infarction; *PCA*, postconceptional age; *TIA*, transient ischemic attack.

ASA Physical Status Classification System, 2020 is reprinted with permission of the American Society of Anesthesiologists, 1061 American Lane, Schaumburg, *Illinois* 60173–4973.

"add-on" urgent and emergent in-patient cases that may represent half of the daily schedule. These "add-on" patients often have extensive medical comorbidities resulting from recent surgery and/or end-of-life palliative care needs. The urgent or emergent need for a procedure often leaves little time for medical optimization; however, the proposed procedure may offer a cure to these acutely debilitated patients. The anesthesiologist caring for this unique patient population outside of the traditional OR must be adept at developing a safe anesthesia plan while maintaining safe clinical practice guidelines.

When anesthesiologists are not involved, the procedure suite is typically staffed with the proceduralist, a circulating registered nurse (RN), and technologists qualified to manage various equipment. Guidelines for sedation given without anesthesia services are commonly defined by specific institutional sedation policies, and the sedation process is overseen by the proceduralist performing the procedure. RNs are responsible for sedating and monitoring the patient while the technologist assists with the positioning and technical aspects to optimize the success of the procedure.[11]

The integration of the anesthesia care team consisting of anesthesiologists and Certified Registered Nurse Anesthetists (CRNAs) or anesthesia residents alters this traditional model. The anesthesia care team training and experience is based upon the OR and surgical procedures. The NORA suite, with its equipment and diversity of procedures, is often unfamiliar ground for the anesthesia care team. The anesthesiologist is often uneasy outside of the traditional, well-equipped OR, and the presence of competent anesthesia technical support is essential in NORA locations. Anesthesia supplies, suction, oxygen supply, medications, and an anesthesia ventilator are necessary items in a NORA suite.[12,13] The additional anesthesia equipment and supplies potentially create space and logistical issues and concerns in the procedure suite, and communication becomes essential to a successful program. It is critical for the proceduralist to explain the procedures being performed to the anesthesia team as well as the potential complications and the depth of anesthesia required. The anesthesia team must describe the differences, indications, risks, and benefits between monitored anesthesia care (MAC) and general anesthesia (GA). The patient's history, associated comorbidities, and required position during the procedure should also be discussed among the teams.

Adverse events are unexpected situations that occur during clinical activities and may result in temporary or permanent, physical and/or mental damage to the patient, and increased health care costs to society. In 2008 the World Health Organization (WHO) launched "Safe Surgery Saves Lives" and developed a "Surgical Safety Checklist" (Fig. 18.1).[14] NORA suites, with their varied and complex procedures, rapid patient turnovers, and patient populations with increased comorbidities would also benefit from a process that incorporates a safety checklist. Three important safety goals of TJC are improving accuracy in patient identification, improving communication between health care coworkers, and eliminating all wrong-site, wrong-patient, and wrong-procedure interventions.[10]

Many facilities have adopted checklists to satisfy regulatory requirements and perform a "Time Out" prior to the start of any procedure. During the "Time Out" there is verbal communication between all team members in the NORA suite: proceduralist, RN, technologist, and anesthesia team member. The entire NORA team typically makes their way through a checklist:

- Identifying the patient by name and date of birth
- Confirming the procedure site and side
- Confirming correct imaging is on display in the suite
- Presence of consent, allergies, need for antibiotics, anticipated critical events, anesthesia concerns, and other pertinent information that each institution has deemed important and essential.

The use of the "Time Out" provides for an introduction between team members and is a way to maximize and share concerns regarding patient safety.

The traditional OR is designed with the anesthesia machine situated on the right side of the patient and anesthesiologist at the head of the OR table. Anesthesia care providers learn to ventilate patients while holding a face mask with the left hand and utilizing the right hand to squeeze the reservoir bag. Direct laryngoscopy is taught with the left hand and endotracheal (ET) tubes are inserted using the right hand. Physiologic monitors are typically attached to the anesthesia machine with cables, wires, and tubing also arising from the right side of the patient. The OR table is controlled with a remote control allowing the table to be manipulated into multiple positions such as tilting from side to side, Trendelenburg, reverse Trendelenburg, flexion, extension, or a combination of these maneuvers. Patients may be positioned supine, prone, lateral, or even sitting up. The patient's arms may be tucked at the side or placed on arm boards and positioned at an angle of less than 90 degrees.

NORA suites are not typically designed with the intent of having anesthesia services. The ASA issued a statement on NORA locations delineating guidelines that apply to all anesthesia care for anesthesia personnel when procedures are performed outside of a traditional OR.[2] Every NORA location should have adequate and reliable sources of oxygen and suction, a self-inflating hand resuscitator bag capable of delivering at least 90% oxygen as a means to deliver positive pressure ventilation, and adequate monitoring equipment to comply with the ASA's "Standard for Basic Monitoring." There should be space to accommodate essential anesthesia equipment and personnel. In addition, every NORA location should have electrical outlets to satisfy the anesthesia machine and monitoring equipment, as well as clearly labeled outlets connected to an emergency power supply. Adequate illumination of the patient, anesthesia machine, and monitoring equipment is essential, and a battery-powered flashlight should be available. NORA suites should also have immediate availability and access to an emergency cart with a defibrillator, emergency drugs, and other equipment to provide cardiopulmonary resuscitation. In addition to a ventilator, standard monitoring, and equipment carts,

Surgical Safety Checklist

Patient Safety
A World Alliance for Safer Health Care

Before induction of anaesthesia

(with at least nurse and anaesthetist)

Has the patient confirmed his/her identity, site, procedure, and consent?

- ☐ Yes

Is the site marked?

- ☐ Yes
- ☐ Not applicable

Is the anaesthesia machine and medication check complete?

- ☐ Yes

Is the pulse oximeter on the patient and functioning?

- ☐ Yes

Does the patient have a:

Known allergy?

- ☐ No
- ☐ Yes

Difficult airway or aspiration risk?

- ☐ No
- ☐ Yes, and equipment/assistance available

Risk of >500ml blood loss (7ml/kg in children)?

- ☐ No
- ☐ Yes, and two IVs/central access and fluids planned

Before skin incision

(with nurse, anaesthetist and surgeon)

- ☐ **Confirm all team members have introduced themselves by name and role.**
- ☐ **Confirm the patient's name, procedure, and where the incision will be made.**

Has antibiotic prophylaxis been given within the last 60 minutes?

- ☐ Yes
- ☐ Not applicable

Anticipated Critical Events

To Surgeon:

- ☐ What are the critical or non-routine steps?
- ☐ How long will the case take?
- ☐ What is the anticipated blood loss?

To Anaesthetist:

- ☐ Are there any patient-specific concerns?

To Nursing Team:

- ☐ Has sterility (including indicator results) been confirmed?
- ☐ Are there equipment issues or any concerns?

Is essential imaging displayed?

- ☐ Yes
- ☐ Not applicable

Before patient leaves operating room

(with nurse, anaesthetist and surgeon)

Nurse Verbally Confirms:

- ☐ The name of the procedure
- ☐ Completion of instrument, sponge and needle counts
- ☐ Specimen labelling (read specimen labels aloud, including patient name)
- ☐ Whether there are any equipment problems to be addressed

To Surgeon, Anaesthetist and Nurse:

- ☐ What are the key concerns for recovery and management of this patient?

This checklist is not intended to be comprehensive. Additions and modifications to fit local practice are encouraged.

Revised 1 / 2009

• **Fig. 18.1** WHO surgical safety checklist.

there must be availability and easy access to code carts and emergency airway equipment including fiberoptic bronchoscope with light source, video glide scopes, and laryngeal mask airways (LMAs). This emergency equipment needs to be maintained and checked regularly, ideally by anesthesia technologists who are familiar and adept at staffing NORA locations.[13] In any NORA location where inhalational anesthesia is to be administered, there should be an anesthesia machine that is well maintained and has a system for scavenging anesthetic gas waste.

However, in many NORA suites, the procedure table is often fixed, with much less flexibility than a traditional OR table. There is often the presence of cumbersome imaging or radiation equipment that makes it difficult for the anesthesia team to get adequately situated. A fixed table increases the challenge of appropriate patient positioning, and if not considered, may lead to position-related injuries. The anesthesia team must do their best to replicate their usual OR setup but may have to extend intravenous tubing, monitoring cables, and inspiratory and expiratory limbs of the ventilatory circuit due to the lack of proximity and limited access to the patient. Wall oxygen is usually available but gases such as nitrous oxide and air are not typically part of the NORA suite design. To provide a safe environment, communication of patient positioning and other needs between the proceduralist, RNs, technologists, anesthesiologist, and the anesthesia support staff is vital. Proper barrier shielding, lead aprons, and thyroid shields must also be provided for the anesthesia staff.

Anesthesia care providers rely on OR pharmacies for distribution of medications. Omnicell and Pyxis are examples of standalone medication cart systems that allow medication management to occur in the OR. These systems are monitored and stocked by the OR pharmacy. In NORA locations, the anesthesiologist and pharmacist may need to collaborate in order to assemble a portable kit that anticipates the potential medication needs of the anesthesia care team.

The communication needs in remote NORA locations is an important consideration. Emergency situations and equipment malfunctions may occur, necessitating a well-planned communication and service strategy. Anesthesia providers and support staff should be familiar with the NORA sites and phones, pagers, or other two-way communication devices should be reliable and maintained on a regular basis.

Basic Anesthesia Monitoring

The ASA issued standards for Basic Anesthetic Monitoring.[15]

Standard I: Qualified anesthesia personnel shall be present in the room throughout the conduct of all general anesthetics, regional anesthetics, and monitored anesthesia care.

Standard II: During all anesthetics the patient's oxygenation, ventilation, circulation, and temperature shall be continually evaluated.

These standards are intended for all types of anesthesia. The ASA does recognize that at times during "rare" or "unusual circumstances," some methods of monitoring may be clinically impractical or personnel may need to briefly leave the procedure room. For example, anesthesia staff may need to exit the procedure room during high-dose radiation exposure but the monitoring standards should still be upheld. Physiologic monitoring standards remain, and there must be a way to visualize both the patient and monitor during such an event. There should also be a plan in place for anesthesia personnel to quickly gain access to the patient in an emergent situation.

During all NORA procedures, adequacy of ventilation must be ensured. Clinical signs, such as chest excursion, observation of the reservoir bag, and auscultation of breath sounds, are useful. Continuous monitoring of expired carbon dioxide (end-tidal CO_2) should always be used and should be easily observed unless the procedure, patient, or equipment prohibits its use, which should be an extremely rare occurrence. The patient's circulatory function should be assessed continuously from the beginning to the end of the anesthetic with an electrocardiogram (ECG). Blood pressure measurement and heart rate must be assessed and documented at least every 5 min. Pulse oximetry, with its pulse tracing and distinctive tone, is an invaluable monitor and allows for circulatory function to be continuously assessed. Body temperature should be maintained and continuously monitored if significant alteration in temperature is intended, anticipated, or expected.

Intraprocedural Anesthetic Plan

Proceduralists perform a wide array of diagnostic, therapeutic, and palliative care procedures that may be elective, urgent, or emergent. The population cared for may range from healthy, ASA I patients to critically ill, ASA V patients with severe systemic disease that is a constant threat to life. Anesthesiologists must account for all of these factors while formulating an anesthetic plan. In addition, there must be communication and coordination with the proceduralist when finalizing this plan. The anesthetic plan may be GA, MAC, or rarely, regional anesthesia. Table 18.2 demonstrates the differences between the various levels of sedation and GA.

GA is a drug-induced loss of consciousness with a loss of gag and cough reflex. Patients are not arousable by painful stimuli. The ability to maintain normal ventilatory status is impaired, and the patients often require assistance to maintain a patent airway with placement of an ET tube or placement of an LMA. Positive pressure ventilation with a ventilator is often required since spontaneous respiration may be impaired or depressed by neuromuscular blocking agents or other medications. GA can be divided into three phases consisting of induction, maintenance, and emergence from anesthesia. Intravenous agents such as benzodiazepines, hypnotics, analgesics, and muscle relaxants are often given to induce anesthesia, while inhalational agents provide for maintenance of anesthesia. At emergence of anesthesia, the patient is awoken by decreasing the inhalational agent

TABLE 18.2 Continuum of Depth Sedation: Definition of General Anesthesia and Levels of Sedation/Analgesia[16]

	Minimal Sedation ("Anxiolysis")	Moderate Sedation/ Analgesia ("Conscious Sedation")	Deep Sedation/ Analgesia	General Anesthesia
Responsiveness	Normal response to verbal stimulation	Purposeful response to verbal or tactile stimulation	Purposeful response following repeated or painful stimulation	Unarousable even with painful stimulus
Airway	Unaffected	No intervention required		Intervention often required
Spontaneous ventilation	Unaffected	Adequate		Frequently inadequate
Cardiovascular function	Unaffected	Usually maintained		May be impaired

concentration to zero and by utilizing reversal agents for neuromuscular blockade and removing airway devices. Analgesics may be given throughout the procedure and titrated so that patients awaken with minimal discomfort. Cardiovascular function may also be affected requiring a vasoactive substance to normalize heart rate and blood pressure. At times, patients may require prolonged intubation in the PACU if cardiopulmonary status remains compromised.

MAC is a broad term that includes minimal, moderate, and deep sedation. Medications are administered to provide varying levels of sedation, analgesia, and anxiolysis. The anesthesiologist must be adept and prepared to convert to GA if necessary. The anesthesiologist must continuously assess the patient's level of consciousness while maintaining an adequate level of analgesia and anxiolysis.[18]

Table 18.3 highlights the commonly used medications available to the anesthesiologist to accomplish an appropriate level of sedation for a given procedure.

The goals for sedation and analgesia should be to provide patients with an increased pain threshold, anxiolysis, and amnesia while providing hemodynamic stability. Sedation should be titrated so that if indicated, there is cooperation with appropriate response to tactile stimuli and verbal commands. The provider should be able to maintain a patent airway and be alert to the potential for loss of protective airway reflexes. Since levels of sedation can be unpredictable, the provider of monitored anesthesia care must be prepared and qualified to convert to GA if necessary.[5] The anesthetic plan may be impacted by the proceduralist's approach to the procedure. Some procedures are extremely painful or compromise ventilation, requiring GA, while others can

TABLE 18.3 Commonly Used Drugs to Achieve Minimal to Deep Sedation in the IR Suite[7]

IV Drug	Pharmacologic Class	Onset (minutes)	Duration (minutes)	Initial Dosing	Continuous Dosing	Repeat Dosing/ Titration	Reversal
Midazolam	Benzodiazepine	1–3	30–80	0.08 mg/kg IV	NA	May repeat every 3–5 min (max 0.2 mg/kg IV total)	Flumazenil
Dexmedetomidine	Alpha2-receptor agonist	15 (once infusion is started)	60–120	NA	0.6–0.7 μg/kg/h IV	Usual range: 0.2–1.5 μg/kg/h	NA
Fentanyl	Opioid	1–2	30–60	0.5–1 μg/kg	1–2 μg/kg/h	May repeat every 10–30 min	Naloxone
Remifentanil	Opioid	1–1.5	3–10	Loading dose: 0.5 μg/kg	After loading dose: 0.025 μg/kg/min	Adjust infusion by 0.025 μg/kg/min every 5–10 min as needed. Max: 0.2 μg/kg/min	Discontinue infusion
Propofol	Sedative hypnotic	1	5–10	0.5–1 mg/kg	5–10 μg/kg/min	Usual range: 5–50 μg/kg/min	NA
Ketamine	Dissociative anesthetic	0.5	5–10	1–2 mg/kg	NA	0.2–0.5 mg/kg every 10 min as needed	NA

be performed with MAC. Communication between the anesthesiologist and proceduralist is critical in forming the appropriate anesthesia plan.

Positioning

Extreme vigilance and frequent positioning checks are required to make sure all body parts of the patient are properly padded and positioned. As mentioned earlier, the NORA procedure table is fixed and has a hard surface and patients may be supine, prone, or lateral for any given procedure. Patients requiring GA or deep sedation will not be able to react if placed in a painful position. During the anesthesia preprocedural evaluation, the extremity and joints must be assessed for limitation in range of motion or presence of artificial joints. Patients requiring GA should have their ET tubes well secured. The head, eyes, nose, and other facial structures should be well padded and protected. The neck should be in a neutral position to prevent cervical spine complications. Chest rolls and abdominal rolls should be placed for the prone position to allow for uncompromised ventilation. The legs should be slightly flexed, the knees padded, and a pillow placed so the feet rest comfortably preventing peroneal and pressure-related injuries. The arms should be placed in a neutral position and not extended to prevent brachial plexus injuries (Figs. 18.2 and 18.3).[17] Care must be taken when moving patients to prevent skin abrasions and breakdown. An advantage of minimal or moderate sedation is that patients can alert the care team to procedural pain or pain due to their position.

Respiratory Compromise

Analysis of the data from the ASA Closed Claims Projects Database that explored patterns of injury and liability associated with anesthesia provided in NORA locations compared with the standard OR setting documented that respiratory events were twice as likely to occur in remote locations as in the traditional OR.[19,20] The most common event was inadequate oxygen/ventilation. In 30% of the remote location claims an absolute or relative overdose of a sedative, hypnotic, and/or analgesic drug led to respiratory depression. Seventy percent of the cases that occurred in radiology involved excessive sedation. The remaining occurrences were esophageal intubation, difficult intubation, and aspiration of gastric contents. NORA claims were judged as having been substandard and being preventable with better monitoring.[19]

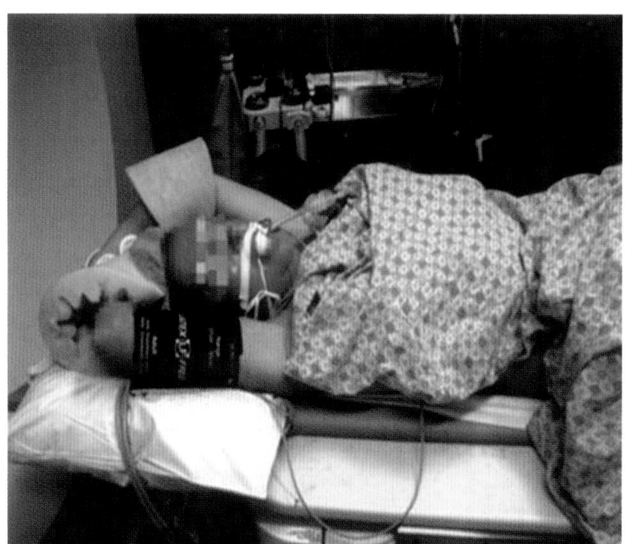

• **Fig. 18.2** Example of incorrect position with risk to brachial plexus.

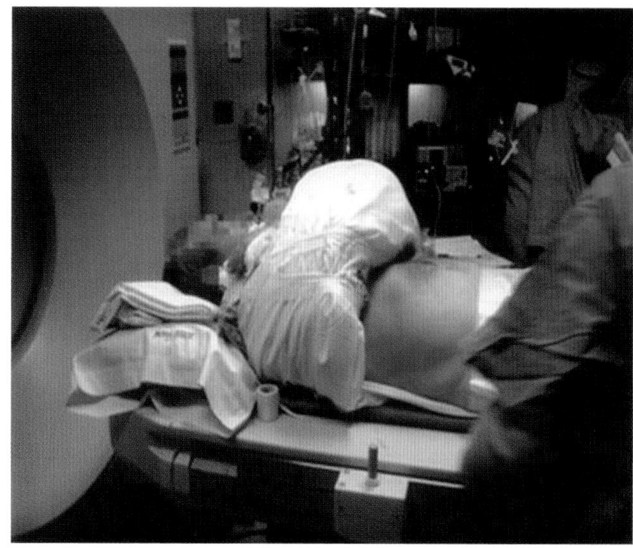

• **Fig. 18.3** Example of correct arm position.

In preparation for procedures outside of the traditional OR, the anesthesia care team must be well prepared and have a set-up that provides all necessary airway equipment, monitors, anesthesia supplies, and medications. There should also always be easy access to emergency airway supplies and code carts.[22]

Post procedure Recovery

After completion of a procedure with anesthesia services, patients should be routinely transferred to and cared for in a PACU until institutional discharge criteria have been met. The ASA has issued standards for postanesthesia care.[21]

Standard I

All patients who have received GA, regional anesthesia, or monitored anesthesia care shall receive postanesthesia care management.

Standard II

A patient transported to the PACU shall be accompanied by a member of the anesthesia care team who is knowledgeable regarding the patient's condition. The patient shall be continually evaluated and treated during transport with monitoring and support appropriate to the patient's condition.

Standard III

Upon arrival in the PACU, the patient shall be reevaluated and a verbal report provided to the responsible PACU nurse by the member of the anesthesia care team who accompanies the patient.

Standard IV

The patient's condition shall be evaluated continually in the PACU.

Standard V

A physician is responsible for the discharge of the patient from the PACU.

It is helpful for a member of the procedure team to accompany the anesthesia care team to the PACU to provide a detailed procedural report to the PACU staff. Common postprocedural issues that may occur in the PACU include but are not limited to: procedural pain, pneumothorax, urosepsis bowel perforation, hemothorax, postdural spinal headache, and contrast allergy reactions.

Conclusion

It is important for anesthesiologists, proceduralist, and oncologists to work together to offer a safe NORA environment for an increasing cancer patient population that requires diagnostic, therapeutic, and palliative care procedures. Optimizing the cancer patient's comorbidities, being familiar with the many NORA procedures and locations, and creating a safe anesthesia work area outside the traditional OR are necessary measures to lower anesthetic risk. With the increasing number of cancer patients requiring procedures and therapies outside of the traditional OR, it is imperative that anesthesiologists caring for this patient population can adapt to this challenging environment. For successful outcomes, it is essential that anesthesiologists are able to navigate complex cases outside of the OR, develop safe anesthetic plans, and communicate with their medical colleagues performing procedures, ordering scans, or providing therapies.

References

1. American College of Radiology. ACR–SIR Practice Parameter for Minimal and/or Moderate Sedation/Analgesia. 2015. Available at https://www.acr.org/-/media/ACR/Files/Practice-Parameters/Sed-Analgesia.pdf
2. American Society of Anesthesiologists Task Force on Sedation and Analgesia by Non-Anesthesiologists. Practice guidelines for sedation and analgesia by non-anesthesiologists. *Anesthesiology*. 2002;96:1004–1007.
3. Apfelbaum JL, Connis RT, Nickinovich DG, et al. Practice advisory for preanesthesia evaluation: an updated report by the American Society of Anesthesiologists Task Force on Preanesthesia Evaluation. *Anesthesiology*. 2012;116(3):522–538. doi:10.1097/ALN.0b013e31823c1067.
4. Twersky R. To be an outpatient, or not to be — selecting the right patients for ambulatory surgery. *Ambulatory Surg*. 1993;1(1):5–14. doi:10.1016/0966-6532(93)90062-T.
5. Chung F, Mezei G, Tong D. Pre-existing medical conditions as predictors of adverse events in day-case surgery. *Br J Anaesth*. 1999;83(2):262–270. doi:10.1093/bja/83.2.262.
6. ASA Committee on Standards and Practice Parameters. Statement on non-operative room anesthetizing locations. 1994. 2018. Available at https://www.asahq.org/standards-and-guidelines/statement-on-nonoperating-room-anesthetizing-locations#/.
7. Lichtor JL. Anesthesia for Ambulatory Surgery, Clinical Anesthesia. 5th ed. Philadelphia: Lippincott Williams & Wilkins; 2006:1230–1245.
8. Corso R, Vacirca F, Patelli C, Leni D. Use of "Time-Out" checklist in interventional radiology procedures as a tool to enhance patient safety. *Radiol Med*. 2014;119(11):828–834. doi:10.1007/s11547-014-0397-9.
9. Beyea SC. 2009 Patient safety goals: a perioperative nursing priority. *AORN J*. 2008;88(3):459–462. doi:10.1016/j.aorn.2008.08.008.
10. https://www.jointcommission.org/standards_information/jcfaqdetails.aspx?StandardsFaqId=1639&ProgramId=46
11. Kotin A., Mascarenhas J., Fischer M. Principles of sedation and analgesia. In: Pua B.B., Covey A.M., Madoff D.C., eds. *Interventional Radiology: Fundamentals of Clinical Practice*: Oxford University Press; 2019:64–74.
12. Goudra B, Alvarez A, Singh PM. Practical considerations in the development of a non-operating room anesthesia practice. *Curr Opin Anaesthesiol*. 2016;29(4):526–530. doi:10.1097/ACO.0000000000000344.
13. Arora L, Weiss LE, Rambhia M, Goff K, Khanna AK. Non-operating room anesthesia (NORA): humbug if not careful. *ASA Monitor*. 2019;83(9):66–68.
14. WHO. Surgical Saftey Checklist. Available at https://apps.who.int/iris/bitstream/handle/10665/44186/9789241598590_eng_Checklist.pdf;jsessionid=BF572276E8529FEE48AFBF37FAFA27DD?sequence=2.
15. ASA. Standards for Basic Anesthetic Monitoring. 1986. 2015. Available at https://www.asahq.org/standards-and-guidelines/standards-for-basic-anesthetic-monitoring.
16. Continuum of Depth of Sedation: Definition of General Anesthesia and Levels of Sedation/Analgesia. 1999. 2014. Available at https://www.asahq.org/standards-and-guidelines/continuum-of-depth-of-sedation-definition-of-general-anesthesia-and-levels-of-sedationanalgesia.
17. Shankar S., Vansonnenberg E., Silverman S.G., et al. Brachial plexus injury from CT guided radiofrequency ablation under general anesthesia. *Cardiovasc Intervent Radiol*. 2005;28:646–648.
18. Position on Monitored Anesthesia Care. 2005. 2018. Available at https://www.asahq.org/standards-and-guidelines/position-on-monitored-anesthesia-care
19. Chang B, Kaye AD, Diaz JH, Westlake B, Dutton RP, Urman RD. Complications of non-operating room procedures: outcomes from the national anesthesia clinical outcomes registry. *J Patient Safety*. 2018;14(1):9–16.
20. Metzner J, Posner KL, Domino KB. The risk and safety of anesthesia at remote locations: the US closed claims analysis. *Curr Opin Anaesthesiol*. 2009;22(4):502–508. doi:10.1097/ACO.0b013e32832dba50.
21. Standards for Postanesthesia Care. 2004. 2014. Available at https://www.asahq.org/standards-and-guidelines/standards-for-postanesthesia-care
22. Walls JD, Weiss MS. Safety in non-operating room anesthesia (NORA). *APSF Newsletter*. 2019;34(1):3–4, 28.

19

Perioperative Care of the Surgical Patient: Brain

ANH QUYNH DANG AND SALLY RADELAT RATY

Introduction

Cancer of the central nervous system is the 10th leading cause of death in the United States. An estimated 23,820 adults and 3720 children under the age of 15 years will be diagnosed with a primary tumor of the brain or spine in 2019.[1] Primary tumors from the lung, breast, kidney, and bladder, and melanoma, leukemia, and lymphoma frequently metastasize to the brain, creating a secondary tumor.[1] The treatment for both primary and metastatic brain tumors includes chemotherapy, radiation therapy, and surgery.

There are many anesthetic challenges for patients undergoing craniotomy for tumor resection. Depending on the size and location of the tumor, these patients can present with baseline motor or sensory neurologic deficits as well as seizures that may be poorly controlled. Intraoperatively, craniotomy patients require tight blood pressure control and hemodynamic stability to optimize surgical exposure and minimize blood loss. At the conclusion of surgery, a smooth and rapid emergence is desirable to decrease the risk of intracranial hemorrhage and allow for an immediate assessment of the patient's neurologic status. Postoperatively, judicious use of pain medication must be undertaken to achieve adequate pain control while minimizing associated side effects, which may mask or mimic the signs and symptoms of postoperative surgical complications.

Preoperative Assessment

Preoperative assessment of the patient scheduled for craniotomy should include a complete history and physical examination with meticulous documentation of current neurologic status and evaluation for the presence of elevated intracranial pressure (ICP). Accurate documentation of the patient's baseline neurologic status serves as a benchmark against which postoperative neurologic status can be measured. A significant number of these patients have neurologic findings, including seizure, vision changes, focal motor or sensory deficits, speech difficulties, balance disturbances, confusion, memory lapses, and headache. Tumors involving the pituitary gland can cause endocrine disturbances including muscle weakness, cold intolerance, excessive sweating, irritability, amenorrhea, sexual dysfunction, polyuria, unintended weight change, hypertension, hyperglycemia, easy bruisability, striae, mood change, moon facies, coarsened facial features, enlargement of hands and feet, and increased body hair. A detailed description of the seizure history, including seizure type, associated symptoms, frequency, most recent occurrence, medications tried, successful medications, and recently taken antiepileptics prepares clinicians to diagnose and treat perioperative seizures. Unilateral pupillary dilatation, double or blurred vision, photophobia, oculomotor or abducens palsy, headache, altered mental status, nausea or vomiting, or papilledema on fundoscopic examination should raise concerns for elevated ICP. Patients with severely elevated ICP can present with somnolence and irregular respiration. The appearance of Cushing's triad consisting of systemic hypertension, bradycardia, and irregular respiration heralds impending brain herniation and death (Fig. 19.1, Table 19.1). Nausea and, less frequently, vomiting are common in patients with brain tumors, and many patients are on antiemetics during the preoperative period. Multimodal prophylaxis for postoperative nausea and vomiting (PONV; described later) is indicated for all patients undergoing a craniotomy, as the procedure itself is associated with a high incidence of PONV even if preprocedure symptoms are not present.

Previous cancer diagnoses and treatments, including surgery, chemotherapy, and radiation therapy, are important details of the patient's history. For patients with a primary brain tumor, a prior craniotomy, especially if recent, may make a scalp block (discussed later) unwise. If the brain tumor is metastatic from a melanoma or renal cell primary, blood loss during craniotomy can be significantly higher. Radiation to the neck can create fibrosis and scarring of the soft tissues, making both mask ventilation and direct laryngoscopy extremely difficult or impossible. Radiation to the chest can impair both cardiac and pulmonary function. Chemotherapy agents can affect cardiac, pulmonary, hematopoietic, renal, and hepatic functions. A thorough

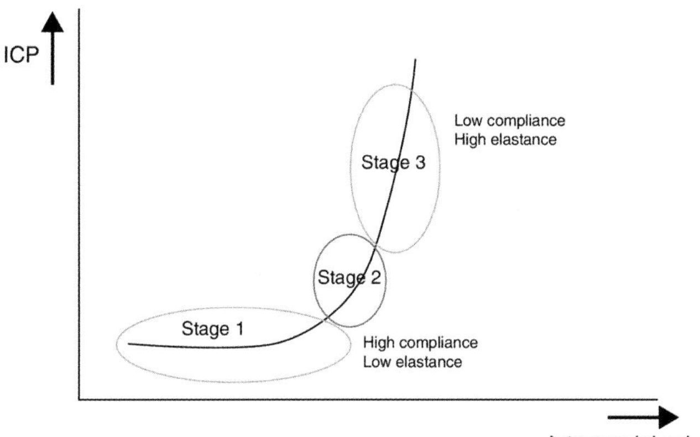

• **Fig. 19.1** Relationship between intracranial pressure (ICP) and intracranial volume. Stages of ICP and intracranial volume changes: (1) The initial stage (stage 1) is characterized by high compliance and low ICP, wherein an increase in volume does not affect ICP. (2) The transition stage (stage 2) is characterized by low compliance and low ICP, wherein an increase in volume translates to a modest increase in ICP. (3) The ascending stage (stage 3) is characterized by a low compliance and high ICP, wherein a slight change in volume results in a significant increase in ICP.[90]

understanding of the impact of each patient's prior chemotherapy regimen on organ function is imperative. Patients frequently use antiepileptics, antiemetics, steroids, and hypoglycemic agents. Antiepileptics should, at a minimum, be continued in the perioperative period, and often an additional dose is administered in the early intraoperative period. A multimodal prophylactic approach to PONV is advised and often includes agents from at least three different drug classes: steroids, 5-HT_3 receptor antagonists, NK-1 receptor antagonists, antihistamines, phenothiazines, and 5-HT_4 receptor agonists. The most common combination used at our institution is a steroid, a 5-HT_3 receptor antagonist, and an NK-1 receptor antagonist. Hyperglycemia secondary to steroid administration and preexisting diabetes is common and should be managed in a systematic manner using an insulin sliding scale with either subcutaneous administration or intravenous infusion of insulin. NK-1 inhibitors interfere with birth control, and alternative means of contraception are advised for 30 days following the last dose of a medication from this drug class.

The mass effect from the brain tumor and the surrounding edema is best quantified with a computed tomography (CT) scan or magnetic resonance imaging (MRI). Findings of flattened gyri, narrowed sulci, or compression of the intracranial ventricles indicate elevated ICP. Preexisting anemia (from chemotherapy) and hyperglycemia (from steroid use) are common laboratory findings. We obtain blood typing and an antibody screen on all craniotomy patients and adhere to a protocol for perioperative glucose management, with treatment indicated for glucose above 180 mg/dL.

Intraoperative Planning

When formulating an intraoperative plan of care, the anesthesiologist should consider the tumor location, surgical positioning, neuromonitoring plans, and bleeding risk. Tumors are classified as either supratentorial or infratentorial, depending on whether they lie above or below the tentorium cerebelli, respectively. In adults primary supratentorial tumors predominate and may involve eloquent areas of the brain responsible for speech generation and comprehension, or motor function. By contrast, infratentorial tumors are more common in pediatric patients and may involve the cerebellum, fourth ventricle, cerebellopontine angle, and brainstem. Due to their locations, supratentorial and infratentorial tumors may present differently.

Positioning surgical patients is often a compromise between optimal surgical exposure and what can actually be physiologically tolerated by the patient. Most craniotomies are performed with the patient in the supine, lateral, or prone positions, with the patient's head elevated by 10–30 degrees. The semisitting or semi-Fowler's position can offer an advantageous surgical exposure for posterior fossa tumors, although the risk of vascular air embolism (VAE) is increased. The risk of VAE and a treatment plan should be discussed with the surgeon for every patient undergoing craniotomy. Transesophageal echocardiography is the most sensitive method for detection of VAE, but it is rarely

TABLE 19.1 Signs and Symptoms of Elevated Intracranial Pressure[92]

General	Tentorial Herniation (Lateral)	Tentorial Herniation (Central)	Tonsillar Herniation

Headache
Vomiting
Visual disturbances
Diplopia
Cushing's triad:
  Increased systolic pressure
  Widened pulse pressure
  Bradycardia
  Irregular breathing
Depressed consciousness
	Third nerve palsy
	False localizing
	Ipsilateral hemiparesis (Kernohan's notch)
	Depressed consciousness
	Homonymous hemianopia
		Upward gaze palsy
		Deteriorating level of consciousness
		Diabetes insipidus
			Neck stiffness
			Elevated blood pressure
			Slowed pulse rate
			Transient losses of vision
			Retinal venous pulsation
			Papilledema
			Unilateral pupillary dilatation
			Kernohans's notch syndrome

employed in craniotomies because of its expense and invasiveness, and the need for special expertise in interpreting images. Precordial Doppler is the most sensitive noninvasive method for detecting VAE and can be placed on the 2nd, 3rd, or 4th intercostal space to the right or left of the sternum, or between the right scapula and spine in prone patients. Other methods of VAE detection that are considered to be highly sensitive include a pulmonary artery catheter and transcranial Doppler, neither of which is routinely used during craniotomies.[2] Treatment for VAE should be readily available during every craniotomy and includes bone wax to seal air entry sites at the cut bone surfaces, normal saline to flood the surgical field, the ability to place the patient in the Trendelenburg position, the application of positive end-expiratory pressure, and manual compression of the jugular veins. Special attention must be paid to the protection of the eyes from both the preoperative skin preparation solution and inadvertent pressure from personnel and equipment. Liberal application of sterile eye ointment followed by eye pads and an occlusive, waterproof cover provides corneal protection, and provider vigilance is necessary to prevent pressure injury to the eyes.

Intraoperative neuromonitoring modalities include somatosensory evoked potentials (SSEPs), motor evoked potentials (MEPs), electroencephalography (EEG), electromyography (EMG), auditory brainstem response (ABR), Hoffmann's reflex testing (H-reflex), and cranial nerve testing, most commonly the facial nerve (CNVII). The selection of which modalities to use is determined by the neurologic pathways at risk of injury during surgery. A detailed description of neuromonitoring modalities is beyond the scope of this chapter. SSEPs and MEPs are the most common neuromonitoring modalities used during craniotomies. SSEPs monitor the integrity of the sensory pathways from the periphery to the brain by measuring both the speed and amplitude of electrical signals traveling from a peripheral sensory nerve through the dorsal root ganglia, along the posterior column of the spinal cord to the brain. MEPs monitor the integrity of the motor pathways from the brain to the periphery by measuring both the speed and amplitude of electrical signals traveling from the motor cortex through the corticospinal tracts through the anterior horn to the peripheral muscle. Both SSEPs and MEPS are commonly used in posterior spine surgery, supratentorial craniotomies, neurovascular surgery, and skull base surgery.

General Anesthesia for Asleep Craniotomy

Inhalational anesthetics and intravenous agents may be used alone or in combination to provide general endotracheal anesthesia for craniotomy surgery. Although the use of inhalational agents alone offers a simple anesthetic approach, may minimize the risk of side effects from polypharmacy, and provide a reliable measure of anesthetic depth, inhalational agents can adversely affect central nervous system physiology. All volatile anesthetics to varying degrees increase cerebral blood flow (CBF), decrease cerebral metabolic rate (CMR), and inhibit or even abolish cerebral autoregulation. Cerebral vasodilation that results from the uncoupling of CBF from CMR can increase ICP in the closed cranium or compromise surgical exposure in an open cranium. While the vasodilatory and ICP effects can be mitigated or even reversed with hypocapnia in a normal brain, eliminating this response may not be possible when intracranial pathology is present.[3,4] Volatile anesthetics also adversely affect intraoperative neuromonitoring of SSEPs, visual evoked potentials (VEPs), and MEPs by increasing cortical latency and decreasing cortical amplitude in a dose-dependent manner. However, volatiles have minimal effects on brainstem potentials, and thus the use of inhalational agents during brainstem monitoring is acceptable.

Total intravenous anesthesia (TIVA) may be clinically indicated for specific craniotomy cases. Given the extreme sensitivity of MEPs to volatile anesthetics, TIVA should be used when neuromonitoring involves MEPs. Additionally, when elevated ICP is of particular concern, TIVA is preferred because inhalational agents can adversely affect ICP. Although ICP may not be an issue in an open cranium, the vasodilatory effects of volatile anesthetics may compromise surgical exposure; therefore if the surgical field is suboptimal, TIVA should be considered.

A combined technique that utilizes both inhalational and intravenous anesthetics offers significant advantages. Although the vasodilatory effects of volatile anesthetics can adversely affect ICP, surgical exposure, and neuromonitoring signals, these effects are usually dose-dependent. For most craniotomy cases, the use of volatile anesthetics at doses of 0.5 MAC or less supplemented with intravenous anesthetics may be acceptable.

Intravenous anesthetics and adjuncts have advantages and disadvantages when used in craniotomy. Propofol is the most commonly used intravenous anesthetic in the setting of a combined general anesthetic technique and is the primary anesthetic for TIVA. Unlike volatile anesthetics, propofol decreases both CBF and CMR without inducing cerebral vasodilation; the result is overall ICP reduction. However, propofol may lower mean arterial pressure (MAP), potentially compromising cerebral perfusion pressure (CPP) and increasing the risk of ischemic injury during craniotomy. Studies have shown that propofol anesthesia, regardless of dose, causes lower jugular bulb oxygen saturation when compared to sevoflurane-nitrous oxide or isoflurane-nitrous oxide anesthesia.[5–7] Improper titration of propofol intraoperatively may contribute to prolonged emergence and postoperative sedation.

Intravenous opioid infusions are commonly used during craniotomy. While administration of opioids provides intraoperative and postoperative analgesia that may facilitate a smooth emergence, their use can delay wake-up, contribute to postoperative sedation, and interfere with an accurate and timely neurologic assessment. To avoid these side effects of longer-acting opioids, remifentanil, an ultrashort-acting opioid, is advantageous for use during craniotomy.

Remifentanil does not provide any postoperative analgesia and may cause postoperative rebound hyperalgesia. According to a literature review that included 21 studies assessing intraoperative remifentanil use and acute or chronic postoperative pain, less than half of the studies found a higher postoperative analgesic requirement in patients who received remifentanil, and only four studies showed a potential association between remifentanil and chronic pain. Remifentanil use with volatile agents was associated with increased pain levels postoperatively compared to its use with TIVA or in a combined inhalation and intravenous technique.[8] The incidence of hyperalgesia with intraoperative remifentanil use may be a function of dose, with higher infusion rates and cumulative doses posing a greater risk.[9]

Lidocaine infusions have been shown to be beneficial in enhanced recovery protocols as adjunct medications. Lidocaine is potentially neuroprotective since it prevents sodium influx, which is the first step in the ischemic cascade, and blocks specific apoptotic cell death pathways to reduce postnecrotic injury. However, local anesthetic toxicity that can induce seizures is a potential risk, while the sedative effects of lidocaine may delay emergence and hinder rapid neurologic assessment postoperatively.[10]

Dexmedetomidine is a selective α_2-adrenergic agonist with anesthetic and analgesic properties. Dexmedetomidine-induced sedation results from indirect upregulation of gamma-aminobutyric acid (GABA) activity in the central nervous system through decreased noradrenergic neuron activity, while its pain-relieving properties are a result of its effects at the spinal cord level and supraspinal sites. Unlike most other sedatives and opioids, dexmedetomidine does not cause respiratory depression. It also does not reduce the latency or amplitude of the intraoperative neuromonitoring signals. Given these advantages and the synergistic effect of dexmedetomidine with various anesthetics, dexmedetomidine may be used as an adjuvant to standard general anesthesia, thereby decreasing the dose requirements of other anesthetics and analgesics that adversely affect intraoperative neuromonitoring.[11] The side effects of dexmedetomidine include hypotension and bradycardia; therefore its use may not be appropriate in patients with significant cardiac disease or hemodynamic compromise.

Ketamine is an *N*-methyl-D-aspartate (NMDA) antagonist that is effective in reducing pain both intraoperatively and postoperatively.[12–14] For craniotomy utilizing neuromonitoring, ketamine enhances SSEPs by increasing the amplitude, but not latency, of these recordings while minimally affecting MEPs. Because ketamine also activates certain cortical areas of the brain, the frequency on EEG is increased, resulting in a higher reading on Bispectral Index (BIS) monitoring. This cerebral stimulatory effect activates subcortical seizure activity in patients with seizure disorders.[15] Furthermore, ketamine increases CBF and CMR, thereby negatively impacting ICP and potentially compromising the surgical exposure. For these reasons, ketamine should be avoided in patients with uncontrolled seizures or elevated ICP. Although ketamine can have psychogenic side effects, the use of subanesthetic doses will mitigate this risk while still providing effective postoperative analgesia.[14,16]

Awake Craniotomy

Introduction

Tumor resection is a balance between extensive tumor removal and the preservation of brain function. The use of preoperative functional MRI, neuronavigation, fluorescent dyes, intraoperative magnetic resonance imaging (iMRI), and intraoperative stimulation mapping (ISM) helps delineate tumors from the functional brain. In awake craniotomy, the patient participates in ISM and neuropsychologic testing during tumor resection. Some centers use both iMRI and ISM to improve resection and minimize functional impairment.

Indications

The awake technique is the gold standard for tumor resection near "eloquent areas" of the brain.[17,18] "Eloquent areas" of the brain if injured lead to motor, sensory, vision, hearing, speech, or language processing deficits. Anatomically, "eloquent areas" of the brain include the primary motor cortex (precentral gyrus), primary sensory cortex (postcentral gyrus), primary visual cortex, primary auditory cortex, left posterior inferior frontal gyrus (Broca's area), and left posterior superior temporal gyrus (Wernicke's area). Tumors in or near the primary motor cortex, primary sensory cortex, or speech areas are often resected under awake conditions. Tumor location is the primary driver for choosing an awake craniotomy technique. During the awake portion of the craniotomy, patient participation in neurocognitive testing assists the surgeon in identifying functional areas of the brain, facilitating a more complete resection of the tumor while preserving brain function. A meta-analysis of 90 published reports of glioma resection with and without ISM concluded that glioma resections using ISM are associated with fewer late severe neurologic deficits and more extensive resection, and they involve eloquent locations more frequently.[19]

Preoperative assessment by an anesthesiologist should occur at least 1 day prior to the planned surgery. A thorough preoperative evaluation and discussion between the anesthesiologist assigned to the case and the patient is strongly recommended to build rapport and trust, document preexisting neurologic deficits, prepare the patient for the surgical events, and appropriately set patient expectations. The discussion must include expected intraoperative body positioning, the possibility of unpleasant sensations (e.g., hip or shoulder pain, dry mouth, headache during resection, nausea, unfamiliar noises from surgical equipment), the tunnel-like view the patient will have due to surgical draping, strategies used to keep the patient as comfortable as possible, and the possibility that an awake technique may be abandoned if safety becomes compromised. The anesthesiologist must assess patient motivation, temperament, ability to cooperate and communicate, and preexisting comorbidities when considering the awake technique. Patients who are claustrophobic, severely anxious, or diagnosed with a psychiatric illness may not be able to stay calm and cooperate during the awake portion of the case. Patients with substantial speech impairment or expressive aphasia may not have a consistent baseline during preoperative testing, making intraoperative testing less reliable. A patient with a difficult airway or sleep apnea poses significant challenges for adequate oxygenation and ventilation.

Techniques

There are two well-described anesthetic techniques for awake craniotomy: asleep-awake-asleep and monitored anesthesia care. The primary differences between the two techniques involve anesthetic management prior to the intraoperative neuropsychologic testing. The asleep-awake-asleep technique includes induction of anesthesia, placement of a supraglottic airway, controlled ventilation during craniectomy and dural opening, awakening, and removal of the supraglottic airway followed by neuropsychologic testing. The advantages of the asleep-awake-asleep technique include a rest period for the patient prior to awake testing and tumor resection, control of ventilation to avoid hypoventilation and brain swelling, and reliable pain control during surgical opening. The monitored anesthesia care technique includes minimal sedation prior to surgical opening with the advantage of avoiding an abrupt, potentially tumultuous transition from fully anesthetized to fully awake. The MAC technique by definition includes spontaneous ventilation, which can lead to hypoventilation, increased CBF, and brain swelling. A third technique, the awake-awake-awake technique, relies on medical hypnosis to avoid all sedation.[20]

Premedications

The choice of premedications should focus on preventing nausea, decreasing the risk of aspiration, and providing analgesia. A common regimen includes oral acetaminophen and aprepitant, and intravenous famotidine. Although transdermal scopolamine is an effective antiemetic, the side effects of mydriasis, blurred vision, and dry mouth are not well suited for patients undergoing awake craniotomy. We avoid administering benzodiazepines to decrease the likelihood of delayed awakening and delirium. However, if the monitored anesthesia care technique is planned, midazolam is commonly administered.

Preinduction

Awake positioning is critical for the success of awake craniotomy. Surgeons should place the patient in the position required for surgery. Significant effort is required to ensure maximum patient comfort in the surgical position prior to induction. Specific areas of concern include the position of the head, neck, and dependent shoulder and hip. The use of Mayfield pins, a three-pin head fixation system, is very common. Although rigid head fixation occurs after induction, the anticipated surgical position of the head and neck should be mimicked during preinduction positioning. Although head position is primarily determined by the required surgical exposure, the patient's gaze direction must allow for participation in neuropsychologic testing. The neck position must allow for effective mask ventilation, insertion of a supraglottic airway, and airway rescue with a video-assisted bronchoscope. Reducing the pressure on the dependent shoulder and hip improves patient comfort, tolerance, and participation in testing. We use a combination of gel rolls, pillows, and foam padding to place the patient in a comfortable "sloppy lateral" position.

Induction

For the asleep-awake-asleep technique, intravenous induction with fentanyl 0.5–1 μg/kg, lidocaine 1.5 mg/kg, and propofol 1.5–2 mg/kg is standard. Following successful mask ventilation with the head and neck in the surgical position, rocuronium 0.6 mg/kg can be administered but this is not mandatory. Soon after induction, infusion of propofol 25–100 μg/kg/min and remifentanil 0.01–0.1 μg/kg/min are started. For younger or more anxious patients, the addition of dexmedetomidine 0.1–0.5 μg/kg/h is useful. Volatile anesthetic can be used if the end-tidal concentration is kept under 0.5 MAC. A supraglottic airway with a port for a gastric tube is placed, and the ability to provide adequate minute ventilation is verified. The inability to maintain an adequate seal or to provide tidal volumes of 4–6 mL/kg at peak inspiratory pressure <20 cmH_2O indicates a poor fit or malposition of the supraglottic airway and will lead to hypoventilation. This problem must be addressed before proceeding with the surgery. The gastric tube should be advanced to a depth indicative of intragastric placement. If oral premedications have been administered, suctioning of the gastric tube is delayed until just before waking up. Following placement of the supraglottic airway, the eyes should be protected with tape to ensure complete closure. An eye lubricant is not used to preserve the clear vision needed for ISM.

For the monitored anesthesia care technique, sedation is initiated with infusions of remifentanil 0.01–0.1 μg/kg/min and either propofol 25–100 μg/kg/min or dexmedetomidine 0.1–0.5 μg/kg/h. The patient's nose can be sprayed with lidocaine and a soft nasal trumpet coated with viscous lidocaine inserted into the most patent nostril. Supplemental oxygen is supplied by attaching the anesthesia circuit to the nasal trumpet.[21]

Regardless of the anesthetic technique, a bilateral scalp block is performed and includes injection of ropivacaine 0.5% with epinephrine 1:200,000 at the supratrochlear, supraorbital, zygomaticotemporal, auriculotemporal, lesser occipital, and greater occipital nerves. A scalp block provides analgesia for both Mayfield pin placement and skin incision. Many surgeons inject additional local anesthetics with epinephrine along the planned incision site.

Head Fixation

The three-pin Mayfield head fixation system is widely used in craniotomies. Shen et al. describe an awake craniotomy protocol used at Stoney Brook that eliminates the need for rigid head fixation using a frameless Brainlab skull-mounted array for stereotactic navigation.[22] The authors describe the use of a soft foam pillow instead of rigid fixation and improved patient comfort and easier access to the airway for the anesthesiologist as advantages.

Access and Monitoring

A second peripheral intravenous line, an arterial catheter, a Foley catheter, and, if available, a BIS monitor should be placed. The intravenous lines and arterial catheter should be placed on the arm ipsilateral to the surgery so that sensory and motor testing on the contralateral side are unimpeded by invasive lines.

Intraoperative Management

Following line and catheter placement, surgeons use neuronavigation, and the patient is prepped and draped. The surgical drapes must be secured in a way that allows a clear visual connection between the patient's eyes and the anesthesiologist and neuropsychologic testing team. The use of surgical drapes containing clear panels allows room light to illuminate the patient's face. A small microphone is secured close to the patient's mouth to facilitate patient-to-surgeon communication.

After the dura is opened, the surgeon will request that the patient be awoken. Intravenous ondansetron should be administered, and a dose of intravenous acetaminophen can be considered. The anesthesiologist discontinues all anesthetic infusions and volatile agents. If a BIS monitor is being used, the anesthesiologist can use the BIS as a rough guide for when the patient is nearing an awake state. If rocuronium has been administered, the response to a train of four should be measured. Reversal of muscle relaxant is indicated if the response is anything less than 4/4 without fade.[23] The patient can be placed on pressure support to elicit spontaneous respiration. The anesthesiologist is positioned in direct line of sight with the patient and should firmly hold each of the patient's hands. The anesthesiologist should begin talking to the patient well before there is objective evidence of the awakened state. Use of a reassuring, repetitive phrase to the patient helps to orient the patient as to where they are for example, "You are in the operating room. Surgery is going well. Don't move. Stay very still. It is time to wake up, just like we talked about. Open your eyes. Squeeze my hands." When the patient is breathing spontaneously with adequate minute ventilation and following commands, the supraglottic airway can be removed. Typically, patients take an additional 5–10 min after airway removal to be able to participate in testing. During this time period, blood pressure often rises and requires treatment to maintain a systolic blood pressure (SBP) of <140 mmHg. Patients may report discomfort that should be promptly addressed with minor repositioning, massage, or a low-dose infusion of remifentanil. Anxiety can be alleviated in most cases with a low-dose infusion of dexmedetomidine. Small ice chips are immensely helpful in treating dry mouth, and patients are grateful for the "treat." When the patient is fully awake, testing can begin and may include object naming, sentence completion, action naming, simple math problems, motor tasks, and sensory identification. We have a neuropsychology team in the operating room to conduct the testing. The advantages of having such a team include quantifiable measurement, precise identification of deficit (e.g., syntax error versus hesitancy versus speech arrest), potentially shorter surgical times, and more frequent gross total resection.[24,25] Additionally, when a neuropsychology team conducts intraoperative testing the anesthesia team can focus on the physical and mental well being of the patient. As the awake time period extends, patients often become fatigued and increasingly notice the discomfort of positioning. The challenges for the patient in enduring through a long awake period cannot be overstated. Throughout the awake period, the anesthesiologist attends to the patient's needs, provides reassurance, addresses pain issues, and communicates with the surgical team regarding the patient's ability to continue in the awake state. At the completion of the resection, the surgeon will inform the anesthesiologist that the patient may "go back to sleep." The anesthesiologist may decide to induce general anesthesia, reinsert the supraglottic airway, and resume controlled ventilation. Alternatively, the anesthesiologist may decide to sedate the patient and allow spontaneous respiration without an airway throughout the closing period. Factors influencing the anesthesiologist's decision include the adequacy of the patient's natural airway, hemodynamic status, anticipated length of closure, and need for additional intraoperative imaging.

Intraoperative Challenges

The intraoperative management plan must consider several common events. Intraoperative seizure is an emergency situation during awake craniotomy and must be managed immediately. Seizures increase cerebral oxygen demand and can cause uncontrolled movement, leading to patient injury. Uncontrolled movement of the head from a seizure can lead to scalp laceration at the pin sites or dislodgement of the head from the head fixation. Ice cold saline placed on the brain by the surgeon during seizures often stops the activity. If this intervention is unsuccessful, propofol is often effective; however, propofol depresses respiration and can lead to patient apnea. Mask ventilation or emergency placement of a supraglottic airway may be necessary; hence positioning is important at the beginning of the case to enable mask ventilation of the patient in the surgical position.

Most patients undergoing awake craniotomy have some level of anxiety, and some patients, upon awakening, develop severe anxiety and simply cannot tolerate the demands of the situation. Low-dose dexmedetomidine can be immensely effective in controlling anxiety. If this intervention fails, and the patient's anxiety makes useful testing nearly impossible, the patient should be returned to an anesthetized state. This scenario should be discussed with every patient scheduled for awake craniotomy.

Many centers use iMRI in combination with the awake craniotomy technique. The use of iMRI usually includes a preincision iMRI, mapping and resection under awake conditions, postresection iMRI with contrast, additional resection if needed, and closure. The use of iMRI precludes the use of a BIS monitor or Foley catheter containing a temperature probe. iMRI following initial resection can be performed with the patient sedated and spontaneously breathing without an artificial airway or after insertion of a supraglottic airway. The significant distance between the anesthesia team and the patient undergoing the iMRI can create a tenuous situation if the patient is sedated without a supraglottic airway. Airway obstruction, respiratory depression, and inadequate sedation leading to movement or anxiety can create a dangerous situation for the patient, and we routinely reinsert the laryngeal mask airway (LMA) and control ventilation for the postresection iMRI.

Intraoperative Considerations and Management

Induction of anesthesia should focus on adequate mask ventilation to avoid hypercarbia and oxygen desaturation. Induction medications should be titrated to avoid large variations in blood pressure during intubation, which can adversely affect ICP and CPP. Succinylcholine has the potential to increase ICP and is best avoided, if possible, in patients undergoing craniotomy. However, if succinylcholine is clinically indicated, pretreatment with a defasciculating dose of a nondepolarizing muscle relaxant blunts the ICP effect.

Vascular Access and Monitoring

Vascular access for patients undergoing craniotomy is dictated by the anticipated blood loss. For the majority of cases, it is sufficient to have two intravenous (IV) lines, preferably with one being a large-bore IV line. If the semisitting position is planned, blood loss is expected to be significant or peripheral access is difficult or impossible, placement of a central venous catheter (CVC) should be strongly considered. Otherwise, a CVC is not necessary. If a CVC is needed, placement in the subclavian vein is preferred over either the internal jugular or femoral veins due to the potential for compromised cerebral venous drainage and infection, respectively.

For intraoperative monitoring, beat-to-beat blood pressure measurements using an arterial line are routine. An arterial line also provides ease of access to blood samples when intraoperative and postoperative laboratory studies are needed. Craniotomy patients benefit from meticulous blood pressure control and hemodynamic stability to minimize fluctuations in CBF that may contribute to changes in ICP or cerebral ischemia.[26] Therefore avoidance of both hypotension and hypertension is important. Arterial hypotension, defined as SBP less than 90 mmHg or MAP less than 70 mmHg,[27] may decrease cerebral perfusion and increase the risk of intracranial ischemic injury. Consequences of arterial hypertension, defined as SBP greater than 140 mmHg or MAP greater than 110 mmHg, include risk of surgical bleeding and increased CBF that may contribute to brain tissue swelling. In treating aberrant blood pressure, consider using vasopressors or antihypertensive medications that are short acting, since surgical stimulation may vary widely during craniotomy. Generally, noxious stimuli are more prevalent during skin incision and closure, bone flap removal and replacement, and dural opening and closure than during the time of tumor resection when stimulation is usually minimal. However, if tumor resection involves areas adjacent to intracranial blood vessels or the dura, elevations in blood pressure and heart rate may occur. Given this dynamic surgical environment, short-acting agents allow the provider to adjust the treatment administered to meet the patient's ever-changing needs. Rhythm disturbances may occur during craniotomy, which warrants vigilant monitoring. Most notably, asystole and bradycardia resulting from surgically induced vagus nerve stimulation or trigeminal cardiac reflex during craniotomy have been reported in the literature; treatment is with cessation of the stimulus.[27–29] If local anesthetics are used, toxicity may occur that could induce both rhythm disturbances and hemodynamic instability. The treatment for local anesthetic toxicity is administration of intralipid and supportive care until the baseline cardiac rhythm and blood pressure are restored.[27]

Measuring the depth of anesthesia using noninvasive tools such as the BIS brain monitor system should be considered when TIVA is used. However, care must be taken to avoid encroaching on the surgical field when placing the BIS electrode sensor on the patient's forehead.

Hyperthermia in the setting of an impaired brain or one at increased risk of injury is associated with poor outcome and higher mortality.[30–32] Additionally, hyperthermia, regardless of severity or duration, can cause both neurologic and cognitive impairment that may persist even after normothermia is established.[33] Mechanistically, hyperthermia negatively impacts the cell structure and function of neurons and can exacerbate neuronal injury resulting from other processes such as ischemia.[34,35] Intraoperative hyperthermia usually results from aggressive patient warming and thus can be avoided by carefully monitoring core temperature and discontinuing active warming and/or removing excessive blankets and drapes when indicated.[36] Ideally, core body temperature for patients undergoing craniotomy should be maintained between 36°C and 37°C.

Head Pinning and Surgical Positioning

A scalp block (discussed later) or infiltration of the pin sites with local anesthetic can dramatically decrease the hemodynamic response to placement of the head fixation pins. If the use of a local anesthetic adjuvant is not possible, pretreatment with propofol, an opioid, nicardipine, and/or esmolol should be administered to control the blood pressure and heart rate during the placement of head pins. Regardless of the drug class used to control the response to the head pins, short-acting agents provide adequate depth without the risk of prolonged hypotension.

Surgical positioning concerns specific to craniotomy include head positioning to optimize surgical exposure and use of the semisitting position. For craniotomy patients positioned horizontally, either supine or in the lateral position, head rotation should be limited to avoid compromising the patient's airway or impeding cerebral venous drainage. As discussed above, the semisitting position is used for surgeries involving tumors in the posterior fossa and cervical region. In addition to providing the neurosurgeon better access to these tumors, the semisitting position facilitates cerebral venous and cerebral spinal fluid (CSF) drainage; consequently, surgical exposure is improved, especially for deeper structures.[37] Anesthetic advantages of the semisitting position include better access to the patient's airway, better access for neuromonitoring, and in the case of a cardiopulmonary event easier access to perform chest compressions.[37–39] The primary risks of the semisitting position are intraoperative VAE, paradoxical air embolism, and hypotension.

The most vulnerable time for VAE occurrence is from skin incision to dural opening. From a surgical standpoint, preventative measures for VAE include applying bone wax along the borders of the intact bone when the bone flap is removed, intermittently irrigating the surgical field, and avoiding dural retraction.[37] Signs of VAE include a millwheel murmur from the Doppler, decline in end-tidal carbon dioxide, and potentially a decline in blood pressure. If VAE is suspected, the immediate goals are prevention of further entrainment of air, identification of the source of the air, maintenance of hemodynamic stability, and repair of open vessels. Placing the patient's bed into the steep Trendelenburg position, initiating positive end-expiratory pressure, and manually compressing the jugular veins increase intracranial venous pressure and prevent the ongoing aspiration of air. If present, the CVC should be used to aspirate any air bubbles that may be present. If hemodynamic compromise occurs, supportive care with fluids and positive inotropic agents should be employed.[37]

Brain Relaxation and Optimizing Surgical Exposure

Intraoperative brain relaxation, defined as the volume of brain tissue relative to the intracranial space in an open cranium, is an important determinant of surgical exposure and overall operating conditions.[40] A variety of strategies may be employed to achieve brain relaxation, a state in which the intracranial tissue is soft, lacks swelling, and the ratio of tissue content to cranial volume is optimized.[40] These strategies include hyperventilation, administration of a hyperosmolar treatment along with judicious use of fluids, placing the patient in the reverse Trendelenburg position, administration of a steroid, and minimizing or eliminating the use of volatile anesthetics.[40]

Hyperventilation results in hypocapnia-induced cerebral vasoconstriction, which decreases cerebral blood volume (CBV) and helps to curtail tissue swelling.[40] Because the reduction in CBV is associated with reduced CBF, the risk of ischemia-induced brain injury may be increased with hyperventilation. Current recommendations are to use hyperventilation only when there is a clinical indication and only as a temporizing measure when brain swelling is present.[40,41] Other side effects of hyperventilation include respiratory alkalosis and potential hypokalemia. Therefore, in the setting of hyperventilation, arterial blood gas (ABG) tests should be performed periodically to monitor the partial pressure of carbon dioxide (Pco_2), pH, and potassium level. If utilizing hyperventilation, the lowest recommended arterial Pco_2 value to target is 30 mmHg; below this threshold, the risks of hyperventilation may outweigh its benefits.

Administration of a hyperosmolar fluid, such as mannitol or hypertonic saline, also aids in brain relaxation. Hyperosmolar agents create an osmotic gradient that displaces free water from brain tissue to the intravascular space, effectively reducing brain tissue edema.[40] However, in the setting of intracranial hypertension, hyperosmolar therapy may cause normal tissue to contract and exacerbate any midline shift or herniation.[40] Risks specifically associated with the use of mannitol include severe diuresis, renal dysfunction, electrolyte disturbances, and transient changes in preload, afterload, and cardiac output.[42–45] Fortunately, these side effects are self-limiting in patients with preserved cardiac and renal function.[46] If there is a disruption in the blood-brain barrier, mannitol may worsen cerebral edema and thus should be avoided in these patients.[47] Potential adverse effects of hypertonic saline include hypernatremia, hypokalemia, central pontine myelinolysis, and pulmonary edema.[44,48,49] In addition to utilizing hyperosmolar treatments, limiting the use of hypotonic fluids can help minimize brain swelling. Although furosemide has traditionally been used to facilitate brain relaxation, recent studies have not demonstrated its efficacy in reducing cerebral edema either alone or in conjunction with hyperosmolar fluids.[50,51]

When feasible, placing the patient in reverse Trendelenburg position can facilitate brain relaxation. In this head-up tilt position, the effect of gravity will translocate cerebral spinal fluid from the intracranial space to the extracranial subarachnoid space and enhance cerebral venous drainage to effectively reduce CBV; as a result, the intracranial tissue volume will be reduced.[40] The risks associated with reverse Trendelenburg include systemic hypotension, cerebral hypoperfusion, VAE, and pneumocephalus.[40,52,53] Limiting the head-up tilt position to 30 degrees or less can reduce ICP and minimize cerebral edema without affecting brain perfusion.[40,54,55]

Administration of glucocorticoids in patients undergoing intracranial tumor resection has become a standard practice to reduce vasogenic edema from tumor-associated disruption of the blood-brain barrier, primarily affecting the white matter.[40] Although the exact mechanism is not known, the effectiveness of glucocorticoids in facilitating brain relaxation is well established.[56–58] The risks of steroid treatment include hyperglycemia and potential immunosuppression that may negatively impact the patient's postoperative outcome and cancer prognosis.[56,59,60]

As discussed above, TIVA, consisting primarily of propofol, reduces ICP through its effect on CBF and CBV compared to volatile anesthetics. This reduction in ICP may translate to improved brain relaxation in the open cranium during craniotomy. Despite the generally accepted premise that TIVA has favorable effects on brain swelling, findings from clinical studies on anesthetic techniques and brain relaxation have not demonstrated a distinct advantage of one anesthetic agent over any other.[40,61–64] Because inhalational anesthetics have a dose-dependent effect on cerebral vasodilation, intravenous anesthetics may confer benefit as an adjunct to limit the dose of the volatile agent to <0.5 MAC.

Emergence From Anesthesia

Emergence from anesthesia is a critical period in which there is a greater chance of intracranial hemorrhage. To reduce this risk, meticulous blood pressure control is crucial, since both hypertension and tachycardia usually occur as the patient awakens. Although these hemodynamic derangements may be brief in duration, they are often severe enough to necessitate treatment. Incremental doses of a short-acting antihypertensive and beta blockers, such as nicardipine and esmolol, respectively, can be used to rapidly treat hypertension and tachycardia while minimizing the risk of prolonged hypotension. For patients with a history of severe hypertension that is refractory to treatment, a continuous infusion of nicardipine may be required and should be titrated to effect. Persistent hypertension that is observed after the extubation of the patient should be treated with a longer-acting antihypertensive medication. The desirable blood pressure and heart rate parameters outside of which the patient will require treatment should be determined based on the patient's baseline preoperative values, comorbidities, and surgical determinants.

An intracranial bleed may also be caused by elevated ICP from coughing or retching during emergence due to endotracheal tube-induced stimulation. Patients with increased airway sensitivity (e.g., smokers and asthmatic patients) or in whom there is an increased risk of surgical bleeding should be considered for either deep extubation or LMA exchange. Deep extubation can decrease the risk of coughing, retching, and bronchospasm, but also has its own risks. Contraindications to deep extubation include known increased risk for aspiration, suspected or proven difficult mask ventilation or intubation, and risk of pneumocephalus if positive pressure mask ventilation is required. Deep extubation leaves the patient at some risk for aspiration because the endotracheal tube is removed before full airway reflexes have returned. Laryngospasm after deep extubation is common and can occur as the patient passes through stage two of anesthesia. Intraoperative fluid administration can cause airway edema, making deep extubation unwise.

An alternative to deep extubation is LMA exchange to facilitate smooth emergence. Similar to deep extubation, LMA exchange requires removal of the endotracheal tube, while the patient is still fully anesthetized. However, after the patient is extubated, an LMA is placed, and the patient can be mechanically ventilated during emergence from anesthesia. The LMA is subsequently removed once the patient meets the extubation criteria. Because LMA is less invasive and better tolerated in most patients than an endotracheal tube, its use may alleviate coughing and retching that might otherwise occur. The main advantage of this technique over deep extubation is the presence of a secured airway. However, it is important to recognize that deep extubation is still required, thus presenting the same risks—aspiration, laryngospasm, and hypoxia. Additionally, there is a potential that the LMA may not seat appropriately to allow adequate ventilation, in which case reintubation with an endotracheal tube is needed.

In addition to a smooth emergence, rapid wake-up from anesthesia is desirable in patients undergoing craniotomy. Intraoperatively, anesthetics and analgesics should be titrated to ensure that patients are awake and alert after extubation, allowing for adequate assessment of the neurologic status. Prolonged sedation from anesthesia can mimic the signs and symptoms of surgical complications and is problematic. While prolonged sedation will resolve with time, the delay in treatment for neurosurgical complications may be life threatening.

Scalp Block

As discussed above, patients undergoing craniotomy present a unique challenge in anesthetic management wherein tight regulation of blood pressure and heart rate is balanced with the need for rapid and smooth emergence. To address such challenges, the use of a regional block, termed a scalp block, can be incorporated in the anesthetic care plan as part of a multimodal approach to perioperative pain control in patients undergoing supratentorial craniotomy. A scalp block selectively targets up to 12 sensory nerves (6 on each side) innervating the forehead and scalp. These include the supraorbital, supratrochlear, zygomaticotemporal, auriculotemporal, greater occipital, and lesser occipital nerves[65] (Fig. 19.2).

This regional anesthesia technique is easy to perform, imparts minimal risk, and has very few contraindications.[65] However, it should not be used in patients who are allergic to local anesthetics or who have compromised skull integrity because of the potential risk of local anesthetic tracking into the subdural space. Additionally, scalp blocks may not be as efficacious in patients who have had multiple previous craniotomies due to the altered anatomy and nerve distribution in these patients.

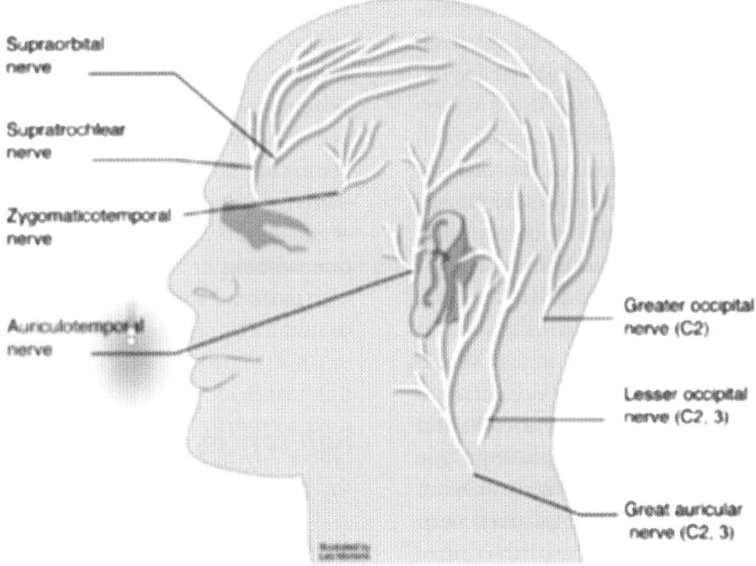

• **Fig. 19.2** Nerve supply to the scalp.[91]

The primary advantage of a scalp block placed prior to the commencement of surgery is its ability to blunt hemodynamic responses to surgical stimulation, including head pinning and skin incision. This may result in greater hemodynamic stability during surgery. Scalp blocks also have the potential to decrease the need for anesthetics and intravenous analgesics, allowing for a more rapid emergence.[65–67] The use of scalp blocks may have important implications in the care of patients undergoing awake craniotomies, minimizing pain and narcotic usage, thus facilitating intraoperative neurologic assessment. The benefits of a scalp block can extend into the postoperative period by providing pain control, reducing opioid consumption, and avoiding increases in CBF and ICP seen with inadequately controlled pain after craniotomy.[68–71]

The most common local anesthetic agents used for scalp blocks are bupivacaine and ropivacaine. Owing to the lower cardiotoxic risk, ropivacaine may be preferable to bupivacaine. The addition of epinephrine to the local anesthetic is recommended to not only extend the duration of action for scalp blockade but also to function as an indicator for inadvertent intravascular injection.

Postoperative Management and Pain Control

Postoperative management of patients undergoing craniotomy should focus on minimizing the risk of intracranial hemorrhage, adequately treating pain, and lessening the incidence or severity of nausea and vomiting. Intraoperative and early postoperative hypertension associated with acute blood pressure elevations may increase the risk of intracranial hemorrhage by nearly five-fold in postcraniotomy patients.[72] Ensuring hemodynamic stability and preventing cerebral hypertension during recovery reduces the risk of bleeding. Patients with baseline hypertension that is exacerbated by surgery should be treated with antihypertensive medications that are titrated to effect.

Alternatively, if pain is the cause of hypertension, additional analgesics must be prescribed. An optimal pain therapy regimen should be multimodal to minimize the use of opioids and their side effects. In addition to intraoperative placement of a scalp block, acetaminophen and Cox-2 inhibitors can be administered as adjuncts. Pharmacologic analgesics that decrease the seizure threshold, induce sedation, or increase the risk of systemic bleeding should be avoided. Decreased opioid consumption reduces the risk of hypercapnia and potential ICP elevation, nausea and vomiting, postoperative sedation, and cognitive dysfunction.[65]

Postoperative nausea and vomiting can be multifactorial and result from patient-related, anesthetic, and surgical factors. The reported incidence of PONV after craniotomy has been as high as 70%.[73] Patient-related risk factors are female sex, a history of PONV or motion sickness, and nonsmoking status.[74] Although age is not a strong determinant in adults, the incidence of PONV is higher in pediatric patients 3 years and older.[74] Anesthesia-associated causes involve the use of volatile anesthetics, nitrous oxide, and opioids.[74] The main surgical consideration is that of the tumor site and whether the resection is infratentorial, as opposed to supratentorial, and whether there is involvement of the ventricles. Although PONV is an undesirable side effect for any surgical patient, vomiting in patients after craniotomy is especially detrimental, since it can cause increased ICP and a potential intracranial bleed or decreased intracranial perfusion.[75] Neurosurgical patients should receive prophylactic multimodal treatment for postoperative emesis.

The most commonly used antiemetics are the serotonin 5-HT_3 receptor antagonists ondansetron, dolasetron, granisetron, and palonosetron, which prevent nausea by inhibiting the action of serotonin on the vomiting center.[74] While the primary advantage of this drug class in neurosurgery is its lack of sedation, be aware that the most common side effect observed is headache, which may also be a presenting symptom of a neurosurgical complication.[74,76] All of the 5-HT_3 receptor antagonists except palonosetron can cause or exacerbate QTc prolongation and have been associated with cardiac arrhythmias.[77–80] Thus palonosetron is the drug of choice for patients with this baseline conduction abnormality. Other perioperative antiemetic adjuncts include aprepitant, scopolamine, promethazine, and dexamethasone.

Aprepitant is an NK-1 receptor antagonist that centrally blocks the action of neurokinin to prevent rather than treat nausea.[81] Therefore it is best administered preoperatively or intraoperatively prior to the onset of PONV. Similar to serotonin 5-HT_3 receptor antagonists, aprepitant is not sedating.[74] Common side effects of aprepitant include fatigue and hiccups.[81] Aprepitant interferes with the effectiveness of oral contraceptives, and female patients must be given both oral and written instructions to use alternative birth control methods for at least 28 days following a dose of aprepitant.

As an anticholinergic, scopolamine prevents PONV by centrally inhibiting muscarinic receptors.[82] Scopolamine has a short half-life and thus is administered via a continuous transdermal route that provides up to 72 h of antiemetic relief.[74] The most common side effect of scopolamine is blurry vision caused by dilated pupils, although dry mouth, decreased sweat secretion, reduced gastrointestinal function, somnolence, and elevated heart rate have been reported.[83–85]

Promethazine, a phenothiazine, is an antihistamine that also has anticholinergic effects. It alleviates nausea by blocking histamine H1 receptors in the vomiting center and vestibular system.[86] Due to its sedative properties, promethazine may contribute to delayed emergence if given at the conclusion of surgery and may not be ideal for use in elderly and/or somnolent patients.[87] Alternatively, it may be given in two divided doses to minimize the risk of sedation. Promethazine is contraindicated in children under 6 years of age and is cautioned in children between the ages of 6 and 12 years.

Dexamethasone is a corticosteroid that is commonly administered to patients undergoing craniotomy to prevent brain edema and inflammation. It is also an antiemetic whose mechanism of action is unclear, although animal studies suggest that dexamethasone's effectiveness against PONV results from central inhibition of the nucleus tractus solitarius.[88] For maximum efficacy, the recommended dose of dexamethasone for PONV prophylaxis is 4–5 mg administered at the time of induction of anesthesia.[89] Dexamethasone may cause elevated blood glucose; therefore close monitoring and treatment of intraoperative and postoperative blood glucose is warranted, especially in patients with preexisting diabetes mellitus.

Conclusion

Patients undergoing craniotomy for tumor resection present numerous anesthetic challenges. To minimize morbidity and mortality, these patients warrant careful preoperative assessment, meticulous intraoperative planning and care, and precise postoperative management. Preoperatively, baseline neurologic deficits as well as signs and symptoms associated with intracranial tumors should be identified and assessed. Intraoperative planning and care should focus on the appropriate anesthetic technique given not only the patient-specific characteristics but also the surgical needs and challenges. Additionally, anesthesia and analgesia medications should be titrated to preserve hemodynamic stability and facilitate rapid emergence. The postoperative strategy should focus on strict blood pressure control and prevention or prompt treatment of PONV.

References

1. Schapira L. Brain tumors: statistics. *Cancer. Net.* 2019; Available at https://www.cancer.net/cancer-types/brain-tumor/statistics.
2. Mirski MA, Lele AV, Fitzsimmons L, Toung TJ. Diagnosis and treatment of vascular air embolism. *Anesthesiology.* 2007;106:164–177.
3. Maekawa T, Tommasino C, Shapiro HM, Keifer-Goodman J, Kohlenberger RW. Local cerebral blood flow and glucose utilization during isoflurane anesthesia in the rat. *Anesthesiology.* 1986;65:144–151.
4. Drummond J, Patel P. Cerebral physiology and the effects of anesthetic techniques. In: Miller R, ed. *Anesthesia.* 5th ed. New York: Churchill Livingstone; 2000:695–734.
5. Muñoz HR, Núñez GE, de la Fuente JE, Campos MG. The effect of nitrous oxide on jugular bulb oxygen saturation during remifentanil plus target-controlled infusion propofol or sevoflurane in patients with brain tumors. *Anesth Analg.* 2002;94:389–392.
6. Jansen GF, van Praagh BH, Kedaria MB, Odoom JA. Jugular bulb oxygen saturation during propofol and isoflurane/nitrous oxide anesthesia in patients undergoing brain tumor surgery. *Anesthesia Analg.* 1999;89:358–363.
7. Iwata M, Kawaguchi M, Inoue S, et al. Effects of increasing concentrations of propofol on jugular venous bulb oxygen saturation in neurosurgical patients under normothermic and mildly hypothermic conditions. *Anesthesiology.* 2006;104:33–38.
8. de Hoogd S, Ahlers SJ, van Dongen EP, et al. Is intraoperative remifentanil associated with acute or chronic postoperative pain after prolonged surgery? An update of the literature. *Clin J Pain.* 2016;32:726–735.
9. Yu EH, Tran DH, Lam SW, Irwin MG. Remifentanil tolerance and hyperalgesia: short-term gain, long-term pain? *Anaesthesia.* 2016;71:1347–1362.
10. Hagan KB, Bhavsar S, Raza SM, et al. Enhanced recovery after surgery for oncological craniotomies. *J Clin Neurosci.* 2016;24:10–16.
11. Obara S. Dexmedetomidine as an adjuvant during general anesthesia. *J Anesth.* 2018;32:313–315.
12. Chou R, Gordon DB, de Leon-Casasola OA, et al. Management of postoperative pain: a clinical practice guideline from the American Pain Society, the American Society of Regional Anesthesia and Pain Medicine, and the American Society of Anesthesiologists' Committee on Regional Anesthesia, Executive Committee, and Administrative Council. *J Pain.* 2016;17:131–157.
13. Brinck EC, Tiippana E, Heesen M, Bell RF, Straube S, Moore RA, Kontinen V. Perioperative intravenous ketamine for acute

postoperative pain in adults. *Cochrane Database Syst Rev.* 2018;12:CD012033.
14. Ban VS, Bhoja R, McDonagh DL. Multimodal analgesia for craniotomy. *Curr Opin Anaesthesiol.* 2019;32:592–599.
15. Modica PA, Tempelhoff R, White PF. Pro- and anticonvulsant effects of anesthetics (Part II). *Anesth Analg.* 1990;70:433–444.
16. Wampole CR, Smith KE. Beyond opioids for pain management in adult critically ill patients. *J Pharm Pract.* 2019;32:256–270.
17. Bilotta F, Rosa G. 'Anesthesia' for awake neurosurgery. *Curr Opin Anaesthesiol.* 2009;22:560–5.
18. Stevanovic A, Rossaint R, Veldeman M, Bilotta F, Coburn M. Anaesthesia management for awake craniotomy: systematic review and meta-analysis. *PLoS One.* 2016;11:e0156448.
19. De Witt Hamer PC, Robles SG, Zwinderman AH, Duffau H, Berger MS. Impact of intraoperative stimulation brain mapping on glioma surgery outcome: a meta-analysis. *J Clin Oncol.* 2012;30:2559–2565.
20. Zemmoura I, Fournier E, El-Hage W, Jolly V, Destrieux C, Velut S. Hypnosis for awake surgery of low-grade gliomas: description of the method and psychological assessment. *Neurosurgery.* 2016;78:53–61.
21. Eseonu CI, ReFaey K, Garcia O, John A, Quiñones-Hinojosa A, Tripathi P. Awake craniotomy anesthesia: a comparison of the monitored anesthesia care and asleep-awake-asleep techniques. *World Neurosurg.* 2017;104:679–686.
22. Shen E, Calandra C, Geralemou S, et al. The Stony Brook awake craniotomy protocol: A technical note. *J Clin Neurosci.* 2019;67:221–5.
23. Naguib M, Brull SJ, Johnson KB. Conceptual and technical insights into the basis of neuromuscular monitoring. *Anaesthesia.* 2017;72(Suppl 1):16–37.
24. DS H. The role of neuropsychology in the assessment and management of CNS tumors. *Clin Oncol.* 2016;1:1065.
25. Kelm A, Sollmann N, Ille S, Meyer B, Ringel F, Krieg SM. Resection of gliomas with and without neuropsychological support during awake craniotomy-effects on surgery and clinical outcome. *Front Oncol.* 2017;7:176.
26. Lassen NA, Christensen MS. Physiology of cerebral blood flow. *Brit J Anaesth.* 1976;48:719–734.
27. Bilotta F, Guerra C, Rosa G. Update on anesthesia for craniotomy. *Curr Opin Anaesthesiol.* 2013;26:517–522.
28. Haldar R, Gyanesh P, Bettaswamy G. Isolated bradycardia due to skull pin fixation: an unusual occurrence. *J Neurosurg Anesthesiol.* 2013;25:206–7.
29. Chowdhury T, West M. Intraoperative asystole in a patient undergoing craniotomy under monitored anesthesia care: is it TCR? *J Neurosurg Anesthesiol.* 2013;25:92–3.
30. Malpas G, Taylor JA, Cumin D, Merry AF, Mitchell SJ. The incidence of hyperthermia during craniotomy. *Anaesth Intensive Care.* 2018;46:368–373.
31. Miller R, Eriksson L, Fleisher L. Temperature regulation and monitoring. In: Miller R. Philadelphia: Churchill Livingstone. *Anesthesia.* 2014:1622–1646, 8th ed.
32. Greer DM, Funk SE, Reaven NL, Ouzounelli M, Uman GC. Impact of fever on outcome in patients with stroke and neurologic injury: a comprehensive meta-analysis. *Stroke.* 2008;39:3029–3035.
33. Walter EJ, Carraretto M. The neurological and cognitive consequences of hyperthermia. *Crit Care.* 2016;20:199.
34. White MG, Luca LE, Nonner D, et al. Cellular mechanisms of neuronal damage from hyperthermia. *Prog Brain Res.* 2007;162:347–371.
35. Kiyatkin EA. Physiological and pathological brain hyperthermia. *Prog Brain Res.* 2007;162:219–243.
36. Bindu B, Bindra A, Rath G. Temperature management under general anesthesia: compulsion or option. *J Anaesthesiol Clin Pharmacol.* 2017;33:306–316.
37. Saladino A, Lamperti M, Mangraviti A, Legnani FG, Prada FU, Casali C, Caputi L, Borrelli P, DiMeco F. The semisitting position: analysis of the risks and surgical outcomes in a contemporary series of 425 adult patients undergoing cranial surgery. *J Neurosurg.* 2017;127:867–876.
38. Beltran SL, Mashour GA. Unsuccessful cardiopulmonary resuscitation during neurosurgery: is the supine position always optimal? *Anesthesiology.* 2008;108:163–4.
39. Gale T, Leslie K. Anaesthesia for neurosurgery in the sitting position. *J Clin Neurosci.* 2004;11:693–696.
40. Li J, Gelb AW, Flexman AM, Ji F, Meng L. Definition, evaluation, and management of brain relaxation during craniotomy. *Brit J Anaesth.* 2016;116:759–769.
41. Talke PO, Sharma D, Heyer EJ, Bergese SD, Blackham KA, Stevens RD. Society for Neuroscience in anesthesiology and Critical Care Expert consensus statement: anesthetic management of endovascular treatment for acute ischemic stroke*: endorsed by the Society of Neurointerventional Surgery and the Neurocritical Care Society. *J Neurosurg Anesthesiol.* 2014;26:95–108.
42. Dostal P, Dostalova V, Schreiberova J, et al. A comparison of equivolume, equiosmolar solutions of hypertonic saline and mannitol for brain relaxation in patients undergoing elective intracranial tumor surgery: a randomized clinical trial. *J Neurosurg Anesthesiol.* 2015;27:51–6.
43. Carney NA. American Association of Neurological Surgeons, Congress of Neurological Surgeons, Joint Section on Neurotrauma and Critical Care, AANS/CNS. Guidelines for the management of severe traumatic brain injury. Methods. *J Neurotrauma.* 2007;24(Suppl 1):S3–S6.
44. Rozet I, Tontisirin N, Muangman S, et al. Effect of equiosmolar solutions of mannitol versus hypertonic saline on intraoperative brain relaxation and electrolyte balance. *Anesthesiology.* 2007;107:697–704.
45. Chatterjee N, Koshy T, Misra S, Suparna B. Changes in left ventricular preload, afterload, and cardiac output in response to a single dose of mannitol in neurosurgical patients undergoing craniotomy: a transesophageal echocardiographic study. *J Neurosurg Anesthesiol.* 2012;24:25–9.
46. Manninen PH, Lam AM, Gelb AW, Brown SC. The effect of high-dose mannitol on serum and urine electrolytes and osmolality in neurosurgical patients. *Can J Anaesth.* 1987;34:442–6.
47. Kaufmann AM, Cardoso ER. Aggravation of vasogenic cerebral edema by multiple-dose mannitol. *J Neurosurg.* 1992;77:584–9.
48. Kleinschmidt-DeMasters BK, Norenberg MD. Rapid correction of hyponatremia causes demyelination: relation to central pontine myelinolysis. *Science.* 1981;211:1068–1070.
49. Qureshi AI, Suarez JI, Bhardwaj A, et al. Use of hypertonic (3%) saline/acetate infusion in the treatment of cerebral edema: effect on intracranial pressure and lateral displacement of the brain. *Crit Care Med.* 1998;26:440–6.
50. Todd MM, Cutkomp J, Brian JE. Influence of mannitol and furosemide, alone and in combination, on brain water content after fluid percussion injury. *Anesthesiology.* 2006;105:1176–1181.
51. Wang LC, Papangelou A, Lin C, Mirski MA, Gottschalk A, Toung TJ. Comparison of equivolume, equiosmolar solutions

of mannitol and hypertonic saline with or without furosemide on brain water content in normal rats. *Anesthesiology.* 2013;118:903–913.
52. Bithal PK, Pandia MP, Dash HH, Chouhan RS, Mohanty B, Padhy N. Comparative incidence of venous air embolism and associated hypotension in adults and children operated for neurosurgery in the sitting position. *Eur J Anaesthesiol.* 2004;21:517–522.
53. Olympio MA, Bell WO. Venous air embolism after craniotomy closure: tension pneumocephalus implicated. *J Neurosurg Anesthesiol.* 1994;6:35–9.
54. Feldman Z, Kanter MJ, Robertson CS, et al. Effect of head elevation on intracranial pressure, cerebral perfusion pressure, and cerebral blood flow in head-injured patients. *J Neurosurg.* 1992;76:207–211.
55. Tankisi A, Rolighed Larsen J, Rasmussen M, Dahl B, Cold GE. The effects of 10 degrees reverse Trendelenburg position on ICP and CPP in prone positioned patients subjected to craniotomy for occipital or cerebellar tumours. *Acta Neurochir.* 2002;144:665–670.
56. Dietrich J, Rao K, Pastorino S, Kesari S. Corticosteroids in brain cancer patients: benefits and pitfalls. *Expert Rev Clin Pharmacol.* 2011;4:233–242.
57. Miller JD, Leech P. Effects of mannitol and steroid therapy on intracranial volume-pressure relationships in patients. *J Neurosurg.* 1975;42:274–281.
58. Ryken TC, McDermott M, Robinson PD, et al. The role of steroids in the management of brain metastases: a systematic review and evidence-based clinical practice guideline. *J Neurooncol.* 2010;96:103–114.
59. Herold MJ, McPherson KG, Reichardt HM. Glucocorticoids in T cell apoptosis and function. *Cell Mol Life Sci.* 2006;63:60–72.
60. Perez A, Jansen-Chaparro S, Saigi I, Bernal-Lopez MR, Miñambres I, Gomez-Huelgas R. Glucocorticoid-induced hyperglycemia. *J Diabetes.* 2014;6:9–20.
61. Sneyd JR, Andrews CJ, Tsubokawa T. Comparison of propofol/remifentanil and sevoflurane/remifentanil for maintenance of anaesthesia for elective intracranial surgery. *Brit J Anaesth.* 2005;94:778–783.
62. Gelb AW, Craen RA, Rao GS. Does hyperventilation improve operating condition during supratentorial craniotomy? A multicenter randomized crossover trial. *Anesth Analg.* 2008;106:585–594 table of contents.
63. Citerio G, Pesenti A, Latini R, et al. A multicentre, randomised, open-label, controlled trial evaluating equivalence of inhalational and intravenous anaesthesia during elective craniotomy. *Eur J Anaesthesiol.* 2012;29:371–9.
64. Chui J, Mariappan R, Mehta J, Manninen P, Venkatraghavan L. Comparison of propofol and volatile agents for maintenance of anesthesia during elective craniotomy procedures: systematic review and meta-analysis. *Can J Anaesth.* 2014;61:347–356.
65. Osborn I, Sebeo J. Scalp block' during craniotomy: a classic technique revisited. *J Neurosurg Anesthesiol.* 2010;22:187–194. doi:10.1097/ANA.0b013e3181d48846.
66. Girvin JP. Neurosurgical considerations and general methods for craniotomy under local anesthesia. *Int Anesthesiol Clin.* 1986;24:89–114.
67. Papangelou A, Radzik BR, Smith T, Gottschalk A. A review of scalp blockade for cranial surgery. *J Clin Anesth.* 2013;25:150–9. doi:10.1016/j.jclinane.2012.06.024.
68. Lee EJ, Lee MY, Shyr MH, et al. Adjuvant bupivacaine scalp block facilitates stabilization of hemodynamics in patients undergoing craniotomy with general anesthesia: a preliminary report. *J Clin Anesth.* 2006;18:490–4.
69. Pinosky ML, Fishman RL, Reeves ST, et al. The effect of bupivacaine skull block on the hemodynamic response to craniotomy. *Anesth Analg.* 1996;83:1256–1261.
70. Geze S, Yilmaz AA, Tuzuner F. The effect of scalp block and local infiltration on the haemodynamic and stress response to skull-pin placement for craniotomy. *Eur J Anaesthesiol.* 2009;26:298–303. doi:10.1097/EJA.0b013e32831aedb2.
71. Gazoni FM, Pouratian N, Nemergut EC. Effect of ropivacaine skull block on perioperative outcomes in patients with supratentorial brain tumors and comparison with remifentanil: a pilot study. *Neurosurg.* 2008;109:44–9. doi:10.3171/JNS/2008/109/7/0044.
72. Basali A, Mascha EJ, Kalfas I, Schubert A. Relation between perioperative hypertension and intracranial hemorrhage after craniotomy. *Anesthesiology.* 2000;93:48–54.
73. Fabling JM, Gan TJ, El-Moalem HE, Warner DS, Borel CO. A randomized, double-blinded comparison of ondansetron, droperidol, and placebo for prevention of postoperative nausea and vomiting after supratentorial craniotomy. *Anesth Analg.* 2000;91:358–361.
74. Fero KE, Jalota L, Hornuss C, Apfel CC. Pharmacologic management of postoperative nausea and vomiting. *Expert Opin Pharmacother.* 2011;12:2283–2296.
75. Habib AS, Keifer JC, Borel CO, White WD, Gan TJ. A comparison of the combination of aprepitant and dexamethasone versus the combination of ondansetron and dexamethasone for the prevention of postoperative nausea and vomiting in patients undergoing craniotomy. *Anesth Analg.* 2011;112:813–8.
76. Goodin S, Cunningham R. 5-HT(3)-receptor antagonists for the treatment of nausea and vomiting: a reappraisal of their side-effect profile. *Oncologist.* 2002;7:424–436.
77. Benedict CR, Arbogast R, Martin L, Patton L, Morrill B, Hahne W. Single-blind study of the effects of intravenous dolasetron mesylate versus ondansetron on electrocardiographic parameters in normal volunteers. *J Cardiovasc Pharmacol.* 1996;28:53–9.
78. Boike SC, Ilson B, Zariffa N, Jorkasky DK. Cardiovascular effects of i.v. granisetron at two administration rates and of ondansetron in healthy adults. *Am J Health Syst Pharm.* 1997;54:1172–6.
79. Baguley WA, Hay WT, Mackie KP, Cheney FW, Cullen BF. Cardiac dysrhythmias associated with the intravenous administration of ondansetron and metoclopramide. *Anesth Analg.* 1997;84:1380–1.
80. Kasinath NS, Malak O, Tetzlaff J. Atrial fibrillation after ondansetron for the prevention and treatment of postoperative nausea and vomiting: a case report. *Can J Anaesth.* 2003;50:229–231.
81. Capsules (Merck) (Aprepitant). USA [Package Insert]. Merck.com/product/usa/pi_circulars/e/emend/emend_pi.pdf; 2006
82. McCarthy BG, Peroutka SJ. Differentiation of muscarinic cholinergic receptor subtypes in human cortex and pons: implications for anti-motion sickness therapy. *Aviat Space Environ Med.* 1988;59:63–6.
83. Apfel CC, Zhang K, George E, et al. Transdermal scopolamine for the prevention of postoperative nausea and vomiting: a systematic review and meta-analysis. *Clin Ther.* 2010;32:1987–2002.
84. Kranke P, Morin AM, Roewer N, Wulf H, Eberhart LH. The efficacy and safety of transdermal scopolamine for the prevention of postoperative nausea and vomiting: a quantitative systematic review. *Anesth Analg.* 2002;95:133–143 table of contents.

85. Gilman AG, Goodman LS, Gilman A. *The Pharmacological Basis of Therapeutics*. Macmillan Publishing Co; 1980. 6th ed.
86. Scuderi PE. Pharmacology of antiemetics. *Int Anesthesiol Clin*. 2003;41:41–66.
87. Carlisle JB, Stevenson CA. Drugs for preventing postoperative nausea and vomiting. *Cochrane Database Syst Rev*. 2006(3):CD004125.
88. Ho CM, Ho ST, Wang JJ, Tsai SK, Chai CY. Dexamethasone has a central antiemetic mechanism in decerebrated cats. *Anesth Analg*. 2004;99:734–9 table of contents.
89. Gan TJ, Diemunsch P, Habib AS, et al. Consensus guidelines for the management of postoperative nausea and vomiting. *Anesth Analg*. 2014;118:85–113.
90. Rodríguez-Boto G, Rivero-Garvía M, Gutiérrez-González R, Márquez-Rivas J. Basic concepts about brain pathophysiology and intracranial pressure monitoring. *Neurologia*. 2015;30:16–22.
91. Burnand C, Sebastian J. Anaesthesia for awake craniotomy. *Contin Educ Anaesth Crit Care Pain*. 2014;14:6–11.
92. Lindsay K. *Bone I Neurology and Neurosurgery Illustrated. Churchill Livingstone*. 2001.

20

Anesthesia for Spine Cancer Surgery

AISLING NÍ EOCHAGÁIN, LAUREN ADRIENNE LEDDY, JOSEPH BUTLER, AND CARA CONNOLLY

Introduction

Spinal cancer is primarily a metastatic disease with >90% having originated from another source.[1,2] In addition, osseous spread is the third most common form of metastasis with 30%–70% of cancer patients encountering spinal metastasis.[2] Many primary tumors affect persons of advanced age, with more than 60% of cancer patients being older than 65 years. Consequently, particular consideration for comorbidities, fitness for therapy, and patient preference are fundamental in guiding management plans to provide holistic care.

Surgery for Spinal Metastases

Indications include mechanical instability, neurologic compression, debilitating pain, and removal of local disease to enable the use of other modalities. Most patients have a life expectancy of <1–2 years, and a balance exists between the risks and benefits of surgery.[3] It is generally accepted that surgery might be considered in a patient with a life expectancy >3 months, with goals to optimize quality of life.[2,3]

Staging and Scoring Systems

Various classification systems aid surgical decisions based on the stage of the disease. The Global Spine Tumor Study Group (GSTSG) recommends the use of the Tomita and Tokuhashi staging systems. The Tomita score incorporates the rate of growth of the primary tumor, the number of bone metastases, and the number of visceral metastases.[3] The Tokuhashi score includes the general condition of the patient, the primary site of the cancer, and the presence of palsy and metastasis (Table 20.1). The use of the Spinal Instability Neoplastic Score (SINS) aids clinical diagnosis of spinal instability associated with cancer (Table 20.2). Mechanical instability is an indication for surgical intervention.[4] There are six parameters, including location, pain, alignment, osteolysis, vertebral body collapse, and posterior element involvement. A score of 13–18 indicates the need for surgical stabilization. Additionally, the use of quality of life scores, such as the Euroquol EQ5D, is encouraged by the GSTSG. Scoring systems can aid management plans. If no encroachment of the canal is evident and the vertebral column is stable, surgical intervention is not required.[1]

Hematologic Malignancies

For myeloma, plasmacytoma, and lymphoma, there is a shifting treatment paradigm away from surgery. For myeloma, the mainstay of treatment is systemic chemotherapy, bisphosphonates, and pain control. For spinal involvement, methods including bracing and cement augmentation, radiotherapy or surgery may be used.[5] Patients can develop rapidly progressive, lytic lesions that can cause spinal instability; however, treatment with instrumented stabilization may fail due to poor bone quality and infection.[6] Bracing can provide pain relief and manage fractures. A case report noted successful management of an unstable myelomatous vertebral fracture without neurologic deficit using a thoracolumbar sacral orthosis for 3 months.[6] Thoracic and cervical fractures with and without deficits were also effectively managed conservatively in this report. Such approaches restore stability without the risks of surgery. Patients with multiple myeloma and back pain, or an early clinical spine deformity, must still be screened urgently for spinal lesions.

Most patients with solitary bone plasmacytoma (SBP) develop multiple myeloma. The spine is the main site of SBP, and radical radiotherapy is the treatment of choice.[7] Multiple solitary plasmacytomas are treated with radiotherapy in the absence of systemic disease. However, patients with extensive disease or early relapse may benefit from systemic therapy +/– autologous stem cell transplantation. Surgical intervention is not recommended first-line.[7]

Regarding lymphoma, the National Institute for Health and Care Excellence (NICE) recommends management strategies, including radiotherapy, immunotherapy, chemotherapy, immunochemotherapy, and stem cell transplantation, with no role for surgery.[8] These malignancies should be managed

TABLE 20.1 The Tokuhashi Score

Characteristic	Score
General condition	
Poor (PS 10%–40%)	0
Moderate (PS 50%–70%)	1
Good (PS 80%–100%)	2
Number of Extra Spinal Metastatic Foci	
≥3	0
1–2	1
0	2
Number of Metastases in Vertebral Body	
≥3	0
2	1
1	2
Metastases to Other Internal Organs	
Unresectable	0
Resectable	1
Absent	2
Primary Site of Malignancy	
Lung, osteosarcoma, stomach, bladder, esophagus, pancreas	0
Liver, gallbladder, unidentified	1
Other	3
Kidney, uterus	4
Thyroid, breast, prostate, carcinoid	5
Palsy	
Complete (Frankel A, B)	0
Incomplete (Frankel B, C)	1
None (Frankel D)	2
Total score	**Months**
0–8	>6
9–11	≥6
12–15	≥12

TABLE 20.2 Spinal Instability Neoplastic Score

Parameter	Score
Location	
Junctional (occiput–C2, C7–T2, T11–L1, L5–S1)	3
Mobile spine (C3–C6, L2–L4)	2
Semirigid (T3–T10)	1
Rigid (S2–S5)	0
Pain	
Yes	3
Occasional pain but not mechanical	1
Pain-free lesion	0
Bone Lesion	
Lytic	2
Mixed (lytic/blastic)	1
Blastic	0
Radiographic Spinal Alignment	
Subluxation/translation present	4
De novo deformity (kyphosis/scoliosis)	2
Normal alignment	0
Vertebral Body Collapse	
>50% collapse	3
<50% collapse	2
No collapse with >50% body involved	1
None of the above	0
Posterolateral Involvement of Spinal Elements	
Bilateral	3
Unilateral	1
None of the above	0
Total Score	
Stable	0–6
Indeterminate	7–12
Unstable	13–18

nonoperatively, similar to plasmacytoma and multiple myeloma, with surgery reserved for cases resistant to nonoperative treatment and progressive neurologic compression.

Cement Augmentation, Kyphoplasty, Vertebroplasty

Cement augmentation using balloon kyphoplasty (BKP) and percutaneous vertebroplasty (PV) is useful in reducing pain and restoring strength.[6] It is indicated for patients who are nonambulatory and unable to engage in physical therapy, and patients who cannot tolerate analgesia side effects.[9] Benefits include shorter operative times and hospital stays, and reduced blood loss and postoperative pain.[10] PV and BKP involve the injection of cement under fluoroscopic guidance.[6] The cement stabilizes the fracture and preserves stability. Some rare complications include cement embolus and neurologic dysfunction. Leaking of cement into the intervertebral disc is less rare and can cause fractures of other vertebral bodies.[6] In BKP, a similar approach is taken; however, a balloon is inflated first to restore the vertebral height.[10] BKP reports a lower cement leakage rate.[6] This is performed for osteoporotic fractures; however, it is also a therapeutic option in pathologic fractures.[10] Patients require careful clinical assessment, magnetic resonance imaging (MRI), and computed tomography (CT) in combination with a SINS score. Cement augmentation may be used to decrease pain and enhance stability following a fracture or prophylactically, if a fracture is likely.

Stereotactic Radiosurgery and Intensity-Modulated Radiotherapy

Stereotactic radiosurgery (SRS) and intensity-modulated radiotherapy (IMRT) target radiation precisely to the cancer to reduce injury to normal tissue. They allow for noninvasive, specific, and efficacious treatment.[11] SRS targets a treatment site with multiple radiation beams of equal intensity. IMRT allows for variation of the intensity of each beam. It may be used solitarily or as an adjunct to surgery reducing the need for large resections.[11] Evidence for these modalities is sparse due to small case series and limited follow-up periods. It has been shown to be a safe intervention; however, it has not been compared with existing techniques. Currently it is used for patients with recurrent disease for whom surgery is not available and is only accessible in centers with the appropriate technology and expertise.[10]

Separation Surgery

Spinal surgery aims to achieve circumferential cord decompression. Separation surgery involves a posterolateral approach to obtain ventrolateral access to nerve roots, the posterior longitudinal ligament, and ventral epidural disease.[12] It allows for rapid decompression, stabilization, and postoperative continuation of treatment.[13] The goal is to create a space between the tumor and the spinal cord that enables safe postoperative delivery of SRS.[13] This technique is useful to prepare patients with epidural disease that is too advanced for radiotherapy. This combined approach is also referred to as a "hybrid therapy."[13]

Decompressive and Stabilization Surgery

Decompression is indicated emergently for spinal cord compression and is commonly achieved with laminectomy.[14] Posterior approaches are the most common and enable multilevel vertebral decompression resulting in effective symptom relief.[14] However, complications associated with this are apparent, including the acceleration of instability and wound complications. Anterior approaches are seen more frequently in the cervical spine.[14] Regardless of approach, posterior spinal stabilization is often needed to avoid instability.[14] It is commonly accepted that at least two levels of fixation above and below the affected vertebrae are necessary to achieve adequate stability.

En Bloc Resection

En bloc resection is considered the gold standard in treatment of solitary spinal metastasis confined to the vertebral body.[15] Unfortunately, patients with spinal metastases are frequently referred late and are not candidates. These surgeries have largely fallen out of favor due to the significant complications associated with an aggressive approach.[10] These complications are divided into surgical (wound infections, cerebrospinal fluid [CSF] fistulas), hardware related (broken, migrated), medical (pneumonia), and neurologic (new deficit). As a result, it should be reserved for curative, as opposed to palliative, therapy.[15]

Prognosis

The primary cancer is the key determinant in predicting survival. Median survival time is highest for breast and renal, and lowest for prostate and lung cancers, respectively.[16] Additionally, factors such as having multiple metastases, cervical metastasis, and pathologic fractures have no significant influence on survival. Evidence supports surgery to enhance quality of life in these cases, and it may be used first-line to reduce pain, preserve neurologic function, prevent pathologic fractures, and correct spinal instability.[16]

Anesthetic Considerations

Anesthesia for cancer patients undergoing spinal tumor surgery (STS) can be challenging. As mentioned above, the majority of this patient cohort is elderly (60% are aged >65 years), and preoperative evaluation may identify multiple organ impairment, which can occur in these patients through metastases, comorbid disease, and metabolic derangements, as well as immunosuppression due to chemo/radiotherapy. In addition, surgery can be extensive, involve special positioning, and have the potential for major hemorrhage. Airway management can be difficult both at intubation and extubation, which is compounded by the need for rapid emergence to facilitate neurologic examination. Postoperatively these patients pose challenges in terms of thromboprophylaxis and analgesia management.

Preoperative Evaluation

The challenge with preoperative evaluation for this patient cohort is that it must be comprehensive, with consideration of the patient's comorbidities and disease burden, while also respecting the urgent nature of this surgery. These patients may present with mechanical instability or neurologic symptoms; therefore preoperative assessment should be focused.

Airway evaluation is crucial as patients presenting for spinal surgery may be challenging to intubate, particularly for surgeries involving the upper thoracic or cervical spine. Patient factors may include pathology that distorts the normal airway anatomy, or they may have reduced movement of their jaw or neck secondary to radiotherapy.[17] This patient cohort may also have cervical spine instability. Airway examination should be paired with a full evaluation of preoperative imaging of the cervical spine, thoracic spine, and airway and a discussion with the surgical team about the degree of instability, all of which serves to guide perioperative airway management.

Evaluation of a patient's respiratory function preoperatively is important, particularly in those cases of complex thoracic spine surgery where one-lung ventilation may be required. It is also important to remember that patients with mechanical instability may have been kept lying supine in bed preoperatively for spinal precautions. This may negatively affect the patient's respiratory function.[18] A chest x-ray, careful assessment of the patient's CT images of the thorax, and arterial blood gas are useful adjuncts to a full respiratory examination. Liaising with physiotherapists for assessment of the patient's cough, FEV1 (forced expiratory volume in the first second of expiration), and vital capacity can also be helpful. For scheduled, complex thoracic surgeries, formal pulmonary function tests may also be beneficial. It is worth undertaking these tests in the supine position, as this will give a more accurate reflection of the patient's respiratory physiology in the perioperative period.[18]

A full cardiovascular examination may be challenging in this patient cohort as many of these patients have reduced mobility, making it more difficult to evaluate exercise tolerance. Nonetheless, a full history should be sought, with particular attention to congestive cardiac failure and pulmonary hypertension, both of which have been shown to be associated with perioperative adverse events after spine surgery.[19] Useful investigations which may assist in a patient's cardiovascular evaluation include a 12-lead electrocardiogram (ECG) and echocardiography. Stress testing should be performed only if it is indicated in the absence of the proposed spine surgery. There is no current evidence that further diagnostic evaluation will improve surgical outcomes.

As mentioned above, patients presenting for STS may have symptoms of mechanical instability or neurologic compression; therefore assessment and recording of neurologic function preoperatively is essential to ensure accurate surveillance and diagnosis of new postoperative deficits should they occur.

As well as the system-specific investigations suggested above, patients should have a comprehensive set of blood tests undertaken prior to surgery. This should include a full blood count, urea and electrolytes, calcium, and a type and screen with cross match. A full blood count is particularly useful in patients on chemotherapy to assess for anemia, leukopenia, or thrombocytopenia. Serum calcium levels are important to consider, as these may be elevated in the setting of malignant disease. Cross matching of blood will depend on the extent of the surgery and the patient's individual risk of blood loss and coagulopathy; however, the risk of significant bleeding and need for transfusion in this patient population are significant.

Anesthetic Technique

Standard monitoring for general anesthesia (pulse oximetry, ECG, end expired carbon dioxide, blood pressure, and temperature) is used for spinal surgery patients. STS may result in significant blood loss with the need for rapid infusion of fluids. Two-wide bore IV cannulae should be placed and attached to fluid warming devices. Central venous access is placed if (a) the patient has difficult peripheral IV access, (b) if a need for vasoactive medications is anticipated, or (c) a volatile sparing anesthetic (total intravenous anaesthesia [TIVA]) technique is to be used intraoperatively. We also recommend the use of an invasive arterial pressure monitor, as this facilitates intraoperative blood sampling and rapid assessment of blood pressure, particularly in the setting of hemorrhage. Urinary catheterization and urine output monitoring would allow accurate assessment of fluid balance intraoperatively. For patients receiving a TIVA technique, processed electromyography (EMG) monitoring is recommended.[20]

Intraoperative spinal cord monitoring should be considered in any case where the spinal cord is at risk.[21] Multimodal intraoperative neuromonitoring (IONM), including motor evoked potential (MEP), somatosensory evoked potential (SSEP), and EMG, are often used to monitor spinal cord function during surgery on the cord or the vertebral column. While neurologic injury can cause changes in recorded potentials, other factors can interfere with their interpretation such as the use of inhalational anesthetics, hypothermia, hypoxia, hypotension, anemia, and preexisting neurologic lesions. Inhaled anesthetics, such as sevoflurane, isoflurane, and nitrous oxide, can suppress MEPs completely and diminish the amplitude and extend the latency of SSEPs. Neuromuscular blocking agents (NMBAs) also terminate MEPs and cannot be used when monitoring. Intravenous anesthetics, such as propofol, barbiturates, and opioids, have less of an effect on monitoring, though very deep anesthesia, with propofol, can have dose-dependent effects.[22] Therefore, a TIVA technique is used for patients in whom neuromonitoring is undertaken. Tongue and lip biting injuries are the most common reported complications during MEP monitoring (incidence 0.2%–0.63%).[23] Risk factors for tongue injury during MEP monitoring include C3–4 stimulation that directly activates the temporalis muscle and prone position, as it predisposes to tongue swelling.[23]

Airway Management

Airway management in these patients can prove challenging, particularly in those with cervical spine instability. A suggested airway management algorithm for these patients is shown in Fig. 20.1. Reinforced endotracheal tubes (ETT) are most commonly used in patients undergoing major spinal surgery. For most patients, a single-lumen ETT will be used; however, the lateral approach to the thoracic spine may require lung isolation with a double-lumen ETT. When a double-lumen ETT is used, it may be replaced by a single-lumen ETT if postoperative ventilation is required. Airway edema can be a significant problem on extubation. The incidence of airway compromise requiring reintubation after anterior cervical spine procedures has been reported as up to 1.9%.[24] Risk factors include multiple level surgery, blood loss of >300 mL, duration >5 h, combined anterior and posterior approach, and previous cervical surgery.[22] Hematoma formation or supraglottic edema as a result of venous and lymphatic obstruction may contribute to the development of airway compromise.[25] Symptoms include neck swelling, change in voice, agitation, and signs of respiratory distress that usually develop within 6–36 h postoperatively. Tracheal deviation may occur, and compression of the carotid sinus can cause bradycardia and hypotension. High-risk patients should be monitored in a critical care setting with consideration for a staged extubation using an airway exchange catheter.

Positioning

Patient position for spine surgery depends on the surgical approach and spinal level. Repositioning of the patient may be required during the procedure to facilitate multiple

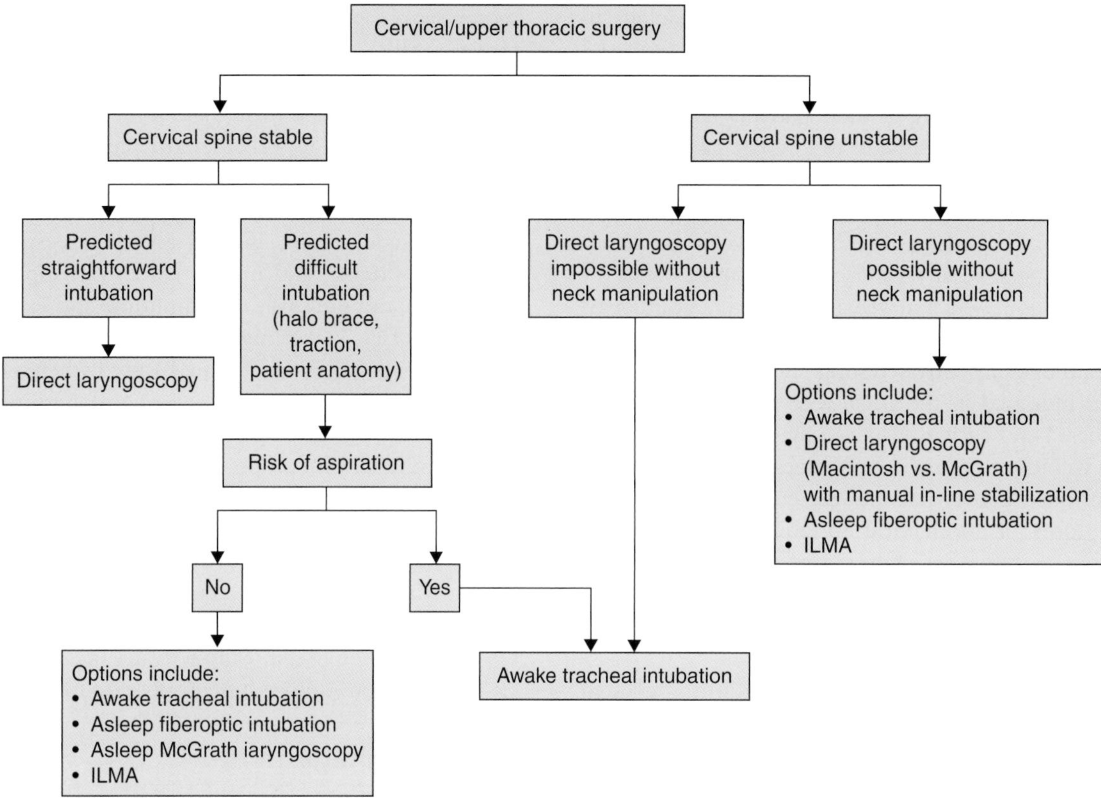

• **Fig. 20.1** Suggested airway management for cervical and upper thoracic spine surgery. *ILMA*, Intubating laryngeal mask airway.

surgical approaches. Appropriate positioning aims to avoid injury, as well as maintenance of low venous pressure at the surgical site.

Cervical spine surgery may involve anterior or posterior approaches. For surgeries involving an anterior approach, the head is placed supine on a padded headrest. For posterior approaches the Mayfield traction device with skull pins is regularly used. Rapid onset analgesia (such as remifentanil or fentanyl) may be required during insertion of pins. The ETT should be secured out of the way of the surgical field and eyes should be taped and padded.[22] Arms should be positioned at the sides ensuring that there are no pressure areas, particularly along the ulnar groove.

Thoracic spine surgery via an anterior approach requires a thoracotomy with the patient in the lateral position. One-lung ventilation may be necessary for surgical exposure. Thoracic spine surgery via the posterior approach is undertaken in the prone position. The head is secured on foam/gel bolsters or in the horseshoe headrest of the Mayfield apparatus. Depending on the level of surgery, arms should be tucked at the sides or in the "surrender position" with arm abduction at <90 degrees.

Lumbar spine surgery via the anterior approach requires a laparotomy, the patient lying supine, with head secured on a padded headrest. Lumbar spine surgery via the posterior approach is performed in the prone position. Positioning into the prone position (for all spine surgery) requires effective teamwork from the surgeons, anesthetists, and other theatre staff. If the head is to be secured in a foam headrest, it should be positioned while the patient is supine to ensure that there are no pressure areas, particularly around the orbital rims. Immediately after proning and also intraoperatively, the nose, mouth, and eyes should be frequently assessed to ensure that they are not compressed and the ETT inspected to ensure that it has not moved or kinked, especially during repositioning or when the neck is flexed. Once proned, it is essential to ensure that the patient's neck is held in a neutral position. The ability to ventilate, bilateral breath sounds, and blood pressure should be confirmed immediately. Arms should be tucked at the sides or in the "surrender position" with arm abduction <90 degrees. Hips and knees should be slightly flexed and supported on pillows or pads. Iliac crests, fibular heads, breasts, and genitalia should be padded to avoid compression. If a Foley catheter is in place, it should be free hanging to avoid traction on genitalia. The Jackson table, which rotates the patient from a supine to a prone position, may be used to help with positioning a prone patient.

Prone positioning is associated with many potential complications, including peripheral neuropathies, postoperative visual loss, direct pressure effects (producing compartment syndromes), cardiovascular instability and increased risk of bleeding, and practical challenges (such as ETT kinking or dislodgment) (Table 20.3).[26]

TABLE 20.3 Complications of Major Spine Surgery

	Nerve Injuries	Opthalmic Complications	Airway Complications	Cardiovascular Complications
Presentation	Ulnar nerve (most common) Brachial plexus Femoral nerve Peroneal nerve	Visual loss in prone position for spine surgery 1:30,000[23] Most common cause posterior ischemic optic neuropathy	Risk of ETT dislodgement or endobronchial intubation Airway and facial edema due to venous congestion	Hemodynamic instability Hypotension Hypertension (and risk of increased blood loss) Increased risk of lower limb thrombosis
Risk factors	Intraoperative: Hypotension Hypovolemia Hypothermia Arms in "surrender" position instead of tucked by side Patient factors Male sex Extremes of body habitus Hypertension Peripheral vascular disease Smokers	Male sex Obesity Use of the Wilson frame Prolonged surgery (>6 h) Greater blood loss Lower percentage of colloid in the non-blood fluid replacement	Prolonged surgery (>6 h) → airway edema Tight ETT tie →venous congestion → airway edema Head positioned below level of heart → venous congestion → airway edema	Preoperative hypovolemia Poorly controlled preop hypertension Change in propofol pharmacokinetics in prone position → increased CVS instability with TIVA (↓cardiac index of 25.9% during TIVA vs. 12.9% during inhalational anesthesia)
Management	Careful patient positioning Avoidance of intraoperative hypotension/ hypovolemia/ hypothermia SSEPs can be used to monitor for impending peripheral nerve injury	If using padding to protect eyes, ensure this does not exert any extra pressure onto the globe → central retinal artery occlusion Avoidance/ management of risk factors	Action plan for management of a dislodged ETT discussed during the theatre time out Corticosteroids may reduce airway edema Avoid/minimize head position below level of the heart	Methods to reduce Intra-abdominal pressure Table that allows for a free hanging abdomen Urinary catheterization Use of inhalational anesthesia over TIVA Regarding risk of lower limb thrombosis: SCDs TED stockings

CVS, Cardiovascular system; *ETT*, endotracheal tube; *SCD*, sudden cardiac death; *SSEP*, somatosensory evoked potentials; *TED*, thromboembolus deterrent; *TIVA*, total intravenous anesthesia.

Bleeding

Major spine surgery can result in significant blood loss. The extent of blood loss is dependent on many factors, including the vascularity of the tumors, age >50 years, obesity, prone position, and the performance of transpedicular osteotomy.[27] A meta-analysis found an average estimated blood loss of 2180 mL during STS.[28]

Methods to reduce intraoperative blood loss include meticulous surgical technique and careful positioning to avoid venous congestion at the surgical site. The use of antifibrinolytic agents such as tranexamic acid and epsilon-aminocaproic acid has been shown to decrease blood loss and intraoperative transfusion without an increase in morbidity or incidence of thromboembolic events.[29,30] Due to the vascularity of spinal metastases (particularly renal or thyroid cancers), preoperative tumor embolization can be beneficial in reducing perioperative blood loss.[31] Allogenic hemodilution may be useful in certain circumstances such as Jehovah's Witness patients who may consent to the technique if the blood is kept in a closed-circuit system. Induced hypotension is no longer recommended for patients having spine surgery due to the potential for end organ ischemia.[32]

Multiple factors guide the decision to transfuse, including patient comorbidities and the rate of blood loss. Studies of allogenic transfusion have shown an increased risk of postoperative infection and progression of tumor growth associated with blood transfusion, thought to be secondary to the associated immunosuppression.[33] We recommend that a restrictive transfusion strategy can be adopted for most hemodynamically stable patients considering transfusion at a hemoglobin level of 7–8 g/dL.

Other techniques to minimize blood transfusion include autologous predonation and cell salvage. Patients who undergo autologous predonation have a higher incidence of perioperative anemia and transfusion in spite of similar differences in blood loss. Autologous transfusions have also been implicated in transfusion-related immunomodulation and decreased disease-free survival.[34] There is interest in the use of cell salvage surgery in STS. There are theoretical risks that cell salvage may induce metastases; however, this is counterbalanced by the proven reduced risk of immunomodulation from allogenic transfusion. Based on this, many clinicians offer cell salvage with a leucodepletion filter for patients undergoing major cancer surgery. Most recent recommendations state that risks and benefits should be discussed with patients before surgery, and specific consent should be obtained.[35]

Postoperative Considerations

Complex spinal surgery involves extensive surgical wounds, and in patients who may have ongoing cancer pain, perioperative analgesia can be challenging. Patients may be on complex analgesic regimes, and these should be continued during the perioperative period. Opioids, often in the form of patient-controlled analgesia (PCA) or intravenous infusions, form the mainstay of treatment; however, using a multimodal approach may help to reduce total opioid consumption and lower the incidence of opioid side effects.

Administration of acetaminophen may be of benefit as part of a multimodal analgesic regime. A meta-analysis of randomized controlled trials found that acetaminophen used in addition to morphine after major surgery resulted in small, but statistically significant reductions in total morphine requirements postoperatively.[36] The perioperative administration of nonsteroidal antiinflammatory drugs (NSAIDs) has been shown to reduce postoperative opioid consumption and opioid side effects.[37] Concerns regarding the effect of NSAIDs on bone healing do not show a significant increase in nonunion.[38] We advise that NSAIDs use should be considered in consultation with surgeons, and on a patient-specific basis taking into account predicted blood loss.

The use of ketamine used in subanesthetic doses has been proven to reduce postoperative opioid requirements and to significantly reduce pain in opioid-tolerant patients undergoing STS. Ketamine can be administered as a bolus intraoperatively or as an IV infusion intraoperatively or postoperatively; it is particularly useful for opioid-tolerant patients undergoing spine surgery.[39]

Gabapentinoids reduce postoperative pain and opioid consumption when used as a preoperative adjunctive analgesic. However, they are associated with increased risks of sedation, respiratory depression, and potentiation of the respiratory depressive effects of opioids. In general, we do not routinely administer gabapentinoids as part of our standard analgesic regimen for major spine surgery patients; however, for patients chronically taking gabapentinoids, we continue to administer their regular medications.[40]

In STS, the use of neuraxial anesthesia for intraoperative and postoperative analgesia may be considered. Intraoperative instillation of intrathecal morphine has been proven to provide improved visual analogue pain scores (VAS) and opioid-sparing properties after spine surgery. It has been shown to provide improved analgesia with no respiratory depressive effects at doses up to 0.4 mg bolus. Epidural analgesia has been shown to reduce opioid requirements after major spine surgery. However, epidural administration of local anesthetic can cause motor block, which can complicate postoperative neurologic assessment resulting in reduced infusion rates or discontinuation of the infusion.[41] Erector spinae plane (ESP) block serves to anesthetize the dorsal rami of spinal nerves that innervate the paraspinal muscles and bony vertebrae. The use of bilateral ESP blocks and ESP catheters has shown benefit in reducing pain scores in patients undergoing thoracic and lumbar spine surgery, and reports of opioid-free postoperative analgesic regimes have been described in patients who received ESP blocks.[42,43]

Venous Thromboembolism

Twenty percent of all newly diagnosed venous thromboembolisms (VTEs) are in patients with malignancy and carry a significant associated mortality. A case series of more than 230 patients undergoing surgery for spinal metastases identified deep venous thrombosis (DVT) in 10% of all patients, and in 24% of nonambulatory patients.[44] Measures to decrease the risk of VTE include antiembolism stockings, intermittent pneumatic calf compression devices, and pharmacologic treatment such as low-molecular-weight heparin (LMWH). The use of specific VTE prophylaxis measures and the timing of their introduction will differ depending on the risk profile created by patient and surgical factors, balancing the individualized risk of VTE with the potentially catastrophic complications of bleeding around the operative site. Prophylactic LMWH must not be given in the 12 h preceding surgery and should be withheld until at least 48 h following surgery when the risk of VTE versus postoperative bleeding must be considered.[45] Multidisciplinary input into the timing of LMWH is important.

Conclusion

There is no proven curative treatment for metastatic spinal disease, and therefore the goals are pain control and functional preservation.[15] Consequently, the clinician should be mindful to tailor management using a patient-specific, risk-benefit analysis. Oncologic spine surgeries vary in length and complexity, and the potential for massive blood loss and hemodynamic instability must be considered. Pain control in the postoperative setting can be challenging and usually requires a multimodal approach. Advances in regional techniques show promise in reducing reliance on opioids and in reducing opioid-related side effects. Laboratory and retrospective clinical research have suggested that certain anesthetic techniques may minimize metastatic spread in the perioperative period. These include the use of TIVA and regional anesthesia techniques (and avoidance of opioids), use of IV lidocaine, and the avoidance of blood transfusion. However, robust prospective clinical data are lacking, and currently there are no trials evaluating the association between anesthetic technique and metastasis after spinal cancer surgery. These principles have been discussed more generally elsewhere in this book. In the management of these complex patients, a well-formulated perioperative plan and effective communication between the multidisciplinary team are essential to ensure optimal patient outcomes.

References

1. Ziu E, Mesfin FB. *Cancer, Metastasis, Spinal*: StatPearls Publishing; 2017.
2. Ciftdemir M, Kaya M, Selcuk E, Yalniz E. Tumors of the spine. *World J Orthop*. 2016;7(2):109.
3. Choi D, Crockard A, Bunger C, et al. Review of metastatic spine tumour classification and indications for surgery: the consensus statement of the Global Spine Tumour Study Group. *Eur Spine J*. 2010;19(2):215–222.
4. Laufer I, Rubin DG, Lis E, et al. The NOMS framework: approach to the treatment of spinal metastatic tumors. *Oncologist*. 2013;18(6):744–751.
5. NICE. Overview. Myeloma: diagnosis and management. 2019. Available at NICE.org.uk.
6. Malhotra K, Lui DF, Butler JS, Selvadurai S, Molloy S. Successful nonsurgical treatment for highly unstable fracture subluxation of the spine secondary to myeloma. *Spine J*. 2016;16(8):e547–e551.
7. Hughes M, Soutar R, Lucraft H, Owen R, Bird J. *Guidelines on the diagnosis and management of solitary plasmacytoma of bone, extramedullary plasmacytoma and multiple solitary plasmacytomas: 2009 update*. London, UK: British Committee for Standards in Haematology; 2009:14.
8. NICE. Non-Hodgkin's lymphoma: diagnosis and management. 2019. Available at NICE.org.uk.
9. Ontario HQ. Vertebral augmentation involving vertebroplasty or kyphoplasty for cancer-related vertebral compression fractures: a systematic review. *Ont Health Technol Assess Ser*. 2016;16(11):1.
10. Galgano M, Fridley J, Oyelese A, et al. Surgical management of spinal metastases. *Expert Rev Anticancer Ther*. 2018;18(5):463–472.
11. Harel R, Pfeffer R, Levin D, et al. Spine radiosurgery: lessons learned from the first 100 treatment sessions. *Neurosurg Focus*. 2017;42(1):E3.
12. Robin AM, Yamada Y, McLaughlin LA, et al. Stereotactic radiosurgery: the revolutionary advance in the treatment of spine metastases. *Neurosurgery*. 2017;64(CN suppl 1):59–65.
13. Barzilai O, Laufer I, Robin A, Xu R, Yamada Y, Bilsky MH. Hybrid therapy for metastatic epidural spinal cord compression: technique for separation surgery and spine radiosurgery. *Oper Neurosurg*. 2018;16(3):310–318.
14. Horn SR, Dhillon ES, Poorman GW. Epidemiology and national trends in prevalence and surgical management of metastatic spinal disease. *J Clin Neurosci*. 2018;53:183–187.
15. Dunning EC, Butler JS, Morris S. Complications in the management of metastatic spinal disease. *World J Orthop*. 2012;3(8):114.
16. Yao A, Sarkiss CA, Ladner TR, Jenkins AL 3rd. Contemporary spinal oncology treatment paradigms and outcomes for metastatic tumors to the spine: a systematic review of breast, prostate, renal, and lung metastases. *J Clin Neurosci*. 2017;41:11–23.
17. Law J, Broemling N, Cooper R, et al. The difficult airway with recommendations for management—Part 2—The anticipated difficult airway. *Can J Anesth*. 2013;60(11):1119–1138.
18. Shikma K, Nissim A, Ariel R, Yacov Z, Esther-Lee M. The effect of body position on pulmonary function: a systematic review. *BMC Pulm Med*. 2018;18(1):1–16.
19. Memtsoudis GS, Vougioukas IV, Ma KY, Gaber-Baylis PL, Girardi PF. Perioperative morbidity and mortality after anterior, posterior, and anterior/posterior spine fusion surgery. *Spine*. 2011;36(22):1867–1877.
20. Nimmo S, Payne S, Shreeve K, Smith J, Torella F. Association of Anaesthetists guidelines: cell salvage for peri-operative blood conservation 2018. *Anaesthesia*. 2018;73(9):1141–1150.
21. Fehlings MG, Brodke DS, Norvell DC, Dettori JR. The evidence for intraoperative neurophysiological monitoring in spine surgery: does it make a difference? *Spine*. 2010;35(9S suppl):S37–S46.
22. Nowicki RW. Anaesthesia for major spinal surgery. *Anaesth Crit Care Pain Med*. 2014;14(4):147–152.
23. Tamkus A, Rice K. The incidence of bite injuries associated with transcranial motor-evoked potential monitoring. *Anesth Analg*. 2012;115(3):663–667.
24. Sagi HC, Beutler W, Carroll E, Connolly PJ. Airway complications associated with surgery on the anterior cervical spine. *Spine*. 2002;27(9):949–953.
25. Carr E, Benjamin E. In vitro study investigating post neck surgery haematoma airway obstruction. *J Laryngol Otol*. 2009;123(6):662–665.
26. Kamel I, Barnette R. Positioning patients for spine surgery: avoiding uncommon position-related complications. *World J Orthop*. 2014;5(4):425.
27. Lee TC, Yang LC, Chen HJ. Effect of patient position and hypotensive anesthesia on inferior vena caval pressure. *Spine (Phila Pa 1976)*. 1998;23:941.
28. Chen Y, Tai BC, Nayak D, et al. Blood loss in spinal tumour surgery and surgery for metastatic spinal disease: a meta-analysis. *Bone Jt J*. 2013;95(5):683–688.
29. Soroceanu HA, Oren SJ, Smith IJ, et al. Effect of antifibrinolytic therapy on complications, thromboembolic events, blood product utilization, and fusion in adult spinal deformity surgery. *Spine*. 2016;41(14):E879–E886.
30. Feng DJ, Gill JB, Chin Y, Levin A. The use of antifibrinolytic agents in spine surgery. a meta-analysis. *J Bone Joint Surg*. 2008;90(11):2399.
31. Prince EA, Ahn SH. *Interventional Management of Vertebral Body Metastases. Seminars in Interventional Radiology*: Thieme Medical Publishers; 2013.
32. Walsh JM, Devereaux XP, Garg NA, et al. Relationship between intraoperative mean arterial pressure and clinical outcomes after noncardiac surgery: toward an empirical definition of hypotension. *Anesthesiology*. 2013;119(3):507–515.
33. Kumar N, Chen Y, Zaw AS, et al. Use of intraoperative cell-salvage for autologous blood transfusions in metastatic spine tumour surgery: a systematic review. *Lancet Oncol*. 2014;15(1):e33–e41.
34. Weber RS, Jabbour N, Martin II RCG. Anemia and transfusions in patients undergoing surgery for cancer. *Ann Surg Oncol*. 2008;15(1):34–45.
35. Klein AA, Bailey CR, Charlton AJ, et al. Association of Anaesthetists guidelines: cell salvage for peri-operative blood conservation 2018. *Anaesthesia*. 2018;73(9):1141–1150.

36. Remy C, Marret E, Bonnet F. Effects of acetaminophen on morphine side-effects and consumption after major surgery: meta-analysis of randomized controlled trials. *Br J Anaesth*. 2005;94(4):505–513.
37. De Oliveira GS, Agarwal D, Benzon HT. Perioperative single dose ketorolac to prevent postoperative pain: a meta-analysis of randomized trials. *Anesth Analg*. 2012;114(2):424–433.
38. Clarke S, Lecky F. Do non-steroidal anti-inflammatory drugs cause a delay in fracture healing? *J Emerg Med*. 2005;22(9):652–653.
39. Pendi A, Field R, Farhan S-D, Eichler M, Bederman SS. Perioperative ketamine for analgesia in spine surgery: a meta-analysis of randomized controlled trials. *Spine*. 2018;43(5):E299–E307.
40. Ho K-Y, Gan TJ, Habib AS. Gabapentin and postoperative pain–a systematic review of randomized controlled trials. *Pain*. 2006;126(1–3):91–101.
41. Brown M. Anaesthesia for elective spine surgery in adults. M. Jeffrey J Pasternak. UpToDate. 2019. Available at https://www.uptodate.com/contents/anesthesia-for-elective-spine-surgery-in-adults.
42. Chin KJ, Lewis S. Opioid-free analgesia for posterior spinal fusion surgery using erector spinae plane (ESP) blocks in a multimodal anesthetic regimen. *Spine*. 2019;44(6):E37 9–E383.
43. Finnerty D, Ní Eochagáin A, Ahmed M, Poynton A, Butler JS, Buggy DJ. A randomised trial of bilateral erector spinae plane block vs. no block for thoracolumbar decompressive spinal surgery. *Anaesthesia*. 2021;76:1499–1503. doi:10.1111/anae.15488.
44. Zacharia BE, Kahn S, Bander ED, et al. Incidence and risk factors for preoperative deep venous thrombosis in 314 consecutive patients undergoing surgery for spinal metastasis. *J Neurosurg Spine*. 2017;27(2):189–197.
45. National Institute for Health and Care Excellence. Venous thromboembolism in over 16s: reducing the risk of hospital-acquired deep vein thrombosis or pulmonary embolism. 2018.

21

Anesthesia for Head and Neck Cancer Surgeries

SHEILA NAINAN MYATRA AND SUSHAN GUPTA

Introduction

Head and neck malignancies are a heterogeneous group of malignancies extending from the upper aerodigestive tract up to the larynx, including the thyroid gland, salivary glands, and paranasal sinuses. They account for more than 650,000 cases worldwide. Considering the current burden of head and neck malignancies and increasing survival, most anesthesiologists would be faced with providing anesthesia to these patients for both oncologic and nononcologic procedures. Difficult airway management, intraoperatively shared airway, prolonged duration of the surgery, and postoperative airway management are the main concerns for the anesthesiologist. The management of head and neck cancer patients is constantly evolving with respect to the type of surgery, reconstruction, and newer adjuvant therapies. Hence, it is imperative that we understand the anatomic and physiologic changes related to the head and neck cancer itself and its associated therapies. In this chapter, we will discuss the various anesthetic and other considerations during head and neck cancer surgery. These recommendations should supplement the routine evaluation and management of a patient undergoing major surgeries.

Cancer Surgery

Surgery remains the mainstay of treatment in head and neck cancer surgeries. Depending on the extent of surgeries and the stage of tumor, radiation or cisplatin/cetuximab-based chemotherapy may also be administered.[1] Debulking surgery may be performed for palliation of symptoms and airway patency.[2] The main goal of cancer surgery is to obtain disease-free margins. Hence unlike nononcologic procedures, surgical excision may often be extensive and accompanied by lymph node dissection, and often require reconstructive procedures.

Neck Dissection

The most common site of cancer spread is the cervical group of lymph nodes, which are commonly excised during head and neck cancer surgery. The patient may undergo a partial/selective, modified, or radical neck dissection along with the removal of the surrounding muscles, nerves, and veins.

Reconstructive Procedures

Plastic flap reconstructions are often required for cosmetic purposes and to help with chewing and swallowing. These may be pedicle flaps where the original blood supply of the structure is retained or they may be free flaps, which require microvascular anastomosis.

Applied Anatomy

One of the main concerns for the anesthesiologist following head and neck cancer surgery is the maintenance of a patent airway after surgical resection. Thus it is important to have an understanding of the role of various structures in maintaining a viable and patent airway. The mandible, maxilla, and the tongue form the external boundary of the airway. The genial tubercle over the mandible provides attachment to genioglossus and geniohyoid muscles, which maintain airway patency. Any loss of these structures may lead to the collapse of the airway, similar to that seen during rapid eye movement sleep.[3,4]

The pharyngeal muscles are crucial in ensuring that the food bolus enters safely into the esophagus. This is accompanied by the simultaneous anterior movement of the epiglottis to close the laryngeal inlet. Superior constrictors close the soft palate and the middle and inferior constrictors contract to push food into the esophagus. In addition, pharyngeal muscles also act as sphincters preventing regurgitation of food from the esophagus.[5]

Preoperative Assessment and Optimization

Other than the routine assessment and optimization prior to major surgery, there are some special considerations in head and neck cancer patients.

Airway Assessment

A careful history of the signs and symptoms related to the airway is vital. The presence of progressive dysphagia, hoarseness of voice, or breathlessness/discomfort on lying supine may be a sign of a compromised airway. Laryngeal cancers may present with stridor and difficulty in breathing. These may present as emergencies and may sometimes require an immediate tracheostomy.

Apart from routine airway examination such as Malampatti grading, thyromental distance, and so on, there are special considerations during airway assessment in head and neck cancer patients that need to be evaluated carefully.

Primary Tumor

Proliferative intraoral lesions along the airway may add to difficulty at both bag-mask ventilation and laryngoscopy. These tumors can also bleed during laryngoscopic manipulation, especially tumors involving the base of the tongue and the vallecula. A thorough examination of the oral cavity should be performed to examine the size, location, and extent of oral tumor. In addition to looking at dentition, check for the presence of fibrous bands and any other conditions in the oral cavity. Lesions lower down in the airway can be assessed by viewing the imaging.

Facial Defects

Previous surgeries, the external proliferation of tumors, radiation, and so on, may lead to improper fit/seal of a face mask, making mask ventilation difficult, and sometimes even lead to bleeding due to manipulation.

Trismus

Fibrosis along the temporomandibular joint, due to radiation therapy of the primary tumor itself, submucous fibrosis due to tobacco chewing, and so on, may hinder mouth opening (Fig. 21.1) Unlike trismus secondary to inflammation, this may not be relieved after induction of general anesthesia, thus making orotracheal intubation and supraglottic airway insertion often impossible. Trismus may be graded as follows: interincisal mouth opening up to or greater than 35 mm (M1), between 25 and 35 mm (M2), between 15 and 25 mm (M3), and opening less than 15 mm (M4).[6]

Ankyloglossia

As the tumor infiltrates the root of the tongue, it hinders the protrusion of the tongue. Due to the restricted tongue movement, lateral displacement of the tongue may not be possible during direct laryngoscopy (DL), which may lead to poor glottis view and failed intubation.[7]

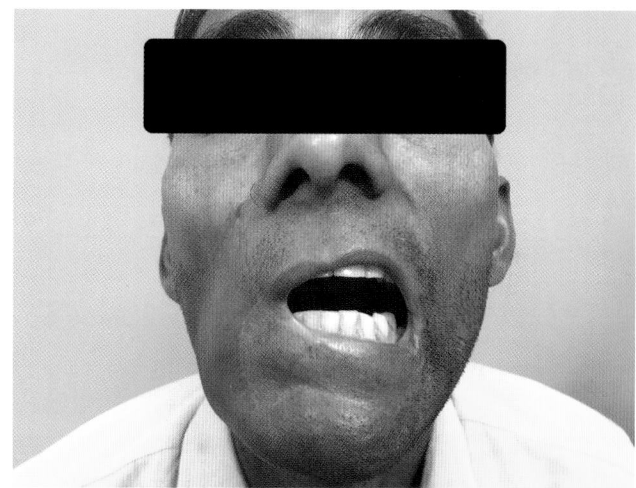

• **Fig. 21.1** A patient with trismus.

Dentition

The tumor, radiation, tobacco chewing, and so on, may lead to loosening, weakening, and destruction of the teeth. Both mask ventilation and laryngoscopy may be difficult in edentulous patients.[7]

Selection of the Nostril for Tracheal Intubation

The presence of intranasal anomalies such as spurs, septal deviation, nasal polyps, concha bullosa, and increased size of the turbinates should be ruled out both clinically and using imaging (computed tomography [CT] scan or anterior/posterior rhinoscopy) to select the more suitable nare for smooth passage of the tracheal tube nasally.[8] Patient history and clinical examination should be performed to assess comfort while breathing and the blast of air on the back of the hand while alternately occluding the nare should be felt after administration of a nasal vasoconstrictor. This may also help in preventing trauma during nasal intubation. In case of equal patency, the nostrils opposite to the side of surgery should be selected especially for maxillectomies where the hard palate will be excised. Moreover, if there is no surgical preference, the right nostril should be preferred over the left, as in the case of the right nostril the bevel faces the nasal septum. This reduces the risk of damage to the nasal turbinates.[8–10]

Tracheomalacia

A long-standing large thyroid mass may weaken the tracheal cartilage and longitudinal elastic fibers. The trachea becomes soft and susceptible to collapse in such cases. A narrowing of >50% along the posterior wall is significant and such patients may have a complete collapse of the airway under anesthesia, and may require tracheostomy or intraoperative aortopexy/bronchopexy to maintain a patent airway postoperatively.[11] Patients commonly present with asthma-like symptoms which may be continuous or intermittent. Symptoms include prolonged and labored breathing, wheezing, or coughing. A thorough clinical examination and pulmonary function test should be performed to rule out respiratory conditions. Bronchoscopy, fluoroscopy, multislice helical CT imaging, or magnetic resonance imaging can be used to confirm the diagnosis preoperatively.

Airway Imaging

History and clinical examination should be complemented with reviewing the airway imaging. Most patients with head and neck cancer have had some prior airway imaging performed for disease evaluation.

X-ray helps determine the site and size of the mass and presence of compression or deviation of the airway, especially when anterior-posterior and lateral views are compared. Further investigations may be required to confirm the findings.

CT scan findings help assess the extent of disease and airway compromise. The CT scan can also be used to assess the patency of either nostril and the presence of aberrant spurs, which could cause tracheal cuff damage during a nasotracheal intubation.

An ultrasound of the neck performed preoperatively, especially in patients with difficult airways, helps identify the cricothyroid membrane, its anatomy, and any associated aberrant vessels. This might be extremely helpful if the need for emergency cricothyroidotomy arises.

Virtual endoscopy is a radiologic simulation of the anatomy of the airway extending from the oropharynx up to the carina. Previous CT scan images are reconstructed to create a video (3D "fly-through") of the airway anatomy. This further improves our interpretation of the 2D CT scan images and helps better identify a difficult airway to make an appropriate airway management plan.[12]

Diagnostic Airway Procedures

Patients may often be subjected to diagnostic procedures prior to major surgeries such as an indirect laryngoscopy (IDL) or awake fiberoptic laryngoscopy (FOL) in the outpatient department, or short diagnostic procedures such as direct- or microlaryngoscopy usually under general anesthesia, to assess the extent of the disease and obtain a diagnosis. These are extremely vital procedures that help to delineate the disease and decide on the further course of management. Findings from these procedures will help the anesthesiologist to plan for airway management.

Anemia

Malnutrition, dysphagia, chronic inflammation, and chemotherapy may cause anemia in these patients. Anemia has been associated with poor postoperative outcomes, in particular delayed recovery, intensive care unit (ICU) admission, hospital readmission, and postoperative complications, especially surgical site infection and flap failures (associated with hemoglobin <10 gm% or hematocrit <30%).[13,14] Depending on the available time prior to the surgery, anemia should be corrected prior to surgery.

Nutrition

Tumors along the aerodigestive tract, dysphagia, radiation-induced mucositis, ulcers, chemotherapy, and cancer cachexia add to the poor nutritional status of patients with head and neck cancer. Improving the nutrition preoperatively is associated with better postoperative outcomes in terms of wound healing, rate of infection, and postoperative complications. Malnutrition can be defined by a BMI of less than 18.5 and/or weight loss greater than 5%–10% of body weight.[15] Nutritional assessment should be performed for all patients prior to surgery and high-risk patients should be referred to a dietician for early intervention. Patients with severe nutritional risk should receive nutritional support for 10–14 days prior to major surgery. All patients should consume a nutritionally balanced diet for at least 5 days prior to surgery.[16]

Previous Cancer Therapies

Previous Surgery

The airway should be carefully evaluated in patients who have undergone previous surgery. The presence of flaps, mandibulectomy, previous tracheostomy, airway defects, and so on, may make both mask ventilation and tracheal intubation challenging. Awake tracheal intubation (ATI) may often be required in these cases.

Radiation

Radiation can significantly alter the airway making airway management difficult. Radiation can lead to fibrosis of the temporomandibular joint leading to trismus. It also affects dentition leading to loss of teeth. Edema secondary to radiation affects the tongue (glossomegaly, glossitis), glottis, and epiglottis. Kheterpal et al. found radiation to the neck an independent risk factor in patients with difficult bag-mask ventilation.[17] Radiation-induced fibrosis in the oropharyngeal region makes the tissue extremely rigid and noncompliant, which presents as poor submental compliance (Fig. 21.2). Obtaining a satisfactory glottic view might be difficult in such patients. Patients receiving head and neck radiation may also have limited neck movement. In addition, considering the possible laryngeal edema and increased risk of bleeding, the anesthesiologist should prefer to use smaller-sized endotracheal tubes (ETTs) in such patients.[17,18]

Radiation to the neck may lead to atherosclerosis and the risk of carotid artery stenosis, which increases the risk of stroke in these patients. In addition, radiation to the neck region may affect the thyroid follicles leading to hypothyroidism. It may also lead to damage of the baroreceptors, which may lead to extreme hemodynamic instability during the procedure.[19] These effects of radiation may not always be

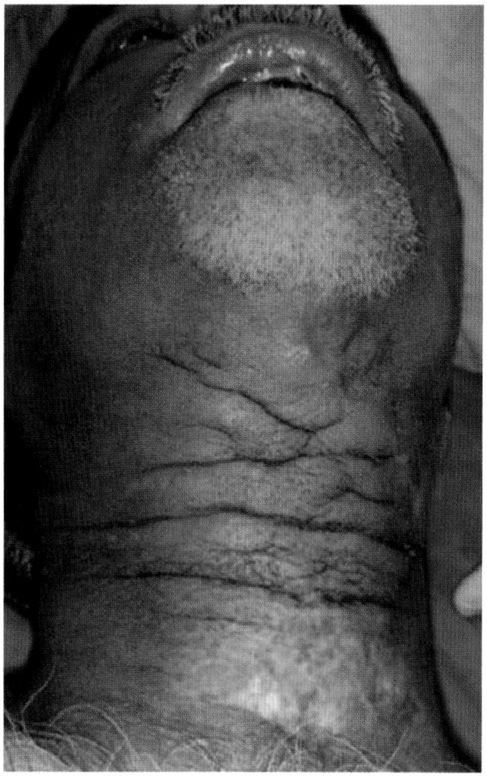

• **Fig. 21.2** A patient following neck radiation therapy.

visible, hence anesthesiologists should keep these changes in mind while managing such patients.

Chemotherapy

The two most common chemotherapeutic agents used in head and neck cancer are cisplatin and cetuximab.[20] Other agents include the taxane group (paclitaxel, docetaxel), fluorouracil, and methotrexate. While platinum-based chemotherapy agents, in particular cisplatin, can adversely affect renal functions, the risk with newer agents such as oxaliplatin is lower. After platinum-based chemotherapy, patients should be assessed for renal and electrolyte imbalance, and in cases of significant impairment a nephrologist's opinion should be sought. A complete blood count should be performed for all head and neck cancer patients to check for anemia and myelosuppression. Neutropenia (counts $<1500/mm^3$) increases the risk of postoperative infection and thrombocytopenia adds to the risk of intraoperative bleeding and should be corrected prior to surgery.

Geriatric Issues

The average age of head and neck cancer patients at presentation is 50–70 years. Hence geriatric considerations during assessment for surgery are essential in these patients. In addition to cardiac and other organ-related dysfunction specific to age, cancer-associated and chemotherapy-related cognitive dysfunction should also be assessed in the geriatric age group.

Effect of Tobacco and Smoking

Respiratory. Chronic obstructive pulmonary disease (COPD) is common in these patients secondary to chronic smoking. The reversible component of the disease should be optimized prior to surgery to reduce the risk of postoperative pulmonary complications. Any superimposed lung infection should also be treated. While it is desirable to stop smoking 8 weeks prior to surgery, it may not always be possible, and hence a minimum of a 12-h cessation is sufficient to reduce carboxyhemoglobin levels. Further cessation will improve mucociliary clearance and reduce airway reactivity.[21]

Cardiovascular. Smoking is strongly associated with a higher risk of ischemic heart disease, hypertension, and atherosclerosis. It also increases the blood viscosity secondary to hypoxia-induced polycythemia in addition to increasing the number of white blood cells and platelets and fibrinogen levels in the blood.[21] A cardiac assessment in these patients is essential.

Preoperative Pain Assessment and Management

Patients with head and neck cancer may present with preoperative pain secondary to cancer itself or due to therapy. The pain is higher as the cancer grows within the confines of a small space and due to the rich innervation of the region. In fact, 25%–60% of patients with head and neck cancer also suffer from neuropathic pain.[22] Compression of the glossopharyngeal and vagal nerve leads to referred pain in the form of otalgia, tinnitus, and dental pain. The neuropathic component can be addressed using antiepileptics such as gabapentin and pregabalin and antidepressants such as amitriptyline and nortriptyline. Systemic analgesics such as opioids can reduce the severity of pain; however, consideration should be given to minimizing dosing to reduce the risk of side effects. Oral mucositis secondary to chemotherapy/radiation therapy also adds to the acute pain. Associated musculoskeletal pain responds well to nonsteroidal antiinflammatory agents (both systemic and topical) and antispasmodics.[23] In addition, almost 30% of head and neck cancer patients suffer from chronic pain, which is associated with the advanced nature of the disease and associated therapies. Patients may even experience long-term musculoskeletal pain due to fibrosis involving the jaw.[23,24]

Anesthetic and analgesic requirements are much higher in these patients. Preoperative pain and the use of opioids are risk factors for the misuse of opioids in the postoperative period. Signs of opioid addiction should be identified. These patients should be flagged and monitored closely in the perioperative period. In addition, appropriate investigations should also be ordered to rule out complications secondary to long-term use of medications such as renal function test with the use of nonsteroidal antiinflammatory drugs (NSAIDs). Education regarding the possible ways to identify, prevent, and treat opioid misuse and overdose, starting in the preanesthesia room itself, should be imparted to clinicians.

Patient Education and Counseling

Patient education and counseling should encompass the perioperative period. This includes counseling regarding the surgery, anesthesia, and the recovery process. This improves patient satisfaction and compliance with recuperation. In addition, efforts to educate patients regarding opioid use in the postoperative period and after discharge, methods of safe disposal, and drug-return policies should be undertaken.

Intraoperative Management

Monitoring

The American Society of Anesthesiologists' (ASA) recommendations for monitoring should be instituted for all patients prior to the induction of anesthesia. This includes continuous electrocardiogram (ECG) monitoring, pulse oximeter monitoring, and noninvasive blood pressure monitoring. BIS monitoring is recommended especially if total intravenous anesthesia (TIVA) is being planned to titrate anesthetic doses. Peripheral nerve stimulation (PNS) is also recommended to titrate muscle relaxant dosing and reversal. More invasive monitoring such as arterial cannulation and central venous cannulation should be reserved for patients with cardiac conditions or when extensive blood loss is anticipated.

Cardiac Output Monitoring

While cardiac output monitoring has shown benefit in other cancer surgeries, the data are comparatively scarce in head and neck cancer patients. Studies have shown the benefit of goal-directed fluid therapy (GDFT) in microvascular free flap surgeries for head and neck cancer patients. While the use of the transesophageal Doppler may be difficult due to proximity with the operating area, pulse contour analysis devices such as LiDCO or FloTrac may be used for dynamic cardiac output monitoring and assessing fluid responsiveness.[25,26]

Temperature Monitoring

Head and neck cancer surgeries, especially with free flap reconstruction, are long duration surgeries, which may involve significant blood loss, and temperature fluctuations may be expected. In addition, since only the head area of the body is exposed during the surgery, there exists a risk of hyperthermia. Nasopharyngeal or esophageal monitoring might be difficult with the risk of displacement of the monitoring device during surgery.

Periintubation Oxygenation

Preoxygenation

Patients with head and neck cancer are anticipated difficult airways and hence preoxygenation is vital. One could use a face mask, or in some cases where the adequate fitting of a face mask is not possible due to facial defects, alternate methods of preoxygenation like high-flow nasal cannula oxygen (HFNCO) may be used.

Apneic Oxygenation

Apneic oxygenation is a technique to constantly replete oxygen stores during the period of apnea. This helps prolong the safe apnea time during which the airway can be secured. Apneic oxygenation can be delivered using a high-flow nasal oxygenation technique called Transnasal Humidified Rapid-Insufflation Ventilatory Exchange (THRIVE)[27] or alternately by supraglottic jet oxygenation and ventilation (SJOV).[28]

Commonly Used Tracheal Tubes

RAE Tubes

The North Pole endotracheal tube made of ivory, which curves away from the surgical site, is the most commonly used ETT for nasal intubation in head and neck cancer surgeries.[29] These tubes are much softer than the routine polyvinyl chloride (PVC) tubes and cause less trauma during insertion. However, they are opaque and obscure any tube blockade and due to the preformed curve, suctioning is not easily performed through the ETT. Moreover, the length, narrower lumen, and preformed curve add to the resistance during spontaneous breathing. Hence it is recommended to cut these tubes along the prelabeled black mark to reduce airway resistance and facilitate suctioning in the postoperative period.[30] The insertion of North Pole ETT over the fiberoptic bronchoscope is also difficult due to the curvature. The North Pole tube needs to be straightened manually to be loaded over the bronchoscope. Due to some of the limitations mentioned above, some prefer to use PVC tubes for tracheal intubation, though they are stiffer.

Flexometallic Tubes

The advantage of flexometallic ETTs is that they are nonkinkable and less traumatic. However, these tubes are floppy making them difficult to insert. These tubes are particularly useful during laryngectomy surgery when the end stoma is being fashioned, to keep away from the field of surgery.

Electromyographic Tube

Intraoperative nerve monitoring (IONM) is being increasingly used to help identify nerves. The common indication includes thyroid surgery, partial laryngectomy, neck dissection, carotid endarterectomy, and so on. These are standard PVC tubes with conductive silver ink electrodes. There is a dark black crossband that guides in electromyographic (EMG) tube placement. These tubes have a minimum outer diameter of 8.8 mm and hence are preferentially used for oral intubation.[31]

Plan for Airway Management—Awake Versus Asleep

It is essential to make a plan for airway management prior to the induction of anesthesia. The decision of whether to secure the airway awake or asleep is crucial. This planning should include careful history taking, assessment of the airway with a review of airway imaging, and a discussion with the surgeon. If the airway management is planned under general anesthesia, a backup plan for rescue ventilation in case of inability to perform tracheal intubation, including equipment and preparedness for performing an emergency cricothyroidotomy, in case of complete ventilation failure should be made. Patients with intraoral surgery usually require a nasal ETT. Skull base fractures and bleeding disorders (risk of epistaxis) are relative contraindications.

Tracheostomy Under Local Anesthesia

In patients in whom there is a prior plan for tracheotomy, for example, a laryngectomy where the glottic opening is severely reduced or a plan for extensive resection where the airway patency is likely to be compromised postoperatively, the patient may undergo tracheostomy under local anesthesia prior to administration of general anesthesia.

Awake Tracheal Intubation

ATI is considered the gold standard in patients with an anticipated difficult airway. It is prudent to familiarize oneself with various available techniques. The recent guidelines for ATI in adults help practitioners to better plan, perform, and address complications related to the procedure. A combination of sedation, topicalization, oxygenation throughout the procedure, and proper performance of the procedure is key to success.[32]

Premedication

To reduce the risk of bleeding in case of nasal intubation, topical vasoconstrictor agents such as pure alpha-agonist agents (oxymetazoline, xylometazoline) can be used. Antisialagogue agents such as glycopyrrolate given intravenously reduce the amount of secretions and ensure a dry field for better visibility during the procedure. In addition, it prevents the local anesthetic from getting diluted with secretions and aids better absorption. These agents should be administered at least 15 min prior to the procedure giving enough time for its action.[33]

Sedation

Patients with head and neck malignancies might have a compromised airway, and hence anesthesiologists should be judicious with the use of sedation. However, mild sedation helps in tolerating awake intubation and increases the success of the procedure. The preferred sedatives for awake intubation include intravenous infusion of dexmedetomidine or remifentanil, mainly due to shorter duration of action, easy titrability, and an increased safety margin. Proper patient counseling prior to the procedure is paramount and increases patient tolerability, often with no requirement for sedation.

Anesthetizing the Airway

Intranasal 2% lignocaine jelly, viscous lignocaine gargle (concentration, 2%), pressurized bottles using 10% lignocaine, and atomizers can be used to anesthetize parts of the airway for awake intubation. The airway can further be anesthetized using the "SprAY as you GO (SAYGO)" technique. This is, however, performed while performing fiberoptic bronchoscopy. The local anesthetic is injected through the suction port of the scope using a syringe or via an epidural catheter passed through the suction port with the tip distal to the tip of the bronchoscope. It anesthetizes the part of the airway distal to scope. More invasive techniques include translaryngeal injection of lidocaine and regional nerve blocks such as glossopharyngeal nerve block, and superior laryngeal nerve block can also be used to anesthetize the airway prior to performing awake intubation. However, these invasive techniques are not routinely recommended or required when good topical anesthesia is used.

Oxygenation

During ATI, nasal oxygen should be continued throughout the procedure. The use of HFNCO especially when sedation is administered can increase the margin of safety.

Types of Awake Tracheal Intubation

i. Intubation With the Flexible Bronchoscope. Most patients, especially with oral pathologies, require a nasal ETT. The flexible bronchoscope (FB) can be used to intubate these patients nasally. A retromolar technique of insertion may also be used. The ETT is mounted over the scope after adequate lubrication, and the scope is introduced along the base of the nose in case of nasal intubation, and between the molars and cheeks in case of retromolar intubation, and guided through the vocal cords. This procedure takes time and requires a skilled operator. The passage of the ETT over the scope through the vocal cords is not performed under vision. Combining this technique with a videolaryngoscopy (VL) or DL can overcome this limitation. Excess secretions, bleeding, or difficulty in maneuvering the scope around the tumor may make this procedure challenging

ii. Awake Video-laryngoscopy. Awake VL is gaining popularity as an alternate technique to awake FB intubation because it is easier to perform and takes less time. A meta-analysis comparing awake intubation using VL and FB found VL to be associated with shorter intubation time.[34] There was no reported difference between the two techniques regarding the first attempt success rate, rate of complication, and level of patient satisfaction. However, most studies in this meta-analysis did not include patients with trismus or intraoral cancers where the use of VL may not always be feasible and FB-guided intubation still remains the gold standard.[35]

iii. Retrograde Intubation. This involves the passage of an ETT over a guide (epidural catheter/guide wire) passed in a retrograde manner through the cricothyroid membrane/transtracheal puncture using an epidural needle or intravenous cannula (16/18 G) into the nasal or oral cavity. This procedure needs patient cooperation and at least 0.5 cm of mouth opening to retrieve the retrograde guide.[36] Though the intubation is completely blind, the success rate is higher than blind nasal as the ETT is railroaded over a guide present in the trachea. Complications include injury to vocal cords, bleeding secondary to aberrant vessels from superior thyroid artery, and injury to the thyroid gland.[36,37]

iv. Blind Nasal Intubation. This involves blindly guiding the ETT through the nose towards the larynx. The ETT passage is guided by the help of the patient's breath sounds or an $Etco_2$ trace during spontaneous breathing. This procedure requires skill and experience and has a low success rate. Complications include trauma to oral, pharyngeal, and laryngeal structures, as the tube is passed blindly into the trachea.

Blind techniques should be discouraged in the era of VL- and FB-guided intubations to avoid complications and improve intubation success rates.

Tracheal Intubation After General Anesthesia

Depending on the plan of airway management, the induction of general anesthesia may vary. More commonly used techniques include TIVA or balanced anesthesia using a combination of inhaled and intravenous anesthetics, analgesics such as opioids, and sedatives such as benzodiazepine. Muscle relaxants should be used at the time of induction of anesthesia to improve glottis view during DL. Since head and neck surgeries are superficial surgeries, they do not require profound relaxation during the further course of the surgery.

Fluid Management

A large-bore venous cannula is essential to rapidly replace lost volume when required. Current studies indicate that GDFT using dynamic markers of fluid resuscitation, such as stroke volume variation (SVV), pulse pressure variation (PPV), and so on, help in reducing the amount of fluid given intraoperatively, postoperative complications, and hospital stay especially in free flap surgeries.[38] The most commonly used fluids include PlasmaLyte-A and Ringer's lactate.

Blood Transfusion

The need for intraoperative blood transfusion depends on the preoperative hemoglobin values and intraoperative blood loss. Concerns exist regarding blood transfusion and increased incidence of flap failure. Although a study by Stahel et al. found that keeping a hematocrit trigger as low as 25% did not increase the risk of flap-related complications,[39] this still remains a bone of contention. A recent study by Kim et al. found on multivariate analysis that the lowest perioperative hemoglobin was independently associated with flap failure, and that blood itself was not associated with the increased flap failure rate. A transfusion trigger value of 7 gm% for is usually practiced in stable patients.[40]

Vasopressor Use

For most major resections, the inability to maintain normal blood pressures despite adequate fluid resuscitation is an indication for starting vasopressors, which are slowly tapered as the blood pressure normalizes. The real concern with the use of vasopressors is flap failure due to vasospasm when used in free flap surgeries. Physiologically, hypoperfusion will reduce oxygen delivery across the organ and also increase the risk of flap failure. However, a recent study by Fagin and Petrisor, found that 85% of cases undergoing free flap surgeries require vasopressor boluses, and use of vasopressor intraoperatively was not associated with an increase in flap failure or pedicle compromise rate.[41,42]

Analgesia

Opioids form the mainstay of intraoperative analgesia in these patients. In addition, they also improve tube tolerance. Other adjuvants such as NSAIDs, acetaminophen, and so on, add to multimodal analgesia. With the recent shift towards opioid-free anesthesia, the role of N-methyl-D-aspartate (NMDA) antagonists, such as ketamine, and alpha-2 agonists such as dexmedetomidine, gabapentin, pregabalin, and lidocaine is increasing to reduce perioperative opioid requirements.

Nerve Blocks[43,44]

Inferior alveolar nerve block may be given intraoperatively for mandibular surgeries. In addition, there are various intraoral and extraoral techniques for maxillary and mandibular nerve blocks used for maxillofacial surgeries. Superficial cervical plexus block can be used for neck dissection surgeries. However, these techniques are rarely practiced.

Prophylaxis for Postoperative Nausea and Vomiting

Depending on the risk factors for postoperative nausea and vomiting (PONV), prophylaxis should be administered. Anesthetic management using TIVA reduces the risk of nausea and vomiting intraoperatively. 5-HT_3 receptor antagonists, steroids, scopolamine patch, and NK-1 receptor antagonists can also be used to reduce the incidence of PONV.

Postoperative Airway Management Plan: Tracheostomy Versus Tracheal Tube

Tracheostomy was traditionally considered a safer technique for airway management in patients undergoing

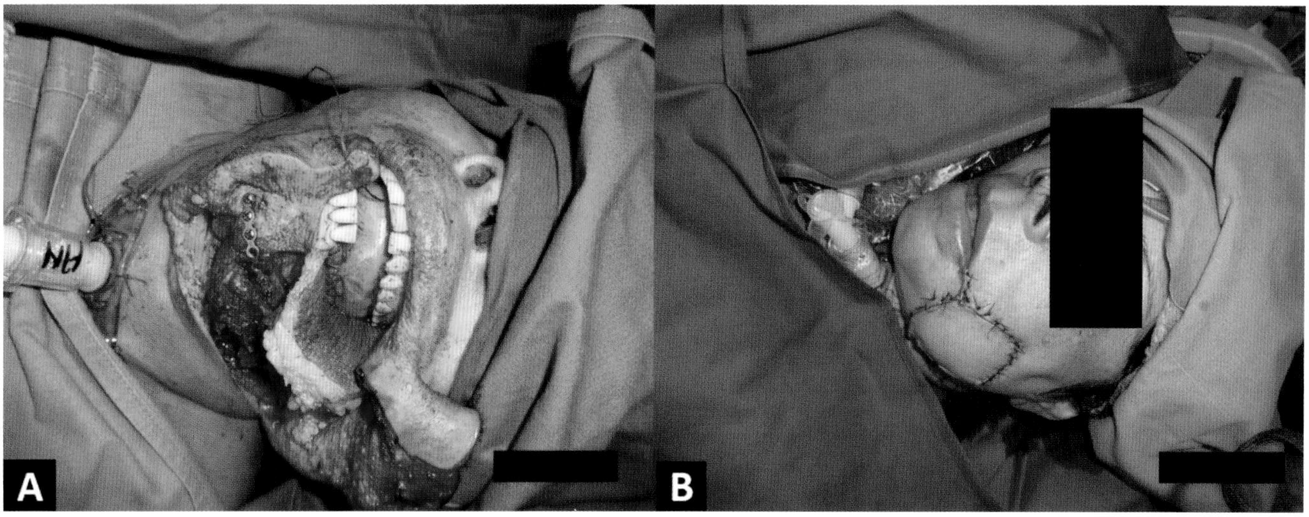

• **Fig. 21.3** (A) A patient undergoing extended mandibulectomy with a bulky flap reconstruction. (B) Postoperative airway management in the same patient using a tracheostomy.

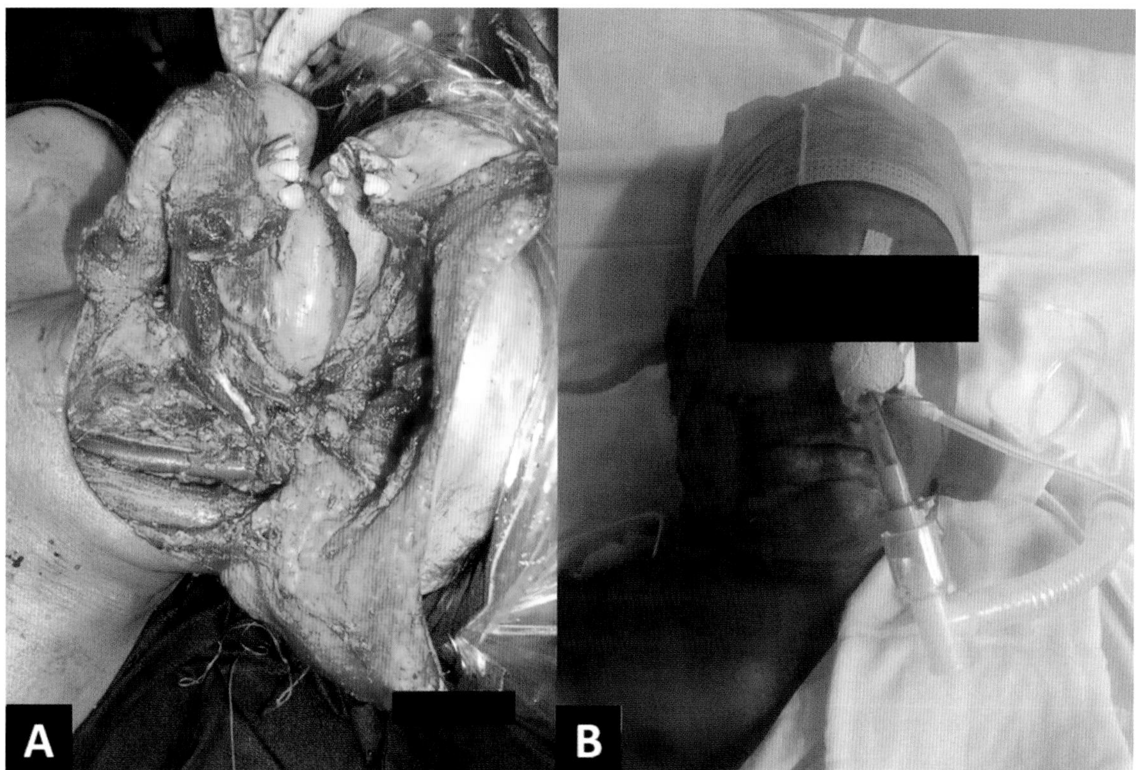

• **Fig. 21.4** (A) A patient undergoing marginal mandibulectomy with reconstruction. (B) Postoperative airway management of the same patient using a tracheal tube overnight.

head and neck cancer surgeries. Postoperative edema, reduced airway caliber, altered anatomy, and postoperative bleeding are the main reasons for advocating a tracheostomy (Fig. 21.3). However, airway complications are high in patients with a tracheostomy. The alternative to tracheostomy is a delayed extubation strategy in select patients, where the ETT is kept overnight, allowing the edema to settle and the patient is extubated the next morning (Fig. 21.4).

The delayed extubation strategy is associated with fewer complications and faster recovery compared to tracheostomy. However, it carries the risk of airway compromise postextubation if not performed in an appropriate patient. Myatra et al. in a recent prospective study in 722 patients showed that a delayed extubation strategy after major oral cancer surgery is a safe and effective alternative for airway management in select patients, with a faster return of speech and oral intake compared to performing a tracheostomy.

Patients with tumor stage (T1 and T2), absence of extensive resection, primary closure or reconstruction using a fasciocutaneous flap, absence of preoperative radiation, unilateral or no neck dissection were independently associated with a decision to manage patients safely with a delayed extubation strategy.[45] Throat pack removal prior to the transfer to the post anesthesia care unit (PACU) should be confirmed.

Postoperative Management

Monitoring

These patients should be closely monitored in the PACU. ECG, pulse oximetry, and blood pressure monitoring must be instituted in all patients postoperatively. The patients should be nursed in a semirecumbent position. Vigilant monitoring is essential for any airway obstruction, ETT malposition, airway patency, hypoventilation, or apnea with sedation or opioids and bleeding. In the case of free flap surgeries, the goal is to ensure normotension and normothermia with close monitoring of the flap.

Airway Management

On arrival to the PACU, the nurse should ensure the tube is in the proper position, free of secretions, and well secured. Patients can be maintained overnight on a T-piece or a mechanical ventilator with spontaneous breathing using pressure support (PS) ventilation, depending on the available resources. Humidification is a must to ensure tube tolerance. Dry oxygen might irritate the airway causing coughing, sloughing of the mucosa, and thickening and retention of secretions with impaired mucociliary clearance, increasing the risk of tube blockage.[46] Humidification may be provided passively using heat and moisture exchanger (HME) filters or actively using nebulizers.[47]

Sedation

Sedation may be required for tolerating the artificial airway postoperatively. The presence of an ETT requires more sedation compared to tracheostomy. Lignocaine nebulization, opioids such as morphine, infusion of dexmedetomidine, and remifentanil can be used for sedation and tube tolerance. Close monitoring is required postoperatively especially in patients not receiving mechanical ventilation, especially if opioids are used for sedation as the action may be compounded by the residual anesthetic effects.

Pain Management

Pain management in head and neck cancer surgery patients is generally suboptimal.[48] The amount of pain is multifactorial depending on the extent and duration of surgery and the presence of preoperative pain,[49] with maximum pain on the day of surgery and decreasing considerably after that.[50] Multimodal analgesia should be used postoperatively with special emphasis on reducing the amount of opioids required for pain management. Recent French guidelines advocate the use of multimodal analgesia along with morphine-patient controlled analgesia (PCA) for postoperative pain management. In addition, pain should be adequately managed during procedures such as tracheostomy tube change and nasogastric tube insertion in the postoperative period.[51]

Extubation

In addition to a preoperatively difficult airway, laryngopharyngeal edema due to surgical handling, bulky flaps encroaching into the oral cavity, and the risk of postoperative bleeding may make resecuring these airways after extubation extremely difficult. Hence, extubation in these patients is considered high risk.[52] Extubation being an elective procedure should be performed with careful planning in these patients. Airway edema can be checked either by performing laryngoscopy or by performing a cuff-leak test. Steroids can be administered on admission to the recovery unit to reduce airway edema.[53,54] Some centers advocate the use of steroids 4 h prior to extubation. If used they should be continued at least until 12 h postextubation.[55] Adrenaline nebulization may also be used to reduce airway obstruction secondary to edema.

Extubation should be performed with a plan to resecure the airway in case of extubation failure, preferably in the daytime and when there is adequate staffing. In case of bleeding from the surgical site or severe edema, extubation should be delayed. Once the patient is completely awake with intact airway reflexes, extubation should be attempted. Suctioning of the ETT followed by the oropharynx should be performed prior to extubation.

In borderline cases where there is a high possibility of extubation failure, the surgeon should be present during extubation to perform a tracheostomy if needed.[52] In such cases extubation may be performed over an airway exchange catheter (AEC) or bronchoscope. Care should be taken to keep the AEC well above the carina and no ventilation should be provided through this catheter. The patient may be oxygenated using a face mask or nasal cannula when the AEC is in place. The AEC should be removed as soon as there are no concerns regarding airway patency.

Reconfirm that the throat pack has been removed prior to extubation. Postextubation, patients should receive oxygen via simple nasal cannula and be monitored for airway compromise. Patients should be encouraged to take deep breaths and perform incentive spirometry, if feasible.

Postoperative Nutrition

Postsurgery, due to altered anatomy, the swallowing functions in these patients may be severely compromised. Hence it is extremely important to ensure that a Ryles tube (RT) is positioned before the patient is shifted out of the operating room (OR), as altered anatomy in the postoperative period along with the risk of disrupting surgical sutures might make it difficult to insert an RT later. Tube feeding should be initiated within 24 h of surgery.[16] Oral feeding should be considered for patients with a primary laryngectomy. Aim for an energy intake of 30 kcal/kg/day and a protein intake of 1.2 g/kg/day, especially if malnutrition exists or the patient will be unable to eat for more than 7 days.

Enhanced Recovery After Surgery (ERAS)

This is a multidisciplinary approach for improving surgical outcomes. For anesthesiologists, it includes nutritional optimization, limiting the fasting period before surgery, preoperative carbohydrate treatment, perioperative antibiotics in clean-contaminated procedures, corticosteroids and antiemetic medications, minimizing the use of anxiolytics or long-acting sedating agents, thromboprophylaxis, use of TIVA techniques, minimizing the use of opioids in the perioperative period, GDFT, and adequate glucose and temperature control. It also includes avoiding the use of tracheostomy as much as possible. Postoperative emphasis must be on a specific pain management protocol, early feeding, and early mobilization. Many studies have found head and neck cancer patients managed with ERAS protocols to recover earlier with fewer postoperative complications and a shorter length of stay.[25,56–58]

Postoperative Complications

Airway Complications

Airway patency should be closely monitored following extubation or decannulation of tracheostomy. Most tracheostomies performed for head and neck cancer surgeries are temporary. On the other hand, laryngostomas for laryngectomies are permanent. Airway complications with tracheostomy include obstructed tube, displaced tube, infection at tracheostomy site, and lower respiratory tract infection.[59] Long-term complications include trachea-cutaneous fistula, tracheal stenosis, and a blocked tube.[60] In patients managed with delayed extubation, tube-blockade secondary to airway secretions or collected blood and inability to maintain a patent airway postextubation are the two most important complications. The rate of airway complications is, however, more common with tracheostomy.[61]

Surgical Complications

Watch for bleeding in the immediate postoperative period. Surgical flaps should be carefully monitored. Delayed wound healing, flap necrosis, and infectious complications may occur in the course of the recovery and should be carefully monitored. Life-threatening hemorrhage may occur following a carotid or major neck vessel blow out, often due to infection.

Troponitis in Head and Neck Cancer Surgery

A study reported that 15% of patients undergoing major head and neck cancer resection had elevated levels of troponin I, of which 20% developed myocardial infarct in the postoperative period.[61] It is important to keep in mind that hypercoagulability secondary to both surgery and cancer increases the risk of perioperative cardiac complications in head and neck cancer patients.

Care of the Patient With a Tracheostomy

Temporary tracheostomy care includes humidification, secure fixation, and regular cleaning of the inner cannula in a productive chest (4 h) with an 8-h gap at night and for mechanically ventilated patients. A separate cannula should be placed at the bedside, allowing for a quick change if required. The entire assembly should be changed after 30 days. If the tube is suspected to be blocked, the suction catheter should be passed; failure to do so suggests a possibility of a tube block or misplacement. While changing the tube, methods of confirmation such as capnography should be readily available. Every ward having patients with a tracheostomy tube should have staff experienced with tracheostomy care, daily checks at the time shift change, and clear procedure guidelines in case of emergencies.

In the case of a blocked tube, one must remember that bag-mask ventilation may not be possible, and changing the cannula or suction in case of laryngostoma will most often relieve the obstruction. It is always better to replace a partially displaced tube rather than attempt to reposition it. To buy time, one can deflate the cuff allowing the patient to breathe around the tube.[62,63] Patients with laryngostomas are "neck only" breathers, and there should be general awareness, patient bands, or signs in patient care areas to avoid face mask ventilation or oral intubation in these patients during an airway emergency.

Postoperative Rehabilitation

Following surgery, head and neck cancer patients require training regarding vocalization and swallowing to improve quality of life. Rehabilitation programs also include mouth opening exercises using jaw stretchers, especially in patients with trismus. Patients with delayed extubation have faster return to daily activities compared with tracheostomy.[59,64]

Special Considerations for Specific Surgeries

Laryngectomy

Total laryngectomy involves en-bloc removal of laryngeal structures including the epiglottis, hyoid, and variable part of the trachea with the creation of a permanent tracheostome for breathing.

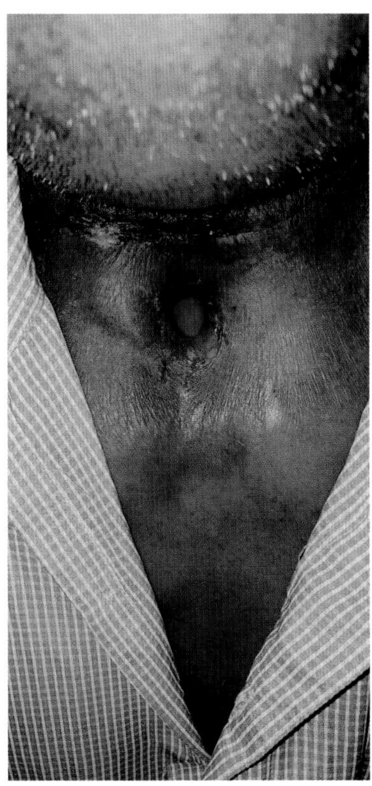

• **Fig. 21.5** A patient with laryngectomy end-stoma.

Preoperative Considerations

Airway assessment should focus on clinical signs related to change in voice, dysphagia, stridor, and difficulty sleeping, which might be clues to difficult airway and the probability of airway obstruction under anesthesia. Patients presenting with stridor require emergency tracheostomy. Tracheostomy is usually avoided in the elective setting due to concerns regarding the seeding of disease at the stoma site. Adrenaline nebulization, heliox, and steroids can help buy time while an airway plan is formulated.

Intraoperative Considerations

Tracheal intubation is usually easy; however, smaller sized ETTs are required due to disease-associated airway narrowing. FB-guided intubation might not be a suitable choice as it may cork an already narrow airway leading to catastrophic occlusion of the narrow laryngeal aperture. When the laryngostoma (end tracheostomy) is created, the oral ETT should be removed and a flexometallic ETT placed within the laryngostoma to continue general anesthesia (Fig. 21.5). The ETT should be properly secured with sutures, and inserted just enough so that cuff is visible at the laryngostoma to avoid endobronchial intubation and leakage of gases.

Postoperative Considerations

A pediatric mask or tracheostomy mask should be placed over laryngostoma for oxygen delivery. A tracheostomy tube should always be available beside the patient in the event of an emergency for ventilation and oxygenation. Other considerations are detailed in the section on tracheostomy care.

Endolaryngeal Vocal Fold Surgery

This is performed with the use of a laser or by means of a microlaryngeal endoscope. Indications include vocal cord nodule, polyp, leukoplakia, and so on. In terms of surgery, it is not a morbid procedure, but due to a shared airway, it is extremely challenging for the anesthesiologist. There is an added concern of airway fire when these surgeries are performed using the laser technique.

Airway Management and Ventilation

Mechanical ventilation can be performed continuously with the use of smaller-diameter ETTs such as the microlaryngoscopy tubes that have a smaller diameter and a longer length with a cuff placed distally to avoid rupture secondary to the surgical instruments. These are good for surgeries of the anterior region of the vocal cords, as the posterior regions are obscured by the tube. Laser-resistant tubes can also be used during laser surgery with minimal risk of airway fire. Intermittent jet ventilation through a jet catheter or via the side port of the MLscope or intermittent tracheal intubation and ventilation are other techniques used for ventilation. A recent method of oxygenation described as a part of tubeless surgery is apneic ventilation using the HFNCO technique called THRIVE. The advantage of this technique is that there is no tube in the field of the surgery and no interruptions for ventilation either. However, during laser surgery THRIVE should be used by those experienced in laser surgery, who understand the fire triangle well. In addition to the type of tubes, recommendations regarding the safety of OR personnel and patient, and preventing laser fire should be strictly followed in the OR.

Thyroid Surgery

Anesthesia of thyroid surgery includes a preoperative assessment of airway compromise and thyroid function, a careful airway management plan in case of retrosternal extension of the thyroid, and postoperative management of thyroid functions and serum calcium in addition to understanding the management of complications specifically related to bilateral vocal cord palsy and bilateral hematoma. While the use of intraoperative neuromonitoring has significantly reduced recurrent laryngeal nerve (RLN) injury, it may still occur due to poor placement of electrodes or inadequate reversal from muscle relaxants at the time of monitoring.

Airway Assessment

Assessment of tracheomalacia is important in the case of a long-standing and large-size thyroid mass. In addition, thyroid function needs to be assessed preoperatively. In the case of neuromonitoring, the correct placement of the ETT electrode is essential with respect to vocal cords. Videolaryngoscopes might especially be of assistance as they might help in better cord visualization and documentation of the position of the ETT. In the case of expected tracheomalacia or retrosternal goiter, where the collapse of the airway might be expected, it is better to maintain spontaneous breathing in patients until a secured airway is established. The use of reinforced tubes is preferred to prevent compression of the ETT due to external compression. FB might be used to ensure the ETT is pushed beyond the point of extrinsic compression. In the case of extrinsic compression, a normal-sized tube might be used. However, in cases where tumor infiltrates the trachea, it might be a fixed deformity, and smaller sized tubes might be required. In a consensus statement for the management of tracheomalacia, the consensus was that a rigid bronchoscope should always be present in the OR in case of airway collapse.[65]

Postoperative Considerations

The incidence of PONV is much higher for thyroid surgeries, and it is recommended to use more than two interventions in patients with high risk. Hypothyroidism might not present for up to a week due to the half-life of preexisting thyroid hormone (T3, 1 day; T4, 5–7 days), in which case they need to be replaced. In the case of thyroidectomy, patients may also develop hypoparathyroidism due to trauma or excision of parathyroids or ischemia secondary to the devascularization of glands. Such cases will present with hypocalcemia (20%–30%) and there may be associated signs such as Chvostek and Trousseau. Intravenous calcium gluconate boluses to acutely settle symptoms of acute hypocalcemia are required. In addition, vitamin D and calcium supplements are provided for long-term management of hypocalcemia (at least 10 days). RLN palsy may also be transient or permanent.

Most cases of RLN palsy tend to recover and do not call for intervention unless the patient goes into stridor, in which case one might have to resort to performing a tracheostomy. In the case of bilateral neck hematoma leading to airway compromise, neck sutures can be removed in the PACU itself to relieve airway compression while preparing for hemostatic surgery.[66]

Microvascular Surgery

Flap failures are associated with patients having increased age, smokers, associated medical conditions, low preoperative hemoglobin levels, and poor perioperative fluid management.

Preoperative Considerations

Comorbidities such as diabetes, hypothyroid, malnutrition, and anemia (hemoglobin <10 gm%) can have adverse effects on flap outcomes and need to be corrected preoperatively.

Intraoperative Considerations

A free flap is sensitive to excess fluid administration due to increased risk of edema, which might be due to lack of lymphatic drainage or the ability to reabsorb interstitial fluid. While excess fluid has been associated with flap failure, negative fluid balance and hemodilution risk thrombosis of the flap. No difference has been seen between crystalloids or colloids. Excess fluid is independently associated with poor flap outcomes. Hypothermia may be associated with vasoconstriction and poor flap outcomes. Sevoflurane has been shown to improve endothelial cell progenitor cell function and may improve vascular healing.[14,41,67,68] Vasopressors should be preferred over fluid overload to maintain blood pressure.

Postoperative Considerations

Zhong et al. found 3.5–6 mL/kg/h to be the sweet spot for fluid administration on postoperative day 1.[69] Vasopressors, in particular norepinephrine used to maintain normotension in the postoperative period, have been shown to improve flap outcomes.[42] Studies have shown blood transfusion to be associated with poor flap outcomes secondary to increased viscosity and immunosuppression.[70] Some centers practice normovolemic hemodilution. Early oral postoperative feeding has shown significantly reduced hospital stay without increasing flap-related complications. However, surgeons may be concerned about restarting an oral diet with the theoretic risk of compromising the suture line and fistula formation.

Surgeries Requiring Neuromuscular Monitoring

The two most common surgeries in head and neck cancer that require neuromonitoring are thyroid surgeries for RLN identification and parotid surgery for facial nerve branch identification.

Thyroid Surgery

The incidence of RLN injury varies from 0.3% to 18.9% even amongst the most experienced surgeons. IOM helps in nerve identification and dissection without causing nerve injury. For anesthesiologist, the induction should be carried out using an intermediate or short-acting muscle relaxant, such that the effects of a relaxant completely wear off at the time of intraoperative monitoring. Special ETTs with conductive silver ink electrodes that have a dark black cross-band positioned between the vocal cords are used. During the time of dissection and RLN stimulation, the patient should not be under the effect of any muscle relaxant. Muscle relaxants reduce the amplitude of evoked responses, making IOM a less sensitive technique to prevent RLN injury. Anesthesia may be maintained using a continuous infusion of intravenous anesthetic agents such as propofol, dexmedetomidine, remifentanil, lidocaine, and so on. At very high doses, propofol might suppress the compound muscle action potential. Adjuvant agents help to minimize the dose of propofol to maintain anesthesia. Ventilation can be maintained using air and oxygen. Inhalational agents if used should be at a minimum alveolar concentration less than one. The neuromuscular

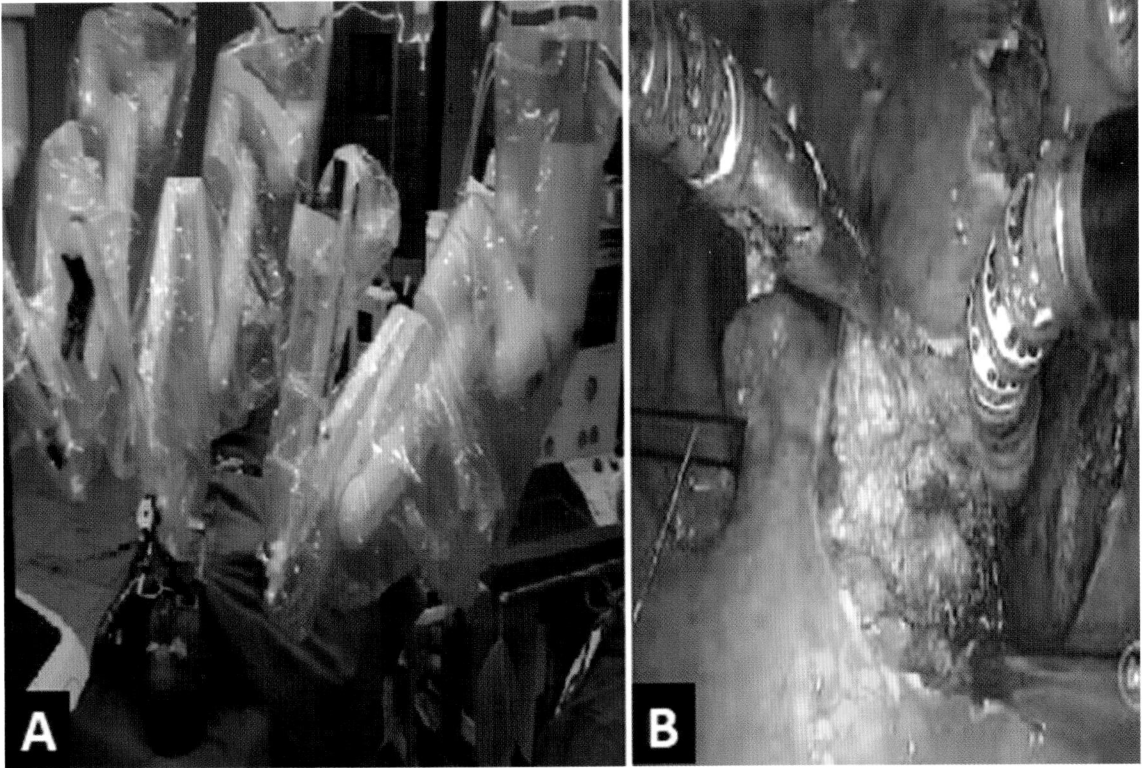

• **Fig. 21.6** (A) A patient undergoing robotic tonsillectomy with the anesthesia station positioned at the foot-end. (B) Robotic tonsillectomy surgery.

monitor should be used to check the action of the adductor pollicis.

Parotid Surgery

Intra-Operative Neuro Monitoring (IONM) is used during parotid surgery to avoid dissection of facial nerve branches, which are closely associated with the parotid gland. The electrodes are placed according to the facial nerve distribution on the face. The basic physiology and anesthetic management are very similar to thyroid surgery.

Transoral Robotic Surgeries (TORS)

Minimally invasive robotic surgery may be performed for oropharyngeal tumors. The Da Vinci robot is remotely controlled by the surgeon who sits at a console, while one robotic arm holds the camera (endoscope) and the other two hands hold left- and right-hand instruments. The surgery is carried out with the patient's feet toward the anesthesia machine, and the robot is moved into position, with the arms positioned over the patient's chest (Fig. 21.6). This limits access to the patient's face, neck, and chest. The anesthesia plan is similar to that described before. Nasal RAE tubes are preferred, and a longer anesthesia circuit is required. The face should be well padded, eyes covered using eyeglasses, and adequate muscle relaxation provided to avoid injury due to the robotic arms. If extensive airway edema is suspected, delayed extubation or tracheostomy may be performed.

References

1. Docampo LI, Arrula VA, Rotllan NB, et al. SEOM clinical guidelines for the treatment of head and neck cancer (2017). *Clin Transl Oncol*. 2018;20(1):75–83.
2. Homer J, Fardy M. Surgery in head and neck cancer: United Kingdom national multidisciplinary guidelines. *J Laryngol Otol*. 2016;130(S2):S68–S70.
3. Wiegand DA, Latz B, Zwillich CW, Wiegand L. Upper airway resistance and geniohyoid muscle activity in normal men during wakefulness and sleep. *J Appl Physiol*. 1990;69(4):1252–1261.
4. Cunningham DP, Basmajian JV. Electromyography of genioglossus and geniohyoid muscles during deglutition. *Anat Rec*. 1969;165(3):401–409.
5. Albahout KS, Waheed A. Anatomy, Head and Neck, Pharynx-*StatPearls*: StatPearls Publishing; 2019.
6. More CB, Das S, Patel H, Adalja C, Kamatchi V, Venkatesh R. Proposed clinical classification for oral submucous fibrosis. *Oral Oncol*. 2012;48(3):200–202.
7. Dougherty TB, Clayman GL. Airway management of surgical patients with head and neck malignancies. *Anesthesiol Clin North Am*. 1998;16(3):547–562.
8. Prasanna D, Bhat S. Nasotracheal intubation: an overview. *J Oral Maxillofac Surg*. 2014;13(4):366–372.
9. Smith J, Reid A. Identifying the more patent nostril before nasotracheal intubation. *Anesthesia*. 2001;56(3):258–262.
10. Thota RS, Doctor JR. Evaluation of paranasal sinuses on available computed tomography in head and neck cancer patients: An assessment tool for nasotracheal intubation. *Indian J Anaesth*. 2016;60(12):960.

11. Murgu SD, Colt HG. Tracheobronchomalacia and excessive dynamic airway collapse. *Respirology*. 2006;11(4):388–406.
12. Ahmad I, Keane O, Muldoon S. Enhancing airway assessment of patients with head and neck pathology using virtual endoscopy. *Indian J Anaesth*. 2017;61(10):782.
13. Busti F, Marchi G, Ugolini S, Castagna A, Girelli D. Anemia and iron deficiency in cancer patients: role of iron replacement therapy. *Pharmaceuticals*. 2018;11(4):94.
14. Hill JB, Patel A, Del Corral GA, et al. Preoperative anemia predicts thrombosis and free flap failure in microvascular reconstruction. *Ann Plastic Surg*. 2012;69(4):364–367.
15. Luma HN, Eloumou SAFB, Mboligong FN, Temfack E, Donfack O-T, Doualla M-S. Malnutrition in patients admitted to the medical wards of the Douala General Hospital: a cross-sectional study. *BMC Res Notes*. 2017;10(1):238.
16. Talwar B, Donnelly R, Skelly R, Donaldson M. Nutritional management in head and neck cancer: United Kingdom National Multidisciplinary Guidelines. *J Laryngol Otol*. 2016;130(S2):S32–S40.
17. Kheterpal S, Martin L, Shanks AM, Tremper KK. Prediction and outcomes of impossible mask ventilation. A review of 50,000 anesthetics. *Anesthesiology*. 2009;110(4):891–897.
18. Sroussi HY, Epstein JB, Bensadoun RJ, et al. Common oral complications of head and neck cancer radiation therapy: mucositis, infections, saliva change, fibrosis, sensory dysfunctions, dental caries, periodontal disease, and osteoradionecrosis. *Cancer Med*. 2017;6(12):2918–2931.
19. Steele SR, Martin MJ, Mullenix PS, Crawford JV, Cuadrado DS, Andersen CA. Focused high-risk population screening for carotid arterial stenosis after radiation therapy for head and neck cancer. *Am J Surg*. 2004;187(5):594–598.
20. Adelstein D, Gillison ML, Pfister DG, et al. NCCN guidelines insights: head and neck cancers, version 2.2017. *J Natl Compr Canc Netw*. 2017;15(6):761–770.
21. Fielding JE. Smoking: health effects and control. *N Engl J Med*. 1985;313(8):491–498.
22. Potter J, Higginson IJ, Scadding JW, Quigley C. Identifying neuropathic pain in patients with head and neck cancer: use of the Leeds Assessment of Neuropathic Symptoms and Signs Scale. *J R Soc Med*. 2003;96(8):379–383.
23. Mirabile A, Airoldi M, Ripamonti C, et al. Pain management in head and neck cancer patients undergoing chemo-radiotherapy: Clinical practical recommendations. *Crit Rev Oncol Hematol*. 2016;99:100–106.
24. Terkawi AS, Tsang S, Alshehri AS, Mulafikh DS, Alghulikah AA, AlDhahri SF. The burden of chronic pain after major head and neck tumor therapy. *Saudi J Anaesth*. 2017;11(Suppl 1):S71.
25. Coyle M, Main B, Hughes C, et al. Enhanced recovery after surgery (ERAS) for head and neck oncology patients. *Clin Otolaryngol*. 2016;41(2):118–126.
26. Chalmers A, Turner MW, Anand R, Puxeddu R, Brennan PA. Cardiac output monitoring to guide fluid replacement in head and neck microvascular free flap surgery—what is current practice in the UK? *Br J Oral Maxillofac Surg*. 2012;50(6):500–503.
27. Patel A, Nouraei S. Transnasal Humidified Rapid-Insufflation Ventilatory Exchange (THRIVE): a physiological method of increasing apnea time in patients with difficult airways. *Anesthesia*. 2015;70(3):323–329.
28. Wu C, Wei J, Cen Q, et al. Supraglottic jet oxygenation and ventilation-assisted fiber-optic bronchoscope intubation in patients with difficult airways. *Intern Emerg Med*. 2017;12(5):667–673.
29. Chauhan V, Acharya G. Nasal intubation: A comprehensive review. *Indian J Crit Care Med*. 2016;20(11):662.
30. Hall C, Shutt L. Nasotracheal intubation for head and neck surgery. *Anesthesia*. 2003;58(3):249–256.
31. Atlas G, Lee M. The neural integrity monitor electromyogram tracheal tube: Anesthetic considerations. *J Anaesthesiol Clin Pharmacol*. 2013;29(3):403.
32. Aziz M, Kristensen M. From variance to guidance for awake tracheal intubation. *Anaesthesia*. 2020;75(4):442–446.
33. Ramkumar V. Preparation of the patient and the airway for awake intubation. *Indian J Anaesth*. 2011;55(5):442.
34. Alhomary M, Ramadan E, Curran E, Walsh S. Videolaryngoscopy vs. fibreoptic bronchoscopy for awake tracheal intubation: a systematic review and meta-analysis. *Anaesthesia*. 2018;73(9):1151–1161.
35. Rosenstock CV, Thøgersen B, Afshari A, Christensen A-L, Eriksen C, Gätke MR. Awake fiberoptic or awake video laryngoscopic tracheal intubation in patients with anticipated difficult airway management. A randomized clinical trial. *Anaesthesiology*. 2012;116(6):1210–1216.
36. Dhara SS. Retrograde tracheal intubation. *Anesthesia*. 2009;64(10):1094–1104.
37. Bennett J, Guha S, Sankar A. Cricothyrotomy: the anatomical basis. *J R Coll Surg Edinb*. 1996;41(1):57–60.
38. Lahtinen SL, Liisanantti JH, Poukkanen MM, Laurila PA. Goal-directed fluid management in free flap surgery for cancer of the head and neck. *Minerva Anestesiol*. 2017;83(1):59–68.
39. Stahel PF, Moore EE, Schreier SL, Flierl MA, Kashuk JL. Transfusion strategies in postinjury coagulopathy. *Curr Opin Anesthesiol*. 2009;22(2):289–298.
40. Kim MJ, Woo K-J, Park BY, Kang SR. Effects of transfusion on free flap survival: searching for an optimal hemoglobin threshold for transfusion. *J Reconstr Microsurg*. 2018;34(8):610–615.
41. Fagin AP, Petrisor D. Controversies in microvascular maxillofacial reconstruction. *Oral Maxillofac Surg Clin North Am*. 2017;29(4):415–424.
42. Fang L, Liu J, Yu C, Hanasono MM, Zheng G, Yu P. Intraoperative use of vasopressors does not increase the risk of free flap compromise and failure in cancer patients. *Ann Surg*. 2018;268(2):379–384.
43. Kanakaraj M, Shanmugasundaram N, Chandramohan M, Kannan R, Perumal SM, Nagendran J. Regional anesthesia in faciomaxillary and oral surgery. *J Pharm Bioallied Sci*. 2012;4(Suppl 2):S264.
44. Takasugi Y, Furuya H, Moriya K, Okamoto Y. Clinical evaluation of inferior alveolar nerve block by injection into the pterygomandibular space anterior to the mandibular foramen. *Anesth Prog*. 2000;47(4):125.
45. Myatra SN, Gupta S, D'Cruz AK et al. Identification of patients for a delayed extubation strategy versus elective tracheostomy for postoperative airway management in major oral cancer surgery: a prospective observational study in seven hundred and twenty patients. *Oral Oncol*. 2021;121:105502. doi:10.1016/j.oraloncology.2021.105502. 34450455.
46. Chalon J. Low humidity and damage to tracheal mucosa. *Bull N Y Acad Med*. 1980;56(3):314.
47. Restrepo RD, Walsh BK. Humidification during invasive and noninvasive mechanical ventilation: 2012. *Respir Care*. 2012;57(5):782–788.
48. Sommer M, Geurts JW, Stessel B, et al. Prevalence and predictors of postoperative pain after ear, nose, and throat surgery. *Arch Otolaryngol Head Neck Surg*. 2009;135(2):124–130.

49. Inhestern J, Schuerer J, Illge C, et al. Pain on the first postoperative day after head and neck cancer surgery. *Eur Arch Otorhinolaryngol.* 2015;272(11):3401–3409.
50. Bianchini C, Malago M, Crema L, et al. Post-operative pain management in head and neck cancer patients: predictive factors and efficacy of therapy. *Acta Otorhinolaryngol Ital.* 2016;36(2):91.
51. Espitalier F, Testelin S, Blanchard D, et al. Management of somatic pain induced by treatment of head and neck cancer: postoperative pain. Guidelines of the French Oto-Rhino-Laryngology–Head and Neck Surgery Society (SFORL). *Eur Ann Otorhinolaryngol Head Neck Dis.* 2014;131(4):249–252.
52. Kundra P, Garg R, Patwa A, et al. All India Difficult Airway Association 2016 guidelines for the management of anticipated difficult extubation. *Indian J Anaesth.* 2016;60(12):915.
53. Hartley M, Vaughan R. Problems associated with tracheal extubation. *Br J Anaesth.* 1993;71(4):561–568.
54. Kriner EJ, Shafazand S, Colice GL. The endotracheal tube cuff-leak test as a predictor for postextubation stridor. *Resp Care.* 2005;50(12):1632–1638.
55. Jaber S, Jung B, Chanques G, Bonnet F, Marret E. Effects of steroids on reintubation and post-extubation stridor in adults: meta-analysis of randomised controlled trials. *Crit Care.* 2009;13(2):1.
56. Dort JC, Farwell DG, Findlay M, et al. Optimal perioperative care in major head and neck cancer surgery with free flap reconstruction: a consensus review and recommendations from the enhanced recovery after surgery society. *JAMA Otolaryngol Head Neck Surg.* 2017;143(3):292–303.
57. Bianchini C, Pelucchi S, Pastore A, Feo CV, Ciorba A. Enhanced recovery after surgery (ERAS) strategies: possible advantages also for head and neck surgery patients? *Eur Arch Otorhinolaryngol.* 2014;271(3):439–443.
58. Simpson JC, Bao X, Agarwala A. Pain management in Enhanced Recovery after Surgery (ERAS) protocols. *Clin Colon Rectal Surg.* 2019;32(2):121–128.
59. Coyle MJ, Tyrrell R, Godden A, et al. Replacing tracheostomy with overnight intubation to manage the airway in head and neck oncology patients: towards an improved recovery. *Br J Oral Maxillofac Surg.* 2013;51(6):493–496.
60. Anehosur VS, Karadiguddi P, Joshi VK, Lakkundi BC, Ghosh R, Krishnan G. Elective tracheostomy in head and neck surgery: our experience. *J Clin Diagn Res.* 2017;11(5):ZC36.
61. Nagele P, Rao LK, Penta M, et al. Postoperative myocardial injury after major head and neck cancer surgery. *Head Neck.* 2011;33(8):1085–1091.
62. Bodenham A, Bell D, Bonner S, et al. Standards for the care of adult patients with a temporary tracheostomy; Standards and Guidelines. *J Intensive Care Soc.* 2014;1:3.
63. McGrath B, Bates L, Atkinson D, Moore J. Multidisciplinary guidelines for the management of tracheostomy and laryngectomy airway emergencies. *Anesthesia.* 2012;67(9):1025–1041.
64. Moore MG, Bhrany AD, Francis DO, Yueh B, Futran ND. Use of nasotracheal intubation in patients receiving oral cavity free flap reconstruction. *Head Neck.* 2010;32(8):1056–1061.
65. Lu I-C, Lin I-H, Wu C-W, et al. Preoperative, intraoperative and postoperative anesthetic prospective for thyroid surgery: what's new. *Gland Surg.* 2017;6(5):469.
66. Christou N, Mathonnet M. Complications after total thyroidectomy. *J Visc Surg.* 2013;150(4):249–256.
67. Vincent A, Sawhney R, Ducic Y. Perioperative care of free flap patients. Paper presented at: Seminars in Plastic Surgery, 2019.
68. Ettinger KS, Arce K, Lohse CM, et al. Higher perioperative fluid administration is associated with increased rates of complications following head and neck microvascular reconstruction with fibular free flaps. *Microsurgery.* 2017;37(2):128–136.
69. Zhong T, Neinstein R, Massey C, et al. Intravenous fluid infusion rate in microsurgical breast reconstruction: important lessons learned from 354 free flaps. *Plast Reconstr Surg.* 2011;128(6):1153–1160.
70. Brinkman JN, Derks LH, Klimek M, Mureau MA. Perioperative fluid management and use of vasoactive and antithrombotic agents in free flap surgery: a literature review and clinical recommendations. *J Reconstr Microsurg.* 2013;29(6):357–366.

22

Perioperative Care of the Surgical Patient: Heart, Lung, and Mediastinum Procedures

ALEXANDRA L. LEWIS AND ANAHITA DABO-TRUBELJA

This chapter consists of three major sections, each of which addresses different aspects of the perioperative management of cancer patients requiring thoracic surgery. Over the last decade, the field of thoracic surgery has advanced in many ways, for example, the rise of minimally invasive surgery, the introduction of immunotherapy drugs, and a growing trend toward standardization of care with enhanced recovery protocols. With these advancements, this chapter is designed to provide recommendations for anesthesiologists to refine their knowledge base of thoracic procedures.

Anesthetic Management for Thoracic Procedures in the Cancer Patient

Lung cancer remains the leading cause of cancer-related deaths in the United States. Recent cancer data have estimated a total of 239,320 new cases of lung cancer each year and 161,250 deaths resulting from lung cancer in the United States in 2010.[1–3] The most common modifiable risk factors influencing the development of lung cancer include cigarette smoking, occupational exposure (i.e., asbestos, arsenic, beryllium silica, and diesel fumes), diet, and ionizing radiation.[4] While there are several risk factors for lung cancer, cigarette smoking is linked to 90% of lung cancer deaths.[5,6] Public health campaigns and physician intervention remain the most effective strategies for promoting smoking cessation. In recent years, there has been a growing effort to encourage early screening among high-risk patients. In 2013, the National Lung Screening Trial (NLST) demonstrated a 20% reduction in mortality with low-dose computed tomographic (LDCT) screening, and the guidelines recommend annual LDCT for high-risk patients.[7,8] As more patients undergo screening, we expect higher detection rates and a growing need for surgical intervention.

Over the last decade, advances in surgical techniques, along with the development of newer immunotherapy agents, have both prolonged survival and improved postoperative outcomes. These advances have introduced new challenges in the perioperative management. In this chapter, we discuss the important elements of preoperative assessment with attention to diagnosis and emerging therapies used in the management of lung cancer. We provide recommendations for intraoperative management during open and minimally invasive thoracic surgeries. We conclude with a discussion on postoperative management to reduce morbidity and mortality after lung resection.

Oncologic Management of Lung Cancer

A clear understanding of the clinical features, staging, and treatment is important to optimize the perioperative care of the lung cancer patient. Lung cancer is classified into two major categories: non–small cell lung cancer (NSCLC) and small cell lung cancer (SCLC). NSCLC and SCLC account for 85% and 15% of all lung cancers, respectively. There are three major subtypes of NSCLC, including adenocarcinoma, squamous cell carcinoma, and large cell carcinoma. Among all lung cancers, adenocarcinoma remains the most common type of lung cancer, with an incidence of 40%.[9]

With a confirmed diagnosis, medical oncologists utilize the TNM staging system (Fig. 22.1) to devise a suitable treatment plan.

It is paramount for anesthesiologists to become familiar with chemotherapy agents and emerging therapies that medical oncologists use in the management of NSCLC and SCLC.

Until recently, chemotherapy and surgery remained the mainstay of management. Platinum-based chemotherapy with carboplatin or cisplatin is the mainstay for NSCLC and SCLC. Platinum-based chemotherapy has been used in combination with other classes of chemotherapy agents to allow for a durable immune response against cancer cells.

Classifications

Primary Tumor (T) Classification

- **TX** Primary tumor cannot be assessed, or tumor proven by the presence of malignant cells in sputum or bronchial washings but not visualized by imaging or bronchoscopy
- **T0** No evidence of primary tumor
- **Tis** Carcinoma in situ
- **T1** Tumor 3 cm or less in greatest dimension, surrounded by lung or visceral pleura, without bronchoscopic evidence of invasion more proximal than the lobar bronchus
- **T1a** Tumor 2 cm or less in greatest dimension
- **T1b** Tumor more than 2 cm but 3 cm or less in greatest dimension
- **T2** Tumor more than 3 cm but 7 cm or less or tumor with any of the following features (T2 tumors with these features are classified T2a if 5 cm or less): involves main bronchus, 2 cm or more distal to the carina; invades visceral pleura (PL1 or PL2); associated with atelectasis or obstructive pneumonitis that extends to the hilar region but does not involve the entire lung
- **T2a** Tumor more than 3 cm but 5 cm or less in greatest dimension
- **T2b** Tumor more than 5 cm but 7 cm or less in greatest dimension
- **T3** Tumor more than 7 cm or one that directly invades any of the following: parietal pleural (PL3), chest wall (including superior sulcus tumors), diaphragm, phrenic nerve, mediastinal pleura, parietal pericardium; or tumor in the main bronchus less than 2 cm distal to the carina[1] but without involvement of the carina; or associated atelectasis or obstructive pneumonitis of the entire lung or separate tumor nodule(s) in the same lobe
- **T4** Tumor of any size that invades any of the following: mediastinum, heart, great vessels, trachea, recurrent laryngeal nerve, esophagus, vertebral body, carina, separate tumor nodule(s) in a different ipsilateral lobe

Distant Metastasis (M) Classification

- **M0** No distant metastasis
- **M1** Distant metastasis
- **M1a** Separate tumor nodule(s) in a contralateral lobe, tumor with pleural nodules or malignant pleural (or pericardial) effusion
- **M1b** Distant metastasis (in extrathoracic organs)

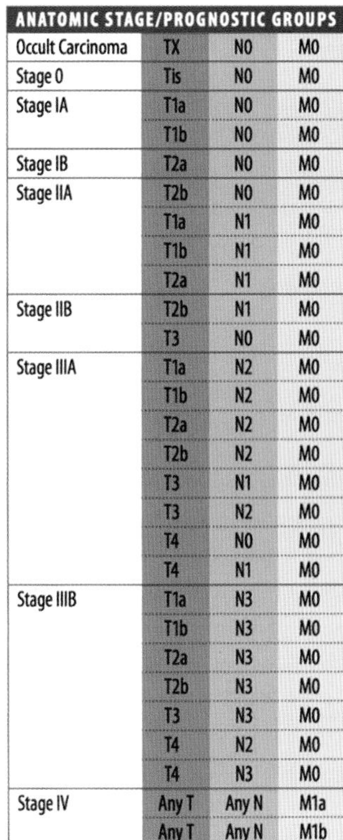

ANATOMIC STAGE/PROGNOSTIC GROUPS			
Occult Carcinoma	TX	N0	M0
Stage 0	Tis	N0	M0
Stage IA	T1a	N0	M0
	T1b	N0	M0
Stage IB	T2a	N0	M0
Stage IIA	T2b	N0	M0
	T1a	N1	M0
	T1b	N1	M0
	T2a	N1	M0
Stage IIB	T2b	N1	M0
	T3	N0	M0
Stage IIIA	T1a	N2	M0
	T1b	N2	M0
	T2a	N2	M0
	T2b	N2	M0
	T3	N1	M0
	T3	N2	M0
	T4	N0	M0
	T4	N1	M0
Stage IIIB	T1a	N3	M0
	T1b	N3	M0
	T2a	N3	M0
	T2b	N3	M0
	T3	N3	M0
	T4	N2	M0
	T4	N3	M0
Stage IV	Any T	Any N	M1a
	Any T	Any N	M1b

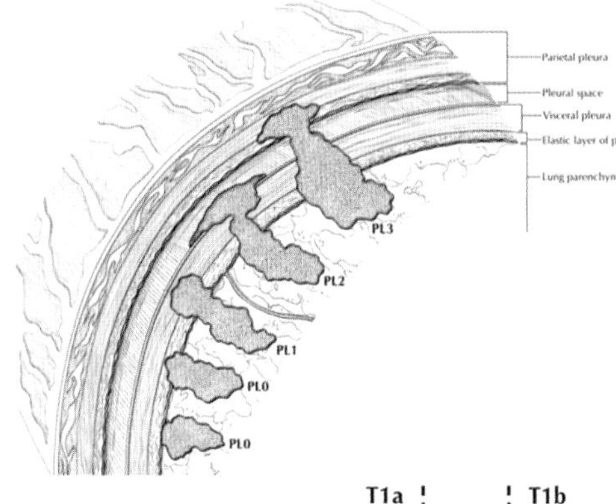

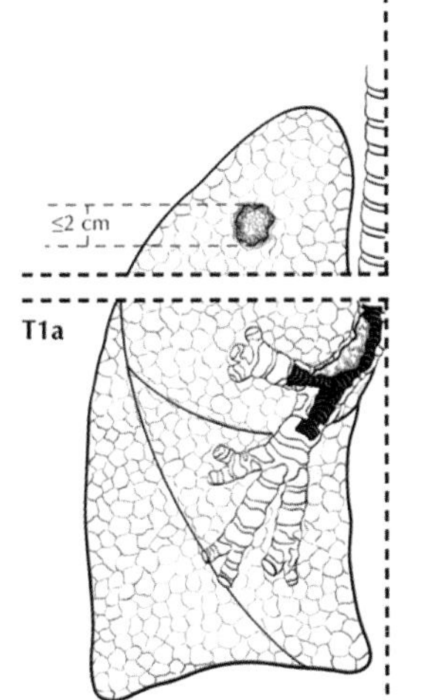

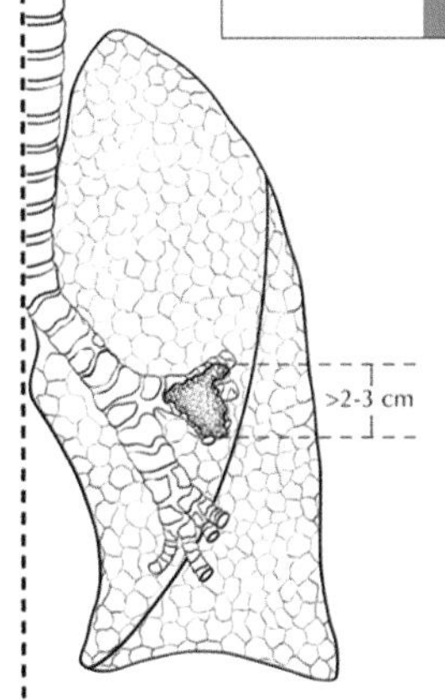

• **Fig. 22.1** American Joint Committee on Cancer: Lung Cancer Staging 7th ed.

The disadvantage of many chemotherapeutic agents, however, is the failure to discriminate between normal and cancer cells, thus leading to major systemic toxicities (Table 22.1).

Cancer immunotherapy has emerged as a new therapy, and these drugs direct the immune system to exclusively target tumor cells, thereby minimizing the harmful effects of systemic chemotherapy. Immunotherapy for lung cancer encompasses a broad class of drugs, including:

- Immune checkpoint inhibitors
- Chimeric antigen receptor (CAR) -T cells
- Monoclonal antibodies
- Nonspecific immunotherapy
- Cancer vaccines

Each class of drugs has a specific mechanism to harness the immune system against tumor cells and their mechanism of action, as detailed in Table 22.2.

Preoperative Evaluation

Thoracic surgical patients often present with complex medical histories and require comprehensive assessment to elicit pertinent medical history. Preoperative assessment of thoracic surgical patients should be divided into three major components: (a) an assessment of pulmonary function, (b) evaluation of comorbidities and major risk factors, and (c) the development of a strategy for optimization.

TABLE 22.1 Chemotherapy for Non–small and Small Cell Lung Cancer

Chemotherapy	Drugs	Common Side Effects
Alkylating agent (platinum-based)	Carboplatin Cisplatin	Nausea, vomiting, anemia, neutropenia, neurotoxicity, nephrotoxicity
Taxanes	Paclitaxel Docetaxel	Ventricular dysfunction, arrhythmias, pneumonitis, peripheral neuropathies, fluid retention, cutaneous toxicity
Anthracyclines	Doxorubicin Adriamycin	Cardiotoxicity (pericarditis, left ventricular dysfunction, heart failure)
Vinca alkaloids	Vincristine Vinblastine Vinorelbine	Myelosuppression, peripheral neuropathy, myalgias, rare weakness

The preoperative assessment of pulmonary function should include a thorough physical examination along with pertinent tests and imaging to assess respiratory mechanics, gas exchange, and cardiopulmonary interaction. During the physical examination, an assessment of general appearance, muscle wasting, neck circumference, digit clubbing, cyanosis, respiratory rate and pattern, respiratory effort during conversation, and movement provide important information about the patient's pulmonary status.[10] Symptoms of cough (i.e., frequency), sputum production, dyspnea with and without activity, and recent pulmonary infections can reveal the severity of pulmonary disease.

Pulmonary function tests (PFTs) provide useful information regarding respiratory mechanics and gas exchange. Specific measurements from the PFT correlate with poor postoperative outcomes. The most valid test for postthoracotomy respiratory complications is the predicted postoperative FEV_1.[11] The FEV_1 is a measurement of the volume of air expelled from a person's lung in 1 s. The predicted postoperative FEV_1 ($ppoFEV_1$) is calculated by determining the amount of functional lung remaining after lung resection. A simple approach to calculating the postoperative FEV_1 is using the following formula[12]:

$ppoFEV_1\ \% = \text{preoperative } FEV_1\% \times (1 - \%\text{ functional lung tissue removed}/100)$.

$ppoFEV_1$ is used primarily for risk stratification. A $ppoFEV_1$ value <40% has consistently been associated with an increased risk of respiratory complications. The diffusing capacity for carbon monoxide (DLCO) is another measurement from the PFTs that can predict postoperative outcomes. DLCO represents the gas exchange capacity across the alveolar-capillary membrane. Similar to FEV_1, the predicted postoperative DLCO can be calculated as:

$ppoDLCO\ \% = \text{preoperative } DLCO\% \times (1 - \%\text{ functional lung tissue removed}/100)$.

Brunelli et al. demonstrated that the assessment of DLCO and ppoDLCO was predictive of postoperative morbidity and respiratory complications, even in the presence of normal airflow.[13,14] Of these parameters, a low DLCO is one of the strongest predictors of postoperative pulmonary complications, whereas FEV_1 is not an independent predictor at all.[15] Some investigators argue that the DLCO should be used regardless of the FEV_1.

An additional benefit of PFTs is the ability to demonstrate the presence of reactive airway disease, which can improve with bronchodilators. The use of bronchodilators is warranted in patients with a favorable response to bronchodilators in PFTs. A cardiopulmonary exercise test (CPET) may be performed to assess oxygen uptake as well as cardiopulmonary reserve and is notably a better predictor of postoperative pulmonary complications than resting cardiac and pulmonary function tests alone.[16] A maximum oxygen consumption (Vo_{2max}) <10 mL/kg/min is associated with a postoperative mortality rate of 4% after thoracic surgery and a cutoff value of 20 mL/kg/min is strongly recommended for pneumonectomy.[17]

Further investigation with special imaging studies is suggested for large pulmonary resections (bilobectomy and pneumonectomy). The use of a ventilation/perfusion lung scan (V/Q scan) provides detailed information about the distribution of perfusion to both lungs. The scan is achieved with the inhalation of radioactive xenon along with the injection of technetium-labeled macroaggregates, and the percentage of radioactivity taken up by each lung correlates with the contribution of that lung to overall function.[18] FEV_1 can also be determined from a V/Q scan and a predicted postoperative FEV_1 value can be calculated from these.

Imaging plays an important role in the preoperative assessment of endobronchial invasion and the involvement of vascular structures. Chest radiography is typically performed as the initial imaging modality. This imaging modality provides an assessment of irregularities in the lung parenchyma, pleural effusions, and mediastinal shift. CT scans provide detailed information about the lung parenchyma (i.e., presence of bullae), the presence of airway compression, and/or endobronchial lesions. A review of multiple imaging modalities can assist in developing a concrete anesthetic plan.

A major component in the preoperative evaluation is preparing a risk-reduction strategy based on the patient's comorbidities and risk factors to prevent postoperative complications. Beyond pulmonary evaluation, an assessment of cardiac history should be performed. Perioperative

TABLE 22.2 Immunotherapy for Lung Cancer

Immunotherapy	Mechanism of Action	Example of Drugs
Immune checkpoint inhibitors	Monoclonal antibodies target specific receptor-ligand pathways on T cells.	Nivolumab Durvalumab Pembrolizumab Atezolizumab
CAR-T cells	T cells are removed from the patient and genetically modified to express specific chimeric antigen receptors. Modified cells are cloned and given back to the patient to elicit an immune response.	PD-L1 CAR-T cells (currently under investigation)[a]
Monoclonal antibodies	Antibodies targeting specific antigens (growth factors).	Cetuximab (EGF) Bevacizumab (VEGF) Erlotinib (VEGF) Gefitinib (EGFR)
Nonspecific immunotherapies	No specific targets. Use of cytokines to boost immune system or slow angiogenesis.	IL-2 Interferon α & β
Cancer vaccines	Exposure to tumor antigens activates memory T cells and B cells.	CIMAvax Epidermal Growth Factor vaccine[a]

CAR-T cells, Chimeric antigen receptor T cells; *EGF*, epidermal growth factor; *EGFR*, EGF receptor; IL, interleukin; PD-L1, programmed-death ligand 1; *VEGF*, vascular epidermal growth factor.

[a]No FDA approval.

cardiovascular risk factors should be assessed and evaluated with further testing, if required. Patients with good functional capacity (>4 metabolic equivalents [METS]) do not require further testing. Patients with poor functional capacity (<4 METS) and/or a known history of ischemic heart disease or heart failure should undergo a pharmacologic stress test. The results of the stress test will determine whether coronary revascularization is necessary.

Other pathologic conditions associated with increased perioperative risks, that can be treated and optimized while awaiting surgery include anemia, malnutrition, frailty, chronic obstructive pulmonary disease, alcohol consumption, and active smoking.[19,20] Anemia and malnutrition are common among cancer patients, and the correction of these derangements can significantly improve clinical outcomes. The underlying causes of anemia should be investigated and appropriately treated. Oral iron supplementation and the use of erythropoietin may benefit specific populations but are not without risk. In most cases, immune-enhancing nutritional supplements may be sufficient to address anemia and malnutrition if initiated in advance. Additionally, preoperative smoking cessation and inspiratory muscle training are encouraged to optimize pulmonary function prior to surgery. A comprehensive review of modifiable and nonmodifiable risk factors should be performed to optimize perioperative planning.

Intraoperative Management

The intraoperative management of lung cancer patients continues to present a unique set of challenges for anesthesiologists. The use of protective ventilation strategies, analgesia, and judicious fluid management is essential to permit fast and functional recovery after surgery. In this section we discuss intraoperative management with special attention to airway management, ventilation strategies, analgesia, and fluid management.

Monitoring

Thoracic surgery requires the use of standard ASA monitors and adequate intravenous access prior to anesthesia induction. Large-bore intravenous access is required, and a central venous catheter (CVC) should be strongly considered in patients with poor peripheral access to ensure adequate fluid resuscitation. The use of invasive monitoring depends on the extent of lung resection and the presence of significant comorbidities. An arterial line is generally indicated for major anatomic lung resections (i.e., lobectomy, bilobectomy, and pneumonectomy). An arterial line is highly recommended in patients with a significant history of cardiac or pulmonary disease (i.e., history of myocardial ischemia or congestive heart failure), regardless of the extent of lung resection. An arterial line permits the measurement of dynamic indices to assess fluid responsiveness. In thoracic surgery, the interpretation of dynamic indices may alter with changes in intrathoracic pressure with an open chest and chest insufflation. Transesophageal echocardiography (TEE) is a valuable imaging modality that can be combined with dynamic indices from the arterial line to provide additional information on fluid status and ventricular function in patients with significant coronary artery disease and/or low ejection fractions.

Airway Management

Airway management for thoracic surgery requires substantial planning prior to anesthesia induction. A thorough history and physical examination may predict the degree of difficulty in airway management. A history of head and neck cancer is common in lung cancer patients. Prior head and neck surgery and radiation can distort the airway anatomy, posing a challenge for airway management. The presence of a tracheostomy or a preexisting stoma may preclude the use of specific airway devices.

Double-lumen tubes are the preferred airway devices for one-lung ventilation (OLV) for thoracic surgery. Left- and right-sided double-lumen tubes are available but left-sided double-lumen tubes are preferred because the right upper lobe orifice remains unobstructed. Right-sided lumen tubes offer the advantage of an additional orifice to ventilate the right upper lobe but they can inadvertently obstruct the right upper lumen if not directly positioned. Anatomic variations of the right upper lobe bronchus contribute to the difficult positioning of a right-sided double-lumen tube. While the use of double-lumen tubes is common, there are clinical circumstances that prevent their use. Double-lumen tubes are relatively contraindicated in the following conditions[21]:

- A difficult airway
- Preexisting stoma from tracheostomy
- Tracheal narrowing
- Distorted anatomy from an obstructing lesion in the airway
- Limited mouth opening

Bronchial blockers are an alternative to the double lumen and should be considered in the clinical circumstances above. Bronchial blockers are used with a single-lumen tube and can be inserted on the inside or outside of the endotracheal tube depending on the size of the endotracheal tube. Bronchial blockers offer distinct advantages in the following clinical cases:

- Pediatric patients (small airway)
- Difficult airways (i.e., head and neck radiation, cervical spine injury)
- A long surgical duration (i.e., esophagectomy) with the potential risk of postoperative ventilation, minimizing the loss of airway from an airway exchange
- Patients unable to tolerate prolonged apnea (i.e., a ventilated ICU patient)

The disadvantages are the difficult placement, risk of displacement, slow collapse of the isolated lung, and inability to suction the operative lung. Both airway devices have advantages and disadvantages. The ultimate choice of a double-lumen tube compared to a bronchial blocker will depend on multiple factors, and the use of specific airway devices should be discussed with the surgeon prior to induction of anesthesia.

Induction and Maintenance

The choice of anesthetic drugs for induction and maintenance should decrease the stress response to surgery and allow for fast recovery times. The use of volatiles over an intravenous anesthetic in thoracic surgery is a contentious issue. Inflammatory markers are known to increase in the ventilated lung after the initiation of OLV but the evidence on whether the choice of volatile or intravenous agents contributes to inflammation during thoracic surgery remains unclear. Schilling et al. demonstrated the comparative effect of sevoflurane, desflurane, or propofol on patients undergoing OLV and found that patients receiving either desflurane or sevoflurane experienced lower levels of inflammatory markers in bronchoalveolar lavage (BAL) samples compared to those receiving propofol.[22,23] The use of desflurane and sevoflurane suppresses the local alveolar but not the systemic inflammatory response to OLV. Based on these findings, there is no clear advantage from a clinical standpoint, and the use of intravenous versus inhalation agents should be made at the discretion of the anesthesiologist.

Pain Management

Pain after thoracic surgery is one of the most severe types of postoperative pain. Inadequate pain relief can lead to immobility, ineffective breathing, and poor clearing of secretions, resulting in an increased incidence of postoperative atelectasis, pneumonia, and pulmonary embolism.[24] Effective analgesia improves respiratory mechanics and increases the success of extubation after surgery. The use of regional anesthesia and opioid and non-opioid pharmacologic agents provides a diverse range of options for pain control. Epidural analgesia has long been established as the gold standard for pain management during thoracic surgery, and an epidural confers a variety of benefits. A major advantage of thoracic epidural analgesia (TEA) is the reduction of systemic opioids during surgery, which decreases the risk of opioid-induced respiratory depression. Respiratory depression suppresses the cough reflex and increases the risk of pulmonary infections due to retention of secretions. The risk of respiratory depression is low in the presence of an epidural catheter. Epidural analgesia provides effective pain relief and increases patient participation in controlled cough techniques. Potential complications of TEA include the development of a hematoma or abscess and should be carefully monitored during the postoperative period.

Although epidural catheter placement remains the gold standard for pain control in lung surgery, the use of peripheral nerve blocks is gaining increasing popularity for pain management, including paravertebral nerve blocks, serratus anterior plane (SAP) block, erector spinae plane (ESP) block, midtransverse process to pleura (MTP) block, and intercostal (ICB) nerve blocks. The benefit of peripheral nerve blocks is the ability to perform a unilateral block with minimal risk of bleeding. Of these nerve blocks, paravertebral nerve blocks have been well studied in the literature. When pain was compared between paraverterbral block (PVB) and TEA at rest and during coughing, results showed that there was a significant difference in favor of PVB up to 72 h after thoracotomy.[25] Studies have consistently demonstrated that paravertebral nerve blocks are an effective alternative to epidural analgesia for postthoracotomy pain but with a more beneficial side effect profile.[26,27] A 2016 systematic review confirmed that PVB had a better minor complication profile than thoracic epidural including hypotension (8 studies, 445 participants; relative risk [RR], 0.16; 95% confidence interval [CI], 0.07–0.38, $P < 0.0001$), nausea and vomiting

(6 studies, 345 participants; RR, 0.48; 95% CI, 0.30–0.75; $P = 0.001$), pruritus (5 studies, 249 participants; RR, 0.29; 95% CI, 0.14–0.59; $P = 0.0005$), and urinary retention (5 studies, 258 participants; RR, 0.22; 95% CI, 0.1–0.46, $P < 0.0001$).[28] Paravertebral nerve blocks have also been described in pain management for minimally invasive thoracic surgery. However, serratus nerve blocks and erector spinae nerve blocks are emerging as suitable alternatives for minimally invasive thoracic surgery because these blocks are safe and easier to perform with distinct landmarks. Few studies on the use of ultrasound-guided serratus nerve blocks have demonstrated a significant reduction in intraoperative opioid consumption and emergence time compared to general anesthesia alone in patients who underwent video-assisted thoracic surgery (VATS) lobectomy.[29] The literature on erector spinae blocks in thoracic surgery is limited, and more research is needed. Intercostal nerve blocks are not frequently performed in the preoperative setting but are easily performed by surgeons under direct visualization for thoracotomy and minimally invasive surgery in patients with major contraindications for neuraxial anesthesia. Finally, these newer fascial blocks can be reserved for use as a rescue block in the event of a conversion of a minimally invasive surgery to an open thoracotomy until an epidural can be placed safely in the postoperative period.

Besides the use of regional anesthesia, non-opioid adjuvants are favored to further minimize the use of opioids. The addition of dexmedetomidine and ketamine infusions enhances analgesia. Dexmedetomidine has been shown to reduce opioid consumption in patients after minimally invasive and open thoracic surgery. Lee et al. showed that pain scores, opioid consumption, the incidence of postoperative nausea and vomiting as well as emergence agitation were significantly reduced with the addition of a dexmedetomidine infusion during VATS.[30] A recent randomized controlled study confirmed that the use of dexmedetomidine in conjunction with a thoracic epidural amplified its effect after open thoracotomy with a reduction in pain scores and total analgesic dose.[31] Intravenous acetaminophen and ketorolac are routinely administered to reduce the use of opioids provided no renal and liver abnormalities are present. In summary, the management of pain in thoracic surgical patients requires a multifaceted approach with the concomitant use of opioids, nonopioid adjuvants, and regional anesthesia to ensure optimal pain control.

Ventilation Strategies

Pulmonary complications have been a leading cause of significant morbidity and mortality after thoracic surgery.[32] Pulmonary complications include atelectasis, pneumonia, empyema, pulmonary embolism, bronchopleural fistulas, and acute respiratory failure. Many of these complications have declined with the use of antibiotic prophylaxis, improvements in analgesia, implementation of protective ventilation strategies, and postoperative chest physiotherapy. Among pulmonary complications, acute lung injury (ALI) remains high, with an incidence reported as 2%–7% in large cohort studies.[33–35] The mortality associated with lung injury is reported to be as high as 50%.[36] The causes of ALI are often multifactorial, with surgical trauma, ventilator-induced injury, and fluid overload identified as contributing factors.

Mechanical ventilation is consistently recognized as an important risk factor for perioperative ALI. Lung overinflation, hypoxia/hyperoxia with oxidative stress, and reperfusion injuries from mechanical ventilation increase the release of proinflammatory mediators contributing to alveolar injury.[37–39] The use of protective ventilation is paramount to reducing the risk of complications after thoracic surgery. The use of lower tidal volumes, recruitment maneuvers, and the application of peak-end expiratory pressure (PEEP) have been widely recognized as core elements in protective ventilation for two-lung ventilation. It has long been established that protective lung strategies reduce pulmonary complications in nonthoracic surgery. Research on protective lung strategies for OLV has lagged, but significant advances have been made over the last decade.

The basic principles of protective ventilation strategies are to minimize barotrauma, atelectrauma, and biotrauma related to OLV. Licker et al. evaluated the impact of a protective lung strategy protocol using a combination of tidal volumes <8 mL/kg predicted body weight, inspiratory plateau pressures <35 cmH_2O, PEEP 4–10 cmH_2O, and the use of recruitment maneuvers on clinical outcomes. This study revealed a lower incidence of ALI in the protective ventilation group than in the conventional ventilation group (0.9% vs. 3.7%, $P < 0.01$).[40] These findings provide a foundation for further research on OLV. Blank et al. demonstrated that the concomitant use of low tidal volumes and sufficient PEEP to prevent overdistension, atelectasis and decruitment protected the lung from iatrogenic injury.[41] Within this study, the authors also explored the relationship between driving pressure and respiratory outcome.

Driving pressure is a surrogate for dynamic lung strain and can be defined as the difference between the plateau pressure of the airways at end-inspiration ($P_{PLAT,rs}$) and PEEP.[42,43] Alternatively, driving pressure is calculated as $\Delta P = V_T$/compliance of the respiratory system or lung. Blank et al. demonstrated that for every unit increase in driving pressure (~ 1 cmH_2O), there was a 3.4% increase in the risk of major morbidity. The incidence of postoperative pulmonary complications was reported to be 5.5% in driving pressure-guided ventilation compared to 12.2% in patients with conventional protective ventilation during thoracic surgery.[44] These research findings will change the current recommendations for protective lung ventilation and encourage anesthesiologists to use driving pressure-guided ventilation.

Special attention should be given to ventilator settings for specific patient populations. Cancer patients with prior exposure to bleomycin have a risk of lung injury during OLV. A higher FiO_2 is often required to prevent hypoxemia during

OLV, and anesthesiologists may need to tolerate a lower oxygen saturation with a lower Fio_2 in patients on bleomycin. Patients with restrictive lung disease may require the addition of PEEP to reduce atelectasis and pulmonary shunting during OLV. In contrast, chronic obstructive pulmonary disease (COPD) may develop auto-PEEP during OLV, increasing the risk of hyperinflation and increased shunt.[45] The presence of bulla within lung parenchyma may require the avoidance of nitrous oxide, ventilation at lower pressures and tidal volumes, increased expiratory time, and permissive hypercapnia.[46] Permissive hypercapnia is generally well-tolerated and anesthesiologists should refrain from adjusting ventilator settings to normalize end-tidal CO_2. Wei et al. demonstrated that therapeutic hypercapnia during OLV not only improves respiratory function but also mitigates the OLV-related local and systemic inflammation in patients undergoing lung resection.[47] Hypercapnia may not be safe in specific patient populations. Hypercarbia increases tachycardia, contractility, and systolic blood pressure, and decreases systemic vascular resistance, which could be detrimental to patients with a significant cardiac history. Therefore, a protective lung strategy during OLV should be carefully performed to minimize complications in patients with significant comorbidities.

Fluid Management

While ventilation strategies impact postoperative outcomes, proper fluid management is equally important to consider during thoracic surgery. Fluid management during thoracic surgery remains a challenge for anesthesiologists. The risk of fluid overload and tissue edema must be balanced against the risk of hypovolemia and end-organ ischemia.[48] Fluid restriction protects against pulmonary complications after thoracic surgery but increases the potential risk of acute kidney injury. Wu et al. performed a retrospective study to examine the impact of the following fluid regimens on postoperative outcomes: restrictive (Q1) ≤9.4 mL/kg/h; moderate (Q2) =9.4–11.8 mL/kg/h, moderately liberal (Q3) ≥11.8–14.2 mL/kg/h, and liberal (Q4) >14.2 mL/kg/h.[49] The study found that restrictive and liberal fluid regimens were associated with poor outcomes, and that a moderate administration rate (9.4–11.8 mL/kg/h) had the lowest incidence of postoperative pneumonia and postoperative pulmonary complications.

The use of crystalloids and colloids in thoracic surgery remains controversial. Ishikawa et al. showed that colloids increase postoperative acute kidney injury, leading to a higher rate of pulmonary complications and prolonged hospitalization.[50,51] In contrast, Wu et al. demonstrated that an intraoperative colloid infusion of hetastarch at a rate of >3.8 mL/kg/h was associated with a lower incidence of postoperative pulmonary complications without increasing the risk of postoperative acute kidney injury. The research on fluid management does not provide clear evidence to support the use of crystalloid or colloid alone. The best approach is to maintain a balanced use of colloids and crystalloids during surgery.

There has been a growing interest in goal-directed fluid therapy to assess fluid status and reduce the risk of fluid overload. Static and dynamic indices (stroke volume, cardiac output, pulse pressure variation, and stroke volume variation) are used to assess fluid status. These dynamic indices should be interpreted with caution during thoracic surgery because an open chest, chest insufflation, depth of tidal volume, and the presence of PEEP can disrupt the heart-lung interaction, which is the major determinant of these indices.

Special Considerations

Minimally Invasive/Robotic-Assisted Thoracic Surgery

As the volume of minimally invasive surgery increases, anesthesia management deserves special consideration. During minimally invasive surgery and robotic surgery, the thoracic cavity is insufflated with carbon dioxide, creating an artificial pneumothorax. The insufflation of carbon dioxide impairs ventilation and increases intrathoracic pressure, posing a challenge for ventilation. Higher inspiratory pressure may be necessary to achieve a suitable tidal volume. Therefore protective ventilation strategies should be implemented. In some cases, the absorption of carbon dioxide from the chest cavity can lead to significant hypercarbia, requiring an increase in minute ventilation. Physiologic changes from carbon dioxide insufflation increase tachycardia. If hypercarbia does not decrease with an increase in ventilation rate, the anesthesiologist should notify the surgeon and consider immediate desufflation to reduce the accumulation of carbon dioxide.

Perioperative fluid administration should be maintained at a minimum. If hypotension occurs, anesthesiologists should first assess the surgical field to rule out mechanical compression of cardiac structures from surgical manipulation, which can precipitate sudden hypotension and arrhythmias. The use of crystalloids and colloids should be used judiciously under these circumstances but vasopressors should be initiated if adequate fluid resuscitation is achieved.

The major benefit of minimally invasive surgery is a reduction in pain due to smaller surgical incisions. The use of epidural analgesia for these procedures has declined and the use of novel regional techniques is increasing.

Postoperative Management

Prior to admission to the postoperative anesthesia care unit (PACU), patients should meet standard criteria for extubation. Prior to extubation, patients may require bronchoscopy for suction and irrigation of excessive secretions. The combination of albuterol and ipratropium in nebulizer treatment may benefit patients after extubation. The fluid should be carefully titrated to further reduce the risk of ALI. Vasopressors should be used judiciously to avoid excessive fluid administration. A range of complications can develop shortly after thoracic surgery, including hemorrhage, lobar torsion, pulmonary edema, ischemia, cardiac herniation, and heart failure. These complications vary in presentation and require vigilance during the postoperative period. The most common complication after thoracic surgery is the development of arrhythmias, with 20% of patients developing atrial fibrillation.[52,53] Atrial fibrillation develops on postoperative day 3 and is typically transient. Electrical cardioversion is generally recommended for patients with hemodynamic instability. Otherwise, atrial fibrillation should be managed with pharmacologic agents and the goal should be rate control with the use of beta blockers and calcium channel blockers. Persistent atrial fibrillation may require chemical cardioversion with amiodarone or flecainide.

During the postoperative period, a multimodal approach to pain should continue with the use of regional anesthesia and nonopioid adjuvants (gabapentin, acetaminophen, and ibuprofen). The use of intravenous opioid patient-controlled analgesia is an option for rescue breakthrough pain but opioids should be used with caution to avoid excessive sedation and respiratory complications. In addition to effective analgesia, chest physiotherapy and early mobilization are important to reduce the risk of atelectasis, pneumonia, and deep vein thrombosis (DVT). DVT prophylaxis with subcutaneous heparin should be initiated as soon as it is safe after surgery.

Mediastinal Masses

Introduction

Advancements in chemotherapy, radiation, and other treatment modalities have led to improved care for cancer patients in the perioperative period. Many mediastinal tumors previously perceived as incurable have a good prognosis. Therefore it is not uncommon to encounter a patient with a mediastinal mass for a diagnostic procedure or staging either in the operating or nonoperating room setting. There are many challenges presented to anesthesiologists, especially the exacerbation of airway compromise and cardiovascular collapse, which can lead to a fatal outcome. Knowledge of anatomy, pathophysiology, understanding the anesthetic implications, and potential complications are key to successful perioperative management of the patient with a mediastinal mass.

Normal Anatomy and Pathology

The mediastinum is a wide space between the two pleural sacs of the chest cavity and extends from the thoracic inlet to the diaphragm. It is divided into the upper or superior mediastinum and lower, which contains the anterior, middle, and posterior mediastinum (Fig. 22.2).

The superior mediastinum is bounded superiorly by the thoracic inlet at the sternal notch, laterally by the mediastinal pleura of the lungs, anteriorly by the manubrium sternum, posteriorly by the thoracic vertebrae, and inferiorly to the level of the 4th thoracic vertebra at the manubriosternal joint. It contains the great vessels, trachea, esophagus,

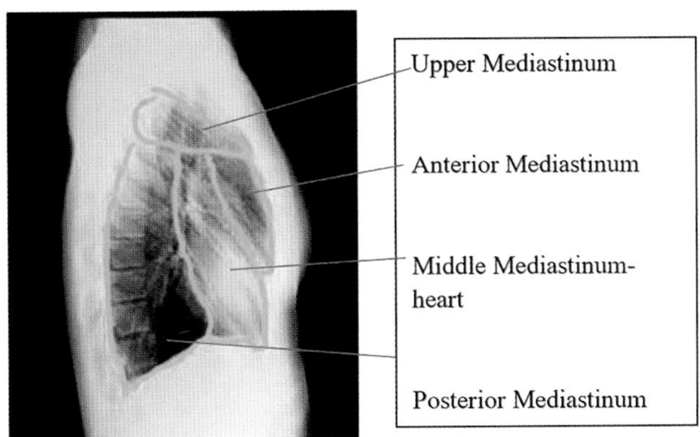

• **Fig. 22.2** Compartments of the mediastinum. American Joint Committee on Cancer: Lung Cancer Staging 7th ed.

thoracic duct, thymus, recurrent laryngeal and phrenic nerves, and lymph nodes.

The anterior mediastinum forms the space between the body of the sternum anteriorly, parietal pericardium posteriorly, and diaphragm inferiorly. It contains the lymph nodes and remnants of the thymus and thyroid glands.

The middle mediastinum contains the heart at the beginning of the great vessels and phrenic nerves.

The posterior mediastinum extends from the posterior pericardium and lower diaphragm anteriorly, posteriorly from the 4th to 12th thoracic vertebrae, and laterally to the mediastinal pleura on both sides. It contains the thoracic descending aorta, azygos veins, tracheal bifurcation and main bronchi, esophagus, thoracic duct, and lymph nodes.[54–60]

Incidence and Location

The incidence of mediastinal masses and locations by compartments are shown in Fig. 22.3.[61–63]

Clinical Presentation

The clinical presentation of a patient with a mediastinal mass can range from asymptomatic to life threatening. The most common presenting symptoms are chest pain, dyspnea, cough, and fever. Cardiovascular compromise depends on the location of the mass. Right heart and pulmonary artery compression can manifest as acute right heart failure, hypotension, arrhythmia, dyspnea, and syncope.[64] Left heart compression by a tumor manifests as hemodynamic instability.[65] Superior vena cava (SVC) syndrome is a serious complication caused by obstruction of venous drainage, resulting in symptoms of headache, visual changes, acute facial swelling, dyspnea, and cough. Compression of the bronchial tree can result in respiratory distress; the symptoms vary with different positions and increase when supine.[66]

Systemic manifestations of a mediastinal mass such as myasthenia gravis or thyroid disease may occur. Lesser symptoms can occur from esophageal compression, dysphagia, Horner's syndrome from compression of the sympathetic chain, or a range of neurologic symptoms when

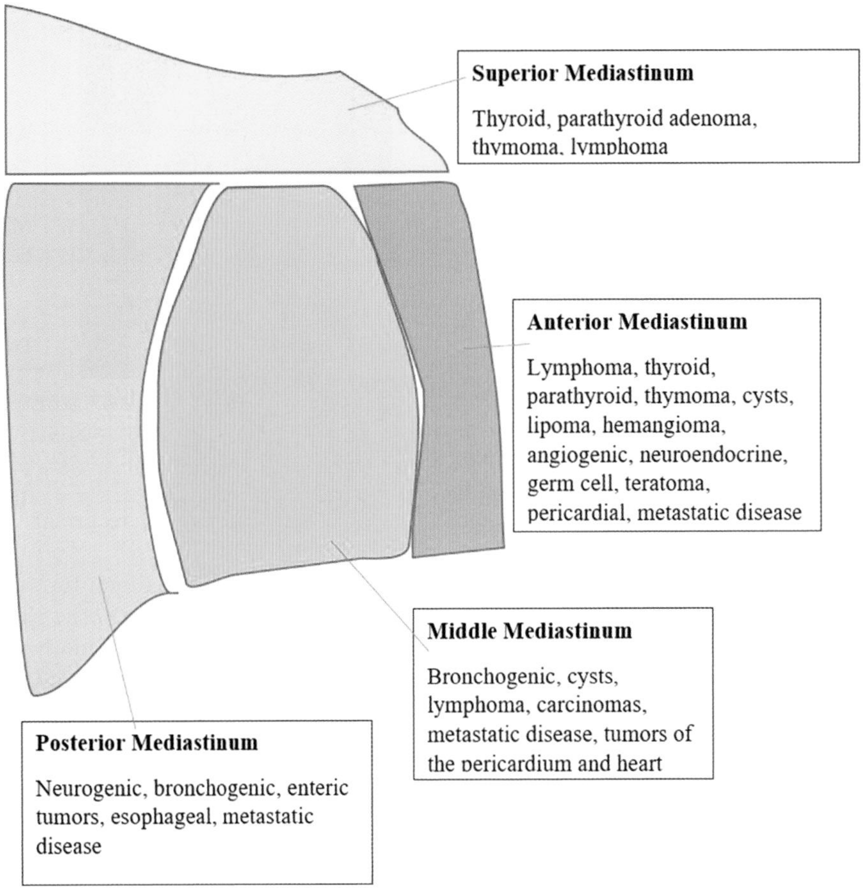

• **Fig. 22.3** Tumors of the mediastinum; incidence and location by compartments.

compression involves the spinal cord. If the recurrent laryngeal nerve is involved, vocal cord paralysis with voice changes may be the presenting symptom.[67,68]

Preoperative Evaluation

Initial evaluation of the above presenting symptoms will be via chest x-ray. Once a mediastinal mass is suspected, a CT scan best evaluates the size, location, compression, extent, and invasiveness of the disease in correlation with the bronchial tree, vascular structures, and chambers of the heart. MRI is indicated if contrast material for CT scan is contraindicated. Transthoracic echocardiography to evaluate cardiac function should be performed if pericardial effusion or invasion of cardiac structures is observed on CT scan. Lung function tests differentiate extrathoracic from intrathoracic obstruction; however, in patients with mediastinal masses, these studies poorly correlate with the degree of airway obstruction and do not influence anesthetic management.[69–74]

Diagnostic Techniques and Anesthetic Implications

Obtaining a tissue diagnosis is paramount to guide treatment. In a symptomatic patient with a large anterior mediastinal mass, a percutaneous CT-guided biopsy performed under local anesthesia is a relatively safe and effective approach.[75] Other procedures under local anesthesia are equally effective at obtaining a tissue diagnosis but may be more invasive: anterior mediastinotomy, endobronchial ultrasound-guided transbronchial (EBUS) needle aspiration. It is occasionally necessary to perform a biopsy through a surgical incision requiring general anesthesia, in which case anesthetic considerations and cardiopulmonary risk factors are the same as those for mediastinoscopy. The risk of cardiopulmonary collapse is significant with a large mediastinal mass.[76] In these patients, pretreatment with radiation therapy or steroids to reduce the mass effect on the cardiopulmonary system may be considered. However, studies have shown that performing these pretreatment modalities before obtaining a tissue diagnosis can affect histologic accuracy before starting treatment. The risk of cardiopulmonary collapse under general anesthesia for a diagnostic procedure must be weighed against the risk of an imprecise histologic diagnosis in the setting of pretreatment.

Anesthetic Management

Anesthetic management starts with a detailed assessment of the mass effect on the cardiopulmonary system, PFTs if applicable, and echocardiographic findings if cardiac involvement is suspected. All comorbidities should be evaluated.

A discussion is had with the surgeon regarding the type of tumor, the degree of cardiopulmonary compromise, surgical approach, anesthetic technique, placement of central venous catheter access, and other options available. The guiding principle is that general anesthesia reduces lung volumes and that neuromuscular blockers lead to the relaxation of bronchial smooth muscles, making the airway more susceptible to compression from the mass. Paralysis of the diaphragm by muscle relaxants leads to a decrease in airway diameter because the normal transpleural pressure keeping the airway open is reduced. As a result, the airway is more susceptible to collapse from extrinsic compression by the mass.[77–79] A preinduction A-line should be placed for invasive monitoring of blood pressure in the setting of possible hemodynamic instability. Induction proceeds in a position that is most comfortable for the patient, preferably with mild head elevation. Induction and intubation techniques should consider the degree of respiratory compromise, as well as preserve right ventricular filling and cardiac contractility.[80] If the patient is asymptomatic, routine intravenous induction with direct laryngoscopy for intubation is acceptable. Ketamine is a good choice as it maintains cardiac function and acts as a bronchodilator. In symptomatic patients, inhalational or awake fiberoptic is the technique of choice. Maintaining spontaneous ventilation throughout the induction phase is the safest airway management technique, without the detrimental effects of general anesthesia. This avoids complete airway obstruction by upholding normal transpulmonary pressure and preserving airway patency. Inhalational induction should be used with caution as it may trigger total or partial supraglottic airway obstruction, initiating negative pressure large enough to cause collapse of the trachea. In obese patients this technique may be limited.[81] Awake fiberoptic intubation allows for the assessment of the airway, the level of tracheobronchial compression, and identification of the least compressed bronchus in case of rescue ventilation due to severe pulmonary compromise. Intubation distal to the obstruction achieves adequate ventilation using a single lumen endotracheal tube or a double-lumen tube if lung isolation during surgery is required. Occasionally, this is not possible and other measures are considered. Rigid bronchoscopy by an experienced surgeon and jet ventilation should always be on standby to assess the possible stenting of the most patent airway. In cases of severe respiratory compromise maintaining spontaneous ventilation and bronchoscopy-guided intubation through a laryngeal mask airway is an option. Airway obstruction, hypoxemia, and hemodynamic instability may develop after intubation, and a return to spontaneous ventilation and/or a change in the position of the patient relieves the symptoms. Occasionally, this is unsuccessful, in which case the surgeon may be required to perform an emergent sternotomy and lift the mass away from the airway and heart to relieve the symptoms. The maintenance of spontaneous ventilation cannot be overemphasized if there is uncertainty in achieving successful endotracheal intubation. If spontaneous ventilation is tolerated, gradual manual overventilation should be attempted. If this is well tolerated, a neuromuscular blocking agent and positive pressure ventilation may proceed. If there is doubt, continue with spontaneous ventilation and occasional assisted ventilation.[82–84]

Special Considerations

Anesthesia for Mediastinoscopy

Cervical mediastinoscopy and anterior mediastinoscopy are two surgical procedures used to access the anterior mediastinum to obtain tissue for the histologic diagnosis of mediastinal masses. Anterior mediastinoscopy is performed via the left second rib interspace through a small incision just lateral to the sternum and may be performed under local or general anesthesia. Cervical mediastinoscopy is performed with an incision at the suprasternal notch, and a mediastinoscope is inserted under the manubrium sterni. The mediastinoscope is inserted near major vessels, trachea, and nerves, and can cause severe complications. General anesthesia should be performed using standard monitoring and a single-lumen endotracheal tube. The noninvasive blood pressure cuff should be placed on the left arm with access to palpate the right radial artery in case of compression of the innominate artery, which can lead to cerebrovascular events if left undetected. For this reason, perfusion of the right arm should be monitored with a pulse oximeter or placement of an arterial catheter line for invasive blood pressure monitoring. If there is a potential for hemorrhage, large-bore intravenous or central venous access in the lower extremities and invasive blood pressure monitoring should be placed, as well as blood available for transfusion. Although the incidence of major hemorrhage is low, it can be life threatening. The most commonly injured blood vessels are the azygos, innominate, and pulmonary arteries. Emergency sternotomy or thoracotomy may be necessary in cases of massive bleeding. Initial control may be achieved through packing by the surgeon, while massive transfusion protocols and resuscitative efforts are undertaken. If necessary, lung isolation may be achieved with a bronchial blocker through the endotracheal tube, especially in a patient with a difficult airway, as a change to a double-lumen tube may not be the best option in an urgent situation.[85,86]

Other complications of mediastinoscopy include compression of the trachea, compression of the aorta leading to reflex bradycardia, recurrent laryngeal nerve injury, pneumothorax, esophageal injury, and air embolism. Uncomplicated mediastinoscopy procedures may be extubated, a routine chest x-ray performed to rule out pneumothorax, and after meeting the discharge criteria, the patient may be discharged home on the same day.

Superior Vena Cava Syndrome

SVC syndrome is defined as obstruction of venous flow from the head and neck and upper extremities and engorgement of veins that drain into the SVC. The increased pressure in the veins causes decreased flow into the right atrium and an increased incidence of venous thrombosis.

Anesthetic implications vary depending on the patient's symptoms. Cough and dyspnea are common respiratory symptoms. The following should be considered in the perioperative period [66,87–91]:

- Careful airway assessment. Consider preoperative radiotherapy to decrease head and neck and airway edema.
- Induction with head elevation as these patients are at an increased risk of severe airway compromise in the supine position.
- Vascular access to the lower extremities is preferable. Upper extremity vascular access that drains into the SVC should be avoided. Radial arterial monitoring is recommended for all but mild instances of SVC syndrome.
- Induction of anesthesia may lead to decreased venous return and compromised cardiac function. Consider ketamine as an induction agent and have vasopressors readily available.
- Blood available for transfusion.
- Avoid coughing and straining on induction and emergence as this increases venous pressure, leading to cardiorespiratory compromise.

Myasthenia Gravis

Perioperative considerations for patients with myasthenia gravis are the same as those for any mediastinal mass. Specific neurologic considerations related to myasthenia gravis are elaborated on in another chapter.

Perioperative Considerations

The perioperative course can be complicated by airway obstruction, which can occur at any time on induction, during the intraoperative period, and postoperatively. The compressive effects of the mediastinal mass on the airway and heart structures can cause severe hypoxia and hypotension. The more symptomatic the patient the higher the perioperative complication rate. Postoperatively, upper airway edema and stridor are significant risks, especially in patients with SVC syndrome. Extubation of the airway should proceed with the patient fully awake, obeying commands, and fully recovered from muscle relaxants. Postsurgical risks, including hemorrhage and respiratory dysfunction requiring re-intubation and potential supportive measures, have been reported to be as high as 10.5%. Attempts to identify risk factors for predicting perioperative complications in patients with a mediastinal mass have been inconsistent. However, respiratory symptoms, especially preoperative stridor, have been correlated with an increased risk of airway compromise and general anesthesia. Preoperative tracheal compression of more than 50% on preoperative CT scan combined with an obstructive and restrictive pattern on PFTs are significant risk factors for postoperative respiratory complications. Preoperative symptomatic patients may benefit from intensive care monitoring in the postoperative period.[91–94]

Conclusion

Anesthesia for mediastinal masses remains a challenge for anesthesiologists. A thorough discussion with the patient, surgeon, and anesthesiologist as to the perioperative plan is vital to minimize risk in the perioperative period. A summary of anesthetic considerations for a patient presenting with a mediastinal mass is shown in Fig 22.4.[77,95–97]

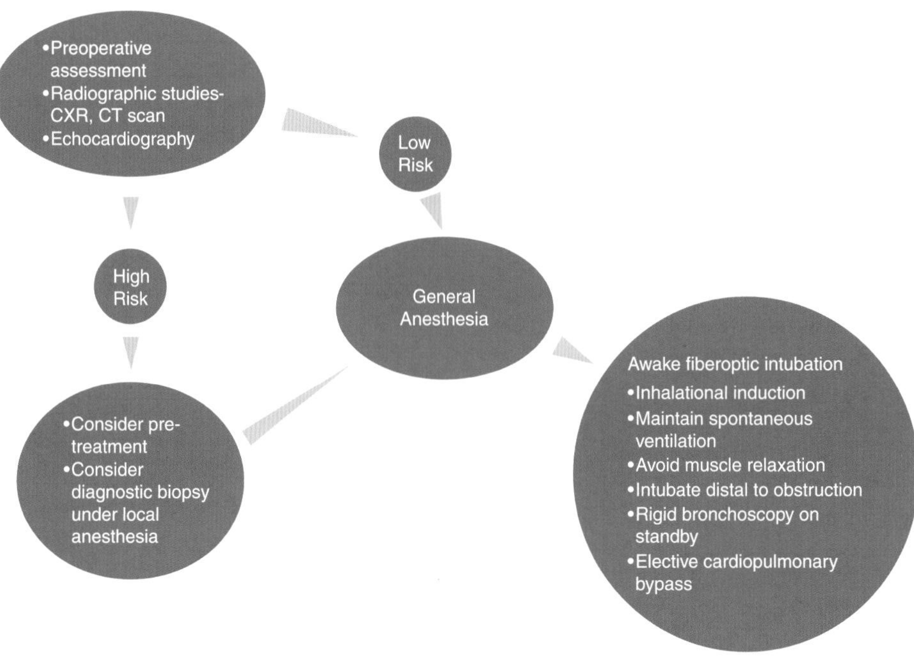

• **Fig. 22.4** Anesthetic consideration for mediastinal masses.

References

1. Jemal A, Bray F, Center MM, et al. Global cancer statistics. *CA Cancer J Clin*. 2011;61:69–90.
2. Siegel R, Ward E, Brawley O, et al. Cancer statistics, 2011: The impact of eliminating socioeconomic and racial disparities on premature cancer deaths. *CA Cancer J Clin*. 2011;61:212–236.
3. Dela Cruz CS, Tanoue LT, Matthay RA. Lung cancer: Epidemiology, etiology, and prevention. *Clin Chest Med*. 2011;32: 605–644.
4. de Groot P, Munden RF. Lung cancer epidemiology, risk factors and prevention. *Radiol Clin North Am*. 2012;50(5):862–876.
5. *The Health Consequences of Active Smoking: A Report of the Surgeon General*. Atlanta, GA: Department of Health and Human Services, Centers for Disease Control and Prevention, National Center for Chronic Disease Prevention and Health Promotion, Office on Smoking and Health; 2004.
6. Alberg AJ, Brock MV, Ford JG, Samet JM, Spivack SD. Epidemiology of lung cancer: Diagnosis and management of lung cancer, 3rd ed: American College of Chest Physicians evidence-based clinical practice guidelines. *Chest*. 2013;143(5):e1S–e29S.
7. Midthun DE. Early detection of lung cancer. *F1000Research*. 2016;5:F1000 Faculty Rev-739.
8. Aberle DR, Aberle DR, et al. National Lung Screening Trial Research Team Reduced lung-cancer mortality with low-dose computed tomographic screening. *N Engl J Med*. 2011;365:395–409.
9. Sharma D, Newman TG, Aronow WS. Lung cancer screening: history, current perspectives, and future directions. *Arch Med Sci*. 2015;11(5):1033–1043.
10. Bevacqua BK. Preoperative pulmonary evaluation in the patient with suspected respiratory disease. *Indian J Anaesth*. 2015;59:542–549.
11. Preanesthetic assessment for thoracic surgery. In: P. Slinger, ed. *Principles and Practice of Anesthesia for Thoracic Surgery*. Springer; 2011.
12. Lederman D, Easwar J, Feldman J, Shapiro V. Anesthetic considerations for lung resection: preoperative assessment, intraoperative challenges and postoperative analgesia. *Ann Transl Med*. 2019;7(15):356.
13. Brunelli A, Refai MA, Salati M, Sabbatini A, Morgan-Hughes NJ, Rocco G. Carbon monoxide lung diffusion capacity improves risk stratification in patients without airflow limitation: evidence for systematic measurement before lung resection. *Eur J Cardiothorac Surg*. 2006;29:567–570.
14. Brunelli A, Kim AW, Berger KI, et al. Physiologic evaluation of the patient with lung cancer being considered for resectional surgery: diagnosis and management of lung cancer, 3rd ed: American College of Chest Physicians evidence-based clinical practice guidelines. *Chest*. 2013;143(5): Supple166S–e190S.
15. Amar D, Munoz D, Shi W, Zhang H, Thaler HT. A clinical prediction rule for pulmonary complications after thoracic surgery for primary lung cancer. *Anesth Analg*. 2010;110:1343–1348.
16. Van Tilburg PMB, Stam H, Hoogsteden HC, van Klaveren RJ. Pre-operative pulmonary evaluation of lung cancer patients: A review of the literature. *Eur Respir J*. 2009;33:1206–1215.
17. Bechard D, Wetstein L. Assessment of exercise oxygen consumption as preoperative criterion for lung resection. *Ann Thorac Surg*. 1987;44:344–349.
18. Gould G, Pearce A. Assessment of suitability for lung resection. *Contin Educ Anaesth Crit Care Pain*. 2006;6:97–100.
19. Eagle KA, Berger PB, Calkins H, et al. ACC/AHA guideline update for perioperative cardiovascular evaluation for noncardiac surgery—executive summary a report of the American College of Cardiology/American Heart Association Task Force on Practice Guidelines (Committee to Update the 1996 Guidelines on Perioperative Cardiovascular Evaluation for Noncardiac Surgery). *Circulation*. 2002;105:1257–1267.
20. Gagné S, McIsaac DI. Modifiable risk factors for patients undergoing lung cancer surgery and their optimization: a review. *J Thorac Dis*. 2018;10(supple 32):S3761–S3772.
21. Campos JH. Lung isolation techniques for patients with difficult airway. *Curr Opin Anaesthesiol*. 2010;Feb23:12–17 .
22. Schilling T, Kozian A, Senturk M, et al. Effects of volatile and intravenous anesthesia on the alveolar and systemic inflammatory response in thoracic surgical patients. *Anesthesiology*. 2011;115:65–74.
23. O'Gara B, Talmor D. Lung protective properties of the volatile anesthetics. *Intensive Care Med*. 2016;42:1487–1489.
24. Broseta AM, Errando C, De Andrés J, Díaz-Cambronero O, Ortega-Monzó J. Serratus plane block: the regional analgesia technique for thoracoscopy? *Anaesthesia*. 2015;70:1329–1330.
25. Raveglia F, Rizzi A, Leporati A, et al. Analgesia in patients undergoing thoracotomy: epidural versus paravertebral technique. A randomized, double-blind, prospective study. *J Thorac Cardiovasc Surg*. 2014;147:469–474.
26. Davies RG, Myles PS, Graham JM. A comparison of the analgesic efficacy and side-effects of paravertebral vs epidural blockade for thoracotomy—a systematic review and meta-analysis of randomized trials. *Br J Anaesth*. 2006;96:418–426.
27. Ibrahim AI, Mamdouh NM. Comparison between continuous thoracic epidural block and continuous thoracic paravertebral block for thoracotomy pain relief. *Ain Shams J Anesthesiol*. 2009;2:16–26.
28. Yeung JH, Gates S, Naidu BV, Wilson MJ. Gao Smith F. Paravertebral block versus thoracic epidural for patients undergoing thoracotomy. *Cochrane Database Syst Rev*. 2016;2:CD009121.
29. Lee J, Kim S. The effects of ultrasound-guided serratus plane block, in combination with general anesthesia, on intraoperative opioid consumption, emergence time, and hemodynamic stability during video-assisted thoracoscopic lobectomy: a randomized prospective study. *Medicine*. 2019;98:e15385.
30. Lee SH, Lee CY, Lee JG, Kim N, Lee HM, Oh YJ. Intraoperative dexmedetomidine improves the quality of recovery and postoperative pulmonary function in patients undergoing video-assisted thoracoscopic surgery: a CONSORT-prospective, randomized, controlled trial. *Medicine (Baltimore)*. 2016;95:e2854.
31. Choi EJ, Yoon JP, Choi YM, Park JY, Kim HY, Byeon GJ, et al. Intravenous infusion of dexmedetomidine amplifies thoracic epidural analgesic effect after open thoracotomy: a prospective, double-blind, randomized controlled trial. *Medicine*. 2019;98:e17983.
32. Lawrence VA, Cornell JE, Smetana GW. American College of Physicians. Strategies to reduce postoperative pulmonary complications after noncardiothoracic surgery: systematic review for the American College of Physicians. *Ann Intern Med*. 2006;144:596–608.
33. Eichenbaum KD, Neustein SM. Acute lung injury after thoracic surgery. *J Cardiothorac Vasc Anesth*. 2010;24:681–690.

34. Licker M, de Perrot M, Spiliopoulos A, et al. Risk factors for acute lung injury after thoracic surgery for lung cancer. *Anesth Analg*. 2003;97:1558–1565.
35. Licker M, Fauconnet P, Villiger Y, et al. Acute lung injury and outcomes after thoracic surgery. *Curr Opin Anaesthesiol.* 2009;22:61–67.
36. Tandon SP, Batchelor A, Bullock R, et al. Peri-operative risk factors for acute lung injury after elective oesophagectomy. *Br J Anaesth*. 2001;86:633–638.
37. Kilpatrick B, Slinger P. Lung protective strategies in anesthesia. *Br J Anaesth*. 2010;105:i108–i116.
38. Jordan S, Mitchell JA, Quinlan GJ, et al. The pathogenesis of lung injury following pulmonary resection. *Eur Respir J*. 2000;15:790–799.
39. Della Rocca G, Coccia C. Acute lung injury in thoracic surgery. *Curr Opin Anaesthesiol*. 2013;26:40–46.
40. Licker M, Diaper J, Villiger Y, et al. Impact of intraoperative lung-protective interventions in patients undergoing lung cancer surgery. *Crit Care*. 2009;13:R41.
41. Blank RS, Colquhoun DA, Durieux ME, et al. Management of one-lung ventilation: impact of tidal volume on complications after thoracic surgery. *Anesthesiology*. 2016;124:1286–1295.
42. Pelosi P, Ball L. Should we titrate ventilation based on driving pressure? Maybe not in the way we would expect. *Ann Transl Med*. 2018;6:389.
43. Amato MB, Meade MO, Slutsky AS, et al. Driving pressure and survival in the acute respiratory distress syndrome. *N Engl J Med*. 2015;372:747–755.
44. Park M, Ahn HJ, Kim JA, et al. Driving pressure during thoracic surgery: a randomized clinical trial. *Anesthesiology*. 2019;130:385–393.
45. Slinger PD, Kruger M, McRae K, Winton T. Relation of the static compliance curve and positive end-expiratory pressure to oxygenation during one-lung ventilation. *Anesthesiology*. 2001;95:1096–1102.
46. Myles PS, Moloney J. Anesthetic management of a patient with severe bullous lung disease complicated by air leak. *Anaesth Intensive Care*. 1994;22:201–203.
47. Gao W, Liu D-D, Li D, Cui GX. Effect of therapeutic hypercapnia on inflammatory responses to one-lung ventilation in lobectomy patients. *Anesthesiology*. 2015;122:1235–1252.
48. Chau EHL, Slinger P. Perioperative fluid management for pulmonary resection surgery and esophagectomy. *Semin Cardiothorac Vasc Anesth*. 2014;18:36–44.
49. Wu Y, Yang R, Xu J, et al. Effects of intraoperative fluid management on postoperative outcomes after lobectomy. *Ann Thorac Surg*. 2019;107:1663–1669.
50. Ishikawa S, Griesdale DE, Lohser J. Acute kidney injury after lung resection surgery: incidence and perioperative risk factors. *Anesth Analg*. 2012;114:1256–1262.
51. Batirel HF. Fluid administration during lung resection: what is the optimum? *J Thorac Dis*. 2019;11:1746–1748.
52. Amar D. Cardiac arrhythmias. *Chest Surg Clin N Am*. 1998;8:479–493.
53. Asamura H, Naruke T, Tsuchiya R, Goya T, Kondo H, Suemasu K. What are the risk factors for arrhythmias after thoracic operations? A retrospective multivariate analysis of 267 consecutive thoracic operations. *J Thorac Cardiovasc Surg*. 1993;106:1104–1110.
54. Fraser RS, Müller NL, Colman N, Paré PD. The mediastinum. *Fraser and Paré's Diagnosis of Diseases of the Chest*. 4th ed. Philadelphia, PA: Saunders; 1999:pp 196–234.
55. Fraser RG, Paré PA. The normal chest. *Diagnosis of Diseases of the Chest*. 2nd ed. Philadelphia, PA: Saunders; 1977:pp 1–183.
56. Carter BW, Benveniste MF, Madan R., et al. ITMIG classification of mediastinal compartments and multidisciplinary approach to mediastinal masses. Radiographics. 2017;37(2):413–436.
57. Warren WH. Chapter 122. Anatomy of the mediastinum with special reference to surgical access. *Pearson's Thoracic and Esophageal Surgery*. 3rd ed.: Elsevier; 2009:1472.
58. Yoneda KY, Louie S, Shelton DK. Mediastinal tumors. *Curr Opin Pulm Med*. 2001;7:226–233.
59. Juanpere S, Cañete N, Ortuño P, Martínez S, Sanchez G, Bernado L. A diagnostic approach to the mediastinal masses. *Insights Imaging*. 2013;4:29–52.
60. Shields TW. Primary tumors and cysts of the mediastinum. In: Shields TW, ed. *General Thoracic Surgery*. Philadelphia, PA: Lea & Febiger; 1983:pp 927–954.
61. Shahrzad M, Le TSM, Silva M, et al. Anterior mediastinal masses. *Am J Roentgenol*. 2014;203:W128–W138.
62. Dubashi B, Cyriac S, Tenali SG. Clinicopathological analysis and outcome of primary mediastinal malignancies—a report of 91 cases from a single institute. *Ann Thorac Med*. 2009;4:140–142.
63. Davis RDJ, Oldham HNJ, Sabiston DCJ. Primary cysts and neoplasms of the mediastinum: recent changes in clinical presentation, methods of diagnosis, management, and results. *Ann Thorac Surg*. 1987;44:229–237.
64. Dasan J, Littleford J, McRae K, Farine D, Winton T. Mediastinal tumor in a pregnant patient presenting as acute cardiorespiratory compromise. *Int J Obstet Anesth*. 2002;11:52–56.
65. Türköz A, Gülcan O, Tercan F, Koçum T, Türköz R. Hemodynamic collapse caused by a large unruptured aneurysm of the ascending aorta in an 18 year old. *Anesth Analg*. 2006;102:1040–1042.
66. Szokol JW, Alspach D, Mehta MK, Parilla BV, Liptay MJ. Intermittent airway obstruction and superior vena cava syndrome in a patient with an undiagnosed mediastinal mass after cesarean delivery. *Anesth Analg*. 2003;97:883–884.
67. Robie DK, Gursoy MH, Pokorny WJ. Mediastinal tumors—airway obstruction and management. *Semin Pediatr Surg*. 1994;3:259–266.
68. Russell JC, Lowry KG. Presentation of non-Hodgkin's lymphoma as acute hypoxia caused by right ventricular compression. *Anesth Analg*. 2003;96:1768–1771.
69. Slinger PD, Campos JH. Anesthesia for thoracic surgery. In: Miller RD, Eriksson LI, Fleisher LA, Young WL, Wiener-Kronish JP, eds. *Miller's Anesthesia*. 7th ed. Amsterdam: Elsevier; 2009:1856.
70. Shamberger RC, Holzman RS, Griscom NT, Tarbell NJ, Weinstein HJ, Wohl ME. Prospective evaluation by computed tomography and pulmonary function tests of children with mediastinal masses. *Surgery*. 1995;118:468–471.
71. Vander Els NJ, Sorhage F, Bach AM, Straus DJ, White DA. Abnormal flow volume loops in patients with intrathoracic Hodgkin's disease. *Chest*. 2000;117:1256–1261.
72. Hnatiuk OW, Corcoran PC, Sierra A. Spirometry in surgery for anterior mediastinal masses. *Chest*. 2001;120:1152–1156.
73. Kulkarni S, Kulkarni A, Roy D, Thakur MH. Percutaneous computed tomography-guided core biopsy for the diagnosis of mediastinal masses. *Ann Thorac Med*. 2008;3:13–17.
74. Hnatiuk OW, MCLTC, Corcoran PC, Sierra A. Spirometry in surgery for anterior mediastinal masses. *Chest*. 2001;120(4):1152–1156.

75. Dvorak P, Hoffmann P, Kocova E, Habal P, Nova M. CT-guided biopsy of the mediastinal masses. Can anatomical relationships predict complications? *Biomed Pap Med Fac Univ Palacky Olomouc Czech Repub.* 2019; Sep163:220–226 .
76. Béchard P, Letourneau L, Lacasse Y et al., Perioperative cardiorespiratory complications in adults with mediastinal mass: incidence and risk factors. *Anesthesiology.* 2004;100(4):826–834 discussion 5A.
77. Gothard JW. Anesthetic considerations for patients with anterior mediastinal masses. *Anesthesiol Clin.* 2008;26:305–314.
78. Westbrook PR, Stubbs SE, Sessler AD, Rehder K, Hyatt RE. Effects of anesthesia and muscle paralysis on respiratory mechanics in normal man. *J Appl Physiol.* 1973;34:81–86.
79. Bergman NA. Reduction in resting end-expiratory position of the respiratory system with induction of anesthesia and neuromuscular paralysis. *Anesthesiology.* 1982;57:14–17.
80. Sharifian Attar A, Jalaeian Taghaddomi R, Bagheri R. Anesthetic management of patients with anterior mediastinal masses undergoing chamberlain procedure (anterior mediastinostomy). *Iran Red Crescent Med J.* 2013;15:373–374.
81. Abdelmalak B, Marcanthony N, Abdelmalak J, Machuzak MS, Gildea TR, Doyle DJ. Dexmedetomidine for anesthetic management of anterior mediastinal mass. *J Anesth.* 2010;24: 607–610.
82. Slinger P, Karsli C. Management of the patient with a large anterior mediastinal mass: recurring myths. *Curr Opin Anaesthesiol.* 2007;20:1–3.
83. Scher CS, Gitlin MC. Dexmedetomidine and low-dose ketamine provide adequate sedation for awake fibreoptic intubation. *Can J Anaesth.* 2003;50:607–610.
84. Gardner JC, Royster RL. Airway collapse with an anterior mediastinal mass despite spontaneous ventilation in an adult. *Anesth Analg.* 2011;113:239–242.
85. Park BJ, Flores R, Downey RJ, Bains MS, Rusch VW. Management of major hemorrhage during mediastinoscopy. *J Thorac Cardiovasc Surg.* 2003;126:726–731.
86. Lohser J, Donington JS, Mitchell JD, Brodsky JB, Raman J, Slinger P. Case 5-2005 Anesthetic management of major hemorrhage during mediastinoscopy. *J Cardiothorac Vasc Anesth.* 2005;19:678–683.
87. Galatoudis Z, Soumpasis IG, Vretzakis G. Anesthetic considerations for surgery involving clamping of superior vena cava. *Greek J Perioper Med.* 2005;3:49–59.
88. Chaudhary K, Gupta A, Wadhawan S, Jain D, Bhadoria P. Anesthetic management of superior vena cava syndrome due to anterior mediastinal mass. *J Anaesthesiol Clin Pharmacol.* 2012;28:242–246.
89. Wilson LD, Detterbeck FC, Yahalom J. Clinical practice. Superior vena cava syndrome with malignant causes. *N Engl J Med.* 2007;356:1862–1869.
90. Rowell NP, Gleeson FV. Steroids, radiotherapy, chemotherapy and stents for superior vena caval obstruction in carcinoma of the bronchus. *Cochrane Database Syst Rev.* 2001;4:CD001316.
91. Wan JF, Bezjak A. Superior vena cava syndrome. *Emerg Med Clin North Am.* 2009;27:243–255.
92. Kafrouni H, Saroufim J, Abdel Massih M. Intraoperative tracheal obstruction management among patients with anterior mediastinal masses. *Case Rep Med.* 2018;2018:4895263.
93. Thakur P, Bhatia PS, Sitalakshmi N, Virmani P. Anaesthesia for mediastinal mass. *Indian J Anaesth.* 2014;58:215–217.
94. Ku CM. Anesthesia for patients with mediastinal masses. *Princ Pract Anesth Thorac Surg.* 2011;14:201–210.
95. Li WW, van Boven WJ, Annema JT, Eberl S, Klomp HM, De Mol BA. Management of large mediastinal masses: surgical and anesthesiological considerations. *J Thorac Dis.* 2016;8:E175–E184.
96. Chow L. Anesthesia for patients with mediastinal masses. In: Slinger P., ed. Principles and Practice of Anesthesia for Thoracic Surgery, 2nd ed. Cham, Switzerland: Springer; 2019:251–264.
97. Tempe DK, Arya R, Dubey S, et al. Mediastinal mass resection: femorofemoral cardiopulmonary bypass before induction of anesthesia in the management of airway obstruction. *J Cardiothorac Vasc Anesth.* 2001;15:233–236.

23

Perioperative Care of the Cancer Patient: Breast Procedures

THAIS O. POLANCO, TRACY-ANN MOO, JONAS A. NELSON, AND HANAE K. TOKITA

Background

In the United States breast cancer is the most commonly diagnosed cancer in women and accounts for over 260,000 new cases each year.[1] A woman living in the United States has a 12% lifetime risk of being diagnosed with breast cancer. Although mortality rates have been declining, it is the second most common cause of death in women and responsible for over 40,000 deaths.[1]

Risk Factors

Multiple risk factors are associated with breast cancer development. Increased exposure to estrogen is associated with an elevated risk of developing breast cancer, whereas reducing exposure is thought to be protective.[2–4] Correspondingly, factors that increase the number of menstrual cycles such as early menarche, nulliparity, older age at first pregnancy, and late menopause are associated with increased risk. Additionally, obesity is associated with long-term heightened exposure to estrogen.[5–7] Nonhormonal risk factors include older age, family history, genetic predisposition, and radiation exposure (particularly mantle radiation during adolescence). Seventy-five percent of breast cancer cases occur in patients aged >50 years. A family history of breast cancer, particularly in a first-degree relative, increases the risk twofold in the case of one affected relative, and up to fourfold in the case of more than one affected relative compared to women without a family history.

Five to ten percent of breast cancers are caused by inheritance of germline mutations in genes such as BRCA1 and BRCA2.[8–10] Compared to women in the general population, BRCA1 and BRCA2 mutation carriers are estimated to have as high as 70% risk of developing breast cancer by the age of 80 years. Other inherited conditions associated with an increase in breast cancer risk include Li-Fraumeni and Cowden syndromes.[8,11] Lobular carcinoma in situ (LCIS) is characterized by abnormal cell growth within and expanding the terminal duct lobular units. Women with LCIS are 7 to 12 times more likely to develop invasive cancer in either breast compared to women without LCIS, with 65% of those being ductal in origin.[12] As such, LCIS is generally not thought to be a precursor for invasive cancer but regarded as a strong marker of increased risk.

Screening

The American Cancer Society (ACS) recommendations for the early detection of breast cancer vary depending on a woman's age and underlying risk factors.[13] Screening modalities include mammography and magnetic resonance imaging (MRI) for women who are at high risk. For women at average risk of developing breast cancer, the ACS recommends that women 40 to 44 years of age have the option to begin annual mammography, those aged 45 to 54 years should undergo annual mammography, and those aged 55 years and older may transition to biennial mammography or continue to have the option of annual mammograms. Furthermore, women should continue breast cancer screening as long as their overall health is good, and they have a life expectancy of 10 years or more. For women with a high lifetime risk (~20%–25%) of breast cancer, recommendations include an annual screening MRI in addition to mammography beginning at 30 years of age.

Staging

All patients diagnosed with breast cancer should be assigned a clinical stage based on the involvement of the breast and/or nodal regions. Staging allows for efficient identification/guidance of local and systemic therapy options and provides baseline prognostic information for patients and providers. TNM is an internationally accepted system used to determine the disease stage. The TNM classification uses information on tumor size and local spread (T), the extent of spread to nearby lymph nodes (N), the presence or absence of distant metastases (M), and additional biological factors.[14,15] A breast cancer stage of 0–IV is assigned, ranging from locally contained disease to advanced disease.

Types of Breast Cancers

Breast cancer cells are considered to be in situ or invasive depending on whether they invade the basement membrane. Ductal carcinoma in situ (DCIS) is characterized by abnormal proliferation of the epithelium that lines the milk ducts. Approximately 20% of breast cancer cases diagnosed in the United States are DCIS. There is a significant risk (nearly fivefold) of invasive breast cancer in women with DCIS. Invasive cancer is usually observed in the ipsilateral breast, suggesting that DCIS is an anatomic precursor for more invasive diseases.

Although invasive breast cancer is generally referred to as a single disease, there are several distinct histologic subtypes[16] and at least four different molecular subtypes that differ in terms of risk factors, presentation, response to treatment, and outcomes.[17,8] Invasive ductal carcinoma accounts for approximately 70%–80% of invasive lesions. This type of carcinoma presents with macroscopic or microscopic axillary lymph node metastases in up to 25% of screen-detected cases and 60% of symptomatic cases. Invasive lobular carcinoma accounts for approximately 8% of all breast cancers. The histopathologic features of this cancer include small cells that infiltrate the mammary stroma and adipose tissue individually and in a single-file pattern. Mixed histology, comprising both ductal and lobular characteristics, occurs in approximately 7% of invasive cancers. Other histologic subtypes include mixed, medullary, papillary, tubular, and mucinous, which account for less than 5% of invasive breast cancers.

Routine identification of the presence or absence of specific hormones or growth factor receptors is utilized in gene profiling. Hormone (estrogen [ER] or progesterone [PR]) receptors, excess levels of human epidermal growth factor receptor 2 (HER2), and/or extra copies of the HER2 gene (HER2+/HER2–) are routinely identified in invasive cancers. Molecular subtypes are identified based on these analyses. The main types include luminal, HER2-enriched, and basal.[18]

Prognosis

The prognosis of patients depends on the stage of the tumor at the time of diagnosis. Influencing factors include tumor size, histologic grade, axillary lymph node status, and hormone receptor status. The majority of breast cancer recurrences occur within the first 5 years of diagnosis, particularly with hormone receptor-negative disease.[19] The overall 5-year relative survival rate is 99% for localized disease, 85% for regional disease, and 27% for distant-stage disease.[20]

Future Aims in the Approach to Breast Cancer

Up to 50% of women in the United States will consult a surgeon about breast disease at some point in their lives. Twenty-five percent of women will undergo breast biopsy for the diagnosis of an abnormality, and 12% will develop some variant of breast cancer. Considerable progress has been made in the integration of surgery, radiation therapy, and systemic therapy to control local-regional disease, enhance survival, and improve the quality of life (QoL) of breast cancer survivors.[21] Potential areas for further research and improvement in breast cancer include: (1) increasing patient access to education regarding breast cancer treatment options with the goal of improving decision-making, (2) health-related quality of life (HR-QoL) outcomes research, (3) prompt dissemination and adoption of new treatment options, and (4) strategies to curb the rising costs of health care for patients.[22,23]

In the next section we present an overview of the medical and surgical management of the breast cancer patient.

Management of the Breast Cancer Patient

Nonsurgical Management of Breast Cancer

Systemic Treatment

Systemic therapy refers to the medical treatment of breast cancer using endocrine therapy, chemotherapy, and/or biologic therapy prior to or following definitive local treatment. To determine the risk of recurrence and the effectiveness of systemic therapy, one must assess factors, such as age, life expectancy, comorbidities, pathologic findings in the breast and axilla, and biological behavior of the tumor.[24] Systemic therapy may be offered based on primary tumor characteristics, such as tumor size, grade, number of involved lymph nodes, status of ER and PR receptors, and expression of HER2 receptor.

Neoadjuvant Chemotherapy

Neoadjuvant chemotherapy is utilized in cases of locally advanced and potentially inoperable breast cancer to render the disease amenable to resection. Clinical criteria for inoperability include inflammatory carcinoma, tumors that are fixed to the bony chest wall (e.g., ribs and sternum), extensive skin involvement with ulceration or satellite skin nodules, fixed or matted axillary lymphadenopathy, involvement of neurovascular structures of the axilla, or lymphedema of the ipsilateral arm. In these cases, systemic therapy may be administered as an initial treatment to reduce tumor burden and will subsequently improve the rate of operability to 80%.[25] Neoadjuvant chemotherapy is also used in cases of operable tumors to downstage disease in the breast and axilla. This may facilitate breast conservation surgery (BCS), improve cosmetic outcome, and in some instances allow patients to avoid axillary lymph node dissection (ALND) and the associated morbidity with this procedure.[26–28] Last, neoadjuvant therapy may be utilized in women who may have a temporary contraindication to surgery such as women diagnosed with breast cancer during pregnancy.

Chemotherapy remains the standard neoadjuvant approach in most patients, including those with hormone receptor-positive disease; however, endocrine therapy may be used in a certain subset of these patients. For patients with HER2-positive breast cancer, a HER2-directed agent (i.e., trastuzumab with or without pertuzumab) is typically administered in addition to the chemotherapy regimen. For patients with hormone receptor-negative and HER2-negative disease, neoadjuvant therapy consists of chemotherapy alone. Overall, in selected patients, neoadjuvant therapy reduces the rate of axillary lymph node metastases, increases the rate of breast conservation, and has comparable long-term disease-free survival and overall survival compared to patients undergoing primary surgery followed by adjuvant systemic therapy.[29,30]

Adjuvant Chemotherapy

Generally, adjuvant chemotherapy is indicated for patients with triple-negative breast cancer and either a tumor size >0.5 cm or pathologically involved lymph nodes (regardless of tumor size). Common regimens utilized for HER2-negative disease include anthracycline-based regimens such as doxorubicin and cyclophosphamide. These are typically administered for four cycles of dose-dense treatment (every 2 weeks) followed by paclitaxel administered either weekly for 12 weeks or every 2 weeks for four cycles. With the use of an anthracycline-containing regimen compared with no treatment, there is a reduction in the risk of recurrence from 47% to 39%. Furthermore, breast cancer mortality also decreases from 36% to 29% and overall mortality from 40% to 35%, respectively.[31]

Meta-analyses have demonstrated the benefits of adjuvant chemotherapy in reducing recurrence and breast cancer mortality. There is a greater magnitude of benefit in those with HR-negative disease (21%–25% relative risk reduction) compared to those with HR-positive disease (8%–12%).[31,32] For patients with HR-positive and node-negative breast cancer, Oncotype DX provides an estimate of chemotherapy benefit.[33] Patients with high Oncotype recurrence scores (≥31) have a large reduction in risk of recurrence with chemotherapy, while those with low scores derive minimal if any benefit from chemotherapy. Chemotherapy for patients in this group may consist of either anthracycline-containing or anthracycline-sparing regimens. In patients with low Oncotype recurrence scores, endocrine therapy alone is sufficient, as these patients have a favorable outcome with a 5-year overall survival of 98% with endocrine therapy alone.[33]

HER2-Directed Therapy

Approximately 20% of patients with early breast cancer have tumors that exhibit overexpression, amplification, or a combination of these characteristics of the HER2 receptor or oncogene. Adjuvant HER2-targeted therapy (trastuzumab and/or pertuzumab) is now the standard of care for these patients. Several large trials[34–36] have demonstrated that a year of adjuvant trastuzumab after chemotherapy reduces recurrence (about 50%) and increases 10-year disease-free survival (9%) in patients with this type of early breast cancer.[37]

Endocrine Therapy

Hormone receptor-positive breast cancer represents the vast majority of breast cancers around the world; approximately 60%–75% of women with invasive breast cancer are ER-positive and 65% are PR-positive.[38] Endocrine therapy is recommended for most patients with hormone-positive disease. Patients may be treated with endocrine therapy for 5–10 years and possibly longer, as a longer duration of therapy may confer additional benefits. If women are pre- or perimenopausal or if menopausal status is unknown, they should be offered tamoxifen for a total duration of 10 years. Aromatase inhibitors (anastrozole, letrozole, and exemestane) are used in postmenopausal women but may also be prescribed sequentially with tamoxifen. Adjuvant tamoxifen reduces the risk of recurrence by nearly 50% during years 0–4 with continued risk reduction of over 30% in years 5–9.[39,40] Furthermore, after 5 years of tamoxifen treatment, an additional 5 years of aromatase inhibitors provides an additional 40% relative risk reduction in recurrence.[41]

Surgical Management of Breast Cancer

Breast-Conserving Therapy

Successful breast-conserving therapy (BCT) entails complete, cosmetically acceptable surgical removal of the tumor (lumpectomy with negative surgical margins defined as no ink on tumor) followed by radiotherapy (RT) to eradicate any residual disease. Among women with operable breast cancer, randomized trials have demonstrated equivalent disease-free and overall survival between mastectomy and BCT.[42–46] Advances in neoadjuvant therapy, surgical and radiation therapy techniques, and pathologic assessment of the tumor have increased patient eligibility for this approach.[47] Inability to obtain adequate surgical margins or patient intolerance of adjuvant RT may preclude BCT. Additional contraindications include inflammatory breast cancer, multicentric disease, diffuse malignant microcalcifications on mammography, prior history of chest RT, pregnancy, and connective tissue disease (i.e., scleroderma or lupus erythematosus).[48,49]

Radiotherapy in Breast-Conserving Therapy

In patients opting for BCT, it is important to determine preoperatively whether the patient is a candidate for adjuvant radiation. For the majority of women treated with lumpectomy, including those who have received neoadjuvant therapy with a complete response to treatment, whole-breast radiation therapy (WBRT) is recommended.

WBRT following BCT reduces the locoregional recurrence rate and risk of breast cancer death. The benefits were demonstrated in a meta-analysis performed by the Early

Breast Cancer Trialists' Collaborative Group (EBCTCG),[50] which included over 10,000 women (known to be either pathologically node-negative or -positive) in 17 trials. Lumpectomy followed by WBRT resulted in a nearly 50% reduction in the 10-year risk of any first recurrence compared with lumpectomy alone and showed an absolute reduction in the 15-year risk of breast cancer death by 3.8%.[50] The conventional dose of WBRT delivered to the entire breast is 1.8–2 Gy in daily fractions over 5 to 7 weeks for a total dose of 45–50 Gy, with a 10–14 Gy boost for most patients. A more current, patient-preferred method of delivery is hypofractionated WBRT. A greater amount of RT is delivered per dose, but the overall treatment duration is shorter, with 40–42.5 Gy administered in approximately 3–5 weeks with or without a boost. This newer approach has been associated with equivalent tumor control, has fewer toxicities, has comparable overall survival, and improved cosmetic outcomes compared to traditional WBRT.[51–53]

Accelerated partial breast irradiation (APBI) refers to the use of focused RT centered around the tumor cavity. Options for the delivery of APBI include brachytherapy, intraoperative RT, or external beam radiation. Compared with WBRT, APBI delivers a higher dose of RT per day over a shorter period of time (i.e., 5 days) and potentially fewer breast symptoms and late skin side effects. This approach may be reasonable in patients >50 years of age with small (<2 cm) node-negative breast cancer. However, in preliminary trials, it is still unclear if APBI is as effective as traditional or hypofractionated WBI in terms of local control, survival, and cosmesis.[54,55]

Last, in a subgroup of women aged >65 years with node-negative, early stage, and hormone receptor-positive breast cancer who are treated with endocrine therapy, omission of RT may be a reasonable option depending on the preferences of the patient as the risk of in-breast recurrence is low.[56,57]

Mastectomy

Mastectomy is an option for breast cancer patients with contraindications to BCT, as well as prophylaxis, to reduce the risk of breast cancer in high-risk women. The rate of mastectomy has been increasing in the United States over the past decades as patients may choose to undergo mastectomy, rather than BCT. This is due to various reasons, including fear of recurrence and a desire to avoid the need for postoperative radiation or future biopsies.[58] Mastectomy options include modified radical mastectomy, total mastectomy (simple mastectomy), skin-sparing mastectomy, and nipple-areolar- sparing mastectomy (NSM). A modified radical mastectomy involves complete removal of the breast and the underlying fascia of the pectoralis major muscle along with the removal of level I and II axillary lymph nodes. With the adoption of sentinel lymph node biopsy (SLNB) for axillary staging in patients with clinically negative axillary lymph nodes, modified radical mastectomy is performed less frequently. Total mastectomy removes most of the overlying skin and the entire breast parenchyma, with preservation of the pectoral muscles and axillary contents. Total mastectomy is generally performed when the patient does not undergo immediate reconstruction.

For skin-sparing mastectomy, the majority of the natural breast skin envelope is preserved, which facilitates immediate reconstructive procedures such as preservation of the skin, and the inframammary fold provides the reconstructed breast with a more natural shape and contour.[59–61] Multiple studies have demonstrated this procedure to be oncologically safe with comparable local recurrence rates to total mastectomy ranging from 0% to 7%.[62–65] NSM preserves the nipple-areolar complex and skin envelope but removes the major ducts from within the nipple lumen.[66] This approach was initially used as an option for patients having prophylactic mastectomy with immediate reconstruction; however, this approach is increasingly used in the therapeutic setting as well. There are no randomized trials comparing NSM to other mastectomy techniques, and long-term follow up in clinical series is limited, reporting local recurrence rates of 2%–5%, with a median follow up ranging from 2 to 5 years.[66–69] As such, patients undergoing therapeutic mastectomy should be carefully selected for a nipple-sparing procedure. Indications for NSM in patients with invasive carcinoma vary by institution. At a large, tertiary, designated cancer institute, the current criteria include patients with tumors <3 cm and at a distance of at least 1 cm from the nipple with no extensive calcifications.[70]

Role of Postmastectomy Radiotherapy

Postmastectomy radiotherapy (PMRT) has been shown to decrease rates of locoregional recurrence and increase long-term breast cancer-specific and overall survival for certain patient populations.[71,72] Indications for PMRT include patients with four or more involved lymph nodes and a tumor greater than 5 cm.[24] PMRT in women with between one and three positive lymph nodes and T1-2 breast cancers is an area of ongoing debate.[71,73–75] In this subset of patients, the decision to administer PMRT should be approached in a multidisciplinary setting.

Axillary Staging

The status of the axillary lymph nodes is one of the most important prognostic factors as it is usually the initial site of metastasis. Preoperative evaluation of axillary lymph nodes separates patients into two categories: patients with clinically positive nodes and patients with clinically negative nodes. SLNB has replaced ALND as the initial assessment of axillary lymph nodes in patients with clinically negative axillary lymph nodes.[76,77] ALND is indicated for most patients with clinically positive ipsilateral axillary lymph nodes either by fine needle aspirate or SLNB. Based on the pathologic results obtained by SLNB, no further axillary treatment is indicated for patients who meet all of the following criteria: clinically negative nodes based on clinical evaluation, T1 or T2 (≤5 cm) primary breast cancer, less than three metastatic sentinel lymph nodes (SLNs), and plan for lumpectomy procedure followed by WBRT. A completion ALND is indicated for patients who have three or more metastatic nodes on SLNB, matted nodes found intraoperatively, or those with one or two metastatic SLNs who do not desire WBRT.[78,79]

The next section will describe plastic surgery reconstructive approaches for breast cancer surgery.

Plastic and Reconstructive Surgery

Postmastectomy Breast Reconstruction

Along with increasing rates of mastectomies,[58,80] more women are undergoing postmastectomy reconstruction (PMR).[81,82] A critical consequence of mastectomy is the psychosocial effect of the physical and esthetic deformity leading to anxiety, depression, and negative effects on body image and sexual function.[83–85] As such, the goal of PMR is to restore a breast mound and to maintain the quality of life without affecting the prognosis or detection of recurrence of cancer.[86]

Women have three main options following mastectomy: (1) no reconstruction, (2) prosthetic-based breast reconstruction using tissue expanders or implants, or (3) tissue-based, autologous breast reconstruction using the patient's own tissue. Most women are considered reasonable candidates for either implant-based or flap-based breast reconstruction. The choice of reconstruction technique is dictated by a variety of factors, including the size and shape of the native breast, the location and type of cancer, the availability of breast and donor site tissue, patient age and comorbidities, additional neo- and adjuvant therapies, and personal choice.

In general, breast reconstruction can be performed at the time of mastectomy (immediate) or during a subsequent operation at some point after mastectomy (delayed). Many patients undergoing mastectomy are candidates for immediate reconstruction. This includes patients having prophylactic mastectomy and mastectomy for invasive or in situ carcinoma. Delayed reconstruction may be preferred in certain patients, such as those with inflammatory breast cancer or those who are at an increased risk for adverse outcomes due to comorbidities. Surgeons and patient preferences also dictate the timeline for reconstruction. The disadvantages of delayed reconstruction include the need for additional surgery and the negative psychologic effects of body disfigurement for a period of time.[85]

Types of Breast Reconstruction Modalities

Prosthetic-Based Breast Reconstruction

Implant-based reconstruction is currently the most common choice for PMR.[80] Current options for implant-based reconstruction include immediate reconstruction with a standard or adjustable implant (single-stage implant), two-stage reconstruction with a tissue expander followed by an implant, or reconstruction with a combination of an implant and autologous tissue. The ideal candidate is a thin female undergoing bilateral mastectomy or a thin female undergoing unilateral mastectomy with little to no ptosis on the remaining breast where obtaining symmetry is easier.[87] An absolute contraindication to tissue expansion/implant reconstruction is the lack of an available skin envelope for tension-free coverage. Although not absolute contraindications, smoking, obesity, hypertension, and radiation therapy age have been implicated in complications after implant-based reconstruction.[88]

Immediate, Single-Stage Implant Reconstruction

Single-stage immediate breast reconstruction creates a definitive breast mound at the time of oncologic resection. In general, single-stage implant reconstruction is appropriate for women with small, non-ptotic breasts whose mastectomy preserves an adequate amount of skin envelope and pectoralis muscle. In this case, the implant is placed at the time of the mastectomy. A remote, removable port may be left in place to allow for the subsequent addition of volume. The port is removed at a later date, leaving the initial implant in situ as the final product. Another option for single-stage reconstruction is to incorporate an acellular dermal matrix (ADM) with an implant.[89,90] In this method, the ADM offers additional support and implant soft-tissue coverage to allow for appropriate healing. The disadvantages of the single-stage approach include the view that esthetic outcomes tend to be inferior compared to two-stage reconstruction, and in many cases, the need for a second, revisionary procedure. Consequently, this approach is not used for the majority of implant-based reconstruction, although it may be successful in select patients.[90]

Immediate or Delayed Two-Staged Implant Reconstruction

The most common technique for implant breast reconstruction is two-stage reconstruction. Traditionally, total submuscular coverage has been used in which a tissue expander is placed in a plane under the pectoralis muscle medially with lateral coverage with a portion of the serratus anterior muscle. Although cosmetic results have been described to be excellent, total submuscular reconstruction can be associated with significant postoperative pain, potential for breast animation deformity, lateral deviation of the breast mound, and insufficient lower pole fullness.[91,92] To reduce manipulation of the pectoralis muscle and associated morbidity, partial subpectoral or partial sub-ADM reconstruction was popularized. This dual-plane reconstruction is performed by release of the inferior and medial inferior insertions of the pectoralis with placement of a tissue expander under the muscle with the inferior portion of the implant supported by an ADM sling. This obviates the need for elevation of the serratus anterior, which may make subsequent expansion less painful and has been shown to have comparable cosmetic outcomes, similar safety profiles, better early fill volumes, and less postoperative pain compared with total submuscular coverage.[91,93]

In properly selected patients, a tissue expander may be placed in a prepectoral position. This method avoids the morbidity associated with muscle elevation and muscular distortion of the implant in the final reconstruction and has gained increasing popularity in the past decade. Furthermore, patients may experience less pain due to the avoidance of pectoral muscle disruption, there is minimal breast animation deformity with pectoral muscle contraction, and a natural breast contour can be maintained.[94,95] Comparative studies between prepectoral and total muscle coverage breast reconstruction have demonstrated similar complication profiles with regard to infection, superficial skin necrosis, and seroma. There is also the potential benefit of decreased rate of capsular contracture.[96,97] Prepectoral tissue expander potentially presents an opportunity to improve upon current reconstructive methods; however, currently available studies are retrospective in nature with limited cohort size and lack of long-term follow up in patients. As such, the associated risks have yet to be fully described, warranting a large multicenter prospective trial to provide better guidance.

Mixed Implant and Autologous Reconstruction

Many patients who are candidates for implant reconstruction have a skin-muscle envelope that is inadequate for expansion. Contributing factors include large skin resection at the time of mastectomy and/or multiple scars and radiation injury to the skin or muscle, resulting in a nonexpandable pocket.[98] In such cases, the addition of autologous tissue (most commonly a latissimus dorsi myocutaneous flap) may be required for adequate coverage of the expander and implant. The addition of autologous tissue to implant reconstruction increases the length and complexity of the procedure, as well as the risk of potential morbidity at the donor site (i.e., on the back).[99] Thus the combination of both reconstruction modalities is generally reserved for select patients.

Tissue Expander Expansion

The expansion process begins at approximately 2 weeks postoperatively. Saline is injected into the integrated port of the expander on a weekly or biweekly basis, depending on patient tolerance, until the expander reaches its final volume (usually after 6 to 8 weeks). The main drawbacks of skin expansion are frequent outpatient visits to gradually fill the expander, the need for an additional procedure (i.e., expander removal for permanent implant or flap), and the relatively high rate of complications, including infection, capsular contracture, and skin perforation.[100] The exchange of the tissue expander to the final implant is then performed as an outpatient procedure and should occur no earlier than 4 to 6 weeks after the final expansion or completion of adjuvant therapy.

Types of Implants

Implant selection is based on dimensional planning and should involve the patient's input. The patient's skin laxity and desired shape are considered when deciding on the type of implant, as well as details of height, width, and projection. In the United States, saline-filled and silicone gel-filled breast implants with a silicone shell are predominantly used. The major difference between the implants is the fill material, and the need for subsequent monitoring for rupture. If a saline implant ruptures, the implant deflates and physical exam can diagnose the defect. Silicone implants, on the other hand, maintain their shape for the most part, should a rupture occur. Radiologic imaging, typically with MRI, is required to detect rupture. Silicone implants generally provide a more natural feel, and appearance, while saline implants tend to be firmer, provide less natural fullness in the upper portion of the breast, and are more likely to lead to visible rippling. Overall, patient satisfaction appears to be higher when silicone implants are used for reconstruction, as opposed to saline.[101] In addition, the surface of the breast implants is either smooth or textured. Regardless of the implant chosen, the exchange usually requires capsulectomy for adequate symmetry and cosmesis.

Autologous Breast Reconstruction

Although autologous approaches remain less common than prosthetic reconstruction, the use of a patient's own tissue has distinct advantages. Autologous reconstruction has the benefit of replacing "like with like," which may lead to a softer, more ptotic and natural-appearing breast mound in a single procedure. In addition, methods using abdominal tissue donation have the added benefit of concomitant abdominoplasty, which many patients find appealing.

Ample tissue at the desired donor site is necessary for successful autologous reconstruction. Prior failed implant reconstruction, history of previous abdominal surgeries, and thin body habitus may make autologous reconstruction challenging. A variety of donor sites have been described for breast reconstruction, including the abdomen, back, buttocks, and thighs. Skin, fat, and muscle are transferred either as a pedicled flap, with its own vascular supply, or as a free flap that requires microvascular reattachment of the blood vessels. For patients who desire autologous reconstruction but who have a paucity of donor site tissue, stacked flaps may be considered in which two flaps are used to create one breast.[102,103]

Autologous reconstruction can be performed in either an immediate or delayed fashion. Immediate reconstruction has several advantages, including the need for only one operation and potential ease for surgeons who are presented with a more predictable mastectomy skin flap envelope. Precise planning of the location of the skin island may be designed on the abdomen before transfer, thus improving the efficiency and precision of the operation. Delayed reconstruction requires reelevation of the skin flaps, which can be scarred and less compliant, and commonly requires replacement of skin to create a naturally appearing, ptotic breast.

Techniques

Over the last few decades, autologous breast reconstruction techniques have evolved to achieve acceptable morbidity and superior esthetic outcomes. The most commonly considered gold standard donor site is the abdomen. The benefits of using abdominal tissue are the availability of ample tissue to form and shape the tissues to recreate the breast and contouring the abdomen for an abdominoplasty-type effect. Current modalities include a pedicled transverse rectus abdominis myocutaneous (pTRAM) flap, free TRAM flap, deep inferior epigastric artery perforator (DIEP) flap, and superficial inferior epigastric artery (SIEA) flap.

The most common pedicled myocutaneous flap is the pTRAM flap.[104] This flap consists of excising excess skin and soft tissue in the infraumbilical area overlying the rectus abdominis muscle together with the rectus muscle itself along with its supply of superior epigastric vessels.[105] However, this procedure has significant disadvantages, including a high tissue-to-blood supply ratio of the flap; protracted recovery time; and abdominal wall morbidity, including weakness, bulging, and herniation. To overcome the drawbacks and associated morbidity of the pTRAM flap, further refinements led to techniques, including the muscle-sparing free TRAM flap and perforator flaps (DIEP and SIEA). The free TRAM flap technique[106] requires a more limited harvest of the rectus abdominis muscle, safer transfer due to improved perfusion originating from the larger caudal pedicle (deep inferior epigastric artery instead of deep superior epigastric artery), and an improved medial breast contour due to the lack of tunneling of the flap's cranial pedicle compared to pedicle TRAM flap.[107,108] The DIEP flap is based on perforating vessels that pass from the inferior epigastric vessels through the rectus muscle into the fat and skin.[109] The DIEP flap has become the gold standard for autologous breast reconstruction because it maximizes the amount of tissue transfer without sacrificing the rectus muscle. Furthermore, it results in less donor site morbidity and excellent esthetic results compared to the traditional TRAM flap.[110–113] Other advantages include decreased pain, quicker recovery, preservation of abdominal wall function, lower incidence of hernia, shorter hospital stay, and decreased cost.[114]

Given that not every woman is suitable for breast reconstruction using abdominal skin and fat, several more donor sites have been recently described to harvest the most suitable microvascular flap to best personalize breast reconstruction. These flaps include the superior gluteal artery perforator flap,[115] the inferior gluteal artery perforator flap[116] from the gluteal region, fasciocutaneous infragluteal flap, profunda femoral artery perforator flap[117] from the infragluteal region, and the transverse myocutaneous gracilis flap from the inner thigh region.[118] The latissimus dorsi myocutaneous flap also remains an option for autologous breast reconstruction. It is typically not used for initial reconstruction because of the lack of appropriate volume; however, it may serve as a salvage flap or a combined prosthetic approach, as previously discussed.

Nipple Reconstruction

Following the completion of breast reconstruction, women are given the option of nipple-areolar reconstruction. The goal of nipple and areolar reconstruction is to achieve symmetry of the position of the nipple-areolar complex in the contralateral breast with comparable appearance and color. Multiple techniques can be used to create a nipple and areola. Surgical methods involve local tissue rearrangement procedures or skin grafts, while others use donor sites that are primarily closed. Nipple projection varies among different techniques, but adequate results can be achieved with most. An alternative to surgical reconstruction of the nipple is a three-dimensional tattoo. The tattooing of a surgically created nipple includes tattooing of the nipple and the creation of a new areola with pigmentation.[119,120]

Advantages and Disadvantages of Modalities

Implant-based reconstruction has the advantages of being a less invasive procedure, technically easier, does not require any special equipment, and may be performed by most plastic surgeons. The procedure itself is short, avoids significant donor site morbidity and additional scar formation, and results in a shorter recovery time. Important disadvantages of implant-based reconstruction include the prolonged time to achieve a breast mound and the need for multiple visits for inflation of the tissue expander. Early complications after placement of the tissue expander include infection, hematoma, and extrusion of the implant.[100] Late complications may occur after insertion of the final implant, including capsular contracture (scarring and contracture around the implant causing deformity), leak or rupture, and infection, all of which can potentially lead to removal or exchange of the implant.[99,100] The incidence of complications is significantly increased in patients with a history of radiation and in those who receive radiation after mastectomy.[121,122] For many of these patients, autogenous tissue may be a better option for reconstruction.

The advantage of reconstruction with autologous tissue includes the creation of a softer, more ptotic and natural-appearing breast mound in a single procedure. Disadvantages include a longer duration of anesthesia (5 to 10 h), more blood loss, a longer recovery period, risk of necrosis of portions of the transferred fat and skin, and problems at the donor site, which include wide, unsightly scars, abdominal weakness, and abdominal bulge or hernia.[99,122] The risk of complications tends to be higher in older and more obese patients, as well as those with compromised vascular microcirculation such as smokers and patients with diabetes.[123–125]

All procedures for breast reconstruction are associated with an increase in morbidity beyond that associated with mastectomy alone. Each procedure has advantages and disadvantages that must be weighed by the patient and physician to reach an appropriate decision. In multiple studies assessing overall complications and reoperative complications comparing modalities, autologous reconstruction is associated with significantly higher odds of complications compared with prosthetic techniques.[122,126,127] However, failure rates were low across both procedure types. As such, reconstruction may be associated with a high risk of complications, but successful reconstruction may still be achieved in most patients.

Special Considerations

Radiation Therapy

Radiation is an essential component of breast cancer treatment, but it often has a detrimental effect on reconstructive results. Women who require postmastectomy radiation therapy present a unique reconstructive challenge. Radiation therapy leads to fibrosis, which compromises the quality of the skin and underlying tissue, resulting in a higher incidence of complications from the reconstructive procedure, and ultimately may produce a less esthetically pleasing result. Patients who undergo radiation prior to reconstruction experience high rates of prosthetic device loss. Postmastectomy radiation therapy can also cause prosthetic device loss, capsular contracture, and higher rates of infection. Although autologous reconstruction may be better able to withstand radiation-induced damage, these patients still have high rates of intraoperative microvascular issues[121,128] and related complications including fat necrosis, flap shrinkage, and contour deformities. Revision rates, however, are unchanged.[128–130]

Regarding patient-reported outcome measures (PROM), irradiated patients have lower HR-QoL outcomes compared to those who did not receive radiation. However, few differences have been elucidated between or within reconstructive modalities, with studies suggesting higher PROM in autologous patients. To date, the best method of integrating radiation therapy into any reconstruction method remains controversial.[128,131]

Breast Implant-Associated Anaplastic Large Cell Lymphoma

BIA-ALCL is an important public health concern because the use of breast implants has increased over the past two decades in the United States and internationally. It is estimated that as of 2015, more than 3 million textured devices have been used in patients in the United States. The risk of developing BIA-ALCL appears to be associated with prolonged exposure to textured implants, with most case series documenting a median exposure time ranging from 6.4 to 15.5 years, although shorter times of 0.4–2 years have also been reported.[132–135] However, a recent study estimated the current incidence at 1.79 per 1000 patients and 1.15 per 1000 implants—a higher incidence than previously thought.[136–138] The US Food and Drug Administration (FDA) has recently recalled certain textured breast implants.[139] Patients who are interested in textured implants should be counseled about these risks prior to surgery.

The FDA does not currently recommend breast implant removal for asymptomatic women who already have this type of implant. The recall does not include smooth surface devices that use either saline or silicone gel as the filler material. Management options for patients with textured devices include continued implant monitoring, exchange for smooth devices, or conversion to autologous tissue reconstruction. It is unknown how the removal of a textured device impacts the likelihood of future BIA-ALCL, although it is reasonable to hypothesize that removal of the implant capsule substantially decreases the risk.

Patient-Reported Outcomes

Breast reconstruction offers significant quality-of-life benefits in many patients undergoing mastectomy. PMR is an essential component in the therapeutic course following breast cancer and mastectomy and enhances postmastectomy quality of life by improving a woman's sense of sexuality, body image, and self-esteem, compared with mastectomy alone.[82,84,85] Differences in surgical outcomes, complications, and costs between these two modalities have been well characterized, yet these outcomes may not correlate with a patient's perception of outcomes of care.[122,126] Several studies have assessed patient-reported outcomes (PROs) in breast reconstruction patients, demonstrating that the type of reconstructive modality appears to affect postoperative satisfaction outcomes.[140,141] A recent study of PROs using the BREAST-Q demonstrated that autologous breast reconstruction patients have higher long-term satisfaction compared to implant breast reconstruction patients. However, this study also found that patients who received implant-based reconstruction had satisfaction scores that remained stable over a long-term period.[142] With a growing focus on health outcomes research and a move toward value-based medicine, patients and surgeons must now not only evaluate clinical differences between implant-based and autologous techniques but also consider a deeper understanding of PROM within each modality.

The decision to choose or decline breast reconstruction should be made by the patient after she has had the opportunity to learn about, discuss, and consider possible options. Contributions from the patient's care providers, including breast oncologic surgeons, medical oncologists, radiation oncologists, and plastic surgeons, may aid the patient in the decision-making process. Studies report that a patient's satisfaction with the decision about reconstruction is highest when the patient has been adequately informed and when their level of involvement in the decision is consistent with their own wishes and expectations.[143,144]

The final section is an overview of perioperative anesthesia considerations for breast cancer surgery.

Anesthesia for Breast Surgery

Perioperative Anesthesia Considerations for Breast Cancer Surgery

Anesthesia and Type of Breast Cancer Surgery

The preoperative assessment should take into account: (1) patient comorbidities and whether the patient is medically optimized prior to surgery, and (2) type of procedure being performed with an understanding of the incision sites, extent of dissection and tissue trauma, and expected postoperative pain. As described in the previous sections, breast cancer surgeries include a wide range of procedure types from breast-conserving surgery with or without sentinel and/or ALND to mastectomy with or without reconstruction. Breast reconstruction may entail temporary placement of a tissue expander, placement of a permanent implant, or autologous flap reconstruction.

For minimally invasive outpatient procedures such as partial mastectomy or lumpectomy, monitored anesthesia care with a continuous propofol infusion in conjunction with surgeon infiltration of local anesthesia is generally appropriate. ALND involves deeper tissue invasion and typically requires general anesthesia with a laryngeal mask airway. Because of the proximity of the brachial plexus and its branches to the axilla, breast surgeons often prefer avoidance of muscle relaxant medications in order to monitor nerve response during dissection. Consideration should be given to placing the intravenous catheter and blood pressure cuff on the arm opposite to the side of the planned surgery.

Reconstruction after mastectomy may be an immediate or delayed procedure. When immediate reconstruction is planned after mastectomy, general endotracheal anesthesia is generally preferred, particularly if the placement of the tissue expander is subpectoral which may be facilitated by muscle relaxation. Tissue expander reconstruction is a risk factor for worse pain after breast reconstruction compared to autologous flap approaches[206]; hence an optimal multimodal analgesic regimen should be planned. Patients undergoing exchange of tissue expanders with permanent implants, which typically occurs at least 3 months but not sooner than 6 weeks after initial tissue expander placement, usually require general endotracheal anesthesia due to frequent upright positioning changes to enable surgeons to assess for symmetry, which limits access to the airway.

General endotracheal anesthesia is standard for patients undergoing autologous flap reconstruction. Due to the prolonged nature of these procedures, the anesthesia team should be mindful of noninvasive blood pressure (NIBP) cuff pressure injuries and consider rotating between two separate sites for NIBP measurement, using invasive blood pressure monitoring, or a continuous NIBP monitoring technique. Pressure point checks of the head and extremities at regular intervals throughout the procedure should also be performed.

Neoadjuvant Chemotherapy

During preoperative evaluation, it is important to understand the cardiac implications of neoadjuvant chemotherapy. Chemotherapy-related cardiac dysfunction has been classified as type I and type II.[145] Type I is associated with anthracycline drugs (e.g., doxorubicin) and may lead to cardiomyopathy with significant morbidity and mortality.[146] The diagnosis of anthracycline-induced cardiotoxicity is confirmed in a patient with new symptoms of heart failure or significant decline in left ventricular ejection fraction following exposure to anthracycline after exclusion of other causes. Risk factors include extremes of age, preexisting cardiovascular disease, hypertension, smoking, hyperlipidemia, obesity, diabetes, and high cumulative anthracycline exposure.[147,148] Additional risk factors include combined treatment with radiation therapy and trastuzumab. There is no established treatment other than supportive measures for patients who have developed doxorubicin heart failure.[147]

Type II cardiac dysfunction is typically associated with trastuzumab, an agent that targets HER2. For 15%–20% of patients with breast cancer whose tumors overexpress HER2, trastuzumab therapy is important in the treatment of both early and advanced disease. However, its use may place patients at a modest risk for cardiotoxicity which is typically manifested by an asymptomatic decrease in left ventricular ejection fraction and less often by overt heart failure.[149–151] In contrast to cardiotoxicity from anthracyclines, trastuzumab-related cardiotoxicity does not appear to be related to cumulative dose. It is often reversible with treatment discontinuation and rechallenge is often tolerated after recovery. Risk factors associated with a higher likelihood of developing trastuzumab-related cardiotoxicity include older age and previous or concurrent anthracycline use.[151]

Limited data are available to guide the assessment and surveillance of patients receiving anthracycline and trastuzumab. Recommendations include obtaining a comprehensive clinical history, electrocardiogram, and cardiac examination prior to initiation of anthracycline-based chemotherapy. Patients should be evaluated at least every 3 months during treatment. For patients who develop symptoms or signs of heart failure, repeat echocardiography should be performed. After completion of anthracycline therapy, monitoring should be performed yearly. Increased vigilance for signs and symptoms of cardiotoxicity is appropriate for high-risk patients. In the adjuvant setting, a baseline evaluation of cardiac function with monitoring every 3 months thereafter is recommended.

The preoperative evaluation of patients who have received neoadjuvant chemotherapy should include an assessment of clinical status, focused examination, and review of electrocardiogram, echocardiography, and any other pertinent data to assess for signs or symptoms of heart failure. New concerning ECG changes or an acute reduction in left ventricular ejection fraction with poor functional status warrants further investigation prior to surgery.

Enhanced Recovery After Surgery (ERAS) for Breast Procedures

In a health care climate increasingly focused on optimizing quality and patient experience clinical settings are increasingly incorporating Enhanced Recovery After Surgery (ERAS) programs as quality improvement initiatives in perioperative care. ERAS is a multidisciplinary, evidence-based, and protocol-driven approach to the management of surgical patients.[152,153] Main principles include preoperative optimization of the patient, avoidance of prolonged fasting, standardized multimodal analgesic and anesthetic regimens, early resumption of diet, and early mobilization in the post-operative period. While ERAS is not a new concept, it is not yet widely described in breast surgery. Suggested elements for breast surgery include preadmission counseling, anxiolysis, optimal pain management including regional anesthesia when feasible, prevention of postoperative nausea and vomiting (PONV), early mobilization, and physical therapy with arm exercises postoperatively.[154] More studies are needed to determine the clinical efficacy of each of these interventions, including analgesic medications, in breast surgery-specific trials.

While ERAS is not yet the standard of care in breast cancer surgery, there is growing evidence of its benefits. Compared with conventional care models, ERAS programs have been shown to reduce morbidity, hospital length of stay, and opioid consumption in patients undergoing microvascular breast reconstruction.[155–158] Implementation of an ERAS program for patients undergoing mastectomy with immediate reconstruction at a single short-stay facility was associated with improved PONV postoperative nausea and vomiting and pain control.[159] Despite these promising findings and the potential for ERAS to optimize perioperative care, gaps in education and execution call for future studies on implementation. In a meta-analysis assessing ERAS pathways in breast reconstruction patients, inconsistent and incomplete implementation of all elements of the ERAS program was observed across the nine included studies.[158]

Pain, Regional Anesthesia, and Breast Surgery

Postoperative pain is a major challenge for patients undergoing complex breast cancer surgery and reconstruction. Suboptimally treated pain results in prolonged hospitalizations, additional resource utilization, and a decrease in HR-QoL outcomes.[160,161] Furthermore, approximately 50% of all patients undergoing mastectomy and breast reconstruction experience chronic postoperative pain syndromes.[160] Poorly controlled pain in the acute postoperative period has been demonstrated to be one of the largest contributors to chronic pain syndromes and disability in breast surgery patients.[160,162–165] While opioid medications are the traditional approach to perioperative pain management, there are several disadvantages to their use in breast surgery patients. Opioids contribute to PONV in this high-risk patient population and there is ongoing concern about the current opioid crisis in the United States. Regional anesthesia as a component of a multimodal opioid-minimizing approach to pain management should be considered for patients undergoing complex breast cancer surgery.

Paravertebral Blocks

A variety of regional anesthetic techniques have been described for breast surgery, including thoracic epidural anesthesia, intercostal blocks, and thoracic paravertebral blocks. Paravertebral blocks are considered the gold standard regional anesthetic technique for breast surgery and have been shown to decrease postoperative pain, limit PONV, and reduce length of stay.[166,167,207] The technique involves injecting local anesthesia in the paravertebral space to anesthetize the thoracic spinal nerves as they emerge from the intervertebral foramina.[168] Thoracic dermatomal coverage of levels T1–T6 (Fig. 23.1) is required for mastectomy surgery, particularly if axillary node dissection is planned. Using an ultrasound-guided approach, the spinous process at the appropriate thoracic level is identified. In a transverse or parasagittal orientation, the probe is moved laterally to identify the transverse process, pleura, and costotransverse ligament (Fig. 23.2). The block needle is advanced beneath the costotransverse ligament and successful placement is confirmed by visualization of pleural depression as local anesthesia is infiltrated into the paravertebral space. The clinician may choose to perform a single injection, multilevel injections, or place an indwelling catheter in the paravertebral space. Pneumothorax remains the most significant concern for clinicians; however, this complication is rare.[169]

"Novel" Plane Blocks

In recent years, novel plane blocks, including PECS,[208] serratus,[170] and erector spinae[171] blocks, have emerged as potential alternatives to paravertebral blocks PECS I block targets the medial pectoral (C8–T1) and lateral pectoral (C5–C7) nerves while PECS II additionally targets the intercostobrachial nerve, long thoracic nerve (C5–C7), thoracodorsal nerve (C6–C8), and upper intercostal nerves (T2–T6) (Fig. 23.1). PECS II block is performed by injecting local anesthetic between pectoralis minor and serratus anterior by the third and fourth ribs in the mid-axillary line and an injection between the pectoralis major and minor (PECS I block) (Fig. 23.3). The serratus block, in which local anesthesia is injected above and/or below the serratus anterior muscle, anesthetizes the lateral cutaneous branches of the thoracic intercostal nerves to provide analgesia to the lateral and anterior chest wall (Fig. 23.4).[170] The erector spinae block, which was first described as a regional anesthetic technique for thoracic neuropathic pain,[171] involves injection at the transverse process below the erector spinae muscle with a purported mechanism of diffusion of local anesthesia into the paravertebral space (Fig. 23.5).

While there is much enthusiasm about these newer fascial plane blocks, high-quality randomized trials comparing various techniques are still needed to determine clinical efficacy. A recent meta-analysis comparing PECS II blocks to systemic analgesia alone and to paravertebral blocks in patients undergoing breast cancer surgery under general anesthesia found that PECS II was superior to systemic analgesia in reducing pain intensity and opioid consumption post-operatively and was noninferior to paravertebral blocks.[172]

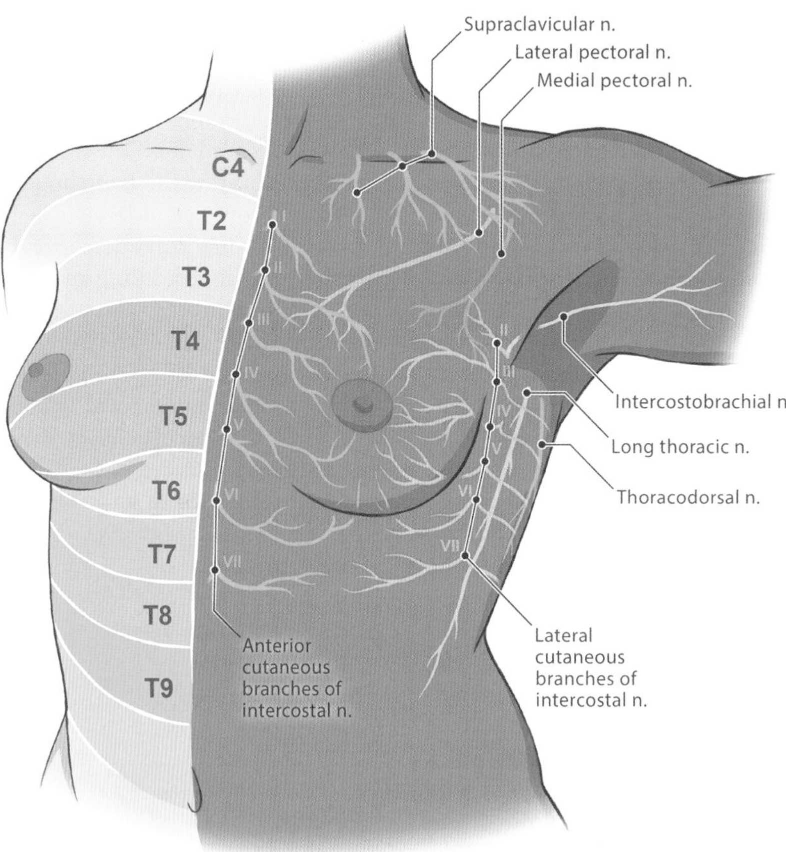

• **Fig. 23.1** Chest wall innervation.

Surgical concerns with fascial plane blocks must also be considered as regional anesthesia approaches evolve. Injection of local anesthesia above the serratus muscle may cause potential blockade of the long thoracic and thoracodorsal nerves which the breast surgeon may want to monitor during a difficult dissection. Injection of local anesthesia between the pectoralis minor and serratus anterior in a PECS II block has the theoretical concerns of distorting axillary anatomy, causing tumor seeding, and rendering electrocautery less effective. Patient-related factors, such as morbid obesity, coagulopathy, or the presence of rods in the spine may also influence choice of regional anesthetic approach. Appropriate patient evaluation, communication with the surgical team, and understanding of the planned surgical approach are necessary to determine the optimal regional anesthetic technique.

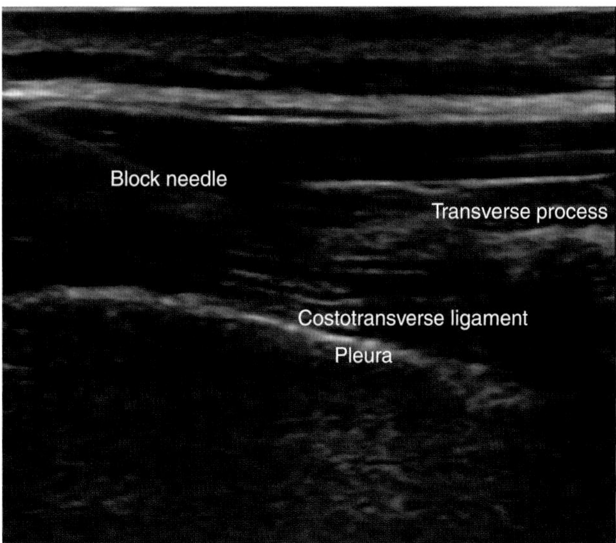

• **Fig. 23.2** Paravertebral block, transverse orientation (transverse process, pleura, needle).

Blue Dye Reactions

SLN mapping was first described in the 1990s and has significantly reduced the rate of women undergoing more invasive ALND and the morbidity associated with this procedure. However, administering blue dye is not without risk. Isosulfan blue carries a 0.3%–0.9% incidence of adverse reactions.[173,174] Three types of allergic reactions have been reported, ranging from hives and rash to transient hypotension to hypotension requiring vasopressor treatment and severe anaphylaxis. A retrospective study found that prophylaxis with steroids, diphenhydramine, and famotidine

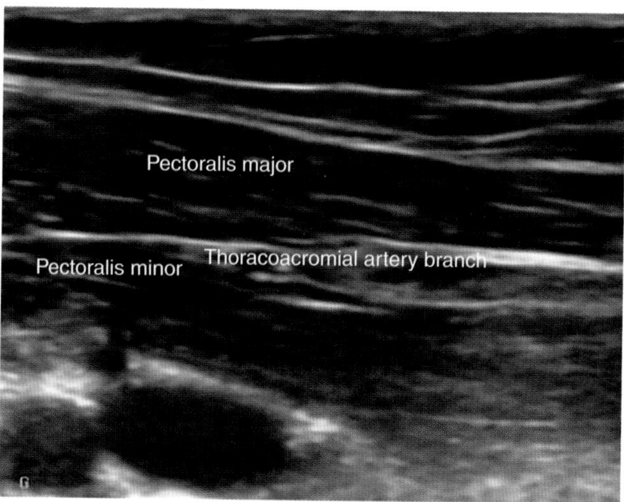

• **Fig. 23.3** PECS I anatomy (pectoralis major and minor, branch of thoracoacromial artery).

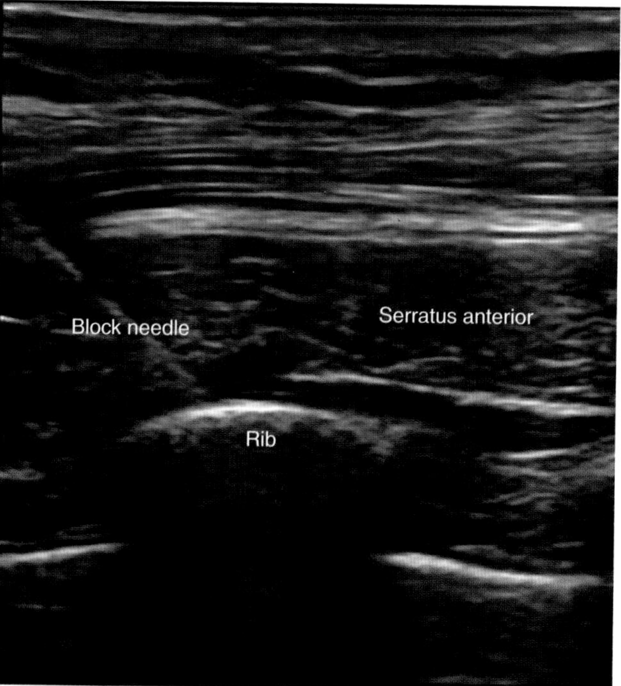

• **Fig. 23.4** Serratus block (serratus anterior muscle, rib, pleura).

did not change the incidence of adverse reactions to isosulfan blue but did reduce the severity of reaction.[174] Routine prophylaxis is not routinely performed in many practices, however. Methylene blue may be a potentially safer alternative in terms of anaphylaxis risk.[175] Side effects may include pain, skin necrosis, or induration and erythema at the injection site. Pulmonary edema and serotonin syndrome in patients taking serotonergic medications have also been reported.[176,177] In addition, methylene blue causes a transient artifact on pulse oximetry and may cause a blue tinge to the skin. Skin and systemic side effects may be minimized by diluting methylene blue with normal saline.[178]

Recognizing and promptly treating blue dye reactions is critical for the anesthesia team to prevent adverse outcomes in patients undergoing breast surgery. Appropriate staff, resuscitation equipment, and emergency medications, including epinephrine, should always be readily available.

Anesthesia and Breast Cancer Recurrence

The question of whether anesthesia technique plays a role in cancer recurrence remains an area of ongoing investigation. Surgical stress is considered a pro-inflammatory state and is thought to reduce host-cell immune function while promoting growth of cancer cells.[179–181] It has been hypothesized that certain anesthetic agents may either contribute to or protect against cancer recurrence.[182] While there has been much enthusiasm in the literature on this topic, much of the evidence to support these theories is derived from in vitro and animal studies and few retrospective clinical trials.

Opioids in particular have been suggested as a risk factor for cancer recurrence. Opioids inhibit the function of natural killer (NK) cells and may stimulate cancer cell proliferation by promoting angiogenesis.[181,183,184] In a murine model of breast cancer, morphine caused increased concentrations of substance P and cytokines and stimulated mast cell activation, which may cause cancer progression.[184] The current evidence for opioids and breast cancer growth, however, remains limited.[179,184–186]

The use of nonsteroidal antiinflammatory drugs (NSAIDs), on the other hand, has been suggested as protective in cancer surgery. Several retrospective studies suggest that intraoperative administration of NSAIDs may reduce cancer recurrence and improve survival. A retrospective, single-institution study of 720 women who underwent breast lumpectomy with or without ALND found an association between intraoperative administration of ketorolac or diclofenac and a longer disease-free and overall survival.[187] Similarly, a retrospective study of 327 women who underwent mastectomy with ALND reported lower cancer recurrence rates in patients who received ketorolac prior to surgery.[187,188] Despite these findings, expert opinion recommends prospective randomized trials are needed in this area.[189]

Volatile anesthetics have been suggested as immunosuppressive agents that may increase the risk of cancer recurrence. The proposed mechanism is a proinflammatory effect and upregulation of hypoxia-inducible factors that protect cancer cells.[190,191] In contrast, propofol has demonstrated immunoprotective effects by exhibiting antiinflammatory and antioxidative properties, and preserving NK cell function in laboratory studies.[179,185,192,193] In studies of breast cancer cell lines, propofol reduced the expression of neuroepithelial cell transforming gene 1,[194] which is associated with promoting migration of adenocarcinoma in vitro and increased cell apoptosis.[195]

Clinical studies comparing total intravenous anesthesia (TIVA) with propofol and inhalation agents have reported mixed results, with some showing a beneficial effect of TIVA and others showing no effect compared with inhalational anesthetic.[196–198] A 2019 meta-analysis of six studies (five

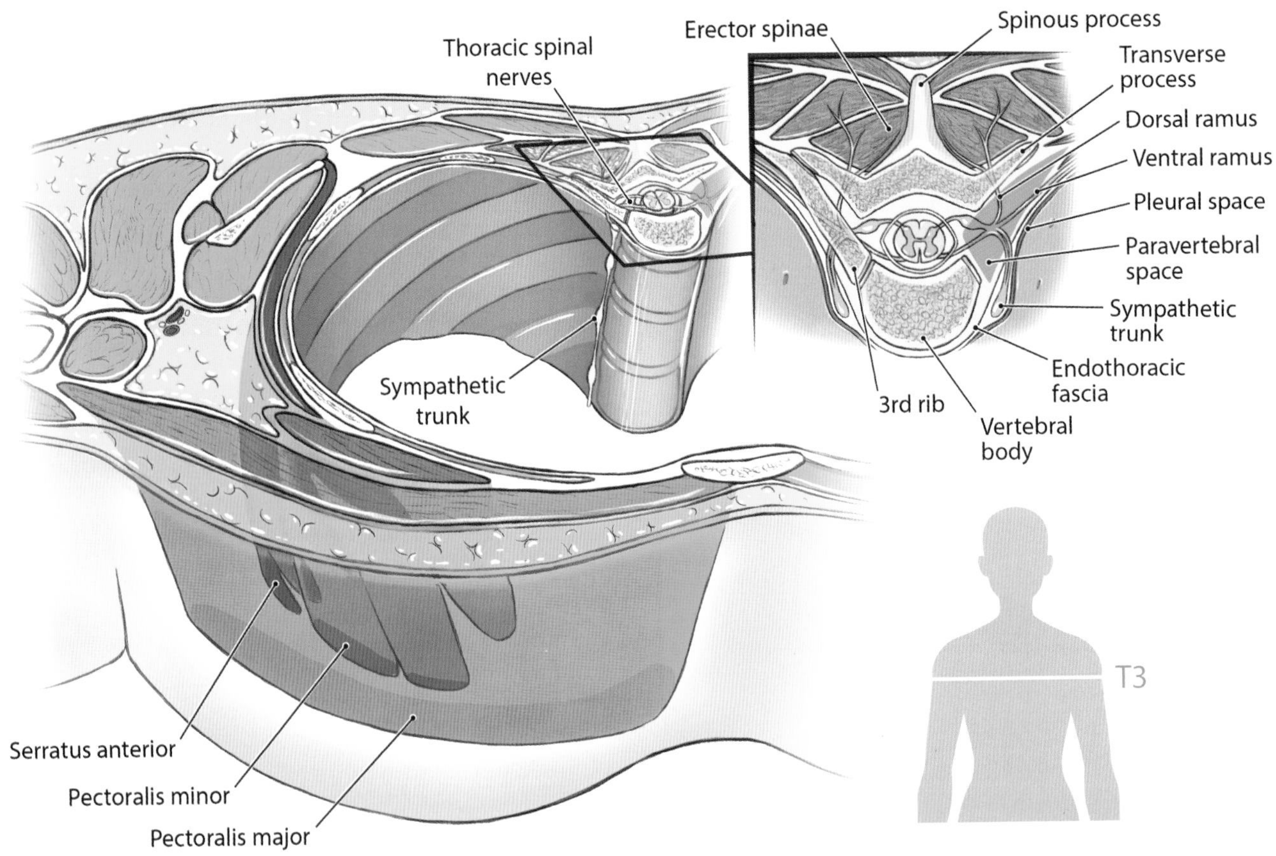

• **Fig. 23.5** Anatomical targets for regional anesthesia for breast surgery.

retrospective, one small randomized controlled trial), including over 7800 patients who underwent cancer surgery, found that the use of TIVA was associated with improved recurrence-free survival compared with volatile anesthesia.[199] However, interpretation of these results was limited due to heterogeneity with respect to the extent of surgery, types of cancers treated, patient characteristics, as well as other limitations associated with the retrospective nature of most of the studies. In contrast, a large, retrospective, propensity-matched cohort study of patients who underwent breast cancer surgery (BCT or total mastectomy) grouped according to whether TIVA or inhalational anesthesia was administered found no difference in the rate of cancer recurrence between the two groups.[200] The conflicting findings indicate that anesthetic techniques may have a greater impact on cancer recurrence in patients undergoing more complex and invasive surgeries.

The effects of regional anesthesia on cancer recurrence remain unclear. Regional anesthesia reduces cancer recurrence through several proposed mechanisms: attenuating the stress response to surgery (by pain control and sympathetic blockade), reducing the need for opioids and volatile agents, and/or by direct effects of absorbed local anesthetics.[201,202] A 2014 meta-analysis with data from over 3000 patients found no associated difference in cancer recurrence or survival in patients who received general epidural anesthesia versus general anesthesia alone.[203] A retrospective study of 129 patients undergoing mastectomy with or without axillary clearance using either paravertebral block and general anesthesia or general anesthesia and postoperative morphine patient-controlled anesthesia (PCA) found a longer time to cancer recurrence (P = 0.013) and overall lower recurrence rate (P = 0.012) in patients who received a paravertebral block in the 2.5–4-year follow up period.[204] More recently, Sessler et al. published the results of a large, multicenter trial in which they randomized patients to a paravertebral block and propofol arm or general anesthesia with sevoflurane and opioid analgesic arm. The primary outcome was local or metastatic recurrence, and the secondary outcome was pain at 6 and 12 months. They found no difference in breast cancer recurrence rate or in chronic pain outcomes between the two groups.[205] Currently, there is no evidence to suggest a superior anesthetic approach for reducing cancer recurrence in breast surgery. However, optimizing short-term outcomes, including PONV, acute postoperative pain, and quality of recovery, should remain a priority for the perioperative team.

Conclusions

- To optimize the care and outcomes of the breast cancer patient, an experienced multidisciplinary cancer team is needed.
- A patient's expectations for treatment and surgery should be discussed in advance in order to make informed decisions based on the risks of procedures as well as the potential esthetic outcomes.
- Breast-conserving therapy and mastectomy are well-established local therapies for early-stage invasive breast cancer and have equivalent survival and recurrence outcomes.
- Neoadjuvant chemotherapy is increasingly used to downstage disease in the breast and axilla.
- Adjuvant medical therapies are administered after breast surgery to eradicate clinically and radiographically occult micrometastatic disease.
- For women who choose mastectomy as part of their approach to breast cancer therapy or prevention, breast reconstruction may be offered.
- The goal of breast reconstruction is to restore a breast mound and maintain the quality of life without affecting the prognosis or detection of cancer recurrence.
- Methods for breast reconstruction include prosthetic and autogenous tissue approaches.
- Preoperative assessment should consider the type of breast cancer surgery performed, anticipated postoperative pain, and patient comorbidities.
- Clinicians should understand the cardiac implications of neoadjuvant chemotherapy.
- ERAS is not yet widely used in breast surgery but these protocols are likely to benefit patients and optimize care.
- Regional anesthesia may provide excellent postoperative pain control in breast surgery.
- Intraoperative blue dye reactions range in severity and should be promptly recognized and treated by the perioperative team.
- The link between anesthetic technique and breast cancer recurrence remains controversial.

References

1. Siegel RL, Miller KD, Jemal A. Cancer statistics, 2019. *CA Cancer J Clin.* 2019;69(1):7–34.
2. Key TJ, Appleby PN, Reeves GK, et al. Steroid hormone measurements from different types of assays in relation to body mass index and breast cancer risk in postmenopausal women: reanalysis of eighteen prospective studies. *Steroids.* 2015;99(A):49–55.
3. Sieri S, Krogh V, Bolelli G, et al. Sex hormone levels, breast cancer risk, and cancer receptor status in postmenopausal women: the ORDET cohort. *Cancer Epidemiol Biomarkers Prev.* 2009;18(1):169–176.
4. Beattie MS, Costantino JP, Cummings SR, et al. Endogenous sex hormones, breast cancer risk, and tamoxifen response: an ancillary study in the NSABP Breast Cancer Prevention Trial (P-1). *J Natl Cancer Inst.* 2006;98(2):110–115.
5. Morimoto LM, White E, Chen Z, et al. Obesity, body size, and risk of postmenopausal breast cancer: the Women's Health Initiative (United States). *Cancer Causes Control.* 2002;13(8):741–751.
6. Lahmann PH, Hoffmann K, Allen N, et al. Body size and breast cancer risk: findings from the European Prospective Investigation into Cancer and Nutrition (EPIC). *Int J Cancer.* 2004;111(5):762–771.
7. Lauby-Secretan B, Scoccianti C, Loomis D, et al. Body fatness and cancer—viewpoint of the IARC working group. *N Engl J Med.* 2016;375(8):794–798.
8. Turnbull C, Rahman N. Genetic predisposition to breast cancer: past, present, and future. *Annu Rev Genomics Hum Genet.* 2008;9:321–345.
9. Tung N, Lin NU, Kidd J, et al. Frequency of germline mutations in 25 cancer susceptibility genes in a sequential series of patients with breast cancer. *J Clin Oncol.* 2016;34(13):1460–1468.
10. Kuchenbaecker KB, Hopper JL, Barnes DR, et al. Risks of breast, ovarian, and contralateral breast cancer for BRCA1 and BRCA2 mutation carriers. *JAMA.* 2017;317(23):2402–2416.
11. Michailidou K, Beesley J, Lindstrom S, et al. Genome-wide association analysis of more than 120,000 individuals identifies 15 new susceptibility loci for breast cancer. *Nat Genet.* 2015;47(4):373–380.
12. Morrow M, Schnitt SJ, Norton L. Current management of lesions associated with an increased risk of breast cancer. *Nat Rev Clin Oncol.* 2015;12(4):227–238.
13. Oeffinger KC, Fontham ET, Etzioni R, et al. Breast cancer screening for women at average risk: 2015 guideline update from the American Cancer Society. *JAMA.* 2015;314(15):1599–1614.
14. Amin MB, Greene FL, Edge SB, et al. The 8th Edition AJCC Cancer Staging Manual: Continuing to build a bridge from a population-based to a more "personalized" approach to cancer staging. *CA Cancer J Clin.* 2017;67(2):93–99.
15. Giuliano AE, Connolly JL, Edge SB, et al. Breast cancer—Major changes in the American Joint Committee on Cancer eighth edition cancer staging manual. *CA Cancer J Clin.* 2017;67(4):290–303.
16. Li CI, Uribe DJ, Daling JR. Clinical characteristics of different histologic types of breast cancer. *Br J Cancer.* 2005;93(9):1046–1052.
17. Tamimi RM, Colditz GA, Hazra A, et al. Traditional breast cancer risk factors in relation to molecular subtypes of breast cancer. *Breast Cancer Res Treat.* 2012;131(1):159–167.
18. Cancer Genome Atlas Network. Comprehensive molecular portraits of human breast tumours. *Nature.* 2012;490(7418):61–70.
19. Colleoni M, Sun Z, Price KN, et al. Annual hazard rates of recurrence for breast cancer during 24 years of follow-up: results from the International Breast Cancer Study Group trials I to V. *J Clin Oncol.* 2016;34(9):927–935.
20. Howlader N, Na KM, Miller D, et al. (eds). SEER Cancer Statistics Review, 1975–2017, National Cancer Institute. Bethesda, MD, https://seer.cancer.gov/csr/1975_2017/, based on November 2019 SEER data submission, posted to the SEER web site, April 2020.
21. Kesson EM, Allardice GM, George WD, et al. Effects of multidisciplinary team working on breast cancer survival: retrospective, comparative, interventional cohort study of 13 722 women. *BMJ.* 2012;344:e2718.
22. Tripathy D. Multidisciplinary care for breast cancer: barriers and solutions. *Breast J.* 2003;9(1):60–63.

23. Roughton MC, Shenaq D, Jaskowiak N, et al. Optimizing delivery of breast conservation therapy: a multidisciplinary approach to oncoplastic surgery. *Ann Plast Surg*. 2012;69(3):250–255.
24. Recht A, Comen EA, Fine RE, et al. Postmastectomy radiotherapy: an American Society of Clinical Oncology, American Society for Radiation Oncology, and Society of Surgical Oncology focused guideline update. *Pract Radiat Oncol*. 2016;6(6):e219–e234.
25. Hortobagyi GN. Comprehensive management of locally advanced breast cancer. *Cancer*. 1990;66(6):1387–1391.
26. Mamtani A, Barrio AV, King TA, et al. How often does neoadjuvant chemotherapy avoid axillary dissection in patients with histologically confirmed nodal metastases? Results of a prospective study. *Ann Surg Oncol*. 2016;23(11):3467–3474.
27. Kaufmann M, Hortobagyi GN, Goldhirsch A, et al. Recommendations from an international expert panel on the use of neoadjuvant (primary) systemic treatment of operable breast cancer: an update. *J Clin Oncol*. 2006;24(12):1940–1949.
28. Gralow JR, Burstein HJ, Wood W, et al. Preoperative therapy in invasive breast cancer: pathologic assessment and systemic therapy issues in operable disease. *J Clin Oncol*. 2008;26(5):814–819.
29. Mieog JS, van der Hage JA, van de Velde CJ. Neoadjuvant chemotherapy for operable breast cancer. *Br J Surg*. 2007;94(10):1189–1200.
30. Fisher B, Bryant J, Wolmark N, et al. Effect of preoperative chemotherapy on the outcome of women with operable breast cancer. *J Clin Oncol*. 1998;16(8):2672–2685.
31. Early Breast Cancer Trialists' Collaborative Group (EBCTCG)Peto R, Davies C, Godwin J, Gray R, Pan HC, Clarke M, Cutter D, Darby S, McGale P, Taylor C, Wang YC, Bergh J, Di Leo A, Albain K, Swain S, Piccart M, Pritchard K. Comparisons between different polychemotherapy regimens for early breast cancer: meta-analyses of long-term outcome among 100,000 women in 123 randomised trials. *Lancet*. 2012;379(9814):432–444.
32. Paik S, Tang G, Shak S, et al. Gene expression and benefit of chemotherapy in women with node-negative, estrogen receptor-positive breast cancer. *J Clin Oncol*. 2006;24(23):3726–3734.
33. Sparano JA, Gray RJ, Makower DF, et al. Prospective validation of a 21-gene expression assay in breast cancer. *N Engl J Med*. 2015;373(21):2005–2014. doi:10.1056/NEJMoa1510764.
34. Piccart-Gebhart MJ, Procter M, Leyland-Jones B, et al. Trastuzumab after adjuvant chemotherapy in HER2-positive breast cancer. *N Engl J Med*. 2005;353(16):1659–1672.
35. Romond EH, Perez EA, Bryant J, et al. Trastuzumab plus adjuvant chemotherapy for operable HER2-positive breast cancer. *N Engl J Med*. 2005;353(16):1673–1684.
36. Slamon D, Eiermann W, Robert N, et al. Adjuvant trastuzumab in HER2-positive breast cancer. *N Engl J Med*. 2011;365(14):1273–1283. doi:10.1056/NEJMoa0910383.
37. Cameron D, Piccart-Gebhart MJ, Gelber RD, et al. 11 years' follow-up of trastuzumab after adjuvant chemotherapy in HER2-positive early breast cancer: final analysis of the HERceptin Adjuvant (HERA) trial. *Lancet*. 2017;389(10075):1195–1205.
38. Burstein HJ, Temin S, Anderson H, et al. Adjuvant endocrine therapy for women with hormone receptor-positive breast cancer: American Society of Clinical Oncology clinical practice guideline focused update. *J Clin Oncol*. 2014;32(21):2255–2269.
39. Davies C, Godwin J, Gray R, et at., Early Breast Cancer Trialists' Collaborative Group (EBCTCG). Relevance of breast cancer hormone receptors and other factors to the efficacy of adjuvant tamoxifen: patient-level meta-analysis of randomised trials. *Lancet*. 2011;378(9793):771–784.
40. Davies C, Pan H, Godwin J, et al. Long-term effects of continuing adjuvant tamoxifen to 10 years versus stopping at 5 years after diagnosis of oestrogen receptor-positive breast cancer: ATLAS, a randomised trial. *Lancet*. 2013;381(9869):805–816.
41. Goss PE, Ingle JN, Martino S, et al. Randomized trial of letrozole following tamoxifen as extended adjuvant therapy in receptor-positive breast cancer: updated findings from NCIC CTG MA.17. *J Natl Cancer Inst*. 2005;97(17):1262–1271.
42. Veronesi U, Cascinelli N, Mariani L, et al. Twenty-year follow-up of a randomized study comparing breast-conserving surgery with radical mastectomy for early breast cancer. *N Engl J Med*. 2002;347(16):1227–1232.
43. Litière S, Werutsky G, Fentiman IS, et al. Breast conserving therapy versus mastectomy for stage I-II breast cancer: 20 year follow-up of the EORTC 10801 phase 3 randomised trial. *Lancet Oncol*. 2012;13(4):412–419.
44. van Maaren MC, de Munck L, de Bock GH, et al. 10 year survival after breast-conserving surgery plus radiotherapy compared with mastectomy in early breast cancer in the Netherlands: a population-based study. *Lancet Oncol*. 2016;17(8):1158–1170.
45. Agarwal S, Pappas L, Neumayer L, et al. Effect of breast conservation therapy vs mastectomy on disease-specific survival for early-stage breast cancer. *JAMA Surg*. 2014;149(3):267–274.
46. Blichert-Toft M, Nielsen M, Düring M, et al. Long-term results of breast conserving surgery vs. mastectomy for early stage invasive breast cancer: 20-year follow-up of the Danish randomized DBCG-82TM protocol. *Acta Oncol*. 2008;47(4):672–681.
47. Newman LA. Decision making in the surgical management of invasive breast cancer-part 2: expanded applications for breast-conserving surgery. Oncology (Williston Park). 2017;31(5):415–420.
48. Moran MS, Schnitt SJ, Giuliano AE, et al. Society of Surgical Oncology-American Society for Radiation Oncology consensus guideline on margins for breast-conserving surgery with whole-breast irradiation in stages I and II invasive breast cancer. *Int J Radiat Oncol Biol Phys*. 2014;88(3):553–564.
49. Gradishar WJ, Anderson BO, Balassanian R, et al. Breast Cancer, Version 4.2017, NCCN Clinical Practice Guidelines in Oncology. *J Natl Compr Canc Netw*. 2018;3:310–320.
50. Early Breast Cancer Trialists' Collaborative Group (EBCTCG)Darby S, McGale P, Correa C, Taylor C, Arriagada R, Clarke M, Cutter D, Davies C, Ewertz M, Godwin J, Gray R, Pierce L, Whelan T, Wang Y, Peto R. Effect of radiotherapy after breast-conserving surgery on 10-year recurrence and 15-year breast cancer death: meta-analysis of individual patient data for 10,801 women in 17 randomised trials. *Lancet*. 2011;378(9804):1707–1716.
51. Hopwood P, Haviland JS, Sumo G, et al. Comparison of patient-reported breast, arm, and shoulder symptoms and body image after radiotherapy for early breast cancer: 5-year follow-up in the randomised Standardisation of Breast Radiotherapy (START) trials. *Lancet Oncol*. 2010;11(3):231–240.
52. Haviland JS, Owen JR, Dewar JA, et al. The UK Standardisation of Breast Radiotherapy (START) trials of radiotherapy hypofractionation for treatment of early breast cancer: 10-year follow-up results of two randomised controlled trials. *Lancet Oncol*. 2013;14(11):1086–1094.

53. Whelan TJ, Pignol JP, Levine MN, et al. Long-term results of hypofractionated radiation therapy for breast cancer. *N Engl J Med.* 2010;362(6):513–520. Doi:10.1056/NEJMoa0906260.
54. Whelan T, Julian J, Levine M, et al. RAPID: a randomized trial of accelerated partial breast irradiation using 3-dimensional conformal radiotherapy (3D-CRT). San Antonio Breast Cancer Symposium; San Antonio, TX, USA; Dec 4–8, 2018. (abstr GS4-03).
55. Vicini FA, Cecchini RS, White JR, et al. Primary results of NSABP B-39/RTOG 0413 (NRG Oncology): a randomized phase III study of conventional whole breast irradiation versus partial breast irradiation for women with stage 0, I, or II breast cancer. San Antonio Breast Cancer Symposium; San Antonio, TX, USA; Dec 4–8, 2018. (abstr GS4-04).
56. Hughes KS, Schnaper LA, Bellon JR, et al. Lumpectomy plus tamoxifen with or without irradiation in women age 70 years or older with early breast cancer: long-term follow-up of CALGB 9343. *J Clin Oncol.* 2013;31(19):2382–2387.
57. Kunkler IH, Williams LJ, Jack WJ, et al. Breast-conserving surgery with or without irradiation in women aged 65 years or older with early breast cancer (PRIME II): a randomised controlled trial. *Lancet Oncol.* 2015;16(3):266–273.
58. Cemal Y, Albornoz CR, Disa JJ, et al. A paradigm shift in U.S. breast reconstruction: Part 2. The influence of changing mastectomy patterns on reconstructive rate and method. *Plast Reconstr Surg.* 2013;131(3):320e–326e.
59. Kroll SS, Khoo A, Singletary SE, et al. Local recurrence risk after skin-sparing and conventional mastectomy: a 6-year follow-up. *Plast Reconstr Surg.* 1999;104(2):421–425.
60. Cocquyt VF, Blondeel PN, Depypere HT, et al. Better cosmetic results and comparable quality of life after skin-sparing mastectomy and immediate autologous breast reconstruction compared to breast conservative treatment. *Br J Plast Surg.* 2003;56(5):462–470.
61. Gerber B, Krause A, Reimer T, et al. Skin-sparing mastectomy with conservation of the nipple-areola complex and autologous reconstruction is an oncologically safe procedure. *Ann Surg.* 2003;238(1):120–127.
62. Warren Peled A, Foster RD, Stover AC, et al. Outcomes after total skin-sparing mastectomy and immediate reconstruction in 657 breasts. *Ann Surg Oncol.* 2012;19(11):3402–3409.
63. Lanitis S, Tekkis PP, Sgourakis G, et al. Comparison of skin-sparing mastectomy versus non-skin-sparing mastectomy for breast cancer: a meta-analysis of observational studies. *Ann Surg.* 2010;251(4):632–639.
64. Medina-Franco H, Vasconez LO, Fix RJ, et al. Factors associated with local recurrence after skin-sparing mastectomy and immediate breast reconstruction for invasive breast cancer. *Ann Surg.* 2002;235(6):814–819.
65. Carlson GW, Styblo TM, Lyles RH, et al. The use of skin sparing mastectomy in the treatment of breast cancer: the Emory experience. *Surg Oncol.* 2003;12(4):265–269.
66. Chung AP, Sacchini V. Nipple-sparing mastectomy: where are we now? *Surg Oncol.* 2008;17(4):261–266.
67. Smith BL, Tang R, Rai U, et al. Oncologic safety of nipple-sparing mastectomy in women with breast cancer. *J Am Coll Surg.* 2017;225(3):361–365.
68. Moo TA, Pinchinat T, Mays S, et al. Oncologic outcomes after nipple-sparing mastectomy. *Ann Surg Oncol.* 2016;23(10):3221–3225.
69. Orzalesi L, Casella D, Santi C, et al. Nipple sparing mastectomy: surgical and oncological outcomes from a national multicentric registry with 913 patients (1006 cases) over a six year period. *Breast.* 2016;25:75–81.
70. Moo TA, Sanford R, Dang C, et al. Overview of breast cancer therapy. *PET Clin.* 2018;13(3):339–354.
71. EBCTCG (Early Breast Cancer Trialists' Collaborative Group)McGale P, Taylor C, Correa C, Cutter D, Duane F, Ewertz M, Gray R, Mannu G, Peto R, Whelan T, Wang Y, Wang Z, Darby S. Effect of radiotherapy after mastectomy and axillary surgery on 10-year recurrence and 20-year breast cancer mortality: meta-analysis of individual patient data for 8135 women in 22 randomised trials. *Lancet.* 2014;383(9935):2127–2135.
72. Recht A, Gray R, Davidson NE, et al. Locoregional failure 10 years after mastectomy and adjuvant chemotherapy with or without tamoxifen without irradiation: experience of the Eastern Cooperative Oncology Group. *J Clin Oncol.* 1999;17(6):1689–1700.
73. Moo TA, McMillan R, Lee M, et al. Selection criteria for postmastectomy radiotherapy in t1-t2 tumors with 1 to 3 positive lymph nodes. *Ann Surg Oncol.* 2013;20(10):3169–3174.
74. Huo D, Hou N, Jaskowiak N, et al. Use of postmastectomy radiotherapy and survival rates for breast cancer patients with T1-T2 and one to three positive lymph nodes. *Ann Surg Oncol.* 2015;22(13):4295–4304.
75. Sharma R, Bedrosian I, Lucci A, et al. Present-day locoregional control in patients with t1 or t2 breast cancer with 0 and 1 to 3 positive lymph nodes after mastectomy without radiotherapy. *Ann Surg Oncol.* 2010;17(11):2899–2908.
76. Lyman GH, Somerfield MR, Bosserman LD, et al. Sentinel lymph node biopsy for patients with early-stage breast cancer: American Society of Clinical Oncology clinical practice guideline update. *J Clin Oncol.* 2017;35(5):561–564.
77. Lyman GH, Giuliano AE, Somerfield MR, et al. American Society of Clinical Oncology guideline recommendations for sentinel lymph node biopsy in early-stage breast cancer. *J Clin Oncol.* 2005;23(30):7703–7720. Doi:10.1200/JCO.2005.08.001.
78. Giuliano AE, Hunt KK, Ballman KV, et al. Axillary dissection vs no axillary dissection in women with invasive breast cancer and sentinel node metastasis: a randomized clinical trial. *JAMA.* 2011;305(6):569–575.
79. Giuliano AE, Ballman K, McCall L, et al. Locoregional recurrence after sentinel lymph node dissection with or without axillary dissection in patients with sentinel lymph node metastases: long-term follow-up from the American College of Surgeons Oncology Group (Alliance) ACOSOG Z0011 randomized trial. *Ann Surg.* 2016;264(3):413–420.
80. Albornoz CR, Bach PB, Mehrara BJ, et al. A paradigm shift in U.S. Breast reconstruction: increasing implant rates. *Plast Reconstr Surg.* 2013;131(1):15–23.
81. Farhangkhoee H, Matros E, Disa J. Trends and concepts in post-mastectomy breast reconstruction. *J Surg Oncol.* 2016;113(8):891–894.
82. Morrow M, Li Y, Alderman AK, et al. Access to breast reconstruction after mastectomy and patient perspectives on reconstruction decision making. *JAMA Surg.* 2014;149(10):1015–1021.
83. Rowland JH, Desmond KA, Meyerowitz BE, et al. Role of breast reconstructive surgery in physical and emotional outcomes among breast cancer survivors. *J Natl Cancer Inst.* 2000;92(17):1422–1429.
84. Ng SK, Hare RM, Kuang RJ, et al. Breast reconstruction post mastectomy: patient satisfaction and decision making. *Ann Plast Surg.* 2016;76(6):640–644.

85. Wellisch DK, Schain WS, Noone RB, et al. Psychosocial correlates of immediate versus delayed reconstruction of the breast. *Plast Reconstr Surg.* 1985;76(5):713–718.
86. Murphy Jr RX, Wahhab S, Rovito PF, et al. Impact of immediate reconstruction on the local recurrence of breast cancer after mastectomy. *Ann Plast Surg.* 2003;50(4):333–338.
87. Nahabedian MY. Breast reconstruction: a review and rationale for patient selection. *Plast Reconstr Surg.* 2009;124(1):55–62.
88. McCarthy CM, Mehrara BJ, Riedel E, et al. Predicting complications following expander/implant breast reconstruction: an outcomes analysis based on preoperative clinical risk. *Plast Reconstr Surg.* 2008;121(6):1886–1892.
89. Ganske I, Verma K, Rosen H, et al. Minimizing complications with the use of acellular dermal matrix for immediate implant-based breast reconstruction. *Ann Plast Surg.* 2013;71(5):464–470.
90. Namnoum JD. Expander/implant reconstruction with AlloDerm: recent experience. *Plast Reconstr Surg.* 2009;124(2):387–394.
91. Vardanian AJ, Clayton JL, Roostaeian J, et al. Comparison of implant-based immediate breast reconstruction with and without acellular dermal matrix. *Plast Reconstr Surg.* 2011;128(5):403e–410e.
92. Harless C, Jacobson SR. Current strategies with 2-staged prosthetic breast reconstruction. *Gland Surg.* 2015;4(3):204–211.
93. Sbitany H, Sandeen SN, Amalfi AN, et al. Acellular dermis-assisted prosthetic breast reconstruction versus complete submuscular coverage: a head-to-head comparison of outcomes. *Plast Reconstr Surg.* 2009;124(6):1735–1740.
94. Sigalove S, Maxwell GP, Sigalove NM, et al. Prepectoral implant-based breast reconstruction: rationale, indications, and preliminary results. *Plast Reconstr Surg.* 2017;139(2):287–294.
95. Woo A, Harless C, Jacobson SR. Revisiting an old place: single-surgeon experience on post-mastectomy subcutaneous implant-based breast reconstruction. *Breast J.* 2017;23(5):545–553.
96. Zhu L, Mohan AT, Abdelsattar JM, et al. Comparison of subcutaneous versus submuscular expander placement in the first stage of immediate breast reconstruction. *J Plast Reconstr Aesthet Surg.* 2016;69(4):e77–e86.
97. Walia GS, Aston J, Bello R, et al. Prepectoral versus subpectoral tissue expander placement: a clinical and quality of life outcomes study. *Plast Reconstr Surg Glob Open.* 2018;6(4):e1731.
98. DeLong MR, Tandon VJ, Rudkin GH, et al. Latissimus dorsi flap breast reconstruction-a nationwide inpatient sample review. *Ann Plast Surg.* 2017;78(5 Suppl 4):S185–S188.
99. Fischer JP, Nelson JA, Au A, et al. Complications and morbidity following breast reconstruction—a review of 16,063 cases from the 2005-2010 NSQIP datasets. *J Plast Surg Hand Surg.* 2014;48(2):104–114.
100. Cordeiro PG, McCarthy CM. A single surgeon's 12-year experience with tissue expander/implant breast reconstruction: Part I. A prospective analysis of early complications. *Plast Reconstr Surg.* 2006;118(4):825–831.
101. McCarthy CM, Klassen AF, Cano SJ, et al. Patient satisfaction with postmastectomy breast reconstruction: a comparison of saline and silicone implants. *Cancer.* 2010;116(24):5584–5591.
102. DellaCroce FJ, Sullivan SK, Trahan C. Stacked deep inferior epigastric perforator flap breast reconstruction: a review of 110 flaps in 55 cases over 3 years. *Plast Reconstr Surg.* 2011;127(3):1093–1099.
103. Stalder MW, Lam J, Allen RJ, et al. Using the retrograde internal mammary system for stacked perforator flap breast reconstruction: 71 breast reconstructions in 53 consecutive patients. *Plast Reconstr Surg.* 2016;137(2):265e–277e.
104. Serletti JM. Breast reconstruction with the TRAM flap: pedicled and free. *J Surg Oncol.* 2006;94(6):532–537.
105. Mathes SJ, Nahai F. Classification of the vascular anatomy of muscles: experimental and clinical correlation. *Plast Reconstr Surg.* 1981;67(2):177–187.
106. Feller AM. Free TRAM. Results and abdominal wall function. *Clin Plast Surg.* 1994;21(2):223–232.
107. Grotting JC, Urist MM, Maddox WA, et al. Conventional TRAM flap versus free microsurgical TRAM flap for immediate breast reconstruction. *Plast Reconstr Surg.* 1989;83(5):828–841 discussion 842–844.
108. Arnez ZM, Smith RW, Eder E, et al. Breast reconstruction by the free lower transverse rectus abdominis musculocutaneous flap. *Br J Plast Surg.* 1988;41(5):500–505.
109. Allen RJ, Treece P. Deep inferior epigastric perforator flap for breast reconstruction. *Ann Plast Surg.* 1994;32(1):32–38.
110. Guerra AB, Metzinger SE, Bidros RS, et al. Bilateral breast reconstruction with the deep inferior epigastric perforator (DIEP) flap: an experience with 280 flaps. *Ann Plast Surg.* 2004;52(3):246–252.
111. Blondeel N, Vanderstraeten GG, Monstrey SJ, et al. The donor site morbidity of free DIEP flaps and free TRAM flaps for breast reconstruction. *Br J Plast Surg.* 1997;50(5):322–330.
112. Nahabedian MY, Momen B, Galdino G, et al. Breast reconstruction with the free TRAM or DIEP flap: patient selection, choice of flap, and outcome. *Plast Reconstr Surg.* 2002;110(2):466–475 discussion 476–477.
113. Garvey PB, Buchel EW, Pockaj BA, et al. DIEP and pedicled TRAM flaps: a comparison of outcomes. *Plast Reconstr Surg.* 2006;117(6):1711–1719 discussion 1720–1721.
114. Kaplan JL, Allen RJ. Cost-based comparison between perforator flaps and TRAM flaps for breast reconstruction. *Plast Reconstr Surg.* 2000;105(3):943–948.
115. Allen RJ, Tucker Jr C. Superior gluteal artery perforator free flap for breast reconstruction. *Plast Reconstr Surg.* 1995;95(7):1207–1212.
116. Paletta CE, Bostwick J 3rd. Nahai F. The inferior gluteal free flap in breast reconstruction. *Plast Reconstr Surg.* 1989;84(6):875–883 discussion 884–885.
117. Ahmadzadeh R, Bergeron L, Tang M, et al. The posterior thigh perforator flap or profunda femoris artery perforator flap. *Plast Reconstr Surg.* 2007;119(1):194–200 discussion 201–202.
118. Fansa H, Schirmer S, Warnecke IC, et al. The transverse myocutaneous gracilis muscle flap: a fast and reliable method for breast reconstruction. *Plast Reconstr Surg.* 2008;122(5):1326–1333.
119. Cordeiro PG. Breast reconstruction after surgery for breast cancer. *N Engl J Med.* 2008;359(15):1590–1601.
120. Serletti JM, Fosnot J, Nelson JA, et al. Breast reconstruction after breast cancer. *Plast Reconstr Surg.* 2011;127(6):124e–135e.
121. Jagsi R, Momoh AO, Qi J, et al. Impact of radiotherapy on complications and patient-reported outcomes after breast reconstruction. *J Natl Cancer Inst.* 2018;110(2).
122. Bennett KG, Qi J, Kim HM, et al. Comparison of 2-year complication rates among common techniques for postmastectomy breast reconstruction. *JAMA Surg.* 2018;153(10):901–908.
123. Schaverien MV, McCulley SJ. Effect of obesity on outcomes of free autologous breast reconstruction: a meta-analysis. *Microsurgery.* 2014;34(6):484–497.

124. Fischer JP, Nelson JA, Kovach SJ, et al. Impact of obesity on outcomes in breast reconstruction: analysis of 15,937 patients from the ACS-NSQIP datasets. *J Am Coll Surg*. 2013;217(4):656–664.
125. Fischer JP, Nelson JA, Sieber B, et al. Free tissue transfer in the obese patient: an outcome and cost analysis in 1258 consecutive abdominally based reconstructions. *Plast Reconstr Surg*. 2013;131(5):681e–692e.
126. Wilkins EG, Hamill JB, Kim HM, et al. Complications in postmastectomy breast reconstruction: one-year outcomes of the Mastectomy Reconstruction Outcomes Consortium (MROC) study. *Ann Surg*. 2018;267(1):164–170.
127. Alderman AK, Wilkins EG, Kim HM, et al. Complications in postmastectomy breast reconstruction: two-year results of the Michigan Breast Reconstruction Outcome Study. *Plast Reconstr Surg*. 2002;109(7):2265–2274.
128. Nelson JA, Disa JJ. Breast reconstruction and radiation therapy: an update. *Plast Reconstr Surg*. 2017;140:60S–68S.
129. Berbers J, van Baardwijk A, Houben R, et al. 'Reconstruction: before or after postmastectomy radiotherapy?' A systematic review of the literature. *Eur J Cancer*. 2014;50(16):2752–2762.
130. Tsoi B, Ziolkowski NI, Thoma A, et al. Safety of tissue expander/implant versus autologous abdominal tissue breast reconstruction in postmastectomy breast cancer patients: a systematic review and meta-analysis. *Plast Reconstr Surg*. 2014;133(2):234–249.
131. Cordeiro PG, Albornoz CR, McCormick B, et al. What is the optimum timing of postmastectomy radiotherapy in two-stage prosthetic reconstruction: radiation to the tissue expander or permanent implant? *Plast Reconstr Surg*. 2015;135(6):1509–1517.
132. Miranda RN, Aladily TN, Prince HM, et al. Breast implant–associated anaplastic large-cell lymphoma: long-term follow-up of 60 patients. *J Clin Oncol*. 2014;32(2):114–120.
133. McCarthy CM, Loyo-Berríos N, Qureshi AA, et al. Patient registry and outcomes for breast implants and anaplastic large cell lymphoma etiology and epidemiology (PROFILE): initial report of findings, 2012-2018. *Plast Reconstr Surg*. 2019;143:65S–73S.
134. Brody GS, Deapen D, Taylor CR, et al. Anaplastic large cell lymphoma occurring in women with breast implants: analysis of 173 cases. *Plast Reconstr Surg*. 2015;135(3):695–705.
135. Loch-Wilkinson A, Beath KJ, Knight RJW, et al. Breast implant-associated anaplastic large cell lymphoma in Australia and New Zealand: high-surface-area textured implants are associated with increased risk. *Plast Reconstr Surg*. 2017;140(4):645–654.
136. Nelson JA, Dabic S, Mehrara BJ, et al. Breast implant-associated anaplastic large cell lymphoma incidence: determining an accurate risk. Ann Surg. 2020;1272(3):403–409.
137. Nelson JA, Allen RJ Jr., Polanco T, et al. Long-term patient-reported outcomes following postmastectomy breast reconstruction: an 8-year examination of 3268 patients. *Ann Surg*. 2019 Sep;270(3):473–483.
138. de Jong D, Vasmel WL, de Boer JP, et al. Anaplastic large-cell lymphoma in women with breast implants. *JAMA*. 2008;300(17):2030–2035.
139. US Food and Drug Administration. FDA takes action to protect patients from risk of certain textured breast implants; requests Allergan voluntarily recall certain breast implants and tissue expanders from market. FDA News Release. 2019, July 24. https://www.fda.gov/news-events/press-announcements/fda-takes-action-protect-patients-risk-certain-textured-breast-implants-requests-allergan.
140. Pusic AL, Matros E, Fine N, et al. Patient-reported outcomes 1 year after immediate breast reconstruction: results of the mastectomy reconstruction outcomes consortium study. *J Clin Oncol*. 2017;35(22):2499–2506.
141. Santosa KB, Qi J, Kim HM, et al. Long-term patient-reported outcomes in postmastectomy breast reconstruction. *JAMA Surg*. 2018;153(10):891–899.
142. Nelson JA, Allen RJ Jr, Polanco T, et al. Long-term patient-reported outcomes following postmastectomy breast reconstruction: an 8-year examination of 3268 patients. *Ann Surg*. 2019;270(3):473–483.
143. Sheehan J, Sherman KA, Lam T, et al. Association of information satisfaction, psychological distress and monitoring coping style with post-decision regret following breast reconstruction. *Psychooncology*. 2007;16(4):342–351.
144. Lantz PM, Janz NK, Fagerlin A, et al. Satisfaction with surgery outcomes and the decision process in a population-based sample of women with breast cancer. *Health Serv Res*. 2005;40(3):745–767.
145. Ewer MS, Lippman SM. Type II chemotherapy-related cardiac dysfunction: time to recognize a new entity. *J Clin Oncol*. 2005;23(13):2900–2902.
146. Khouri MG, Douglas PS, Mackey JR, et al. Cancer therapy-induced cardiac toxicity in early breast cancer: addressing the unresolved issues. *Circulation*. 2012;126(23):2749–2763.
147. Chatterjee K, Zhang J, Honbo N, et al. Doxorubicin cardiomyopathy. *Cardiology*. 2010;115(2):155–162.
148. Swain SM, Whaley FS, Ewer MS. Congestive heart failure in patients treated with doxorubicin: a retrospective analysis of three trials. *Cancer*. 2003;97(11):2869–2879.
149. Keefe DL. Trastuzumab-associated cardiotoxicity. *Cancer*. 2002;95(7):1592–1600.
150. Perez EA, Rodeheffer R. Clinical cardiac tolerability of trastuzumab. *J Clin Oncol*. 2004;22(2):322–329.
151. Slamon DJ, Leyland-Jones B, Shak S, et al. Use of chemotherapy plus a monoclonal antibody against HER2 for metastatic breast cancer that overexpresses HER2. *N Engl J Med*. 2001;344(11):783–792.
152. Kehlet H. Multimodal approach to control postoperative pathophysiology and rehabilitation. *Br J Anaesth*. 1997;78(5):606–617.
153. Ljungqvist O, Scott M, Fearon KC. Enhanced Recovery After Surgery: a review. *JAMA Surg*. 2019;152(3):292–298.
154. Arsalani-Zadeh R, ElFadl D, Yassin N, et al. Evidence-based review of enhancing postoperative recovery after breast surgery. *Br J Surg*. 2011;98(2):181–196.
155. Afonso A, Oskar S, Tan KS, et al. Is enhanced recovery the new standard of care in microsurgical breast reconstruction? *Plast Reconstr Surg*. 2017;139(5):1053–1061.
156. Bonde C, Khorasani H, Eriksen K, et al. Introducing the fast track surgery principles can reduce length of stay after autologous breast reconstruction using free flaps: a case control study. *J Plast Surg Hand Surg*. 2015;49(6):367–371.
157. Batdorf NJ, Lemaine V, Lovely JK, et al. Enhanced recovery after surgery in microvascular breast reconstruction. *J Plast Reconstr Aesthet Surg*. 2015;68(3):395–402.
158. Offodile 2nd AC, Gu C, Boukovalas S, et al. Enhanced recovery after surgery (ERAS) pathways in breast reconstruction: systematic review and meta-analysis of the literature. *Breast Cancer Res Treat*. 2019;173(1):65–77.

159. Chiu C, Aleshi P, Esserman LJ, et al. Improved analgesia and reduced post-operative nausea and vomiting after implementation of an enhanced recovery after surgery (ERAS) pathway for total mastectomy. *BMC Anesthesiol.* 2018;18(1):41.
160. Wallace MS, Wallace AM, Lee J, et al. Pain after breast surgery: a survey of 282 women. *Pain.* 1996;66(2-3):195–205.
161. Nelson JA, Fischer JP, Pasick C, et al. Chronic pain following abdominal free flap breast reconstruction: a prospective pilot analysis. *Ann Plast Surg.* 2013;71(3):278–282.
162. Fassoulaki A, Melemeni A, Staikou C, et al. Acute postoperative pain predicts chronic pain and long-term analgesic requirements after breast surgery for cancer. *Acta Anaesthesiol Belg.* 2008;59(4):241–248.
163. Poleshuck EL, Katz J, Andrus CH, et al. Risk factors for chronic pain following breast cancer surgery: a prospective study. *J Pain.* 2006;7(9):626–634.
164. Caffo O, Amichetti M, Ferro A, et al. Pain and quality of life after surgery for breast cancer. *Breast Cancer Res Treat.* 2003;80(1):39–48.
165. Fortner BV, Stepanski EJ, Wang SC, et al. Sleep and quality of life in breast cancer patients. *J Pain Symptom Manage.* 2002;24(5):471–480.
166. Tokita HK, Polanco TO, Shamsunder MG, et al. Non-narcotic perioperative pain management in prosthetic breast reconstruction during an opioid crisis: a systematic review of paravertebral blocks. *Plast Reconstr Surg Glob Open.* 2019;7(6):e2299.
167. Schnabel A, Reichl SU, Kranke P, et al. Efficacy and safety of paravertebral blocks in breast surgery: a meta-analysis of randomized controlled trials. *Br J Anaesth.* 2010;105(6):842–852.
168. Woodworth GE, Ivie RMJ, Nelson SM, et al. Perioperative breast analgesia: a qualitative review of anatomy and regional techniques. *Reg Anesth Pain Med.* 2017;42(5):609–631.
169. Pace MM, Sharma B, Anderson-Dam J, et al. Ultrasound-guided thoracic paravertebral blockade: a retrospective study of the incidence of complications. *Anesth Analg.* 2016;122(4):1186–1191.
170. Blanco R, Parras T, McDonnell JG, et al. Serratus plane block: a novel ultrasound-guided thoracic wall nerve block. *Anaesthesia.* 2013;68(11):1107–1113.
171. Forero M, Adhikary SD, Lopez H, et al. The erector spinae plane block: a novel analgesic technique in thoracic neuropathic pain. *Reg Anesth Pain Med.* 2016;41(5):621–627.
172. Hussain N, Brull R, McCartney CJL, et al. Pectoralis-II myofascial block and analgesia in breast cancer surgery: a systematic review and meta-analysis. *Anesthesiology.* 2019;131(3):630–648.
173. Krag DN, Anderson SJ, Julian TB, et al. Technical outcomes of sentinel-lymph-node resection and conventional axillary-lymph-node dissection in patients with clinically node-negative breast cancer: results from the NSABP B-32 randomised phase III trial. *Lancet Oncol.* 2007;8(10):881–888.
174. Raut CP, Hunt KK, Akins JS, et al. Incidence of anaphylactoid reactions to isosulfan blue dye during breast carcinoma lymphatic mapping in patients treated with preoperative prophylaxis: results of a surgical prospective clinical practice protocol. *Cancer.* 2005;104(4):692–699.
175. Ramin S, Azar FP, Malihe H. Methylene blue as the safest blue dye for sentinel node mapping: emphasis on anaphylaxis reaction. *Acta Oncol.* 2011;50(5):729–731.
176. Bleicher RJ, Kloth DD, Robinson D, et al. Inflammatory cutaneous adverse effects of methylene blue dye injection for lymphatic mapping/sentinel lymphadenectomy. *J Surg Oncol.* 2009;99(6):356–360.
177. Teknos D, Ramcharan A, Oluwole SF. Pulmonary edema associated with methylene blue dye administration during sentinel lymph node biopsy. *J Natl Med Assoc.* 2008;100(12):1483–1484.
188. Zakaria S, Hoskin TL, Degnim AC. Safety and technical success of methylene blue dye for lymphatic mapping in breast cancer. *Am J Surg.* 2008;196(2):228–233.
179. Kim R. Anesthetic technique and cancer recurrence in oncologic surgery: unraveling the puzzle. *Cancer Metastasis Rev.* 2017;36(1):159–177.
180. Stollings LM, Jia LJ, Tang P, et al. Immune modulation by volatile anesthetics. *Anesthesiology.* 2016;125(2):399–411.
181. Byrne K, Levins KJ, Buggy DJ. Can anesthetic-analgesic technique during primary cancer surgery affect recurrence or metastasis? *Can J Anaesth.* 2016;63(2):184–192.
182. Heaney A, Buggy DJ. Can anaesthetic and analgesic techniques affect cancer recurrence or metastasis? *Br J Anaesth.* 2012;109(suppl 1):i17–i28.
183. Wall T, Sherwin A, Ma D, et al. Influence of perioperative anaesthetic and analgesic interventions on oncological outcomes: a narrative review. *Br J Anaesth.* 2019;123(2):135–150.
184. Nguyen J, Luk K, Vang D, et al. Morphine stimulates cancer progression and mast cell activation and impairs survival in transgenic mice with breast cancer. *Br J Anaesth.* 2014;113(suppl 1):i4–i13.
185. Jaura AI, Flood G, Gallagher HC, et al. Differential effects of serum from patients administered distinct anaesthetic techniques on apoptosis in breast cancer cells in vitro: a pilot study. *Br J Anaesth.* 2014;113(suppl 1):i63–i67.
186. Buckley A, McQuaid S, Johnson P, et al. Effect of anaesthetic technique on the natural killer cell anti-tumour activity of serum from women undergoing breast cancer surgery: a pilot study. *Br J Anaesth.* 2014;113(suppl 1):i56–i62.
187. Forget P, Bentin C, Machiels JP, et al. Intraoperative use of ketorolac or diclofenac is associated with improved disease-free survival and overall survival in conservative breast cancer surgery. *Br J Anaesth.* 2014;113(suppl 1):i82–i87.
188. Forget P, Vandenhende J, Berliere M, et al. Do intraoperative analgesics influence breast cancer recurrence after mastectomy? A retrospective analysis. *Anesth Analg.* 2010;110(6):1630–1635.
189. Sherwin A, Buggy DJ. The effect of anaesthetic and analgesic technique on oncological outcomes. SpringerLink. 2019.
190. Tavare AN, Perry NJ, Benzonana LL, et al. Cancer recurrence after surgery: direct and indirect effects of anesthetic agents. *Int J Cancer.* 2012;130(6):1237–1250.
191. Kurosawa S, Kato M. Anesthetics, immune cells, and immune responses. *J Anesth.* 2008;22(3):263–277.
192. Chen Y, Liang M, Zhu Y, et al. [The effect of propofol and sevoflurane on the perioperative immunity in patients under laparoscopic radical resection of colorectal cancer]. *Zhonghua Yi Xue Za Zhi.* 2015;95(42):3440–3444.
193. Liu TC. Influence of propofol, isoflurane and enflurance on levels of serum interleukin-8 and interleukin-10 in cancer patients. *Asian Pac J Cancer Prev.* 2014;15(16):6703–6707.
194. Ecimovic P, Murray D, Doran P, et al. Propofol and bupivacaine in breast cancer cell function in vitro—role of the NET1 gene. *Anticancer Res.* 2014;34(3):1321–1331.
195. Yu B, Gao W, Zhou H, et al. Propofol induces apoptosis of breast cancer cells by downregulation of miR-24 signal pathway. *Cancer Biomark.* 2018;21(3):513–519.
196. Lee JH, Kang SH, Kim Y, et al. Effects of propofol-based total intravenous anesthesia on recurrence and overall survival in pa-

tients after modified radical mastectomy: a retrospective study. *Korean J Anesthesiol.* 2016;69(2):126–132.
197. Lai HC, Lee MS, Lin C, et al. Propofol-based total intravenous anaesthesia is associated with better survival than desflurane anaesthesia in hepatectomy for hepatocellular carcinoma: a retrospective cohort study. *Br J Anaesth.* 2019;123(2):151–160.
198. Wigmore TJ, Mohammed K, Jhanji S. Long-term survival for patients undergoing volatile versus IV anesthesia for cancer surgery: a retrospective analysis. *Anesthesiology.* 2016;124(1):69–79.
199. Yap A, Lopez-Olivo MA, Dubowitz J, et al. Anesthetic technique and cancer outcomes: a meta-analysis of total intravenous versus volatile anesthesia. *Can J Anaesth.* 2019;66(5):546–561.
200. Yoo S, Lee HB, Han W, et al. Total intravenous anesthesia versus inhalation anesthesia for breast cancer surgery: a retrospective cohort study. *Anesthesiology.* 2019;130(1):31–40.
201. Hahnenkamp K, Herroeder S, Hollmann MW. Regional anaesthesia, local anaesthetics and the surgical stress response. *Best Pract Res Clin Anaesthesiol.* 2004;18(3):509–527.
202. O'Riain SC, Buggy DJ, Kerin MJ, et al. Inhibition of the stress response to breast cancer surgery by regional anesthesia and analgesia does not affect vascular endothelial growth factor and prostaglandin E2. *Anesth Analg.* 2005;100(1):244–249.
203. Pei L, Tan G, Wang L, et al. Comparison of combined general-epidural anesthesia with general anesthesia effects on survival and cancer recurrence: a meta-analysis of retrospective and prospective studies. *PLoS One.* 2014;9(12):e114667.
204. Exadaktylos AK, Buggy DJ, Moriarty DC, et al. Can anesthetic technique for primary breast cancer surgery affect recurrence or metastasis? *Anesthesiology.* 2006;105(4):660–664.
205. Sessler DI, Pei L, Huang Y, et al. Recurrence of breast cancer after regional or general anaesthesia: a randomised controlled trial. *Lancet.* 2019;394(10211):1807–1815.
206. Kulkarni A, Pusic A, Hamill J, et al. Factors associated with acute postoperative pain following breast reconstruction. *JPRAS Open.* 2017;11:1–13. doi:10.1016/j.jpra.2016.08.005.
207. Coopey S, Specht M, Warren L, et al. Use of preoperative paravertebral block decreases length of stay in patients undergoing mastectomy plus immediate reconstruction. *Ann Surg Oncol.* 2013;20:1282–1286. doi:10.1245/s10434-012-2678-7.
208. Blanco R. The 'pecs block': a novel technique for providing analgesia after breast surgery. *Anaesthesia.* 2011;66(9):847–848. doi:10.1111/j.1365-2044.2011.06838.x.

24

Intraoperative Care of the Surgical Patient: Upper Gastrointestinal Cancers

ALESSANDRO R. DE CAMILLI AND DANIELA MOLENA

Introduction

The upper gastrointestinal (GI) tract comprises the mouth, esophagus, stomach, and duodenum. The incidence of such cancers is rising, and improved operative safety and successes of neoadjuvant chemotherapy have increased the number of patients who are candidates for curative resection. Resection of tumors involving the upper GI tract carries high intraoperative risk, and due to shared anatomy, close concert between the anesthesiologist and surgeon. The goals of intraoperative management include optimal fluid management, appropriate multimodal analgesia, reduction of postoperative pulmonary complications, and optimizing the physiologic milieu to promote anastomotic healing.

Chemotherapeutic Toxicity

Patients receiving neoadjuvant chemotherapy for upper esophageal cancer may suffer from chemotherapeutic toxicity of which the intraoperative team should be aware. Chemotherapeutic agents can cause dysrhythmias (anthracycline, pembrolizumab), myocarditis (cyclophosphamide, busulfan), dilated cardiomyopathy (doxorubicin), and prolonged QT interval (oxaliplatin, tamoxifen, anthracycline, 5-fluorouracil, paclitaxel). Patients receiving these agents may have pericardial effusions, restrictive cardiomyopathy, and congestive heart failure. All patients who have received chemotherapy agents and who express symptoms of dyspnea on exertion should receive a preoperative echocardiogram to screen for cardiomyopathy.

Esophageal Cancer

Epidemiology

The incidence of esophageal cancer in the United States is 0.7% in men and 0.2% in women, making it the 18th most common type of cancer and the 11th in terms of risk of death.[1] Ninety-five percent of esophageal cancers are squamous cell carcinoma (SCC) and adenocarcinoma. The incidence of adenocarcinoma, once considered to be quite rare, now accounts for more than 60% of esophageal cancers, largely due to the increase in incidence of Barrett's esophagus. In southern and eastern Africa and eastern Asia, the incidence of esophageal cancer is much higher and predominantly due to SCC. Small cell cancers, leiomyosarcomas, leiomyomas, and GI stromal tumors account for a very small portion of esophageal cancers. Due to improved treatment modalities, the 5-year survival rate has increased from 5% in the 1960s to 20% in the modern day.

Behavioral risk factors for squamous cell esophageal cancer include smoking and alcohol consumption. Dietary factors include red meat consumption, low fiber diets, hot beverage consumption, zinc deficiency, and selenium deficiency. History of achalasia or caustic injury are additional predisposing factors.[2] Human papilloma virus (HPV) has not been definitively linked to esophageal cancer.[3] The increasing prevalence of adenocarcinoma is linked to higher rates of obesity, gastroesophageal reflux disease, and diets low in fruits and vegetables. A history of Barrett's esophagus increases the risk of developing esophageal cancer by 30-fold.[4] Adenocarcinoma is more prevalent among Caucasians, and six times more prevalent in males than females.

The most common location of SCC in the esophagus is at the midportion, arising from small plaques that can be missed on endoscopy. Local lymph node infiltration occurs early due to the close proximity of the lymph nodes to the lamina propria of the esophagus. It eventually progresses to invade adjacent organs, including the celiac artery and aorta, which can present with massive upper GI bleeding.

Adenocarcinoma most commonly arises in the gastroesophageal junction and most commonly spreads to the celiac and perihepatic nodes.

Diagnosis and Staging

Early esophageal cancer is usually asymptomatic and only detected during endoscopy for alternative purposes or during surveillance for Barrett's esophagus. Symptoms for more advanced cancers are usually dysphagia (often manifested in the early stage by the "sticking" of hard foods), weight loss, and iron-deficiency anemia. Severely advanced cases can progress to cause tracheobronchial fistulas. Rarely, recurrent laryngeal nerve involvement can cause hoarseness. Endoscopic biopsy is required to confirm the diagnosis.

At the time of presentation, 22% of esophageal cancers are localized to the esophagus. Regional spread is present 30% of the time, and the remaining present as advanced disease.[5]

Staging to evaluate regional and advanced spread is done via endoscopic ultrasound (EUS, which can diagnose local lymph nodes and liver metastases), bronchoscopy, and whole-body positron emission tomography (PET), and occasionally diagnostic laparoscopy. Laparoscopy is reserved for patients who have responded to chemotherapy and are surgical candidates but the extent of disease is unknown, or in whom extent of peritoneal disease is unclear from imaging. Tumor extending into the stomach for more than 5 cm is considered unresectable.

Treatment

Disease that is limited to the mucosa or submucosa is of a diameter of <2 cm, and does not involve the entire circumference of the esophagus can be treated with surgery or endoscopic therapy. For cancers that have invaded into the esophageal wall or are node-positive, treatment involves chemotherapy and surgery.

Endoscopic Ultrasound

Endoscopy with the use of ultrasound is becoming standard of care for diagnosis, biopsy, and occasionally treatment of small, localized esophageal tumors. Deep sedation may be appropriate for a small subset of patients who are asymptomatic at the time of presentation; general anesthesia with a protected airway is the method of choice due to aspiration risk.

Surgical Treatment and Intraoperative Considerations

Surgical Candidacy

Patients with stage T4b disease that is invasive to the aorta, trachea, or spine are considered unresectable, as are those who present with tracheoesophageal fistula. These patients can be candidates for radiation and chemotherapy, and reassessed for candidacy after demonstrating the appropriate response.

For early esophageal cancer, surgery is the mainstay of treatment, with or without neoadjuvant chemotherapy and radiation. Chemotherapy and/or radiation are considered before surgery for patients with full thickness involvement of the esophagus, or with local invasion to structures that can be easily resected. These patients undergo posttreatment radiologic staging to reassess resectability and undergo surgery 4–6 weeks after. Severe cardiac or pulmonary comorbid disease and advanced age are relative contraindications to surgery. Chronic obstructive pulmonary disease portends a higher risk of postoperative pulmonary complications, but several prehabilitation guidelines have been proposed to reduce this risk.[6] Preoperative nutrition optimization is critical, as malnutrition is immunosuppressive and negatively impacts survival.[7]

Relevant Anatomy

The esophagus consists of four layers: the mucosa, submucosa, muscularis propria, and adventitia. The arterial supply consists of the thyroid artery, the left gastric artery, the inferior phrenic artery, and the aorta. Lymphatic drainage is to the cervical, tracheobronchial, gastric, celiac, and mediastinal nodes.[8]

Type of Surgery

Esophageal cancers involving more than two-thirds of the esophagus or the proximal portion of the esophagus typically require resection of the entire esophagus. Distal tumors, or tumors at the level of the gastroesophageal junction, can be treated with a partial resection, using intraoperative surgical pathology to ensure that the margins do not contain carcinoma or Barrett's esophagus changes.

A gastric interposition is the most common organ used to reconstruct the esophagus, although a colonic or jejunal segment can also be used. The latter is suboptimal when compared with a gastric interposition because it requires multiple anastomoses and involves a more complex surgical resection. Additionally, blood supply via the mesenteric arteries limits the distance that this segment can be moved.

There are three commonly used approaches. The **Ivor Lewis esophagectomy (ILE)** starts with a laparotomy for mobilization of gastric structures and conduit construction. This is followed by a right thoracotomy for esophageal mobilization, resection, and intrathoracic anastomosis. This approach is intended for lower-third esophageal cancers, and allows for a full visualization of the thoracic esophagus and full thoracic lymphadenectomy. For tumors involving the gastroesophageal junction (GEJ), a thoracoabdominal approach can be used in which the entire procedure is performed via a left thoracic incision. This limits visualization of the proximal esophagus.

The **three-hole approach** (also known as the McKeown method) involves an abdominal incision, thoracic incision, and a cervical incision. In this approach, the esophageal anastomosis is made via the cervical incision. In this approach, the left neck should be free of invasive lines to make room for surgical dissection of the neck.

A **transhiatal esophagectomy (THE)** uses a midline upper laparotomy incision to mobilize the stomach and esophagus and a cervical incision to pull up the stomach. This does not require a thoracotomy and instead mobilizes the esophagus via dissection from the neck. This technique does not allow for extensive lymph node dissection in the chest and is not ideal for patients with cancers in the mid-esophagus. It is advantageous for patients with crippling pulmonary disease owing to its lack of a thoracotomy.

Outcomes for the above techniques are roughly similar, with a postoperative mortality rate of around 3% at high-volume centers.[9] These approaches can be performed partially or completely using a laparoscopic or video-assisted thoracoscopic (VATS) approach. A laparoscopic and video-thoracoscopic esophagectomy is referred to as minimally invasive esophagectomy (MIE). Studies comparing MIE to the open approach have demonstrated a reduced rate of pulmonary infections,[10] intensive care unit (ICU) length of stay, improved quality of life scores, improved physical function, superior analgesia, and decreased fluid requirements. The TIME trial (traditional invasive vs. minimally invasive esophagectomy) demonstrated superior postoperative outcomes for patients undergoing MIE as compared with open esophagectomy, and similar oncologic outcomes to open esophagectomy when patients were followed up within 3 years for cancer recurrence.[11,12] Additionally, it had equivalent specimen quality and a similar number of lymph nodes removed. Similar studies have demonstrated improved postoperative outcomes, or noninferior outcomes, as well as similar 3-year survival rates.[13] At this time, MIE is recognized as a safe and ideal option to reduce the physiologic impact of esophageal surgery. However, data are not yet sufficient to recommend MIE as a full replacement for open esophagectomy.

Lymph node dissection is standard in all esophagectomies; however, the extent to which this is performed is subject to debate. Lymph node dissection is typically performed in the mediastinum, upper abdomen, and occasionally cervical nodes (for thoracic esophageal cancers). Paratracheal and paraaortic lymph nodes are commonly dissected.

A feeding jejunostomy is placed for the purpose of nutritional support during chemotherapy and radiation therapy.

Cervical esophageal cancer (between the posterior pharynx and upper one-third of the esophagus) is usually treated with radiation and chemotherapy, but those who fail may be candidates for surgical resection. Surgical resection is highly complex and involves a bilateral neck dissection, potential tracheostomy (if laryngectomy is required), and a thoracic and abdominal incision. It may also require removal of the pharynx, larynx, and thyroid gland.

Intraoperative Considerations

Induction and Airway Management

Patients with esophageal carcinoma often have symptoms of reflux and dysphagia, but these are not often bothersome when presenting for elective surgery. However, gastric outlet obstruction from GEJ tumors can lead to residual gastric volumes. Additionally, reflux symptoms in patients with Barrett's esophagus may be more pronounced when lying flat. For this reason, intubation should be performed with slight head of bed elevation at 30 degrees, and mask ventilation should not exceed pressures of 20 mmHg. Patients with significant upper GI symptoms should additionally be considered for a rapid sequence intubation.

Mask ventilation, as well as noninvasive positive pressure ventilation (NIPPV) via mask, is contraindicated in the immediate postesophagectomy phase due to risk of air insufflation into the newly anastomosed esophagus. Patients with esophageal leaks or anastomotic complications who return to the operating room after esophagectomy should be treated with similar caution. At all times in the perioperative phase, even after discharge, patients with esophageal conduits are considered to be at high risk of aspiration.

Clear communication must occur between the anesthesiologist and surgeon at all times with regard to any foreign bodies in the esophagus. Orogastric tube insertion may be requested by the surgeon at the start of the case, which may be placed via endoscopic guidance. Care should be taken when removing the orogastric tube during the abdominal phase, and it should not be removed under suction to prevent esophageal shearing. Placement of the nasogastric tube during the thoracic portion should be performed under surgical instruction and very slowly to prevent esophageal rupture. Avoidance of any other monitoring devices (temperature probe, pressure monitors, etc.) in the oropharynx or esophagus is essential. Communication regarding orogastric and nasogastric tube placement and timing is perhaps the most critical element to esophagectomy (Fig. 24.1).

One-lung ventilation is necessary for the thoracic portion of the procedure and is best achieved via the placement of a double-lumen endotracheal tube. In most cases, it is desirable to place the double-lumen endotracheal tube at the start of the case; however, in the appropriate patient, a single-lumen tube may be used for the abdominal portion and exchanged for a double-lumen tube for the thoracic portion.

Maintenance of Anesthesia

Controversy has emerged regarding volatile anesthetics versus total intravenous agents, with some evidence that volatile agents may impair function of neutrophil and T-cell activity, making them a desirable choice for cancer resection.[14] Other studies have correlated improved cancer-free survival rates with total intravenous agents.[15] Neither volatile anesthetics nor intravenous anesthetics has any clinically significant effect on oxygenation during one-lung ventilation. Complete pharmacologic muscle paralysis is required for all portions of esophagectomy.

Intravenous Access

Large bore intravenous access and radial arterial monitoring are necessary. Central line insertion is indicated if adequate peripheral large bore access is unattainable, or if a patient's cardiac comorbidity makes vasopressor use more likely. Central venous pressure (CVP) measurement has not been demonstrated to be accurate for volume status assessment and is confounded by an open chest cavity, one-lung

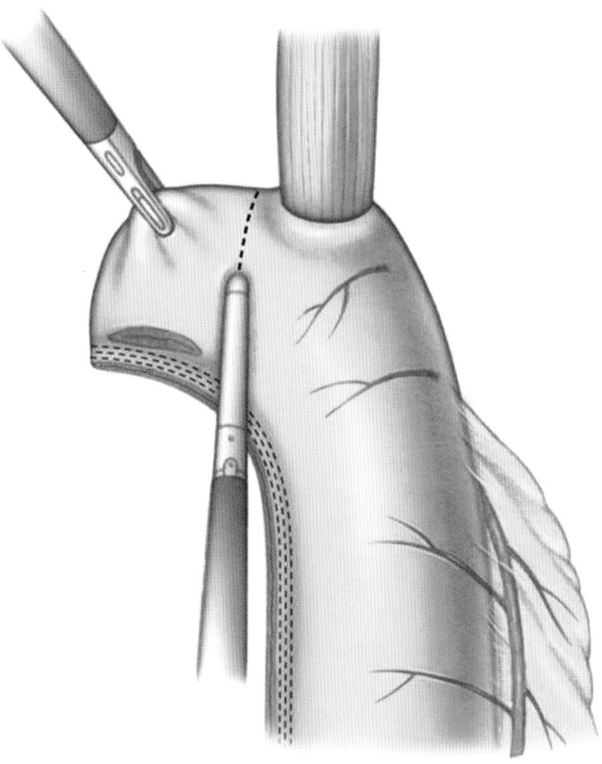

• **Fig. 24.1** In minimally invasive esophagectomy, the gastric conduit is connected to the esophagus using a stapler and proper nasogastric tube placement, and communication is vital. Nasogastric manipulation can perforate the anastomosis.

ventilation, and occasional surgical manipulation of the inferior vena cava (IVC).

Fluid

Surgical resection involving a major body cavity is associated with major fluid shifts. Patients with upper GI cancers may experience prolonged periods of poor oral intake, and those with advanced cancer may be undernourished. Complications such as anastomotic leak and pulmonary infections may cause a vasodilatory state and relative intravascular hypovolemia. Surgical stress is associated with a release of vasopressin, aldosterone, catecholamines, and acute-phase reactants that cause a proinflammatory state. Tachycardia, hypotension, and oliguria can make it difficult to distinguish between surgical-related inflammation and true hypovolemia.

Open esophagectomy with thoracotomy puts the fluid-sparing approach at odds with appropriate fluid resuscitation to compensate for evaporative losses from the abdomen. Evidence-based practice suggests a general trend toward minimizing fluid[16,17]; however, studies are highly variable in what constitutes a "sparing" or "liberal approach."[18] For esophageal surgery, evidence suggests a trend toward a restrictive fluid management approach in which fluid is only administered for signs of hypovolemia, rather than utilizing a predetermined calculation for "fluid deficit."[19] Avoidance of volume overload has been clearly associated with fewer infectious complications, improved wound healing, faster extubation times, and thinner bronchoscopic secretions.

As it has become clear that invasive pressure measurements in the form of central venous and Swan-Ganz catheters carry far higher risk than benefit (and additionally confer the risk of misinterpretation), newer, less invasive approaches are recommended. Systolic pressure variation, FloTrac, and transthoracic echocardiography have been demonstrated to be useful for intraoperative fluid management, but these may be of limited benefit in the setting of an open chest, an open abdomen, and the presence of chest tubes. Esophageal Doppler measurements of cardiac output are clearly contraindicated in surgery involving the esophagus.

The first stage of esophagectomy, particularly during use of the minimally invasive laparoscopic technique, often requires steep reverse Trendelenburg position. This pooling of the blood in the lower extremities can cause postural hypotension over time and, in prolonged cases, lead to metabolic acidosis. Judicious use of fluids and vasopressors, as well as frequent arterial blood gas measurements, are warranted to prevent this.

Vasopressor Use

Phenylephrine and norepinephrine, due to their selective alpha-1 receptor agonism, are commonly used intraoperatively as vasoconstrictors to counteract anesthetic-induced vasodilation. In euvolemic patients, for whom vasopressors are used solely for this purpose, perfusion to peripheral vascular beds is maintained. However, in the setting of hypovolemia, vasopressors can impair microvascular perfusion.[20] In patients who are bleeding or dry, efforts should be taken to restore intravascular volume prior to initiating vasopressor therapy. Fluid restrictive strategies should be used with careful titration to avoid "masking" hypovolemia with vasopressors.

Patients who are elderly, frail, or have significant cardiovascular disease may have increased susceptibility to the vasodilatory effects of anesthesia. Furthermore, evidence exists to suggest that intraoperative deviations of more than 20% from a patient's baseline blood pressure are associated with increased perioperative mortality.[21] After optimization of volume status, it is appropriate to use vasopressors to maintain appropriate perfusion pressure to satisfy these demands.

Pain Management

Use of thoracic epidural catheters for open esophagectomy is considered standard of care, with clear benefits for pain control, more rapid extubation times, decreased ICU length of stay, and possibly improved blood flow to the anastomosis due to local anesthetic-mediated vasodilatory effects.[22,23] There is also evidence that neuraxial anesthesia, with or without general anesthesia, is associated with prolonged survival in patients undergoing cancer resection.[24] Thoracic epidurals are generally placed at the T7/8 level to provide adequate coverage of abdominal and thoracic incisions.

The goal of intraoperative epidural management serves to minimize opiate administration and ensure proper spread of local anesthetic to produce an effective block upon

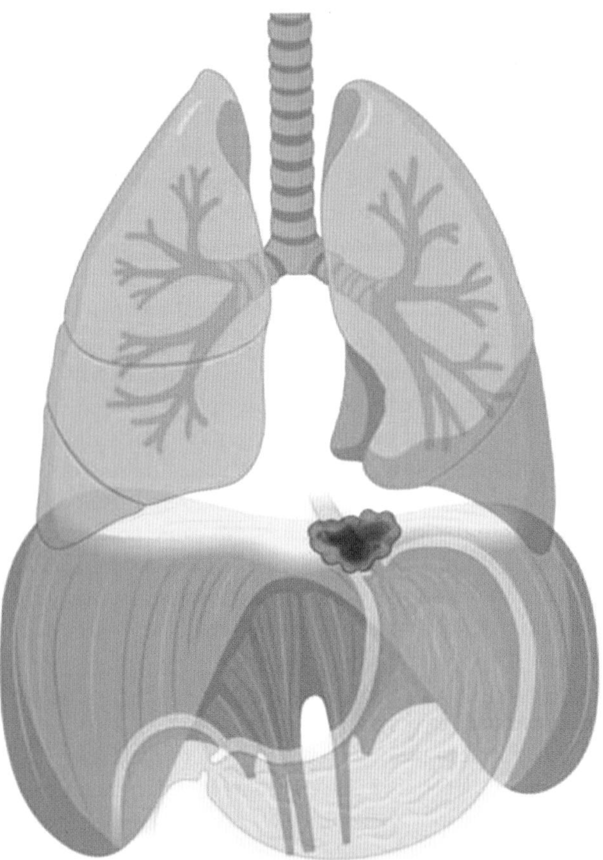

• **Fig. 24.2** Pneumothorax can occur during the abdominal phase, particularly if the tumor is adherent to the diaphragm. Treat with 100% FiO_2, flattening table, and vasopressors and reduce insufflation pressure (if laparoscopic).

extubation. The addition of an opioid to the epidural solution is recommended to allow for lower doses of local anesthetic to prevent excess epidural-mediated sympathectomy. It may be prudent to delay initiation of the epidural infusion until closure to minimize hypotension during the case. Close monitoring of epidural analgesia should be provided by an acute pain service, in conjunction with the surgical and postanesthetic recovery room team. Epidural-mediated sympathectomy resulting in undesirable hypotension should be mitigated by dilution or cessation of the epidural infusion, rather than continuous fluid-bolusing.

Additional regional anesthetic techniques for patients who have contraindications for neuraxial anesthesia or in whom attempts were unsuccessful include paravertebral, erector spinae, serratus, and intercostal blocks. Transversus abdominus plane (TAP) blocks have demonstrated success for laparotomy incisions in one study showing similar efficacy to epidurals with regard to reduction in pulmonary complications.[25] Serratus anterior blocks have also been shown to be comparable to neuraxial anesthesia in terms of postoperative opiate consumption in patients undergoing thoracotomy and thus in conjunction with TAP blocks represent an ideal backup choice for those who are not candidates for neuraxial anesthesia.[26]

Minimally invasive surgical techniques allow for smaller, less painful incision sites. For such cases, multimodal anesthetic techniques using acetaminophen, gabapentinoids, intercostal nerve blocks, and intravenous opioids are appropriate.

Emergence

Provided there is no significant acidosis and usual extubation criteria are met, efforts should be taken to extubate in the operating room. This is achievable in most esophagectomy patients. Early extubation is paramount to preventing pulmonary infections, early ambulation, and pulmonary toilet.

Intraoperative Complications

Pneumothorax is common during the abdominal portion of esophagectomy (Fig. 24.2). The esophagus is covered by the pleura on both sides, and bulky tumors can be adherent. A pneumothorax is most often first noted by the surgeon and then followed by increased airway pressure. Hypotension and tachycardia herald the progression to tension pneumothorax. This is more common during laparoscopic surgery due to the increased intraabdominal pressures from carbon dioxide (CO_2) insufflation. Upon detection of tension pneumothorax, fraction of inspired oxygen should be increased to 100%, the table should be flattened, insufflation pressures reduced, and hemodynamics supported with vasopressors.

Recurrent laryngeal nerve injury, which can be asymptomatic and transient, occurs in approximately 10%–15% of patients after esophageal resection. It carries a higher rate of pulmonary infections, respiratory failure, and longer hospital length of stay. It is most common with three-hole esophagectomy due to the creation of the anastomosis in the left neck. Injury to either the left or right recurrent laryngeal nerve can occur via thermal damage, stretching, or compression during paratracheal lymph node resection, owing to its path around the trachea (Fig. 24.3).

Bleeding is a complication during the abdominal phase, particularly from the short gastric vessels. During the thoracic portion, major bleeding can occur due to injury to the inferior pulmonary vein, the azygos (which courses along the thoracic vertebrae), or esophageal branches of the aorta (Fig. 24.4). Type and screen should be available for all patients, in addition to large bore intravenous access and arterial line monitoring.

Prevention of Pulmonary Complications

Approximately one-third of esophagectomy patients develop pulmonary complications.[27] The most common are pneumonia, acute respiratory distress syndrome (ARDS), and acute lung injury (ALI). Risk factors for pulmonary complications include advanced age, reduced lung capacity, elevated creatinine, poor functional status, smoking status, high blood loss surgery, and open surgery.[28] Modifiable risk factors include nutritional optimization, early enteral feeding, adequate pain control, fluid restriction, lung-protective ventilation, preoperative lung physiotherapy, and minimally invasive surgery when feasible.

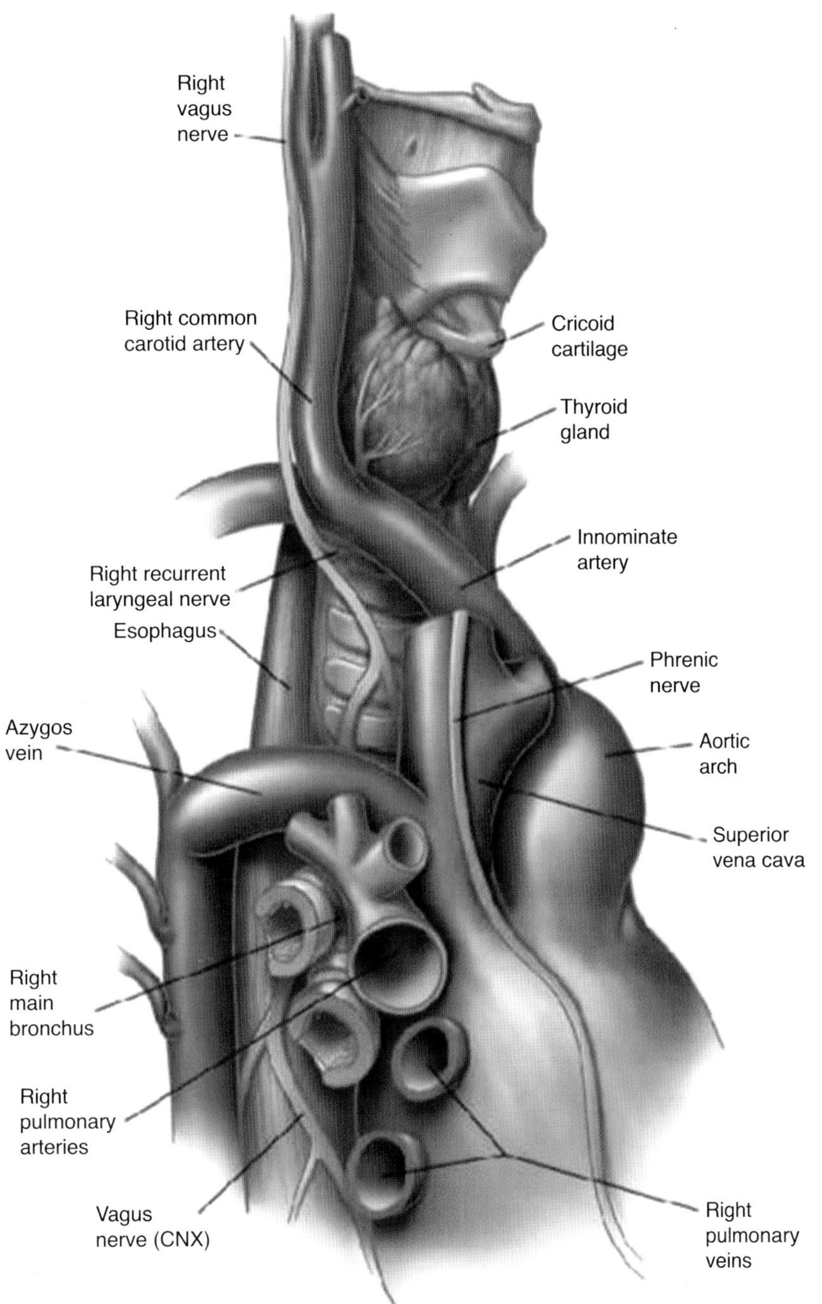

• **Fig. 24.3** The close proximity of the esophagus to the azygos vein, pulmonary vein, and recurrent laryngeal nerve makes for a delicate dissection during the thoracic portion of the case. Rapid bleeding and phrenic nerve injury can occur.

A strategy of "lung-protective ventilation" has long been recognized to be beneficial in ARDS. This strategy traditionally employs tidal volumes of 6–8 mL/kg for two-lung ventilation, 4–6 mL/kg for one-lung ventilation, positive end-expiratory pressure (PEEP), and avoidance of plateau pressures greater than 30 mmHg. This has not been clearly demonstrated to translate to the operating room, with studies suggesting no decrease in pulmonary complications with lung-protective ventilation during major surgery.[29] However, there is evidence that decreased tidal volumes lead to lower levels of barotrauma and release of acute-phase reactants when compared with high-tidal volume strategies,[30] and it is unlikely that this strategy causes harm.

Enhanced Recovery After Surgery Protocols

Enhanced Recovery After Surgery (ERAS) protocols have been shown to be an effective strategy to streamline perioperative care and improve patient outcomes (Fig. 24.5).

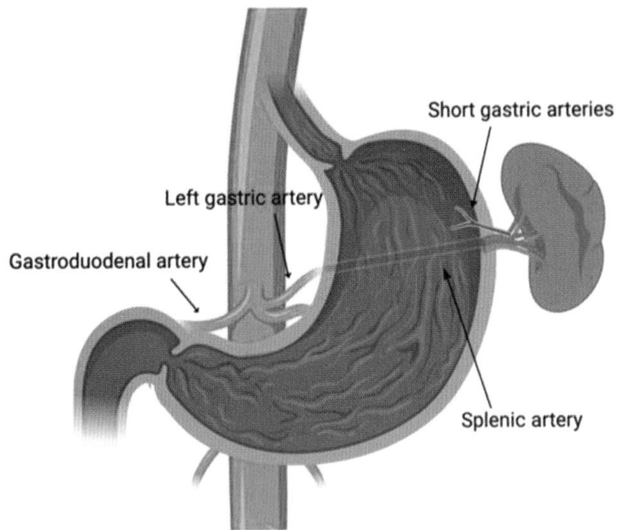

• **Fig. 24.4** Injury to the short gastric vessels can occur during manipulation/retraction of the stomach in the abdominal phase.

Prevention of Atrial Fibrillation

The incidence of atrial arrhythmias after esophageal resection is approximately 15%, with risk factors, including older age and preoperative worsened diffusion capacity of CO_2.[31] This complication portends a higher rate of pulmonary complications, ICU stays, hospital length of stay, and overall mortality.[32] Clinical trials investigating the optimal prophylactic agent are ongoing, but thus far evidence suggests that amiodarone or scheduled intravenous metoprolol in the immediate postoperative period is prudent to reduce this risk.[33]

Repair of Tracheoesophageal Fistula

Tracheoesophageal fistula formation is a rare complication of esophagectomy, or as sequelae of esophageal cancer. Patients often present with coughing, recurrent pneumonia, or purulent bronchitis. Ideal treatment strategies are tracheal and/or esophageal stent placement, depending on the location of the lesion. Tracheal stent placement requires induction of general anesthesia and rigid bronchoscopy with jet ventilation. Paralysis is ideal to decrease respiratory compliance and facilitate rigid bronchoscopy. Esophageal stent placement in a patient with no active upper GI symptoms can be performed with deep sedation and a natural airway.

Gastric Cancer

Gastric cancer was the leading cause of cancer deaths worldwide until the end of the 20th century, when it is postulated that treatment for the bacteria *Helicobacter pylori*, improved food sanitation, and a greater variety of fruits and vegetables led to a decreased carcinogenic milieu in the digestive system. There are approximately 20,000 cases in the United States annually.[34] Risk factors for gastric cancer in the United States include male sex, non-White race, and advanced age. However, despite the decrease in incidence overall, the number of cases is increasing due to increasing life expectancy. Mortality for gastric cancer is high because of the late stage in which it is typically diagnosed; early gastric cancer is typically asymptomatic.

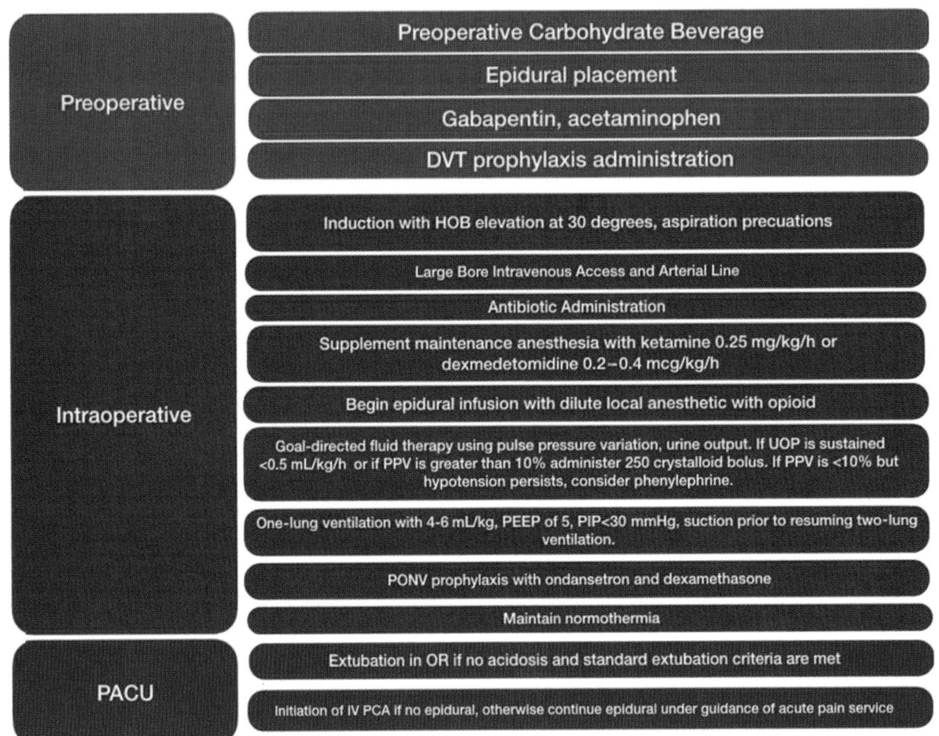

• **Fig. 24.5** Sample Enhanced Recovery After Surgery protocol for esophagogastrectomy. *PEEP*, Positive end-expiratory pressure; *PPV*, positive pressure ventilation.

Abdominal pain and unintentional weight loss are the most common presenting symptoms of gastric cancer, and upper endoscopy is highly sensitive for diagnosis. Staging is performed via PET scan and EUS. Most patients with high-grade tumors require staging laparoscopy due to the insensitivity of imaging to detect peritoneal disease. Metastatic spread is most often to the left supraclavicular nodes, ovaries, liver, and peritoneum. Positive peritoneal cytology portends a much graver prognosis and often precludes gastrectomy.

Esophagogastric junction tumors are classified as esophageal cancers unless they invade more than 2 cm into the stomach, in which case they are classified as gastric cancers.

Surgical candidates for gastric cancer resection do not have distant metastases, peritoneal carcinomatosis, extensive lymphadenopathy, or involvement of major vascular structures (not including gastric and splenic vasculature). Linitis plastica is a histologic subtype of gastric cancer that invades and thickens the gastric wall and, due to its aggressive and advanced nature at the time of diagnosis, is typically nonoperable.

The stomach derives its vascular supply from the gastric arteries, the splenic artery, and the gastroepiploic arteries, which are all branches of the celiac trunk.

Gastric malignancies that involve the proximal stomach typically require complete gastrectomy. Lesions that involve the lower two-thirds of the stomach are candidates for partial gastrectomy, which may involve a wedge or sleeve resection. Laparoscopic resection of gastric cancer has been shown to have comparable outcomes to open surgery in terms of short-term outcomes, as well as long-term survival.[35]

Intraoperative Management

Patients with gastric tumors involving the GEJ should be treated as an aspiration risk due to impaired gastric emptying and tumor involvement of the lower esophageal sphincter. Patients presenting for surgery after gastrectomy should be treated similarly, since there is no longer tonic contraction of the stomach to prevent reflux.

Thoracic epidurals are standard for postoperative pain control for open gastrectomy. Traditionally epidural anesthesia for GI surgery has been shown to offer superior pain control with a reduced rate of respiratory complications when compared with intravenous opioid-based regimens.[36] TAP blocks and rectus sheath blocks are additional options. Laparoscopic gastrectomy can be managed with multimodal analgesia with postoperative patient-controlled opioid delivery devices. Large bore intravenous access is required for all gastric tumor resections, while arterial and central access is dependent upon patient comorbidities.

Cancers of the Duodenum

Isolated duodenal cancers are rare, comprising 0.3% of all GI tumors. They are more common in patients with genetic predisposition to colon cancer, such as familial adenomatous polyposis, Gardner syndrome, Lynch syndrome, as well as patients with chronic inflammatory bowel disease. The most common type of duodenal tumor is adenocarcinoma, followed by lymphoma, carcinoid, gastrointestinal stromal tumors, and leiomyosarcomas.

At presentation, approximately half of duodenal cancers have spread to local lymph nodes, though most are without distant metastases. Pancreaticoduodenectomy is often indicated for tumors in the proximal third of the duodenum, while segmental resection with locoregional lymph node dissection can be performed for tumors in the distal duodenum.

Segmental resection of the duodenum can be performed laparoscopically and does not often require invasive access. Pancreaticoduodenectomy most often involves open resection of the head of the pancreas and the duodenum. This procedure involves significant fluid shifts and works around major arteries and thus requires large bore intravenous access, arterial line monitoring, and a thoracic epidural.

Cancers of the Oropharynx

SCC is the most common type of oropharyngeal carcinoma and, compared to other cancers of the GI tract, is quite rare. The most common risk factors are HPV infection, and alcohol and tobacco use. The most advanced oropharyngeal cancers are subject to neoadjuvant chemotherapy and radiation therapy prior to surgery.

Surgical options for oropharyngeal cancer include transoral robotic surgery and laser microsurgery, and the more invasive mandibulectomy.

Oropharyngeal cancer that has been irradiated presents a high risk for difficult intubation due to radiation-induced tissue fibrosis of the soft tissues of the neck. For tumors in the posterior oropharynx, even slight airway manipulation may lead to bleeding of friable mucosa. Direct laryngoscopy can induce tumor bleeding. Preoperatively, patients will have had a flexible nasolaryngoscopy exam and computed tomography results. This allows for additional insight into airway planning. Any involvement of tumor in the periglottic area warrants an awake intubation due to the risk of complete airway obstruction with sedation. Topicalization of the airway is necessary, though sometimes difficult if the tumor is so obstructive it absorbs attempts at spraying the vocal cords with local anesthetic. Nasal intubation is typically warranted for ease of surgical access to the oropharynx. Intubation should be performed cautiously, with preservation of spontaneous ventilation, and with surgical airway equipment nearby. Awake intubation should be accompanied by an antisialagogue such as glycopyrrolate. Ominous predictive factors for the presence of a difficult airway include dysphagia, odynophagia, hoarseness, and orthopnea.

After cautious induction and securing of the airway, anesthesia should be maintained with efforts to avoid excessive hypertension, and to minimize coughing upon extubation. Airway surgery can be extremely stimulating. Propofol and remifentanil offer ease of titratability, a predictably smoother wakeup, and the added advantage of avoiding volatile gas leaks during airway manipulation or in tracheostomy placement. Robotic oral surgery requires careful positioning of the robot and the patient's head to avoid compression of the face by robot arms. Intraoperative fraction of inspired oxygen should not exceed 30% to reduce the risk of airway fire. Deep paralysis is required for optimal surgical visualization. Recurrent laryngeal nerve injury can cause postextubation stridor, so care should be taken to extubate an awake, adequately breathing patient. Throat pack removal reminders should be set.

For tumors with invasion into the mandible, radiation alone is not sufficient to reduce tumor infiltration and prolonged radiation can cause osteoradionecrosis. For such cases, mandibulectomy is indicated. Mandibulectomy is a complex surgery that includes neck dissection and carries high risk for rapid blood loss. Preoperative airway exam should evaluate for trismus and mouth opening. Patients with dysphagia may suffer from prolonged periods of poor oral intake and present intravascularly dry. Large bore and arterial access are necessary. Maneuvers that can reduce surgical blood loss include reducing venous pressure (slight head-up position), preventing arterial pressure in excess of the patient's baseline, and local infiltration of the tissue with epinephrine-containing solutions. Cessation of paralysis after induction may be required for certain cases to identify tissue innervation of the facial nerve. Exchange of the endotracheal tube for a surgically placed tracheostomy must be done with extreme caution, and preoxygenation with 100% oxygen for a few minutes will help lengthen the time to desaturation. Increased airway pressures and lack of end-tidal CO_2 after tracheostomy placement are indicative of the tracheostomy placed in a false passage. For this reason, intubation equipment should be continuously available in case of need for reintubation.

As with resections for other upper GI tumors, oropharyngeal tumor resection has been shown to benefit from ERAS pathways that include multimodal analgesia, early ambulation, and fluid restriction. Pain control with acetaminophen, gabapentin, nonsteroidal antiinflammatory drugs (NSAIDs), and opioids are usually appropriate for postoperative pain.[37]

Other Upper Gastrointestinal Tumors

A subset of GI tumors that involve the mesenchymal cells of Cajal are called gastrointestinal stromal tumors (GISTs). These malignancies most commonly spread to local lymph nodes, liver, omentum, and peritoneum. GISTs may obstruct and compress other structures, but rarely invade them, making surgical resection more feasible than with adenocarcinomas.

Approximately half of neuroendocrine tumors (NETs) arise in the GI tract and are typically found distal to the ileum. However, some may arise in the stomach or proximal small bowel. These tumors, which arise from enterochromaffin cells, are characterized as low grade or high grade. The typical symptoms of carcinoid (flushing, diarrhea, hypotension) occur only when the tumor has metastasized, and the hormones are not first metabolized via the liver. This syndrome should be suspected in patients with NET who report episodes of flushing, wheezing, palpitations, or dizziness. To suppress these episodes intraoperatively, appropriate anxiolysis should occur, as well as preventing extremes of blood pressure. In the event of a crisis, octreotide (a somatostatin analogue), ondansetron, and vasopressors should be used. Etomidate, epinephrine, and drugs that release histamine should be avoided.

Conclusion

Cancers of the upper GI tract carry significant patient morbidity and mortality, and neoadjuvant therapy followed by surgical resection can be curative. The goals of intraoperative management are to protect the airway and reduce the risk of pulmonary complications, provide adequate oxygen delivery to the anastomoses, prophylaxis against cardiac complications, reduce the risk of nerve injury, and provide adequate postoperative analgesia to promote early ambulation. Clear communication with the surgical team and the use of evidence-based pathways are essential to providing excellent care.

References

1. American Cancer Society. Key Statistics for Esophageal Cancer. *American Cancer Society*. 2020. Available at https://www.cancer.org/cancer/esophagus-cancer/about/key-statistics.html.
2. Appelqvist P, Salmo M. Lye corrosion carcinoma of the esophagus: a review of 63 cases. *Cancer*. 1980;45(10):2655–2658. doi:10.1002/1097-0142(19800515)45:10<2655::aid-cncr2820451028>3.0.co;2-p.
3. IARC Monographs Working Group. IARC Monographs on the Evaluation of Carcinogenic Risks to Humans: International Agency for Research on Cancer. Biological Agents. IARC; 2011.
4. Eckardt VF, Kanzler G, Bernhard G. Life expectancy and cancer risk in patients with Barrett's esophagus: a prospective controlled investigation. *Am J Med*. 2001;111(1):33–37. doi:10.1016/s0002-9343(01)00745-8.
5. Cancer Stat Facts: Esophageal Cancer. National Cancer Institute. 2020. Available at seer.cancer.gov/statfacts/html/esoph.html#survival.
6. Gillinov AM, Heitmiller RF. Strategies to reduce pulmonary complications after transhiatal esophagectomy. *Dis Esophagus*. 2017;11(1):43–47. doi:10.1093/dote/11.1.43.
7. Grimm JC, Valero V. III, Molena D. Surgical indications and optimization of patients for resectable esophageal malignancies. *J Thorac Dis*. 2014;6(3):249–257. doi:10.3978/j.issn.2072-1439.2013.11.18.
8. Rice TW, Kelsen D, Blackstone EH, et al. Esophagus and esophagogastric junction. In: Amin MB, ed. *AJCC Cancer Staging Manual*. AJCC; 2017:85. 8th ed. Corrected at 4th printing, 2018.
9. Greene CL, Demeester SR, Worrell SG, Oh DS, Hagen JA, Demeester TR. Alimentary satisfaction, gastrointestinal symptoms, and quality of life 10 or more years after esophagectomy with gastric pull-up. *J Thorac Cardiovasc Surg*. 2014;147(3):909–914.

10. Straatman J, Van der wielen N, Cuesta MA, et al. Minimally invasive versus open esophageal resection: three-year follow-up of the previously reported randomized controlled trial: the TIME trial. *Ann Surg.* 2017;266(2):232–236.
11. Biere SS, Maas KW, Bonavina L, et al. Traditional invasive vs. minimally invasive esophagectomy: a multi-center, randomized trial (TIME-trial). *BMC Surg.* 2011;11:2.
12. Tan L, Tang H. Oncological outcomes of the TIME trial in esophageal cancer: is it the era of minimally invasive esophagectomy? *Ann Transl Med.* 2018;6(4):85. doi:10.21037/atm.2017.10.30.
13. Mariette C, Markar SR, Dabakuyo-Yonli TS, et al. Hybrid minimally invasive esophagectomy for esophageal cancer. *N Engl J Med.* 2019;380(2):152–162.
14. Stollings LM, Jia LJ, Tang P, Dou H, Lu B, Xu Y. Immune modulation by volatile anesthetics. *Anesthesiology.* 2016;125(2):399–411. doi:10.1097/ALN.0000000000001195.
15. Yap A, Lopez-Olivo MA, Dubowitz J, Hiller J, Riedel B. Anesthetic technique and cancer outcomes: a meta-analysis of total intravenous versus volatile anesthesia. *Can J Anaesth.* 2019;66(5):546–561.
16. Eng OS, Arlow RL, Moore D, et al. Fluid administration and morbidity in transhiatal esophagectomy. *J Surg Res.* 2016;200(1):91–97. doi:10.1016/j.jss.2015.07.021.
17. Casado D, López F, Martí R. Perioperative fluid management and major respiratory complications in patients undergoing esophagectomy. *Dis Esophagus.* 2010;23(7):523–528.
18. Chau EH, Slinger P. Perioperative fluid management for pulmonary resection surgery and esophagectomy. *Semin Cardiothorac Vasc Anesth.* 2014;18(1):36–44.
19. Neal JM, Wilcox RT, Allen HW, Low DE. Near-total esophagectomy: the influence of standardized multimodal management and intraoperative fluid restriction. *Reg Anesth Pain Med.* 2003;28(4):328–334.
20. De Backer D, Orbegozo Cortes D, Donadello K, Vincent JL. Pathophysiology of microcirculatory dysfunction and the pathogenesis of septic shock. *Virulence.* 2014;5(1):73–79. doi:10.4161/viru.26482.
21. Monk TG, Bronsert MR, Henderson WG, et al. Association between intraoperative hypotension and hypertension and 30-day postoperative mortality in noncardiac surgery. *Anesthesiology.* 2015;123(2):307–319. doi:10.1097/ALN.0000000000000756.
22. Michelet P, Roch A, D'Journo XB, et al. Effect of thoracic epidural analgesia on gastric blood flow after oesophagectomy. *Acta Anaesthesiol Scand.* 2007;51(5):587–594.
23. Theodorou D, Drimousis PG, Larentzakis A, Papalois A, Toutouzas KG, Katsaragakis S. The effects of vasopressors on perfusion of gastric graft after esophagectomy. An experimental study. *J Gastrointest Surg.* 2008;12(9):1497–1501.
24. Chen WK, Miao CH. The effect of anesthetic technique on survival in human cancers: a meta-analysis of retrospective and prospective studies. *PLoS One.* 2013;8(2):e56540. doi:10.1371/journal.pone.0056540.
25. Levy G, Cordes MA, Farivar AS, Aye RW, Louie BE. Transversus abdominis plane block improves perioperative outcome after esophagectomy versus epidural. *Ann Thorac Surg.* 2018;105(2):406–412.
26. Khalil AE, Abdallah NM, Bashandy GM, Kaddah TA. Ultrasound-guided serratus anterior plane block versus thoracic epidural analgesia for thoracotomy pain. *J Cardiothorac Vasc Anesth.* 2017;31(1):152–158.
27. Weijs TJ, Ruurda JP, Nieuwenhuijzen GA, van Hillegersberg R, Luyer MD. Strategies to reduce pulmonary complications after esophagectomy. *World J Gastroenterol.* 2013;19(39):6509–6514. doi:10.3748/wjg.v19.i39.6509.
28. Yoshida N, Watanabe M, Baba Y, et al. Risk factors for pulmonary complications after esophagectomy for esophageal cancer. *Surg Today.* 2014;44(3):526–532.
29. Futier E, Constantin JM, Paugam-Burtz C, et al. A trial of intraoperative low-tidal-volume ventilation in abdominal surgery. *N Engl J Med.* 2013;369(5):428–437.
30. Park SH. Perioperative lung-protective ventilation strategy reduces postoperative pulmonary complications in patients undergoing thoracic and major abdominal surgery. *Korean J Anesthesiol.* 2016;69(1):3–7. doi:10.4097/kjae.2016.69.1.3.
31. Amar D, Burt ME, Bains MS, Leung DH. Symptomatic tachydysrhythmias after esophagectomy: incidence and outcome measures. *Ann Thorac Surg.* 1996;61(5):1506–1509.
32. Stawicki SP, Prosciak MP, Gerlach AT, et al. Atrial fibrillation after esophagectomy: an indicator of postoperative morbidity. *Gen Thorac Cardiovasc Surg.* 2011;59(6):399–405. doi:10.1007/s11748-010-0713-9.
33. Tisdale JE, Wroblewski HA, Wall DS, et al. A randomized, controlled study of amiodarone for prevention of atrial fibrillation after transthoracic esophagectomy. *J Thorac Cardiovasc Surg.* 2010;140(1):45–51.
34. National Cancer Institute. Cancer Stat Facts: Stomach Cancer. National Cancer Institute. 2020. Available at https://seer.cancer.gov/statfacts/html/stomach.html.
35. Honda M, Hiki N, Kinoshita T, et al. Long-term outcomes of laparoscopic versus open surgery for clinical stage I gastric cancer: the LOC-1 study. *Ann Surg.* 2016;264(2):214–222.
36. Rigg JR, Jamrozik K, Myles PS, et al. Epidural anaesthesia and analgesia and outcome of major surgery: a randomised trial. *Lancet.* 2002;359(9314):1276–1282.
37. Coyle MJ, Main B, Hughes C, et al. Enhanced recovery after surgery (ERAS) for head and neck oncology patients. *Clin Otolaryngol.* 2016;41(2):118–126.

25

Perioperative Care of the Colorectal Cancer Patient

TOM WALL, RONAN CAHILL, AND DONAL J. BUGGY

Introduction

Colorectal cancer is the third most commonly diagnosed cancer worldwide with an estimated 1.8 million new cases in 2018, but ranks second in terms of mortality (after lung cancer) with an estimated 881,000 associated deaths per annum.[1] Approximately 50% of all colorectal cancer patients die from metastatic disease, with around 20% found to have metastases at time of presentation.[2] A higher incidence of colorectal cancer is found in developed societies, with evidence that elements of lifestyle common in developed countries such as higher consumption of processed foods, red meat, and alcohol, as well as obesity increase the risk of colorectal cancer development.[3] However, incidence and mortality rates have been declining in developed countries in recent years due to improvements in public health programs, screening, early diagnosis, and treatment.[4] Worryingly, incidence rates are increasing in those under 50 years of age, particularly for rectal cancers, and cancers are more likely to be detected at an advanced stage in this cohort.[5]

Presentation, Diagnosis, and Treatment

Asymptomatic colorectal cancer may be detected by screening, or patients may present with a constellation of symptoms, including passing blood per rectum, abdominal pain, altered bowel habit, and symptomatic anemia.[6] Occasionally, advanced cancers may present as surgical emergencies with bowel obstruction, perforation, or massive bleeding. Diagnosis is typically performed via endoscopy and biopsy of the lesion, with determination of the extent of local and distant disease spread requiring radiologic investigation in the form of CT, MR, and/or PET imaging. Pathologic staging uses the TNM (tumor, nodal involvement, metastasis) system and provides the most important factor in determining patient prognosis.[7] The depth of tumor invasion of the bowel wall determines the T stage, regional lymph node involvement determines the N stage, and presence or absence of metastases determines the M stage (see Fig. 25.1). Aside from the TNM stage, other factors affecting prognosis include poorly differentiated histology, perineural, or lymphovascular invasion; aneuploid DNA chromosomal patterns; and elevated serum carcinoembryonic antigen (CEA).[8] In 20% of patients with metastatic disease at the time of presentation, the most commonly affected sites are the liver, lungs, and peritoneum.[9] Eighty percent of newly diagnosed colorectal cancers are localized to the colon and/or local lymph nodes.[10]

Surgical excision is the appropriate treatment modality for localized disease, with the aim of surgery of curative intent being the removal of the diseased segment of bowel attached to its vascular pedicle and the associated lymphatic drainage system (see Fig. 25.2). For rectal cancers, total mesorectal excision (TME), which entails complete en bloc resection of the rectum along with the mesorectum containing the rectal blood supply and lymphatics, results in reduced recurrence rates.[11] Primary anastomosis to restore bowel continuity is generally appropriate in straightforward elective procedures, with formation of proximal defunctioning colostomy or ileostomy reserved for emergency or complex cases or for those with low rectal resection (<8 cm from anal canal). Lesions invading or attached to adjacent structures or organs frequently require more complex resection requiring multispecialty surgical involvement. Patients with metastatic disease at time of presentation are typically treated with chemotherapy; however, if metastases are limited to isolated lesions in the liver or lung, then metastasectomy can be considered and can significantly improve survival. Radiotherapy is infrequently used in the treatment of colon cancer, but it often plays an important role in the neoadjuvant or adjuvant treatment of rectal cancer where it has been shown to reduce local recurrence in stage III tumors.[12] Neoadjuvant radiotherapy is often given concomitantly with low-dose chemotherapy and commonly causes bowel and bladder dysfunction, rectal bleeding, dermatitis, and increases the risk of leakage from surgical anastomoses.[13] In some patients, a complete pathologic response may result from such therapy giving consideration to rectal

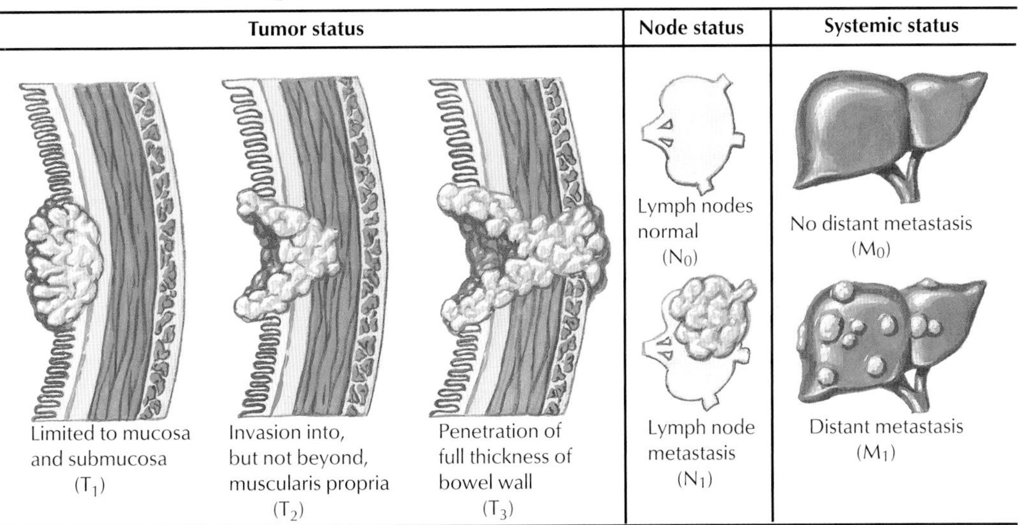

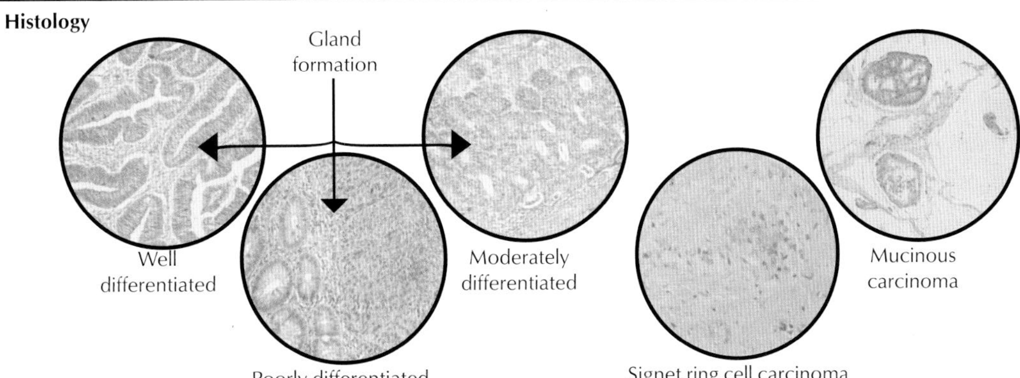

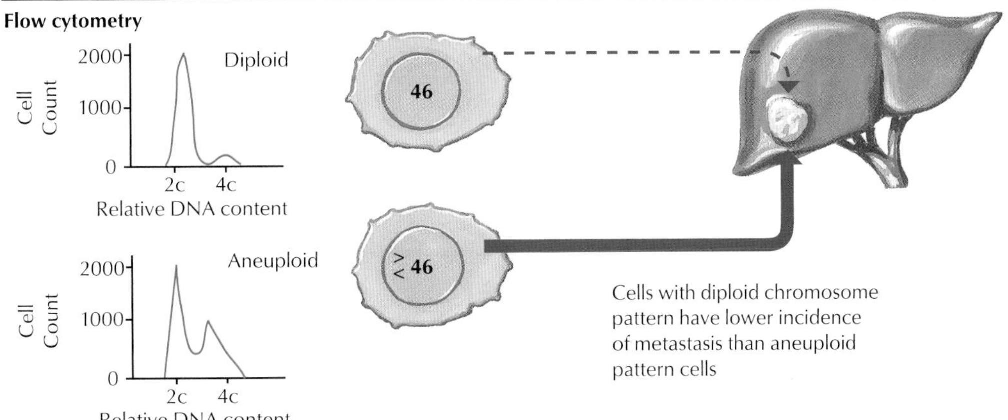

• **Fig. 25.1** Prognostic indicators in colorectal cancer. (From NetterImages.com Image ID: 5851, Reg ID: C0495.)

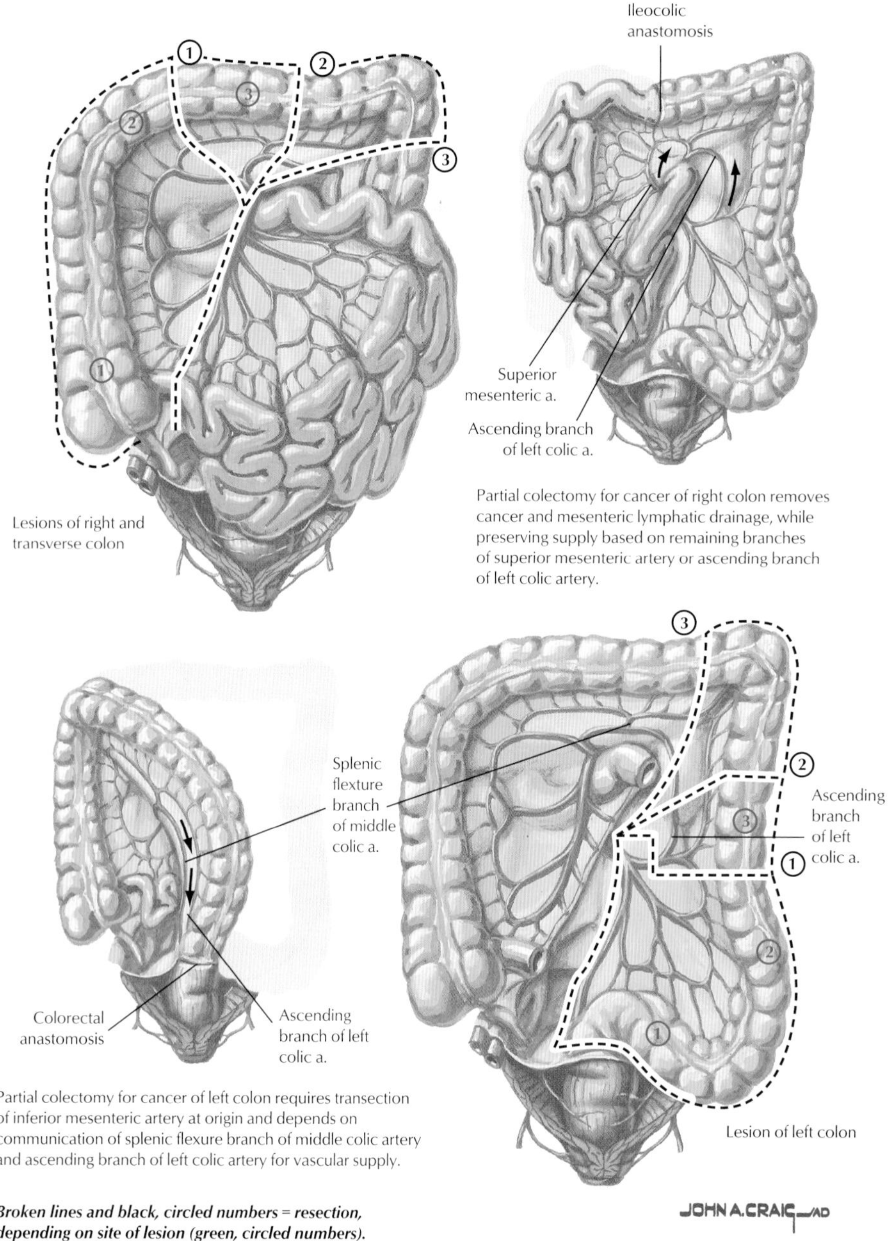

Ileocolic
anastomosis
Superior
mesenteric a.
Ascending branch
of left colic a.
Lesions of right and
transverse colon
Partial colectomy for cancer of right colon removes
cancer and mesenteric lymphatic drainage, while
preserving supply based on remaining branches
of superior mesenteric artery or ascending branch
of left colic artery.
Splenic
flexture
branch
of middle
colic a.
Ascending
branch
of left
colic a.
Colorectal
anastomosis
Ascending
branch of left
colic a.
Partial colectomy for cancer of left colon requires transection
of inferior mesenteric artery at origin and depends on
communication of splenic flexure branch of middle colic artery
and ascending branch of left colic artery for vascular supply.
Lesion of left colon
Broken lines and black, circled numbers = resection,
depending on site of lesion (green, circled numbers).
JOHN A.CRAIG—AD

• **Fig. 25.2** Surgical resection of colon cancer. (From NetterImages.com Image ID: 10179, Reg ID: C0497.)

preservation (i.e., avoidance of surgery) in association with "watchful waiting," although precise selection criteria are yet to be determined.

Perioperative Considerations of Neoadjuvant Chemotherapy

In addition to the patient's general physiologic status, preexisting comorbidities, and the pathologic effects of the malignant process, the perioperative physician must take into account the multisystem effects of neoadjuvant chemotherapy, if it has been employed. Patients should be assessed preoperatively for the presence of symptoms and signs suggestive of concerning systemic toxicity, particularly with respect to the cardiac, respiratory, hematologic, and immune systems. 5-Fluorouracil (5-FU) has provided the mainstay of chemotherapy for metastatic colorectal cancer for decades and is used in combination with other agents in a variety of treatment protocols. Perhaps the most familiar regime is FOLFOX (5-fluorouracil, oxaliplatin, leucovorin—otherwise known as folinic acid); FOLFIRI consists of 5-FU in combination with the cytotoxic alkaloid irinotecan, with FOLFIRINOX adding leucovorin and oxaliplatin; CAPOX replaces 5-FU with its prodrug capecitabine administered alongside oxaloplatin.[14]

Oxaliplatin is a third-generation platinum agent and is infrequently associated with nephrotoxicity, with reported cases of acute tubular necrosis, renal tubular acidosis, hemolytic anemia, and acute kidney injury.[15] Hypertension may also develop as a result. Serial renal function tests may demonstrate a deteriorating trend during or after oxaliplatin treatment. Perioperative physicians managing patients presenting with oxaliplatin-related kidney injury should of course avoid causing further perioperative deterioration in renal function by paying particular care to preventing hypotension and hypovolemia, and avoiding concomitant use of nephrotoxins (e.g., nonsteroidal antiinflammatory drugs [NSAIDs]) where possible.

5-FU is a pyrimidine analogue and is associated with commonly occurring adverse effects on the heart and bone marrow. Myelosuppression typically occurs within 7 days of commencing treatment, reaching a nadir at 14 days and recovering at 20 days. Extreme vigilance is required for the potential development of infection during this period, with a low threshold for commencing antimicrobial treatment. Full recovery from 5-FU-related anemia and thrombocytopenia might not have occurred prior to the patient presenting for surgery. 5-FU causes the second-highest incidence of cardiotoxicity of all chemotherapeutic agents (anthracyclines having the highest incidence). ECG changes, angina, and myocardial infarction may complicate 5-FU treatment, with induced coronary vasospasm suspected of being the underlying cause.[16] 5-FU-induced cardiotoxicity usually resolves spontaneously following cessation of treatment, although in the acute phase the patient may require symptomatic treatment with calcium channel blockade or nitrates.[17] However, the perioperative physician should have a high index of suspicion and further investigate patient-reported cardiac symptoms as appropriate (with cardiology referral for ECG, exercise stress testing, cardiac perfusion imaging, coronary angiography, etc., as appropriate). Although patients are likely to have completed 5-FU therapy prior to surgery, in the event of patients on current 5-FU therapy presenting for emergency surgery, it should be noted that several drugs interact with 5-FU and may precipitate cardiac toxicity; these include (but are not limited to) metronidazole, cimetidine, phenytoin, fosphenytoin, and hydrochlorothiazide.

Capecitabine is an orally administered prodrug of 5-FU and is selectively converted to 5-FU mostly within cancer cells. It has a more favorable side effect profile than intravenous 5-FU in terms of a lower incidence of myelotoxicity.[18] However, it causes cardiotoxicity with a frequency as high as 5-FU, and perhaps even higher when coadministered with oxaliplatin.[19] Management as before is cessation of capecitabine treatment with symptomatic treatment as required.

Irinotecan is a camptothecin derivative, commonly used as a second-line agent in patients with 5-FU-resistant disease. It commonly causes neutropenia and has significant gastrointestinal side effects with vomiting, diarrhea, and abdominal pain occurring frequently.[20] More rarely it can cause pulmonary, hepatic, or skin toxicity.

Anemia and Perioperative Blood Transfusion

The majority of colorectal cancer patients are iron deficient at time of presentation, with many of these being overtly anemic. Indeed symptomatic anemia is a common presenting complaint with patients reporting fatigue, lethargy, or dyspnea. Iron deficiency has been found to be present in 60% of colorectal cancer patients at presentation with 40% meeting the diagnostic criteria for iron-deficiency anemia (hemoglobin below 12 g/dL in females and 13 g/dL in males as per the WHO definition); iron-deficiency is particularly common in right-sided colonic tumors, with an incidence of up to 80%.[21,22] Although gastrointestinal bleeding is the most obvious cause of anemia, malnutrition, anemia of chronic disease, and neoadjuvant chemotherapy-induced bone marrow suppression may also contribute to the anemic state.[23]

Evidence points to an independent correlation between the severity of preoperative anemia and perioperative morbidity and mortality.[24,25] Allogeneic blood transfusion (ABT) is well known to carry its own risks and has a proven impact on clinical outcomes (including increasing the risk of postoperative infection, surgical intervention, and death).[26] ABT has also been suspected of having a detrimental effect on colorectal cancer recurrence—a 2006 Cochrane meta-analysis of trials that examined the influence of ABT on oncologic outcomes following colorectal cancer surgery reported an overall odds ratio (OR) for cancer recurrence of 1.42 (95% CI, 1.20–1.67), although the authors stated that study heterogeneity and poor quality data on surgical techniques prevented the definitive establishment of a causal relationship.[27] Given the risks associated with ABT, it should not be considered a "quick fix" to correct anemia on the day of surgery, and all efforts should be made to restore hemoglobin levels by safer means prior to surgery.

The concept of a perioperative blood management (PBM) program has evolved in recent years with the aim of preoperative correction of iron-deficiency anemia in order to significantly reduce clinical risk for colorectal cancer patients. Given the urgency of proceeding with surgical resection of a primary tumor the time in which iron-deficiency anemia can be treated preoperatively by a PBM program is limited. A recent trial randomized colorectal cancer patients to receive either oral or intravenous iron for at least 2 weeks preoperatively. Mean hemoglobin rise was significantly higher in the intravenous group (1.55 g/dL) compared to the oral group (0.50 g/dL, $P < 0.001$), although there was no significant difference in transfusion requirements between the two groups.[28]

Intravenous iron provides a favorable risk-benefit profile in terms of speed of replenishment of iron stores and recovery of hemoglobin concentration with very low risks of significant allergic reaction to the infusate. Given the risks associated with ABT, it appears prudent (as well as cost effective) to minimize patient exposure to transfusion by considering intravenous iron deficiency treatment even if the allowed time period before surgery is short.

Preoperative Exercise and Prehabilitation

Preoperative exercise programs are being developed and evaluated for patients planned for elective colorectal operations. Such programs can be hospital- or community-based with the former often using cardiopulmonary exercise testing (CPEX) as an assessment tool. In general, compliance and completion rates are high with objective improvements in exercise capability occurring with six sessions over a 2-week period.[29] Improved postoperative outcomes are expected but not yet conclusively proven, and more expansive programs now include nutrition and psychology preparation for patients facing this major intervention.

Enhanced Recovery After Surgery (ERAS) Protocols

Enhanced Recovery After Surgery (ERAS) protocols are combinations of evidence-based, multidisciplinary perioperative interventions that are applied to patient care with the aim of improving patient outcomes, hastening recovery, and reducing costs in the early postoperative period. ERAS as a concept in colorectal surgery was promoted by the surgeon Henrik Kehlet in Denmark in the 1990s, who hypothesized that a key factor underlying the development of serious postoperative complications (e.g., cardiac, pulmonary, infective) was the deleterious effects of the physiologic stress response to surgery.[30] By inhibiting this metabolic stress response via a multifaceted approach, Kehlet suggested that the incidence of postoperative complications could be reduced, thereby improving patient morbidity and mortality, reducing length of stay, and reducing health care–related costs. Such an approach requires highly organized, protocolized care with coordinated delivery of the various elements between surgery, anesthesia, nursing, physiotherapy, and other disciplines involved in perioperative patient care.

The ERAS Society was founded in 2010 to guide the education and research of ERAS principles. The guidelines initially published in 2012 were for enhanced recovery for colonic resection patients, followed shortly after by guidelines for rectal resection. The ERAS Society published the fourth edition of the guidelines for colorectal surgery in 2018.[31] The guidelines list 24 ERAS elements with each being given a recommendation grade from weak to strong depending on the nature and quality of the evidence base underlying each element (see Table 25.1). Compliance with ERAS protocols has been shown to significantly reduce the incidence of postoperative nonsurgical complications and

TABLE 25.1 Guidelines for Perioperative Care in Elective Colorectal Surgery: Enhanced Recovery After Surgery (ERAS) Society Recommendations, 2018

No.	ERAS Recommendation	Aim	Notes
	Preadmission		
1	Cessation of smoking and excessive intake of alcohol	Reduce complications	Quality of evidence of outcome improvement with smoking cessation is especially high.
2	Preoperative nutritional screening, assessment, and support	Reduce complications	Patients at risk of malnutrition should receive preoperative oral nutritional treatment for at least 7–10 days.
3	Medical optimization of chronic disease	Reduce complications	Preoperative medical optimization is intuitively important, but for specified risk assessment tools, the evidence of clinical accuracy is low.
	Preoperative		
4	Structured preoperative information for patient and caregivers	Reduce anxiety, involve the patient to improve compliance with protocol	Patients should receive dedicated preoperative counseling routinely.
5	Preoperative carbohydrate treatment	Reduce insulin resistance, improve well being, possibly faster recovery	Elective surgical patients should be allowed to eat up to 6 h, and take clear fluids up until 2 h before surgery.
6	Preoperative prophylaxis against thrombosis	Reduce thromboembolic complications	Patients undergoing major colorectal surgery should have (i) mechanical thromboprophylaxis by compression stockings and/or intermittent pneumatic compression until discharge and (ii) receive pharmacologic prophylaxis with low-molecular-weight heparin (LMWH) daily for 28 days after surgery.
7	Preoperative prophylaxis against infection	Reduce infection rates	IV antibiotic prophylaxis should be given within 60 min of skin incision.

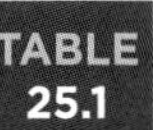

TABLE 25.1 Guidelines for Perioperative Care in Elective Colorectal Surgery: Enhanced Recovery After Surgery (ERAS) Society Recommendations, 2018—cont'd

No.	ERAS Recommendation	Aim	Notes
8	Prophylaxis against nausea and vomiting	Minimize postoperative nausea and vomiting	Patients with 1–2 risk factors should receive two-drug prophylaxis. Patients with >2 risk factors should receive 2–3 antiemetics.
	Intraoperative		
9	Minimal invasive surgical (MIS) techniques	Reduce complications, faster recovery, reduce pain	High quality evidence that MIS improves outcomes.
10	Standardized anesthesia, avoiding long-acting opioids	Avoid or reduce postoperative ileus	Avoid routine sedation.
11	Maintaining fluid balance to avoid over- or underhydration, administer vasopressors to support blood pressure control	Reduce complications, reduce postoperative ileus	Avoid prolonged preoperative fasting, avoid routine bowel preparation. Goal-directed fluid therapy is strongly recommended.
12	Thoracic epidural analgesia (TEA) for open surgery	Reduce stress response and insulin resistance Reduce complications	TEA using low dose of local anesthetic and opioids is recommended in open colorectal surgery to minimize the stress response and provide postoperative analgesia.
13	Restrictive use of pelvic and peritoneal drains	Support mobilization, reduce pain and discomfort, no proven benefit of use	Drains have no effect on outcome and should not be used routinely.
14	Removal of nasogastric tubes before reversal of anesthesia	Reduce the risk of pneumonia, support oral intake of solids	Postoperative nasogastric tubes should not be used routinely; if inserted during surgery, they should be removed before reversal of anesthesia.
15	Control of body temperature using warm air flow blankets and warmed IV infusions	Reduce complications	Even mild hypothermia is associated with increased bleeding and transfusion risk.
	Postoperative		
16	Early mobilization (day of surgery)	Support return to normal movement	Prolonged immobilization is associated with a variety of adverse effects.
17	Early intake of oral fluids and solids (offered the day of surgery)	Support energy and protein supply, reduce starvation-induced insulin resistance	Most patients can and should be offered food and oral nutritional supplementation from the day of surgery.
18	Early removal of urinary catheters and IV fluids (morning after surgery)	Support ambulation and mobilization	Patients at low risk of urinary retention should have urethral catheters removed on the 1st day postoperative, while patients at moderate-to-high risk require catheterization for up to 3 days.
19	Use of chewing gums and laxatives and peripheral opioid-blocking agents (when using opioids)	Support return of gut function	Peripherally acting l-opioid receptor antagonists, chewing gum, bisacodyl, magnesium oxide, and coffee have some indications for affecting an established ileus.
20	Intake of protein and energy-rich nutritional supplements	Increase energy and protein intake in addition to normal food	Perioperative immunonutrition in malnourished patients is beneficial in colorectal cancer surgery.
21	Multimodal approach to opioid-sparing pain control	Pain control reduces insulin resistance, supports mobilization	Avoid opioids and apply multimodal analgesia in combination with spinal/epidural analgesia or fascial plane blocks when indicated.
22	Multimodal approach to control of nausea and vomiting	Minimize postoperative nausea and vomiting and support energy and protein intake	Use of one or more antiemetics depending on symptoms.
23	Prepare for early discharge	Avoid unnecessary delays in discharge	Setting discharge criteria and daily goals is critical.
24	Audit of outcomes and process in a multiprofessional, multidisciplinary team on a regular basis	Control of practice (a key to improve outcomes)	Outcomes (complications and mortality at 30 days) and processes should be audited on a regular basis when implementing ERAS programs, as well as for sustaining improvements.

shorten primary hospital admission in pooled data from randomized control trials (RCTs) and also international multicenter registry data.[32,33]

Not all ERAS programs incorporate all 24 recommendations, and some may incorporate other elements not included in the ERAS Society guidelines. It remains unclear which elements exert the greatest impact on clinical outcomes and whether a reduced set of ERAS protocol elements may provide substantially the same effect. However, compliance of 70% or greater with the elements of the ERAS protocol appears to be important in maximizing outcome improvements, regardless of whether open or laparoscopic approaches are examined.[34–36] Overall, as a consensus-based formula derived from frequently updated clinical evidence, the ERAS guidelines provide an invaluable framework for optimizing the perioperative care of the colorectal cancer patient.

Operative Risk Assessment

In addition to standard preoperative categorization, some specialty-specific risk scores exist aimed at stratifying patients according to the likelihood of postoperative complications. One such score is CR-POSSUM (a specialty-specific adaption of the standard POSSUM score), which utilizes six physiologic criteria and four operative measures.[37] The Association of Coloproctology of Great Britain and Ireland (ACPGBI) has also developed a score of four measurements (age, ASA, cancer stage, and operative urgency) in an equation to predict postoperative mortality.[38] Both scales need contextualization within an individual unit, as variation between centers exists. With regard to both general and specific postoperative complications, online scoring systems exist to guide practice (e.g., the ACS NSQIP surgical risk calculator, and the colon leakage score and anastomoticleak.com) but again need individual center validation.[39–41]

Surgery—Open, Laparoscopic-Assisted, or Robotic-Assisted Laparoscopic Approaches

The advent of laparoscopic surgical techniques has transformed colorectal cancer surgery over the past 30 years. Though technically more challenging and requiring a longer and steeper learning curve for trainees to master, laparoscopic colorectal cancer surgery has been shown in RCTs to be superior to open surgery in terms of improving short-term outcomes, including postoperative pain, opioid requirements, blood loss, recovery of bowel function, and length of hospital stay.[42] As smaller incisions conceptually reduce the severity of the surgical stress response, which is the key aim underlying the creation of enhanced recovery programs, laparoscopic surgery forms a key recommendation of ERAS programs.[30] A significant disadvantage of laparoscopic surgery is the longer procedure time, which may impact negatively on surgical caseload. Although some researchers have reported trial data suggesting laparoscopic-assisted colectomy (LAC) surgery is associated with an improvement in longer-term outcomes including mortality and cancer recurrence,[43] a Cochrane review in 2008 found that there is no conclusive evidence that long-term outcomes (including cancer recurrence) are better with LAC than open colectomy.[44]

Robotic-assisted colorectal surgery (RACS) has been increasing in popularity with the spread of robotic surgical systems in recent years. RACS procedures increased from 2.6% to 6.6% of all colorectal surgeries performed in the United States between 2011 and 2015.[45] Overall complication rates are similar for robotic-assisted colectomy compared with laparoscopic colectomy, albeit with a higher risk of iatrogenic complications, with the higher costs and longer procedure times asso associated with robotic surgery leading some to question its role.[46,47]

Rectal cancers can be resected via open, laparoscopic, robotic-assisted laparoscopic or transanal approaches. From accumulated evidence to date, there is little difference between the techniques in terms of perioperative morbidity and overall survival, but open and transanal approaches appear possibly superior in terms of oncologic resection, while postoperative patient recovery is better with laparoscopic and robotic approaches.[48] Laparoscopic rectal resection is technically demanding with a higher rate of conversion to an open procedure than LAC, which is unsurprising given the limited anatomic space and the low margin for error involved in pelvic dissection for rectal cancer.[49] Robotic-assisted techniques appear well suited for working in the confined space of the pelvis and provide the surgeon with greater maneuverability and visibility. Robotic-assisted laparoscopic rectal resection is in its infancy relative to conventional laparoscopic resection; however, meta-analysis of the small number of relevant trials completed to date suggests that both techniques have similar rates of perioperative complications and mortality, with a lower risk of conversion to open and longer operating times for robotic-assisted procedures.[50] Robotic technology will undoubtedly improve further, and future trial evidence may eventually prove RACS to be superior to laparoscopic surgery in terms of clinical outcomes.

Choice of Anesthesia and Analgesia and Effect on Clinical Outcomes

Propofol Versus Inhalational Anesthesia

The 2018 ERAS Society guidelines recommend the avoidance of benzodiazepines and the use of short-acting general anesthetic agents and opioids in order to "allow rapid awakening with minimal residual effects" to facilitate faster recovery and progression along the ERAS pathway.[31] The ERAS guideline authors acknowledge the paucity of evidence to recommend one anesthetic technique over another in terms of optimizing short-term clinical outcomes. Sevoflurane-based anesthesia for laparoscopic surgery (in patients over 65 years of age) may result in faster awakening, tracheal extubation, and return of bowel function than a propofol-based technique.[51] In contrast, propofol total intravenous anesthesia (TIVA) has been associated with a shorter hospital stay in data on over 2000 patients from an international, multicenter ERAS registry.[32]

Propofol may possess beneficial antiinflammatory and immune-stimulating properties, while volatile anesthetic agents are suspected of having harmful proinflammatory and angiogenesis-stimulating effects, although in vitro and in vivo evidence is conflicting and the influence on clinical outcomes is unclear.[52,53] Evidence from retrospective studies points to a beneficial effect of propofol-based TIVA techniques on improving overall survival compared to inhalational techniques for a variety of cancer surgery types, including colorectal cancer.[54–56] One retrospective cohort study comparing propofol-based intravenous versus desflurane-based inhalational anesthesia for colon cancer surgery detected improved survival in the propofol group, with a hazard ratio of 0.27 (95% confidence interval [CI], 0.22–0.35; $P < 0.001$).[57] Such a dramatic improvement in survival has not been replicated in other studies, and in any event, any association between an anesthetic agent and survival has yet to be conclusively proven in an appropriately powered RCT.

Epidural Analgesia

Thoracic epidural analgesia (TEA) has been considered the gold standard for postoperative analgesia for open colorectal procedures. Physiologically, TEA should inhibit the stress response to surgery by blocking the pain stimulus that activates catecholamine release, allowing for reduced patient exposure to inhalational anesthetic agents and opioids; thus its role in supporting the concepts underpinning ERAS programs is clear. TEA has been associated in meta-analysis of trial data with a reduction in risk of postoperative venous thromboembolism, respiratory depression and pneumonia, as well as improved recovery of bowel function.[58,59] All of these benefits have not been conclusively demonstrated in other meta-analyses, however, and despite its "gold standard" label, TEA is associated with significant failure rates, pruritus, and hypotension, and may produce only modestly better pain scores than IV patient-controlled analgesia (PCA).[60] The move away from open surgery toward minimally invasive approaches has reduced the role of TEA, with epidural techniques generally considered unnecessary for providing effective analgesia following laparoscopic procedures given the rare but significant complications associated with TEA (including vertebral canal hematoma, epidural abscess, and spinal cord ischemia).[61,62]

Fascial Plane Regional Anesthesia

Regional anesthetic techniques for blockading the branches of the intercostal nerves that supply the anterior abdominal wall are frequently used to provide analgesia following open colorectal surgery when TEA is unsuccessful or contraindicated, or for analgesia after laparoscopic procedures. Various fascial plane blocks are performed, the most popular being transversus abdominis plane (TAP) and rectus sheath (RS) blocks. Although considered a relatively safe and straightforward block to perform, meta-analysis of trial evidence to date shows that TAP blocks provide only a small reduction in postoperative opioid requirements following open or laparoscopic abdominal procedures, although heterogeneity in study design complicates analysis.[63] Single-shot blocks or catheters for prolonged infusion can be placed bilaterally in the RSs or in the erector spinae plane, generally under ultrasound guidance, although RS catheters can be placed by the surgeon under direct vision. Initial evidence for the analgesic efficacy of these techniques is promising, although more rigorous trial analysis is required.[64–67] Whichever technique is chosen, abdominal wall blocks are unlikely to provide comparative postoperative analgesia to TEA and should be viewed as just one component within a broader multimodal analgesic regime.[68]

Multimodal Analgesia

All colorectal surgery patients will require systemic analgesics at some point in their postoperative course; even well-functioning thoracic epidurals will need to be removed, generally by postoperative day 5. Opioids are typically used for moderate-to-severe postoperative pain and are effective analgesic agents; unfortunately, they come at the cost of significant risks, including nausea, vomiting, ileus, delirium, and slower mobilization.[69] Several of the ERAS recommendations (including the promotion of minimally invasive surgery and the use of neuraxial/regional analgesia) are designed to minimize the amount of opioids required. Multimodal analgesia also plays an important role with the aim being to modulate the transduction and transmission of pain signals at multiple points, and so provide effective analgesia at lower doses than would be required if any agent was used on its own, thereby reducing the risks of encountering any side effects.[70] Paracetamol (acetaminophen) plays an important role for the vast majority of ERAS patients as it provides significant analgesic effects with a minimal side effect profile when dosed appropriately. Other analgesic agents that can be considered in multimodal regimes include NSAIDs, COX-2 inhibitors, gabapentinoids, ketamine, alpha-2 agonists (clonidine or dexmedetomidine), magnesium sulfate, and intravenous lidocaine.[71]

Neuromuscular Blocking Agents

A meta-analysis of 12 studies showed that use of neuromuscular blocking agents (NMBAs) during laparoscopic- or robotic-assisted procedures to produce "deep" neuromuscular block improves surgical space conditions, lowers pneumoperitoneum pressures, and reduces postoperative pain scores.[72] Such "deep" blockade should be used with caution, however, as a higher cumulative dose of NMBA is associated with an increased risk of postoperative pulmonary complications, although it is a risk which is ameliorated by the use of appropriate neuromuscular transmission monitoring to guide the administration of reversal agents (such as neostigmine or sugammadex).[73]

Dexamethasone

Use of dexamethasone to prevent postoperative nausea and vomiting (PONV) is a routine component of anesthesia practice in many centers worldwide. Corticosteroids have an unknown clinical effect on outcomes after colorectal cancer surgery and on cancer recurrence in particular. To date, the only prospectively collected data come from the post hoc analysis of a small (n = 60) study of colorectal cancer patients randomized to dexamethasone or placebo presurgery, which showed an increased risk of metastasis with dexamethasone.[74] Only future RCT evidence will provide clarity as to whether perioperative dexamethasone influences cancer recurrence.

Intravenous Lidocaine

Perioperative intravenous lidocaine infusions have been used for their supposed beneficial effects not only as analgesic agents, but also to hasten the postoperative recovery of bowel function. The most recent Cochrane review in 2015 found low-to-moderate evidence that lidocaine infusion improves early postoperative pain scores, as well as nausea, but limited evidence of a beneficial effect on recovery of bowel function.[75] The optimal dose and duration of infusion remain unclear. Lidocaine is an inexpensive agent and commonly used in clinical practice but does pose the risk of arrhythmia and seizures that mandates continuous patient monitoring during infusion.

NSAIDs

Regular NSAID use has been shown in some observational and randomized control studies to reduce the incidence of colorectal cancer and improve recurrence-free survival postoperatively.[76] However, perioperative NSAIDs have also been associated with increasing the risk of anastomotic leak by some authors.[77] More recent publications have failed to detect an association with anastomotic leak.[78] A review of 16 studies of perioperative NSAID use published up to 2017 found the evidence to be too heterogeneous or of poor quality to attempt a meta-analysis, with the authors concluding that the evidence supporting a link between perioperative NSAID use, and either cancer recurrence or anastomotic breakdown, remains equivocal.[79]

Effect of Anesthetic and Analgesic Agents on Cancer Recurrence

In recent years, it has become increasingly recognized that events occurring during the perioperative phase (including the surgical insult itself, hypothermia, and blood transfusion) may have an important role to play in modulating the risk of postoperative cancer recurrence.[80] These factors have been suspected, largely in laboratory studies, of positively or negatively influencing the human immune system, inflammation, or cancer cells themselves—all factors that play a crucial role in determining whether residual cancer cells will develop into clinically relevant metastatic disease. Anesthetic and analgesic agents are also suspected of influencing cancer recurrence risk.[81] The overall weight of evidence from laboratory and largely retrospective clinical studies is suggestive of a possibly harmful, prometastatic effect with inhalational agents and opioids, with possibly beneficial, antimetastatic effects attributed to regional/neuraxial anesthesia, propofol, and NSAIDs.[82] To date, however, the only suitably powered RCT to examine the effects of anesthesia on cancer recurrence compared a propofol-paravertebral technique to a inhalational-opioid technique in breast cancer surgery patients and found no difference in cancer recurrence between the two groups.[83] Given the widely varying pathophysiologic behavior of different cancer types, it is unclear how applicable the results of this RCT are to colorectal cancer patients. While we await the completion of further RCTs in the coming years, the consensus opinion remains that there is currently no evidence to recommend any change in anesthetic practice to alter postoperative cancer recurrence risk.[84]

References

1. Bray F, Ferlay J, Soerjomataram I, Siegel RL, Torre LA, Jemal A. Global cancer statistics 2018: GLOBOCAN estimates of incidence and mortality worldwide for 36 cancers in 185 countries. *CA Cancer J Clin*. 2018;68(6):394–424. doi:10.3322/caac.21492.
2. White A, Joseph D, Rim SH, Johnson CJ, Coleman MP, Allemani C. Colon cancer survival in the United States by race and stage (2001-2009): findings from the CONCORD-2 study. *Cancer*. 2017;123(Suppl 24):5014–5036. doi:10.1002/cncr.31076.
3. Clinton SK, Giovannucci EL, Hursting SD. The World Cancer Research Fund/American Institute for Cancer Research Third Expert Report on Diet, Nutrition, Physical Activity, and Cancer: Impact and Future Directions. *J Nutr*. 2020;150(4):663–671. doi:10.1093/jn/nxz268.
4. Arnold M, Sierra MS, Laversanne M, Soerjomataram I, Jemal A, Bray F. Global patterns and trends in colorectal cancer incidence and mortality. *Gut*. Apr 2017;66(4):683–691. doi:10.1136/gutjnl-2015-310912.
5. Ahnen DJ, Wade SW, Jones WF, et al. The increasing incidence of young-onset colorectal cancer: a call to action. *Mayo Clin Proc*. 2014;89(2):216–224. doi:10.1016/j.mayocp.2013.09.006.
6. Thompson MR, O'Leary DP, Flashman K, Asiimwe A, Ellis BG, Senapati A. Clinical assessment to determine the risk of bowel cancer using symptoms, age, mass and iron deficiency anaemia (SAMI). *Br J Surg*. 2017;104(10):1393–1404. doi:10.1002/bjs.10573.
7. Wolpin BM, Mayer RJ. Systemic treatment of colorectal cancer. *Gastroenterology*. 2008;134(5):1296–1310. doi:10.1053/j.gastro.2008.02.098.

8. Hveem TS, Merok MA, Pretorius ME, et al. Prognostic impact of genomic instability in colorectal cancer. *Br J Cancer*. 2014;110(8):2159–2164. doi:10.1038/bjc.2014.133.
9. Riihimaki M, Hemminki A, Sundquist J, Hemminki K. Patterns of metastasis in colon and rectal cancer. *Sci Rep*. 2016;6:29765. doi:10.1038/srep29765.
10. van der Geest LG, Lam-Boer J, Koopman M, Verhoef C, Elferink MA, de Wilt JH. Nationwide trends in incidence, treatment and survival of colorectal cancer patients with synchronous metastases. *Clin Exp Metastasis*. 2015;32(5):457–465. doi:10.1007/s10585-015-9719-0.
11. Zaheer S, Pemberton JH, Farouk R, Dozois RR, Wolff BG, Ilstrup D. Surgical treatment of adenocarcinoma of the rectum. *Ann Surg*. 1998;227(6):800–811. doi:10.1097/00000658-199806000-00003.
12. Kapiteijn E, Marijnen CA, Nagtegaal ID, et al. Preoperative radiotherapy combined with total mesorectal excision for resectable rectal cancer. *N Engl J Med*. 2001;345(9):638–646. doi:10.1056/NEJMoa010580.
13. Qin Q, Ma T, Deng Y, et al. Impact of preoperative radiotherapy on anastomotic leakage and stenosis after rectal cancer resection: post hoc analysis of a randomized controlled trial. *Dis Colon Rectum*. 2016;59(10):934–942. doi:10.1097/dcr.0000000000000665.
14. Assenat E. FOLFIRINOX for the treatment of colorectal cancer: latest evidence from clinical trials. *Colorect Cancer*. 2012;1(3):181–184.
15. Ulusakarya A, Misra S, Haydar M, et al. Acute renal failure related to oxaliplatin-induced intravascular hemolysis. *Med Oncol*. 2010;27(4):1425–1426. doi:10.1007/s12032-009-9263-3.
16. Saif WBJ, Köhne C-H. Fluoropyrimidine-associated cardiotoxicity: incidence, clinical manifestations, mechanisms, and management. UpToDate. 2019. Available at https://www.uptodate.com/contents/fluoropyrimidine-associated-cardiotoxicity-incidence-clinical-manifestations-mechanisms-and-management?search=Cardiotoxicity%20in%20patients%20receiving%20chemotherapy&topicRef=2812&source=see_link.
17. Chong JH, Ghosh AK. Coronary artery vasospasm induced by 5-fluorouracil: proposed mechanisms, existing management options and future directions. *Interv Cardiol*. 2019;14(2):89–94. doi:10.15420/icr.2019.12.
18. Saif MW, Katirtzoglou NA, Syrigos KN. Capecitabine: an overview of the side effects and their management. *Anticancer Drugs*. 2008;19(5):447–644. doi:10.1097/CAD.0b013e3282f945aa.
19. Keramida K, Charalampopoulos G, Filippiadis D, Tsougos E, Farmakis D. Cardiovascular complications of metastatic colorectal cancer treatment. *J Gastrointest Oncol*. 2019;10(4):797–806. doi:10.21037/jgo.2019.03.04.
20. Paulik A, Nekvindova J, Filip PS. Irinotecan toxicity during treatment of metastatic colorectal cancer: focus on pharmacogenomics and personalized medicine. *Tumori*. 2018:300891618811283. doi:10.1177/0300891618811283.
21. Beale AL, Penney MD, Allison AC. The prevalence of iron deficiency among patients presenting with colorectal cancer. *Colorectal Dis*. 2005;7(4):398–402. doi:10.1111/j.1463-1318.2005.00789.x.
22. Ludwig H, Van Belle S, Barrett-Lee P, et al. The European Cancer Anaemia Survey (ECAS): a large, multinational, prospective survey defining the prevalence, incidence, and treatment of anaemia in cancer patients. *Eur J Cancer*. 2004;40(15):2293–2306. doi:10.1016/j.ejca.2004.06.019.
23. Aapro M, Osterborg A, Gascon P, Ludwig H, Beguin Y. Prevalence and management of cancer-related anaemia, iron deficiency and the specific role of i.v. iron. *Ann Oncol*. 2012;23(8):1954–1962. doi:10.1093/annonc/mds112.
24. Munoz M, Gomez-Ramirez S, Kozek-Langeneker S, et al. 'Fit to fly': overcoming barriers to preoperative haemoglobin optimization in surgical patients. *Br J Anaesth*. 2015;115(1):15–24. doi:10.1093/bja/aev165.
25. Shander A, Javidroozi M, Ozawa S, Hare GM. What is really dangerous: anaemia or transfusion? *Br J Anaesth*. 2011;107(Suppl 1):i41–i59. doi:10.1093/bja/aer350.
26. Acheson AG, Brookes MJ, Spahn DR. Effects of allogeneic red blood cell transfusions on clinical outcomes in patients undergoing colorectal cancer surgery: a systematic review and meta-analysis. *Ann Surg*. 2012;256(2):235–244. doi:10.1097/SLA.0b013e31825b35d5.
27. Amato A, Pescatori M. Perioperative blood transfusions for the recurrence of colorectal cancer. *Cochrane Database Syst Rev*. 2006(1):Cd005033. doi:10.1002/14651858.CD005033.pub2.
28. Keeler BD, Simpson JA, Ng O, Padmanabhan H, Brookes MJ, Acheson AG. Randomized clinical trial of preoperative oral versus intravenous iron in anaemic patients with colorectal cancer. *Br J Surg*. 2017;104(3):214–221. doi:10.1002/bjs.10328.
29. Heger P, Probst P, Wiskemann J, Steindorf K, Diener MK, Mihaljevic AL. A systematic review and meta-analysis of physical exercise prehabilitation in major abdominal surgery (PROSPERO 2017 CRD42017080366). *J Gastrointest Surg*. 2019;24(6):1375–1385. doi:10.1007/s11605-019-04287-w.
30. Kehlet H. Multimodal approach to control postoperative pathophysiology and rehabilitation. *Br J Anaesth*. 1997;78(5):606–617. doi:10.1093/bja/78.5.606.
31. Gustafsson UO, Scott MJ, Hubner M, et al. Guidelines for perioperative care in elective colorectal surgery: Enhanced Recovery After Surgery (ERAS®) Society Recommendations: 2018. *World J Surg*. 2019;43(3):659–695. doi:10.1007/s00268-018-4844-y.
32. ERAS Compliance Group. The impact of enhanced recovery protocol compliance on elective colorectal cancer resection: results from an international registry. *Ann Surg*. Jun 2015;261(6):1153–1159. doi:10.1097/sla.0000000000001029.
33. Greco M, Capretti G, Beretta L, Gemma M, Pecorelli N, Braga M. Enhanced recovery program in colorectal surgery: a meta-analysis of randomized controlled trials. *World J Surg*. 2014;38(6):1531–1541. doi:10.1007/s00268-013-2416-8.
34. Gustafsson UO, Hausel J, Thorell A, Ljungqvist O, Soop M, Nygren J. Adherence to the enhanced recovery after surgery protocol and outcomes after colorectal cancer surgery. *Arch Surg*. 2011;146(5):571–577. doi:10.1001/archsurg.2010.309.
35. Pisarska M, Pedziwiatr M, Malczak P, et al. Do we really need the full compliance with ERAS protocol in laparoscopic colorectal surgery? A prospective cohort study. *Int J Surg*. 2016;36(Pt A):377–382. doi:10.1016/j.ijsu.2016.11.088.
36. Messenger DE, Curtis NJ, Jones A, Jones EL, Smart NJ, Francis NK. Factors predicting outcome from enhanced recovery programmes in laparoscopic colorectal surgery: a systematic review. *Surg Endosc*. 2017;31(5):2050–2071. doi:10.1007/s00464-016-5205-2.
37. Tekkis PP, Prytherch DR, Kocher HM, et al. Development of a dedicated risk-adjustment scoring system for colorectal surgery (colorectal POSSUM). *Br J Surg*. 2004;91(9):1174–1182. doi:10.1002/bjs.4430.

38. Ferjani AM, Griffin D, Stallard N, Wong LS. A newly devised scoring system for prediction of mortality in patients with colorectal cancer: a prospective study. *Lancet Oncol.* 2007;8(4):317–322. doi:10.1016/s1470-2045(07)70045-1.
39. Dekker JW, Liefers GJ, de Mol van Otterloo JC, Putter H, Tollenaar RA. Predicting the risk of anastomotic leakage in left-sided colorectal surgery using a colon leakage score. *J Surg Res.* 2011;166(1):e27–e34. doi:10.1016/j.jss.2010.11.004.
40. Bilimoria KY, Liu Y, Paruch JL, et al. Development and evaluation of the universal ACS NSQIP surgical risk calculator: a decision aid and informed consent tool for patients and surgeons. *J Am Coll Surg.* 2013;217(5):833–842. doi:10.1016/j.jamcollsurg.2013.07.385.
41. Sammour T, Lewis M, Thomas ML, Lawrence MJ, Hunter A, Moore JW. A simple web-based risk calculator (www.anastomoticleak.com) is superior to the surgeon's estimate of anastomotic leak after colon cancer resection. *Tech Coloproctol.* 2017;21(1):35–41. doi:10.1007/s10151-016-1567-7.
42. Schwenk W, Haase O, Neudecker J, Muller JM. Short term benefits for laparoscopic colorectal resection. *Cochrane Database Syst Rev.* 2005(3):Cd003145. doi:10.1002/14651858.CD003145.pub2.
43. Lacy AM, Delgado S, Castells A, et al. The long-term results of a randomized clinical trial of laparoscopy-assisted versus open surgery for colon cancer. *Ann Surg.* 2008;248(1):1–7. doi:10.1097/SLA.0b013e31816a9d65.
44. Kuhry E, Schwenk WF, Gaupset R, Romild U, Bonjer HJ. Long-term results of laparoscopic colorectal cancer resection. *Cochrane Database Syst Rev.* 2008(2):Cd003432. doi:10.1002/14651858.CD003432.pub2.
45. Damle A, Damle RN, Flahive JM, et al. Diffusion of technology: Trends in robotic-assisted colorectal surgery. *Am J Surg.* 2017;214(5):820–824. doi:10.1016/j.amjsurg.2017.03.020.
46. Yeo HL, Isaacs AJ, Abelson JS, Milsom JW, Sedrakyan A. Comparison of open, laparoscopic, and robotic colectomies using a large national database: outcomes and trends related to surgery center volume. *Dis Colon Rectum.* 2016;59(6):535–542. doi:10.1097/dcr.0000000000000580.
47. Tyler JA, Fox JP, Desai MM, Perry WB, Glasgow SC. Outcomes and costs associated with robotic colectomy in the minimally invasive era. *Dis Colon Rectum.* 2013;56(4):458–466. doi:10.1097/DCR.0b013e31827085ec.
48. Simillis C, Lal N, Thoukididou SN, et al. Open versus laparoscopic versus robotic versus transanal mesorectal excision for rectal cancer: a systematic review and network meta-analysis. *Ann Surg.* 2019;270(1):59–68. doi:10.1097/sla.0000000000003227.
49. Jayne DG, Thorpe HC, Copeland J, Quirke P, Brown JM, Guillou PJ. Five-year follow-up of the Medical Research Council CLASICC trial of laparoscopically assisted versus open surgery for colorectal cancer. *Br J Surg.* 2010;97(11):1638–1645. doi:10.1002/bjs.7160.
50. Prete FP, Pezzolla A, Prete F, et al. Robotic versus laparoscopic minimally invasive surgery for rectal cancer: a systematic review and meta-analysis of randomized controlled trials. *Ann Surg.* 2018;267(6):1034–1046. doi:10.1097/sla.0000000000002523.
51. Nishikawa K, Nakayama M, Omote K, Namiki A. Recovery characteristics and post-operative delirium after long-duration laparoscope-assisted surgery in elderly patients: propofol-based vs. sevoflurane-based anesthesia. *Acta Anaesthesiol Scand.* 2004;48(2):162–168. doi:10.1111/j.0001-5172.2004.00264.x.
52. Jiang S, Liu Y, Huang L, Zhang F, Kang R. Effects of propofol on cancer development and chemotherapy: potential mechanisms. *Eur J Pharmacol.* 2018;831:46–51. doi:10.1016/j.ejphar.2018.04.009.
53. Stollings LM, Jia LJ, Tang P, Dou H, Lu B, Xu Y. Immune modulation by volatile anesthetics. *Anesthesiology.* 2016;125(2):399–411. doi:10.1097/aln.0000000000001195.
54. Yap A, Lopez-Olivo MA, Dubowitz J, Hiller J, Riedel B. Anesthetic technique and cancer outcomes: a meta-analysis of total intravenous versus volatile anesthesia. *Can J Anaesth.* 2019;66(5):546–561. doi:10.1007/s12630-019-01330-x.
55. Wigmore TJ, Mohammed K, Jhanji S. Long-term survival for patients undergoing volatile versus IV anesthesia for cancer surgery: a retrospective analysis. *Anesthesiology.* 2016;124(1):69–79. doi:10.1097/aln.0000000000000936.
56. Enlund M, Berglund A, Andreasson K, Cicek C, Enlund A, Bergkvist L. The choice of anaesthetic–sevoflurane or propofol–and outcome from cancer surgery: a retrospective analysis. *Ups J Med Sci.* 2014;119(3):251–261. doi:10.3109/03009734.2014.922649.
57. Wu ZF, Lee MS, Wong CS, et al. Propofol-based total intravenous anesthesia is associated with better survival than desflurane anesthesia in colon cancer surgery. *Anesthesiology.* 2018;129(5):932–941. doi:10.1097/aln.0000000000002357.
58. Popping DM, Elia N, Van Aken HK, et al. Impact of epidural analgesia on mortality and morbidity after surgery: systematic review and meta-analysis of randomized controlled trials. *Ann Surg.* 2014;259(6):1056–1067. doi:10.1097/sla.0000000000000237.
59. Guay J, Nishimori M, Kopp SL. Epidural local anesthetics versus opioid-based analgesic regimens for postoperative gastrointestinal paralysis, vomiting, and pain after abdominal surgery: a Cochrane review. *Anesth Analg.* 2016;123(6):1591–1602. doi:10.1213/ane.0000000000001628.
60. Salicath JH, Yeoh EC, Bennett MH. Epidural analgesia versus patient-controlled intravenous analgesia for pain following intra-abdominal surgery in adults. *Cochrane Database Syst Rev.* 2018;8:Cd010434. doi:10.1002/14651858.CD010434.pub2.
61. Joshi GP, Bonnet F, Kehlet H. Evidence-based postoperative pain management after laparoscopic colorectal surgery. *Colorectal Dis.* 2013;15(2):146–155. doi:10.1111/j.1463-1318.2012.03062.x.
62. Cook TM, Counsell D, Wildsmith JA. Major complications of central neuraxial block: report on the Third National Audit Project of the Royal College of Anaesthetists. *Br J Anaesth.* 2009;102(2):179–190. doi:10.1093/bja/aen360.
63. Baeriswyl M, Kirkham KR, Kern C, Albrecht E. The analgesic efficacy of ultrasound-guided transversus abdominis plane block in adult patients: a meta-analysis. *Anesth Analg.* 2015;121(6):1640–1654. doi:10.1213/ane.0000000000000967.
64. Tudor EC, Yang W, Brown R, Mackey PM. Rectus sheath catheters provide equivalent analgesia to epidurals following laparotomy for colorectal surgery. *Ann R Coll Surg Engl.* 2015;97(7):530–533. doi:10.1308/rcsann.2015.0018.
65. Godden AR, Marshall MJ, Grice AS, Daniels IR. Ultrasonography guided rectus sheath catheters versus epidural analgesia for open colorectal cancer surgery in a single centre. *Ann R Coll Surg Engl.* 2013;95(8):591–594. doi:10.1308/003588413x13629960049270.
66. Yassin HM, Abd Elmoneim AT, El Moutaz H. The analgesic efficiency of ultrasound-guided rectus sheath analgesia compared

with low thoracic epidural analgesia after elective abdominal surgery with a midline incision: a prospective randomized controlled trial. *Anesth Pain Med.* 2017;7(3):e14244. doi:10.5812/aapm.14244.

67. Tsui BCH, Fonseca A, Munshey F, McFadyen G, Caruso TJ. The erector spinae plane (ESP) block: a pooled review of 242 cases. *J Clin Anesth.* 2019;53:29–34. doi:10.1016/j.jclinane.2018.09.036.
68. Chin KJ, McDonnell JG, Carvalho B, Sharkey A, Pawa A, Gadsden J. Essentials of our current understanding: abdominal wall blocks. *Reg Anesth Pain Med.* 2017;42(2):133–183. doi:10.1097/aap.0000000000000545.
69. Benyamin R, Trescot AM, Datta S, et al. Opioid complications and side effects. *Pain Physician.* 2008;11(Suppl 2):S105–S120.
70. Beverly A, Kaye AD, Ljungqvist O, Urman RD. Essential elements of multimodal analgesia in Enhanced Recovery After Surgery (ERAS) Guidelines. *Anesthesiol Clin.* 2017;35(2):e115–e143. doi:10.1016/j.anclin.2017.01.018.
71. Carmichael JC, Keller DS, Baldini G, et al. Clinical practice guidelines for enhanced recovery after colon and rectal surgery from the American Society of Colon and Rectal Surgeons and Society of American Gastrointestinal and Endoscopic Surgeons. *Dis Colon Rectum.* 2017;60(8):761–784. doi:10.1097/dcr.0000000000000883.
72. Bruintjes MH, van Helden EV, Braat AE, et al. Deep neuromuscular block to optimize surgical space conditions during laparoscopic surgery: a systematic review and meta-analysis. *Br J Anaesth.* 2017;118(6):834–842. doi:10.1093/bja/aex116.
73. McLean DJ, Diaz-Gil D, Farhan HN, Ladha KS, Kurth T, Eikermann M. Dose-dependent association between intermediate-acting neuromuscular-blocking agents and postoperative respiratory complications. *Anesthesiology.* 2015;122(6):1201–1213. doi:10.1097/aln.0000000000000674.
74. Singh PP, Lemanu DP, Taylor MH, Hill AG. Association between preoperative glucocorticoids and long-term survival and cancer recurrence after colectomy: follow-up analysis of a previous randomized controlled trial. *Br J Anaesth.* 2014;113(Suppl 1):i68–i73. doi:10.1093/bja/aet577.
75. Kranke P, Jokinen J, Pace NL, et al. Continuous intravenous perioperative lidocaine infusion for postoperative pain and recovery. *Cochrane Database Syst Rev.* 2015(7):Cd009642. doi:10.1002/14651858.CD009642.pub2.
76. Rigas B, Tsioulias GJ. The evolving role of nonsteroidal anti-inflammatory drugs in colon cancer prevention: a cause for optimism. *J Pharmacol Exp Ther.* 2015;353(1):2–8. doi:10.1124/jpet.114.220806.
77. Klein M. Postoperative non-steroidal anti-inflammatory drugs and colorectal anastomotic leakage. NSAIDs and anastomotic leakage. *Dan Med J.* 2012;59(3):B4420.
78. Impact of postoperative non-steroidal anti-inflammatory drugs on adverse events after gastrointestinal surgery. *Br J Surg.* Oct 2014;101(11):1413–1423. doi:10.1002/bjs.9614.
79. Cata JP, Guerra CE, Chang GJ, Gottumukkala V, Joshi GP. Non-steroidal anti-inflammatory drugs in the oncological surgical population: beneficial or harmful? A systematic review of the literature. *Br J Anaesth.* 2017;119(4):750–764. doi:10.1093/bja/aex225.
80. Hiller JG, Perry NJ, Poulogiannis G, Riedel B, Sloan EK. Perioperative events influence cancer recurrence risk after surgery. *Nat Rev Clin Oncol.* 2018;15(4):205–218. doi:10.1038/nrclinonc.2017.194.
81. Byrne K, Levins KJ, Buggy DJ. Can anesthetic-analgesic technique during primary cancer surgery affect recurrence or metastasis? *Can J Anaesth.* 2016;63(2):184–192. doi:10.1007/s12630-015-0523-8.
82. Wall T, Sherwin A, Ma D, Buggy DJ. Influence of perioperative anaesthetic and analgesic interventions on oncological outcomes: a narrative review. *Br J Anaesth.* 2019;123(2):135–150. doi:10.1016/j.bja.2019.04.062.
83. Sessler DI, Pei L, Huang Y, et al. Recurrence of breast cancer after regional or general anaesthesia: a randomised controlled trial. *Lancet.* 2019;394(10211):1807–1815. doi:10.1016/s0140-6736(19)32313-x.
84. Buggy DJ, Borgeat A, Cata J, et al. Consensus statement from the BJA workshop on cancer and anaesthesia. *Br J Anaesth.* 2015;114(1):2–3.

26

Perioperative Care of the Surgical Patient: Genitourinary Cancers

JO-LYNN TAN, ELLEN O'CONNOR, SAMANTHA KOSCHEL, NIRANJAN SATHIANATHEN, NATHAN LAWRENTSCHUK, AND DECLAN G. MURPHY

Introduction

Good perioperative planning, which begins at the time the decision is made to perform surgery and continues through the postoperative recovery phase after discharge, is crucial to achieving successful outcomes in urological cancer surgery. Improvements in surgical technology and technique paired with enhanced recovery and perioperative optimization programs have been shown to reduce patient morbidity and mortality following major urological surgery.[1,2]

Common urological malignancies and surgical management options are outlined in Table 26.1. Frequent endoscopic procedures are common in the treatment of bladder cancer; however, owing to the aging population that this condition affects, perioperative morbidity can be misleadingly high. Patients at risk of anesthetic and surgical complications can be identified via predictive indices, such as the Charlson Comorbidity Index (CCI), patient Eastern Cooperative Oncology Group (ECOG) status, and American Society of Anesthesiology (ASA) scores.[3] Early identification of common issues, such as anticoagulation, diabetic control, and pain management needs, allows for adequate preparation and better control when issues arise.

The practice landscape in urological cancer surgery has changed dramatically over the last 15 years, where a significant rise in the adoption of minimally invasive approaches has been seen.[4,5] This has resulted in a change in the nature of complications following major urological cancer surgery. Radical prostatectomy (RP) was previously considered a procedure that carried significant morbidity and risks, whereas most centers that practice robotic RP now only require their patients to have overnight admissions. Radical cystectomy (RC), on the other hand, has surpassed RP as having the highest surgical complication rate. This has led to a strong body of research looking at the impact of Enhanced Recovery After Surgery (ERAS) protocols in RC surgery.[6,7]

Perioperative Assessment and Optimization

Perioperative assessment commences the moment surgical intervention for treatment of the given malignancy is proposed. This is initiated by the urologist or other treating clinician upon meeting the patient, however, can quickly expand to include a much larger multidisciplinary team. Establishing fitness for surgery is a complex and multifactorial decision that can be made within moments in some instances or take months in others. In the first instance, a thorough history of the presenting complaint, past medical history, and medications, as well as physical examination, are essential.[3]

Cardiopulmonary evaluation is important prior to any major urological surgery. Pulmonary function testing may be beneficial for patients with chronic obstructive pulmonary disease (COPD) to determine their baseline function prior to surgery or to assess those with undiagnosed COPD; however, spirometry alone does not determine postoperative risk.[3] Particular attention should be paid to patients with germ-cell tumors who have undergone neoadjuvant chemotherapy with bleomycin, etoposide, and cisplatin (BEP). Pulmonary fibrosis is a well-documented side effect of bleomycin; therefore preoperative pulmonary function tests should be considered prior to proceeding with anesthetic for retroperitoneal lymph node dissection (RPLND).[9] Many patients undergoing urological cancer surgery have preexisting risk factors for cardiovascular disease. Furthermore, it may also be necessary to cease preventative antiplatelet and anticoagulant therapy prior to surgery due to risk of intra- and postoperative bleeding. Guidelines highlight the need for clinicians to weigh up these risks on an individual basis.[10] Bridging anticoagulation should be used for patients at especially high risk in the perioperative period.

TABLE 26.1 Common Urological Malignancies and Surgical Management

Urological Malignancy	Surgical Management	Patient Demographic[8]
Renal	Radical nephrectomy Open, laparoscopic, robotic Partial nephrectomy Open, laparoscopic, robotic inferior vena cava thrombectomy	1.5:1 male predominance Peak incidence 60–70 years *Risk factors:* smoking, obesity, hypertension
Urothelial	Cystectomy (and urinary diversion) Endoscopic procedures Transurethral resection of bladder tumor Rigid cystoscopy and diathermy Endoscopic laser ablation Ureterectomy	4:1 male predominance *Risk factors:* smoking, occupational exposure, radiotherapy
Prostate	Radical prostatectomy Open, laparoscopic, robotic Pelvic lymph node dissection	Second most commonly diagnosed cancer in men Prevalence 59% by age >79 years
Testicular	Orchidectomy Partial orchidectomy Retroperitoneal lymph node dissection	Most common solid malignancy in men aged 20–40 years *Risk factors:* undescended testis, family history
Penile	Radical penectomy Partial penectomy Lymph node dissection	Peak incidence at ages 60–70 years *Risk factors:* human papilloma virus

• BOX 26.1 Validated Perioperative Assessment Scoring Systems

Assessment Tools

American Society of Anesthesiology (ASA) Physical Classification[12]
Charlson Comorbidity Index (CCI)[13]
Functional Status[3]
Fried Frailty Score[14]
Surgical Risk Calculator[15]

Validated perioperative assessment scoring systems are now widely used across all surgical specialties as a guide to surgical planning, perioperative care interventions, and as an adjunct to informed patient decision-making (Box 26.1). A range of nonsurgical management options exist for some urooncological conditions, most commonly radiotherapy used for the treatment of prostate and bladder cancer, as well as ablative options for renal cancer. As such, perioperative consideration together with the patient serves an important role in guiding the best standard of care. The multidisciplinary team meeting (MDTM) is recognized as a gold standard for cancer care delivery globally. It provides a forum for interdisciplinary discussion regarding patient care and involves surgeons, medical oncologists, radiation oncologists, pathologists, radiologists, and specialty cancer nurses, among others. Decision-making at the MDTM can be significantly impacted, however, in the event of lack of patient-specific information or knowledge of the patient's wishes.[11]

Assessment of global "surgical fitness" is a deviation from the traditional approach of preoperative assessment based on organ system. This can be particularly useful in an elderly demographic of patients and has been studied with regard to those undergoing RC.[16,17] Functional status and frailty are both associated with increased postoperative morbidity and mortality.[14] Frailty is a distinct syndrome separate to comorbidity and disability, resulting in decreased physiologic reserve and resistance to stressors. Combined, this results in increased vulnerability and poorer health outcomes. Frailty has been shown to be an independent predictor of complications following RC.[16,17]

Enhanced Recovery and Postoperative Care

ERAS protocols are a seasoned concept in the postoperative care of urological patients.[2] These are standardized, evidence-based programs designed to accelerate recovery times, improve outcomes, and reduce health care costs. Broadly, ERAS protocols are multimodal, and integrate preoperative, intraoperative, and postoperative care principles with the goal of minimizing the surgical stress response, thereby optimizing recovery.[18–20] They utilize the expertise of a multidisciplinary team, while simultaneously providing clear guidance for progression of postoperative management to the clinical team involved. This includes aspects of postoperative care, such as diet initiation and progression, fluid management, early ambulation, and urinary catheter management to list a few.

There is a large body of research investigating the efficacy of ERAS protocols in the setting of RC[6,7,21,22] and RP surgeries.[2,23] In urological surgery, ERAS pathways have been demonstrated to reduce duration of hospital stay by up to 30% and without increasing postoperative complications or readmission rates.[6,18] The early success of ERAS protocols can be seen in the trajectory of care for patients who have undergone RP and partial nephrectomy (PN). Evidence-based perioperative care pathways in urology were introduced with the aim of reducing hospital length of stay (LOS). RP, which was once thought to be a considerably morbid operation, previously required an average LOS of 6 days. Today, robotic approaches often involve only overnight hospital admissions. ERAS protocols have since been studied and adopted in partial nephrectomy (PN), radical nephrectomy (RN), and radical cystectomy (RC).[7,24–27] These studies have demonstrated the feasibility of ERAS protocols in reducing hospital LOS in the setting of these major urological surgeries. Additionally, hospital readmission and complication rates were not increased with the implementation of ERAS protocols regardless of surgical approach.[22,28,29] Elements of ERAS pertaining to urological surgery are summarized in Table 26.2.

Few studies have explored the relationship between intensive care unit (ICU) admission and adherence to ERAS protocols.[31,32] Evidence supporting planned ICU admission following RC is currently lacking. Cheng et al.[31] studied the drivers of ICU admission following RC with ERAS protocols. Although the rate of unplanned ICU admissions after

TABLE 26.2 Urology-Specific Enhanced Recovery After Surgery (ERAS) Elements (from Saidian and Nix[30])

	ERAS Item	Unique Application to Urological Surgery
Preoperative	Patient education and counseling	Detailed counseling about urinary diversion and expectations
	Patient selection and optimization	Most of the cystectomy patients are malnourished to some degree
	Oral bowel preparation	No benefit to oral bowel preparation in cystectomy patients No high-level evidence for prostatectomy patients
	Preoperative fasting and carbohydrate load	None
	Alvimopan administration	Earlier first bowel movement, shorter LOS, and decreased incidence of ileus in cystectomy patients
	Preanesthesia medications	May consider use of preoperative gabapentin or oxybutynin for reducing catheter-related bladder pain
	Antibiotic recommendations	Clean-contaminated procedure; recommend second- or third-generation cephalosporin
Intraoperative	Anesthesia recommendations	None
	Surgical approach	Decreased LOS in robotic vs. open approach
	Perioperative fluid management	Goal-directed fluid therapy in RC patients shows decreased incidence of ileus and postoperative nausea and vomiting
	Intraoperative hypothermia prevention	None
	Resection site drainage	Peritoneal drainage is not necessary in patients undergoing RARP, even with extended PLND
	NG tube	Routine NG tube removal after RC surgery
Postoperative	Urinary drainage	In RP patients, cystogram must be considered prior to catheter removal or longer catheter times in patients with high risk of urinary anastomotic leakage May be short-term benefits of suprapubic vs. urethral catheter; however, no long-term functional differences seen Neobladder: recommend frequent irrigation of any newly formed neobladder. No official recommendations for catheter during or after surgery; however most, recommend 2 weeks minimum
	Early ambulation	Early ambulation can decrease thromboembolic events, pulmonary complications, and ileus risk
	Early diet initiation	No specific studies in urological surgery
	Postoperative pain management	Opioid-sparing protocols have been shown to reduce LOS in RC patients Consideration of antimuscarinics of gabapentinoids for catheter-related bladder pain

LOS, Length of stay; *NG*, nasogastric tube; *PLND*, peritoneal lymph node dissection; *RARP*, robotic-assisted radical prostatectomy; *RC*, radical cystectomy; *RP*, radical prostatectomy.

RC was low, they found that advanced age and CCI ≥ 3 were significantly associated with unplanned ICU admission after RC. In their cohort, a significantly higher proportion of past myocardial infarctions and congestive heart failure were seen in those who had unplanned ICU admissions. This highlights the importance of identification and optimization of cardiac disease during preoperative patient workup, particularly in older patients. Specific age cutoffs are not identified in the current literature.

Present data demonstrate the benefit and value of ERAS protocols in the setting of major urological cancer surgery. Gaps lie in the lack of procedure-specific ERAS guidelines.[33] Further studies focusing on refining current protocols for urology, specifically preoperative medical optimization, perioperative nutritional management, management of urinary drainage, e.g., timing of stent removal in ileal conduits, earlier catheter removal in robotic-assisted radical prostatectomy (RARP), and the use of anesthetic alternatives such as spinal epidural anesthesia may further improve outcomes, reduce ICU admissions, and reduce overall hospital LOS.

TABLE 26.3 Top Causes of Readmission by Surgery Type (Schmid et al.[34])

Surgery Type	Most Common Causes of Readmission
Radical cystectomy Open or minimally invasive	Renal/genitourinary (15.5%) Wound (14.8%) Sepsis/infection (14.1%) Gastrointestinal (11.1%) General symptoms, e.g., nausea, pain, hypotension (9.2%) Thromboembolic (8.5%)
Radical prostatectomy Open or minimally invasive	Thromboembolic (13.6%) Wound issues (12.2%) Renal/genitourinary (12.2%) Gastrointestinal (11.8%) Sepsis/infection (8.6%)
Radical nephrectomy Open or minimally invasive	Wound issues (12.9%) Gastrointestinal (12.9%)
Partial nephrectomy Open or minimally invasive	Renal/genitourinary (19.6%) Cardiovascular (9.8%) Bleeding/hematoma (9.8%) Wound (7.8%)

Common Complications and Causes for Readmission

Hospital LOS and the rate of unplanned hospital readmissions are key indicators of health care costs and funding, as well as being important indicators of successful patient outcomes. For major urological surgeries, the hospital readmission rate has been reported to range from 5.5% for all urological cancer surgeries to up to 25% in RC alone.[34,35] The majority of readmissions occur within the first 2 weeks after discharge, and in the case of RC, almost a quarter of patients are readmitted within 30 days of discharge.[34–36]

Common causes of complications and readmissions are thromboembolic events; wound breakdown; bleeding and hematoma; and renal/genitourinary, gastrointestinal, and infection/sepsis.[34,37,38] Schmid et al.[34] further break these complications down by type of surgery; their data demonstrated that RC carries the highest rates of complications and readmission, followed by RP and RN, then PN (Table 26.3). Many other studies show similar findings to RC, regardless of surgical approach.[39–44] Additionally, open procedures for RP or PN are more likely to experience hospital readmissions compared with their minimally invasive equivalents.

Berger et al.[29] examined specific factors associated with postdischarge complications and readmission within the first 30 days after surgery. They found that obesity, COPD, diabetes, steroid use, dependent functional status, a continent diversion, and longer operation duration were all significantly and independently associated with hospital readmission or postoperative complications.[29] In the RC population, low preoperative serum albumin has also been identified as a risk factor for postoperative complications and higher 90-day mortality.[45] A common thread seen in these risk factors is the presence of reduced physiological conditioning and reserve, and impaired immune status. This bears important clinical relevance, as it highlights the value of early identification and preoperative optimization of patients at risk. Patients who are prediabetic can be managed early and steroid use can be tapered with a clear medical plan laid out for the perioperative period. Functional conditioning and high or low body mass indices may be optimized with the involvement of dieticians and physiotherapists, or exercise physiologists. Smoking cessation programs, particularly in patients with COPD, can be instituted early on in the preoperative stages. Although current data lack detail on patients undergoing neoadjuvant chemotherapy, it would seem logical that this also poses a threat to patients' immune status in the perioperative recovery period.

Nursing follow up, such as with hospital in the home services and timely postoperative review in the outpatient setting, may help to avert readmissions by identifying and managing potential issues early. Primary care physicians also play an important role in the early identification and management of issues in the postoperative phase, and any potential issues should be communicated to ensure early follow up.

Thromboprophylaxis

Venous thromboembolism (VTE) is the most common modifiable cause of readmission following urological cancer surgery.[34] As a result of the hypercoagulable state during surgery and active malignancy, both pulmonary embolism (PE) and deep vein thrombosis (DVT) are serious complications in this patient group. Timing and duration of thromboprophylaxis following urological cancer surgery is

TABLE 26.4 Venous Thromboembolism (VTE) Risk Stratification for Major Urological Surgery (Tikkinen et al. [51])

VTE Risk Stratification for Major Urological Surgery		
Low risk	No risk factors	Onefold
Medium risk	Any one of the following: – Age >75 years – Body mass index >35 kg/m^2 – VTE in first-degree relative (parent, full sibling, or child)	Twofold
High risk	Personal history of VTE Patients with any combination of two or more risk factors	Fourfold

counterbalanced against the risk of bleeding. This risk versus benefit depends on both patient and surgical factors.[46,47] Current guidelines highlight a lack of high-quality evidence to guide practice in this area; however, it is essential to consider VTE thromboprophylaxis in all patients undergoing urological cancer surgery.[46–50]

Patient risk for VTE after major urological cancer surgery can be stratified based upon well-documented risk factors for VTE. Tikkinen et al.[51] developed a simple model for VTE risk in the context of urological, general, and gynecological surgery (Table 26.4). Bleeding risk is more difficult to quantify due to the lack of a universal measure defining bleeding risk and the heterogeneity of outcomes reported in current literature. However, this risk remains highest following PN and RP with extended lymph node dissection.[51] Risk of major bleeding is greatest within the first 24 h following surgery, with >90% occurring within the first 4 postoperative days.[52] In contrast, VTE risk remains constant over the first 4 weeks postoperatively.

VTE incidence varies among urological cancer operations, with RP, RC, and RPLND carrying the highest documented risk and renal surgery carrying a lower risk.[34,48] Pelvic lymph node dissection doubles the risk of VTE following RP compared to without.[51] Patients who receive neoadjuvant chemotherapy prior to RC may also have increased risk of VTE when compared to those who received adjuvant or no chemotherapy.[53] Surgical approach, patient positioning (lithotomy vs. supine), and time to ambulation influence VTE risk. Both mechanical (graduated compression stockings and intermittent pneumatic compression) and pharmacological (low-dose unfractionated heparin and low-molecular-weight heparin) therapies have been found to significantly reduce the risk of VTE and should be considered in all patients.[49,51]

Extended thromboembolism prophylaxis (ETP) involves ongoing pharmacological therapy upon patient discharge for a duration of 28 days after the operation. European Association of Urology (EAU) and National Institute for Health and Care Excellence (NICE) guidelines stratify need for ETP against bleeding risk in all urological cancer operations.[48,54] This includes strong recommendations for ETP following RC and open RP with pelvic lymph node dissection (Table 26.5). Despite these guidelines, there remains a lack of high-quality urology-specific evidence to aid clinicians in navigating management.[48] A number of recently published literature reviews have highlighted the absence of randomized controlled trials in current literature.[51,55] Current best practice thus relies on clinicians balancing the

TABLE 26.5 Procedure-Specific Recommendations for Extended Thromboembolism Prophylaxis (ETP) Based on Low-Risk Patient (European Association of Urology Guidelines 2019, Tikkinen et al.[48]).

Surgery Type	Risk of Bleeding Among 1000 Patients	Risk of VTE Among 1000 Patients	Recommendation for ETP
Radical cystectomy			
Open	3.0	29	Strong—for
Robotic	3.0	26	Weak—for
Radical prostatectomy			
Open (with/without PLND)	1.0–2.0	10–20	Weak—for
Open with extended PLND	2.0	39	Strong—for
Robotic (with/without PLND)	4.0–8.0	2.0–9.0	Strong—against
Laparoscopic (with/without PLND)	7.0–10	4.0–8.0	Strong—against
Radical nephrectomy			
Open	0.5	11	Weak—for
Laparoscopic	5.0	7.0	Weak—against
With thrombectomy	20	29	Weak—for
Partial nephrectomy			
Open	1.0	10	Weak—for
Laparoscopic/robotic	5.0–17	10–11	Weak—against
Primary retroperitoneal lymph node dissection	2.0	23	Weak—for

PLND, Peritoneal lymph node dissection; *VTE*, venous thromboembolism.

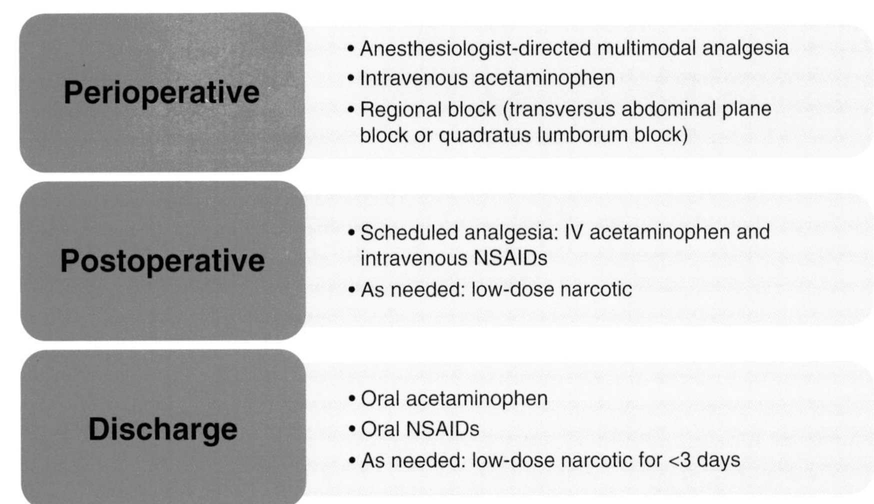

Perioperative
• Anesthesiologist-directed multimodal analgesia
• Intravenous acetaminophen
• Regional block (transversus abdominal plane block or quadratus lumborum block)
Postoperative
• Scheduled analgesia: IV acetaminophen and intravenous NSAIDs
• As needed: low-dose narcotic
Discharge
• Oral acetaminophen
• Oral NSAIDs
• As needed: low-dose narcotic for <3 days

• **Fig. 26.1** A proposed pathway for management of perioperative pain while limiting narcotic needs. (From Theisen KM, et al. Excessive opioid prescribing after major urologic procedures. *Urology*. 2019;123:101–107.)

known risks of bleeding versus VTE within the context of each procedure and consideration of individual patient profiles.

Limited evidence provides guidance regarding choice of agent used for pharmacological prophylaxis; however, options include low-molecular-weight heparins, low-dose unfractionated heparin, and direct-acting oral anticoagulations.[49,54] Special consideration should be taken for those with renal impairment and dosage adjustment is required.

Overall, the decision to use ETP after major urological cancer surgery is not straightforward and requires the complex balancing of surgical factors, VTE risk factors, bleeding risk, and mortality risk. For patients already anticoagulated the decision for bridging therapy generally relies on evaluating patient and surgical risks, and decisions are made on a case-by-case basis. Individual patient factors and the changing landscape of urological surgery must be considered when general recommendations are made.

Opioid-Sparing Surgery

As the landscape of urological cancer surgery shifts toward more minimally-invasive approaches, and ERAS protocols become more refined, procedures such as RP that were once considered highly morbid are now requiring only overnight hospital admissions. A key factor requiring postprostatectomy patients to stay overnight in hospital at present is pain management.

It has been shown that RP patients have minimal requirements for opioid analgesia when multimodal analgesia is used.[56,57] Effective pain management begins in the preoperative assessment clinics where early education and counseling regarding the use of simple analgesia, paracetamol (acetaminophen), and nonsteroidal antiinflammatory drugs (NSAIDs) can empower patients with self-management strategies and reduce anxiety relating to postoperative pain. Furthermore, patients at risk of poor pain control such as those with prior opioid exposure or chronic pain syndromes can be identified early and management plans put in place.

Recent studies highlight the benefits of multimodal pain management approaches, and there is a current shift toward "opioid-sparing" or opioid reduction in RP.[58,59] The main sources of discomfort experienced by patients following RARP are abdominal/incisional, penile, urethral catheter, and bladder spasm related. Most patients experience mild-to-moderate abdominal discomfort that declines gradually over days. Additionally, surgical approach has not been shown to correlate with higher opioid use in RP; therefore those undergoing open or minimally invasive RP should be similar in their analgesic requirements.[59] A number of other analgesic approaches for improving RP-specific pain include penile block for improved catheter tolerance, although this was not found to make a difference[60]; intravesical ropivacaine, although this did not demonstrate improved pain control[61]; antimuscarinic medications such as oxybutynin and tolteridine that have been shown to improve catheter-related bladder discomfort[62]; and gabapentinoids (a single preoperative 900 mg dose) have been shown to improve pain without reducing opioid requirements.[63]

The issues and complications relating to opioid overuse are well documented, yet across specialties the patterns of prescribing do not reflect acknowledgement of these risks.[64,65] Well-described complications include respiratory depression, somnolence resulting in decreased early mobilization, constipation, postoperative ileus, nausea, and delirium, especially in the elderly. It is also useful to note that a single perioperative exposure to opioids can result in opioid dependence and abuse; thus caution with physician opioid prescribing is paramount.

Studies are underway examining the use of multimodal pain management protocols for RP (Fig. 26.1).[64] Procedure-specific pain management can also facilitate recovery and complement ERAS protocols. More studies assessing the use of pain management protocols in a number of major urological cancer surgeries and consensus recommendations are needed.

Conclusion

Like all surgical specialties, the perioperative management of the patient undergoing major urological cancer surgery requires a multidisciplinary approach. Assessment and optimization of patient factors can be performed in a preoperative assessment clinic involving anesthesiologists, urologists, nurses, pharmacists, and other allied health professionals. Considerations must be made for patients already on anticoagulation and clear plans laid out for the peri- and postoperative periods. Baseline renal function should be assessed particularly for those patients undergoing partial or radical nephrectomy. Patients at high risk of unplanned ICU admissions should be identified. Risk stratification of patients can be performed using well-validated indices. This is also the ideal opportunity for patients to be educated about smoking cessation, diet and nutrition, and diabetes management. Factors that may hinder timely discharge may be flagged early. Further, pain management in the postoperative period can be addressed so that opioid use in the postoperative phase can be rationalized. Patients with chronic pain conditions should be identified, so that early pain management strategies can be implemented. Finally, ERAS protocols are a familiar practice in urological surgery, and patients can be educated early regarding recovery milestones in the early postoperative period.

References

1. Dy GW, Gore JL, Forouzanfar MH, Naghavi M, Fitzmaurice C. Global burden of urologic cancers, 1990–2013. *Eur Urol.* 2017;71(3):437–446. doi:10.1016/j.eururo.2016.10.008.
2. Azhar RA, Bochner B, Catto J, et al. Enhanced recovery after urological surgery: a contemporary systematic review of outcomes, key elements, and research needs. *Eur Urol.* 2016;70(1):176–187.
3. Stoffel JT, Montgomery JS, Suskind M, Tucci C, Vanni AJ. American Urological Association (AUA). Optimizing outcomes in urologic surgery : pre-operative care for the patient undergoing urologic surgery or procedure. 2018. Available at www.auanet.org/guidelines/stoma-marking.
4. Imkamp F, Herrmann TRW, Stolzenburg JU, et al. Acceptance and indication for robot assisted laparoscopy limited to few indications-results of a 2012 survey among urologists in Germany, Austria and Switzerland. *Eur Urol Suppl.* 2014;95(3):336–345.
5. Ghani KR, Sukumar S, Sammon JD, Rogers CG, Trinh QD, Menon M. Practice patterns and outcomes of open and minimally invasive partial nephrectomy since the introduction of robotic partial nephrectomy: results from the nationwide inpatient sample. *J Urol.* 2014;191(4):907–912.
6. Tyson MD, Chang SS. Enhanced recovery pathways versus standard care after cystectomy: a meta-analysis of the effect on perioperative outcomes. *Eur Urol.* 2016;70(6):995–1003.
7. Dunkman WJ, Manning MW, Whittle J, et al. Impact of an enhanced recovery pathway on length of stay and complications in elective radical cystectomy: a before and after cohort study. *Perioper Med.* 2019;22(8):9.
8. EAU. EAU Guidelines, presented at the EAU Annual Congress Copenhagen 2019 [Internet]. Arnhem, The Netherlands: EAU Guidelines Office. Available at http://uroweb.org/guidelines/compilations-of-all-guidelines/.
9. Lauritsen J, Gry M, Kier G, Bandak M, Mortensen MS. Pulmonary function in patients with germ cell cancer treated with bleomycin, etoposide, and cisplatin. *J Clin Oncol.* 2016;34(13):1492–1499.
10. Dimitropoulos K, Omar MI, Chalkias A, Arnaoutoglou E, Douketis J, Gravas S. Perioperative antithrombotic (antiplatelet and anticoagulant) therapy in urological practice : a critical assessment and summary of the clinical practice guidelines. *World J Urol.* 2020; 38(11):2761–2770. doi:10.1007/s00345-020-03078-2.
11. Soukup T, Lamb BW, Arora S, Darzi A, Sevdalis N, Green JSA. Successful strategies in implementing a multidisciplinary team working in the care of patients with cancer: an overview and synthesis of theavailable literature. *J Multidiscip Healthc.* 2018;11:49–61.
12. Doyle D, Garmon E. American Society of Anesthesiologists Classification (ASA Class). StatPearls. 2019. Available at https://www.ncbi.nlm.nih.gov/books/NBK441940/.
13. Charlson M, Szatrowski TP, Peterson J, Gold J. Validation of a combined comorbidity index. *J Clin Epidemiol.* 1994; Nov;47(11):1245–1251. doi:10.1016/0895-4356(94)90129-5. PMID:7722560.
14. Fried LP, Ferrucci L, Darer J, Williamson JD, Anderson G. Untangling the concepts of disability, frailty, and comorbidity: implications for improved targeting and care. *J Gerontol A Biol Sci Med Sci.* 2004;59(3):255–263.
15. American College of Surgeons National Surgical Quality Improvement Program. Surgical Risk Calculator. American College of Surgeons website. 2017. Available at http://www.riskcalculator.facs.org/RiskCalculator/about.html.
16. Burg ML, Clifford TG, Bazargani ST, et al. Frailty as a predictor of complications after radical cystectomy: A prospective study of various preoperative assessments. *Urol Oncol.* 2019: 37(1):40–47. doi:10.1016/j.urolonc.2018.10.002.
17. Chappidi MR, Kates M, Patel HD, et al. Frailty as a marker of adverse outcomes in patients with bladder cancer undergoing radical cystectomy. *Urol Oncol.* 2016;34(6):256.e1–6. doi:10.1016/j.urolonc.2015.12.010.
18. Varadhan KK, Lobo DN, Ljungqvist O. Enhanced recovery after surgery: the future of improving surgical care. *Crit Care Clin.* 2010;26:527–547.
19. Kehlet H, Wilmore DW. Multimodal strategies to improve surgical outcome. *Am J Surg.* 2002;183(6):630–641.
20. Kehlet H. Multimodal approach to control postoperative pathophysiology and rehabilitation. *Br J Anaesth.* 1997;78(5):606–617.
21. Mir MC, Zargar H, Bolton DM, Murphy DG, Lawrentschuk N. Enhanced Recovery After Surgery protocols for radical cystectomy surgery: review of current evidence and local protocols. *ANZ J Surg.* 2015;85(7–8):514–520.
22. Baack Kukreja JE, Kiernan M, Schempp B, et al. Quality improvement in cystectomy care with enhanced recovery (QUICCER) study. *BJU Int.* 2017;119(1):38–49.
23. Chang SS, Cole E, Smith JA, Baumgartner R, Wells N, Cookson MS. Safely reducing length of stay after open radical retropubic prostatectomy under the guidance of a clinical care pathway. *Cancer.* 2005;104(4):747–751.

24. Hwang YJ, Minnillo BJ, Kim SP, Abouassaly R. Assessment of healthcare quality metrics: length-of-stay, 30-day readmission, and 30-day mortality for radical nephrectomy with inferior vena cava thrombectomy. *J Can Urol Assoc*. 2015;9(3–4):114–121.
25. Autorino R, Zargar H, Butler S, Laydner H, Kaouk JH. Incidence and risk factors for 30-day readmission in patients undergoing nephrectomy procedures: a contemporary analysis of 5276 cases from the national surgical quality improvement program database. *Urology*. 2015;85(4):843–849.
26. Tarin T, Feifer A, Kimm S, et al. Impact of a common clinical pathway on length of hospital stay in patients undergoing open and minimally invasive kidney surgery. *J Urol*. 2014;191(5):1225–1230.
27. Chen J, Djaladat H, Schuckman AK, et al. Surgical approach as a determinant factor of clinical outcome following radical cystectomy: does enhanced recovery after surgery (ERAS) level the playing field? *Urol Oncol*. 2019;37(10):765–773.
28. Patel A, Golan S, Razmaria A, Prasad S, Eggener S, Shalhav A. Early discharge after laparoscopic or robotic partial nephrectomy: care pathway evaluation. *BJU Int*. 2014;113(4):592–597.
29. Berger I, Xia L, Wirtalla C, Dowzicky P, Guzzo TJ. Kelz RR. 30-day readmission after radical cystectomy: identifying targets for improvement using the phases of surgical care. *Can Urol Assoc J*. 2019;20:E190–E201.
30. Saidian A, Nix JW. Enhanced recovery after surgery: urology. *Surg Clin North Am*. 2018;98(6):1265–1274.
31. Cheng KW, Shah A, Bazargani S, et al. Factors influencing ICU admission and associated outcome in patients undergoing radical cystectomy with enhanced recovery pathway. *Urol Oncol*. 2019;37(9):572.e13–572.e19. doi:10.03248/j.urolonc.2019.06.019.
32. Nabhani J, Ahmadi H, Schuckman AK, et al. Cost analysis of the Enhanced Recovery After Surgery protocol in patients undergoing radical cystectomy for bladder cancer. *Eur Urol Focus*. 2016;2(1):92–96.
33. Vukovic N, Dinic L. Enhanced recovery after surgery protocols in major urologic surgery. *Front Med*. 2018;5:93. doi:10.3389/fmed.2018.00093.
34. Schmid M, Chiang HA, Sood A, et al. Causes of hospital readmissions after urologic cancer surgery. *Urol Oncol*. 2016; 34(5):236.e1-e11. doi:10.03248/j.urolonc.2019.06.019.
35. Skolarus TA, Jacobs BL, Schroeck FR, et al. Understanding hospital readmission intensity after radical cystectomy. *J Urol*. 2015;193(5):1500–1506.
36. Saluk JL, Blackwell RH, Gange WS, et al. The LACE score as a tool to identify radical cystectomy patients at increased risk of 90-day readmission and mortality. *Curr Urol*. 2018;12:20–26.
37. Lavallée LT, Schramm D, Witiuk K, et al. Peri-operative morbidity associated with radical cystectomy in a multicenter database of community and academic hospitals. *PLoS One*. 2014;9(10):e111281.
38. Sood A, Kachroo N, Abdollah F, et al. An evaluation of the timing of surgical complications following radical cystectomy: data from the American College of Surgeons National Surgical Quality Improvement Program. *Urology*. 2017;103:91–98.
39. Schiavina R, Borghesi M, Guidi M, et al. Perioperative complications and mortality after radical cystectomy when using a standardized reporting methodology. *Clin Genitourin Cancer*. 2013;11(2):189–197.
40. Shabsigh A, Korets R, Vora KC, et al. Defining early morbidity of radical cystectomy for patients with bladder cancer using a standardized reporting methodology. *Eur Urol*. 2009;55(1):164–174.
41. Yuh BE, Nazmy M, Ruel NH, et al. Standardized analysis of frequency and severity of complications after robot-assisted radical cystectomy. *Eur Urol*. 2012;62(5):806–813.
42. Johar RS, Hayn MH, Stegemann AP, et al. Complications after robot-assisted radical cystectomy: results from the International Robotic Cystectomy Consortium. *Eur Urol*. 2013;64(1):52–57.
43. Moschini M, Simone G, Stenzl A, Gill IS, Catto J. Critical review of outcomes from radical cystectomy: can complications from radical cystectomy be reduced by surgical volume and robotic surgery? *Eur Urol Focus*. 2016;2(1):19–29.
44. Li K, Lin T, Fan X, et al. Systematic review and meta-analysis of comparative studies reporting early outcomes after robot-assisted radical cystectomy versus open radical cystectomy. *Cancer Treat Rev*. 2013;9(6):551–560.
45. Garg T, Chen LY, Kim PH, Zhao PT, Herr HW, Donat SM. Preoperative serum albumin is associated with mortality and complications after radical cystectomy. *BJU Int*. 2014;113(6):918–923.
46. Violette PD, Cartwright R, Briel M, Tikkinen KAO, Guyatt GH. Guideline of guidelines: thromboprophylaxis for urological surgery. *BJU Int*. 2016;118(3):351–358. doi:10.1111/bju.13496.
47. Gould MK, Garcia DA, Wren SM, et al. Prevention of VTE in nonorthopedic surgical patients: Antithrombotic Therapy and Prevention of Thrombosis, 9th ed: American College of Chest Physicians Evidence-Based Clinical Practice Guidelines. *Chest*. 2012;141(2):e227S–e277S. doi:10.1378/chest.11-2297.
48. Tikkinen K, Cartwright R, Gould M, et al. Thromboprophylaxis in urological surgery. European Association of Urology Guidelines Office, 2019.
49. Forrest JB, Clemens JQ, Finamore P, et al. AUA best practice statement for the prevention of deep vein thrombosis in patients undergoing urologic surgery. *JURO*. 2009;181(3):1170–1177. doi:10.1016/j.juro.2008.12.027.
50. Violette P.D, Lavallée L.T, Kassouf W, Gross P.L, Shayegan B. Canadian Urological Association guideline: perioperative thromboprophylaxis and management of anticoagulation. *Can Urol Assoc J*. 2019;13(4):105–114. . doi:10.5489/cuaj.5828.
51. Tikkinen KAO, Craigie S, Agarwal A, et al. Procedure-specific risks of thrombosis and bleeding in urological cancer surgery: systematic review and meta-analysis. *Eur Urol*. 2018;73(2):242–251.
52. Tikkinen KAO, Agarwal A, Craigie S, et al. Systematic reviews of observational studies of risk of thrombosis and bleeding in urological surgery (ROTBUS): Introduction and methodology. *Syst Rev*. 2014;23(3):150.
53. Brennan K, Karim S, Doiron RC, Siemens DR. Venous thromboembolism and peri-operative chemotherapy for muscle-invasive bladder cancer: a population-based study. *Bladder Cancer*. 2018;4:419–428.
54. NICE. Venous thromboembolism in over 16s: reducing the risk of hospital-acquired deep vein thrombosis or pulmonary embolism. NICE Guideline. 2018. Available at https://www.nice.org.uk/guidance/ng89.
55. Naik R, Mandal I, Hampson A, et al. The role of extended venous thromboembolism prophylaxis for major urological cancer operations. *BJU Int*. 2019;124(6):935–944.
56. Cacciamani GE, Menestrina N, Pirozzi M, et al. Impact of combination of local anesthetic wounds infiltration and ultrasound transversus abdominal plane block in patients undergoing robot-assisted radical prostatectomy: perioperative results of a double-blind randomized controlled trial. *J Endourol*. 2019;33(4):295–301.

57. Wang VC, Preston MA, Kibel AS, et al. A prospective, randomized, double-blind, placebo-controlled trial to evaluate intravenous acetaminophen versus placebo in patients undergoing robotic-assisted laparoscopic prostatectomy. *J Pain Palliat Care Pharmacother*. 2018;32(2–3):82–89.
58. Joshi GP, Jaschinski T, Bonnet F, et al. PROSPECT collaboration. Optimal pain management for radical prostatectomy surgery: what is the evidence? *BMC Anesthesiol*. 2015;15:159. doi:10.1186/s12871-015-0137-2.
59. Patel HD, Faisal FA, Patel ND, et al. Effect of a prospective opioid reduction intervention on opioid prescribing and use after radical prostatectomy: results of the Opioid Reduction Intervention for Open, Laparoscopic, and Endoscopic Surgery (ORIOLES) Initiative. *BJU Int*. 2020;125(3):426–432. doi:10.1111/bju.14932.
60. Weinberg AC, Woldu SL, Bergman A, et al. Dorsal penile nerve block for robot-assisted radical prostatectomy catheter related pain: a randomized, double-blind, placebo-controlled trial. *Springerplus*. 2014;7(3):181.
61. Fuller A, Vanderhaeghe L, Nott L, Martin PR, Pautler SE. Intravesical ropivacaine as a novel means of analgesia post-robot-assisted radical prostatectomy: a randomized, double-blind, placebo-controlled trial. *J Endourol*. 2013;27(3):313–317.
62. Agarwal A, Dhiraaj S, Singhal V, Kapoor R, Tandon M. Comparison of efficacy of oxybutynin and tolterodine for prevention of catheter related bladder discomfort: a prospective, randomized, placebo-controlled, double-blind study. *Br J Anaesth*. 2006;96(3):377–380.
63. Deniz MN, Sertoz N, Erhan E, Ugur G. Effects of preoperative gabapentin on postoperative pain after radical retropubic prostatectomy. *J Int Med Res*. 2012;40(6):2362–2369.
64. Theisen KM, Myrga JM, Hale N, et al. Excessive opioid prescribing after major urologic procedures. *Urology*. 2019;123:101–107.
65. Fiore JF, Olleik G, El-Kefraoui C, et al. Preventing opioid prescription after major surgery: a scoping review of opioid-free analgesia. *Br J Anaesth*. 2019;123(5):627–636.

27

Perioperative Care of the Surgical Cancer Patient: Gynecologic Cancers

PÉREZ-GONZÁLEZ OSCAR RAFAEL

Introduction

According to the American Cancer Society (ACS), there will be >900,000 new all-cause cancer cases in American women by 2020, approximately a third of whom will die as a result.[1] The most prevalent gynecologic cancers among women are ovarian cancer, endometrial cancer, cervical cancer, and vulval cancer.[2] Cancer therapies are increasingly complex, and for solid tumors, surgical management remains the cornerstone of treatment.[3] The perioperative period is considered a time of maximum vulnerability in patients with cancer, as outlined in most enhanced recovery protocols.[4]

Ovarian Cancer

An estimated 23,000 new cases of ovarian cancer were diagnosed in the United States in 2020.

Most (90%) were epithelial ovarian cancers, the most common of which is serous carcinoma (52%).[5] Ovarian cancer incidence rates have decreased by approximately 1% per year in the past 50 years among women aged <65 years, but only since the early 1990s in older women. An estimated 14,000 deaths occurred in 2020—accounting for 5% of cancer deaths among women—more than any other gynecologic cancer.[5]

The most important risk factor besides age is a strong family history of breast or ovarian cancer. Women who have tested positive for inherited mutations in cancer susceptibility genes such as *BRCA1* or *BRCA2* are at increased risk. Modifiable factors associated with increased risk include excess body weight, menopausal hormone therapy (estrogen alone or combined with progesterone), and cigarette smoking. Factors associated with lower risk include pregnancy, fallopian tube ligation or removal (salpingectomy), and use of oral contraceptives.[5]

At first presentation, 75% have metastatic cancer to the peritoneal cavity or liver, corresponding to stage 3 cancer (according to the International Federation of Gynecology and Obstetrics [FIGO]). Surgery aims to achieve maximal reduction of tumor volume. The degree to which this can be achieved correlates with survival[6]; therefore surgery needs to be extensive. Surgery is often accompanied by 3–6 cycles of prior (neoadjuvant) platinum-based chemotherapy.[7] Second laparotomy (or "interval debulking") may be required for resection of recurrent disease, or where optimal tumor debulking could not be achieved initially. Survival from ovarian cancer depends on the extent of disease, but currently women with stage 3 disease might only expect 30%–35% survival at 5 years. Women predisposed to ovarian cancer (e.g., carriers of *BRCA* gene mutations) are increasingly being offered prophylactic salpingo-oophorectomy.[8]

Debulking of ovarian cancer is normally performed via a full mid-line laparotomy. The need for optimal cytoreduction often requires prolonged surgery. Excision of the uterus, ovaries, and adnexa is standard, accompanied by omentectomy and sampling of peritoneal deposits and lymph node chains. Wider spread of disease may necessitate bowel resection and/or splenectomy and can involve difficult dissections.[9]

Cervical Cancer

An estimated 13,500 cases of invasive cervical cancer were diagnosed in the United States in 2020, and there were an estimated 4250 deaths. Almost all cervical cancers are caused by persistent infection with certain types of human papillomavirus (HPV). Several factors are known to increase the risk of both persistent HPV infection and progression to cervical cancer, including a suppressed immune system, a high number of childbirths, and cigarette smoking.[5] Long-term use of oral contraceptives is also associated with increased risk that gradually declines after cessation. Precancerous cervical lesions may be treated with a loop electrosurgical excision procedure (LEEP), which removes abnormal tissue with a

TABLE 27.1 Common Chemotherapy Toxicities

Organic System	Chemotherapeutic Agents	Common Concerns
Pulmonary toxicity[7]	Vinca alkaloids, antitumor antibiotics, alkylating agents, antimetabolites, biological response modifiers	Pneumonitis, ARDS, interstitial lung disease, pulmonary fibrosis, capillary leak syndrome, pulmonary hypertension
Cardiac toxicity[8]	Antitumor antibiotics, vinca alkaloids, metal salts, biological response modifiers	Tachycardia, bradycardia, arrhythmia, hemorrhagic myocarditis, acute pericarditis, myocardial ischemia
Hepatic toxicity[9]	Nitrosoureas, antimetabolites, antitumor antibiotics, vinca alkaloids, topoisomerase inhibitors, tyrosine kinase inhibitors, immunotherapy, metal salts	Hepatitis, cholestasis, biliary stricture, steatosis, nodular hyperplasia fibrosis, veno-occlusive disease
Renal toxicity[10]	Nitrosoureas, metal salts, antitumor antibiotics, antimetabolites, immunotherapy, biological response modifiers	Capillary leak syndrome, glomerulosclerosis, acute tubular necrosis, Fanconi syndrome, acute interstitial nephritis, crystal nephropathy

ARDS, Acute respiratory distress syndrome.

wire loop heated by electric current. Precancerous lesions may also be surgically treated by cryotherapy (the destruction of cells by extreme cold), laser ablation (destruction of tissue using a laser beam), or conization (the removal of a cone-shaped piece of tissue containing the abnormal tissue). Invasive cervical cancers are generally treated with surgery or radiation combined with chemotherapy. Chemotherapy alone is often used to treat advanced disease.[5]

Endometrial Carcinoma

An estimated 62,000 cases of cancer of the uterine corpus were diagnosed in the United States in 2020. Cancer of the uterine corpus is often referred to as endometrial cancer because more than 90% occurs in the endometrium. Many of these tumors are associated with excess body weight and insufficient physical activity.[5]

Obesity is the main risk factor for uterine cancer, as well as factors that increase estrogen exposure, including the use of postmenopausal estrogen, late menopause, nulliparity, and a history of polycystic ovary syndrome. Tamoxifen, which may be given as treatment for breast cancer, slightly increases risk of endometrial cancer because it has estrogen-like effects on the uterus. Medical conditions that increase risk include Lynch syndrome and type 2 diabetes.[5]

Surgical management ranges from simple hysterectomy with oophorectomy and lymph node sampling to radical hysterectomy. Adjuvant pelvic radiotherapy and brachytherapy are commonly used in women with residual cancer or patients deemed unfit for surgery.[10]

Vulval Cancer

Vulvar cancer comprises approximately 6% of gynecologic cancers and less than 1% of all cancers in women. It is estimated that 1300 deaths from vulvar cancer occur in a given year. The 5-year survival rate for women with vulvar cancer is 71%. Survival rates depend on several factors, including the type of vulvar cancer and the stage of disease at the time it is diagnosed. Incidence peaks in patients aged >65 years and older patients present with later stage disease. Surgical strategies range from laser therapy to wide local excision and radical vulvectomy with groin node dissection.[11]

Perioperative Considerations

Preoperative

Preoperative assessment should include a general approach for underlying pathologies, paying particular interest to general risk factors, including obesity, advanced age, and smoking.

Cancer staging should be assessed, as well as the need for adjuvant therapy that requires specific treatments with a variable impact on the patient's overall status.[12]

Particular focus on cardiac and pulmonary function is warranted because chemotherapeutic agents may result in toxicity. Commonly observed chemotherapy toxicities are summarized in Table 27.1.[13–18]

Gynecologic cancers may present paraneoplastic syndromes, such as cerebellar degeneration, nephrotic syndrome, retinopathy, and cauda equina syndrome, and are most likely to appear in ovarian cancer patients. On the other hand, hypercalcemia, retinopathy, peripheral neuropathy, encephalitis, myelitis, and dermatomyositis are more occasionally seen in uterine cancers.[13]

Preoperative investigations should routinely include a full blood count, a clotting screen, urea and electrolyte analyses, liver function tests, group and save or cross-match for blood product transfusion, chest x-ray, and electrocardiogram. However, if specific cardiac, lung, or renal toxicity are suspected, further investigation should be performed in order to accurately establish chemotherapy or radiotherapy-induced organ dysfunction.[12]

Preoperative counseling is important to set expectations regarding surgical and anesthetic procedures, and provide information regarding a care plan in the postoperative period. This can also reduce anxiety and increase patient satisfaction, which may improve fatigue and facilitate early discharge.[19–21]

Radiotherapy

Radiotherapy for gynecologic cancers may be associated with short-term toxicity and long-term consequences. Short-term adverse effects occur during therapy or within 3 months afterwards. Short-term or acute toxicity (e.g., mucositis) generally heals within weeks. Later effects, such as fibrosis, are generally considered irreversible and progressive over time. The early and late effects of radiotherapy toxicity are strongly dependent on the tissue targeted and can include acute gastritis, cardiac toxicity, cognitive impairment, reproductive disorders, deformity and impairments to bone growth, hair loss, and secondary malignancy.[22]

Prehabilitation

Prehabilitation aims to optimize patients' physical and mental well-being in anticipation of an upcoming stress, e.g., tumor resection surgery, rather than being a reactive process to restore wellness. Prehabilitation uses aerobic and resistance exercises to improve physical function, body composition, and cardiorespiratory fitness; dietary interventions to support exercise-induced anabolism and treatment-related malnutrition; and psychological interventions to reduce stress, support behavior change, and encourage overall well-being.[23] Certain patients may benefit with improved postoperative outcomes due to prehabilitation; however, results may vary in different cancer diagnoses and stages.

Preoperative Fasting

Patients should be encouraged to eat a light meal up to 6 h and consume clear fluids, including oral carbohydrate drinks, up to 2 h before initiation of anesthesia. Patients with delayed gastric emptying should fast overnight or for 8 h before surgery. Oral carbohydrate ingestion reduces insulin resistance and improves well-being, and should be used routinely (extrapolated from nongynecologic surgery data). There are insufficient data to make recommendations in diabetic patients.[20,21]

Venous Thromboembolism Prophylaxis

Chemotherapy leads to a 2–6-fold increase in thromboembolic risk, most likely as a result of endothelial damage, reduced concentrations of circulating plasma protein C and S, and release of inflammatory cytokines. Radiotherapy has inflammatory effects on the vasculature with endothelial disruption, cytokine release, and increased platelet aggregation.

Patients at increased risk of venous thromboembolism (VTE) should receive dual mechanical prophylaxis to their lower limbs and chemoprophylaxis with either low-molecular-weight heparin or unfractionated heparin. The use of mechanical prophylaxis, specifically pneumatic compression devices, has been shown to decrease the rate of VTE when compared with no prophylaxis within the first 5 postoperative days.[22,23] Prophylaxis should be initiated preoperatively and continued postoperatively. Extended chemoprophylaxis (28 days postoperative) should be prescribed to patients who meet high-risk criteria, including patients with advanced ovarian cancer. Prophylactic anticoagulation has not been shown to increase the risk of intraoperative bleeding, thrombocytopenia, or epidural hematoma; therefore epidural catheter placement and removal should be timed according to the last dose.

Surgical Site Infection Prevention

Surgical site infection (SSI) adversely affects outcomes and is associated with increased morbidity and mortality among cancer patients. The rate for SSI following surgery for gynecologic malignancy has been estimated to be 10%–15%. Many institutions implement a "bundle" of interventions aimed at decreasing the rate of SSI, rather than a single intervention.[24] SSI prevention bundles include antimicrobial prophylaxis, skin preparation, avoiding hypothermia during surgery, avoiding surgical drains, and reducing perioperative hyperglycemia.[4]

Inadequate perioperative glucose control is associated with increased risk of developing SSIs in both diabetic and nondiabetic patients undergoing surgery, and current recommendations suggest that blood glucose levels should be maintained at <10 mmol/L regardless of diabetic status. Hypoglycemia must be avoided, as well as hyperglycemia, as both extremes have been associated with higher mortality risk.[25,26]

Evidence suggests that peritoneal and subcutaneous drains and nasogastric tubes should be removed as soon as possible because their routine use can increase the rate of postoperative complications.[27]

Showering before surgery with a chlorhexidine-based antimicrobial soap and a chlorhexidine-alcohol skin preparation in the operating room before surgery reduces skin SSI.[27]

Antimicrobial prophylaxis with the administration of a first-generation cephalosporin and metronidazole reduces SSI if the bowel is inadvertently opened during gynecologic surgery. It should be given 1 h before skin incision in order to obtain the highest drug levels. Intraoperative repeat dosing should be observed depending on surgical duration and blood loss.[28]

Preoperative recommendations are summarized in Table 27.2.

Intraoperative Considerations

The proximity of the gynecologic tumor to other abdominal structures, such as the kidneys or rectum, may require input from other surgical specialties. Neurovascular bundles and lymph nodes often adhere to the pelvic sidewall making dissection difficult.[29]

These procedures usually require general anesthesia in the lithotomy position for extended periods, with attendant risks of common peroneal nerve injury and compartment syndrome in the legs, or pressure injuries in the arms.

TABLE 27.2 Preoperative Recommendations

Preoperative
Patient education: anesthetic and surgical procedure related information.
Smoking: smoking cessation at least 4 weeks before the procedure.
Alcohol: alcohol cessation at least 4 weeks before the procedure.
Anemia: diagnose and treat before surgery if possible.
Preoperative bowel preparation: no longer recommended.
Fasting: light meal up to 6 h before surgery, carbohydrate load up to 2 h before induction.
Preanesthetic medication: routine administration of sedatives to reduce anxiety preoperatively should be avoided.
Venous thromboembolism prophylaxis: oral contraceptives should be suspended before surgery; use of stockings, pneumatic compression devices, low-molecular-weight heparin.
Surgical site infection reduction: antimicrobial prophylaxis (first-generation cephalosporin 1 h before surgery), skin preparation, prevention of hypothermia, avoidance of drains/tubes, control of perioperative hyperglycemia.

Careful positioning and padding of all vulnerable points are essential. Head down positioning may also result in facial or airway edema. Supine hypotensive syndrome and abdominal compartment syndrome have also been reported in association with sizeable tumours.[29]

Finally, surgical staging is required for most cancers intraoperatively because microscopic disease cannot always be determined only through radiologic investigations. Maximal surgical debulking may involve radical oophorectomy, bowel resection, splenectomy, diaphragmatic peritonectomy, omentectomy, and partial liver resection.[29]

As a general approach, intraoperative management should consider multimodal analgesia, use of regional anesthesia and nonsteroidal antiinflammatory drugs (NSAIDs), minimization of blood transfusions, and implementation of enhanced recovery protocols.

Minimally Invasive Surgery

The use of laparoscopy and, more recently, robotic surgery has led to substantial improvements in patient outcomes by decreasing intraoperative blood loss, length of stay, analgesic requirements, return of bowel function, length of hospitalization, and return to normal daily activities.[30]

Older age, blood loss, perioperative blood transfusion, and postoperative complications have been associated with prolonged length of stay after laparoscopic gynecologic surgery. Oncologic outcomes have been found to be equivalent in women undergoing minimally invasive surgery and open procedures for endometrial cancer, but not for early-stage cervical cancer.[30]

Given the improvements in surgical recovery in patients undergoing minimally invasive surgery procedures compared with open surgery, minimally invasive surgery is recommended for suitable patients when long-term oncologic outcomes are similar, and where expertise and resources are available. All laparoscopic procedures carry a possible need for conversion to an open procedure, which should be anticipated at 5%–10% risk.[30]

Anesthetic Technique

Multimodal analgesia is recommended. A number of intravenous anesthetic agents may be used in combination with propofol to provide an effective total intravenous anesthesia regimen (TIVA). In addition to its direct sedative-analgesic properties, dexmedetomidine also reduces opioid requirements and minimum alveolar concentration levels for inhalational anesthetics.[29] Ketamine has benefits in reducing chronic postoperative pain, although the optimum treatment duration and dose are yet to be identified.[30]

Intravenous lidocaine infusion in the perioperative period decreases intraoperative anesthetic requirements, lowers pain scores, reduces postoperative analgesic requirements, and improves return of bowel function with decreased length of hospital stay.[31] There is also evidence that ketamine, lidocaine, propofol, and avoidance of inhalational anesthetic agents may lead to a reduction in cancer recurrence.

Regional anesthetic techniques can be a major component of reducing the stress response and diminishing opioid consumption. Some studies have proposed that regional anesthesia could impact on clinical outcomes such as overall survival and recurrence-free survival; however, recent evidence has demonstrated that use of regional anesthesia or analgesia did not reduce breast cancer recurrence after potentially curative surgery compared with volatile anesthesia and opioids. The frequency and severity of persistent incisional breast pain were unaffected by anesthetic technique.[32] Multimodal nonopioid analgesia use decreases postoperative nausea and vomiting (PONV) and allows more rapid recovery.[33]

Fluid Management

Maintaining proper fluid management in the postoperative period and avoiding fluid overload are just as important as in the preoperative period. The aim of intravenous fluid therapy is to maintain normovolemia and reduce flux across

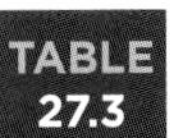

Intraoperative Recommendations

Intraoperative
Minimally invasive surgery: recommended for appropriate patients if feasible.
Anesthetic protocol: use of short-acting agents, use of BIS and combination with regional anesthesia/analgesia if feasible, monitoring of neuromuscular block.
Ventilation: protective strategy, tidal volume 5–7 mL/kg of predicted body weight and positive end expiratory pressure 6–8 cmH_2O.
Venous thromboembolism prophylaxis: stockings, pneumatic compression devices.
Nausea and vomiting prevention: multimodal approach according to risk factors, dexamethasone, 5HT3 antagonists, NK-1 antagonists.
Drains and tubes: routine use should be avoided; if placed, should be removed as soon as possible after surgery.
Hypothermia prevention: forced air mattress and fluid warmer, together with continuous temperature monitoring should be used in every case.
Fluid management: goal-directed fluid therapy in major abdominal surgery in patients with high comorbidities or high blood loss surgery.
Opioid sparing strategy: combination of acetaminophen and nonsteroidal antiinflammatory drugs, incisional bupivacaine infiltration, intravenous lidocaine, patient-controlled analgesia.

the extracellular space. Enhanced recovery protocols and modern surgical techniques reduce the need for both total volume and duration of intravenous fluid therapy.[34] While salt and fluid overload in the postoperative period is a major cause of morbidity, very restrictive fluid regimes also lead to increased morbidity and mortality.[35]

Most important is the prevention of unwanted complications related to fluid overload and excessive intravenous hydration, ranging from improved pulmonary function, tissue oxygenation, gastrointestinal motility, and wound healing.[36–38]

Postoperative hydration provides an improved method of fluid delivery, and it is recommended that patients receive 25–35 mL/kg water per day in the recovery period. Early transition to oral hydration postoperatively improves conditions for healing and recovery from surgery, allowing for an improved patient experience and earlier discharge without an increase in morbidity.[39,40]

Goal-Directed Fluid Therapy

Goal-directed fluid therapy (GDT) has been associated with improvements in short- and long-term outcomes. GDT extrapolates a patient's fluid responsiveness from measurable hemodynamic changes. Fluid responders will demonstrate an increase in stroke volume (SV) by ≥10%–15% after a fluid challenge. However, larger clinical studies have not demonstrated a benefit of GDT over zero balance or moderately positive fluid balance.[41]

Nausea and Vomiting Prevention

A multimodal approach to Postoperative Nausea and Vomiting (PONV) prevention is quickly becoming standard of care. Antiemetics are classified into the following categories: 5HT3 antagonists, NK-1 antagonists, corticosteroids, butyrophenones, antihistamines, anticholinergics, and phenothiazines.[41] Combinations of two or more classes of antiemetics may enhance potency (e.g., aprepitant, ondansetron, midazolam, or haloperidol combined with dexamethasone).[42,43]

Drains and Tubes

It has been suggested that nasogastric intubation increases the risk of postoperative pneumonia (6% vs. 3%) after elective abdominal surgery, while nasogastric decompression does not reduce the risk of wound dehiscence.[44] Only 10% of the early feeding arm required nasogastric tube insertion because of subocclusive symptoms. Conversely, 88% of patients who had a nasogastric tube experienced moderate-to-severe discomfort. One exception where gastric decompression may be of benefit is during laparoscopic or robotic surgery, whereby decompression may be used to reduce the risk of gastric perforation by trochar or Veress needle insertion.[4]

Hypothermia Prevention

Inadvertent perioperative hypothermia during prolonged surgery has been shown to impair drug metabolism, adversely affect coagulation, and increase bleeding, cardiac morbidity, and wound infection. Temperature monitoring should always be used. Forced convective air warming devices are the most effective intervention to prevent this.[45] Underbody warming mattresses are also effective particularly in robotic surgery.[46] Intravenous fluids should be warmed.[47] Patients who have prolonged surgery with a likelihood of a systemic inflammatory response (SIRS), such as open debulking procedures, could possibly extend to hyperpyrexia as surgery progresses if warming is not monitored.[47]

Intraoperative recommendations are summarized in Table 27.3.

TABLE 27.4 **Postoperative Recommendations**

Postoperative
Venous thromboembolism prophylaxis: extend prophylaxis up to 28 PO days, preferably LMWH, except if minimally invasive with low risk.
Fluid management: 1–2 mL/kg balanced crystalloids IV, 25–35 mL/kg oral, start oral intake before 24 h if indicated.
Nutrition: early oral intake, up to 2.0 g protein/kg/day and 25–30 kcal/kg/day.
Ileus prevention: drinking coffee, euvolemia, opioid-sparing analgesia, and early feeding.
Glucose control: glucose levels should be maintained at less than 200 mg/dL in diabetics and nondiabetics.
Postoperative analgesia: multimodal approach is recommended, NSAID, acetaminophen, gabapentin, wound infiltration and regional anesthesia if possible, avoid high opioid dosing.
Urinary catheter: should be removed within 24 h if possible.
Early mobilization: recommended within 24 h after surgery, adequate analgesia should be achieved, falling risk exists thus special attention is required.

LMWH, Low-molecular-weight heparin; *NSAID*, nonsteroidal antiinflammatory drug.

Postoperative Considerations

Venous Thromboembolism Prophylaxis

VTE is a major risk in gynecologic oncology patients with rates up to 3%–4% in cervical cancer, 4%–9% in endometrial cancer, and 17%–38% in ovarian cancer. The risk of VTE extends beyond the traditional 30-day postoperative complication window in these patients[48,49] and is inherently present among those undergoing neoadjuvant chemotherapy for ovarian cancer.[49] Low-molecular-weight heparin has been shown in two randomized, placebo controlled trials in solid tumors to reduce VTE during chemotherapy by 50%.[50,51]

Women undergoing gynecologic cancer surgery meet the high-risk American College of Chest Physicians (ACCP) criteria, and National Comprehensive Cancer Network guidelines[48,49] recommend extended, 28-day chemoprophylaxis. While the role of extended prophylaxis in minimally invasive gynecologic surgery remains the subject of debate, VTE rates are 0.5% or less and do not appear to be modulated based on whether or not prophylaxis was given.[52] However, current evidence suggests that use of minimally invasive surgery without extended prophylaxis provides improved patient experience and earlier discharge, without an increase in morbidity.[39,40]

Postoperative Nutrition

The main goals of perioperative nutritional support are to minimize negative protein balance by avoiding starvation, with the purpose of maintaining muscle, immune, and cognitive function, and to enhance postoperative recovery.[53] The small bowel recovers normal function 4–8 h after laparotomy; early enteral feeding after abdominal surgery is tolerated, and the feed is well absorbed.[53]

Some degree of insulin resistance develops after all kinds of surgery, but its severity is related to the magnitude of the surgery and development of complications.

Early normal food, including clear liquids on the first or second postoperative day, does not cause impairment of healing of anastomoses and leads to significantly shortened hospital length of stay, compared with delayed postoperative feeding practices.[54] The energy and protein requirements can be estimated using 25–30 kcal/kg and 1.5 g/kg ideal body weight, respectively.[53] If the energy and nutrient requirements cannot be met by oral and enteral intake alone (<50% of caloric requirement) for more than 7 days, a combination of enteral and parenteral nutrition is recommended.[55]

Postoperative Ileus Prevention

Factors that influence the return of bowel function include, but are not limited to, exposure to opioids, fluid balance, extent of peritoneal disease and complexity of surgery, receipt of transfusion, and postoperative abdominopelvic complications.[56]

Intravenous infusion of lidocaine reduces ileus by reducing pain and therefore sympathetic stimulation. Some Enhanced Recovery After Surgery (ERAS) protocols have recently introduced intravenous lidocaine as a therapeutic measure.[56,57]

NSAIDs act on phase 2 of ileus and are intended to reduce postoperative inflammation by their action on cyclooxygenase (COX)2 (and COX1 for nonspecific NSAIDs), having a promising theoretical mode of action on the pathophysiology of postoperative ileus.[58] This should be balanced against the risk of NSAID-induced acute kidney injury and gastritis.

Intravenous magnesium was studied in a randomized controlled trial that demonstrated a decrease in the interval to return of bowel function without any side effects. Magnesium sulfate was administered as a bolus of 40 mg/kg, followed by an infusion of 10 mg/kg during the operative period.[59] The main mechanism of postoperative ileus is the inflammatory response to bowel manipulation. The clinical literature also reports improvement in gastrointestinal motility related to the use of the laparoscopic approach.[60] Mastication of chewing gum mimics dietary intake. Chewing stimulates vagal tone, which has an antiinflammatory effect (phase 3 of ileus). The use of chewing gum has been discussed in the literature with regard to all surgical specialties.[61] Early feeding decreases the risk of infectious complications, protein wasting, and leaky intestinal mucosa.[62] It also reduces the need for IV hydration and potential electrolyte imbalance.[63] Reducing the volume of IV fluids reduces the incidence of postoperative ileus (POI).[63]

Postoperative Pain Management

For open procedures, a combined multimodal systemic and regional analgesia regimen is recommended. Gabapentin and NSAIDs may improve pain scores while sparing opioid consumption, particularly if administered with oral acetaminophen.[64]

Strong opioids are the cornerstone of acute pain management. Experimental data suggest that opioid use is associated with adverse oncologic outcome, but the evidence remains equivocal in clinical studies. Opioids should continue to be given postoperatively for gynecologic cancer patients where needed for pain relief.[64]

Particular Considerations

The most extensive procedures performed in gynecologic oncology surgery are pelvic exenteration and hyperthermic intraperitoneal chemotherapy.

Relevant fluid, blood, and protein losses, increased intraabdominal pressure, systemic hypo- or hyperthermia, and increased metabolic rate should be expected and treated in patients undergoing these procedures.[65]

Postoperative recommendations are summarized in Table 27.4.

Conclusion

Perioperative management in patients presenting gynecologic cancers requires a multidisciplinary approach to preoperative evaluation. Many of these patients require complex, prolonged surgery, and are at high risk of postoperative complications. Competent perioperative care can reduce this risk and promote early postoperative recovery. Ongoing observational research will determine whether optimizing short-term postoperative outcomes can improve longer-term oncologic sequelae.

References

1. Siegel RL, Miller KD, Jemal A. Cancer statistics, 2019. *CA Cancer J Clin.* 2019;69:7–34. doi:10.3322/caac.21551.
2. Sekandarzad MW, van Zundert AAJ, Lirk PB, Doonerbal CW, Hollmann MW. Perioperative anesthesia care and tumor progression. *Anesth Analg.* 2017;124:1697–1708.
3. Cata JP. Can the perioperative anesthesia care of patients with cancer affect their long-term oncological outcomes? *Anesth Analg.* 2017;125(5):1383–1384.
4. Nelson G, Bakkum-Gamez J, Kalogera E, et al. Guidelines for perioperative care in gynecologic/oncology: Enhanced Recovery After Surgery (ERAS) Society recommendations—2019 update. *Int J Gynecol Cancer.* 2019;29(4):651–658. doi:10.1136/ijgc-2019-000356.
5. American Cancer Society. *Cancer Facts & Figures 2019*: American Cancer Society; 2019.
6. Bristow RE, Tomacruz RS, Armstrong DK, Trimble EL, Montz FJ. Survival effect of maximal cytoreductive surgery for advanced ovarian carcinoma during the platinum era: a meta-analysis. *J Clin Oncol.* 2002;20:1248–1259.
7. Fader AN, Rose PG. Role of surgery in ovarian carcinoma. *J Clin Oncol.* 2007;25:2873–2883.
8. Cannistra SA. Cancer of the ovary. *N Engl J Med.* 2004;351: 2519–2529.
9. Yap OW, Husain A, Kapp DS, Teng NN, Carroll I, Rosenthal MH. Gynecologic oncology. In: Jaffe RA, Samuels S, eds. *Anesthesiologists' Manual of Surgical Procedures.* 3rd ed.: Lippincott Williams & Wilkins; 2004:591–629. 3rd ed.
10. Amant F, Moerman P, Neven P, Timmerman D, Van Limbergen E, Vergote I. Treatment modalities in endometrial cancer. *Curr Opin Oncol.* 2007;19:479–485.
11. Moore J, McLeod A. Anaesthesia for gynaecological oncology surgery. *Curr Anaesth Crit Care.* 2009;20:8–12.
12. Sahai SK. Perioperative assessment of the cancer patient. *Best Pract Res Clin Anaesthesiol.* 2013;27(4):465–480.
13. Grigorian A, O'Brien CB. Hepatotoxicity secondary to chemotherapy. *J Clin Transl Hepatol.* 2014;2:95–102.
14. Perazella MA. Onco-nephrology: renal toxicities of chemotherapeutic agents. *Colin J Am Soc Nephrol.* 2012;7:1713–1721.
15. Waller A, Forshaw K, Bryant J, et al. Preparatory education for cancer patients undergoing surgery: a systematic review of volume and quality of research output over time. *Patient Educ Couns.* 2015; 98:1540–1549 doi:10.1016/j.pec.2015.05.008.
16. Powell R, Scott NW, Manyande A, et al. Psychological preparation and postoperative outcomes for adults undergoing surgery under general anaesthesia. *Cochrane Database Syst Rev.* 2016;5; 18–28.
17. Wang F, Li C-B, Li S, et al. Integrated interventions for improving negative emotions and stress reactions of young women receiving total hysterectomy. *Int J Clin Exp Med.* 2014;7:331–336.
18. De Ruysscher D, Niedermann G, Burnet NG, Siva S, Lee AWM, Hegi-Johnson F. Radiotherapy toxicity. *Nat Rev Dis Prim.* 2019;5:13. doi:10.1038/s41572-019-0064-5.
19. Carli F, Silver JK, Feldman LS, et al. Surgical prehabilitation in patients with cancer: state-of-the-science and recommendations for future research from a panel of subject matter experts. *Phys Med Rehabil Clin N Am.* 2017;28:49–64:26–28
20. Brady M, Kinn S, Stuart P. Preoperative fasting for adults to prevent perioperative complications. *Cochrane Database Syst Rev.* 2003;4:26–28.
21. Nygren J, Thorell A, Ljungqvist O. Preoperative oral carbohydrate therapy. *Curr Opin Anaesthesiol.* 2015;28:364–369.
22. Horlocker TT, Wedel DJ, Rowlingson JC, et al. Regional anesthesia in the patient receiving antithrombotic or thrombolytic therapy: American Society of Regional Anesthesia and Pain Medicine evidence-based guidelines (third edition). *Reg Anesth Pain Med.* 2010;35:64–101.

23. Gogarten W, Vandermeulen E, Van Aken H, et al. Regional anaesthesia and antithrombotic agents: recommendations of the European Society of Anaesthesiology. *Eur J Anaesthesiol.* 2010;27:999–1015.
24. Tran CW, McGree ME, Weaver AL, et al. Surgical site infection after primary surgery for epithelial ovarian cancer: predictors and impact on survival. *Gynecol Oncol.* 2015;136(2):278–284.
25. Van den Berghe G, Wouters P, Weekers F, et al. Intensive insulin therapy in critically ill patients. *N Engl J Med Overseas Ed.* 2001;345:1359–1367.
26. van den Boom W, Schroeder RA, Manning MW, et al. Effect of A1C and glucose on postoperative mortality in noncardiac and cardiac surgeries. *Diabetes Care.* 2018;41:782–788.
27. Novetsky AP, Zighelboim I, Guntupalli SR, et al. A phase II trial of a surgical protocol to decrease the incidence of wound complications in obese gynecologic oncology patients. *Gynecol Oncol.* 2014;134:233–237.
28. Berríos-Torres SI, Umscheid CA, Bratzler DW, et al. Centers for Disease Control and Prevention guideline for the prevention of surgical site infection. *JAMA Surg.* 2017;152:784–791.
29. Blaudszun G, Lysakowski C, Elia N, et al. Effect of perioperative systemic α2 agonists on postoperative morphine consumption and pain intensity: systematic review and meta-analysis of randomized controlled trials. *Anesthesiology.* 2012;116:1312–1322.
30. Elia N, Tramèr MR. Ketamine and postoperative pain–a quantitative systematic review of randomised trials. *Pain.* 2005; 113:61–70.
31. Weibel S, Jelting Y, Pace NL, et al. Continuous intravenous perioperative lidocaine infusion for postoperative pain and recovery in adults. *Cochrane Database Syst Rev.* 2018;6:23–34
32. Sessler DI, Pei L, Huang Y, et al. Recurrence of breast cancer after regional or general anaesthesia: a randomised controlled trial. *Lancet.* 2019;394:1807–1815. doi:10.1016/S01406736(19)32313X.
33. Carey ET, Moulder JK. Perioperative management and implementation of enhanced recovery programs in gynecologic surgery for benign indications. *Obstet Gynecol.* 2018;132:137–146.
34. Raghunathan K, Singh M, Lobo DN. Fluid management in abdominal surgery: what, when, and when not to administer. *Anesthesiol Clin.* 2015;33(1):51–64.
35. Lobo DN, Bostock KA, Neal KR, Perkins AC, Rowlands BJ, Allison SP. Effect of salt and water balance on recovery of gastrointestinal function after elective colonic resection: a randomised controlled trial. *Lancet.* 2002;359(9320):1812–1818.
36. Christopherson R, Beattie C, Frank SM, et al. Perioperative morbidity in patients randomized to epidural or general anesthesia for lower extremity vascular surgery. Perioperative Ischemia Randomized Anesthesia Trial Study Group. *Anesthesiology.* 1993;79(3):422–434.
37. Hartmann M, Jonsson K, Zederfeldt B. Effect of tissue perfusion and oxygenation on accumulation of collagen in healing wounds. Randomized study in patients after major abdominal operations. *Eur J Surg.* 1992;158:521e6.
38. Jonsson K, Jensen JA, Goodson WH, et al. Tissue oxygenation, anemia, and perfusion in relation to wound healing in surgical patients. *Ann Surg.* 1991;214:605e13.
39. Miller TE, Roche AM, Mythen M. Fluid management and goal-directed therapy as an adjunct to Enhanced Recovery after Surgery (ERAS). *Can J Anaesth.* 2015;62:158e68.
40. Miller TE, Thacker JK, White WD, et al. Reduced length of hospital stay in colorectal surgery after implementation of an enhanced recovery protocol. *Anesth Analg.* 2014;118:1052e61.
41. Kendrick JB, Kaye AD, Tong Y, et al. Goal-directed fluid therapy in the perioperative setting. *J Anaesthesiol Clin Pharmacol.* 2019;35(Suppl 1):S29–S34. doi:10.4103/joacp.JOACP_26_18.
42. Pan PH, Lee SC, Harris LC. Antiemetic prophylaxis for postdischarge nausea and vomiting and impact on functional quality of living during recovery in patients with high emetic risks: a prospective, randomized, double-blind comparison of two prophylactic antiemetic regimens. *Anesth Analg.* 2008;107:429–438.
43. Gan TJ, Meyer TA, Apfel CC, et al. Society for Ambulatory Anesthesia guidelines for the management of postoperative nausea and vomiting. *Anesth Analg.* 2007;105:1615–1628.
44. Cheatham ML, Chapman WC, Key SP, Sawyers JL. A meta-analysis of selective versus routine nasogastric decompression after elective laparotomy. *Ann Surg.* 1995;221(5):469–476, discussion 476–478.
45. Galvão CM, Liang Y, Clark AM. Effectiveness of cutaneous warming systems on temperature control: meta analysis. *J Adv Nurs.* 2010;66(6):1196–1206.
46. Perez-Protto S, Sessler DI, Reynolds LF, et al. Circulating-water garment or the combination of a circulating-water mattress and forced-air cover to maintain core temperature during major upper-abdominal surgery. *Br J Anaesth.* 2010;5(4):466–470.
47. Campbell G, Alderson P, Smith AF, Warttig S. Warming of intravenous and irrigation fluids for preventing inadvertent perioperative hypothermia. *Cochrane Database Syst Rev.* 2015;(4):CD009891. doi:10.1002/14651858.CD009891.pub2.
48. Schmeler KM, Wilson GL, Cain K, et al. Venous thromboembolism (VTE) rates following the implementation of extended duration prophylaxis for patients undergoing surgery for gynecologic malignancies. *Gynecol Oncol.* 2013;128:204–208.
49. Greco PS, Bazzi AA, McLean K, et al. Incidence and timing of thromboembolic events in patients with ovarian cancer undergoing neoadjuvant chemotherapy. *Obstet Gynecol.* 2017; 129:979–985.
50. Agnelli G, Gussoni G, Bianchini C, et al. Nadroparin for the prevention of thromboembolic events in ambulatory patients with metastatic or locally advanced solid cancer receiving chemotherapy: a randomised, placebo-controlled, double-blind study. *Lancet Oncol.* 2009;10:943–949.
51. Agnelli G, George DJ, Kakkar AK, et al. Semuloparin for thromboprophylaxis in patients receiving chemotherapy for cancer. *N Engl J Med.* 2012;366:601–609.
52. Bouchard-Fortier G, Geerts WH, Covens A, et al. Is venous thromboprophylaxis necessary in patients undergoing minimally invasive surgery for a gynecologic malignancy? *Gynecol Oncol.* 2014;134:228–322.
53. Varadhan KK, Lobo DN. A meta-analysis of randomised controlled trials of intravenous fluid therapy in major elective open abdominal surgery: getting the balance right. *Proc Nutr Soc.* 2010;69:488e98.
54. Osland E, Yunus RM, Khan S, Memon MA. Early versus traditional postoperative feeding in patients undergoing resectional gastrointestinal surgery: a meta-analysis. *J Parenter Enteral Nutr.* 2011;35:473e87.
55. McClave SA, Taylor BE, Martindale RG, et al. A.S.P.E.N. Board of Directors, American College of Critical Care Medicine, Society of Critical Care Medicine. Guidelines for the provision and assessment of nutrition support therapy in the adult critically ill patient: Society of Critical Care Medicine (SCCM) and American Society for Parenteral and Enteral Nutrition (A.S.P.E.N.). *J Parenter Enteral Nutr.* 2016;40:159e211.

56. Vigneault L, Turgeon AF, Côté D, et al. Perioperative intra-venous lidocaine infusion for postoperative pain control: a meta-analysis of randomized controlled trials. *Can J Anaesth*. 2011;58:22–37.
57. Kranke P, Jokinen J, Pace NL, et al. Continuous intravenous perioperative lidocaine infusion for postoperative pain and recovery. *Cochrane Database Syst Rev*. 2015;7:CD009642.
58. Schlachta CM, Burpee SE, Fernandez C, et al. Optimizing recovery after laparoscopic colon surgery (ORAL-CS): effect of intravenous ketorolac on length of hospital stay. *Surg Endosc*. 2007;21:2212–2219.
59. Shariat Moharari R, Motalebi M, Najafi A, et al. Magnesium can decrease postoperative physiological ileus and post- operative pain in major non laparoscopic gastrointestinal surgeries: a randomized controlled trial. *Anesthesiol Pain Med*. 2014;4:e12750.
60. Pitiakoudis M, Fotakis SN, Zezos P, et al. Alterations in colonic transit time after laparoscopic versus open cholecystectomy: a clinical study. *Tech Coloproctol*. 2011;15(Suppl 1):S37–S41.
61. Su'a BU, Pollock TT, Lemanu DP, et al. Chewing gum and post-operative ileus in adults: a systematic literature review and meta-analysis. *Int J Surg*. 2015;14:49–55.
62. Bragg D, El-Sharkawy AM, Psaltis E, et al. Postoperative ileus: recent developments in pathophysiology and management. *Clin Nutr*. 2015;34:367–376.
63. Thacker JKM, Mountford WK, Ernst FR, et al. Perioperative fluid utilization variability and association with outcomes: considerations for enhanced recovery efforts in sample US surgical populations. *Ann Surg*. 2016;263:502–510.
64. Pérez-González O, Cuéllar-Guzmán LF, Soliz J, Cata JP. Impact of regional anesthesia on recurrence, metastasis, and immune response in breast cancer surgery: a systematic review of the literature. *Reg Anesth Pain Med*. 2017;42:751.
65. Raspé C, Flöther L, Schneider R, Bucher M, Piso P. Best practice for perioperative management of patients with cytoreductive surgery and HIPEC. *Eur J Surg Oncol*. 2017;43(6):1013–1027.

28

Anesthesiology and Perioperative Management of Patients Presenting for Surgical Excision of Endocrine Tumors

MEGHAN CARTON AND DONAL J. BUGGY

General Introduction

Surgical excision of endocrine tumors ranges from relatively common thyroid cancer surgery to rare conditions such as removal of pheochromocytoma and hypophysectomy for pituitary adenoma.

A comprehensive evaluation of the perioperative management of all endocrine tumors is beyond the scope of this chapter. Therefore this chapter focuses on the perioperative management of the following endocrine tumors:

- Thyroid tumors
- Pheochromocytoma
- Cushing's disease
- Carcinoid syndrome
- Hypophysectomy for pituitary adenomas

Perioperative Management of Thyroid Tumor Resection

Epidemiology

Thyroid cancer is now the most common endocrine malignancy worldwide. The incidence increased from 1.5 cases per 100,000 in 1953 to 7.5 cases per 100,000 in 2002.[1] Developments in diagnostic capabilities, including neck ultrasonography, fine needle aspiration, computed tomography, and magnetic resonance imaging, may have contributed to this apparent increase in the diagnosis of thyroid cancer.[1] Ninety percent of all thyroid tumors are indolent, with the estimated mortality rate at just 0.6 deaths per 100,000 person years.[2] Benign thyroid disease requires treatment only in the presence of dysfunction or local compressive symptoms.[3]

Preoperative Management

A comprehensive history and examination should assess for signs of severe hypothyroidism hyperthyroidism, or complications of thyroid disease, as outlined in Table 28.1.

Enlarged thyroid glands or goiters as seen in Fig. 28.1 can lead to tracheal compression and difficult airway management. Airway assessment should include thyromental distance, assessment of neck movement, and visualization of pharyngeal structures.

Investigations recommended prior to thyroid surgery are outlined in Table 28.2.

Interpretation of the Thyroid Function Test

Euthyroid Sick Syndrome

Significant physiological stress, such as critical illness, starvation, or surgery, results in hypothalamic adjustment of thyroid homeostasis.

Thyroid function tests reveal a decreased triiodothyronine (T3) level occasionally accompanied by a fall in circulating thyroxine (T4); however, thyroid stimulating hormone (TSH) levels remain within normal limits. Of note, patients remain clinically euthyroid throughout. As this is an adaptive response to physiological stress, no treatment is needed.

Clinical judgment is thus required in the interpretation of abnormal thyroid results in patients with a significant acute or chronic illness.

TABLE 28.1 Signs and Symptoms of Thyroid Disease

Pathology	Signs and Symptoms
Hypothyroidism	Low respiratory rate, hypothermia Weight gain, atrial fibrillation, myxedematous facies, delayed reflexes
Hyperthyroidism	Hyperthermia, atrial fibrillation, tachyarrhythmias, sweating, anxiety, weight loss, diarrhea
Large Goiter (may be hypo- or hyper thyroid)	Positional dyspnea or dysphagia, neck swelling

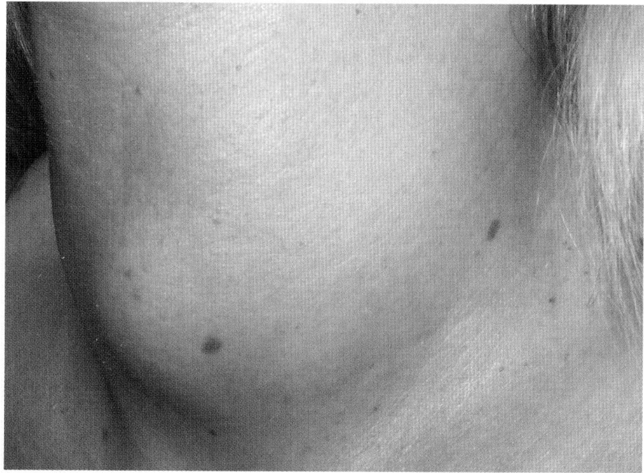

• **Fig. 28.1** A goiter.

Corticosteroids

High doses of glucocorticoids inhibit the deiodination of T4 to T3, resulting in a decrease in circulating T3 levels. Corticosteroids also act on the hypothalamic-hypophyseal-thyroid axis by suppressing the pituitary's production of TSH.

These interactions result in abnormal thyroid function tests and the administration of high-dose or long-term exogenous glucocorticoids. Such changes rarely reach clinical significance, with patients for the most part remaining euthyroid throughout their treatment course.

Intraoperative Management

Thyroid surgery is almost always performed under general anesthesia with tracheal intubation. General anesthesia may be induced in a standard manner. Awake fiberoptic intubation should be considered with a large goiter if it is causing tracheal compression, or in a retrosternal goiter with compressive symptoms, or vocal cord dysfunction.

Regarding the endotracheal tube itself, as the surgical field is focused on the head and neck, a simple endotracheal tube could potentially be at risk of kinking under the pressure of surgical handling in the upper neck. For this reason, some anesthesiologists prefer to use a wire-reinforced endotracheal tube, but there is no evidence that this affects patient outcomes.[4]

TABLE 28.2 Investigations Recommended Prior to Thyroid Surgery and Their Indications

Investigation	Indication
Full blood count	Antithyroid medications can cause agranulocytosis and aplastic anemia. Hypothyroidism may be associated with anemia of chronic disease
Urea and electrolytes	Hyperthyroidism can lead to diarrhea that can result in electrolyte abnormalities
Liver function tests	Antithyroid medications can cause hepatitis
Thyroid function test	Hypothyroidism: high TSH, low T4 Hyperthyroidism: low TSH, high T4
Chest x-ray	Assessing for tracheal compression or deviation
CT scan	Assessing for a retrosternal goiter and tracheal compresssion
Laryngoscopy	Assessing for vocal cord dysfunction

T4, Thyroxine; *TSH*, thyroid stimulating hormone.

A study of over 3000 thyroidectomies found that difficult intubation occurred in 6% of cases.[5] Patients undergoing thyroid surgery are at risk of injury to the recurrent laryngeal nerve.

Short acting muscle relaxants can be used to facilitate tracheal intubation and allow for recurrent laryngeal nerve monitoring during the surgery.[6]

Patients are positioned for surgery in neck extension with a head-up table tilt of 25% to reduce blood loss. As visualizing the patient's face is often not possible intraoperatively, careful attention must be paid to securing the endotracheal tube and protecting the eyes.

Intraoperative monitoring of blood loss is required, via regular assessment of estimated blood loss and weighted swabs, especially in patients with large goiters.

Surgical technique involves raising of skin flaps, muscle retraction, superior pedicle mobilization, ligation and dissection of vessels, and hemostasis and wound closure.

Complications include the following.

Recurrent Laryngeal Nerve Damage

This can occur via ischemia, contusion, or inadvertent dissection. Incidence of recurrent laryngeal nerve (RLN) damage and vocal cord dysfunction ranges from 0% to 7.2% of all patients undergoing thyroidectomies. There is a higher incidence of RLN injury during repeat surgery for recurrent goiter or surgery for thyroid malignancy.[7] Signs of vocal cord dysfunction, including stridor, dyspnea, and hoarseness, should be monitored in the postoperative period.[8] Intraoperative electromyography can be used to protect the RLN from inadvertent surgical injury, whereby intramuscular vocal cord electrodes are placed into the laryngeal muscles and connected to the neuromonitoring device, which emits sound and displays graphics, so the surgical team remain aware of their proximity to the RLN.

Postoperatively vocal cords may be visualized directly using laryngoscopy. Visualization of both vocal cords moving is reassuring that RLN function is preserved, but this can be difficult to achieve safely in the reemerging patient. Surgical experience remains the most effective prognostic indicator of preservation of RLN. A vocal cordectomy may be necessary if vocal cord dysfunction does not improve after 4–6 weeks.[9]

Cervical Hematoma

Signs include stridor (abnormal high-pitched breath sounds, especially on inspiration) occurring within 6 hours of tracheal extubation. Bleeding leads to compression of the trachea and potentially acute airway obstruction. Intraoperative Valsalva maneuvers can identify potential sites of early postoperative bleeding for the surgical team.[8] Management of a suspected postoperative hematoma involves reexploring the cervical incision with removal of the hematoma, local hemostasis, and surgical revision. In this circumstance, tracheal reintubation may be extremely difficult because of airway tissue edema from venous congestion.[9]

Hypocalcemia

Due to the small size of the parathyroid glands and firm adherence to the thyroid, patients undergoing thyroidectomy are at high risk of parathyroid gland disruption or removal, leading to postoperative hypocalcemia. Signs include numbness in the hands, feet and lips, muscle cramps, and rarely, seizures occurring within 36 hours postoperatively. Postoperative monitoring of serial calcium and parathyroid hormone levels is crucial. Reimplantation of at least one of the parathyroid glands intraoperatively, combined with supplemental calcium and vitamin D in the postoperative period, can reduce the risk of hypocalcemia.[9]

Postoperative Management

Measures should be undertaken to prevent straining on tracheal extubation where possible, because this can cause venous engorgement of airway tissues and hence airway edema. It can also rupture small blood vessels directly, leading to hematoma formation and airway compromise. Options to prevent this include tracheal extubation under deep anesthesia, topical use of lidocaine, and the use of an intravenous narcotic such as remifentanil.[8]

Pheochromocytoma

Epidemiology

A Danish population-based study found that the incidence of pheochromocytomas has doubled in the last two decades (0.2 per 100,000 person years to 0.4 per 100,000 person years). Similarly, a systematic review in the Netherlands found that the incidence rate increased from 0.29 to 0.46 per 100,000 over the same time period, while age at diagnosis increased.[10] These trends are likely related to improved diagnosis, including imaging studies and advances in biochemical testing, with up to 40% of all pheochromocytomas now diagnosed incidentally on imaging.[11,12]

TABLE 28.3 Diagnosis of Pheochromocytoma

Biochemical testing	Plasma free metanephrines 24-hour urinary fractionated metanephrines and catecholamines[15]
Imaging	High-resolution computed tomography to localize tumor

Approximately 40% of pheochromocytomas are hereditary and more likely to be bilateral and present at a younger age. The 5-year survival rate for localized and metastatic pheochromocytomas is 95% and 60%, respectively.[13] Biochemical diagnosis and precise tumor localization are required, and the definitive treatment is complete surgical excision (see Table 28.3).[14]

Preoperative Management

Pheochromocytomas cause symptoms in approximately 50% of patients. A comprehensive history and clinical exam should include the following[16]:

- Signs and symptoms of a pheochromocytoma
  - Episodic headaches
  - Diaphoresis
  - Abdominal pain
  - Vomiting or diarrhea
  - Weakness
  - Weight loss
- Cardiorespiratory signs of pheochromocytomas
  - Tachycardia
  - Dyspnea
  - Palpations
  - Hypertension
  - Orthostatic hypotension

Preoperative investigations and their clinical indications are included in Table 28.4.

Preoperative Medical Management

Alpha-adrenoceptor Blockade

Catecholamine excess leads to alpha-1 mediated vasoconstriction and hypertension. These effects must be negated with a nonselective, irreversible alpha receptor antagonist such as phenoxybenzamine. This therapy may lead to hypotension, therefore in-hospital monitoring for side effects, such as orthostatic hypotension, tachycardia, dizziness, headaches, and drowsiness, is indicated.[12,15]

Beta-adrenoceptor Blockade

Adrenergic beta-1 mediated tachycardia and ionotropy requires appropriate beta-receptor blockade with agents

TABLE 28.4 Pheochromocytoma and Preoperative Investigations and Their Clinical Indications

Investigations	Indication
Full blood count	To assess for anemia
Blood pressure	Hypertension is often encountered in this cohort
Blood glucose	Hyperglycemia is common due to excess catecholamines
Chest x-ray	To rule out pulmonary edema and cardiomegaly
Electrocardiogram	Left ventricular hypertrophy can occur due to prolonged hypertension
Echocardiography	Where clinical suspicion of cardiomyopathy is high

TABLE 28.5 Preoperative Hemodynamic and Hematological Goals of Pheochromocytoma Treatment

Vital Sign	Aim
Systolic blood pressure	<130 mmHg
Diastolic blood pressure	<80 mmHg
Mean arterial pressure	<100 mmHg
Heart rate	<80 bpm
Hematocrit	45

such as metoprolol or bisoprolol. This must only be initiated after establishing reliable alpha blockade. Alpha blockade causes vasodilation, which reduces arterial blood pressure, and so requires a degree of increased cardiac output in compensation. Introducing beta blockade before alpha blockade could inhibit compensatory cardiac output and lead to acute cardiac insufficiency, syncope, or pulmonary edema.[12]

Vascular Expansion

To counteract the vasodilation caused by alpha-1 blockade, intravenous crystalloids are to be administered until serum hematocrit has decreased by 5%–10%.[12,15]

In total, in-patient preoperative preparation may take up to 5–10 days.

Preoperative hemodynamic and hematological goals of pheochromocytoma treatment are outlined in Table 28.5.

Intraoperative Management

Endotracheal intubation is advised in all patients undergoing surgical removal of a pheochromocytoma because of the extent and duration of surgery and its intraabdominal location. Preoperative alpha and beta blockade regimens should be continued. Laparoscopic adrenalectomy is sufficient in up to 95% of patients; however, large (>6 cm) or invasive tumors may require open resection.[15,17] Where open surgical technique is utilized, epidural anesthesia attenuates intraoperative stress-mediated catecholamine surges and postoperatively reduces pain.[12]

Surgical Technique

Surgery comprises complete tumor resection and minimal tumor manipulation with appropriate control of vascular supply.[14]

Up to 50% of patients will become hemodynamically unstable with tumor manipulation; therefore invasive blood pressure monitoring is essential. Central venous access allows for the administration of rapid fluid resuscitation and vasoactive medication as required.[12]

Case reports describe the use of intraoperative transesophageal echocardiography to guide fluid management; however, level 1 evidence-based clinical trials have not shown any patient-centered benefit to intraoperative goal-directed fluid therapy.[18] In patients diagnosed with catecholamine-induced cardiomyopathy a pulmonary artery catheter may allow for closer monitoring of cardiac index.[12]

Common Intraoperative Issues

Hypertension

Noradrenaline (norepinephrine)-induced alpha-1 vasoconstriction can lead to hypertension intraoperatively. Short-acting potent vasodilators such as sodium nitroprusside and nitroglyceride (nitroglycerine) can be used to manage this effectively.[12]

Tachyarrhythmias

Catecholamine secretions can result in arrhythmias, which may be effectively managed with a short acting beta-blocker if supraventricular in origin or lidocaine if ventricular.[12,14]

Hypotension

Causes of intraoperative hypotension include a reduction in catecholamine levels, residual preoperative alpha blockade, blood loss, or myocardial dysfunction. Fluid replacement, blood products, or vasoactive medication may be required to stabilize the patient.[14]

Postoperative Management

Postoperatively patients require a high dependency bed to monitor blood pressure, heart rate, and blood glucose levels. Some of the common complications that may occur are outlined in Table 28.6.

Cushing's Syndrome

Introduction

The hypothalamus-pituitary-adrenal axis is a major neuroendocrine system, controlling the body's reactions to

TABLE 28.6 Common Postoperative Issues in Pheochromocytoma

Complication	Etiology and management
Hypotension	Caused by decreased catecholamine levels, residual preoperative alpha blockade, blood loss or myocardial dysfunction. Can occur in up to 70% of cases requiring fluid loading and vasopressors.[12]
Hypertension	Caused by residual metastatic disease, intraoperative damage to the renal artery or kidney, or acquired renovascular changes secondary to persistent preoperative hypertension.
Hypoglycemia	Sudden catecholamine withdrawal leads to rebound hyperinsulinemia that can cause hypoglycemia; hourly blood sugar monitoring for 12–24 hours postoperatively is required.
Recurrence	Plasma and urine metanephrines should be checked postoperatively to diagnose persistent disease, with lifelong biochemical testing to assess for disease reoccurrence.[15]

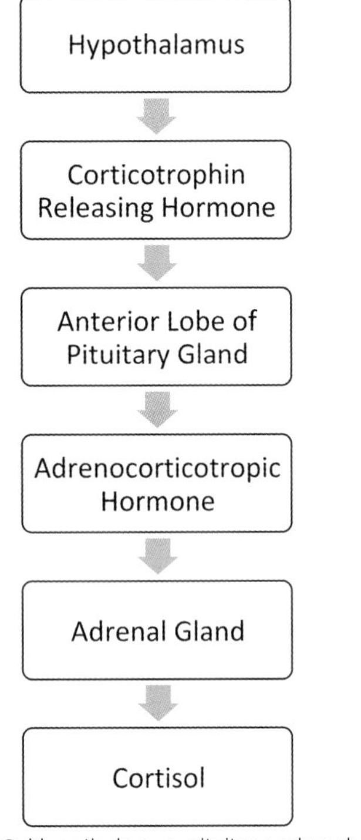

• **Fig. 28.2** Hypothalamus-pituitary-adrenal axis.

stress, digestion, the immune system, mood, and energy levels.[19] The hypothalamus releases corticotrophin-releasing hormone (CRH), which stimulates the anterior pituitary to release adrenocorticotropic hormone (ACTH), which causes the adrenal cortex to release cortisol. High levels of cortisol negatively feedback to both the hypothalamus and anterior pituitary leading to reduced adrenal production of cortisol (see Fig. 28.2). Cushing's disease is due to a pituitary adenoma producing excess ACTH, whereas Cushing's syndrome describes the clinical signs and symptoms of cortisol excess regardless of the cause.[20]

Cushing's syndrome can be ACTH-dependent, including

- Cushing's disease, which is caused by a pituitary adenoma, producing excess ACTH,
- Ectopic ACTH-secreting tumor.

Cushing's syndrome can be independent of ACTH, including

- Benign or malignant adrenal tumors producing cortisol independent of ACTH,
- Other adrenal causes.

This is summarized in Fig. 28.3.

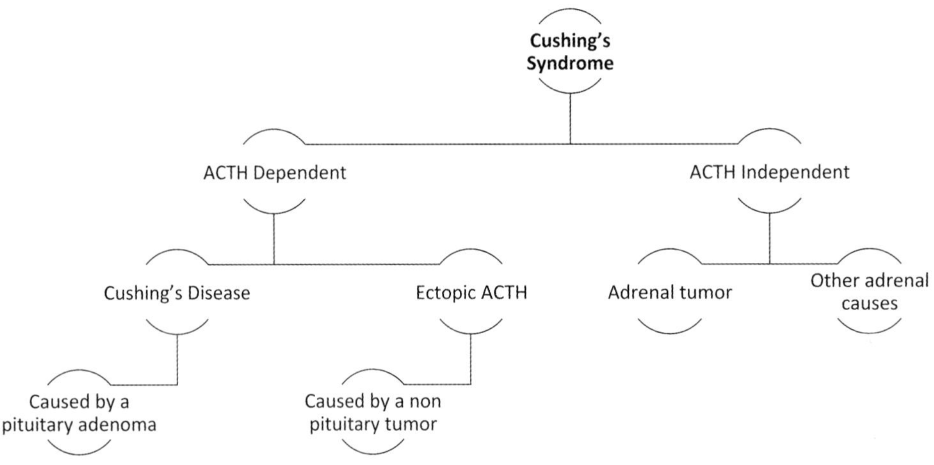

• **Fig. 28.3** Overview of Cushing's syndrome.

Epidemiology

The prevalence of Cushing's disease is 3.9 cases per 100,000 persons, with a yearly incidence estimated at 0.2 per 100,000 persons.[21,22] The mortality ratio (the ratio of observed deaths in the study population to expected deaths in the general population) of patients with Cushing's disease in the UK was found to be 4.8. Vascular disease, including coronary artery disease and stroke, is currently the leading cause of mortality in this patient cohort.[23]

Signs and symptoms of Cushing's disease

- Skin thinning
- Hypertension
- Osteoporosis
- Necrosis of femoral head
- Immunosuppression
- Amenorrhea
- Diabetes

Investigations required for the diagnosis of Cushing's syndrome are outlined as follows.

Twenty-four Hours Urinary Free Cortisol

- Greater than three times the upper limit of normal (which varies in different assays) is indicative of hypercortisolism.

Late-night Salivary Cortisol

- Elevated levels are indicative of hypercortisolism (assay specific norms vary).

Dexamethasone Suppression Test[24]

Low-Dose Dexamethasone Suppression Test

- Failure to suppress plasma cortisol levels is indicative of Cushing's syndrome.

High-Dose Dexamethasone Suppression Test

- Suppression of plasma cortisol levels is indicative of Cushing's disease.
- Failure to suppress plasma cortisol levels is indicative of an adrenal or ectopic etiology of Cushing's syndrome.

Preoperative Management

A full history and exam should be undertaken assessing for signs and symptoms of Cushing's syndrome, which include central obesity, moon facies, supra scapular fat pad, skin thinning, easy bruising, vertebral osteoporosis, myopathy, hypertension, and poor wound healing.[21] Evaluation of signs and symptoms specific to Cushing's disease includes bitemporal hemianopia (caused by the pituitary adenoma compressing the optic chiasm) and headaches.[21] A full list of preoperative investigations and their indications are outlined in Table 28.7.

Conditions commonly associated with Cushing's syndrome include polycystic ovary syndrome, type 2 diabetes mellitus, ischemic heart disease, obstructive sleep apnea, pulmonary hypertension, or any underlying autoimmune disorders requiring long-term glucocorticoid use.

Truncal obesity leads to reduced functional residual capacity and rapid desaturation during tracheal intubation. Adequate preoxygenation is essential and useful adjuncts such as the Oxford Ramp pillow and transnasal humidified rapid insufflation ventilatory exchange should also be considered if there is morbid obesity.[26]

Rapid sequence induction, video laryngoscopy, or awake fiber optic intubation should be considered to reduce the risk of pulmonary aspiration in obese patients. Patients undergoing transsphenoidal microadenomectomy will require a reinforced endotracheal tube.

Intraoperative Management

Angiotensin-converting enzyme inhibitors or angiotensin II receptor blockers should be omitted on the morning of

TABLE 28.7 Preoperative Investigations and their Indications for Cushing's Syndrome

Investigation	Indication
Full blood count	Steroid-induced leukocytosis.
Urea and electrolytes	Hypokalemia, a common consequence of hypercortisolism; this can be managed with preoperative spironolactone.[21]
Arterial blood gas	Metabolic alkalosis is commonly found, as excess corticosteroids have some mineralocorticoid effect leading to a metabolic alkalosis.
Blood glucose	Patients are frequently hyperglycemic due to the antiinsulin effect of corticosteroids. Variable rate insulin infusion is indicated in a type 2 diabetic patient missing more than one meal due to surgery.[25]
Electrocardiogram	Chronic hypertension can lead to left ventricular hypertrophy.
Transthoracic echocardiography	To assess for left ventricular hypertrophy as sleep apnea is associated with increased risk of pulmonary hypertension.

surgery because of increased risk of excessive hypotension due to interaction with vasodilatory general anesthetic agents.[21]

Invasive blood pressure monitoring is advised. Epidural analgesia reduces the requirements for systemic opioids in open procedures; however, most adrenalectomies are performed by laparoscopic technique or by robotic-assisted laparoscopic technique.[26] Short-acting opioids are advised to avoid postoperative respiratory depression. Chronic glucocorticoid exposure leads to immunosuppression and perioperative prophylactic antibiotics should be administered. Patients with Cushing's disease should have steroid supplementation intraoperatively and for up to 5 days postoperatively because of the endogenous steroid suppression induced by the disease process. Long-term steroid supplementation is required in any patient undergoing bilateral adrenalectomy. Consultation with an endocrinologist is essential.[27,28]

Fluid therapy should be guided by blood pressure and urine output, and possibly by goal-directed fluid therapy strategies, if available. Obesity is common in these patients and can lead to reduced chest wall compliance and functional residual capacity. Pneumoperitoneum during laparoscopic surgery can also reduce functional residual capacity, making ventilation more challenging in this patient cohort.

Surgical Technique

In Cushing's syndrome, if adrenal hyperplasia or tumors are found to be the causative pathology, these can be treated by laparoscopic adrenalectomy. In Cushing's disease, where an ACTH-secreting pituitary adenoma is identified as the pathology, the treatment of choice is transsphenoidal microadenomectomy.[21]

Postoperative Management

Potential complications include the following:

Venous Thromboembolism

This cohort is at increased risk due to obesity, hyperglycemia, and hypertension.

Respiratory Depression

Long-acting opioids causing respiratory depression should be used with caution in obese patients or used only in a high-dependency postoperative care environment.

Diabetes Insipidus

Diabetes insipidus can be caused by surgical manipulation of the posterior pituitary gland leading to a reduction or absence of endogenous vasopressin. Diabetes insipidus should be managed with exogenous vasopressin.

Hypoglycemia

Hypoglycemia may be caused by a reduction in circulating corticotrophin hormone. Routine glucose monitoring and adjustment of insulin regime should avoid hypoglycemia.

Electrolyte Abnormalities

Can be effectively managed with regular postoperative monitoring and replacement where required.

Adrenal Insufficiency

Adrenal insufficiency can occur in patients undergoing bilateral adrenalectomies; therefore long-term steroid replacement therapy may be required.

Nelson's Syndrome

Bilateral adrenalectomies cause plasma cortisol levels to decrease, reducing the negative feedback on anterior pituitary production of CRH. This results in a locally invasive CRH-secreting pituitary tumor leading to increased levels of ACTH. Signs and symptoms include hyperpigmentation of the skin, visual disturbances, headaches, and interruption of the menstrual cycle.

Carcinoid Syndrome

Carcinoid tumors are of neuroendocrine origin and derived from enterochromaffin cells, which are disseminated throughout the gastrointestinal and bronchopulmonary system.[29–30] Carcinoid tumors occur most commonly in the gastrointestinal tract (67.5%) and the bronchopulmonary system (25.3%).[31] Serotonin produced by carcinoid tumors may evade hepatic metabolism and can enter into the systemic circulation causing carcinoid syndrome. This results in skin flushing, diarrhea, bronchospasm, and tricuspid or pulmonary valvular dysfunction.[30]

Carcinoid crises is an exaggerated form of carcinoid syndrome characterized by profound flushing, bronchospasm, tachycardia, and fluctuations of blood pressure.[32]

Carcinoid Syndrome: Signs and Symptoms[33]

In 2010 Ellis et al. estimated the clinical incidence of carcinoid tumors at 1.5 cases per 100,000 population, with the incidence on autopsy as high as 650 cases per 100,000.[34] The overall 5-year survival of all carcinoid tumors regardless of location is 67.2%.[31]

The diagnosis comprises biochemical testing, direct imaging, and histology, as outlined in Table 28.8.

TABLE 28.8 Diagnosis of Carcinoid Tumor

Biochemical testing	24-hour urine collection to assess for elevated levels of 5-hydroxyindoleacetic acid (5-HIAA) and serum analysis chromogranin A (CgA).[30]
Imaging	Abdominal computed tomography with contrast is utilized as a means of cross-sectional imaging to localize carcinoid tumors and their metastases.[30]
Histology	Immunohistochemical staining.

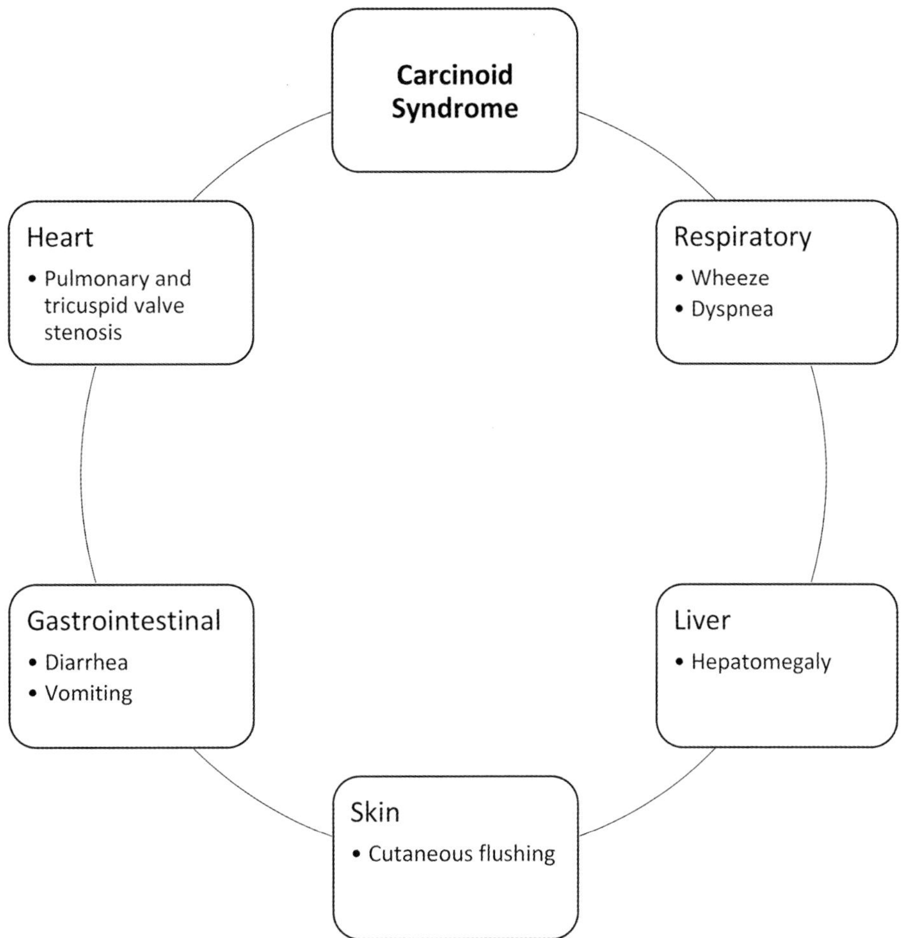

• **Fig. 28.4** Carcinoid syndrome: signs and symptoms.

Signs and symptoms include:

- Flushing
- Diarrhea
- Wheeze
- Anemia
- Dehydration
- Electrolyte imbalance
- Intestinal obstruction

The preferred treatment for carcinoid tumors remains primarily surgical resection in combination with somatostatin analogues. Definitive treatment plans are individualized to the patient and largely based on the location of metastases and primary tumor.[30]

Significant autonomic stimulus, such as pain and hemodynamic variations, can lead to carcinoid crises. The primary aim of anesthesia in carcinoid surgery is to reduce the impact of such stimuli.[32]

Preoperative Management

A comprehensive history and examination should be undertaken, with careful attention to signs of right heart failure (orthopnea, paroxysmal dyspnea, and peripheral edema) caused by tricuspid or pulmonary valvular dysfunction.[32] A list of the pertinent preoperative investigations to order in a patient with a carcinoid tumor can be found in Table 28.9.

Octreotide is a somatostatin analogue, which binds to receptors on the tumor cells and inhibits the vasoactive products of the tumor.

In patients with serotonergic symptoms, an octreotide infusion at a rate of 50 μg/h for at least 12 hours before surgery is advised. Close monitoring for common side effects of infusions, including QT prolongation, bradycardia, abdominal cramps, nausea, and vomiting, is advised.[32]

Intraoperative Management

Thoracic epidurals are advised in patients undergoing elective laparotomy to reduce the stress response to surgery and the subsequent risk of a carcinoid crises.[32]

Morphine and atracurium should be used with caution because of the potential for histamine release. Remifentanil infusion has been reported to provide titratable

TABLE 28.9 Preoperative Investigations of Carcinoid Tumor

Investigation	Indication
Chest x-ray	To rule out carcinoid lesions or miliary shadowing of a carcinoid lung
Electrocardiogram	Assessing for signs of right ventricular hypertrophy
Full blood count	To check for preexisting anemia
Urea and electrolytes	To identify hypokalemia and hypernatremia associated with chronic diarrhea
Liver function tests	May be altered in the presence of hepatic infiltration
Coagulation screen and group and cross matching	Hepatic resections carry high bleeding risk
Arterial blood gas	Metabolic acidosis associated with chronic diarrhea
Echocardiography	To exclude right side carcinoid cardiac disease

intraoperative blood pressure control during surgery for carcinoid syndrome.[35]

Norepinephrine and epinephrine infusions may lead to stimulation of the autonomic nervous system and provoke a carcinoid crisis. Where necessary, small doses of phenylephrine have been used with good effect.[32] Intravenous bolus of 20–50 µg of the somatostatin analogue octreotide can aid in the attenuation of intraoperative hormone release.

Zero balance fluid therapy, and arterial line and central venous pressure monitoring can help optimize fluid management. Blood loss should be closely monitored throughout surgical resection, with fluid or blood products administered accordingly.

In cases that require surgical resection of hepatic metastases with clamping of the hepatic artery and portal vein, maintaining a low central venous pressure to reduce venous bleeding is advised.[32]

Surgical technique is largely dependent on tumor location and can include endoscopic resection, local resection, cryosurgery, hepatic artery embolization, and ablation.[36] Each technique carries its own specific risks and complications that should be discussed with the patient and their carers in advance.

Postoperative Management

Monitoring in a high dependency unit for the 48 hours immediately postoperatively is advised.[32] The primary aim in the postoperative period is reduced autonomic stimulus by ensuring stable hemodynamic conditions and adequate pain control.

TABLE 28.10 Syndromes of Hormone Hypersecretion in the Pituitary Gland[37]

Anterior Pituitary Hormone	Hormone Hypersecretion Syndrome	Signs and Symptoms
Thyroid stimulating hormone	Thyrotoxicosis	Tachycardia Hypertension Diaphoresis
Adrenocortico-tropic hormone	Cushing's disease	Truncal obesity Skin thinning Immunosuppression Obstructive sleep apnea Proximal myopathy Hypertension Left ventricular hypertrophy Diabetes mellitus Gastric ulceration
Growth hormone	Acromegaly	Macrognathia Macroglossia Obstructive sleep apnea Kyphoscoliosis Proximal myopathy Hypertension Left ventricular hypertrophy Ischemic heart disease
Prolactin	Prolactinoma	Galactorrhea Menstrual dysfunction Erectile dysfunction

Pituitary Adenomas

Definitions

Pituitary adenomas are divided into two main groups: functional and nonfunctional.

Functional pituitary adenomas, including prolactinomas, ACTH-producing tumors, and growth hormone–producing tumors, produce hormones, as outlined in Table 28.10.

Nonfunctional pituitary adenomas produce no hormones but may cause a mass effect. This can present with headaches, cranial nerve palsies, hydrocephalus, and compression of the functional pituitary cells leading to hypopituitarism (see Table 28.11).

Pituitary adenomas can be further categorized by their size. Macroadenomas are those exceeding 10 mm in size and can lead to mass effects as outlined.[37] Microadenomas are those less than 10 mm in size and commonly present with symptoms of hormonal excess, as outlined in Table 28.10.

TABLE 28.11 Hypopituitarism Signs and Symptoms[37]

Anterior Pituitary Hormone	Hormone Hyposecretion Syndrome	Signs and Symptoms
Adrenocorticotropic hormone	Adrenocortical insufficiency	Hypoglycemia Hypotension Nausea Vomiting
Thyroid stimulating hormone	Hypothyroidism	Bradycardia Hyporeflexia
Antidiuretic hormone	Diabetes insipidus	Polyuria Polydipsia

Rarely a patient will present with pituitary apoplexy caused by a hemorrhage into an adenoma. Signs and symptoms include dramatic endocrine alterations, headache, and meningism.[38]

Epidemiology

The incidence of pituitary adenomas is estimated at 8 per 100,000 persons, with pituitary adenomas accounting for 9.1% of all brain tumors.[39]

Preoperative Management

Tests to be ordered preoperatively depend on the primary pituitary pathology as outlined in Table 28.12.

Lumbar drains can be placed preoperatively to allow injection of small volumes of air or saline to encourage descent of the tumor into the surgical field. A similar effect can be achieved with controlled hypoventilation.[37,38]

Post-intubation the posterior pharynx should be packed with saline soaked gauze before surgery to stabilize the tracheal tube and protect the lower airway from blood and secretions.[38]

Intraoperative Management

The primary aim is to maintain stable cerebral oxygenation throughout surgery.

Invasive blood pressure monitoring should be considered. Short-acting opioids such as remifentanil may facilitate intraoperative hemodynamic stability. Patients with acromegaly may have three times the rate of difficult tracheal intubation compared with the general population due to macrognathia and macroglossia, and an awake fiberoptic tracheal intubation may be required.[37,40]

Patients are positioned for surgery supine with a moderate degree of head-up tilt.[38] Ventilation to avoid hypocapnia should be employed to ensure no loss of brain bulk and maintain optimum tumor accessibility throughout.[38]

Surgical Technique

Primarily pituitary surgery is performed using the transsphenoidal approach. This approach requires deliberate nasal septum fracture. Application of ephedrine or cocaine for topical mucosal vasoconstriction may lead to hypertensive reaction in patients with Cushing's disease, and

TABLE 28.12 Preoperative Investigations for Primary Pituitary Pathology and Their Indications

Investigation	Indication
Magnetic resonance imaging	Surgical planning to assess for hydrocephalus
Computerized tomography	To assess for boney invasion of tumor
Full visual acuity test	Visual field defects must be clearly documented prior to any surgical intervention
Hormone levels	
Serum growth hormone and insulin-like growth factor 1	High levels of both hormones indicates a growth hormone–secreting adenoma
Glucose suppression test: 75 g oral glucose	Failure to a reduce plasma growth hormone levels is indicative of a growth hormone–secreting adenoma
Plasma ACTH levels Late-night salivary cortisol levels 24-hour urinary free cortisol level	High levels of each indicates an ACTH-secreting adenoma
Low-dose dexamethasone suppression test	Failure to reduce plasma cortisol levels is indicative of Cushing's syndrome
High-dose dexamethasone suppression test	A reduction in plasma cortisol levels is indicative of Cushing's disease
Plasma prolactin levels	High levels indicate a prolactinoma
Thyroid function test	Elevated thyroid stimulating hormone and low thyroxine levels indicate a TSH-secreting adenoma

cophenylcaine (lidocaine and phenylephrine) is a suitable alternative.[37]

Postoperative Management

All patients require a reducing regime of steroids in the postoperative course. Specific hormone replacement will be defined by the patient's residual hormonal function and in conjunction with a consultant endocrinologist.[37]

Complications include the following.

Vascular Damage

Damage to the carotid artery is rare. Such patients require carotid angiography postoperatively due to increased risk of developing a carotid aneurysm.[38]

Transient Diabetes Insipidus

This usually occurs within the first 24 hours and lasts for up to a week. Biochemical diagnosis includes plasma osmolality of greater than 295 mOsm/kg, urine osmolality of less than 300 mOsm/kg, and a urine output greater than 2 m/kg/h.[38] Persistent diabetes insipidus can be managed with desmopressin.[37]

Airway Obstruction

Post-transsphenoidal pituitary surgery patients are at increased risk of airway obstruction due to blood and packing in the naso- and oropharynx. This patient cohort requires close monitoring in a high dependency unit postoperatively.[37,38]

Intracranial Bleeding

Careful monitoring for alterations in levels of consciousness and pupil size is crucial in the postoperative period, with a low threshold for reimaging the brain.[37]

References

1. Brito J, Morris J, Montori V. Thyroid cancer: zealous imaging has increased detection and treatment of low risk tumors. *Br Med J*. 2013;347:f4706.
2. European Cancer Information System. European Network of Cancer Registries, Thyroid Cancer Factsheet. The European Network of Cancer Registries Factsheets. January 1, 2017. Available at https://www.encr.eu/sites/default/files/factsheets/ENCR_Factsheet_Thyroid_2017-2.pdf.
3. Constantinides V, Palazzo F. Goitre and thyroid cancer. *Medicine*. 2013;41(9):546–550.
4. Bajwa S, Sehgal V. Anesthesia and thryoid surgery: the never ending challenges. *Indian J Enocrinolol Metab*. 2013;17(2):228–234.
5. Lacoste L, Gineste D, Karayan J, et al. Airway complications in thyroid surgery. *Ann Otol Rhinol Laryngol*. 1993;102(6):441–446.
6. Marusch F, Hussock J, Haring G, Hachenberg T, Gastinger I. Influence of muscle relaxation on neuromonitoring of the recurrent laryngeal nerve during thyroid surgery. *Br J Anaesth*. 2005;94:596–600.
7. Rulli F, Ambrogi V, Dionigi G, Amirhassaankhani S, Mineo T, Ottaviani F. Meta-analysis of recurrent laryngeal nerve injury in thyroid surgery with or without nerve monitoring. *Acta Ortorhinolaryngol Ital*. 2014;34(4):223–229.
8. Farling P. Thyroid disease. *Br J Anesth*. 2000;85(1):15–28. doi: 10.1093/bja/85.1.15.
9. Bilard V, Shekih M, Delaport-Hoop S, Raffin Sanson M Anaesthesia for endocrine tumor removal. *Ann Fr Anesth Reanim*. 2009;28(6):549–563. doi:10.1016/j.annfar.2009.04.004.
10. Bernards A, Buitenwerf E, Krijger R, et al. Incidence of pheochromocytoma and sympathetic paraganglioma in the Netherlands: a nationwide study and systematic review. *Eur J Intern Med*. 2018;51:68–73.
11. Ebbehoj A, Sondergaard E, Trolle C, Stochholm K, Poulsen P. The epidemiology of pheochromocytomas: increasing incidence and changing clinical presentation. A population based retrospective study 1977–2015. *Endocr Abstr*. 2017;49(4):e2251–e2261. doi: 10.1530/endoabs.49.OC1.4.
12. Ramachandran R, Rewari V. Current perioperative management of pheochromocytomas. *Indan J Urol*. 2017;33(10):19–25.
13. Cancer.Net Editorial Board. Pheochromocytoma and Paraganglioma: Statistics. December 2018. Available at https://www.cancer.net/cancer-types/pheochromocytoma-and-paraganglioma/statistics.
14. Hanna N, KenadySurgical Treatment D. *Evidence-Based and Problem-Orientated*. Zuckschwerdt; 2001.
15. Lenders J, Duh Q, Eisenhofer G, et al. Pheochromocytoma and paraganglioma: an Endocrine Society Clinical Practice Guidelines. *J Clin Endocrinol Metab*. 2014;99(6):1915–1942.
16. Young W. Clinical Presenation and Diagnosis of Pheochromocytoma. UptoDate. 2019. Available at https://www.uptodate.com/contents/clinical-presentation-and-diagnosis-of-pheochromocytoma.
17. Shen W, Grogan R, Vriens M. One hundred two patients with pheochromocytoma treated at a single institution since the introduction of laparoscopi adrenalectomy. *JAMA Surgery*. 2010;145(9):893–897. doi:10.1001/archsurg.2010.159.
18. Connor D, Bounphrey S. Perioperative care of pheochromocytoma. *BJA Educ*. 2015;16(5):153–158.
19. Grossman A. Cushing's Syndrome. 2019. Available at https://www.epgonline.org/cushings-syndrome-kc/en/disease-overview/symptoms.html.
20. Kairys N, Schwell A. *Cushing Disease*. In: StatPearls [Internet]. StatPearls Publishing; 2019.
21. Roshanov PS, Rochwerg B, Patel A, et al. Withholding or continuing angiotensin converting enzyme inhibitors or angiotensin II receptor blockers before non-cardiac surgery: an analysis of the vascular events in non-cardiac surgery patient's cohort evaluations prospective cohort. *Anesthesiology*. 2017;126:16–27.
22. Sharma S, Nieman L, Feelders R. Cushing's syndrome: epidiomology and developments in disease management. *Clin Epidemiol*. 2015;7:281–293.
23. Clayton R, Raskauskiene D, Reulen R, Jones P. Mortality and morbidity in Cushing's disease over 50 years in Stoke-on-Trent, UK: audit and meta-analysis of literature. *J Clin Endocrinol Metab*. 2011;96(3):632–642. doi:10.1210/jc.2010-1942.
24. Nieman L, Biller B, Findling J, et al. The diagnosis of Cushing's Syndrome: an Endocrine Society Clinical Practice Guideline. *J Clin Endocrinol Metab*. 2008;93(5):1526–1540. doi:10.1210/jc.2008-0125.
25. Association of Anesthetists of Great Britain and Ireland. Perioperative management of the surgical patient with diabetes 2015. *Anesthesia*. 2015;0:1427–1440.

26. Memtsoudis S, Swamidoss C, Psoma M. Anesthesia for adrenal surgery. *Adrenal Glands*. Springer; 2005:287–297.
27. Davies M, Hardman J. Anaesthesia and adrenocortical disease. *Br J Anaesth*. 2005;5(4):122–126.
28. Chilkoti T, Singh A, Mohta M, Saxena A. A perioperative "stress dose" of corticosteroid: Pharmacological and clinical perspective. *J Anaesthesiol Clin Pharmacol*. 2019;35(2):147–152. doi:10.4103/joacp.JOACP_242_17.
29. Ominoe G, Kodish E, Herman R. Neuroendocrine tumors of the appendix in adolescents and young adults. *Clin Oncol*. 2017;2:1318.
30. Pinchot S, Holen K, Sippel R, Chen H. Carcinoid tumors. *Oncologist*. 2010; 13(12):1255–1269. doi:10.1634/theoncologist.2008-0207.
31. Modlin M, Lye K, Kidd M. A 5 decade analysis of 13,715 carcinoid tumors. *Cancer*. 2003;97(4):934–959.
32. Powell B, Mukhtar A, Mills G. Carcinoid: the disease and its implications for anaesthesia. *Br J Anaesth*. 2011;11(1):9–13. doi:10.1093/bjaceaccp/mkq045.
33. National Cancer Institute. Gastrointestinal Carcinoid Tumors Treatment (Adult) (PDQ®). Gastrointestinal Neuroendocrine. (Carcinoid) Tumors. September 14, 2013. Updated August 23, 2021. Available at: https://www.cancer.gov/types/gi-carcinoid-tumors/patient/gi-carcinoid-treatment-pdq.
34. Ellis L, Shale M, Coleman M. Carcinoid tumors of the gastrointestinal tract: trends in incidence in England since 1971. *Am J Gastroenterol*. 2010;105(12):2563–2569.
35. Farling P, Durairaju A. Remifentanil and anaesthesia for carcinoid syndrome. *Br J Anaesth*. 2004;92:893–895.
36. The American Cancer Society Medical and Editorial Content Team. Surgery for Gastrointestinal Carcinoid Tumors. September 24, 2018. Available at https://www.cancer.org/cancer/gastrointestinal-carcinoid-tumor/treating/surgery.html.
37. Menon R, Murphy P, Lindley A. Anaesthesia and pituitary disease. *Br J Anaesth*. 2011;11(4):133–137.
38. Smith M, Hirsch N. Pituitary disease and anaesthesia. *Br J Anaesth*. 2000;85(1):3–14.
39. Ezzat S, Asa S, Couldwell W, Barr C, Dodge W, Vance M. The prevalence of pituitary adenoma: a systematic review. *CA Cancer J Clin*. 2004;101(3):613–619.
40. Nemergut E, Zuo Z. Airway Management in patient with pituitary disease: a review of 746 patients. *J Neurosurg Anesthesiol*. 2006;18(1):73–77.

29

Anesthesia and Surgery for Cytoreductive Surgery With Hyperthermic Intraperitoneal Chemotherapy (HIPEC)

AISLINN SHERWIN, FARAZ KHAN, CONOR SHIELDS, AND DONAL J. BUGGY

Introduction

Cytoreductive surgery (CRS) was initially described in the 1930s for patients with locally advanced gynecologic cancers, especially those with local and peritoneal spread, in an attempt to reduce symptoms arising from tumor burden.[1] The subsequent extensive debulking surgeries developed in the 1960s and 1970s demonstrated an improvement in patient survival in conjunction with postoperative chemotherapy and improved tumor response to adjuvant treatment.[2]

Seeding of tumor cells to the peritoneum is believed to occur as a result of inherent tumor biology; however, spillage of microscopic tumor cells into the peritoneum during surgery is also inevitable. The development of metastatic disease within the abdomen is thought to occur due to the "sticky surface" of the peritoneum, which provides a beneficial environment in which tumor deposits can flourish.[3]

Hyperthermic intraperitoneal chemotherapy (HIPEC) was first reported in 1955 when intraperitoneal nitrogen mustard was administered to seven patients with ovarian cancer.[4] In a landmark paper, Dedrick et al. examined the pharmacokinetic properties of intraperitoneal chemotherapy and found a positive impact on transport across the peritoneal-plasma barrier.[4] Intraperitoneal chemotherapy was found to offer a survival benefit to patients with appendiceal tumors, and phase I and II trials commenced in the 1980s.

HIPEC is thought to improve tumor response in a number of ways. Intraperitoneal perfusion of chemotherapeutic agents was found to have a slower rate of clearance from the body than intravenous chemotherapy.[3] The drugs used are hydrophilic and have a high molecular weight, thereby sequestering the active agent in the peritoneal cavity more effectively.[5]

Tumor cells have less ability to repair DNA and exhibit increased apoptosis when heat is applied, and specific chemotherapeutic agents including cisplatin, doxorubicin, and mitomycin C demonstrate improved cytotoxicity and penetration when combined with hyperthermia, which adds to the effectiveness of the treatment.[6] The application of HIPEC is most effective when administered immediately following the cytoreductive portion of the procedure and prior to reconstruction.[5]

Epidemiology and Cancer Subtypes

CRS combined with HIPEC is predominantly used to treat patients with peritoneal carcinomatosis from appendiceal, colorectal, ovarian, and mesothelioma primary cancers.[7]

Pseudomyxoma peritonei (PMP) primarily arises from mucinous tumors of the appendix or ovary, which rupture and seed within the peritoneal cavity.[8] Systemic treatment is often ineffective for these cancers, and morbidity and mortality are often a result of relentless tumor progression, resulting in intestinal obstruction.[2] Prior to the development of CRS and HIPEC, low-grade appendiceal malignancies were invariably fatal.[3] Low-grade appendiceal tumor recurrence primarily recurs at the original resection site and peritoneal surfaces, while aggressive cancers can also exhibit metastases to the lymph nodes and liver.[3]

Epithelial ovarian cancer affects over 200,000 women worldwide on a yearly basis.[9] Minimal symptoms in the early stages of the disease often result in the presence of distal spread on presentation.[9] Overall survival is poor, with a rate of only 50% at 5 years.[9] A recent analysis highlighted increased survival in patients with ovarian cancer who received HIPEC with CRS compared with those without HIPEC.[10]

TABLE 29.1 Compartmentalization of the Cytoreductive Surgical Approach

Abdominal Region	Peritonectomies	Visceral Resections
Right upper	Right subphrenic	Glisson's capsule dissection
Left upper	Left subphrenic	Splenectomy
Anterolateral	Stripping of paracolic gutters Greater omentectomy	Appendectomy Right colectomy
Subhepatic	Lesser omentectomy Stripping of omental bursa	Gastric antrectomy/total gastrectomy, cholecystectomy
Pelvis	Pelvic peritonectomy	Sigmoidectomy Hysterectomy Bilateral salpingo-oopherectomy

Malignant mesothelioma is a neoplasm of the serosal lining of the body cavities, including the abdomen.[11] Diffuse malignant peritoneal mesothelioma is an aggressive form of the disease and has an annual occurrence rate of 300–400 cases annually in the United States, with many patients dying within a year of diagnosis.[12] HIPEC and CRS have offered an alternative treatment strategy and improved median survival up to 60 months in some patients.[11]

Approximately 10% of patients presenting with colorectal carcinoma will have coexisting peritoneal metastases,[13] while one-quarter of those with recurrent disease have peritoneal metastases.[13] Aggressive treatment with CRS and HIPEC targeting peritoneal metastases has demonstrated significantly improved survival rates.[13]

The incidence of peritoneal dissemination of primary gastric cancer is estimated to be 20%.[3] Patients with peritoneal spread of the disease have an extremely poor prognosis, with median survival estimated at 1–3 months.[14] In select patients HIPEC and CRS can almost double the survival time.[15]

Strategy in Cytoreductive Surgery and HIPEC

CRS involves both visceral and peritoneal resections.[16] CRS can be either primary, intended to completely remove tumors prior to commencement of chemotherapeutic regimens, or secondary, intended to remove residual tumor following chemotherapy.[17] CRS is aimed at removing all macroscopic deposits of the tumor, i.e., >2.5 mm, while HIPEC is designed to target microscopic disease.[16] Palliative debulking surgery can also be performed to relieve symptoms due to disease.[17]

Sugarbaker's Five Peritonectomy Procedures

The cytoreductive surgical technique has been standardized by Sugarbaker et al.[18] (Table 29.1). Current evidence suggests that the removal of all visible tumors should be operative intent. The completeness of cytoreduction is a major prognostic factor in all peritoneal surgeries. The survival advantage of macroscopically complete cytoreduction has been demonstrated in the treatment of sarcomatosis, abdominal mesothelioma, and peritoneal metastases of ovarian, gastric, and colorectal origin. Near-complete cytoreduction, leaving behind small volume residual tumor, should be pursued only when complete CRS is not feasible, and to preserve postoperative organ function.[18] After initial laparotomy, assessment was performed using a standardized scoring system, the peritoneal carcinomatosis index (PCI). PCI is a clinical assessment of both the size and distribution of nodules on the peritoneal surface (Fig. 29.1).[19]

The abdominal cavity is divided into nine regions, while the area of the small bowel from the duodenojejunal flexure to the terminal ileum is subdivided into four areas. The greatest possible extent of tumor burden is assessed within these specific regions and is given a score of 0 to 3 depending on the lesion size (LS). An LS score of 0 means no malignant deposit is visible macroscopically, rising to LS 3, which indicates a cumulative tumor burden of greater than 5.0 cm. A maximum PCI score of 39 is attainable.[19] Regardless of the primary cause of peritoneal carcinomatosis, a lower PCI score is associated with a higher chance of complete CRS and hence curative intent at the time of surgery. A radiographically derived PCI score can be used as a prognostic indicator in advance of surgery, although it can be difficult to accurately assess tumor burden, and consequently PCI, with imaging alone. PCI may also be calculated at staging laparoscopy; however, it remains the case that the most accurate PCI score is obtained during traditional open surgery.[19,20]

Completeness of Cytoreduction Score

The most definitive assessment used to assess the prognosis of patients with peritoneal surface malignancy is the completeness of the cytoreduction (CC) score (Fig. 29.2). The CC score has been shown to accurately predict outcomes in PMP, peritoneal metastases from colorectal, ovarian, and gastric malignancies, and sarcomatosis and peritoneal

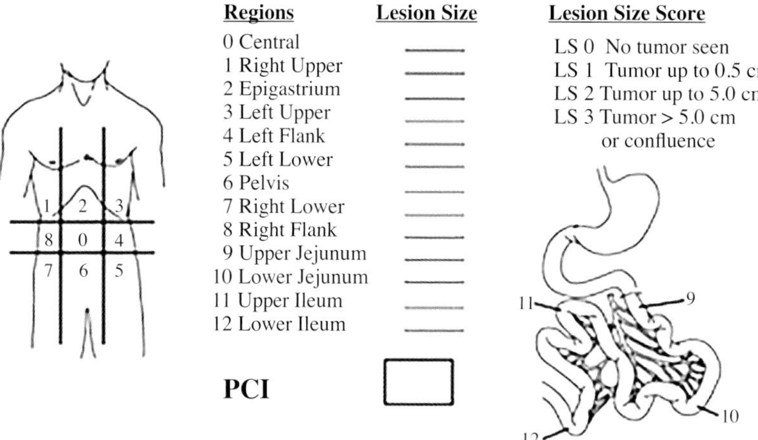

• **Fig. 29.1** Peritoneal carcinomatosis index. (Reprinted from *Cytoreductive Surgery & Perioperative Chemotherapy for Peritoneal Surface Malignancy*, 2nd Edition, Copyright © 2017 with permission, Ciné-Med, Inc.).

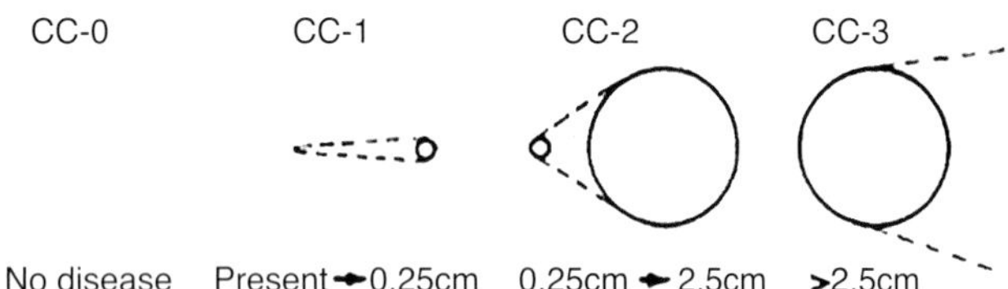

• **Fig. 29.2** Completeness of cytoreduction score. (From Jacquet P., Sugarbaker P.H. Current methodologies for clinical assessment of patients with peritoneal carcinomatosis. *J Clin Exp Cancer Res.* 1996;15(1):49–58).

mesothelioma.[21–23] A CC score of 0 indicates that no visible peritoneal seeding exists following cytoreduction, while a CC score of 3 indicates tumor nodules >2.5 cm or a confluence of unresectable tumor nodules at any site within the abdominal cavity. CC-2 and CC-3 cytoreductions are considered incomplete.

HIPEC Rationale

Locoregional administration of chemotherapy increases the local concentration of the chemotherapeutic agent at the site of action, thereby reducing systemic toxicity. In HIPEC, the carrier solution for chemotherapy is initially heated to a temperature between 40°C and 43°C. The HIPEC solution is administered for 30–120 min depending on the institutional protocol, and the desired chemotherapy agent utilized.[24] For example, in our institution (Peritoneal Malignancy Institute at Mater Misericordiae University Hospital, Dublin, Ireland), heated mitomycin C is administered for 60 min to treat PMP and colorectal and gastric peritoneal metastases. Ovarian peritoneal metastases are commonly treated with cisplatin for 90 min, while a combination of doxorubicin and cisplatin for 60 min is used to treat abdominal mesothelioma. Following HIPEC, the abdominal cavity is lavaged prior to the creation of any anastomoses and abdominal closure with placement of intraabdominal drains.[24,25]

The Dedrick Diffusion Model

The pharmacokinetic rationale of perioperative intraperitoneal chemotherapy is based on dose intensification provided by the direct instillation of chemotherapy into the peritoneal cavity and delayed clearance caused by the peritoneal plasma barrier. The peritoneal permeability of a number of hydrophilic anticancer drugs may be less than that of the same drug.[24,25]

Techniques of HIPEC

Coliseum Technique

This employs a retractor with catheters and temperature probes to secure the edges of the abdominal cavity in an elevated position, creating a "coliseum," to allow perfusion and circulation of the hyperthermic solution.[2] It has the added benefit of allowing manual stirring for a more effective and even distribution of heat and cytotoxic agents; however, it can lead to heat loss, reduced exposure of the anterior wall of the peritoneum to the fluid,[26] and potentially a risk to staff from direct contact with chemotherapeutic agents or aerosolized particles (Fig. 29.3).[2]

Closed Technique

The closed technique employs a similar placement of catheters and temperature probes; however, the edges of the laparotomy wound are sutured in a watertight fashion.[27] This can reduce the risk of drug spillage and heat loss and increase drug penetration due to the positive pressure effect exerted by the closed abdomen.[26] However, there is a risk of uneven distribution of chemotherapeutic agents within

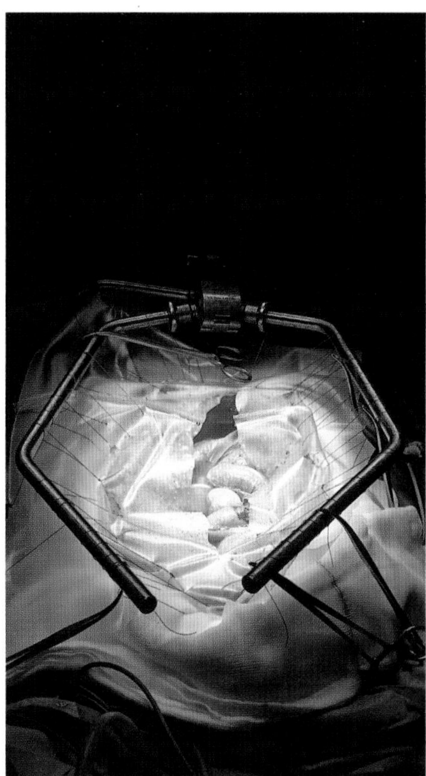

• **Fig. 29.3** The Coliseum technique. Intraoperative photograph—Mater Misericordiae Hospital, Dublin.

the cavity and pooling of fluids, which can result in toxic levels of both heat and cytotoxic agents.[2] Table 29.2 lists the advantages and disadvantages of both techniques.[19]

PIPAC

Pressurized intraperitoneal aerosol chemotherapy (PIPAC) is a further evolution of intraperitoneal chemotherapy, employing a pressurized normothermic aerosol to distribute chemotherapy throughout the peritoneal cavity.[28] This has been shown to affect the rapid, even, and effective spread of chemotherapeutic agents within the abdominal cavity. The procedure involves the use of a nebulizer connected to a high-pressure injector to generate an aerosol of the active agent.[29] This procedure can be repeated throughout the treatment cycles prior to definitive CRS and HIPEC.[28] Although currently employed as a rescue technique in those who have failed other therapeutic options, it has shown promise as a neoadjuvant therapy prior to formal CRS and HIPEC.[28] PIPAC may allow the selection of patients whose tumors are chemosensitive and in whom resection may be favorable.[28]

Chemotherapeutic Agents Employed During HIPEC

Table 29.3 lists some agents that can be used for HIPEC.[19] There is a wide discrepancy in terms of chemotherapy selection. Mitomycin C is classically used in appendiceal PMP and colonic peritoneal metastases. For abdominal mesothelioma cases, a combination of cisplatin and doxorubicin is used. Cisplatin is commonly used for ovarian primaries. In some institutions, bidirectional chemotherapy can also be employed, where systemic 5-fluorouracil (5-FU) is given at the same time as HIPEC.

Conduct of Anesthesia for HIPEC

Preoperative Assessment

Preoperative assessment is vital in patients undergoing CRS and HIPEC. Determining prognosis is important in this cohort; for example, those with colorectal carcinoma and

TABLE 29.2 Comparison of Closed and Open HIPEC Procedures

Features	Open HIPEC	Closed HIPEC
Efficiency	Allows continued cytoreduction of bowel and mesenteric surfaces	No surgery possible during chemotherapy
Environmental hazard	No aerosols detected	Perception of increased safety
Distribution	Uniform distribution of heat and chemotherapy solutions, tissues close to skin edge not immersed	Possible poor distribution to dependent sites and closed spaces
Pressure	No increased intraabdominal pressure	Increased intraabdominal pressure may increase chemotherapy penetration into tissue
Pharmacology	Allows pharmacokinetic monitoring of tumor and normal tissue	Tissue uptake of chemotherapy cannot be determined
Abdominal incisions and suture lines	Treated prior to performing the suturing	Risk of recurrence in abdominal incision and suture lines
Intestinal perforation	Detected by observing immersed bowel loops	Not detected
Hyperthermia	Increased heat necessary to maintain 42°C	Less heat required to maintain 42°C

HIPEC, Hyperthermic intraperitoneal chemotherapy.

TABLE 29.3 Chemotherapeutic Agents Used in HIPEC

Drug	Type	Dose	Heat Stability
Doxorubicin	Antitumor antibiotic	15 mg/m²	42°C
Mitomycin C	Antitumor antibiotic	15 mg/m²	42.5°C
Cisplatin	Alkylator	90 mg/m²	41.5°C
Oxaliplatin	Alkylator	400 mg/m²	46°C
Paclitaxel	Antimitotic	120–180 mg	42.5°C
Melphalan	Alkylator	70 mg/m²	42°C
5-Fluorouracil	Antimetabolite	650 mg/m²	43°C

synchronous peritoneal metastases have a median survival of approximately 36 months, with 1-year mortality as high as 13%.[30] Patients will be exposed to long operating times accompanied by intra- and postoperative fluid shifts, temperature changes, and potential coagulopathies. Therefore a number of factors must be considered prior to the selection of patients for CRS and HIPEC. Factors such as those in the following list must be considered by the team as a whole[31]:

- The primary tumor and its aggressiveness
- Presence or absence of extraabdominal metastases
- Likelihood of complete surgical resection
- Preoperative status and comorbid disease
- Peritoneal cancer index score

Preoperative Assessment and Optimization

Patients should ideally attend a multidisciplinary preoperative assessment clinic for full workup and assessment of both physical and mental status. "Successful surgery" is not solely dependent on the achievement of clear surgical margins—the resumption of normal physiological and physical status is also of prime importance.[32] Preoperative performance status can have a bearing on postoperative outcome, as poorer global function predicts morbidity and mortality.[33] The stress response associated with major surgery reduces lean body mass and aerobic capacity, which can have negative postoperative effects.[32]

There is increasing interest in the use of cardiopulmonary exercise testing (CPET) for the stratification of postoperative outcomes. Primary measures utilized during CPET, such as anaerobic threshold and peak oxygen consumption, can predict the patients' ergometric capacity, i.e., their overall fitness.[34] It is thought that those with a higher level of fitness can cope better with the demand for increased oxygen delivery required during prolonged surgery.[35] Furthermore, it is thought that participation in regular exercise can have a systemic effect similar to ischemic preconditioning for patients.[35] CPET is also an independent predictor of mortality following major elective surgery and can also predict the length of stay.[36]

Recognition of the importance of the preoperative period in the optimization of patients' physical status has increased in the past 10 years.[32] This period allows targeted interventions to improve postoperative outcomes. Enhanced Recovery After Surgery (ERAS) protocols have demonstrated benefits for patients undergoing major gastrointestinal surgery. A Cochrane systematic review found that ERAS protocols can reduce the length of hospital stay in patients following liver, gastrointestinal, and pancreatic surgeries.[37]

Preoperative exercise therapy can reduce the overall complication rate and length of stay of patients undergoing abdominal surgery.[38] In those undergoing liver resections, a planned prehabilitation program undertaken preoperatively can improve overall CPET and quality of life scores.[39] Trimodal prehabilitation programs which include elements of psychological support, nutrition education, and exercise have been shown to reduce the loss of lean body mass in comparison with those who undergo rehabilitation programs after cancer surgery and those who have no such treatment.[40] Preservation of lean body muscle mass can improve overall survival and reduce the complications of chemotherapy.[41] The heterogeneity of trials examining the outcomes of exercise programs for cancer patients has led to difficulty in assessing the utility of exercise programs, with some authors commenting that increases in fitness are difficult to translate into improvements in clinical outcomes.[42]

Preoperative anemia is present in up to 40% of patients undergoing major surgery.[43] Patients with anemia have an increased risk of increased short-term mortality after surgery.[43] In cancer patients, red cell transfusion is associated with increased mortality and the risk of cancer recurrence.[44] Preoperative intravenous iron transfusion is well tolerated by patients and has been proven to increase the preoperative hemoglobin level.[45]

Patients undergoing CRS and HIPEC may present with weight loss and malnutrition. The perioperative period has high catabolic demands and patients who are malnourished can further develop a protein-calorie deficit.[46] Evidence of preoperative hypoalbuminemia and associated malnutrition can highlight patients who may also have poorer outcomes postoperatively.[47] Serum albumin levels have been found to demonstrate a linear relationship with postoperative outcomes in patients with colon cancer.[46] Perioperative nutritional support can also reduce the length of hospitalization and intensive care stay.[48]

The preoperative period allows clinicians to assess patient status and potentially identify those at high risk of complications following a prolonged and intensive surgical course with CRS and HIPEC. Preoperative clinic visits allow discussion with the patient regarding regional anesthesia and analgesia, use of invasive monitoring, potential anesthetic complications, and postoperative analgesic regimes, which may serve to reduce patient anxiety. Interventions to improve outcomes prior to the date of surgery can also be employed during this period.

Intraoperative Management

Fluid Management

Fluid shifts are common during both the cytoreductive portion of the surgery and the instillation of chemotherapeutic agents. Fluid loss has been estimated to be up to 12 mL/kg/h depending on the extent of the debulking surgery being performed.[31] This is further compounded by evaporative fluid loss from high temperatures caused by the systemic inflammatory response syndrome (SIRS) response to chemotherapy agents.[47]

The best choice of intravenous fluid is yet to be determined. Colloid has been discredited as a volume-replacement fluid. Colloids, such as hydroxyethyl starches, dextran, and albumin, have a number of drawbacks in CRS.

The SPLIT trial[49] examined the prevalence rates of acute kidney injury (AKI) in intensive care unit patients receiving normal saline versus buffered crystalloid fluid. The results of this multicenter trial showed no clear benefit of one fluid over the other in the rates of AKI.[49] The larger, more recent SMART trial examined composite outcomes in critically ill adults receiving either normal saline or balanced crystalloid fluids.[50] Major adverse kidney events within 30 days (MAKE30), which included mortality, renal replacement therapy, and persistent creatinine elevation, were studied with an apparent reduction in MAKE30 in the balanced crystalloid group.[50] A 2017 Cochrane review concluded that there was insufficient evidence to demonstrate the effects of buffered versus nonbuffered crystalloid fluids on mortality and organ system function in the perioperative period.[51] However, benefits were noted in postoperative reduction in hyperchloremia and metabolic acidosis in buffered crystalloids.[51]

Restrictive fluid regimes in major abdominal surgery, while initially associated with reduced postoperative morbidity, have been found to have a higher rate of AKI,[52] particularly with nephrotoxic agents used in HIPEC, and reduced tissue- and end-organ perfusion.[53] However, liberal regimes have been associated with fluid overload and abdominal complications such as anastomotic breakdown and tissue edema.[53] While the ideal regime for fluid management during HIPEC is yet to be defined, liberal fluid regimes of up to 16 mL/kg/h have been associated with a significant increase in the complication rate observed in this cohort.[54]

Volume status and fluid responsiveness may be monitored using cardiac output monitoring, pulse pressure variation monitoring, or esophageal Doppler devices. Goal-directed fluid therapy is recommended by a number of authors[26,47,53] for HIPEC and CRS surgery, particularly as interpatient requirements can vary greatly.[55] The requirement for fluid therapy can also vary within the procedure itself, and during CRS, blood loss can cause hypovolemia; during HIPEC, increased abdominal pressure can lead to reduced venous return and preload initially, while hyperthermia and systemic inflammatory response can then lead to a reduction in systemic vascular resistance.[56]

However, major trials on high-risk patients (not including HIPEC patients), such as OPTIMISE and RELIEF, have shown no benefit with goal-directed therapy and compared with a moderately positive fluid balance over the first 24 h postoperatively, as discussed earlier.

Vasopressors can be used to improve hemodynamic management if required. Noradrenaline (norepinephrine) is the primary agent used in our center for blood pressure augmentation. Some authors recommend the use of dopamine for improved splanchnic and renal perfusion and oxygenation[53] and furosemide to improve urine output.[57] However, this is a contentious practice, with others advocating normovolemia and appropriate doses of noradrenaline to maintain end-organ perfusion and oxygenation.[47]

Thermoregulation

Temperature swings are common in CRS and HIPEC procedures. Initial exposure of the abdomen to the environment and evaporation of heat from the bowel surface can lead to a reduction in the core temperature. Hypothermia during this period can be associated with increased blood loss due to coagulopathy, increased surgical wound infection, and impairment in end-organ oxygenation and perfusion.[58]

During the HIPEC phase, which can last up to 90 min, instillation of fluid at 40–43°C can cause significant side effects. Temperature monitoring can indicate core increases of up to 40.5°C, which can cause increased heart rate, metabolic rate, end-tidal CO_2 levels, and metabolic acidosis.[31] Hyperthermia can also cause consumptive coagulopathies, seizures, and liver and renal injury.[5]

Analgesia

Thoracic epidural analgesia (TEA) is favored for both intra- and postoperative pain management. It optimizes postoperative analgesia and improves patient adherence to postoperative physiotherapy regimes, in turn reducing atelectasis and pneumonia.[5] A recent study examining outcomes for those with TEA demonstrated improved outcomes for those with TEA in comparison with opioid patient-controlled analgesia with improved overall morbidity and overall survival following HIPEC.[59] Reduction of opioids during the perioperative period also reduces ventilation time and improves postoperative bowel motility.[5] Evidence from animal studies, laboratory studies, and retrospective work has also demonstrated an association between improved long-term outcomes and the potential for increased disease-free survival.[47]

Hemodynamic changes associated with HIPEC can also be augmented by the sympathetic blockade of TEA. Epidural infusions have been associated with significantly less blood loss and fluid requirements in HIPEC procedures, and associated periods of hypotension can be well tolerated by these patients.[47]

There is concern in some areas that TEA can be associated with epidural hematoma due to relative coagulopathy experienced in the perioperative period. Some studies have demonstrated alterations in international normalized ratio (INR), platelet count, and fibrinogen levels in the perioperative period, which may potentially be associated with blood loss, dilutional effect, and fluid shifts.[60,61] However, studies have demonstrated the safety of epidural analgesia in this cohort of patients with no reported complications in a large cohort of patients undergoing CRS and HIPEC in the United States.[62] On balance, the benefits of TEA in this population in the management of perioperative pain outweigh the risks.[47]

Intrathecal opioids and patient-controlled opioid analgesic regimes are alternatives to thoracic epidurals. As some patients presenting for CRS and HIPEC can have coexisting chronic pain syndromes it is important to provide adequate analgesia in the perioperative period. Continuation of long-term opioids during this period is recommended and supplementation with multimodal analgesia should occur.[31]

Postoperative Management

The transfer of patients to high-dependency level care is the standard of care in our institution. Adequate monitoring of renal indices, analgesic requirements, and coagulopathy is possible on a regular basis in this environment, and early detection and treatment of any issues can occur in a timely fashion.

The majority of patients do not require end-organ support following HIPEC and CRS; however, approximately one-quarter may require postoperative vasopressor support for a short period of time.[60] This requirement is likely due to vasodilation postoperatively, and careful assessment of fluid responsiveness prior to aggressive fluid administration is recommended.[5] The median length of stay in a high dependency or intensive care unit setting for HIPEC and CRS patients is estimated at 5 days.[63]

Patients with diaphragmatic peritonectomy, intraoperative blood transfusion, and a long duration of surgery are all predisposed to higher rates of postoperative complications.[56] Common postoperative complications include anastomotic breakdown, postoperative bleeding, systemic sepsis, wound infection, pneumonia, and renal insufficiency.[33] Complications can arise from the chemotherapeutic agents used during the HIPEC portion of CRS. Mitomycin C, a common agent for pseudomyxoma, can cause elevated transaminases and deranged white cell counts.[5]

Extended surgical time, immobility, and preexisting malignancy all increase the risk of venous thromboembolism in these patients.[64] Thromboprophylaxis, both mechanical and pharmacological, should be prescribed accordingly.

Conclusion

Patients undergoing CRS and HIPEC procedures present unique challenges for the anesthesiologist. They are also surgically challenging and can involve hours of minute resection of tumor deposits prior to the application of heated intraperitoneal chemotherapy.

This technique has improved the overall survival of patients with peritoneal metastasis from a number of sources, particularly appendiceal and ovarian primary carcinomas. HIPEC allows targeted chemotherapeutic treatment of microscopic deposits, which is not achievable with intravenous dosing.

Meticulous preoperative assessment and optimization of patients prior to the day of surgery improves overall outcomes and reduces the length of hospital stay. Enhanced recovery protocols, including nutritional optimization, exercise programs, and psychological support, may offer benefits that have yet to be fully defined.

Intraoperatively, analgesia, fluid management, and thermoregulation require keen attention to detail, with thoracic epidural anesthesia and analgesia offering a safe perioperative modality for pain management despite associated hypotension and alterations to clotting function in this period.

Postoperative management should focus on adequate multimodal analgesia, venous thromboprophylaxis, and prevention and reduction of complications.

CRS and HIPEC can increase the chances of survival in patients with advanced malignancy. Multidisciplinary management of the perioperative period, including pre-, intra-, and postoperative-targeted management, will continue to improve outcomes for patients, including length of stay, morbidity, and overall mortality.

References

1. Vincent MJ. *Tumors of the Female Pelvic Organs*: MacMillan; 1934.
2. Neuwirth MG, Alexander HR, Karakousis GC. Then and now: cytoreductive surgery with hyperthermic intraperitoneal chemotherapy (HIPEC), a historical perspective. *J Gastrointest Oncol.* 2016;7(1):18–28.
3. Sugarbaker PH. Cytoreductive surgery and hyperthermic intraperitoneal chemotherapy in the management of gastrointestinal cancers with peritoneal metastases: progress toward a new standard of care. *Cancer Treat Rev.* 2016;48:42–49.

4. Witkamp AJ, de Bree E, Van Goethem R, Zoetmulder FA. Rationale and techniques of intra-operative hyperthermic intraperitoneal chemotherapy. *Cancer Treat Rev*. 2001;27(6):365–374.
5. Webb CA, Weyker PD, Moitra VK, Raker RK. An overview of cytoreductive surgery and hyperthermic intraperitoneal chemoperfusion for the anesthesiologist. *Anesth Analg*. 2013;116(4):924–931.
6. Sugarbaker PH. Van der Speeten K. Surgical technology and pharmacology of hyperthermic perioperative chemotherapy. *J Gastrointest Oncol*. 2016;7(1):29–44.
7. Mogal H, Chouliaras K, Levine EA., et al. Repeat cytoreductive surgery with hyperthermic intraperitoneal chemotherapy: review of indications and outcomes. *J Gastrointest Oncol*. 2016;7(1):129–142.
8. Rizvi SA, Syed W, Shergill R. Approach to pseudomyxoma peritonei. *World J Gastrointest Surg*. 2018;10(5):49–56.
9. Helm CW. Current status and future directions of cytoreductive surgery and hyperthermic intraperitoneal chemotherapy in the treatment of ovarian cancer. *Surg Oncol Clin N Am*. 2012;21(4):645–663.
10. van Driel WJ, Koole SN, Sikorska K, et al. Hyperthermic intraperitoneal chemotherapy in ovarian cancer. *N Engl J Med*. 2018;378(3):230–240.
11. Yan TD, Deraco M, Baratti D, et al. Cytoreductive surgery and hyperthermic intraperitoneal chemotherapy for malignant peritoneal mesothelioma: multi-institutional experience. *J Clin Oncol*. 2009;27(36):6237–6242.
12. Jang HJ, Lee HS, Burt BM, et al. Integrated genomic analysis of recurrence-associated small non-coding RNAs in oesophageal cancer. *Gut*. 2017;66(2):215–225.
13. Verwaal VJ, van Ruth S, Witkamp A, et al. Long-term survival of peritoneal carcinomatosis of colorectal origin. *Ann Surg Oncol*. 2005;12(1):65–71.
14. Gill RS, Campbell S, Shi X, Haase E, Schiller D. Treatment of gastric cancer with peritoneal carcinomatosis by cytoreductive surgery and HIPEC: a systematic review of survival, mortality, and morbidity. *J Surg Oncol*. 2011;104(6):692–698.
15. Yang XJ, Mei LJ, Yang GL, et al. Cytoreductive surgery and hyperthermic intraperitoneal chemotherapy improves survival of patients with peritoneal carcinomatosis from gastric cancer: final results of a phase III randomized clinical trial. *Ann Surg Oncol*. 2011;18(6):1575–1581.
16. Mehta SS, Bhatt A, Glehen O. Cytoreductive surgery and peritonectomy procedures. *Indian J Surg Oncol*. 2016;7(2):139–151.
17. Harter P, du Bois A. The role of surgery in ovarian cancer with special emphasis on cytoreductive surgery for recurrence. *Curr Opin Oncol*. 2005;17(5):505–514.
18. Sugarbaker PH. Cytoreductive surgery using peritonectomy and visceral resections for peritoneal surface malignancy. *Transl Gastrointest Cancer*. 2013;2(2):54–74.
19. Sugarbaker P. Cytoreductive Surgery & Perioperative Chemotherapy for Peritoneal Surface Malignancy. 2nd ed. *Cine-Med*. 2017.
20. Sugarbaker PH. Epithelial appendiceal neoplasms. *Cancer J*. 2009;15(3):225–235.
21. Jacquet P, Sugarbaker PH. Current methodologies for clinical assessment of patients with peritoneal carcinomatosis. *J Clin Exp Cancer Res*. 1996;15(1):49–58.
22. Fagotti A, Vizzielli G, Fanfani F, et al. Introduction of staging laparoscopy in the management of advanced epithelial ovarian, tubal and peritoneal cancer: impact on prognosis in a single institution experience. *Gynecol Oncol*. 2013;131(2):341–346.
23. Portilla AG, Sugarbaker PH, Chang D. Second-look surgery after cytoreduction and intraperitoneal chemotherapy for peritoneal carcinomatosis from colorectal cancer: analysis of prognostic features. *World J Surg*. 1999;23(1):23–29.
24. Dedrick RL. Theoretical and experimental bases of intraperitoneal chemotherapy. *Semin Oncol*. 1985;12(3 Suppl 4):1–6.
25. Flessner MF, Fenstermacher JD, Dedrick RL, Blasberg RG. A distributed model of peritoneal-plasma transport: tissue concentration gradients. *Am J Physiol*. 1985;248(3 Pt 2):F425–F435.
26. Kearsley R, Egan S, McCaul C. Anaesthesia for cytoreductive surgery with hyperthermic intraperitoneal chemotherapy (HIPEC). 2018. Available at https://www.wfsahq.org/components/com_virtual_library/media/3d34b517333f05b627444cb24a38be2e-atow-379-00-01.pdf.3.
27. González-Moreno S, González-Bayón LA, Ortega-Pérez G. Hyperthermic intraperitoneal chemotherapy: rationale and technique. *World J Gastrointest Oncol*. 2010;2(2):68–75.
28. Girshally R, Demtröder C, Albayrak N. et al. Pressurized intraperitoneal aerosol chemotherapy (PIPAC) as a neoadjuvant therapy before cytoreductive surgery and hyperthermic intraperitoneal Chemotherapy. *World J Surg Oncol*. 2016;14(1):253.
29. Solaß W, Hetzel A, Nadiradze G. et al. Description of a novel approach for intraperitoneal drug delivery and the related device. *Surg Endosc*. 2012;26(7):1849–1855.
30. Simkens GA, Rovers KP, Nienhuijs SW., de Hingh IH. Patient selection for cytoreductive surgery and HIPEC for the treatment of peritoneal metastases from colorectal cancer. *Cancer Manag Res*. 2017;9:259–266.
31. Raspe C, Piso P, Wiesenack C, Bucher M. Anesthetic management in patients undergoing hyperthermic chemotherapy. *Curr Opin Anaesthesiol*. 2012;25(3):348–355.
32. Scheede-Bergdahl C, Minnella EM, Carli F. Multi-modal prehabilitation: addressing the why, when, what, how, who and where next? *Anaesthesia*. 2019;74 (Suppl 1):20–26.
33. Newton AD, Bartlett EK, Karakousis GC. Cytoreductive surgery and hyperthermic intraperitoneal chemotherapy: a review of factors contributing to morbidity and mortality. *J Gastrointest Oncol*. 2016;7(1):99–111.
34. National Guideline Centre UK. Routine preoperative tests for elective surgery. NICE guideline [NG45] Published: April 05, 2016. https://www.nice.org.uk/guidance/ng45.
35. Moran J, Wilson F, Guinan E, et al. Role of cardiopulmonary exercise testing as a risk-assessment method in patients undergoing intra-abdominal surgery: a systematic review. *Br J Anaesth*. 2016;116(2):177–191.
36. Snowden CP, Anderson H, Manas D, Jones D, Trenell M. Cardiorespiratory fitness predicts mortality and hospital length of stay after major elective surgery in older people. *Ann Surg*. 2013;257(6):999–1004.
37. Giles B-S, Belgaumkar Ajay P, Davidson Brian R, Selvan GK. Enhanced recovery protocols for major upper gastrointestinal, liver and pancreatic surgery. *Cochrane Database Syst Rev*. 2016;2.
38. Valkenet K, van de Port IG, Dronkers JJ. et al. The effects of preoperative exercise therapy on postoperative outcome: a systematic review. *Clin Rehabil*. 2011;25(2):99–111.
39. Dunne DF, Jack S, Jones RP, et al. Randomized clinical trial of prehabilitation before planned liver resection. *Br J Surg*. 2016;103(5):504–512.

40. Gillis C, Fenton TR, Sajobi TT, et al. Trimodal prehabilitation for colorectal surgery attenuates post-surgical losses in lean body mass: a pooled analysis of randomized controlled trials. *Clin Nutr.* 2019;38(3):1053–1060.
41. Pin F, Couch ME, Bonetto A. Preservation of muscle mass as a strategy to reduce the toxic effects of cancer chemotherapy on body composition. *Curr Opin Support Palliat Care.* 2018;12(4):420–426.
42. Boereboom C, Doleman B, Lund JN, Williams JP. Systematic review of pre-operative exercise in colorectal cancer patients. *Tech Coloproctol.* 2016;20(2):81–89.
43. Fowler AJ, Ahmad T, Phull MK. et al. Meta-analysis of the association between preoperative anaemia and mortality after surgery. *Br J Surg.* 2015;102(11):1314–1324.
44. Munting KE, Klein AA. Optimisation of pre-operative anaemia in patients before elective major surgery – why, who, when and how? *Anaesthesia.* 2019;74(Suppl 1):49–57.
45. Wilson MJ, Dekker JW, Bruns E. et al. Short-term effect of preoperative intravenous iron therapy in colorectal cancer patients with anemia: results of a cohort study. *Transfusion.* 2018;58(3):795–803.
46. Haskins IN, Baginsky M, Amdur RL, Agarwal S. Preoperative hypoalbuminemia is associated with worse outcomes in colon cancer patients. *Clin Nutr.* 2017;36(5):1333–1338.
47. Raspé C, Flöther L, Schneider R., et al. Best practice for perioperative management of patients with cytoreductive surgery and HIPEC. *Eur J Surg Oncol.* 2017;43(6):1013–1027.
48. Ali Abdelhamid Y, Chapman MJ, Deane AM. Peri-operative nutrition. *Anaesthesia.* 2016;71(Suppl 1):9–18.
49. Young P, Bailey M, Beasley R. et al. Effect of a buffered crystalloid solution vs saline on acute kidney injury among patients in the intensive care unit: the split randomized clinical trial. *JAMA.* 2015;314(16):1701–1710.
50. Semler MW, Self WH, Rice TW. Balanced crystalloids versus saline in critically ill adults. *N Engl J Med.* 2018;378(20):1951.
51. Bampoe S, Odor PM, Dushianthan A. et al. Perioperative administration of buffered versus non-buffered crystalloid intravenous fluid to improve outcomes following adult surgical procedures. *Cochrane Database Syst Rev.* 2017;9:CD004089.
52. Myles PS, Bellomo R, Corcoran T. et al. Restrictive versus liberal fluid therapy for major abdominal surgery. *N Engl J Med.* 2018;378(24):2263–2274.
53. Colantonio L, Claroni C, Fabrizi L. et al. A randomized trial of goal directed vs. standard fluid therapy in cytoreductive surgery with hyperthermic intraperitoneal chemotherapy. *J Gastrointest Surg.* 2015;19(4):722–729.
54. Eng OS, Dumitra S, O'Leary M. et al. Association of fluid administration with morbidity in cytoreductive surgery with hyperthermic intraperitoneal chemotherapy. *JAMA Surg.* 2017;152(12):1156–1160.
55. Esteve-Pérez N, Ferrer-Robles A, Gómez-Romero G., et al. Goal-directed therapy in cytoreductive surgery with hyperthermic intraperitoneal chemotherapy: a prospective observational study. *Clin Transl Oncol.* 2019;21(4):451–458.
56. Malfroy S, Wallet F, Maucort-Boulch D., et al. Complications after cytoreductive surgery with hyperthermic intraperitoneal chemotherapy for treatment of peritoneal carcinomatosis: risk factors for ICU admission and morbidity prognostic score. *Surg Oncol.* 2016;25(1):6–15.
57. Schmidt C, Creutzenberg M, Piso P, et al. Peri-operative anaesthetic management of cytoreductive surgery with hyperthermic intraperitoneal chemotherapy. *Anaesthesia.* 2008;63(4):389–395.
58. Torossian A. Thermal management during anaesthesia and thermoregulation standards for the prevention of inadvertent perioperative hypothermia. *Best Pract Res Clin Anaesthesiol.* 2008;22(4):659–668.
59. Lorimier G, Seegers V, Coudert M, et al. Prolonged perioperative thoracic epidural analgesia may improve survival after cytoreductive surgery with hyperthermic intraperitoneal chemotherapy for colorectal peritoneal metastases: a comparative study. *Eur J Surg Oncol.* 2018;44(11):1824–1831.
60. Cooksley TJ, Haji-Michael P. Post-operative critical care management of patients undergoing cytoreductive surgery and heated intraperitoneal chemotherapy (HIPEC). *World J Surg Oncol.* 2011;9:169.
61. Korakianitis O, Daskalou T, Alevizos L., et al. Lack of significant intraoperative coagulopathy in patients undergoing cytoreductive surgery and hyperthermic intraperitoneal chemotherapy (HIPEC) indicates that epidural anaesthesia is a safe option. *Int J Hyperthermia.* 2015;31(8):857–862.
62. Owusu-Agyemang P, Soliz J, Hayes-Jordan A., et al. Safety of epidural analgesia in the perioperative care of patients undergoing cytoreductive surgery with hyperthermic intraperitoneal chemotherapy. *Ann Surg Oncol.* 2014;21(5):1487–1493.
63. Kapoor S, Bassily-Marcus A, Alba Yunen R. et al. Critical care management and intensive care unit outcomes following cytoreductive surgery with hyperthermic intraperitoneal chemotherapy. *World J Crit Care Med.* 2017;6(2):116–123.
64. Padmakumar AV. Intensive care management of patient after cytoreductive surgery and HIPEC – a concise review. *Indian J Surg Oncol.* 2016;7(2):244–248.

30

Perioperative Care: Sarcoma and Melanoma

JENNIFER S. DOWNS AND DAVID E. GYORKI

Perioperative Care: Sarcoma

Introduction

Sarcoma is an umbrella term for malignant neoplasms of mesenchymal origin. A wide variety of underlying cell types can become neoplastic, and so these cancers are best understood by division into histologic subtype and anatomic location.

Sarcomas are rare cancers in adulthood, making up less than 1% of all adult malignancies. Approximately 10% are of bony origin and the remainder originate in soft tissues. The occurrence of soft tissue sarcomas is lowest amongst young adults and slowly increases as patients get older, with a dramatic increase in incidence over the age of 50 years. Incidence of bony sarcomas has a bimodal distribution, with a peak in adolescents and young teens, and a second smaller peak in incidence in the elderly.[1,2]

Risk factors for sarcomas are not well understood. There are certain genetic syndromes that predispose to the development of soft tissue and bone sarcomas. Germline mutation in *TP53* causing Li–Fraumeni syndrome, loss of function of the *NF1* gene causing neurofibromatosis, and *RB1* gene-causing retinoblastoma and secondary malignancies are some of the more well-known syndromes.[1] Geographic and race distribution of certain sarcomas, for example, Ewing sarcoma, being more common in Caucasian populations indicate further unidentified genetic links.

Environmental exposures have also been implicated in the development of sarcomas, but studies are small and results conflicting. Radiation exposure is clearly understood to increase the risk of sarcoma, and certain chemicals.[1] However, there is currently insufficient evidence to generate guidelines on limiting exposure.

General Principles

Presentation of the sarcoma patient is determined both by the anatomic location of the tumor and the histologic subtype.

Extremity soft tissue tumors can present with a self-identified mass and symptoms due to invasion or compression of surrounding structures. Patients can complain of worsening pain or pain in a specific neurologic distribution. Persistent unexplained bone pain, recurrent limp, and pathologic fractures are all features of bony sarcomas.[2]

Retroperitoneal tumors tend to present later, with larger tumors, due to the large area for the tumor to expand into before beginning to compress structures and cause symptoms. These patients often describe a prolonged course of vague abdominal symptoms, which are difficult to classify or correlate, prior to undergoing diagnostic scanning.[3]

Diagnosis is usually confirmed by image-guided core biopsy, which permits targeting specific areas of the lesion that are most likely to provide diagnostic tissue.[4] Core needle biopsy is used to reduce the risk of tumor seeding.[5] However, should open incisional biopsy be required, it is advisable that this be done by the team who will perform the definitive resection, as open biopsies have a higher risk of tumor seeding. This incision must be carefully placed to allow later excision.[2]

Retroperitoneal sarcomas provide their own challenges in terms of diagnosis and provision of tissue. The biopsy should be performed by a unit that regularly undertakes such biopsies, as sampling of tissue that is more likely to yield a diagnosis is important (for example, areas of increased density or metabolic activity on scanning). Peritoneal breaches and intraabdominal tumor seeding should be avoided wherever possible. Therefore all core biopsies should be performed via a retroperitoneal approach.[5] Advice should be requested from a high-volume team as to the best method of proceeding. Core biopsy under direct vision can be considered but is at risk of being nondiagnostic and causing vascular injury.[4]

When planning definitive treatment, cross-sectional imaging to assess the relationship of the primary tumor to adjacent organs, as well as to assess for the presence of metastatic disease, is required. Good quality imaging is useful for diagnosis and planning resection. Choice of imaging modality is based on surgeon preference, but CT for central tumors and MRI for skeletal and extremity masses are widely used as the starting point. Functional imaging such as ^{18}fluorine-labeled fluorodeoxyglucose positron emission tomography (FDG-PET) provides added information about tumor activity and distant disease.[2,4,6,7]

Histology

The WHO classification of soft tissue tumors includes more than 100 histologic subtypes.[8] Tumor diagnostics are dependent on histologic appearance, patterns of immunohistochemistry (IHC) staining, and molecular pathology. Specific mutations in genes, for example, *EWSR1* in Ewing sarcoma, are commonly used to definitively diagnose certain tumors.

In general, sarcomas are named based on the presumed tissue of origin, for example, liposarcomas, leiomyosarcomas, angiosarcoma. This does not apply to all sarcomas and this can cause diagnostic dilemmas. Synovial sarcoma does not originate in synovium but was named because those were the cells that the tumor most closely resembled. IHC patterns are not always definitive. Histologic diagnosis is essential to allow for accurate prognostication and tailored therapy, both surgical and adjuvant. Tumor histology can predict both risk of local recurrence and distant metastasis, and this varies widely across different subtypes. Diagnosis also allows for consideration of added adjuvant or neoadjuvant therapy if benefit has been demonstrated. For example, different treatment strategies will be used when considering a patient with an undifferentiated pleomorphic sarcoma of the extremity, a tumor with a high risk of distant metastases compared to a myxofibrosarcoma, a locally aggressive tumor that has a high rate of local recurrence.

Natural History and Prognosis

The natural history of sarcoma depends on the histologic subtype, with a variety of disease trajectories. In general, the natural history of sarcoma is as a locally aggressive tumor with risk of hematogenous metastasis. Approximately 50% of soft tissue sarcomas (STS) will develop metastatic disease, most commonly in the lungs.[9] Important prognostic factors include histologic grade, subtype, tumor size, pathologic stage, anatomic site, and age. Current American Joint Committee on Cancer (AJCC) staging (8th edition) also separates extremity and retroperitoneal tumours.[10]

Management

Once histology has been confirmed and the intent of treatment has been assessed as curative or palliative, a management plan can be determined. As with other solid malignancies, the aim of treatment is to minimize the risk of local recurrence and distant metastasis while maximizing the functional outcome. Choice of treatment varies according to histology and lesion location, but many types of sarcoma will receive neoadjuvant chemotherapy or radiotherapy prior to definitive surgical resection.[11]

Neoadjuvant Therapy

The aim of neoadjuvant therapy is to improve local control, assist in lower morbidity resection by decreasing tumor size and viability of margins, and decrease the risk of distant metastases.[12] This therapy can comprise chemotherapy, radiation therapy, or a combination thereof, and varies between institutions according to local preference.

Neoadjuvant Chemotherapy

Most soft tissue regimens are based around use of doxorubicin (anthracycline) with or without added ifosfamide.[11] The key adverse effect of anthracycline-based regimens is the risk of cardiotoxicity. This cardiotoxicity occurs with the first dose and is cumulative. Myelosuppression is also a common side effect of doxorubicin and ifosfamide.[13] Bone sarcomas rely on neoadjuvant chemotherapy prior to surgery, and patients can receive high doses of methotrexate, cisplatin, and doxorubicin. Nephrotoxicity and gastrointestinal side effects are also well documented for methotrexate and cisplatin.[14] Nephrotoxicity can be a particular problem for patients with retroperitoneal sarcoma if patients are scheduled for nephrectomy.

Neoadjuvant Radiotherapy

Radiotherapy is widely used in the neoadjuvant setting for soft tissue sarcomas both in the extremity and retroperitoneum. The standard protocol involves patients receiving 50.4 Gy in 28 fractions over approximately 5 weeks. Side effects are mostly limited to the area being irradiated, with edema and inflammation of those local tissues. General effects such as fatigue are also well described.[15] Local effects causing nausea and loss of appetite become specifically relevant in neoadjuvant irradiation of retroperitoneal tumors. These patients can rapidly become deconditioned during radiation therapy and require specific interventions and nutritional support to minimize these effects prior to surgery.

Targeted Therapies

The utility of molecular targeted therapies in sarcoma is minimal. Few tumors carry mutations that have available therapies. The exception to this are gastrointestinal stromal tumors (GISTs), the vast majority of which harbor mutations that respond to tyrosine kinase inhibitors (TKIs).[16] TKIs can be used in the neoadjuvant, adjuvant, and advanced setting, and improve resectability, progression-free survival, and overall survival.[17] Side effects include fatigue, gastrointestinal disturbances, skin changes, hypertension, and rarely cardiotoxicity.[18]

Preoperative Care

Altering surgical stressors preoperatively can have an impact on postoperative morbidity and recovery. Obesity, poor glycemic control, smoking, and poor nutritional status increase the risk of postoperative complications. Interventions to improve these stressors and manage comorbidities prior to surgery, such as those parts of an Enhanced Recovery After Surgery (ERAS) program, or in isolation, should be considered in the sarcoma patient.[19]

Prehabilitation

Prehabilitation has been likened to preparation for a marathon—working through all aspects around surgery to try and make the patient as "fit" as possible. Input from exercise physiologists, physicians, dieticians, and psychologists, and social support are all important. Interventions range from a single 30-min education session to structured exercise, and nutritional, medical, and psychologic support plans over multiple weeks. These interventions have been shown in small trials to halve the risk of postoperative complications.[20] However, the benefits of prehabilitation should always be balanced by the possibility that the patient's cancer could progress to being irresectable in the time to surgery and worsen the overall prognosis. Clear communication between team members is vital for good decision-making.

Intraoperative blood transfusion adversely affects overall cancer prognosis and independently increases postoperative morbidity.[21] Although intraoperative strategies can be employed, every effort should be made to minimize the need for intraoperative blood transfusion by treating preoperative anemia, which is common in cancer patients.[22] This can be in the form of intravenous iron infusion if time allows, or preoperative autologous blood transfusion. Preoperative allogenic blood transfusion can also be considered in extensive surgery if there is a poor response to iron infusion and a high likelihood of needing blood intraoperatively. Management of preoperative anemia may also improve the patient's ability to exercise and therefore increase the benefit of prehabilitation.[20]

Intraoperative Considerations

The main determinant of prognosis in surgically resectable sarcomas is that of a negative margin at resection, and this dictates the surgical strategy.

Bone

Over time, neoadjuvant therapies, imaging, and improved medical technology in the form of bone implants, prostheses and computer-assisted orthopedic surgery (CAOS) have allowed for more limb salvage surgeries rather than amputation.[23] However, these remain extensive and challenging surgeries. Currently, approximately 85% of bony sarcoma surgery is limb salvage surgery.[12] These procedures involve prolonged operations, requiring soft tissue and bone resection, replacement with prosthetic or grafted bone, and may need vascularized soft tissue reconstruction to cover the defect.[23] Occasionally vascular resections are also involved. Blood loss can be significant. Postoperative intensive care support is often required.

Extremity Soft Tissue

Although these tumors can be simpler resections than primary bone tumors, they can also result in prolonged operative times due to the need for soft tissue reconstruction to fill defects. As with bone tumor surgery, the aim of surgery is to clear the tumor with a margin of normal surrounding tissue. The amount of normal tissue required depends on the type of tissue margin and the tumor histology. Studies have demonstrated that certain tissue types, more resistant to invasion, form the "equivalent of centimeters" of skeletal muscle or fat when determining the resection margin, thus allowing for salvage of abutting vital structures.[24]

Retroperitoneal

As previously mentioned, retroperitoneal tumors tend to present late when relatively advanced due to the nature of such tumors to remain asymptomatic for prolonged periods. This means that they tend to be large tumors closely related to multiple organs at surgery. Commonly resected organs include the colon and kidney.[3] Recent data from high-volume centers suggest that resection of adjacent organs where imaging does not necessarily show organ invasion is associated with improved disease control, as microscopic organ invasion is not readily seen on cross-sectional imaging.

Histologic Tailored Surgery

As previously mentioned, accurate histological diagnosis can change surgical planning based on the behavior of the sarcoma subtype. Tumors with higher risk of local recurrence require more aggressive local surgery with wider margins. An example of this is surgery for retroperitoneal liposarcoma, where high rates of recurrence make clear margins crucial. Improved prognosis for these tumors has been gained by more extensive multiorgan resection for these tumors, including ipsilateral kidney, colon, and mesocolon, to improve the chances of an R0 resection.[4] In contrast, other retroperitoneal tumors such as leiomyosarcoma may require more extensive vascular resection, but surrounding structures can often be preserved.

Isolated Limb Infusion/Perfusion

Although limb salvage surgery is the standard of care in extremity sarcoma, there remains a group of patients without distant metastases whose sarcoma is not initially amenable to limb salvage. These patients could be considered for attempted limb salvage using isolated limb infusion/perfusion (ILI/P). ILI/P allows for high-dose locoregional therapy to the primary while allowing the patient to retain the affected limb and limiting the potential for systemic toxicity. This can reduce the disease sufficiently for it to become locally resectable and does not appear to be associated with worse overall outcomes (in a disease with a high propensity to metastasize).[25] Infusion requires chemotherapy (typically melphalan based) to be circulated via radiologically placed catheters in a tourniqueted limb.[26] Perfusion requires open surgical insertion of catheters, and the hyperthermic chemotherapy with added tumor necrosis factor-alpha (TNF-α) is circulated via an oxygenated extracorporeal perfusion circuit. Early complications include limb edema, skin loss, and rarely compartment syndrome and myoglobin-induced kidney injury.[26]

Other intraoperative considerations are as follows.

Intraoperative Blood Loss

Intraoperative blood loss is a significant risk for patients undergoing sarcoma surgery. Hemostatic devices are commonly used to limit blood loss, but tumors are extensive and can be highly vascular. Certain anatomic locations such as pelvic dissection also predispose the patient to hemorrhage, and preoperative planning, including massive transfusion protocols, should be agreed upon in advance. Use of a cell salvage device to reduce the need for allogeneic blood can be considered but remains controversial in the setting of cancer surgery. There is concern that there may be viable tumor cells in the salvaged blood that could put the patient at higher risk of metastasis. Leucodepletion filters can be used to reduce the number of cells in the salvaged blood. However, this significantly increases the time it takes for salvaged blood to become available, which can limit its usefulness. It is advised that if cell salvage is considered, the patient specifically consents to the risks and benefits.[27]

Bypass

Veno-venous, veno-arterial, and full cardiopulmonary bypass are rarely used in sarcoma surgery, but are options if facilities are available. Full bypass is usually reserved for cardiac sarcoma resection.[28] Veno-venous or veno-arterial perfusion can be considered for retroperitoneal sarcoma resections that will require prolonged vascular clamp time, in order to maintain distal organ perfusion, minimize reperfusion injury, and simplify fluid balance during prolonged surgery. All the complications associated with major surgery on bypass, such as acute kidney injury, electrolyte abnormalities, platelet dysfunction, systemic inflammatory response, hyper- and hypothermia, cerebral injury, and immunosuppression, can occur in these patients.[29] There are no current international guidelines for perioperative antibiotics specific to sarcoma surgery. Antibiotics are widely used but choice of antibiotics and regimens differ.[30]

Postoperative Care

The need for intensive care postoperatively is dictated by the length of surgery, type of procedure, and the underlying condition of the patient. With the increase in incidence of soft tissue sarcomas in elderly patients, these are often older patients who can be deconditioned due to neoadjuvant therapy, or simply due to their cancer. Extensive resections and prolonged operations often need intensive care support postoperatively and prolonged hospital stays.

Special Considerations

Enhanced Recovery Programs

There are no direct guidelines from the ERAS society regarding sarcoma surgery. However, gastrointestinal guidelines are easily extrapolated to retroperitoneal sarcoma surgery patients. Most ERAS principles can be applied to extremity surgery too. Programs such as those, including judicious use of intravenous fluid, early mobilization, minimal drainage, and early or no urinary catheter use among other things, have been used in Soft Tissue Sarcoma surgery centers with good results.[31,32]

Extremity Surgery

The operated extremity is often placed in a fixed brace or dressing to limit movement that could damage the reconstruction. Early mobilization and rehabilitation by allied health staff using specific methods is needed, taking into account the surgery and specific reconstruction.[32,33]

Thromboprophylaxis

Recently published international guidelines for venous thromboprophylaxis agree that sarcoma surgery places patients at high risk for venous thromboembolism, although guidelines specific to sarcoma are lacking. The use of postoperative thromboprophylaxis is wide but not standardized. Local protocols for dosing regimens and drug choice should be applied. Extended thromboprophylaxis for 4 weeks or longer is advised for intraabdominal and pelvic surgery.[34]

Pain Control

Postoperative patients require multimodal analgesia beginning at the operative period.[35] Combination analgesia makes use of opioids, nonsteroidal antiinflammatories, regional anesthesia such as blocks and epidurals, and other agents to treat pain in a proactive fashion from the start of the surgical stimulus. Good patient communication and multidisciplinary input from pain and allied health staff also play a role in postoperative pain management.[36]

Conclusion

Sarcomas represent a heterogeneous group of diseases in anatomically varied locations, can be clinically complex to manage, and show a range of biological behaviors. Surgery has been the backbone of management, but a tendency to both local recurrence and distant metastasis in a number of subtypes suggests a poor prognosis. However, multidisciplinary management with a focus on careful and appropriate histologic diagnosis and histology-tailored treatment is associated with the best outcomes for patients.

Perioperative Care: Melanoma

Introduction

Melanoma is a mesenchymal malignancy of melanocytes, occurring wherever melanocytes are found. This leads to three principal subtypes, namely cutaneous, ocular, and mucosal, each with their own distinct tumor biology and behavior. Cutaneous melanoma makes up the large majority of cases. Most patients present with early-stage local disease. However, the management of patients with metastatic melanoma has seen the most dramatic change over the last decade. The introduction of effective systemic therapies both with checkpoint blockade immunotherapy (CBI) and molecular targeted therapies has induced profound responses in patients with metastatic disease.[37] Similar responses are seen using these agents in the adjuvant and neoadjuvant setting.[38] This has similarly resulted in changes in anesthetic and surgical management of later-stage melanoma.

Cutaneous melanoma is a rare skin cancer, with a variable global incidence (worldwide average, 22 per 100,000), and the peak being in Australia and New Zealand at 49 per 100,000 people.[39] There are marked differences in melanoma incidence across different races (and therefore skin types), with the incidence of melanoma in white males in the United States being 27 times higher than in black males.[40] There are also geographic differences, with higher incidences noted at lower latitudes. The geographic effects span skin types.[41] Cutaneous melanoma occurs across all ages, with the incidence increasing with age. It remains rare but not unheard of in the pediatric and adolescent population.

UV exposure is the most important risk factor for melanoma development. Intermittent exposure in early life appears to be the highest risk, with more than five early sunburns increasing the lifetime risk of melanoma twofold.[42] Use of indoor tanning beds also increases the risk of developing melanoma proportional to the amount of use, further reinforcing the association with UV exposure.[43]

Other risk factors include phenotypic traits, such as skin type, and type, and number of naevi.[44] Familial melanoma clusters are thought to be a combination of genetic predisposition, common heavy sun exposure, and phenotypic risk factors.[45] Numerous other risk factors have shown small increases in risk, including immunosuppression, nonmelanomatous skin cancers, and others.[46]

Mucosal melanomas are very rare, occurring most commonly in the upper aerodigestive tract, the vulvovaginal area, and the anorectal tract. They generally have a poor prognosis, present later, and are at high risk of distant metastases.[47] Ocular melanoma develops in the choroid, ciliary body, iris (uvea), or conjunctiva. These often late-presenting tumors can be managed initially with eye conserving local therapies. Patients are at high risk of metastatic disease despite adequate local control, predominantly in the liver.[48] Given the rarity of mucosal and ocular melanoma, the remainder of this review will discuss patients with cutaneous melanoma.

General Principles

Preoperative Workup

After presenting to their general practitioner or dermatologist with a skin lesion, subsequently biopsied, patients will often present to their surgeon with a histologically confirmed diagnosis. The extent of preoperative workup is determined by the tumor Breslow thickness (maximal depth of skin invasion). Axial imaging can be used to rule out metastatic disease at presentation. Evidence of benefit is limited in asymptomatic patients. FDG-PET can be considered for staging in thick melanomas.[49] Clinical evidence of nodal disease (either palpable or found on radiology) requires ruling out of further metastatic disease prior to proceeding to surgery.

Surgical Principles for the Management of Cutaneous Melanoma

Wide excision of the primary site is aimed at preventing local recurrence of the melanoma. The width of the margin around the primary lesion or biopsy site is dictated by the thickness of the melanoma, varying between 1 and 2 cm of normal skin around the lesion. Closure may require local flap reconstruction or skin graft, depending on the location.

Sentinel lymph node biopsy is used to provide lymph node staging and is regarded as one of the most important prognostic stratification tools. Accurate localization of the first draining lymph node in the relevant nodal basins requires the use of intradermal injection of localizing agents. Use of dual tracers combining radiolabeled nanocolloid with patent blue dye decreases the risk of removing a false negative sentinel node.

Radiolabeled nanocolloid is injected, and single photon emission computed tomography (SPECT) imaging with or without the use of low-dose Computerised Tomography (widely used abbreviation) localizes the draining nodal basins and number of sentinel nodes. A small incision is made, and the sentinel node removed. The node is identified by using the gamma probe intraoperatively to identify the radioactive lymph node. Intradermal injection of blue dye at the primary site on the theater table provides visual confirmation by coloring the sentinel node.

Wide excision alone can be performed under local anesthetic. Sentinel lymph node biopsy usually necessitates general anesthetic.

Intraoperative Considerations

Melanoma occurs across all ages, but is more common in the elderly, and this should be borne in mind when considering anesthesia. Most surgery for patients with primary melanoma is a simple day surgery procedure of wide excision with or without sentinel lymph node biopsy. Where sentinel node biopsy is not required, surgery can often be done under local anesthetic alone. Wound closure may require local procedures such as advancement, rotational, or island-type flaps but seldom more than this. Skin grafts may also be required.

Methylene or patent blue is widely used as the second tracer in dual modality sentinel node biopsy, and injected intradermally as the case begins. This carries a 0.9% risk of allergic reactions.[50] Awareness and close monitoring of all cases is essential.

Isolated Limb Infusion/Perfusion

This procedure is used for patients with regionally advanced melanoma with multiple unresectable dermal or subcutaneous metastases. The limb is isolated with an arterial tourniquet and high-dose administration of cytotoxic drugs can provide responses in up to 75% of patients. Limb infusion is simpler than limb perfusion, requiring image-guided cannulation of the relevant vein and artery, tourniquet isolation of the limb and circulation, and then flushing of the cytotoxic agent. Risks include reperfusion injury, rhabdomyolysis, acute kidney injury, vascular injury, and delayed compartment syndrome and skin complications.[51]

Perfusion requires open vascular cannulation and use of bypass equipment to actively circulate oxygenated blood and cytotoxic drugs.

Postoperative care seldom requires intensive care or prolonged hospital stays, and care should be focused on rapid mobilization and return to normal life.

Surgery for "Immune Escape" Lesions

Surgical resection of oligometasatic lesions progressing on CBI is evolving. These lesions may be primary progressors (where all tumor deposits respond to the therapy except for a single lesion that continues to grow) or secondary progressors (where an initial complete or near-complete response is followed by isolated progression).[52–54] Surgical resection of the isolated progressing lesion is associated with a good outcome. This can obtain durable disease control. Importantly, it is likely that patients with this type of progression have other sites of disease that remain in equilibrium under ongoing immune control. Therefore there is a strong theoretical basis for avoiding any immunosuppression in these patients.

Systemic Therapy

Immunotherapy

Although the concept of immunomodulation to treat melanoma has been used for decades, the identification of immune checkpoints such as CTLA4 and PD-1 and the effective inhibition of these have significantly improved the effectiveness of this approach. CBI works by binding and inhibiting specific receptors that downregulate the host immune response to the tumor, releasing the brakes on the immune response. These allow the host's own immune system to identify and eradicate the tumors. Multiple receptors can be targeted by antibody infusions, including PD-1, PD-L1, and CTLA4 amongst others.[1] This is a rapidly expanding field of cancer therapy used across multiple tumor types and the applications are constantly growing. Responses to single agent and combination therapy are 40% and 55%, respectively, with a 15%–20% complete response rate. Up to 80% will have a heterogeneous response to treatment, with lesions responding differently requiring other modalities for treatment.[55]

Complications of immunotherapy, although less commonly severe than those caused by traditional chemotherapy, can be significant. Known as immune-related adverse events (IrAEs), use of checkpoint inhibitors can result in immune infiltrates in almost all organ systems, resulting in autoimmune disorders.[56] These include colitis, pneumonitis, myocarditis, hypophysitis, nephritis, thyroiditis, hepatitis, and skin disorders, amongst others. Although fatal IrAEs are rare, the highest risk of death is from immune-related colitis. The incidence of more severe IrAEs (grades III–V) varies from 10% to 31% depending on the agent used, and combination immunotherapy, although more effective, carries the highest risk of severe adverse events of all. Adverse events are managed by cessation of immunotherapy and initiation of systemic corticosteroids, oral or intravenous, depending on the severity of the IrAE. Steroid requirements can be prolonged following an IrAE and should be borne in mind. Hypophysitis can also result in lifelong steroid dependence and inability to mount an appropriate stress response.[56]

Immunotherapy can also cause flares of previous autoimmune diseases and requires cessation of immunosuppressive treatments. Decision-making and planning can be complicated, and multidisciplinary discussion is mandatory for example, for transplant recipients.

There is currently no evidence that immunotherapy should be paused for surgery, and no clear data on timing of surgery related to dosing in well patients.[57]

Targeted Therapy

Approximately 40% of melanomas carry the driver *BRAF* genetic mutation that can be targeted therapeutically. Patients whose tumors harbor an actionable *BRAF* mutation can be treated with agents targeting BRAF and MEK. Combined blockade results in both higher response rates and lower rates of certain toxicities.[22] In most patients, the tumor will develop resistance mechanisms to therapy. Combination targeted and immunotherapy approaches are under investigation but toxicities are high. Targeted therapy can be used both in the neoadjuvant and adjuvant setting.

Complications commonly include pyrexia, chills, fatigue, diarrhea, and photosensitivity, depending on the agents of choice. Rarer complications more relevant to the surgical population include new-onset hypertension, left ventricular dysfunction, and alteration in liver enzymes. These should be borne in mind during preoperative review.[58]

Neoadjuvant Therapy

Neoadjuvant therapy with either immunotherapy or targeted therapy in appropriately selected stage 3 and resectable stage 4 patients is in its infancy. Early trials show promising relapse-free survival in patients who have received either regimen and had major or complete pathologic responses in their resected specimens. However, this is not a risk-free approach, as the possibility that there could be disease progression in the interval between therapy and surgery remains. There is also a risk of toxicity from the neoadjuvant therapy that could delay surgery. Although early reports do not suggest an increased risk of surgical complications, anecdotal evidence indicates that surgery may be more challenging after neoadjuvant therapy. A number of prospective trials are currently underway.

Modern randomized controlled trials (RCTs) have changed the face of melanoma surgery. Surgery will continue to shift as access and efficacy of immunotherapy and targeted therapies improve. Fewer lymphadenectomies are performed than ever before, simplifying the surgical burden. The majority of melanoma surgery is limited to primary excision with or without complex wound closure and sentinel node staging. This allows for more procedures to be performed under local or regional anesthesia, according to preference and patient factors.

Beta Blockade

A number of observational studies across multiple cancer types show promise for the use of beta blockers to limit cancer progression based on the theory that blocking beta-adrenergic receptors can inhibit pathways that cause progression. Long-term follow-up of one of these cohorts in melanoma shows improved overall and melanoma-specific survival.[59]

However, these results remain controversial with many of the studies being subject to methodological flaws. A large meta-analysis of specific melanoma patients showed an improvement in overall rather than cancer-specific survival, suggesting the benefits are not related to prevention of melanoma progression. Randomized evidence is awaited.[60]

Conclusion

Melanoma management is a rapidly evolving field, undergoing rapid changes as systemic management becomes the mainstay for later-stage melanoma. Early-stage melanoma is still managed by simple surgical and staging procedures. The role of extensive surgery for patients with melanoma is changing as systemic therapies are used in earlier stages of disease.

References

1. Burningham Z, Hashibe M, Spector L, Schiffman JD. The epidemiology of sarcoma. *Clin Sarcoma Res.* 2012;2(1):14.
2. Moore DD, Luu HH. Osteosarcoma. In: Peabody TD, Attar S, eds. *Orthopaedic Oncology: Primary and Metastatic Tumors of the Skeletal System*: Springer International Publishing; 2014:65–92.
3. Fairweather M, Gonzalez RJ, Strauss D, Raut CP. Current principles of surgery for retroperitoneal sarcomas. *J Surg Oncol.* 2018;117(1):33–41.
4. Sarcomas ST. Management of primary retroperitoneal sarcoma (RPS) in the adult: a consensus approach from the Trans-Atlantic RPS Working Group. *Ann Surg Oncol.* 2015;22(1):256–263.
5. Wilkinson MJ, Martin JL, Khan AA, Hayes AJ, Thomas JM, Strauss DC. Percutaneous core needle biopsy in retroperitoneal sarcomas does not influence local recurrence or overall survival. *Ann Surg Oncol.* 2015;853–858.
6. Rutkowski PL, Mullen JT. Management of the "other" retroperitoneal sarcomas. *J Surg Oncol.* 2018;117(1):79–86.
7. Messiou C, Morosi C. Imaging in retroperitoneal soft tissue sarcoma. *J Surg Oncol.* 2018;117(1):25–32.
8. Jo VY, Doyle LA. Refinements in sarcoma classification in the current 2013 World Health Organization classification of tumours of soft tissue and bone. *Surg Oncol Clin N Am.* 2020;25(4):621–643. doi:10.1016/j.soc.2016.05.001.
9. Vincenzi B, Frezza AM, Schiavon G, et al. Bone metastases in soft tissue sarcoma: a survey of natural history, prognostic value and treatment options. *Clin Sarcoma Res.* 2013;3(1):6.
10. Cates JMM. The AJCC 8th edition staging system for soft tissue sarcoma of the extremities or trunk: a cohort study of the SEER database. *J Natl Compr Cancer Netw.* 2018;16(2):144–152.
11. Baldini EH, Le Cesne A, Trent JC. Neoadjuvant chemotherapy, concurrent chemoradiation, and adjuvant chemotherapy for high-risk extremity soft tissue sarcoma. *Am Soc Clin Oncol Educ Book.* 2018;38:910–915. doi:10.1200/EDBK_201421.
12. Chauhan A, Joshi GR, Chopra BK, Ganguly M, Reddy GR. Limb salvage surgery in bone tumors: a retrospective study of 50 aases in a single center. *Indian J Surg Oncol.* 2013;4(3):248–254.
13. Cheong A, Mcgrath S, Cutts S. Anthracyclines. *WikiJournal of Medicine.* 2018;5(1):1–8.
14. de Souza P. Cancer drug toxicities and anaesthesia. *Australas Anaesth.* 2007;1:71–79.
15. Dickie CI, Haas R, O'Sullivan B. Adjuvant radiation for soft tissue sarcomas. *Am Soc Clin Oncol Educ Book.* 2015;35:e634–e642.
16. von Mehren M, Joensuu H. Gastrointestinal stromal tumors. *J Clin Oncol.* 2018;36(2):136–143.
17. Call JW, Wang Y, Montoya D, Scherzer NJ, Heinrich MC. Survival in advanced GIST has improved over time and correlates with increased access to post-imatinib tyrosine kinase inhibitors: results from Life Raft Group Registry. *Clin Sarcoma Res.* 2019;9(1):1–14. doi:10.1186/s13569-019-0114-5.
18. Li J, Wang M, Zhang B, et al. Chinese consensus on management of tyrosine kinase inhibitor-associated side effects in gastrointestinal stromal tumors. *World J Gastroenterol.* 2018; 24(46):5189–5202.
19. Scott MJ, Baldini G, Fearon KCH, et al. Enhanced Recovery after Surgery (ERAS) for gastrointestinal surgery, part 1: pathophysiological considerations. *Acta Anaesthesiol Scand* 2015;59(10):1212–1231.
20. Ismail H, Cormie P, Burbury K, Waterland J, Denehy L, Riedel B. Prehabilitation prior to major cancer surgery: training for surgery to optimize physiologic reserve to reduce postoperative complications. *Curr Anesthesiol Rep.* 2018;8(4):375–385.
21. Goodnough LT, Shander A. Patient blood management. *Anesthesiol J Am Soc Anesthesiol.* 2012;116(6):1367–1376. doi:10.1097/ALN.0b013e318254d1a3.
22. Cata JP, Gottumukkala V. Blood loss and massive transfusion in patients undergoing major oncological surgery: what do we know? *ISRN Anesthesiol.* 2012; 2012:1–11.
23. Yang Y, Han L, He Z, et al. Advances in limb salvage treatment of osteosarcoma. *J Bone Oncol.* 2018;10:36–40. doi:10.1016/j.jbo.2017.11.005.
24. Kawaguchi N, Ahmed AR, Matsumoto S, Manabe J, Matsushita Y. The concept of curative margin in surgery for bone and soft tissue sarcoma. *Clin Orthop Relat Res.* 2004;419:165–172.
25. Neuwirth MG, Song Y, Sinnamon AJ, Fraker DL, Zager JS, Karakousis GC. Isolated limb perfusion and infusion for extremity soft tissue sarcoma: a contemporary systematic review and meta-analysis. *Ann Surg Oncol.* 2017;24(13):3803–3810.
26. Smith HG, Hayes AJ. The role of regional chemotherapy in the management of extremity soft tissue malignancies. *Eur J Surg Oncol.* 2016;42(1):7–17. doi:10.1016/j.ejso.2015.08.165.
27. Klein AA, Bailey CR, Charlton AJ, et al. Association of Anaesthetists guidelines: cell salvage for peri-operative blood conservation 2018. *Anaesthesia.* 2018;73(9):1141–1150.
28. Arif R, Eichhorn F, Kallenbach K, et al. Resection of thoracic malignancies infiltrating cardiac structures with use of cardiopulmonary bypass. *J Cardiothorac Surg.* 2015;10(1):1–8. doi:10.1186/s13019-015-0296-8.
29. López-Ruiz JA, Tallón-Aguilar L, Marenco-de la Cuadra B, López-Pérez J, Oliva-Mompeán F, Padillo-Ruiz J. Leiomyosarcoma of the inferior vena cava. Case report and literature review. *Cir Cir.* 2017;85(4):361–365. doi:10.1016/j.circen.2017.07.003.

30. Baad-Hansen T, Freund SS, Bech BH, Keller J. Is there consensus regarding surgical treatment of bone sarcomas? *World J Orthop*. 2018;9(9):173–179.
31. Bellamy MC. Wet, dry or something else? *Br J Anaesth*. 2006; 97(6):755–757.
32. Michot A, Stoeckle E, Bannel JD, et al. The introduction of early patient rehabilitation in surgery of soft tissue sarcoma and its impact on post-operative outcome. *Eur J Surg Oncol*. 2015;41(12):1678–1684. doi:10.1016/j.ejso.2015.08.173.
33. Shehadeh A, Dahleh M El, Salem A, et al. Standardization of rehabilitation after limb salvage surgery for sarcomas improves patients' outcome. *Hematol Oncol Stem Cell Ther*. 2013;6(3–4): 105–111. doi:10.1016/j.hemonc.2013.09.001.
34. Farge D, Frere C, Connors JM, et al. 2019 International Clinical Practice Guidelines for the treatment and prophylaxis of venous thromboembolism in patients with cancer. *Lancet Oncol*. 2019;20(10):e566–e581.
35. Kehlet H, Dahl JB. The value of "multimodal" or "balanced analgesia" in postoperative pain treatment. *Anesth Analg*. 1993;77(5):1048–1056.
36. Rhodes LA. Pain management for sarcoma patients BT. In: Henshaw RM, ed. *Sarcoma: A Multidisciplinary Approach to Treatment*: Springer International Publishing; 2017.
37. Ascierto PA, Flaherty K, Goff S. Emerging strategies in systemic therapy for the treatment of melanoma. *Am Soc Clin Oncol Educ Book*. 2018;38:751–758.
38. Kwak M, Farrow NE, Salama AKS, et al. Updates in adjuvant systemic therapy for melanoma. *J Surg Oncol*. 2019;119(2):222–231. doi:10.1002/jso.25298.
39. Siegel RL, Miller KD. Jemal A. Cancer statistics, 2018. *CA Cancer J Clin*. 2018;68(1):7–30.
40. Cormier JN, Xing Y, Ding M, et al. Ethnic differences among patients with cutaneous melanoma. *Arch Intern Med*. 2006;166(17):1907–1914. doi:10.1001/archinte.166.17.1907.
41. Eide MJ, Weinstock MA. Association of UV index, latitude, and melanoma incidence in nonwhite populations—US Surveillance, Epidemiology, and End Results (SEER) Program, 1992 to 2001. *Arch Dermatol*. 2005;141(4):477–481. doi:10.1001/archderm.141.4.477.
42. Wu S, Han J, Laden F, Qureshi AA. Long-term ultraviolet flux, other potential risk factors, and skin cancer risk: a cohort study. *Cancer Epidemiol Biomarkers Prev*. 2014;23(6):1080–1089.
43. De Ann L, Vogel RI, Weinstock MA, Nelson HH, Ahmed RL, Berwick M. Association between indoor tanning and melanoma in younger men and women. *JAMA Dermatol*. 2016;152(3): 268–275.
44. Tucker MA, Halpern A, Holly EA, et al. Clinically recognized dysplastic nevi: a central risk factor for cutaneous melanoma. *JAMA*. 1997;277(18):1439–1444. doi:10.1001/jama.1997.03540420035026.
45. Chaudru V, Chompret A, Bressac-de Paillerets B, Spatz A, Avril MF, Demenais F. Influence of genes, nevi, and sun sensitivity on melanoma risk in a family sample unselected by family history and in melanoma-prone families. *J Natl Cancer Inst*. 2004;96(10):785–795.
46. Ascha M, Ascha MS, Tanenbaum J, Bordeaux JS. Risk factors for melanoma in renal transplant recipients. *JAMA Dermatol*. 2017;153(11):1130–1136.
47. Yde SS, Sjoegren P, Heje M, Stolle LB. Mucosal melanoma: a literature review. *Curr Oncol Rep*. 2018;20(3):28.
48. Curtin JA, Busam K, Pinkel D, Bastian BC. Somatic activation of KIT in distinct subtypes of melanoma. *J Clin Oncol*. 2019;24(26):4340–4346.
49. Ortega-Candil A, Rodriguez-Rey C, Cano-Carrizal R, et al. Breslow thickness and (18)F-FDG PET-CT result in initial staging of cutaneous melanoma: can a cut-off point be established? *Rev Esp Med Nucl Imagen Mol*. 2016;35(2):96–101.
50. Manson AL, Juneja R, Self R, Farquhar-Smith P, MacNeill F, Seneviratne SL. Anaphylaxis to patent blue V: a case series. *Asia Pac Allergy*. 2012;2(1):86.
51. Kroon HM, Coventry BJ, Giles MH, et al. Australian multicenter study of isolated limb infusion for melanoma. *Ann Surg Oncol*. 2016;23(4):1096–1103.
52. Gyorki DE, Yuan J, Mu Z, et al. Immunological insights from patients undergoing surgery on ipilimumab for metastatic melanoma. *Ann Surg Oncol*. 2013;20(9):3106–3111.
53. Klemen ND, Wang M, Feingold PL, et al. Patterns of failure after immunotherapy with checkpoint inhibitors predict durable progression-free survival after local therapy for metastatic melanoma. *J Immunother Cancer*. 2019;7(1):196.
54. Bello DM. Indications for the surgical resection of stage IV disease. *J Surg Oncol*. 2019;119(2):249–261.
55. Puza CJ, Bressler ES, Terando AM, et al. The emerging role of surgery for patients with advanced melanoma treated with immunotherapy. *J Surg Res*. 2019;236:209–215. doi:10.1016/j.jss.2018.11.045.
56. Lemiale V, Meert AP, Vincent F, et al. Severe toxicity from checkpoint protein inhibitors: what intensive care physicians need to know? *Ann Intensive Care*. 2019;9(1):1–16. doi:10.1186/s13613-019-0487-x.
57. Elias AW, Kasi PM, Stauffer JA, Thiel DD. The feasibility and safety of surgery in patients receiving immune checkpoint inhibitors: a retrospective study. *Front Oncol*. 2017;7:121.
58. Welsh SJ, Corrie PG. Management of BRAF and MEK inhibitor toxicities in patients with metastatic melanoma. *Ther Adv Med Oncol*. 2015;7(2):122–136.
59. De Giorgi V, Grazzini M, Benemei S, Marchionni N, Geppetti P, Gandini S. β-Blocker use and reduced disease progression in patients with thick melanoma: 8 years of follow-up. *Melanoma Res*. 2017;27(3):268–270.
60. Weberpals J, Jansen L, Carr PR, Hoffmeister M, Brenner H. Beta blockers and cancer prognosis - the role of immortal time bias: a systematic review and meta-analysis. *Cancer Treat Rev*. 2016;47(2016):1–11. doi:10.1016/j.ctrv.2016.04.004.

31

Perioperative Care of the Surgical Patient: Bone and Soft Tissue Tumors

LUIS FELIPE CUELLAR GUZMAN AND DORIAN YARIH GARCÍA-ORTEGA

Introduction

Orthopedic oncology is one of the newest subspecialties in orthopedics that specializes in the management of musculoskeletal tumors, which are slowly increasing globally.[1] The great variability of complexity and duration of oncologic orthopedic surgeries is such that there is no guide that can universalize the management for all patients. Surgery can range from short duration with limited bleeding to more demanding procedures such as sacrectomies or hemipelvectomies that require more complex management. Many procedures often require significant neurovascular dissection, removal of bone and/or significant muscle, replacement of large segments of bone and adjacent joints that may also require significant cement boluses for fixation, and free and rotational flaps. A clear understanding of what surgery implies allows proper positioning, airway management, and postoperative planning.[2–4]

Patients undergoing surgery to remove bone tumors have frequently received diverse preoperative medical treatments such as chemotherapy, radiotherapy, or a combination. The possible side effects of these agents are diverse. For example, doxorubicin, which is commonly used in bone chemotherapy, can cause dilated cardiomyopathy and arrhythmias. Bleomycin can lead to pulmonary fibrosis, and vincristine can contribute to peripheral neuropathy. In addition, patients who have undergone chemotherapy or radiotherapy may have significant anemia and thrombocytopenia, which could require transfusions of red blood cells or platelets. Obtaining adequate intravenous (IV) access and invasive monitors in preparation for resuscitation with fluids and possible transfusions can be a secondary challenge in ongoing cancer treatments. If the possibility of large blood loss due to a highly vascularized tumor is expected, preoperative tumor embolization may be considered.[5,6]

Oncoanesthesia and Some of the Crucial Steps for Better Perioperative Outcomes

Preoperative Evaluation

Patients with cancer, in addition to having many comorbidities, might have received previous treatments of chemotherapy or radiotherapy; therefore the surgical team must be aware of the side effects of these oncologic treatments on different body organs. In addition, it is crucial to be aware of the natural evolution of tumors. Comorbidities, such as diabetes, cardiovascular, pulmonary, cerebrovascular, and renal diseases, should be thoroughly investigated. The presence of previous chronic pain, use of anticoagulants or antiplatelet agents, and history of thromboembolic disease should be identified. In patients who received neoadjuvant therapies, a key question is whether they have experienced a decrease in their tolerance to exercise before and after treatment.[7]

Physical Examination

The surgical and anesthesiology team must pay special attention to the features/findings detected during examination that may complicate the surgery. For example, patients with malignancy in the head and neck area must undergo rigorous examination of the airway. Tumors can cause airway obstruction and injury to the recurrent laryngeal nerve, as well as vascular obstruction, resulting in superior vena cava syndrome, which can be aggravated with the use of positive pressure ventilation. In addition, it is important to consider that these patients may have received neoadjuvant radiotherapy and therefore undergone anatomic changes.[7]

Selecting an Anesthetic Technique

There is increasing evidence (mostly retrospective and in vitro) that anesthesiology techniques might influence the outcomes of oncologic procedures. Laboratory data show some signal toward positive or negative effects depending on the drug or intervention studied. Although there are many variables to consider in the choice of anesthetic technique, perhaps the most important in the cancer patient are anesthetic maintenance (total intravenous anesthesia [TIVA] with propofol or AGB with inhaled agents) and the use of regional anesthesia.

Anesthetic Maintenance

Different research protocols have concluded that volatile anesthetics induce apoptosis of natural killer cells (NK) and T lymphocytes, which might potentially lead to a deleterious influence on tumor metastases.[8] These agents increase angiogenesis by releasing hypoxia-inducible factor 1α (HIF-1α).[9] The increase in HIF correlates directly with the severity of the tumor, the risk of metastasis, and the presence of chemoresistance.[10] Propofol can be an alternative. It exerts its protective effects through several mechanisms, including antiinflammatory effects, type 2 cyclooxygenase (COX-2) inhibition and prostaglandin E_2 (PGE2) reduction, increased antitumor immunity, and preservation of NK cell function.[11] Propofol may also cause inhibition of matrix metalloproteinase (MMP), molecules that promote tumor invasion and dissemination.[12] A retrospective cohort in the UK reported a 5% increase in overall survival in the 5-year follow up among >2600 patients in those who received propofol as an anesthetic technique compared to an inhaled technique. In a retrospective analysis, patients undergoing surgery for breast, colon, and rectal cancer found that after adjustment for all variables, the differences were not statistically significant.[13] In another study in patients undergoing modified radical mastectomy, maintenance with propofol, compared with sevoflurane, reduced the recurrence rate at the 5-year follow up.

Regional Anesthesia

Regional anesthesia is commonly used in orthopedic procedures to prevent or mitigate the response to surgical stress by blocking afferent neural transmission, which prevents the nociceptive stimulus from reaching the central nervous system, while some techniques and anesthetics have been associated with better outcomes.[14,15] In two systematic reviews on the impact of different regional techniques (paravertebral block [PVB] and epidural) in patients with breast and gastroesophageal cancer, no difference was found in cancer outcomes compared to other anesthetic techniques.[15,16]

Orthopedic Cancers

Sarcomas

Regarding mortality due to malignant neoplasms of soft tissue sarcomas (STS), bone and joint sarcomas, people between 30 and 60 years have a mortality rate of 4 deaths per 100,000 inhabitants.[17] STS comprise a group of relatively rare, anatomically and histologically diverse malignancies. They share a common embryologic origin, which arises mainly from tissues derived from mesodermal or ectodermal germ layers.[18] The annual incidence of STS in the United States is approximately 13,130 new cases, with less than 1%–2% of cancer diagnoses.[19]

However, it is estimated that 5000 patients die annually from STS, which is almost 10 times higher than deaths due to testicular cancer. The development of sarcoma after the use of ionizing radiation for the treatment of lymphoma has been reported. Most sarcomas are associated with the use of high rate radiation (87%), and the predominant histologic types include undifferentiated pleomorphic sarcoma, angiosarcoma, and osteosarcoma.[20]

For sarcomas of the extremities, 5-year survival rates remain low, particularly in clinical stages III–IV, where it is 5%–10%.

The WHO classification classifies soft tissue and bone tumors into four categories according to clinical behavior: (1) benign; (2) medium, locally aggressive; (3) medium, rarely with metastases; and (4) malignant (i.e., sarcoma).

Clinical Presentation and Diagnosis

Most patients with STS have a painless mass, although pain is noticeable in the presentation in up to one-third of cases. Physical examination must include an evaluation of the size and mobility of the mass. It is important to note the location of the mass (superficial vs. deep) and nearby neurovascular and bone structures.

Treatment

Chemotherapy and radiation are usually administered before the surgery. These neoadjuvant treatments can reduce the size of the tumor and allow it to be completely removed.

Perfusion of Extremities

A form of hyperthermic intraoperative chemotherapy, using a tumor-containing limb with tumor necrosis factor-alpha (TNF-α), interferon-alpha (IFN-α), and melphalan, has been described. This technique has been used as a neoadjuvant therapy to facilitate tumor resection and as a primary therapy to prevent amputation in patients with STS of unresectable limbs. Regarding side effects, chronic edema is the most common long-term complication.[21]

Bone Tumors

Malignant bone tumors account for a small percentage of cancers nationwide and are much less common than soft tissue malignancies. The most common primary malignant bone tumors, osteosarcoma and Ewing sarcoma, present in childhood. Chondrosarcoma occurs most often in older adults. Rare tumors such as chordoma and adamantinoma have anatomic predilections for the sacrum and tibia, respectively. The main symptom of a patient with a malignant bone tumor is pain, which often occurs at rest or at night. There are also characteristic findings on physical examination such as swelling or decreased range of motion of the joints. Patients with possible malignancy require complete staging to determine the extent of the disease and a well-planned biopsy for an accurate diagnosis. Biopsy may be an image-guided needle biopsy or open incisional biopsy. It is important to know the specific characteristics of the tumor and the treatment options for osteosarcoma, Ewing sarcoma, chondrosarcoma, malignant fibrous histiocytoma, chordoma, and adamantinoma. Patients with resectable osteosarcoma and Ewing sarcoma are treated with chemotherapy followed by surgical resection. Secondary sarcomas can occur in previously benign bone lesions and require aggressive treatment. There are specific techniques for the resection of malignant bone tumors of the upper and lower extremities, pelvis, and spine. Reconstruction options include the use of vascularized allografts, megaprostheses, and autografts. There has been a trend toward more prosthetic reconstructions due to early complications with allografts. The care of patients with primary malignant bone tumors requires a multidisciplinary approach to treatment.[22]

Regional Anesthesia and Cancer

It is important to avoid a prooncogenic environment in patients with an already altered response toward their environment and, consequently, to surgical stimuli. Surgical tumor resection remains the main technique for the treatment of most types of cancer. The anesthesiologist's role is to select appropriate techniques to reduce the release of proinflammatory cytokines in the perioperative period. Regional anesthesia may have a modest role, but there is currently no concrete clinical evidence to support this hypothesis. A well-applied peripheral blockade can positively influence early postoperative outcomes, such as better analgesia and better quality of recovery in patients with cancer.[15,16]

Combining peripheral regional techniques with general anesthesia may reduce the use of IV opioid consumption, which may facilitate earlier postoperative recovery.

Anesthetic Agents and Impact on the Immune System

Volatile Anesthetics

The available evidence is limited, and most of it comes from experimental studies. However, there is a signal toward the suppressive effect of volatile anesthetics on the immune system of patients with cancer.

Sevoflurane induces apoptosis of T lymphocytes, increases HIF-1α, increases plasma levels of protumorigenic cytokines (interleukin [IL]-1β, TNF-α, and IL-6) and MMPs that have been associated with modifications in the oncologic outcomes. It also decreases the amount and activity of NK cells.[8]

In a small retrospective analysis, progression-free survival time for women with ovarian cancer was longer for women who received desflurane than for those who received sevoflurane anesthesia. However, such retrospective analyses are inherently limited and do not warrant a change in practice.[23]

Intravenous Anesthetics

By contrast, propofol inhibits HIF-1α and inhibits the production of prostanoids by suppressing the activity of COX-2, induces apoptosis, and suppresses proliferation, cell adhesion, migration, and angiogenesis in various cancer cell lines.[16–19] Theoretically, these laboratory model characteristics may be beneficial to patients with osteosarcoma and other cancers. Recent experimental data have shown a reduction of IL-6 up to 6 h after surgery, inhibition of nuclear factor kappa B (NF-κB), inhibition of neutrophil activation, and proinflammatory regulation of synthetase oxide and cyclooxygenase.[24]

Regarding the use of alpha-2 agonists, mainly dexmedetomidine, a potential beneficial effect was initially associated with a reduction in the use of volatile opioids and anesthetics, in addition to immunoprotective and antiinflammatory properties.[25,26] However, recent data suggest that dexmedetomidine may promote tumor growth and stimulate prometastatic modification of the tumor microenvironment.[27–29]

Opioids

The impact of opioid use on patients with cancer is controversial. Morphine suppresses both the activity of NK cells and the differentiation of T lymphocytes, promotes lymphocyte apoptosis, and decreases the expression of Toll-like receptor 4 (TLR4).[30–34] Fentanyl and sufentanyl have similar effects decreasing NK cell activity; however, they increase the amount of regulatory T cells.[35–36] Sufentanyl apparently also inhibits leukocyte migration,[37] while alfentanil decreases the activity of NK cells.[30]

It is important to emphasize that the mu opioid receptor (MOR) is expressed in various tumor and nontumor cell types, and despite the predominantly immunosuppressive nature of opioids, it is important to note that their effects depend on the type of opioid administered, total dose, and additional conditions.[31]

Opioids also have immunomodulatory properties; for example, morphine induces changes in macrophages from M1 to M2. This effect is consistent with the increase in COX-2 expression in macrophages.[32]

In murine in vivo models, continuous use of morphine compared to its intermittent use is more likely to inhibit tumor growth and metastasis.[33]

Based on the evidence proposed, it is possible to infer that not only the type of opioid used, but also the dose may influence their effect on cancer cell biology. However, at present, there is no clinical evidence that warrants any change in practice. Therefore cancer patients for whom opioids are indicated for postoperative analgesia should receive them without hesitation.

Nonsteroidal Antiinflammatory Drugs

Few studies have focused on the perioperative effects of nonsteroidal antiinflammatory drug (NSAID) use in terms of possible oncologic effects.

Choi et al. concluded that the use of ketorolac in patients with lung cancer resulted in better disease-free survival, while Forget et al. found that it was independently associated with a lower risk of metastasis and greater survival. Both are inherently limited retrospective studies.[37]

Local Anesthetics

Recent studies have reported that both lidocaine and ropivacaine can inhibit the growth, invasion, and migration of tumor cells in vitro. In addition to inducing apoptosis,[3,8] antiinflammatory properties were evident with IV lidocaine use.[38,39]

In vitro studies of tongue cancer cells found that amide local anesthetics inhibited cancer cell migration by epidermal growth factor receptor (EGFR) inhibition.[40] Other studies involving the use of ropivacaine and bupivacaine reported beneficial effects in specific cancer cell lines such as breast cancer via DNA demethylation.[41]

Conclusions

The complexity of managing orthopedic oncologic patients requires close multidisciplinary collaboration.

As for all tumor types, no specific anesthetic agent or technique is superior to any other at the present state of knowledge.

References

1. Siegel RL, Miller KD, Jemal A. Cancer statistics, 2019. *CA Cancer J Clin*. 2019;69(1):7–34.
2. Puri A. Orthopedic oncology– 'the challenges ahead'. *Front Surg*. 2014;1:27.
3. Trovarelli G, Ruggieri P. Rehabilitation for older patients with musculoskeletal oncologic disease. In: Masiero, G, Carraro, U, eds. *Rehabilitation Medicine for Elderly Patients. Springer, Cham*. 2018:287–291.
4. Henrichs MP, Krebs J, Gosheger G, Streitbuerger A, Nottrott M, Sauer T, Hoell S, Singh G, Hardes J. Modular tumor endoprostheses in surgical palliation of long-bone metastases: a reduction in tumor burden and a durable reconstruction. *World J Surg Oncol*. 2014;12:330.
5. Anderson MR, Leng CJ, Wittig JC, Rosenblatt MA Anesthesia for patients undergoing orthopedic oncologic surgeries. *J Clin Anesth*. 2010;22(7):565–572.
6. Wigmore T, Gottumukkala V, Riedel B. Making the case for the subspecialty of onco-anesthesia. *Int Anesthesiol Clin*. 2016;54(4):19–28.
7. Sahai SK. Perioperative assessment of the cancer patient. *Best Pract Res Clin Anaesthesiol*. 2013;27(4):465–480.
8. Kim R. Effects of surgery and anesthetic choice on immunosuppression and cancer recurrence. *J Transl Med*. 2018;16(1):8.
9. Tavare AN, Perry NJ, Benzonana LL, Takata M, Ma D. Cancer recurrence after surgery: direct and indirect effects of anesthetic agents. *Int J Cancer*. 2012;130(6):1237–1250.
10. Unwith S, Zhao H, Hennah L, Ma D. The potential role of HIF on tumor progression and dissemination. *Int J Cancer*. 2015;136(11):2491–2503.
11. Cassinello F, Prieto I, del Olmo M, Rivas S, Strichartz GR. Cancer surgery: how may anesthesia influence outcome? *J Clin Anesth*. 2015;27(3):262–272.
12. Miao Y, Zhang Y, Wan H, Chen L, Wang F. GABA-receptor agonist, propofol inhibits invasion of colon carcinoma cells. *Biomed Pharmacother*. 2010;64(9):583–588.
13. Enlund M, Berglund A, Andreasson K, Cicek C, Enlund A, Bergkvist L. The choice of anesthetic—sevoflurane or propofol—and outcome from cancer surgery: a retrospective analysis. *Ups J Med Sci*. 2014;119(3):251–261.
14. Pérez-González O, Cuéllar-Guzmán LF, Soliz J, Cata JP. Impact of regional anesthesia on recurrence, metastasis, and immune response in breast cancer surgery: a systematic review of the literature. *Reg Anesth Pain Med*. 2017;42(6):751–756.
15. Pérez-González O, Cuéllar-Guzmán LF, Navarrete-Pacheco M, Ortiz-Martínez JJ, Williams WH, Cata JP. Impact of regional anesthesia on gastroesophageal cancer surgery outcomes: a systematic review of the literature. *Anesth Analg*. 2018;127(3):753–758.
16. Aldaco-Sarvide F. Mortalidad por cáncer en México. *Gac Mex Oncol*. 2018;17:28–34.
17. Potter JW, Jones KB, Barrott JJ. Sarcoma–the standard-bearer in cancer discovery. *Crit Rev Oncol Hematol*. 2018;126:1–5.
18. Siegel RL, Miller KD, Jemal A. Cancer statistics, 2020. *CA Cancer J Clin*. 2020;70(1):7–30.
19. Gladdy RA, Qin LX, Moraco N, Edgar MA, Antonescu CR, Alektiar KM, Brennan MF, Singer S. Do radiation- associated soft tissue sarcomas have the same prognosis as sporadic soft tissue sarcomas? *J Clin Oncol*. 2010;28(12):2064–2069.
20. Jo VY, Doyle LA. Refinements in sarcoma classification in the current 2013 World Health Organization classification of tumors of soft tissue and bone. *Surg Oncol Clin N Am*. 2016;25(4):621–643.
21. Weber K, Damron TA, Frassica FJ, Sim FH. Malignant bone tumors. *Instr Course Lect*. 2008;57:673–688.
22. Elias KM, Kang S, Liu X, Horowitz NS, Berkowitz RS, Frendl G. Anesthetic selection and disease-free survival following optimal primary cytoreductive surgery for stage III epithelial ovarian cancer. *Ann Surg Oncol*. 2015;22(4):1341–1348.
23. Kairaluoma PM, Bachmann MS, Korpinen AK, Rosenberg PH, Pere PJ. Single-injection paravertebral block before general anesthesia enhances analgesia after breast cancer surgery with and without associated lymph node biopsy. *Anesth Analg*. 2004;99(6):1837–1843.
24. Mowbray A, Wong KK, Murray JM. Intercostal catheterization: an alternative approach to the paravertebral space. *Anaesthesia*. 1987;42(9):958–961.
25. Fajardo M, García FJ, López S, Dieguez P, Alfaro P. Bloqueo de las ramas cutáneas laterales y anteriores de los nervios intercostales para analgesia de mama. *Cir Maj Amb*. 2012;17:95–104.
26. Pérez MF, Álvarez SL, García PD, de la Torre PA, Miguel FG. Abordaje ecoguiado de las ramas cutáneas de los nervios intercostales a nivel de la línea axilar para cirugía no reconstructiva de mama. A new ultrasound-guided cutaneous intercostal branches nerves blocked for analgesia after no reconscturctive breast surgery. *Cir May AMB*. 2013;18(1):3–6.

27. López-Matamala B, Fajardo M, Estébanez-Montiel B, Blancas R, Alfaro P, Chana M. A new thoracic interfascial plane block as anesthesia for difficult weaning due to ribcage pain in critically ill patients. *Med Intensiva.* 2014;38(7):463–465.
28. García PD, Pérez MF, Álvarez SL, de la Torre PA, Castiñeiras APP, Ultrasound-assisted approach to blocking the intercostal nerves in the mid-axillary line for non-reconstructive breast and axilla surgery. *Rev Esp Anestesiol Reanim.* 2013;60(7):365–370.
29. Xu YB, Jiang W, Zhao FR, Li G, Du QH, Zhang MY, Guo XG. Propofol suppresses invasion and induces apoptosis of osteosarcoma cell in vitro via downregulation of TGF-beta1 expression. *Eur Rev Med Pharmacol Sci.* 2016;20(7):1430–1435.
30. Das J, Kumar S, Khanna S, Mehta Y. Are we causing the recurrence–impact of perioperative period on long-term cancer prognosis: review of current evidence and practice. *J Anaesthesiol Clin Pharmacol.* 2014;30(2):153–159.
31. Yardeni IZ, Beilin B, Mayburd E, Alcalay Y, Bessler H. Relationship between fentanyl dosage and immune function in the postoperative period. *J Opioid Manag.* 2008;4(1):27–33.
32. Godai K, Hasegawa-Moriyama M, Kurimoto T, et al. Peripheral administration of morphine attenuates post incisional pain by regulating macrophage polarization through COX-2-dependent pathway. *Mol Pain.* 2014;10:36.
33. Afsharimani B, Doornebal CW, Cabot PJ, Hollmann MW, Parat MO. Comparison and analysis of the animal models used to study the effect of morphine on tumor growth and metastasis. *Br J Pharmacol.* 2015;172(2):251–259.
34. Martinet L, Jean C, Dietrich G, Fournié JJ, Poupot R. PGE2 inhibits natural killer and γδ T cell cytotoxicity triggered by NKR and TCR through a cAMP-mediated PKA type I-dependent signaling. *Biochem Pharmacol.* 2010;80(6):838–845.
35. Chattopadhyay S, Bhattacharyya S, Saha B, et al. Tumor-shed PGE (2) impairs IL2Rgammac-signaling to inhibit CD4T cell survival: regulation by theaflavins. *PLoS One.* 2009;4(10):e7382.
36. Ahmadi M, Emery DC, Morgan DJ. Prevention of both direct and cross-priming of antitumor CD8+ T-cell responses following overproduction of prostaglandin E2 by tumor cells in vivo. *Cancer Res.* 2008;68(18):7520–7529.
37. Choi JE, Villarreal J, Lasala J, et al. Perioperative neutrophil: lymphocyte ratio and postoperative NSAID use as predictors of survival after lung cancer surgery: a retrospective study. *Cancer Med.* 2015;4(6):825–833.
38. Wang HW, Wang LY, Jiang L, Tian SM, Zhong TD, Fang XM. Amide-linked local anesthetics induce apoptosis in human non-small cell lung cancer. *J Thorac Dis.* 2016;8(10):2748–2757.
39. Herroeder S, Pecher S, Schönherr ME, et al. Systemic lidocaine shortens length of hospital stay after colorectal surgery: a double-blinded, randomized, placebo-controlled trial. *Ann Surg.* 2007; 246(2):192–200.
40. Sakaguchi M, Kuroda Y, Hirose M. The antiproliferative effect of lidocaine on human tongue cancer cells with inhibition of the activity of epidermal growth factor receptor. *Anesth Analg.* 2006;102(4):1103–1107.
41. Li R, Xiao C, Liu H, Huang Y, Dilger JP, Lin J. Effects of local anesthetics on breast cancer cell viability and migration. *BMC Cancer.* 2018;18(1):666.

32

Perioperative Care of the Surgical Patient: Reconstructive Surgery

CHRISTELLE BOTHA, ANNA LOUISE WAYLEN, AND MICHELLE GERSTMAN

Applied Surgical, Pathologic, and Physiologic Concepts

General

The resection of tumors may cause large aesthetically and functionally unacceptable defects. Similarly, adjuvant therapies may leave functional tissue impairment or chronic nonhealing wounds requiring excision and reconstruction. Reconstructive surgery aims to obliterate dead space, provide structural support for remaining tissues, ensure adequate wound closure and healing, and maintain an aesthetically acceptable appearance.

Flap surgery has improved markedly over the last few decades, with success rates of greater than 95% reported. This is the result of enhanced microsurgical techniques and an evolving appreciation for perioperative optimization. In this setting of progress, however, anesthetic perioperative management of free flap surgery is varied,[1] reflecting the paucity of high-level evidence guiding best practice. Continued critical review of current flap surgery literature and extrapolation from other surgical fields is imperative to improve outcomes.

Surgical Concepts

Autologous flap reconstructions can be categorized as "pedicled" or "free." A pedicled flap remains partially connected to the donor site via an intact vascular pedicle. The pedicle is at most 5 cm long, limiting reconstruction to local defects. A latissimus dorsi flap, used in breast reconstruction, is a commonly used example. Free flaps are completely detached from the donor site and constitute any combination of skin, fat, fascia, muscle, bone, nerves, bowel, or omentum. These flaps are used for more distant reconstructions.

There are several distinct phases during free flap surgery. In the initial phase, donor tissue and its vascular pedicle (artery and vein) are *dissected* or *raised*. The *clamping* and *division* of the pedicle leads to cessation of blood flow to the donor tissue. This *primary ischemic phase* varies in duration but typically lasts between 60 and 90 min. Donor blood vessels are then *anastomosed* to distant recipient blood vessels using microsurgical techniques. Restoration of blood flow and reversal of the effects of anaerobic metabolism occur during this *reperfusion phase*. This phase, also called the *secondary ischemic phase*, is susceptible to ischemic reperfusion injury.

There is a single surgical anastomosis of each vascular pedicle, making free flaps extremely vulnerable to hypoperfusion and venous congestion. Common causes of impaired blood flow include arterial or venous thrombosis at the anastomotic site, arterial vasospasm, and insufficient venous drainage. Ruptured anastomosis with hematoma formation, tightly applied dressings, and poorly positioned equipment can cause external compression on the pedicle. Some vascular pedicles are prone to kinking or stretching with changes in patient positioning. Prolonged ischemic times and flap hypoperfusion secondary to low cardiac output states may exacerbate the secondary ischemic injury.

Pathologic Concepts Associated With Free Flap Complications: The Endothelial Glycocalyx, Inflammation, and Ischemic Reperfusion Injury

The endothelial glycocalyx (EG) is a gel-like structure, lining the intraluminal surface of the endothelial cells of all blood vessels and organs. It has several well-defined functions and plays an integral role in blood vessel wall integrity. It is a delicate structure and can rapidly change under certain metabolic and inflammatory conditions. Lifestyle risk factors (obesity, smoking), adjuvant treatments (radiotherapy), and chronic pathologic conditions (hyperglycemia, renal and cardiovascular disease) predisposes this delicate structure to pathologic insults.[2,3] Acute degradation of the EG has also been observed in patients undergoing major surgery, leading to capillary leak, platelet aggregation, and loss of vascular responsiveness.[4] In the perioperative setting, this can result in tissue edema, detrimental to wound healing, acute kidney injury, increased risk of venous thromboembolism (VTE), and lability of arterial pressure.

Flap surgery has the potential to cause major systemic inflammatory perturbation in the postoperative period. Large, multisite tissue disruption, and ischemic reperfusion injury, seen within the flap microvasculature, can cause disruption to the composition and structure of the fragile EG. Degradation leads to loss of the barrier function between blood components and the underlying vessel wall. The adhesion of circulating immune cells and activation of several proinflammatory pathways cause further disruption and dysfunction within this layer. These pathologic processes may progress and lead to localized effects (flap complications, organ dysfunction) or systemic effects (systemic inflammatory response syndrome, coagulopathies).[2,5]

Following ischemic reperfusion injury, deactivation of some of the protective antioxidative enzymes within the EG leads to oxidative stress. This includes the deactivation of superoxide, a natural antioxidant active within the EG, which keeps reactive oxygen species and free radicals in equilibrium under physiologic conditions. It also has a role in the functionality and release of other antioxidants such as nitric oxide. Nitric oxide causes localized vasodilation in response to increases in shear stress (increased blood flow). Therefore a reduction in its levels will result in loss of microvascular autoregulation, possibly compromising reperfusion.

In addition a degraded and exposed endothelium is vulnerable to platelet adhesion and activation of the coagulation cascade with subsequent thrombus propagation. As previously mentioned, venous and arterial thrombosis can be detrimental to flap viability. Venous thrombosis is more prevalent than arterial thrombosis.

Blood flow and oxygen delivery to free flap tissue may become impaired with a rise in local interstitial tissue pressure. Several factors predispose free flap tissues to this pathologic process.

In its physiologic state, the EG is a protein-rich layer that contributes significantly to intravascular oncotic pressure. According to the revised Starling equation,[5] this oncotic pressure is an important factor opposing fluid filtration across the endothelial layer into the interstitium. With degradation and loss of the protein content of the EG, the layer becomes more permeable with increased filtration of fluid and other intravascular molecules into the interstitium. This is commonly seen in inflammatory states and contributes to a decrease in the half-life of intravenous (IV) crystalloids and colloids alike.[3,6,7] Reabsorption of interstitial fluid relies exclusively on intact lymphatic flow and not on reabsorption from the venous capillaries, as previously stated by the original Starling equation. Transplanted free flap tissues are devoid of an intact lymphatic system and therefore vulnerable to any increase in fluid accumulation.

Perioperative fluid management is known to have a profound impact upon the integrity of the glycocalyx[8]: acute hypervolemic hemodilution causes EG injury by mechanical stress on the vascular wall and via the secretion of atrial natriuretic peptide. This peptide is secreted in response to atrial stretch, which can be a consequence of rapidly infused IV fluid. It also increases microvascular permeability permitting fluid and colloid extravasation into the interstitium.[3] Studies have shown that when 5% human albumin or 6% hydroxyethyl starch (HES) is infused into a normovolemic patient, 60% of the colloid rapidly extravasates into the interstitium.[5]

The combination of the above-mentioned pathologic processes are likely reasons why multiple studies specific to flap surgery have linked high volumes of IV fluids with worse surgical (wound healing, flap failure) and medical (pulmonary congestion) outcomes.[9–12]

Relevant to cancer surgery, the EG layer also acts as a barrier to prevent interaction between the ligands on circulating tumor cells and the adhesion receptors on endothelial cells. Following surgical tissue damage, inflammatory activation of procoagulant and prothrombotic pathways may cause clot formation in the microvasculature and platelet adhesion onto circulating tumor cells. This pathologic process has two consequences. The platelet coat on the circulating tumor cells decreases detection by host defense mechanisms such as natural killer cells. In addition, microvascular occlusion promotes adhesion of these cells onto the degraded endothelium, enabling migration across this layer. In effect, inflammatory mediators may contribute to colonization and lymphatic spread, promoting metastasis.[7,13]

Hyperoxia causes increased levels of reactive oxygen species with increased tissue destruction after ischemic reperfusion injury. Studies looking at outcomes after ischemic events such as cerebral vascular accidents and myocardial infarction have linked hyperoxia with expansion of infarct size and worse outcomes.[14,15] Intraoperative inspired oxygen concentrations should be carefully titrated to the arterial partial pressure of oxygen (Pao_2) deemed appropriate for the clinical setting. Perioperative measures to improve pulmonary function should be employed to reduce the need for and duration of oxygen therapy.

In conclusion, seemingly safe routine perioperative therapies such as IV fluid and oxygen therapy can potentially cause harm by exacerbating the degradation of the EG seen during surgery. Possible strategies to reduce EG breakdown are discussed in the section on Strategies for Hemodynamic Optimization.

Physiology of Flap Perfusion and Relevant Perioperative Factors

The blood supply and drainage of free flap tissue can be complex. One cannot assume that an isolated understanding of the physiologic laws governing blood flow is sufficient. Instead, there is a dynamic and complex interplay between the pathologic and other physiologic processes requiring more complex consideration.

The Hagen-Poiseuille law is frequently used to describe the determinants of flap perfusion/flow:

$$Q = \Delta P \pi r^4 / 8 \eta l$$

where Q (flow) is directly proportional to ΔP (perfusion pressure) and the fourth power of r (radius), and inversely proportional to η (viscosity) and l (length of the tube).

The radius of the blood vessels is an important determinant of blood flow but is not constant and homogeneous within the flap. This can be due to a number of independent factors. Irregularities in the endothelial layer close to the surgical anastomosis will invariably cause turbulence in blood flow and a decrease in the radius of the blood vessel. Reperfusion injury causes localized vasospasm, as well as shedding of the endothelial cells and glycocalyx with resultant microthrombus formation and propagation. Surgical manipulation and cold exposure of the vascular pedicle may also cause vasospasm. In addition, acute denervation of pedicle blood vessels causes an attenuated vasoconstrictor response to systemic catecholamines. As a result, normal physiologic laws do not hold true, and medical interventions aimed at altering the radius of the blood vessels might not reliably lead to improvements of blood flow.

The Hagen-Poiseuille law states that cardiac output is directly related to a pressure differential across a vascular bed. This is one of the reasons why routine intraoperative blood pressure (macrovascular) monitoring is used as a surrogate for tissue perfusion (microvascular). This has several limitations, as follows.

Cardiac output or blood flow is also dependent on systemic vascular resistance, as seen in the following equation:

Cardiac output = (mean arterial pressure – right atrial pressure)/systemic vascular resistance

An increase in peripheral resistance seen after the administration of a vasopressor agent may lead to an increase in blood pressure but a decrease in flow or cardiac output. This may compromise the free flap tissues. Additionally, the physiologic response to a hypovolemic state is to preserve perfusion pressure to vital organs at the expense of nonvital organs (skin and fat in the free flap). As a consequence, a predetermined target blood pressure may not reflect adequate flap perfusion and may be falsely reassuring.

Under physiologic conditions, there is an expectation that microvascular perfusion will improve in parallel with macrovascular optimization. This is referred to as hemodynamic coherence.[16] Loss of hemodynamic coherence has been described in states of infection, inflammation, and reperfusion injury. The resultant impaired function of the endothelium and the EG leads to microvascular obstruction, vasoconstriction, and interstitial edema, despite correction of the macrovascular parameters. Regardless, optimization of the macrovascular parameters should be primarily achieved prior to targeting the microcirculation.

Noninvasive, intraoperative optical techniques may be used in real time to assess the microcirculation of free flap tissue. Novel techniques under investigation include optical coherence tomography (vessel density and decorrelation), side-stream darkfield microscopy (velocity, microvascular flow index, total vessel density, perfused vessel density), laser speckle contrast imaging (perfusion units), and fluorescence imaging (time constant and time to peak measured).[17] Once integrated into standard practice, these bedside measurements may allow for dynamic assessment of medical interventions to optimize macrovascular parameters and flap tissue perfusion.

Strategies for Hemodynamic Optimization

Surgical intervention leads to an increase in oxygen consumption and metabolic demand. The aim of hemodynamic optimization is to reduce tissue hypoperfusion and meet the increased metabolic demands of the tissues. These measures should be instituted in the early preoperative period and may be continued postoperatively to overcome potential oxygen debt.

Preoperative Carbohydrate Drinks

Adequate preoperative hydration starts with minimization of fasting times. Complex carbohydrate drinks up to 2 h prior to surgery are safe and improve metabolism, and decrease insulin resistance and postoperative nausea and vomiting (PONV).[18] Postoperatively, early transition to oral hydration should be encouraged, and IV fluids should be discontinued once the patient is hemodynamically stable.

Goal-Directed Therapy

Perioperative administration of IV fluid plays a pivotal role in patient management and has a direct impact on outcomes. The principles of IV fluid administration are to maintain central normovolemia for optimal cellular perfusion and to avoid interstitial edema from salt and water excess.[19] The utilization of goal-directed therapy (GDT) allows for tailored IV fluid, inotropic, and vasoactive agent administration. Contemporary minimally invasive devices derive measurements such as cardiac index, stroke volume, or stroke volume variation from pulse power analysis, pulse contour analysis, and esophageal Doppler monitoring.[20] Medical therapy is titrated according to these explicit targets that reflect end-organ blood flow.

Although a large number of randomized trials have been conducted investigating the effect of GDT on perioperative outcomes, concerns exist regarding the quality of studies, with the majority being single-center trials with methodological limitations and risk of bias. A systematic review and meta-analysis of 31 studies carried out by the Cochrane group in 2013[21] found no difference in mortality between patients receiving GDT compared with controls, but reported a significant reduction in overall complication rate and a reduced rate of renal and respiratory failure, wound infection, and length of hospital stay (LOHS). Two multicenter studies with larger participant numbers investigating the effects of GDT have been published since this review.[22,23] Addition of the OPTIMISE study,[22] a multicenter randomized trial of high-risk patients undergoing major gastrointestinal surgery, to the original meta-analysis confirmed an overall reduction in complication rates across trials when GDT was utilized. These findings were reproduced in the FEDORA trial, where patients were randomized to GDT with optimization of circulating volume prior to vasopressor use versus standard care[23]: significantly fewer complications were observed in the GDT group, and again a reduction in LOHS was observed. Finally, a recent meta-analysis of 95 randomized controlled trials comparing GDT versus standard hemodynamic care showed a reduction in mortality and complications,[24] although a high risk of bias and poor methodological quality was again present in a number of included studies.

Studies specific to autologous breast flap surgery comparing standard care with GDT in combination with an Enhanced Recovery After Surgery (ERAS) protocol have shown a reduction in LOHS with no difference in complications.[25–28] The average amount of intraoperative fluids used in the GDT group averaged 3.85 L versus 5.5 L in the preimplementation group.

Central line placement in free flap surgery is not indicated unless prolonged vasoactive infusions are anticipated. Central venous pressure monitoring does not improve hemodynamic optimization and has been associated with worse outcomes and complications from line placement.[27,29]

Intraoperative oliguria defined as urine output of less than 0.5 mL/kg/h has not been correlated with acute kidney injury in noncardiac surgery. Oliguria should not be interpreted in isolation. Careful consideration of the patient's comorbidities, the clinical context, and other hemodynamic parameters should be used as a guide for fluid resuscitation.[30]

Choice of Intravenous Fluid Therapy

Consensus has been reached within the anesthesia community that perioperative IV fluid therapy to meet maintenance fluid requirements should consist of the infusion of balanced crystalloid solutions, with the avoidance of 0.9% saline. Administration of saline results in hyperchloremic metabolic acidosis and has been associated with renal dysfunction, increased LOHS, and increased mortality in patients undergoing noncardiac surgery.[31] There is insufficient evidence to preferentially direct the choice of balanced crystalloid specifically for reconstructive surgery. Rate of infusion of maintenance crystalloid is pertinent in the perioperative management of these patients, primarily in the avoidance of iatrogenic fluid overload and the resultant effects on EG disruption previously discussed. A recent systematic review recommended intraoperative volume replacement during autologous tissue transfer surgery to be maintained between 3.5 and 6.0 mL/kg/h.[32]

Ongoing debate continues regarding whether HES colloids are safe to administer in the perioperative period for volume therapy. Significant concerns regarding the use of HES and the risk of acute kidney injury in critically unwell patients have resulted in cautious perioperative use, although evidence from recent trials is challenging this mindset. A systematic review and meta-analysis of the impact of perioperative administration of HES reported no difference in risk of acute kidney injury in the *elective* surgical setting with colloid use, although the authors noted that trials were typically small and underpowered.[33] Results from two larger randomized controlled trials recently published confirm these findings: GDT consisting of colloid versus crystalloid boluses revealed no increased risk of renal toxicity with colloid administration, with one study reporting an increase in disability-free survival in the treatment group.[34,35]

A paucity of studies examining the effect of IV colloid infusion specifically during autologous reconstruction surgery exists. A single study compared the effects of HES and 5% albumin solution for volume replacement therapy during major reconstructive head and neck (HN) surgery,[36] with both colloids effectively maintaining physiologic variables in the perioperative period. No difference in outcome was observed until an excess of 30 mL/kg HES occurred over a 24-h period, which was associated with coagulopathy and increased risk of allogenic blood transfusion. Allogenic blood transfusion has been associated with increased mortality[37] and surgical site infection[38] following free flap reconstructive surgery for oral cancer.

Historically, the rheological properties of dextran, a complex branched glucan polysaccharide, were thought to confer benefit in reconstructive flap surgery for prophylaxis of microvascular thrombosis. This ideology has since been disproved, with a significant increase in risk of flap failure with dextran use observed in high-risk oncologic patients, no observed benefit in flap survival,[39] and an association with higher incidence of systemic complications, including unwanted bleeding, acute renal failure, allergic reactions, and cerebral edema.[40]

Vasoactive and Inotropic Drugs

Utilization of vasopressor support in an attempt to improve end-organ perfusion and reduce perioperative complications requires consideration of not only the resultant mean arterial pressure achieved but also the context in which the vasopressor is used with regard to both circulating intravascular volume and adequacy of flow. Vasopressor use in the setting of hypovolemia may be detrimental to tissue and microcirculatory blood flow, and optimization of circulating volume prior to vasopressor use should be considered in the perioperative period.

It is known that sustained periods of intraoperative hypotension should be avoided due to their association with adverse outcomes: myocardial injury, acute kidney injury, and increased risk of mortality. A recent consensus statement from the perioperative quality initiative stated that even brief durations of systolic blood pressures <100 mmHg or mean arterial pressures <60–70 mmHg are harmful during noncardiac surgery.[41] A novel trial reported that individualized targeting of systolic blood pressure within 10% of baseline value significantly reduced the risk of organ dysfunction compared with standard care.[42]

The use of vasoactive and inotropic drugs during flap surgery remains contentious. Concerns exist that these drugs may cause anastomotic and flap microvascular vasoconstriction, limiting flap tissue perfusion. Multiple studies have demonstrated no link between perioperative vasoactive/inotropic agent use and flap complications, including flap failure.[11,43–47] The acute denervation of pedicle blood vessels changes their response upon exposure to vasoconstrictor agents. Specifically, they have an attenuated response; hence vasoconstriction may not occur at these sites despite the administration of a vasoconstrictor such as noradrenaline. This is in contrast to the vasoconstriction seen in innervated skin blood vessels.[48] Another contributory explanation is the anticipated increase in the cardiac index with appropriate inotropic drug administration in normovolemic patients. This may result in increased flap perfusion.

With respect to choice of agent, noradrenaline increases free flap skin blood flow in hypotensive patients in a dose-dependent manner. Dobutamine increases free flap blood flow to a lesser extent without increasing mean arterial blood pressure. The use of dobutamine may be limited by tachycardia, especially in patients predisposed to ischemic heart disease.[48] Adrenaline and dopexamine both decrease free flap skin blood flow and are not suitable agents for flap surgery. Milrinone, an inodilator, does not improve free flap outcomes and is associated with increased intraoperative use of vasopressor support.[49]

Therapies Targeting the Endothelial Glycocalyx

Therapeutic approaches aimed to protect or restore the EG against injury represent a promising direction in clinical medicine. Strategies to reduce oxidative stress and inflammation may include the perioperative use of glucocorticoids, human plasma, plasma augmented with albumin,[2] and IV lidocaine.[50] There is currently insufficient evidence supporting the routine integration of these modalities into clinical practice.

Perioperative Considerations for Microvascular Free Flap Transfer Procedures

Patient outcomes are broadly determined by an interplay of three major variables: the extent of the surgical insult, the patient's risk factors as determined by acute and chronic medical disease, and the quality of the perioperative care they receive.

The extent of tissue injury during flap reconstruction can be considerable. There may be numerous surgical sites, including the area of cancer ablation surgery, and one or more donor sites for flap harvesting. This may result in significant metabolic and physiologic derangements. Anticipating these disturbances is important for anesthetic planning and potential patient optimization.

Patient risk factors, as determined by their comorbidities and diseases of lifestyle, should be identified and modified where possible. There is emerging evidence that risk factors, such as smoking and hyperglycemia, affect the EG and predispose patients to inflammatory processes in the perioperative period.[2] In addition, cancer burden and neoadjuvant therapies may further contribute to adverse outcomes. Adequate optimization might not be possible in the setting of time-pressured cancer surgery.

Perioperative care is ideally provided by a multidisciplinary team. The implementation of perioperative care bundles reduces variation in practice and aims to address modifiable factors leading to incremental and cumulative improvements in outcomes.[28,51] (See sections on Autologous Breast Reconstruction and Enhanced Recovery After Surgery for Autologous Breast Reconstruction.)

Perioperative Considerations

Identification and Optimization of Risk Factors Associated With Poor Flap Outcomes

Smoking and Nicotine Replacement Therapy

Smoking is an independent risk factor for complications in reconstructive procedures. It has been linked to deep surgical site infections, incisional dehiscence, and a higher return to theater rates.[10,52–54] Smoking causes harm via a number of pathways. Carbon monoxide alters the oxygen-carrying capacity of hemoglobin. Nicotine causes vasoconstriction and promotes the formation of microthrombi via catecholamine and thromboxane A2 release, respectively. Hydrogen cyanide impairs the function of enzymes implicated in cell metabolism. Combined, these factors contribute to impaired wound healing. Each week of abstinence allows reversal of some of these processes, with a significant benefit demonstrated at approximately 4 weeks.[55] Preclinical animal studies link nicotine replacement therapy with wound healing complications; however, it is unclear if this translates into worse outcomes for reconstructive procedures. While nicotine replacement therapy is preferred to active smoking, complete cessation of both is preferable in the perioperative period.

Diabetes Mellitus and HbA1c

There is little research specifically assessing the impact of diabetes in patients undergoing reconstructive surgery. In the field of reconstructive breast surgery, studies have demonstrated a greater incidence of adverse outcomes in diabetic patients undergoing autologous breast reconstruction. This has not been demonstrated with implant-based breast reconstruction.[56]

Current guidelines have been extrapolated from diabetic patients undergoing other major surgeries, cardiac and noncardiac, in which there is a demonstrable increase in both morbidity and mortality. Good preoperative glycemic control, as determined by HbA1c concentrations, is associated with a lower incidence of systemic and surgical complications, decreased mortality, and shorter LOHS.[57]

Radiotherapy

Preoperative radiation to the recipient site causes fibrosis to the vasculature and surrounding tissue with an increased risk of flap-related complications. Complications include poor wound healing, fat necrosis, and flap loss.[53,58] Radiotherapy to the HN region is also a risk factor for a difficult airway.[59]

Anemia

Anemia is defined as a hemoglobin level <13 g/dL for men and <12 g/dL for women. It is diagnosed in almost 50% of cancer patients during the course of their disease[60] and is an independent risk factor for increased 30-day morbidity and mortality in patients undergoing major noncardiac surgery.[61] In the setting of oncosurgery, the causes of anemia include impaired production of red blood cells (systemic inflammation, chemotherapy-related bone marrow suppression, and renal tubular toxicity with decreased erythropoietin production) and iron deficiency anemia (occult bleeding, decreased iron absorption).[60]

Studies specifically assessing preoperative anemia in autologous reconstruction surgery did not show an association with surgical complications, including flap thrombosis or flap loss. Postoperative hemoglobin levels <10 g/dL were associated with increased LOHS and medical complications, but did not increase flap-related complications.[54,62] Intraoperative blood transfusion correlated with postoperative medical complications (mostly respiratory related), but again not with surgical complications.

Anterolateral thigh (ALT) free flaps were associated with more blood loss and have higher rates of intraoperative blood transfusion when compared with radial forearm free flaps (RFFF) and fibular free flaps.[63]

Specific management of preoperative anemia involves a multidisciplinary approach targeting the likely causes of anemia. Proven therapeutic interventions include diet modification and IV iron therapy. Oral iron supplementation has reduced efficacy and does not meet the time constraints of planned surgery.[61] Treatment of anemia with recombinant erythropoietin has been associated with symptomatic venous thrombosis in the setting of chronic inflammation in cancer patients.[64] It is unclear if this translates into a risk for flap thrombosis. The modest benefit in treating anemia with erythropoietin in the short term may not justify this theoretical risk for flap thrombosis. Expert opinion should be sought.

In conclusion, preoperative anemia should be optimized to minimize the risk of transfusion-related medical complications. Anemia and perioperative blood transfusions are not independently associated with flap complications and therefore should not influence the consideration for blood transfusion.

Malnutrition

The prevalence of malnutrition in cancer surgery is reportedly as high as 47%. Causation can be multifactorial: secondary to the inflammatory or neoplastic disease, or due to altered metabolic state, poor access to nutrition, or gastrointestinal tract dysfunction. The Nutrition Risk Screening tool-2002 (NRS-2002) and the Subjective Global Assessment (SGA) tool are currently the most validated nutrition screening tools in the surgical population. The NRS-2002 is a good predictor of postoperative complications and can be used to predict mortality, morbidity, and LOHS.

Key elements of nutritional optimization involve provision of protein and micronutrient supplementation to increase muscle mass and support metabolic functions. There is currently no consensus on the duration of nutritional support. However, a 5- to 7-day duration of preoperative nutrition therapy is reported to reduce postoperative morbidity by 50%.[61] The European Society for Clinical Nutrition and Metabolism guidelines advocate a 7- to 14-day supplementation period for severely malnourished patients.

Autologous Breast Reconstruction

General

Breast cancer is the most frequently diagnosed cancer worldwide, accounting for 23% of global cancer cases.[65] Most will undergo lumpectomy or mastectomy as part of their treatment. Reconstruction timing and type (implant vs. autologous) varies geographically.

Commonly used free flaps for breast reconstruction include deep inferior epigastric perforator (DIEP) and transverse rectus abdominal musculocutaneous (TRAM) flaps. The donor sites for these methods are from the inferior abdominal area with vascular pedicles dissected from the deep inferior epigastric vessels. The internal mammary vessels form the recipient vascular pedicle.

Risk for developing complications after reconstruction depends broadly on patient comorbidities, type of reconstruction, and additional adjuvant therapies. Any combination(s) of risk factors seems to dramatically increase the risk of having poorer outcomes.[53]

Comorbidities

Data extracted from the ACS-NSQIP database (United States) identified that the majority of patients having immediate reconstruction after mastectomy were American Society of Anesthesiologists (ASA) class II. Twenty-three percent of patients had hypertension and almost 5% were diabetic. Thirteen percent were active smokers. In this study factors linked with increased surgical complications were smoking, hypertension, diabetes, and obesity.[54]

Obesity

Obese patients undergoing breast reconstructive procedures experience higher rates of wound-related complications and reconstructive failure.[53,54,66] There is an appreciable increase in complication rates in patients with a body mass index (BMI) >30 kg/m^2, with a significant increase beyond a BMI of 40 kg/m^2. Notably, obese patients having implant-based reconstruction have a greater failure rate than autologous breast reconstruction, especially if the BMI is >35 kg/m^2.

Obese patients undergoing delayed breast reconstruction should be encouraged to lose weight until their BMI is within an acceptable range.

Type of Reconstruction

Compared with implant-based reconstruction, autologous reconstruction involves a more substantial operation with a longer recovery time. It is associated with an increase in surgical complications in the short term, but compared with implant-based reconstruction, this risk diminishes over time.[54]

Adjuvant Therapies

Radiotherapy

Postmastectomy radiotherapy (PMRT) for node-positive breast cancer reduces the risk of local recurrence and improves overall survival.[67] However, it is unfortunately associated with increased reconstruction failure and complications, regardless of the reconstructive method. Compared with implant-based reconstruction, autologous reconstruction is associated with significantly fewer postoperative wound complications. In a study of bilateral autologous reconstruction, there were an increase in complications on the irradiated side. Common complications associated with recipient site radiotherapy include flap fibrosis, fat necrosis, and wound dehiscence.[67]

Radiation-Induced Heart Injury

Radiotherapy to the thorax can cause pathologic changes to the heart, blood vessels, and lung tissue. It causes an acute increase in reactive oxygen and nitrogen species and can lead to acute endothelial dysfunction and long-term tissue fibrosis. Patients who received postoperative radiotherapy for breast cancer have higher rates of mortality associated with ischemic heart disease, and may have signs and symptoms of congestive cardiac failure.[64] Further investigation and referral may be needed.

Hormone Inhibitors

Adjuvant therapy for estrogen receptor-positive breast cancers includes hormone inhibitor (HI) agents such as tamoxifen (selective estrogen receptor modulator) and letrozole (aromatase inhibitor). These drugs decrease the constitutive effects of estrogen in the skin, impacting wound healing and increasing rates of high-grade prosthetic capsular contractures.[69] HI agents have been implicated in microvascular thrombotic events resulting in thrombotic flap complications and total flap loss. There is conflicting evidence regarding the systemic thromboembolic phenomenon; however, there is likely to be a contributory role. Temporary cessation of these agents is recommended, although there is currently no consensus regarding the timing of this. Considering the pharmacodynamic properties of these drugs and timing of postoperative complications, cessation 2–4 weeks prior to surgery and recommencement 2 weeks postoperatively has been suggested. No studies have demonstrated a decrease in cancer survival rate with temporary discontinuation of HIs.[70]

Chemotherapy-Induced Cardiac Toxicity

Systolic dysfunction may develop in breast cancer patients treated with anthracyclines (doxorubicin) and trastuzumab (targets human epidermal growth factor receptor 2 [HER2]).[71] Further investigation and referral may be needed.

Enhanced Recovery After Surgery for Autologous Breast Reconstruction

There is mounting evidence demonstrating the benefits of ERAS implementation within several surgical fields. Currently there are only a few quality studies[25,26,28] evaluating the outcomes after ERAS implementation in autologous breast reconstruction. These studies had several common findings and are summarized below:

- Fasting periods were limited to 2 h preoperatively with early resumption of eating and drinking in the postoperative period. There were no incidences of aspiration reported.
- Multimodal analgesia included regular paracetamol and a nonsteroidal antiinflammatory agent. Regional techniques such as transverse abdominis plane (TAP) blocks were used. The decreased reliance on parenteral opioids and earlier transition to oral analgesia resulted in a reduction in total opioid and antiemetic use. A common finding in these studies was a positive correlation between the total amount of opioids used and LOHS.
- GDT resulted in a reduction of the amount of intraoperative fluid volumes administered. The average amount of intraoperative fluids used in the GDT group was 3.85 L versus 5.5 L in the non-GDT group.
- Thromboprophylaxis was started in the early postoperative period with no significant difference in hematoma formation.

There was no difference in major complications between groups, implying that the above measures are safe and effective. LOHS was decreased by an average of 1 day.

The ERAS Society has published consensus recommendations pertaining to reconstructive procedures. This includes Head and Neck[72] and Breast surgery,[73] respectively.

Head and Neck Cancer Resection With Immediate Flap Reconstruction

General

HN neoplasms form the fifth most common cancer worldwide and originate most frequently from the mucosa of the upper oral cavity, pharynx, larynx, nasal cavity, and sinuses. Less frequently, neoplasms originate from the salivary glands, thyroid, soft tissue, bone, and skin. Squamous cell carcinoma and papillary thyroid cancer are commonly seen.[74]

Etiology

The etiologies of HN cancers are an interplay between host and environmental factors. Many of these factors are dose-dependent and synergistic (e.g., alcohol and tobacco).[75]

Host factors

- Immunosuppression (human immunodeficiency virus infection, chronic immunosuppression after organ transplantation)

Environmental exposure
- Alcohol abuse
- Tobacco
- Infection with human papilloma virus and Epstein-Barr virus
- Ionizing radiation

Demographic

Patients with HN malignancies are most commonly male and elderly. There are, however, an increasing number of younger patients due to exposure to human papilloma virus.[75] A recent review found that the average overall complication rate was 48% with flap success rates nearing 95%. The mortality rate was between 1% and 2%. The incidence of complications was found to be directly related to the comorbid state of the patient, rather than the age. There are several comorbidity scores that can help predict flap survival rates and complications. The Kaplan-Feinstein index (KFI), Adult Comorbidity Evaluation-27 (ACE-27), ASA score, and the Index of Coexistent Diseases (ICED) score correlated well with flap survival and complication rates.[76] Pertinent comorbidities that are strongly associated with flap failure rates include diabetes and chronic obstructive pulmonary disease. Hypertension was present in 64% of patients but was not associated with worse outcomes. Pulmonary and cardiac complications were frequently seen in the postoperative period.[10,77,78]

Commonly Used Free Flaps in HN Reconstruction

Resection of complex tumors in the HN area can have major functional and aesthetic consequences. Flap reconstruction plays a major role in the restoration of form and physiologic function. The most common musculocutaneous free flaps are RFFF and ALT flaps, whereas fibula free flaps are the most common osteocutaneous flaps.[79]

Airway Planning and Postoperative Destination

Patients undergoing surgery for HN tumors should undergo a thorough airway assessment.[71] HN cancer patients have a high rate of difficult intubation compared to other patient groups.[80,81] Distortion of the upper airway by prior surgery, irradiation, or bulky and friable tumors may make oxygenation difficult after induction of anesthesia. Thirty-nine percent of airway cases reported in National Audits Project 4 (NAP4) had HN pathology.[82]

Airway choice and location should be discussed with the surgeon, as this will vary depending on the location and extent of surgery. A tracheostomy may be inserted prior to commencement of resection, or a nasal tube may be required.

HN patients may also be at risk of postoperative airway obstruction. A discussion between surgeon and anesthetist at the end of the case is essential to forming a clear airway plan. Documentation should include the ease of airway management at the start of the case, likely changes after reconstruction, and any airway examination performed at the end of the case. Flap position and potential flap damage from airway maneuvers should also be considered. Surgical procedures that carry greatest risk of postoperative airway occlusion include bilateral neck dissection and resection of the mandible, tongue, and floor of mouth. Free flap edema may cause additional narrowing of the aerodigestive tract. The RFFF is smaller and more pliable than other commonly used flaps and poses less risk. The Cameron tracheostomy scoring system[83] takes surgical risk factors into consideration with a threshold score of more than five points prompting consideration for elective tracheostomy placement. It does not take into consideration the cardiopulmonary reserve of the patient, and this should be evaluated in conjunction with surgical risk factors for the planning of appropriate postoperative destination and ventilation. Patients with adequate cardiopulmonary reserve undergoing free flap reconstruction for unilateral neck dissection may be considered for overnight sedation and delayed extubation, instead of elective tracheostomy placement.[84]

It should be noted that not all HN reconstruction patients will require postoperative ventilation in an intensive care unit. Indeed, the hemodynamic side effects of sedation can have a negative effect on flap perfusion.[68] Carefully selected patients may recover in wards with specialized nursing staff trained to identify flap and airway compromise and escalate management where appropriate.

The Cook Staged Extubation Set includes an airway wire that can be left in the trachea after extubation. This allows insertion of the included reintubation catheter over the wire enabling oxygenation and reinsertion of an endotracheal tube if required. It does, however, require appropriate training of staff and has some limitations.[85]

Analgesia

HN patients have high rates of neuropathic pain due to either direct tumor effect or secondary to cancer treatment.[86] Specialist pain input may be needed. Patients who have had bone harvested generally require a plaster cast and the donor site may be more painful than the reconstruction. Due to limited oral intake, IV analgesia is often required.

Feeding

Oral intake may be limited after a major reconstruction. Some patients will require nasogastric feeding, and if this is the case, a nasogastric tube can be inserted under direct vision at the end of surgery.

Postoperative Delirium

Postoperative delirium is commonly seen after HN reconstruction. It is defined as a reversible neurologic deficit and is characterized by fluctuations in conscious level and a change in cognition. Several risk factors have been identified and include age above 70 years, male sex, prolonged surgery, intraoperative blood transfusions, tracheostomy placement, and ASA physical status above III.[87] It is commonly seen within the first 3 days of surgery. Postoperative agitation and disorientation seen with postoperative delirium may lead to surgical anastomotic disruption and flap compromise. Early identification and specialized intervention are imperative and may include a short period of intubation and ventilation in an intensive care unit.

Patients presenting with HN tumors may have a history of alcohol abuse. Acute alcohol withdrawal may present in the postoperative period as confusion, agitation, and generalized seizures, putting the patient at risk for surgical anastomotic disruption. Patients should be screened and managed appropriately.

Patient Positioning and Pressure Care

The duration of free flap surgery can be long and may exceed 8 h. This brings unique challenges with regards to positioning, access to the patient, and pressure care.[88] To avoid injury of the brachial plexus and ulnar nerve, shoulder abduction should be less than 90 degrees and arms in the neutral position, respectively. The patient needs to be adequately positioned and secured to allow for intraoperative assessment of symmetry. Attention should be paid to avoid focal areas of pressure caused by cables, gown knots, or inadequate cushioning. Vulnerable areas include the heels, sacrum, and occiput.[89] Consider passively moving joints for extended procedures to avoid joint stiffness and pressure areas.

Free Flap Breast Reconstruction

For delayed reconstruction, the patient will be supine with the arms adducted for the duration of the surgery. For patients undergoing simultaneous mastectomy and immediate reconstruction, the arm position may start in the abducted position to allow access to the axilla. The arms are then adducted for the reconstruction part of the procedure.

Distal venous and arterial line access points will not be readily accessible during surgery; therefore extension lines and/proximal access points will be needed. For the same reason, two peripheral venous access sites are advised. Care should be taken to avoid pressure injuries secondary to lines and access points. Central venous access is not routinely used, unless the prolonged use of inotropes or vasoactive drugs is anticipated. It should be noted that peripheral venous access points will not be visible or readily accessible should a total intravenous anesthetic (TIVA) technique be employed. There is ongoing debate on the acceptability of the approach and whether a central venous line with its potential placement complications is justified.

The anterior superior iliac spine should be in line with the break of the table to allow table flexion to assist donor site closure. To minimize tension on the donor site wound, the patient will remain with their hips in flexion for 24–48 h postoperatively. For this reason, the ward bed should be appropriately positioned prior to transfer from the operating table.

HN Reconstruction

Theatre layout will depend on the location of the flap donor site, the backup donor site, and the area of tumor excision. Generally, the head of the patient will be distant to the anesthetic machine with the flap donor site exposed and accessible to the surgical team(s). The eyes should be occluded with a watertight dressing and appropriately shielded if surgery does not include the ocular area. A head ring and shoulder roll are frequently needed to gain adequate access to the HN area. The endotracheal tube and airway connectors will not be readily accessible during the case and should be adequately secured. Long airway circuits are frequently used and arranged either cephalad or caudally depending on the surgery location. Pressure areas caused by circuit, connectors, and heat and moisture filter should be avoided. Particular care should be taken to avoid pressure injuries caused by nasally placed endotracheal tubes. The head may be slightly elevated to avoid venous congestion and venous bleeding from surgical sites.

Central venous access is not routinely placed for HN surgery. If prolonged use of vasoactive agents is anticipated, femoral central lines on the contralateral side to the surgical site are advised. If a radial forearm free flap is considered, vascular access and invasive monitoring should be placed on the contralateral arm.

Monitoring

Routine intraoperative monitoring should be used during free flap reconstruction procedures. In addition, invasive arterial blood pressure monitoring allows for arterial blood gas analysis. The arterial partial pressure of oxygen and carbon dioxide should be kept within physiologic limits. Urine output should be measured via an indwelling catheter. Core temperature may be measured via an indwelling catheter or via a temperature probe placed in the esophagus. Nerve monitoring may be required if resection close to the recurrent laryngeal nerve is undertaken. Optional equipment includes depth of anesthesia monitoring, peripheral nerve stimulation, pulse contour analysis systems, or esophageal Doppler monitoring.

Anesthetic Maintenance

With respect to free flap outcomes, maintenance of anesthesia using propofol as a TIVA agent has not been proven to be superior over inhalational anesthesia. However, anesthetic maintenance with propofol reduces the incidence of PONV,[73,90] possibly reducing the risk of anastomosis disruption due to retching and vomiting. In the setting of oncosurgery, propofol may have a cancer survival benefit by inhibiting cancer cell migration and preserving the function of natural killer and T cells.[13] In a single-center retrospective study of more than 7000 cancer surgery patients there was an increased risk of death in patients receiving an inhalational compared with propofol-based anesthetic.[91]

Multimodal Analgesia

Good analgesia mitigates the surge of stress hormones as well as the vasoconstrictive response to pain. The paradigm of multimodal analgesia is advocated and widely practiced for postsurgical pain.[92] The concept involves the use of combinations of analgesic agents with different modes of action to achieve improved analgesia and reduced opioid requirements. This includes the use of antiinflammatory agents, regional techniques, and other adjuvants in addition to opioids. The concept of preemptive analgesia describes the reduction in magnitude and duration of postoperative pain by applying antinociceptive techniques prior to tissue injury. While there is no definite evidence to show improvement in postsurgical pain control, there may be a role in reducing the development of chronic postsurgical pain.[93]

Lignocaine Infusions

The incidence of chronic postsurgical pain is high in breast surgery, with an incidence up to 65%.[94,95] Even minor procedures such as lumpectomy and sentinel lymph node dissection have a 40% incidence, with mostly a neuropathic component.[96] Perioperative lignocaine infusion is associated with a modestly decreased incidence of chronic postsurgical pain in the setting of mastectomies.[97] Postulated mechanisms include its sodium channel blocking mechanism of action, as well as antiinflammatory and antihyperalgesic properties. Intraoperative IV lignocaine infusion combined with postoperative subcutaneous lignocaine infusion reduces pain at rest, cumulative morphine consumption, and LOHS in the setting of major colorectal, urologic, and neuropathic cancer pain settings.[98–100]

Nonsteroidal Antiinflammatory Drugs and Cyclooxygenase-2 Inhibitors

In a retrospective cohort study of autologous breast reconstruction comparing perioperative ibuprofen versus celecoxib, celecoxib was not associated with an increase in flap failure rates. There was a threefold increase in postoperative hematoma formation in the ibuprofen group. It should be noted that patients in both groups received additional aspirin as an antiplatelet agent.[101] Another autologous breast reconstruction study did not show a correlation between perioperative ketorolac administration and postoperative hematoma formation.[26]

Gabapentinoids

The administration of gabapentinoids such as gabapentin and pregabalin preoperatively improves postoperative acute pain with an opioid-sparing effect, although there is no evidence for prevention of chronic postsurgical pain.[102]

Regional Anesthetic Techniques for Autologous Breast Reconstruction

The abdominal donor site is the major contributor to pain in autologous breast reconstructions.[103]

Epidural

Intraoperative epidural use has been described in a small study of 99 patients.[104] In this study, the group receiving general anesthetic with intraoperative epidural had improved pain scores, a decrease in opioid consumption, and lower PONV scores, compared with the general anesthetic alone. The need for vasopressor support was marginally higher in the epidural group, presumably to correct epidural-associated vasodilatation and hypotension. This study did not compare the total volume of perioperative IV fluid used. There was no significant difference in postoperative complications. Postoperative hypotension and delay in mobilization associated with epidural use may make this technique less favorable.

Transverse Abdominis Plane Blocks and Rectus Sheath Block

TAP and rectus sheath blocks, with or without catheter placement, resulted in reductions in postoperative opioid consumption, better PONV scores, and a reduction in LOHS.[25,26,28,103]

Postoperative Nausea and Vomiting

PONV remain common with an incidence ranging from 25% to 60%.[105] Vomiting can have several detrimental effects on flap outcomes. Complications include wound dehiscence, hematoma formation, and reduced patient satisfaction. The Apfel score is a useful tool that predicts risk of PONV based on the number of patient factors. These factors include the use of postoperative opioids, nonsmoking status, female sex, and history of PONV or motion sickness.[106] Based on the score, the patient would be categorized as low (0–1 risk factor), medium (2 risk factors), or high risk (3 risk factors). The recommendation from the Australian and New Zealand College of Anaesthetists is to monitor for low risk, one to two interventions for medium risk, and more than two interventions for high risk.[107]

Temperature Management

While there is theoretical evidence to suggest hypothermia reduces pedicle thrombosis,[108, 109] this has not been proven in the clinical setting. Instead, intraoperative hypothermia may pose a risk for the development of flap infection with no benefit to anastomotic patency in free tissue transfer.[110] Preoperatively, patients should be actively warmed. Exposure for surgical site marking by the surgical teams should be kept to a minimum, or should be completed the day prior to surgery. Intraoperatively, the patient should be actively warmed, and IV fluid warmers should be utilized. As HN patients often only have a small surface area exposed, these patients have a tendency to develop hyperthermia; thus vigilance with active warming is required.

Venous Thromboembolism Prevention

The 2005 Caprini Risk assessment model is a risk stratification tool that has been validated in reconstructive patients to calculate the 6-day VTE risk.[111] Individualized measures to prevent VTE are recommended according to the risk category and include mechanical (compression stockings) and chemical (enoxaparin/heparin) prophylaxis. Contraindications and potential risk of bleeding should be assessed prior to determining the appropriate method of prophylaxis. Postoperative bleeding into HN surgical sites can have catastrophic consequences and this must be considered when weighing up the risks and benefits of chemical prophylaxis. Most patients undergoing free flap reconstructive procedures in the setting of malignancy will fall into the high-risk category of developing VTE.

On review of the literature, it was noted that there was variation in practice in terms of dosing, duration, and timing of administration of VTE prophylaxis. Doses ranged from 30 to 60 mg enoxaparin daily, adjusted for weight and renal function. Timing of drug administration ranged from 1 h preoperatively to 12 h postoperatively.[112] Duration of drug administration varied according to the risk stratification score. Review of these protocols did not provide sufficient evidence to dictate administration protocols.

In the setting of flap reconstruction, the observed rates of clinically significant reoperative hematoma are not increased with the use of perioperative enoxaparin or unfractionated heparin.[112–114] Dextran is associated with an increase in hematoma formation, cardiac and respiratory complications, anaphylaxis, and flap loss.[115] Aspirin is associated with increased hematoma formation.[115] Of note, postoperative administration of aspirin, dextran, heparin, and low-molecular-weight heparin have no protective effect against the development of pedicel thrombosis and no significant effect on flap survival overall.[115]

Antibiotic Regimen

Systemic antibiotic prophylaxis given preincision and continued for 24 h postoperatively is recommended for breast surgery, and clean-contaminated surgery of the HN. The most commonly isolated organisms in plastic surgery are *Staphylococcus aureus* and streptococci. In clean-contaminated HN surgery, organisms include anaerobic and gram-positive aerobic organisms. Patients with wound infections may have polymicrobial colonization with gram-negative aerobic and anaerobic organisms. Local guidelines should guide antibiotic use due to regional variations in organism sensitivity. Administration of repeat doses of IV antibiotic should be given in prolonged procedures. The overall duration of antibiotic therapy should be limited to less than 24 h as the benefit beyond this has not been demonstrated.[116,117]

Postoperative Considerations

Key aspects for optimal postoperative flap care include:

- Gentle anesthetic emergence
- Optimization of flap perfusion
- Postoperative flap monitoring
- Safe and comfortable recovery

Anesthetic Emergence

Any sudden increases in intrathoracic pressure may disrupt the surgical anastomosis with potential hematoma formation. Measures to minimize coughing, vomiting, shivering, and excessive movement should be employed. Any blood or secretions should be cleared from the airway while the patient is still anesthetized. It may be useful to reexamine the airway at completion of HN surgery. A slow emergence with the patient already transferred onto a ward bed is advised. Humidified air and oxygen might reduce airway irritation and coughing postextubation.

Optimization of Flap Perfusion

Careless postoperative IV fluid administration can negate the meticulous steps taken intraoperatively to optimize the hemodynamic status of the patient. IV fluids can be discontinued once a patient is stable and tolerating oral fluids. A degree of postoperative oliguria can be expected in the early postoperative period. It is a normal neurohormonal response to surgical stress and is a poor indicator of overall fluid status. A low urine output interpreted in isolation should not trigger unnecessary IV fluid administration.

Cardiovascular complications are common in postoperative HN reconstruction patients[118] and should be excluded in hemodynamically unstable patients. Clinical assessment includes urgent review of vital sign trends, wound sites, drain output, and fluid balance charts. The passive leg raise test is a useful bedside maneuver to assess fluid responsiveness.[119] It has been validated in nonventilated patients with or without arrhythmias. Fluid responsiveness is defined as an increase in cardiac output (or its surrogate) of more than 15% following passive leg raise. These patients may benefit from fluid resuscitation to improve hemodynamic status. Ongoing hypotension or low cardiac output despite fluid resuscitation warrants specialist review and treatment.

Specific attention is required to ensure that the flap pedicle is not compressed by equipment or dressings. HN reconstructions may be compromised if neck vessels are kinked, stretched, or compressed by adjacent structures or drains. The head should therefore be maintained in a neutral position postoperatively.

Postoperative Flap Monitoring

Postoperatively, patients require dedicated nursing staff with experience and expertise to diagnose early flap compromise. Microvascular thrombosis occurs most frequently within the first 72 h, reflecting the need for more frequent and intensive flap observations during this time.[73] Subjective assessment of flap health includes observation of color, temperature, turgor, and changes in appearance. More objective monitoring methods include the use of Doppler devices, near infrared spectroscopy, and indocyanine green fluorescent videoangiography.[72,120–122] Insufficiencies of arterial inflow and venous congestion should be diagnosed promptly and may warrant urgent surgical exploration.

Pulmonary Function and Early Mobilization

Postoperative pulmonary complications can be reduced by implementing a multidisciplinary perioperative respiratory care bundle.[123] Components of this bundle include perioperative incentive spirometry; cough and deep breathing exercises; oral care, including perioperative chlorhexidine mouthwashes, patient education, early mobilization, and head of bed elevation. Adequate pain management, prevention of PONV, and timely removal of catheters and drains may promote early mobilization.

Conclusion

Outcomes after autologous free flap reconstruction depend on the interplay between multiple factors. The implementation of perioperative care bundles reduces variation in practice by addressing modifiable factors known to alter outcomes. This may lead to incremental and cumulative improvements in care. Appreciation of the pathophysiologic determinants of flap perfusion and the consequence of therapeutic interventions will permit a more considered approach.

References

1. Gooneratne H, Lalabekyan B, Clarke S, Burdett E. Perioperative anaesthetic practice for head and neck free tissue transfer – a UK national survey. *Acta Anaesthesiol Scand.* 2013;57(10):1293–1300.
2. Cerny Vladimir AD, Florian B. Targeting the endothelial glycocalyx in the acute critical illness as a challenge for clinical and laboratory medicine. *Crit Rev Clin Lab Sci.* 2017;54(5):343–357.
3. Myers GJ, Wegner J. Endothelial glycocalyx and cardiopulmonary bypass. *J Extra Corpor Technol.* 2017;49:174–181.
4. Song JW, Goligorsky MS. Perioperative implication of the endothelial glycocalyx. *Korean J Anesthesiol.* 2018;71(2):92–102.
5. Pillinger NL, KPCA. Endothelial glycocalyx: basic science and clinical implication. *Anaesth Intensive Care.* 2017;45(3):295–307.
6. MacDonald N, Pearse RM. Are we close to the ideal intravenous fluid? *Br J Anaesth.* 2017;119(suppl 1):i63–i71.
7. Bashandy. Implications of recent accumulating knowledge about endothelial glycocalyx on anesthetic management. *J Anaesth.* 2015;29(269–278):269.
8. Alphonsus CS, Rodseth RN. The endothelial glycocalyx: a review of the vascular barrier. *Anaesthesia.* 2014;69(7):777–784.
9. Booi DI. Perioperative fluid overload increases anastomosis thrombosis in the free TRAM flap used for breast reconstruction. *Eur J Plast Surg.* 2011;34(2):81–86.
10. Clark JR, McCluskey S.A., Hall F., et al. Predictors of morbidity following free flap reconstruction for cancer of the head and neck. *Head Neck.* 2007;29(12):1090–1101.
11. Ettinger KS, Moore EJ, Lohse CM, Reiland MD, Yetzer JG, Arce K. Application of the surgical Apgar score to microvascular head and neck reconstruction. *J Oral Maxillofac Surg.* 2016;74(8):1668–1677.
12. Zhong T, Neinstein R, Massey C, et al. Intravenous fluid infusion rate in microsurgical breast reconstruction: important lessons learned from 354 free flaps. *Plast Reconstr Surg.* 2011;128(6):1153–1160.
13. Hiller JG, Perry NJ, Poulogiannis G, Riedel B, Sloan EK Perioperative events influence cancer recurrence risk after surgery. *Nat Rev Clin Oncol.* 2017;15:205–218.
14. Wenk M, Van Aken H, Zarbock A. The New World Health Organization recommendations on perioperative administration of oxygen to prevent surgical site infections: a dangerous reductionist approach? *Anesth Analg.* 2017;125(2): 682–687.
15. Shaefi S, Marcantonio ER, Mueller A, et al. Intraoperative oxygen concentration and neurocognition after cardiac surgery: study protocol for a randomized controlled trial. *Trials.* 2017;18(1):600.
16. Ince C, Ertmer C. Hemodynamic coherence: its meaning in perioperative and intensive care medicine. *Best Pract Res Clin Anaesthesiol.* 2016;30(4):395–397.
17. Jansen SM, de Bruin DM, van Berge Henegouwen MI, et al. Can we predict necrosis intra-operatively? Real-time optical quantitative perfusion imaging in surgery: study protocol for a prospective, observational, in vivo pilot study. *Pilot Feasibility Stud.* 2017;3:65.
18. Makaryus R, Miller TE, Gan TJ. Current concepts of fluid management in enhanced recovery pathways. *Br J Anaesth.* 2018; 120(2):376–383.
19. Myles PS, Andrews S, Nicholson J, Lobo DN, Mythen M. Contemporary approaches to perioperative IV fluid therapy. *World J Surg.* 2017;41(10):2457–2463.
20. Bellamy MC. Wet, dry or something else? *Br J Anaesth.* 2006; 97(6):755–757.
21. Grocott MP, Dushianthan A, Hamilton MA, et al. Perioperative increase in global blood flow to explicit defined goals and outcomes after surgery: a Cochrane Systematic Review. *Br J Anaesth.* 2013;111(4):535–548.
22. Pearse RM, Harrison DA, MacDonald N, et al. Effect of a perioperative, cardiac output-guided hemodynamic therapy algorithm on outcomes following major gastrointestinal surgery: a randomized clinical trial and systematic review. *JAMA.* 2014;311(21):2181–2190.
23. Calvo-Vecino JM, Ripolles-Melchor J, Mythen MG, et al. Effect of goal-directed haemodynamic therapy on postoperative complications in low-moderate risk surgical patients: a multicentre randomised controlled trial (FEDORA trial). *Br J Anaesth.* 2018;120(4):734–744.
24. Chong MA, Wang Y, Berbenetz NM, McConachie I. Does goal-directed haemodynamic and fluid therapy improve perioperative outcomes? A systematic review and meta-analysis. *Eur J Anaesthesiol.* 2018;35(7):469–483.
25. Kaoutzanis C, Kumar NG, O'Neill D, et al. Enhanced recovery pathway in microvascular autologous tissue-based breast reconstruction: should it become the standard of care? *Plast Reconstr Surg.* 2018.
26. Afonso A, Oskar S, Tan KS, et al. Is enhanced recovery the new standard of care in microsurgical breast reconstruction? *Plast Reconstr Surg.* 2017; 139(5):1053–1061.
27. Figus A, Wade RG, Oakey S, Ramakrishnan VV Intraoperative esophageal Doppler hemodynamic monitoring in free perforator flap surgery. *Ann Plast Surg.* 2013; 70(3):301–307.
28. Astanehe A, Temple-Oberle C, Nielsen M, et al. An enhanced recovery after surgery pathway for microvascular breast recon-

struction is safe and effective. *Plast Reconstr Surg Glob Open.* 2018;6(1):e1634.

29. Chalmers A, Turner MW, Anand R, Puxeddu R, Brennan PA. Cardiac output monitoring to guide fluid replacement in head and neck microvascular free flap surgery-what is current practice in the UK? *Br J Oral Maxillofac Surg.* 2012;50(6):500–503.
30. Kunst G, Ostermann M. Intraoperative permissive oliguria - how much is too much? *Br J Anaesth.* 2017;119(6):1075–1077.
31. McCluskey SA, Karkouti K, Wijeysundera D, Minkovich L, Tait G, Beattie WS Hyperchloremia after noncardiac surgery is independently associated with increased morbidity and mortality: a propensity-matched cohort study. *Anesth Analg.* 2013;117(2):412–421.
32. Motakef S, Mountziaris PM, Ismail IK, Agag RL, Patel A Emerging paradigms in perioperative management for microsurgical free tissue transfer: review of the literature and evidence-based guidelines. *Plast Reconstr Surg.* 2015;135(1):290–299.
33. Raiman M, Mitchell CG, Biccard BM, Rodseth RN. Comparison of hydroxyethyl starch colloids with crystalloids for surgical patients: a systematic review and meta-analysis. *Eur J Anaesthesiol.* 2016;33(1):42–48.
34. Joosten A, Delaporte A, Mortier J, et al. Long-term impact of crystalloid versus colloid solutions on renal function and disability-free survival after major abdominal surgery. *Anesthesiology.* 2019;130(2):227–236.
35. Kabon BS, Kurz D. Effect of intraoperative goal-directed balanced crystalloid versus colloid administration on major postoperative morbidity: a randomized trial. *Anesthesiology.* 2019;130:728–744.
36. Arellano R, Gan BS, Salpeter MJ, et al. A triple-blinded randomized trial comparing the hemostatic effects of large-dose 10% hydroxyethyl starch 264/0.45 versus 5% albumin during major reconstructive surgery. *Anesth Analg.* 2005;100(6):1846–1853.
37. Szakmany T, Dodd M, Dempsey GA, et al. The influence of allogenic blood transfusion in patients having free-flap primary surgery for oral and oropharyngeal squamous cell carcinoma. *Br J Cancer.* 2006; 94(5):647–653.
38. Karakida K, Aoki T, Ota Y, et al. Analysis of risk factors for surgical-site infections in 276 oral cancer surgeries with microvascular free-flap reconstructions at a single university hospital. *J Infect Chemother.* 2010;16(5):334–339.
39. Pohlenz P, Blessmann M, Heiland M, Blake F, Schmelzle R, Li L. Postoperative complications in 202 cases of microvascular head and neck reconstruction. *J Craniomaxillofac Surg.* 2007;35(6–7):311–315.
40. Disa JJ, Polvora VP, Pusic AL, Singh B, Cordeiro PG Dextran-related complications in head and neck microsurgery: do the benefits outweigh the risks? A prospective randomized analysis. *Plast Reconstr Surg.* 2003;112(6):1534–1539.
41. Sessler DI, Bloomstone JA, Aronson S, et al. Perioperative Quality Initiative consensus statement on intraoperative blood pressure, risk and outcomes for elective surgery. *Br J Anaesth.* 2019;122(5):563–574.
42. Futier E, Lefrant JY, Guinot PG, et al. Effect of individualized vs standard blood pressure management strategies on postoperative organ dysfunction among high-risk patients undergoing major surgery: a randomized clinical trial. *JAMA.* 2017;318(14):1346–1357.
43. Hand WR, McSwain JR, McEvoy MD, et al. Characteristics and intraoperative treatments associated with head and neck free tissue transfer complications and failures. *Otolaryngol Head Neck Surg.* 2014;152(3):480–487.
44. Chen C, Nguyen MD, Bar-Meir E, et al. Effects of vasopressor administration on the outcomes of microsurgical breast reconstruction. *Ann Plast Surg.* 2010;65(1):28–31.
45. Monroe MM, Cannady SB, Ghanem TA, Swide CE, Wax MK Safety of vasopressor use in head and neck microvascular reconstruction: a prospective observational study. *Otolaryngol Head Neck Surg.* 2011;144(6):877–882.
46. Swanson EW, Cheng HT, Susarla SM, et al. Intraoperative use of vasopressors is safe in head and neck free tissue transfer. *J Reconstr Microsurg.* 2016; 32(2):87–93.
47. Kelly DA, Reynolds M, Crantford C, Pestana IA. Impact of intraoperative vasopressor use in free tissue transfer for head, neck, and extremity reconstruction. *Ann Plast Surg.* 2014;72(6):S135–S138.
48. Eley KA, Young JD, Watt-Smith S. Epinephrine, norepinephrine, dobutamine, and dopexamine effects on free flap skin blood flow. *Plast Reconstr Surg.* 2012;130(3):564–570.
49. Jones SJ, Scott DA, Watson R, Morrison WA. Milrinone does not improve free flap survival in microvascular surgery. *Anaesth Intensive Care.* 2007;35:720–725.
50. Dunn LK, Durieux ME. Perioperative use of intravenous lidocaine. *Anesthesiology.* 2017;126(4):729–737.
51. Cook DA, Pencille LJ, Dupras DM, Linderbaum JA, Pankratz VS, Wilkinson JM. Practice variation and practice guidelines: attitudes of generalist and specialist physicians, nurse practitioners, and physician assistants. *PLoS One.* 2018;13(1): e0191943.
52. Toyoda Y, Fu RH, Li L, Otterburn DM, Rohde CH. Smoking as an independent risk factor for postoperative complications in plastic surgical procedures: a propensity score-matched analysis of 36,454 patients from the NSQIP Database from 2005 to 2014. *Plast Reconstr Surg.* 2018;141(1):226–236.
53. Thorarinsson A, Fröjd V, Kölby L, Lidén M, Elander A, Mark H Patient determinants as independent risk factors for postoperative complications of breast reconstruction. *Gland Surgery.* 2017;6(4):355–367.
54. Fischer JP, Wes AM, Tuggle CT, Serletti JM, Wu LC. Risk analysis and stratification of surgical morbidity after immediate breast reconstruction. *J Am Coll Surg.* 2013;217(5):780–787.
55. Mills E, Eyawo O, Lockhart I, Kelly S, Wu P, Ebbert JO Smoking cessation reduces postoperative complications: a systematic review and meta-analysis. *Am J Med.* 2011;124(2):144–154.
56. Qin C, Vaca E, Lovecchio F, Ver Halen JP, Hansen NM, Kim JY Differential impact of non-insulin-dependent diabetes mellitus and insulin-dependent diabetes mellitus on breast reconstruction outcomes. *Breast Cancer Res Treat.* 2014; 146(2):429–438.
57. Aldam P, Levy N, Hall GM. Perioperative management of diabetic patients: new controversies. *Br J Anaesth.* 2014;113(6):906–909.
58. Loupatatzi A, Stavrianos SD, Karantonis FF, et al. Are females predisposed to complications in head and neck cancer free flap reconstruction? *J Oral Maxillofac Surg.* 2014;72(1):178–185.
59. Wong P, Iqbal R, Light KP, Williams E, Hayward J. Head and neck surgery in a tertiary centre: predictors of difficult airway and anaesthetic management. *Proc Singapore Healthc.* 2015;25(1):19–26.
60. Tzounakas VL, Seghatchian J, Grouzi E, Kokoris S, Antonelou MH. Red blood cell transfusion in surgical cancer patients: targets, risks, mechanistic understanding and further therapeutic opportunities. *Transfus Apher Sci.* 2017;56(3):291–304.
61. Ripolles-Melchor J, Carli F, Coca-Martinez M, Barbero-Mielgo M, Ramirez-Rodriguez JM, Garcia-Erce JA. Committed to be

fit. The value of preoperative care in the perioperative medicine era. *Minerva Anestesiol.* 2018;84(5):615–625.

62. Nelson JA, Fischer JP, Grover R, et al. Intraoperative perfusion management impacts postoperative outcomes: an analysis of 682 autologous breast reconstruction patients. *J Plast Reconstr Aesthet Surg.* 2015;68(2):175–183.
63. Puram SV, Yarlagadda BB, Sethi R, et al. Transfusion in head and neck free flap patients: practice patterns and a comparative analysis by flap type. *Otolaryngol Head Neck Surg.* 2015;152(3):449–457.
64. Tobu Mahmut IO, Fareed D. Erythropoietin-induced thrombosis as a result of increased inflammation and thrombin activatable fibrinolytic inhibitor. *Clin Appl Thromb Hemost.* 2004; 10(3):225–232.
65. Jemal A, Bray F, Center MM, Ferlay J, Ward E, Forman D. Global cancer statistics. *CA Cancer J Clin.* 2011; 61(2):69–90.
66. Mark V, Schaverien SJM. Effect of obesity on outcomes of free autologous breast reconstruction: a meta-anaysis. *Microsurgery.* 2014;34:484–497.
67. Sekiguchi K, Kawamori J, Yamauchi H. Breast reconstruction and postmastectomy radiotherapy: complications by type and timing and other problems in radiation oncology. *Breast Cancer.* 2017;24(4):511–520.
68. Slezak J, Kura B, Babal P, et al. Potential markers and metabolic processes involved in the mechanism of radiation-induced heart injury. *Can J Physiol Pharmacol.* 2017;95(10):1190–1203.
69. Billon R, Bosc R, Belkacemi Y, et al. Impact of adjuvant antiestrogen therapies (tamoxifen and aromatase inhibitors) on perioperative outcomes of breast reconstruction. *J Plast Reconstr Aesthet Surg.* 2017;70(11):1495–1504.
70. Parikh RP, Odom EB, Yu L, Colditz GA, Myckatyn TM. Complications and thromboembolic events associated with tamoxifen therapy in patients with breast cancer undergoing microvascular breast reconstruction: a systematic review and meta-analysis. *Breast Cancer Res Treat.* 2017;163(1):1–10.
71. Glass CK, Mitchell RN. Winning the battle, but losing the war: mechanisms and morphology of cancer-therapy-associated cardiovascular toxicity. *Cardiovasc Pathol.* 2017;30:55–63.
72. Dort JC, Farwell DG, Findlay M, et al. Optimal perioperative care in major head and neck cancer surgery with free flap reconstruction. A consensus review of recommendations from the Enhanced Recovery After Surgery Society. *JAMA Otolaryngol Head Neck Surg.* 2017;143(3):292–303.
73. Temple-Oberle C, Shea-Budgell MA, Tan M, et al. Consensus review of optimal perioperative care in breast reconstuction: Enhanced Recovery After Surgery (ERAS) Society Recommendations. *Plast Reconstr Surg.* 2017;139(5):1056e–1071e.
74. Shah J.P., Patel S.G., Singh B., eds Jatin Shah's Head and Neck Surgery and Oncology. Elsevier; 2012:1–3. 4th ed.
75. Young D, Xiao CC, Murphy B, Moore M, Fakhry C, Day TA. Increase in head and neck cancer in younger patients due to human papillomavirus (HPV). Oral Oncol. 2015;51(8):727–730. doi:10.1016/j.oraloncology.2015.03.015.
76. Hwang K, Lee JP, Yoo SY, Kim H. Relationship of comorbidities and old age with postoperative complications of head and neck free flaps: a review. *J Plast Reconstr Aesthet Surg.* 2016;69(2016):1627–1635.
77. McMahon JD, MacIver C, Smith M, et al. Postoperative complications after major head and neck surgery with free flap repair–prevalence, patterns, and determinants: a prospective cohort study. *Br J Oral Maxillofac Surg.* 2013;51(8):689–695.
78. Patel RS, McCluskey SA, Goldstein DP, et al. Clinicopathologic and therapeutic risk factors for perioperative complications and prolonged hospital stay in free flap reconstruction of the head and neck. *Head Neck.* 2010;2(10):1345–1353.
79. Kim H, Jeong WJ, Ahn SH. Results of free flap reconstruction after ablative surgery in the head and neck. *Clin Exp Otorhinolaryngol.* 2015;8(2):167–173.
80. Mishra S, Bhatnagar S, Jha RR, Singhal AK. Airway management of patients undergoing oral cancer surgery: a retrospective study. *Eur J Anaesthesiol.* 2005;22(7):510–514.
81. Arne J, Descoins P, Fusciardi J, et al. Preoperative assessment for difficult intubation in general and ENT surgery: predictive value of a clinical multivariate risk index. *Br J Anaesth.* 1998;80(2):140–146.
82. Cook TM, Woodall N, Frerk C. Major complications of airway management in the UK: results of the Fourth National Audit Project of the Royal College of Anaesthetists and the Difficult Airway Society. Part 1: Anaesthesia. *Br J Anaesth.* 2011;106(5):617–631.
83. Cameron M, Corner A, Diba A, Hankins M. Development of a tracheostomy scoring system to guide airway management after major head and neck surgery. *Int J Oral Maxillofac Surg.* 2009;38(8):846–849.
84. Singh T, Sankla P, Smith G. Tracheostomy or delayed extubation after maxillofacial free-flap reconstruction? *Br J Oral Maxillofac Surg.* 2016;54(8):878–882.
85. Furyk C, Walsh ML, Kaliaperumal I, Bentley S, Hattingh C. Assessment of the reliability of intubation and ease of use of the Cook Staged Extubation Set–an observational study. *Anaesth Intensive Care.* 2017;45(6):695–699.
86. Macfarlane TV, Wirth T, Ranasinghe S, Ah-See KW, Renny N, Hurman D Head and neck cancer pain: systematic review of prevalence and associated factors. *J Oral Maxillofac Surg.* 2012;3(1):e1 –e1.
87. Zhu Y, Wang G, Liu S, et al. Risk factors for postoperative delirium in patients undergoing major head and neck cancer surgery: a meta-analysis. *Japanese J Clin Oncol.* 2017;47(6):505–511.
88. Nimalan N, Branford OA, Stocks G. Anaesthesia for free flap breast reconstruction. *BJA Education.* 2016;16(5):162–166.
89. Cassorla L., Lee J.-W. Patient positioning and anaesthesia. In: Miller R.D., Eriksson L.I., Fleisher L.A., Wiener-Kronish J.P., Young W.L., eds. Miller's Anaesthesia. Philadelphia, PA: Churchill Livingstone, Elsevier; 2010:1151–1170. 7th ed.
90. Matsuura H, Inoue S, Kawaguchi M. The risk of postoperative nausea and vomiting between surgical patients received propofol and sevoflurane anesthesia: a matched study. *Acta Anaesthesiol Taiwan.* 2016;54(4):114–120.
91. Wigmore TJ, Mohammed K, Jhanji S. Long-term survival for patients undergoing volatile versus IV anesthesia for cancer surgery: a etrospective analysis. *Anesthesiology.* 2016;124(1):69–79.
92. Kehlet H, Dahl JB. The value of "multimodal" or "balanced analgesia" in postoperative pain treatment. *Anesth Analg.* 1993;77(5):1048–1056.
93. Møiniche S, Kehlet H, Dahl JB. A qualitative and quantitative systematic review of preemptive analgesia for postoperative pain relief: the role of timing of analgesia. *Anesthesiology.* 2002;96(3):725–741.
94. Hayes C, Browne S, Lantry G, Burstal R. Neuropathic pain in the acute pain service: a prospective survey. *Acute Pain.* 2002;4(2):45–48.

95. Kehlet H, Jensen TS, Woolf CJ. Persistent postsurgical pain: risk factors and prevention. *Lancet.* 2006;367(9522):1618–1625.
96. Fuzier R, Puel F, Izard P, Sommet A, Pierre S. Prospective cohort study assessing chronic pain in patients following minor surgery for breast cancer. *J Anesth.* 2017;31(2):246–254.
97. Terkawi AS, Sharma S, Durieux ME, Thammishetti S, Brenin D, Tiouririne M. Perioperative lidocaine infusion reduces the incidence of post-mastectomy chronic pain: a double-blind, placebo-controlled randomized trial. *Pain Physician.* 2015;18(2):E139–E146.
98. Weinberg L, Rachbuch C, Ting S, et al. A randomised controlled trial of peri-operative lidocaine infusions for open radical prostatectomy. *Anaesthesia.* 2016;71(4):405–410.
99. Marret E, Rolin M, Beaussier M, Bonnet F. Meta-analysis of intravenous lidocaine and postoperative recovery after abdominal surgery. *Br J Surg.* 2008;95(11):1331–1338.
100. Brose WG, Cousins M. Subcutaneous lidocaine for treatment of neuropathic cancer pain. *Pain.* 1991;45(2):145–148.
101. Bonde C, Khorasani H, Hoejvig J, Kehlet H Cyclooxygenase-2 inhibitors and free flap complications after autologous breast reconstruction: a retrospective cohort study. *J Plast Reconstr Aesthet Surg.* 2017;70(11):1543–1546.
102. Rai AS, Khan JS, Dhaliwal J, et al. Preoperative pregabalin or gabapentin for acute and chronic postoperative pain among patients undergoing breast cancer surgery: a systematic review and meta-analysis of randomized controlled trials. *J Plast Reconstr Aesthet Surg.* 2017;70(10):1317–1328.
103. Zhong T, Wong KW, Cheng H, et al. Transversus abdominis plane (TAP) catheters inserted under direct vision in the donor site following free DIEP and MS-TRAM breast reconstruction: a prospective cohort study of 45 patients. *J Plast Reconstr Aesthet Surg.* 2013;66(3):329–336.
104. Lou F, Sun Z, Huang N, et al. Epidural combined with general anesthesia versus general anesthesia alone in patients undergoing free flap breast reconstruction. *Plast Reconstr Surg.* 2016;137(3):502e–509e.
105. Tolga Eryilmaz AS, Camgoz N, Ak B, Yavuzer R. A challenging problem that concerns the aesthetic surgeon. *Ann Plast Surg.* 2008;61:489–491.
106. Apfel CC, Heidrich FM, Jukar-Rao S, et al. Evidence-based analysis of risk factors for postoperative nausea and vomiting. *Br J Anaesth.* 2012;109(5):742–753.
107. Gan TJ, Diemunsch P, Habib AS Consensus guidelines for the management of postoperative nausea and vomiting. *Anesth Analg.* 2014;118(1):85–113.
108. Liu YJ, Hirsch BP, Shah AA, Reid MA, Thomson JG. Mild intraoperative hypothermia reduces free tissue transfer thrombosis. *J Reconstr Microsurg.* 2011;27(2):121–126.
109. Thomson JG, Mine R, Shah A, et al. The effect of core temperature on the success of free tissue transfer. *J Reconstr Microsurg.* 2009;25(7):411–416.
110. Hill JB, Sexton KW, Bartlett EL, et al. The clinical role of intraoperative core temperature in free tissue transfer. *Ann Plast Surg.* 2015;75(6):620–624.
111. Pannucci CJ, Bailey SH, Dreszer G, et al. Validation of the Caprini risk assessment model in plastic and reconstructive surgery patients. *J Am Coll Surg.* 2011;212(1):105–112.
112. Murphy Jr RX, Alderman A, Gutowski K, et al. Evidence-based practices for thromboembolism prevention: summary of the ASPS Venous Thromboembolism Task Force Report. *Plast Reconstr Surg.* 2012;130(1):168e–175e.
113. Liao EC, Taghinia AH, Nguyen LP, Yueh YH, May Jr JW, Orgill DP. Incidence of hematoma complication with heparin venous thrombosis prophylaxis after TRAM flap breast reconstruction. *Plast Reconstr Surg.* 2008;121(4):1101–1107.
114. Pannucci CJ, Wachtman CF, Dreszer G, et al. The effect of postoperative enoxaparin on risk for reoperative hematoma. *Plast Reconstr Surg.* 2012; 129(1):160–168.
115. Lee KT, Mun GH. The efficacy of postoperative antithrombotics in free flap surgery: a systematic review and meta-analysis. *Plast Reconstr Surg.* 2015;135(4):1124–1139.
116. Busch CJ, Knecht R, Munscher A, Matern J, Dalchow C, Lorincz BB Postoperative antibiotic prophylaxis in clean-contaminated head and neck oncologic surgery: a retrospective cohort study. *Eur Arch Otorhinolaryngol.* 2016;273(9):2805–2811.
117. Ariyan S, Martin J, Lal A, et al. Antibiotic prophylaxis for preventing surgical-site infection in plastic surgery: an evidence-based consensus conference statement from the American Association of Plastic Surgeons. *Plast Reconstr Sur.* 2015;135(6):1723–1739.
118. Haapio E, Kiviniemi T, Irjala H, Koivunen P, Airaksinen JKE, Kinnunen I Incidence and predictors of 30-day cardiovascular complications in patients undergoing head and neck cancer surgery. *Eur Arch Otorhinolaryngol.* 2016;273(12):4601–4606.
119. Cavallaro F, Sandroni C, Marano C, et al. Diagnostic accuracy of passive leg raising for prediction of fluid responsiveness in adults: systematic review and meta-analysis of clinical studies. *Intensive Care Med.* 2010;36(9):1475–1483.
120. Hosein RC, Cornejo A, Wang HT. Postoperative monitoring of free flap reconstruction: a comparison of external Doppler ultrasonography and the implantable Doppler probe. *Plast Surg.* 2016;24(1):1–19.
121. Mucke T, Fichter AM, Schmidt LH, Mitchell DA, Wolff KD, Ritschl LM, Indocyanine green videoangiography-assisted prediction of flap necrosis in the rat epigastric flap using the FLOW® 800 tool. *Microsurgery.* 2017;37(3):235–242.
122. Kagaya Y, Miyamoto S. A systematic review of near-infrared spectroscopy in flap monitoring: current basic and clinical evidence and prospects. *J Plast Reconstr Aesthet Surg.* 2018; 71(2):246–257.
123. Moore JA, Conway DH, Thomas N, Cummings D, Atkinson D. Impact of a peri-operative quality improvement programme on postoperative pulmonary complications. *Anaesthesia.* 2017;72(3):317–327.

33

Perioperative Care of the Surgical Patient: Surgical Emergencies in Cancer

ATUL PRABHAKAR KULKARNI, MADHAVI D. DESAI, AND GOURI H. PANTVAIDYA

Background

Oncologic surgical emergency may be defined as an acute, potentially life-threatening condition arising from cancer pathology, e.g., obstruction of hollow viscera, bleeding from the tumor, or its treatment such as cecal perforation in a neutropenic patient. Understanding the pathophysiology and prognosis of the surgical condition the patient presents with is therefore very important for appropriate management and improving outcomes. Broadly, cancer patients present with three main emergencies: obstruction, infection, and bleeding. The common emergency oncosurgeries are listed in Table 33.1.

Triage

Depending on the anatomic site of the problems and the resultant severity of their symptoms, the urgency of the situation can be decided. The World Society of Emergency Surgery study group initiative on Timing of Acute Care Surgery (TACS) classification described the nature of emergency surgeries and the ideal time for surgery. Prioritizing care of patients in need of surgical interventions is based on the color-coding system (Table 33.2), which is used for injured patients requiring surgery in trauma centers.[1] Similarly, the National Confidential Enquiry into Patient Outcome and Death (NCEPOD) also classified the timing of intervention for emergency surgeries (Table 33.3).[2] Though these classifications and timelines are not meant for emergency oncosurgeries, they can be easily adopted for this purpose. In an excellent review, Eschamann and colleagues note the advantages of TACS classification.[3] It allows continuous feedback via a regularly updated surgical plan, monitoring of the classifying urgency according to patients' clinical condition, and ensures that the patient status is communicated, with the proviso of being time-dependent, i.e., urgent, immediate, etc., in an emergency. The World Society of Emergency Surgery study group notes some limitations of the NCEPOD classification system. The surgery and main symptoms outlined in NCEPOD may not always match the clinical situations. Factors other than pathophysiology processes, such as psychologic factors and quality of life issues, should influence the urgency of the surgery. For example, a body image issue may be the main issue for a young woman scheduled for breast reconstructive surgery for a malignant lesion. The TACS also has the following important advantages: adoption and consistent adherence to the triage system for oncosurgical emergencies will ensure that time to surgery (TTS) can be made into a quality improvement tool. Thus the actual timing to surgery (aTTS) can be checked against the ideal time to surgery (iTTS). This ratio, if lower than 1, indicates that the surgery occurred within the "ideal time." A ratio higher than 1 indicates delayed surgery; the Acute Care Surgery team and management can then take measures to improve compliance and engage in a quality improvement cycle.[1]

While it is recognized that additional categories or subcategories could be defined, it is important that the classification system remains as simple as possible to use.[2]

Risk Stratification

In emergency surgeries the time available to evaluate the patient preoperatively and optimizing for surgery is limited. The key challenge is achieving meaningful improvement in the patient's condition without causing delay in performing time-sensitive surgery. Prompt decision-making by senior caregivers is required to minimize delays. The time taken to correct any physiologic abnormalities needs to be balanced against the urgency for the surgery to be undertaken.

Cancer patients are sometimes cachectic. Cancer cachexia is a syndrome presenting as a significant loss of body weight due to muscle wasting (also called sarcopenia) and

TABLE 33.1 Common Surgical Emergencies in Oncology Patients

Airway Emergencies
Airway obstruction and stridor from upper aerodigestive tract cancers
Tracheobronchial tree obstruction
Hemorrhage from upper aerodigestive tract cancers
Abdominal Problems
Acute intestinal/gastric outlet obstruction
Biliary tract obstruction
Hematemesis from upper GI malignancies
Perforations (GI and hematolymphoid tumors)
Choriocarcinoma leading to hemorrhage
Intraabdominal/intrathoracic leaks/hemorrhage
CNS Problems
Raised intracranial pressure (due to intracranial tumors, intracranial bleed with hematolymphoid malignancies)
Malignant spinal cord compression
Others
Malignant pathologic fractures

CNS, Central nervous system; *GI*, gastrointestinal.

fat loss. The other signs are loss of appetite, anemia, and asthenia. Cachexia cannot be treated with conventional nutritional therapy.[4]

There may be additional comorbidities associated with the particular cancer or related to the treatment (e.g., adriamycin-induced cardiomyopathy, reduced diffusing capacity for carbon monoxide (DLCO) following bleomycin, etc.). Occasionally, emergency surgical procedures may be necessary as a temporary remedy. Various audits have shown that the clinical outcomes of patients with surgical oncologic emergencies are often poor and the surgery is associated with higher short-term mortality (9.8%–13%) compared with elective surgeries.[5–8] Risk factors for poor outcome after emergency oncosurgery are shown in Table 33.4. All these factors have been shown to correlate with higher 30-day postoperative mortality. These predictors can be used for patient counseling and documentation for emergency oncosurgeries.[5–7]

Care Processes to Improve Patient Outcomes

The 4th National Emergency Laparotomy Audit (NELA) in the UK made the following recommendations for this purpose.[9] It must be kept in mind that the NELA report is meant for all patients undergoing emergency laparotomies and may be useful in improving patient care and outcomes, but may not apply to oncosurgical emergencies.[9,10]

1. Improving outcomes and reducing complications: intrahospital variation can be reduced through standardization of processes and modification of systems.
2. Ensuring all patients receive an assessment of their risk of death: preoperative assessment and documentation of risk has been encouraged, initially using the P-POSSUM model and more recently, the NELA risk prediction model.[11]
3. Delivering care within agreed time frames for all patients.
4. Enabling consultant input in the perioperative period for all high-risk patients: consultant-led care—the right intervention, at the right time, and at right place with the right facilities available.

TABLE 33.2 Proposed Ideal Time to Surgery (iTTS) and Color Coding[1]

Timing—iTTS From Diagnosis	Possible Clinical Scenarios (TACS)	Color Code	Note
Immediate surgery	Bleeding emergencies		Immediate life-saving surgical intervention, resuscitative laparotomy.
Within 1 h	Incarcerated hernia, perforated viscus, diffuse peritonitis, soft tissue infection accompanied with sepsis		Surgical intervention as soon as possible, but only after resuscitation (within 1–2 h). Administration of antibiotics upon diagnosis: no delay.
Within 6 h	Soft tissue infection (abscess) not accompanied with sepsis		Administration of antibiotics upon diagnosis: no delay.
Within 12 h	Appendicitis (local peritonitis), cholecystitis (optional)		Administration of antibiotics upon diagnosis: no delay.
Within 24 or 48 h	Second-look laparotomy		Schedule in advance. Intervention should occur during day time.

TACS, Timing of Acute Care Surgery.
Adapted from Kluger Y, Ben-Ishay O, Sartelli M, et al. World Society of Emergency Surgery study group initiative on Timing of Acute Care Surgery classification (TACS). *World J Emerg Surg*. 2013;8(1):17.

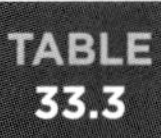

TABLE 33.3 NCEPOD Classification of Interventions[2]

Immediate	Immediate life (1A), limb or organ-saving intervention (1B)—resuscitation simultaneous with intervention. Normally within minutes of decision to operate. Life-saving, other, e.g., limb or organ saving.
Urgent	Intervention for acute onset or clinical deterioration of potentially life-threatening conditions, for those conditions that may threaten the survival of limb or organ, for fixation of many fractures and for relief of pain or other distressing symptoms. Normally within hours of decision to operate.
Expedited	Patient requiring early treatment where the condition is not an immediate threat to life, limb, or organ survival. Normally within days of decision to operate.
Elective	Intervention planned or booked in advance of routine admission to hospital. Timing to suit patient, hospital, and staff.

While it is recognized that additional categories or subcategories could be defined it is important that the classification remains as simple as possible to use. (National confidential enquiry into patient outcome and death. London: The NCEPOD classification of interventions [Online]. 2004. http://www.ncepod.org.uk/pdf/NCEPOD-Classification.pdf)

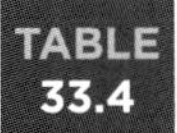

TABLE 33.4 Risk Factors for Poor Outcome After Emergency OncoSurgery[5–7]

Palliative intent of prior cancer treatment
Eastern Cooperative Oncology Group Performance Score (ECOG-PS)
Raised lactate dehydrogenase
Low handgrip strength
Low albumin (<28 g/L)
ASA physical status >3

5. Effective multidisciplinary working. This involves inputs and timely services from three departments/teams, i.e., Radiology, Critical Care, and the Elderly Care group (if required). The radiology services provide timely reports on computed tomography (CT) scans to prevent delays in emergency surgery without discrepancy in the reports. Critical care ensures adequate bed availability such that premature discharges are prevented. When required the Elderly Care group also provides input.
6. Supporting quality improvement. Quality improvement is defined as a formal and systematic approach to analyzing the practice and improving performance to deliver timely, safe, efficient, effective, patient-centered equitable health care.[12,13] Health care managers can support this by adopting one of the quality improvement models such as the Model for Improvement (Plan-Do-Study-Act [PDSA] cycle) described by the Institute for Healthcare Improvement or the Six Sigma model (Define-Measure-Analyze-Improve-Control [DMAIC]) described by the American Society for Quality.[14,15]

Optimizing Patient Condition

Poulton and Murray described the following strategies for improving the patient outcomes in patients undergoing emergency laparotomies.[10] It must be kept in kind that these strategies may not be entirely applicable to emergency oncosurgical patients.

These strategies can be grouped into two categories:

1. Timely Antibiotics: The recommendation for elective surgery is that antibiotic for surgical prophylaxis be administered 60 min before surgical incision. However, patients presenting for emergency surgeries may have signs suggestive of sepsis at the time of admission. In these cases, intravenous antibiotics should be administered as soon as possible. The Surviving Sepsis Guidelines suggest administration of broad-spectrum antibiotics intravenously within 1 h of admission to the intensive care unit (ICU).[16] This recommendation is based on a landmark retrospective study over a 6-year period in ICUs in the United States and Canada. The survival of patients with sepsis improved (79%) when antibiotics were administered before the development of shock. With every 1-h delay in administration of antibiotics after the hypotension set in, there was a decrease in survival by 7.6%.[17]

2. Management of Hypovolemia and Correction of Electrolyte Disturbances: Cancer patients presenting for emergency surgery may have hypovolemia due to either presence of sepsis or hemorrhage due to previous surgery for cancer or from the untreated tumor itself. A patient presenting with abdominal emergency may have vasoplegia due to severe inflammatory response caused by sepsis, lost fluids due to nausea, vomiting or diarrhea, fluid sequestration within the bowel lumen, or intraabdominal hemorrhage. These patients may need administration of high-volume fluid resuscitation in the first 24–72 h of the perioperative period. The cancer patient may therefore present with mixed etiology of hypervolemia. A rapid correction of hypovolemia with appropriate intravenous fluids and/or blood and blood products (if the patient is coagulopathic) is essential. Perioperative blood transfusion has been shown to increase cancer recurrence rates and reduced disease-free survival in patients undergoing surgeries for various solid tumors.[18–21] It is not possible to use the usual measures to reduce transfusion requirements such as autologous blood donation, preoperative erythropoietin therapy, or isovolemic hemodilution in an emergency. A lower transfusion trigger, i.e., 8 g/dL should be aimed at, unless the patient is in shock and needs an increased oxygen-carrying capacity. The transfusion of fresh frozen plasma (FFP) has also been shown to negatively impact patient outcomes.[22,23] Though the transfusion thresholds for blood and blood products in cancer patients remain unknown,[24] in patients with massive blood loss, the only option is to replace the lost volume with blood and aim to correct coagulopathy, guided by viscoelastic hemostatic assays such as TEG or RoTEM.[25]

Target Blood Pressure in Patients Undergoing Emergency Surgery

In a retrospective study of over 33,000 patients undergoing noncardiac surgery, Walsh and colleagues found that mean arterial pressure (MAP) <55 mmHg for increasing durations of time ranging from 5 min to >20 min led to a graded risk of increase in acute kidney injury (AKI) and acute myocardial injury (AMI), both diagnosed by raised biomarkers.[26] Futier et al. (IMPRESS study) compared two strategies in 298 high-risk (of AKI) adults. The first strategy aimed to maintain systolic blood pressure (SBP) within 10% of the patient's resting SBP using noradrenaline infusion. The second was the standard management strategy of treating SBP ≤80 mmHg or lower than 40% of the patient's resting SBP intraoperatively and up to 4 h after the surgery using ephedrine boluses. The primary outcome, i.e., systemic inflammatory response syndrome (SIRS) and at least one organ dysfunction, occurred more commonly in the control group (52% vs. 38%; relative risk [RR], 0.73; 95% confidence interval [CI], 0.56–0.94; *P* = 0.02; AR difference, −14%; 95% CI, −25% to −2%), but there was no difference in mortality.[27] Currently, there is no universally accepted definition of intraoperative hypotension, and in any case a single threshold will not fit all patients.[28] An extensive literature review concluded that blood pressure targets should be decided by the following considerations: the surgery to be performed, the patient's preoperative blood pressure (provided it is not too low or too high), and risk of hypotension-related organ dysfunction and bleeding due to hypertension.[29] In patients with low blood pressure preoperatively, they suggest maintaining MAP between 60 and 65 mmHg unless bleeding is present.[29] Perioperative goal-directed therapy was found to improve outcomes in acutely ill patients, septic or trauma patients, or those undergoing high-risk surgeries (baseline mortality expected to be >20%) when hemodynamic optimization to supranormal values (cardiac index [CI]) >4.5 L/m/m^2, pulmonary artery occlusion pressure <18 mmHg, oxygen delivery of >600 mL/min/m^2, and oxygen consumption of >170 mL/min/m^2) was performed before the development of organ failure.[30] However, more recent trials have shown no benefit of goal-directed fluid therapy either in critically ill or major surgery patients.

1. *Omitting/Optimizing Medication:* Cancer patients may have several comorbidities and may be taking multiple medications. Considering the likelihood of perioperative hypotension and possible presence of AKI, medications such as ACE inhibitors or angiotensin receptor blockers should be avoided and may be changed to some other class of antihypertensive drug class if required. Beta blocker administration should be individualized but none should be added in the immediate preoperative period. The POISE trial evaluated the efficacy of extended release metoprolol, 100 mg administered 2–4 h preoperatively and within 6 h postoperatively, then 200 mg daily for the next 30 days in over 8000 high-risk patients undergoing noncardiac surgery. There was a reduction in cardiovascular deaths, myocardial infarction (MI), or cardiac arrest (5.8% vs. 6.9%, hazard ratio [HR], 0.84; 95% CI, 0.70–0.99, *P* = 0.04) in patients given metoprolol. However, there was an increased incidence of stroke (1.0% vs. 0.5%; HR, 2.17; *P* = 0.0053) and death (3.1% vs. 2.3%; HR, 1.33; *P* = 0.032) as compared with the placebo group. To obtain benefit from beta blocker therapy, it cannot be started in the immediate preoperative period, rather at least 30 days prior to surgery. This is not possible when the patients present for emergency oncosurgery, and therefore unless the patient is already taking beta blockers, they should not be started afresh.[31,32] If the patient is already taking statins, they should be continued. The decision regarding continuing or discontinuing antiplatelet agents and anticoagulants needs to be individualized. In patients with recently inserted drug eluting stents or mechanical valves, bridging therapy with intravenous unfractionated heparin may be required. If it is deemed essential, the effects of newer oral anticoagulants (NOACs) may be reversed using 4-factor prothrombin complex concentrate that contains coagulation factors II, VII, IX, and X, and also protein C and S or appropriate reversal agents such as idarucizumab or andexanet alfa, depending on the urgency of surgery. Idarucizumab is a humanized monoclonal antibody fragment (Fab). It binds to free and thrombin-bound dabigatran, nullifying its effect.[33] Andexanet alfa acts as a decoy receptor for all FXa inhibitors (apixaban, edoxaban, and rivaroxaban) and by binding to them reverses their effect.[34]

2. *Nutrition:* When emergency surgery is required, it is challenging to make a decision regarding initiating nutrition postoperatively. However, the patient's nutritional status should be assessed preoperatively time permitting, and a postoperative nutritional strategy should be planned. The route of nutrition will depend on the nature of surgery and clinical status of the patient in the immediate postoperative period. For example, if the patient undergoes excision of a necrotizing fasciitis-affected area on the periphery or torso, an enteral feeding route may be possible, but not for someone undergoing resection of the colon and anastomosis. If the patient is still in shock postoperatively and needs vasopressor therapy, enteral nutrition should still be tried, at least in the form of trophic feeds for the multiple benefits described recently. Further increases in the amount of feeds to be given will depend on the clinical improvement in the patient condition, improvement in indices of tissue perfusion, and signs of feed intolerance, if any.[35] If enteral feeding does not seem possible, parenteral nutrition may be considered within a week following surgery. In some patients when adequate

nutrition cannot be achieved enterally, partial parenteral nutrition supplementation may be started to meet the goals.

3. *Perioperative Glycemic Control:* Patients with preexisting diabetes mellitus and patients who need emergency surgery will often have hyperglycemia. A study from the Leuven University almost two decades ago in 1548 patients (of which a large proportion were perioperative patients) showed that strict glycemic control (4.44–6.11 mmol/L) improved ICU survival.[36] However, a subsequent study suggested a high incidence of hypoglycemia and no survival benefit of strict glycemic control in medical ICU patients.[37] A large multicenter study from Australia and Canada showed that a blood glucose target of 9.99 mmol/L resulted in lower mortality than intensive sugar control.[38] The current recommendation is to maintain blood glucose level in the preoperative or anesthetized patient at 9.99 mmol/L.[39]

4. *Preoperative Chest Physiotherapy:* A recent multicenter study in more than 400 patients undergoing elective abdominal surgery found that 30 min of preoperative physiotherapy session resulted in a 15% absolute risk reduction in the postoperative pulmonary complications (PPCs).[40] This may not be possible in emergency situations; however, early institution of physiotherapy in the postoperative period with early mobilization should go a long way toward reducing PPCs. The second part of optimization includes minimizing delays in surgery by optimizing the care pathway, which was discussed earlier.

Another study recommended the following strategies for improving outcomes in patients undergoing emergency general surgery: early recognition and resuscitation, early intervention if serum lactate >2 mmol/L, early identification and treatment of sepsis as per surviving sepsis guidelines (as one in five patients requiring emergency laparotomy fulfills sepsis criteria), prioritization to early surgical intervention, use of protocolized fluid management, and using a noninvasive cardiac output monitoring device to measure dynamic fluid response. In addition, postoperative admission of selected patients to ICU or HDU and continued care by the anesthesiologist and surgeon were also recommended.[41]

Preoperative Airway Assessment

The ability to predict a difficult airway is critically important in emergency situations in situ to help identify the optimal approach to airway management. This is particularly important when confronted with a patient with cancer. The airway in a cancer patient may be difficult to secure if the patient is suffering from head and neck cancer or has previously undergone surgery for head and neck cancer, laryngeal tumors, and so on etc. The patient may be at high risk for regurgitation and aspiration of gastric content if a gastric outlet obstruction is present. In hypoxic, hemodynamically unstable, septic patients, the airway becomes physiologically challenging as the cardiopulmonary reserve of the patient reduces. Quick tests, such as the MACOCHA score (Table 33.5), or the HEAVEN criteria (Table 33.6), in addition to the existing difficult airway predicting tools

TABLE 33.5 The MACOCHA Score[42]

Factors	Points
Factors Related to Patient	
Mallampati score III or IV	5
Obstructive sleep apnea syndrome	2
Reduced mobility of cervical spine	1
Limited mouth opening <3 cm	1
Factors Related to Pathology	
Coma	1
Severe hypoxemia (<80%)	1
Factors Related to Operator	
Nonanesthesiologist	1
Total	12

M. **M**allampati score III or IV
A. **A**pnea syndrome (obstructive)
C. **C**ervical spine limitation
O. **O**pening mouth < 3 cm
C. **C**oma
H. **H**ypoxia
A. **A**nesthesiologist nontrained
Coded from 0 to 12
0 = easy, 12 = very difficult

Reprinted with permission of the American Thoracic Society. Copyright © 2022 American Thoracic Society. All rights reserved. Audrey De Jong, Nicolas Molinari, et. al., Early Identification of Patients at Risk for Difficult Intubation in the Intensive Care Unit Development and Validation of the MACOCHA Score in a Multicenter Cohort Study. *Am J Respir Crit Care Med.* 2013; 187(8): 832-9. The American Journal of Respiratory and Critical Care Medicine is an official journal of the American Thoracic Society.

TABLE 33.6 The HEAVEN Criteria[43]

Hypoxemia	Oxygen saturation value ≤93% at the time of initial laryngoscopy
Extremes of size	Pediatric patient ≤8 years of age or clinical obesity
Anatomic challenge	Includes trauma, mass, swelling, foreign body, or other structural abnormality limiting laryngoscopic view
Vomit/blood/fluid	Clinically significant fluid present in the pharynx/hypopharynx at the time of laryngoscopy
Exsanguination	Suspected anemia that could potentially accelerate desaturation during rapid sequence intubation (RSI)-associated apnea
Neck	Limited cervical range-of-motion due to immobilization or arthritis

Kluger Y, Ben-Ishay O, Sartelli M, et al. World Society of Emergency Surgery study group initiative on Timing of Acute Care Surgery classification (TACS). *World J Emerg Surg*. 2013;8(1):17.
Kuzmack E, Inglis T, Olvera D, Wolfe A, Seng K, Davis D. A novel difficult-airway prediction tool for emergency airway management: validation of the HEAVEN criteria in a large air medical cohort. *J Emerg Med*. 2018;54(4):395–401.

like LEMON (Look externally, Evaluate 3-3-2 rule, Mallampati score, Obstruction, Neck mobility), can be useful for assessing the risk of difficult airway and preparation for management.[42,43]

Airway Management in the Emergency Onco-surgical Patient

1. Differences in Emergency Oncosurgical and Other Patients: Airway management of patients in emergency oncosurgery may pose a challenge to the anesthetist due to various reasons.[44] These patients have severe progressive illness, which needs rapid intubation and the time available for preparation is short. The patients also have reduced cardiorespiratory vascular reserve, in particular, respiratory reserve, which means that they can rapidly become hypoxic. They are also at increased risk of profound hypotension or cardiac arrest on anesthetic induction. Due to either the disease itself or medications, such as opiates given earlier for pain, there is an increased risk of pulmonary aspiration of gastric content. Surgery may be required out-of-hours, the person intubating the patient is often inexperienced, and most importantly, emergency surgery cannot be postponed.

2. Preoxygenation: In a nonrandomized controlled study, it was demonstrated that administration of 100% O_2 for 4 min increased Pao_2 by merely 37 mmHg. In 36% of patients the increase was minimal (±5%) from baseline.[45] A French study compared the effect of noninvasive ventilation (NIV) on improving apnea reserve. All patients were given oxygen by high Fio_2 mask for 30 min, and a blood gas sample was collected. The patients were then randomized to receive either 15 L oxygen by bag and mask or NIV in the form of pressure support ventilation (to obtain a tidal volume of 7–10 mL/kg) and positive end-expiratory pressure (PEEP) for 3 min. There was a significant improvement in Pao_2 in patients who were randomized to receive NIV (Pao_2, 12.93 [8.79–21.73]; kPa vs. 27.06 [15.46–36.79]; kPa, $P < 0.01$). This improvement in oxygenation persisted at 5 and 30 min after intubation.[46] It is possible that the significant improvement in oxygenation after NIV, as compared with bag mask ventilation, may be because of the delivery of high oxygen concentration, increase in functional residual capacity (FRC), and end-expiratory lung volume (EELV) due to the recruitment of collapsed alveoli and unloading of the respiratory muscles.[45,46]

3. Risk of Aspiration During Intubation: Pulmonary aspiration is a complication of anesthesia that is associated with significant morbidity and mortality. Recently, Eltorai analyzed incidents of periprocedural pulmonary aspiration from a nationwide database of medical malpractice claims. Of the 43 cases identified to have pulmonary aspiration, the most common causative factor was failure to secure the airway with an endotracheal tube (37%), followed by failure to perform a proper rapid sequence induction and/or failure to place a nasogastric tube for gastric decompression (33%). They concluded that litigation could arise even when the evidence for supporting these practices is weak and that there is a need to develop reliable, high-sensitivity tests for detecting elevated risk.[47]

4. Role of Cricoid Pressure and Rapid Sequence Intubation (RSI): The role of cricoid pressure in RSI is controversial because of the lack of scientific evidence. The classical RSI technique is now seldom used. Gentle mask ventilation is practiced in obese and critically ill patients to prevent hypoxemia during the apneic period.[48] A randomized controlled trial was undertaken to study effectiveness of cricoid and parapharyngeal pressure during RSI and concluded that the relative position of the upper esophageal entrance to the glottis may change after induction of anesthesia and during direct laryngoscopy. Cricoid and paralaryngeal force both decrease the diameter of the upper esophageal entrance in awake and anesthetized states. Occlusion of the esophageal entrance is achieved more frequently with cricoid force compared with paralaryngeal force during direct laryngoscopy.[49]

5. Securing the Airway: To reduce complications in the periintubation period in critically ill patients, Jaber et al. proposed the intubation bundle, which can be extrapolated to and used in emergency oncosurgery patients.[50] The intubation bundle consists of the following three parts:

Preintubation (four elements)

1. Presence of two operators
2. Fluid loading in the absence of cardiogenic pulmonary edema (CPE)
3. Preparation for long-term sedation
4. Preoxygenation for 3 min with noninvasive positive pressure ventilation (NIPPV) in acute respiratory failure (ARF): Fio_2 of 1, PSV of 5–15 cmH_2O to achieve VT_E of 6–8 mL/kg and PEEP of 5 cmH_2O.

During intubation (two elements)

1. Rapid sequence induction: etomidate or ketamine may be used with succinylcholine 1–1.5 mg/kg in the absence of
   - Allergy
   - Hyperkalemia
   - Severe acidosis
   - Acute or chronic neuromuscular disease
   - Burns within 48 h
   - Spinal cord trauma

However, since a rapidly acting, immediately reversible (using sugammadex) neuromuscular blocking drug is now available, intravenous rocuronium (1–1.2 mg/kg) can be used to facilitate tracheal intubation during RSI.

2. Sellick's maneuver

Postintubation (four elements)

1. Immediate confirmation of endotracheal intubation with $ETco_2$
2. Norepinephrine if diastolic blood pressure remains <35 mmHg
3. Initiate long-term sedation
4. Initiate "protective ventilation": tidal volume 6–8 mL/kg predicted body weight, PEEP of 5 cm H_2O, and respiratory rate 10–20 bpm, Fio_2 of 1.0, for a plateau pressure <30 cmH_2O.

Jaber et al. conducted a two-phase, prospective, multicenter controlled study to assess the impact of implementation of intubation bundle on the complications associated with intubation in adult ICU patients. Compared with the control phase, there was a significant decrease in both life-threatening complications (from 34% to 21%, $P = 0.03$) and other complications (from 21% to 9%, $P = 0.01$).

High-frequency nasal cannula (HFNC) has been compared with conventional oxygen therapy (COT) and NIV for preoxygenation in the ICU to prevent desaturation during endotracheal intubation.[51–53] These studies found no difference in the lowest mean Spo_2 during intubation between HFNC and COT. A network meta-analysis of seven randomized trials (959 patients) comparing different modalities (NIV, HFNC, COT) found that in patients with acute hypoxemic respiratory failure, NIV was the best and most effective method of preoxygenation. The incidence of intubation-related complications was lower in the NIV and HFNC groups; however, there was no difference in mortality in patients in whom any of the three modalities were used.[54] The OPTINIV trial compared NIV alone with NIV and HFNC combination for preoxygenation. In the HFNC + NIV group, during the apnea phase (while laryngoscopy and intubation were being carried out), the patients continued to receive HFNC.[55] Since the Spo_2 was better maintained in this group during the apnea phase, the authors concluded that adding HFNC for apneic oxygenation to NIV prior to endotracheal intubation may be more effective than using NIV alone.

Airway Emergencies in Cancer Patients—Anesthetic Management

Upper airway obstruction from upper aerodigestive tract cancers is one of the most common airway emergencies (Table 33.7 and Fig. 33.1). Patients with very large oropharyngeal tumors, hypopharyngeal-laryngeal tumors, and upper esophageal cancer with infiltration of the upper airway can present with stridor, tachypnea, inability to lie down, use of accessory muscles of respiration, restlessness, mental obtundation, and so on. The effects of radiation on the neck leading to fibrosis of the neck, scarring of the neck following previous head neck surgeries and flaps used for reconstruction during previous surgery, and the presence of disease make front of the neck access (tracheostomy and scalpel-bougie cricothyroidotomy technique) challenging. The primary aim of the anesthetist while the airway obstruction is tackled is to maintain oxygenation. Attempting intubation in patients with tumors of the base of the tongue, hypopharynx, pyriform fossa with bleeding, or severe stridor may prove disastrous.[56]

Some patients with severe airway obstruction may have orthopnea, and these patients may obtain enough relief with the use of either HFNC or NIV support that they are able to lie down for the airway to be secured surgically.[57,58]

For the patients in early stridor who are able to lie supine comfortably, conscious sedation can be given safely along with oxygen supplementation. In rare cases, especially in patients with anaplastic carcinoma of the thyroid, the trachea may be displaced and surrounded by the disease, making its identification difficult. Preoperative ultrasonographic assessment of the airway in the neck and illumination of the trachea using a pediatric fiberoptic bronchoscope can help to identify the trachea. A special tracheostomy tube with an adjustable flange that allows the length of the shaft of the tube to be adjusted may be useful in patients with large neck mass or obese patients, since there is a danger of loosing the airway if normal tracheostomy tubes are used (Fig. 33.2).

TABLE 33.7 Causes of Airway Obstruction in Oncology Patients[56]

Causes	Presentation
Upper Airway Obstruction	
Large oropharyngeal tumors	Swelling over face, presence of intraoral tumors, on examination and imaging
Tumors of base of tongue, tonsil, pyriform fossa, epiglottis, upper esophageal tumors	Dysphagia, stridor, pooling of secretions, drooling, breathlessness (depending on the size of the tumor)
Tumors of the laryngeal inlet, including vocal cords	Change in voice, hoarseness of voice, Stridor, orthopnea
Lower Airway Obstruction	
Tracheobronchial tree obstruction due to extrinsic compression by mediastinal masses (of hematolymphoid malignancy), large retrosternal goiter, thymomas, tumors of the pleural cavity, esophagus, primary intratracheal/bronchial tumors (uncommon)	Depends on the pathology, breathlessness, paroxysmal nocturnal dyspnea, inability to lie down on a particular side, inspiratory and/or expiratory stridor
Other Causes	
Vocal cord palsy either due to involvement due to disease or surgery	Change in voice, hoarseness of voice, signs suggestive of upper airway obstruction
Hemorrhage from upper aerodigestive tract cancers	Hemoptysis, breathlessness

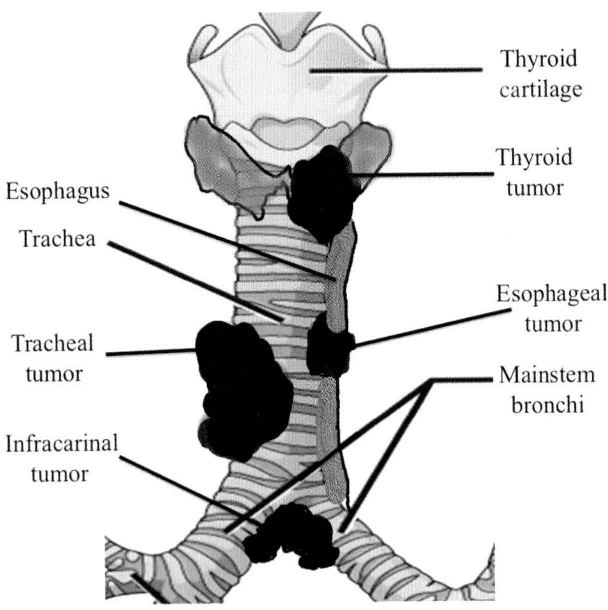

• **Fig. 33.1** Sites of obstructive lesions of central airways.

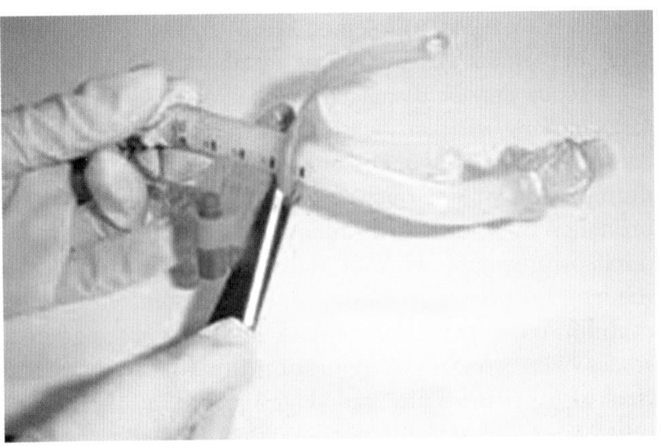

• **Fig. 33.2** Tracheostomy tube with adjustable flange.

Malignant Central Airway Obstruction

Critical obstruction of the intrathoracic airway may be caused by either extraluminal compression by mediastinal mass or by intraluminal tracheobronchial tumors.

The management of patients with lower airway obstruction will depend on the surgical plan. The airway of the patients who have extrinsic compression of trachea, which may or may not end above the level of carina, can be assessed using imaging (CT) and judicious fiberoptic bronchoscopy performed on the operating table. The aim of this assessment is to ascertain whether the airway obstruction can be bypassed by advancing the endotracheal tube beyond the level of obstruction. Further plans for anesthesia are decided after a thorough discussion with the surgical team to understand the surgical intent and the objective of the surgery. A complete discussion of the anesthetic management of these cases, which will vary as per the surgical plan, is beyond the scope of this chapter.

Carotid Blowout Syndrome

Rupture of the common carotid artery (CCA) and the internal carotid artery (ICA) or their major branches is an uncommon but life-threatening complication of head and neck cancer. The overall incidence is 3%–4.5% but is higher in patients who had previously received radiotherapy to the neck (4%–21%). The carotid blowout usually occurs as a result of the necrosis of arterial wall in patients who develop orocutaneous fistula and infection following surgeries for intraoral tumors, and it is more likely if the neck has been radiated preoperatively. Other etiologies include repeat irradiation for a recurrent or second primary tumor and direct invasion of the carotid artery wall by tumor. Three types have been described. In type I (threatened) carotid blowout, carotid artery exposure may be detected on clinical examination or imaging of the neck showing air surrounding the vessel and presence of tumor with fistula and areas of arterial wall disruption. Type II (impending blowout) presents with "herald or sentinel bleeding," which may be controlled temporarily by external compression, but these are warning signs for carotid hemorrhage (type III). It will prove rapidly fatal unless it occurs in the hospital and is witnessed. If it occurs in the postoperative period, after head and neck surgery, the presence of narrowed oral cavity and flaps used for reconstruction may make securing the airway difficult. Surgical tracheostomy is therefore performed under local anesthesia for securing a definitive airway before induction of anesthesia. The patients are often hemodynamically unstable and will need rapid infusion of blood and blood products to achieve some degree of stability. The definitive treatment is surgical ligation of the carotid artery or a branch of the carotid artery. Alternatively, endovascular placement of a covered stent in the ruptured artery or carotid artery embolization can be performed.[59]

Intra-abdominal and Intra-thoracic Surgeries

It is important to emphasize here that apart from surgical control of bleeding or treatment of airway obstruction, the magnitude of the surgery to be undertaken should be such that it will cause the fewest physiologic disturbances. The approach for achieving this is summarized in Table 33.8.

Anesthetic Management of Patients With Anastomotic Leaks Following Gastrointestinal Surgeries

The true incidence of anastomotic leak following gastrointestinal surgeries is difficult to judge due to the large number of definitions used to diagnose the problem. A systematic review assessed the definitions of leaks used and the measurement of anastomotic leaks in patients undergoing surgeries of the gastrointestinal tract for cancer.[60] According to this review

TABLE 33.8 Source Control for Intraabdominal and Thoracic Infections

Intraabdominal Infections
Drainage of abscesses using imaging-guided insertion of pigtail or other catheters
Bedside debridement of infected necrotic tissues
Anastomotic disconnections (in case of leaks) with stoma(s) for cover
Insertion of intercostal catheters or pigtail catheters for decreasing peritoneal inoculum
Thoracic Infections
Bedside imaging with ultrasound with drainage using appropriate drainage catheters including intercostal drains
Anastomotic disconnections (in case of leaks) with stoma(s) for cover
Use laparoscopic or video-assisted (VATS) approach to minimize the need for open surgeries

after upper gastrointestinal surgeries (33 case series, 5303 patients), the incidence of anastomotic leak varied widely. For example, in patients undergoing colorectal surgeries (39 case series), the leak rates varied from 2% to 39%.

The most difficult leaks are postesophagectomy leaks, since they lead to significant morbidity and mortality in the perioperative period. Early fulminant leaks occur within 48 h of surgery due to either necrosis of the gastric tube or a major technical surgical error. The patients are extremely sick and present with manifestations of septic shock, requiring multiorgan support. In spite of anastomotic disconnection, esophagostomy (neck), and gastrostomy (abdomen), the outcomes are dismal, with >90% mortality. The other type of anastomotic leaks that anesthetists may have to deal with is gastrointestinal content in the thoracic tube drains. These patients appear septic and need vasopressor support and ventilation. These patients are generally managed conservatively with CT-guided mediastinal drain placement or a surgical toilet but rarely is the anastomosis disconnected. Other types of leaks may be insidious in onset and the clinical presentation will depend on the site of the leak, preoperative nutritional status of the patient, and preoperative comorbidities.[61]

The principles of preoperative optimization remain the same as described earlier. Fluid resuscitation, immediate administration of broad-spectrum antibiotics, intubation, and controlled mechanical ventilation and vasopressor infusion, if needed to maintain MAP >65 mmHg (unless the patient is previously known to be hypertensive, in which case a higher MAP should be targeted), with normalization of lactate levels are the goals of resuscitation therapy. Vascular access, including arterial pressure monitoring (for beat-to-beat arterial pressure monitoring, frequent arterial blood gas sampling, and cardiac output monitoring if desired) and central venous catheterization (for infusion of vasopressors and monitoring of the central venous pressure), is established. In some patients with severe preexisting cardiorespiratory comorbid conditions, advanced cardiac output monitoring such as pulmonary artery catheterization may be instituted. Intraoperative management is aimed at maintaining the MAP >65 mmHg and replacing blood loss and fluids to maintain adequate urine output.[61] The commonest surgery undertaken in these patients is disconnection of the anastomosis followed by esophagostomy (in the neck) and gastrostomy. In addition, a feeding jejunostomy may be performed for postoperative feeding. These patients need to be managed in the ICU postoperatively with multiple organ support generally being required.

Management of Patients With Emergency Colorectal Surgeries

Acute intestinal obstruction or perforation may be the first presentation of surgical patients with colorectal cancer. These patients are usually elderly with multiple comorbid conditions, though certain types of colorectal tumors may be seen in younger population (such as signet ring carcinoma). Patients who present with subacute intestinal obstruction may be managed conservatively. Depending on the patient's physical status, the surgeon may want to perform colostomy; however, a decision is often made to also excise the malignancy. The principles of resuscitation, monitoring, and intraoperative management in patients presenting with colorectal emergencies such as perforation peritonitis and acute intestinal obstruction remain the same as those undergoing other abdominal emergency surgeries.[62] Fig. 33.3 summarizes the management of patients undergoing complicated colorectal surgeries.[63] One major difference in these patients is that when the resection and anastomosis are carried out following resection of the colorectal tumors, there is a higher susceptibility to anastomotic leaks due to the limited blood supply to the colon. Therefore the anesthetist must be extra careful during fluid management of these patients and use of the Enhanced Recovery After Surgery pathway may be beneficial.[64] Fig. 33.4 shows the problems with excessive fluid therapy in patients undergoing colorectal surgeries, while Fig. 33.5 shows the end points of fluid therapy in these patients.[63] Though this is meant for elective surgeries, the problems remain the same in emergency surgeries. The fluid management of patients undergoing colorectal surgery is a matter of much debate in the literature. Both restrictive and individual optimization of fluid therapy in these patients have their proponents. Myles and colleagues in the randomized controlled RELIEF trial compared intraoperative liberal fluid therapy (median intravenous fluid intake of 6.1 L [interquartile range, 5.0–7.4]) in 1493 with restrictive fluid therapy (3.7 L [interquartile range, 2.9–4.9, $P < 0.001$]) in 3000 patients undergoing major abdominal surgery.[65] The rate of disability-free survival at 1 year was 82.3% in the liberal fluid group versus 81.9% in the restrictive fluid group (HR for death or disability, 1.05;

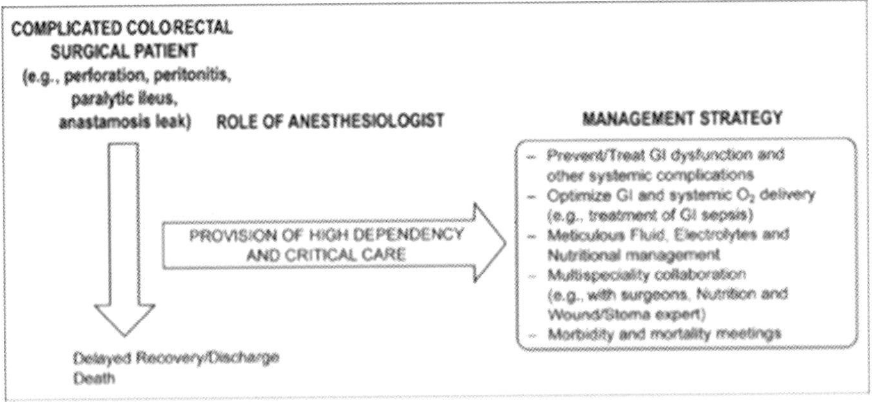

• **Fig. 33.3** Management of complicated colorectal surgical patients.[63]

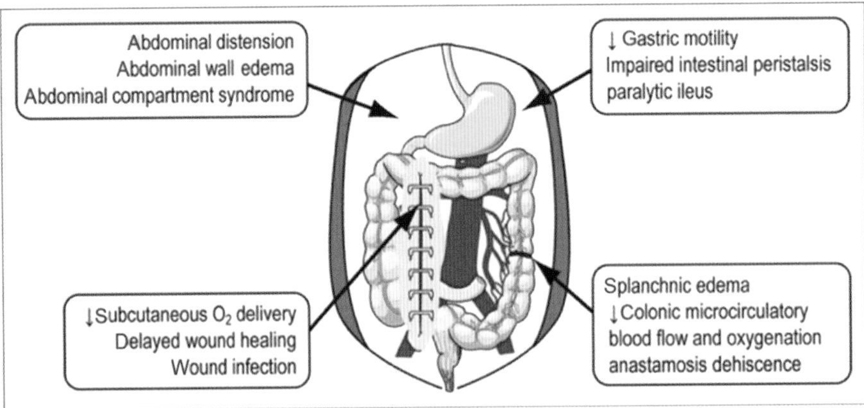

• **Fig. 33.4** Fluid excess in colorectal surgical patients—pathophysiology and complications.[63]

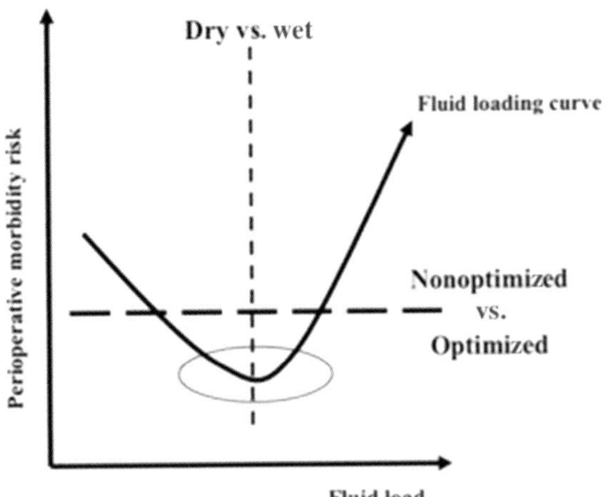

• **Fig. 33.5** End points of fluid therapy in patients undergoing colorectal surgeries.[63]

95% CI, 0.88–1.24; $P = 0.61$). Importantly, the rate of AKI was higher in the restrictive fluid group (8.6% vs. 5.0%, $P < 0.001$). Thus the restrictive fluid strategy caused increased incidence of renal dysfunction without improving survival. This trial shows the limitations of restrictive fluid therapy.

Management of Massive Transfusion in Patients Undergoing Emergency Oncosurgeries

Detailed discussion of the management of massive bleeding and transfusion is beyond the scope of this chapter. Massive transfusion is defined as the "requirement of more than 10 units of packed RBCs within 24 h," the "requirement of more than four packed RBCs in an hour with anticipation of ongoing need," or "the requirement to replace more than 50% of estimated blood volume with blood and blood products within 3 h."[66,67] Massive transfusion aims at both the replacement of the depleted intravascular volume and preventing further blood loss by achieving homeostasis early. Early identification of patients requiring massive transfusion is important as they may rapidly progress to coagulopathy. Implementation of massive transfusion protocol (MTP) guidelines decreases both the mortality and the overall blood requirement due to better resuscitation. A significant difference in mortality was demonstrated by improving the compliance with timely activation and the type of product given.[68] Cotton et al. found that both the short-term and long-term survival increased when MTP was initiated early in the course of bleeding.[69] Massive transfusion

TABLE 33.9 Complications of Massive Transfusion[70]

Transfusion-associated acute lung injury (TRALI) Acute respiratory distress syndrome (ARDS)
Transfusion-associated cardiac overload (TACO)
Transfusion-associated immunomodulation (TRIM)
Transmission of infections
Electrolyte abnormalities—hypokalemia, hyperkalemia, hypocalcemia
Citrate toxicity
Hypothermia
Compartment syndrome
Dilutional coagulopathy
Hemolytic transfusion reactions
Posttransfusion graft-versus-host disease

may be life-saving, but it is also associated with several complications (Table 33.9).[70]

Raised Intracranial Pressure

Raised intracranial pressure (ICP) in cancer patients is caused by primary central nervous system (CNS) tumors, metastatic lesions from other tumors, hematolymphoid malignancies of the CNS, or intracranial hemorrhage (ICH) due to coagulopathy.

ICH is spontaneous bleeding within the parenchyma of the brain. It is potentially lethal, and survival depends on ensuring an adequate airway, proper diagnosis, and early management of several specific issues such as raised blood pressure, coagulopathy reversal, and surgical hematoma evacuation in appropriate patients.

In a study from Memorial Sloan Kettering Cancer Center, it was reported that among cancer patients with ICH, 68% had solid tumors, 16% had primary brain tumors, and 16% had hematopoietic tumors.[71] In adult patients with hematologic malignancies, ICH is the second most common complication with overall incidence of 2.8%. The incidence of ICH in patients with acute myeloid leukemia is higher (6.8%) than patients with other hematologic malignancies (1%). However, in those with intracranial malignant disease, patients with CNS lymphoma were more prone to ICH than patients with CNS lymphoma involving acute leukemia.[72] Sustained intracranial hypertension and acute brain herniation are "brain codes," signifying catastrophic neurologic events that require immediate recognition and treatment to prevent irreversible injury and death. Brain code resuscitation mandates a step-wise approach similar to that in cardiac arrest, which starts with an assessment of circulation, airway patency, and ventilation.

Cadena et al. have recently described the management of intracranial hypertension and herniation.[73]

Tier Zero consists of the following measures:

1. Head elevation to >30 degrees and the head kept in midline to facilitate cerebral venous drainage
2. Minimize stimuli that can increase ICP such as coughing and endotracheal suction
3. Avoid hypotonic intravenous fluids
4. Correct hyponatremia
5. High-dose corticosteroids for vasogenic edema arising from brain tumors
6. CT scan of head after securing the airway and hemodynamic stabilization

Tier One involves:

1. Administration of IV mannitol 0.5–1 g/kg bolus through a peripheral intravenous line, which may be repeated every 4–6 h. No therapeutic benefit is appreciable if serum osmolality >320 mOsm/kg.
2. Hypertonic saline (HTS) 3%–23.4% administered as a bolus, alone or in addition to mannitol. HTS concentrations of 7.5% or more should be given via a central venous catheter.
3. When acute obstructive hydrocephalus is present as determined by neuroimaging, an external ventricular drainage (EVD) system should be placed emergently.
4. If an EVD system is already in place, drain 5–10 mL cerebrospinal fluid (CSF). If the clinical signs of herniation do not resolve with Tier One interventions, review decompressive surgical options.

Tier Two:

1. Increase the target serum sodium concentration to 160 mmol/L.
2. Propofol infusion to sedate the patient; however, the possibility of hypotension and development of propofol infusion syndrome should be kept in mind.
3. If the ICP still remains high, surgical options should be considered, which include the following:
   - Placement of EVD
   - Evacuation of extraaxial lesion (e.g., epidural hematoma)
   - Resection of intracerebral lesion (e.g., lobar hemorrhage)
   - Removal of brain parenchyma (e.g., cerebellar mass)
   - Unilateral or bilateral craniectomies

General principles of neuroprotection, such as normovolemia, normothermia, normotension, and normocapnia, should be followed for adequate cerebral perfusion. If the brain is still herniating after these measures, rescue decompressive craniectomy is considered.

Tier Three:

This is the most aggressive management approach. If the patient is not eligible for surgery, the following may be tried:

1. EEG burst suppression or ICP-directed infusion of pentobarbital. Patients who have had or are at risk for a brain code may benefit from additional neuromonitoring, such as jugular venous oximetry, brain tissue oxygenation, and cerebral microdialysis catheters.

2. Moderate hypothermia (target core temperature 32–34°C) to reduce the ICP may be induced with the administration of cold intravenous fluids, external cooling devices, intravenous devices, or a combination of any of these. Hypothermia can cause arrhythmias, shivering, and make patients prone to infection and electrolyte disturbances.
3. Hyperventilation to achieve mild to moderate hypocapnia ($Paco_2$: 25–35 mmHg) may be tried for a limited period of time (up to 6 h), while other strategies are being considered.

Spinal Cord Compression

Spinal cord compression (SCC) is an oncologic emergency requiring early diagnosis and immediate treatment. The compression can arise from the space-occupying lesion emerging from the meninges of the spine, intra/extraaxial tumors such as Schwannoma, metastatic lesions in spine, deposits of hematolymphoid lesions, or neural crest cell lesions abutting the spinal cord (neuroblastomas in children). The MRI should be carried out within a few hours of acute onset of symptoms, and definitive therapy should be initiated within 24 h.[74,75] Patients with primary spinal cord tumors will benefit from surgery. The spine is the most common site for bone metastasis, and these metastases are frequently seen in patients with prostate, breast, lung, or renal cancers. Between 5% and 10% of cancer patients develop metastatic SCC. Dexamethasone 16 mg OD is started immediately after onset of the symptom of nerve compression, followed by 16 mg/day and is tapered over 4 weeks after radiotherapy or surgery. Chemotherapy is initiated for chemosensitive tumors. Surgery has been a more controversial approach in terms of maximal cytoreduction of the metastatic mass, immediate decompression, pain relief, and stabilization of the spine and most of the time this may be palliative in intent.[75]

Anesthetic management should ensure the following:

1. Log roll for transport and positioning of the patient
2. Wide bore peripheral intravenous access
3. Adequate spinal cord perfusion pressure (MAP-CSF pressure) to prevent secondary ischemic insult
4. Care of patient in the prone position
5. Coagulopathy reversal

Summary

Oncologic surgical emergency may be defined as an acute, potentially life-threatening condition arising from cancer pathology, mainly obstruction of hollow viscera and bleeding from the tumor. Depending on the anatomic site of the problems and the resultant severity of their symptoms, the urgency of the situation needs to be decided. The key challenge is achieving meaningful improvement through preoperative optimization in the patient's condition without causing delay in performing time-sensitive surgery to minimize postoperative morbidity.

Outcomes of patients with surgical oncologic emergencies are often poor, and surgery is associated with higher short-term mortality compared to elective surgeries. Palliative intent of the prior cancer treatment, high Eastern Cooperative Oncology Group Performance Score (ECOG-PS), raised lactate dehydrogenase, low handgrip strength, low albumin (<28 g/L), and American Society of Anesthesiologists physical status >3 have been shown to correlate with higher 30-day postoperative mortality. These predictors can be used for patient counseling and documentation for emergency oncosurgeries.

Upper airway obstruction from upper aerodigestive tract cancers is one of the most common airway emergencies. Critical obstruction of intrathoracic airway may be caused by either extraluminal compression by mediastinal mass or by intraluminal tracheobronchial tumors. Rupture of the CCA and the ICA or their major branches is an uncommon but life-threatening complication of head and neck cancer. Acute intestinal obstruction or perforation may be the first presentation of the surgical patients with colorectal cancer. These patients are usually elderly with multiple comorbid conditions.

Acknowledgment

We gratefully acknowledge the artistic contribution toward Fig. 33.1 of Dr. Ashwini Wanjari, Junior Resident, Department of Anesthesiology, Critical Care & Pain, Tata Memorial Hospital, Parel, Mumbai, India.

References

1. Kluger Y, Ben-Ishay O, Sartelli M, et al. World Society of Emergency Surgery study group initiative on Timing of Acute Care Surgery classification (TACS). *World J Emerg Surg*. 2013;8(1):17.
2. National confidential enquiry into patient outcome and death. London: The NCEPOD classification of interventions [Online]; 2004. Available at: http://www.ncepod.org.uk/pdf/NCEPODClassification.pdf.
3. Eschmann D, Köck M, Bludau F, Obertacke U. Scientific backgrounds for the timing of acute care surgery. *Z Orthop Unfall*. 2019;158(1):104–110. doi:10.1055/a-0862-6065.
4. Dhanapal R, Saraswathi T, Govind RN. Cancer cachexia. *J Oral Maxillofac Pathol*. 2011;15(3):257–260. doi:10.4103/0973-029X.86670.
5. Bosscher M, Bastiaannet E, Leeuwen B, Harald J, Hoekstra H. Factors associated with short-term mortality after surgical oncologic emergencies. *Ann Surg Oncol*. 2016;23:1803–1814.
6. Roses R, Tzeng C, Ross M, Fournier K, Abbott D, You Y. The palliative index: predicting outcomes of emergent surgery in patients with cancer. *J Palliat Med*. 2014;17(1):37–42.
7. Bosscher M, Leeuwen B, Harald J, Hoekstra H. Current management of surgical oncologic emergencies. *PLoS One*. 2015;10(5):e0124641.
8. Oliphant R, Mansouri D, Nicholson GA, et al. Emergency presentation of node-negative colorectal cancer treated with curative surgery is associated with poorer short and longer-term survival. *Int J Colorectal Dis*. 2014;29(5):591–598.
9. NELA Project Team. Fourth Patient Report of the National Emergency Laparotomy Audit RCoA London. 2018 https://

www.hqip.org.uk/wp-content/uploads/2018/11/The-Fourth-Patient-Report-of-the-National-Emergency-Laparotomy-Audit-October-2018.pdf.
10. Poulton TD, Murray D. Pre-optimisation of patients undergoing emergency laparotomy: a review of best practice. *Anaesthesia*. 2019;74(Suppl 1):100–107.
11. Eugene N, Oliver CM, Bassett MG, et al. Development and internal validation of a novel risk adjustment model for adult patients undergoing emergency laparotomy surgery: the National Emergency Laparotomy Audit risk model. *Br J Anaesth*. 2018;121(4):739–748.
12. AAFP. Basics of quality improvement. https://www.aafp.org/family-physician/practice-and-career/managing-your-practice/quality-improvement-basics.html. Accessed October 13, 2021.
13. NHS Health Education England South East. What is quality improvement? https://wessex.hee.nhs.uk/quality/quality-improvement/what-is-quality-improvement. Accessed October 13, 2021.
14. Institute for Healthcare Improvement. How to improve. http://www.ihi.org/resources/Pages/HowtoImprove/ScienceofImprovementEstablishingMeasures.aspx. Accessed October 13, 2021.
15. ASQ. DMAIC guidelines. https://asqasktheexperts.com/tag/six-sigma. Accessed October 13, 2021.
16. Rhodes A, Evans LE, Alhazzani W, et al. Surviving sepsis campaign: international guidelines for management of sepsis and septic shock: 2016. *Intensive Care Med*. 2017;43:304–377.
17. Kumar A, Roberts D, Wood KE, et al. Duration of hypotension before initiation of effective antimicrobial therapy is the critical determinant of survival in human septic shock. *Crit Care Med*. 2006;34(6):1589–1596.
18. Xun Y, Tian H, Hu L, Yan P, Yang K, Guo T. The impact of perioperative allogeneic blood transfusion on prognosis of hepatocellular carcinoma after radical hepatectomy: a systematic review and meta-analysis of cohort studies. *Medicine (Baltimore)*. 2018;97(43):e12911.
19. Boshier PR, Ziff C, Adam ME, Fehervari M, Markar SR, Hanna GB. Effect of perioperative blood transfusion on the long-term survival of patients undergoing esophagectomy for esophageal cancer: a systematic review and meta-analysis. *Dis Esophagus*. 2018;31(4). doi:10.1093/dote/dox134.
20. Qiu L, Wang DR, Zhang XY, et al. Impact of perioperative blood transfusion on immune function and prognosis in colorectal cancer patients. *Transfus Apher Sci*. 2016;54:235–241.
21. Chalfin HJ, Liu JJ, Gandhi N, et al. Blood transfusion is associated with increased perioperative morbidity and adverse oncologic outcomes in bladder cancer patients receiving neoadjuvant chemotherapy and radical cystectomy. *Ann Surg Oncol*. 2016;23:2715–2722.
22. Nakaseko Y, Haruki K, Shiba H, et al. Impact of fresh frozen plasma transfusion on postoperative inflammation and prognosis of colorectal liver metastases. *J Surg Res*. 2018;226:157–165.
23. Shiba H, Ishida Y, Haruki K, et al. Negative impact of fresh-frozen plasma transfusion on prognosis after hepatic resection for liver metastases from colorectal cancer. *Anticancer Res*. 2013;33(6):2723–2728.
24. Cata JP, Gottumukkala V. Blood transfusion practices in cancer surgery. *Indian J Anaesth*. 2014;58(5):637–642.
25. Kozek-Langenecker SA, Ahmed AB, Afshari A, et al. Management of severe perioperative bleeding: guidelines from the European Society of Anaesthesiology: First update 2016. *Eur J Anaesthesiol*. 2017;34(6):332–395.
26. Walsh M, Devereaux PJ, Garg AX, et al. Relationship between intraoperative mean arterial pressure and clinical outcomes after noncardiac surgery: toward an empirical definition of hypotension. *Anesthesiology*. 2013;119(3):507–515.
27. Futier E, Lefrant JY, Guinot PG, et al. Effect of individualized vs standard blood pressure management strategies on postoperative organ dysfunction among high-risk patients undergoing major surgery: a randomized clinical trial. *JAMA*. 2017;318(14):1346–1357.
28. Packiasabapathy KS, Subramaniam B. Optimal perioperative blood pressure management. *Adv Anesth*. 2018;36:67–79.
29. Meng L, Yu W, Wang T, Zhang L, Heerdt PM, Gelb AW. Blood pressure targets in perioperative care. *Hypertension*. 2018;72(4):806–817.
30. Kern JW, Shoemaker WC. Meta-analysis of hemodynamic optimization in high-risk patients. *Crit Care Med*. 2002;30(8):1686–1692.
31. POISE Study GroupDevereaux PJ, Yang H, et al. Effects of extended-release metoprolol succinate in patients undergoing non-cardiac surgery (POISE trial): a randomized controlled trial. *Lancet*. 2008;371(96 27):1839–1847.
32. Blessberger H, Lewis SR, Pritchard MW, et al. Perioperative beta-blockers for preventing surgery-related mortality and morbidity in adults undergoing non-cardiac surgery. *Cochrane Database Syst Rev*. 2019;9:CD013438.
33. Kuramatsu JB, Sembill JA, Huttner HB. Reversal of oral anticoagulation in patients with acute intracerebral hemorrhage. *Crit Care*. 2019;23(1):206.
34. Kaatz S, Bhansali H, Gibbs J, Lavender R, Mahan CE, Paje DG. Reversing factor Xa inhibitors - clinical utility of andexanet alfa. *J Blood Med*. 2017;8:141–149.
35. Wischmeyer PE. Enteral nutrition can be given to patients on vasopressors. *Crit Care Med*. 2019;48(1):122–125. doi:10.1097/CCM.0000000000003965.
36. van den Berghe G, Wouters P, Weekers F, et al. Intensive insulin therapy in critically ill patients. *N Engl J Med*. 2001;345(19):1359–1367.
37. van den Berghe G, Wilmer A, Hermans G, et al. Intensive insulin therapy in the medical ICU. *N Engl J Med*. 2006;354(5):449–461.
38. NICE-SUGAR Study Investigators, Finfer S, Chittock DR, et al. Intensive versus conventional glucose control in critically ill patients. *N Engl J Med*. 2009;360(13):1283–1297.
39. Weimann A, Braga M, Carli F, et al. ESPEN guideline: clinical nutrition in surgery. *Clin Nutr*. 2017;36(3):623–650.
40. Boden I, Skinner EH, Browning L, et al. Preoperative physiotherapy for the prevention of respiratory complications after upper abdominal surgery: pragmatic, double blinded, multicentre randomized controlled trial. *BMJ*. 2018;360:j5916.
41. Aggarwal G, Peden C, Quiney N. Improving outcomes in emergency general surgery patients: what evidence is out there? *Anesth Analg*. 2017;125(4):1403–1405.
42. De Jong A, Molinari N, Terzi N, et al. AzuRéa Network for the Frida-Réa Study Group. Early identification of patients at risk for difficult intubation in the intensive care unit: development and validation of the MACOCHA score in a multicenter cohort study. *Am J Respir Crit Care Med*. 2013;187(8):832–839.
43. Kuzmack E, Inglis T, Olvera D, Wolfe A, Seng K, Davis D. A novel difficult-airway prediction tool for emergency airway management: validation of the HEAVEN criteria in a large air medical cohort. *J Emerg Med*. 2018;54(4):395–401.
44. Nolan JP, Kelly FE. Airway challenges in critical care. *Anaesthesia*. 2011;66(Suppl 2):81–92.

45. Mort TC. Preoxygenation in critically ill patients requiring emergency tracheal intubation. *Crit Care Med.* 2005;33(11): 2672–2675.
46. Baillard C, Fosse JP, Sebbane M, et al. Noninvasive ventilation improves preoxygenation before intubation of hypoxic patients. *Am J Respir Crit Care Med.* 2006;174(2):171–177.
47. Eltorai AS. Periprocedural pulmonary aspiration: an analysis of medical malpractice cases and alleged causative factors. *J Eval Clin Pract.* 2019;25(5):739–743.
48. Algie CM, Mahar RK, Tan HB, Wilson G, Mahar PD, Wasiak J. Effectiveness and risks of cricoid pressure during rapid sequence induction for endotracheal intubation. *Cochrane Database Syst Rev.* 2015(11):CD011656.
49. Kim H, Chang JE, Won D, et al. The effect of cricoid and paralaryngeal force on upper esophageal occlusion during induction of anesthesia: a randomized, crossover study. *Anaesthesia.* 2019;75(2):179–186. doi:10.1111/anae.14873.
50. Jaber S, Jung B, Corne P, et al. An intervention to decrease complications related to endotracheal intubation in the intensive care unit: a prospective, multiple-center study. *Intensive Care Med.* 2010;36(2):248–255.
51. Vourc'h M, Asfar P, Volteau C, et al. High-flow nasal cannula oxygen during endotracheal intubation in hypoxemic patients: a randomized controlled clinical trial. *Intensive Care Med.* 2015;41(9):1538–1548.
52. High-flow nasal cannula versus bag-valve-mask for preoxygenation before intubation in subjects with hypoxemic respiratory failure. *Respir Care.* 2016;61(9):1160–1167.
53. Guitton C, Ehrmann S, Volteau C, et al. Nasal high-flow preoxygenation for endotracheal intubation in the critically ill patient: a randomized clinical trial. *Intensive Care Med.* 2019;45(4):447–458.
54. Fong KM, Au S, Ng GWY. Preoxygenation before intubation in adult patients with acute hypoxemic respiratory failure: a network meta-analysis of randomized trials. *Crit Care.* 2019;23:319.
55. Jaber S, Monnin M, Girard M, et al. Apnoeic oxygenation via high-flow nasal cannula oxygen combined with non-invasive ventilation preoxygenation for intubation in hypoxaemic patients in the intensive care unit: the single-centre, blinded, randomized controlled OPTINIV trial. *Intensive Care Med.* 2016;42(12):1877–1887.
56. Patil V. Airway emergencies in cancer. *Indian J Crit Care Med.* 2007;11(1):36–44.
57. Weingart SD, Levitan RM. Preoxygenation and prevention of desaturation during emergency airway management. *Ann Emerg Med.* 2012;59(3):165–175.
58. Ffrench-O'Carroll R, Fitzpatrick K, Jonker WR, Choo M, Tujjar O. Maintaining oxygenation with high-flow nasal cannula during emergent awake surgical tracheostomy. *Br J Anaesth.* 2017;118(6):954–955.
59. Suárez C, Fernández-Alvarez V, Hamoir M, et al. Carotid blowout syndrome: modern trends in management. *Cancer Manag Res.* 2018;10:5617–5628.
60. Bruce J, Krukowski ZH, Al-Khairy G, Russell EM, Park KG. Systematic review of the definition and measurement of anastomotic leak after gastrointestinal surgery. *Surgery.* 2001;88(9): 1157–1168.
61. Urschel JD. Esophagogastrostomy anastomotic leaks complicating esophagectomy: a review. *B J Surg.* 1995;169(6):634–640.
62. Peden C, Scott MJ. Anesthesia for emergency abdominal surgery. *Anesthesiol Clin.* 2015;33(1):209–221.
63. Patel S, Lutz JM, Panchagnula U, Bansal S. Anesthesia and perioperative management of colorectal surgical patients - specific issues (part 2). *J Anaesthesiol Clin Pharmacol.* 2012;28(3):304–313.
64. Zhu AC, Agarwala A, Bao X. Perioperative fluid management in the enhanced recovery after surgery (ERAS) pathway. *Clin Colon Rectal Surg.* 2019;32(2):114–120.
65. Myles PS, Bellomo R, Corcoran T, et al. Australian and New Zealand College of Anaesthetists Clinical Trials Network and the Australian and New Zealand Intensive Care Society Clinical Trials Group. Restrictive versus liberal fluid therapy for major abdominal surgery. *N Engl J Med.* 2018;378(24):2263–2274.
66. Patil V, Shetmahajan M. Massive transfusion and massive transfusion protocol. *Indian J Anaesth.* 2014;58:590–595.
67. Pham HP, Shaz BH. Update on massive transfusion. *Br J Anaesth.* 2013;111:i71–i82.
68. Bawazeer M, Ahmed N, Izadi H, McFarlan A, Nathens A, Pavenski K. Compliance with a massive transfusion protocol (MTP) impacts patient outcome. *Injury.* 2015;46:21–28.
69. Cotton BA, Dossett LA, Au BK, Nunez TC, Robertson AM, Young PP. Room for (performance) improvement: provider-related factors associated with poor outcomes in massive transfusion. *J Trauma Inj Infect Crit Care.* 2009;67:1004–1012.
70. Sihler KC, Napolitano LM. Complications of massive transfusion. *Chest.* 2010;137:209–220.
71. Navi B, Reichman J, Berlin D, et al. Intracerebral and subarachnoid hemorrhage in patients with cancer. *Neurology.* 2010;74:494–501.
72. Chen CY, Tai CH, Cheng A, et al. Intracranial hemorrhage in adult patients with hematological malignancies. *BMC Med.* 2012;10:97.
73. Cadena R, Shoykhet M, Ratcliff JJ. Emergency neurological life support: intracranial hypertension and herniation. *Neurocrit Care.* 2017;27(S1):82–88.
74. Qurainy R, Collis E. Metastatic spinal cord compression: diagnosis and management. *BMJ.* 2016;353:I2539.
75. Savage P, Sharkey R, Kua T, et al. Malignant spinal cord compression: NICE guidance, improvements and challenges. *Q J Med.* 2014;107:277–278.

34 Palliative Surgery in Cancer Patients

MATTHIAS WILHELM WICHMANN

Introduction

Palliative surgery is "… used with the primary intention of improving quality of life or relieving symptoms caused by advanced disease. Its effectiveness is judged by the presence and durability of patient-acknowledged symptom resolution."[1]

Surgical treatment decisions for patients receiving palliative care are challenging. Often they have to be made within a short period of time, and the outcome expectations may vary significantly between the surgeon on one side and the patient/family on the other side.[2] The goals of surgery and those of good palliative care are, however, directly compatible. They often are shared clinical decisions, an evidence base is usually not available, and the consequences of decision-making are profound. Clinical intuition and experience are therefore very important in this situation.[3]

The major prognostic feature is overall well being rather than the organs in which metastases appear. Increasing global frailty is the hallmark of death approaching.[3] If a person is in a catabolic state, anything that accelerates their deterioration is likely to be irreversible. The trauma of surgery compounds the deterioration of the disease itself.[3] Urgent operations are associated with increased risk and 30-day mortality of up to 28% is seen in patients with disseminated malignancy.[4] Despite these risks, patients may experience significant benefits from palliative procedures, with observational studies demonstrating that 80%–90% of patients undergoing palliative surgery experience symptom improvement or resolution.[5,6] It has also been demonstrated in common solid tumors that the longer a patient survives from the time of diagnosis the more likely they are to survive the next 5 years (conditional survival).[7–9]

These complexities highlight that when weighing the risks and benefits of surgical intervention in a patient with advanced cancer, the nuances of prognostication are best handled by a multidisciplinary team (MDT). MDTs have been shown to be more accurate at predicting survival than individual clinicians.[10] A multidisciplinary approach is beneficial but due to the wide variation of disease presentation and underlying conditions of patients undergoing palliative surgery only very limited or no studies are available to support treatment decisions.[11,12]

There is no doubt that decisions in palliative surgery are very difficult but it is important to make every decision in this challenging area of surgery with profound and humble respect for the person who is dying and for their family.[3]

Preoperative Assessment

The overall condition of the patient must be weighed against the proposed intervention in a multifactorial calculus that has little certainty. What is the overall condition of the person? Where might this person be in their disease trajectory either with or without the intervention proposed? What has been the rate of systemic decline in recent weeks and is it reversible? Rapid decline without a reversible cause is likely to delineate a very short prognosis, while a slower decline is likely to indicate a longer prognosis. Ultimately, is this person otherwise going to tolerate this procedure and live long enough to recover from the effects of the procedure to enjoy the benefits offered?[3]

Prognostication is very difficult and clinicians tend to be too optimistic. Gripp et al.[13] showed that patients suffering from metastatic colorectal and breast cancer had a more favorable prognosis, whereas brain metastases, Karnofsky performance status less than 50%, need for strong analgesics, dyspnea, high lactate dehydrogenase (LDH), and leukocytosis were associated with a poor prognosis.

In the preoperative phase it is important to review and clarify the goals of care with the patient and their caregivers, and this should be actively performed by the treating clinicians.[3]

Interventional Radiology

The interventional radiologist can offer less invasive management of complications occurring in patients receiving palliative care.

Complications from vascular thrombosis are the second leading cause of death in patients with malignancy.[14] For larger vessel venous disease, stenting is an option, such as in superior vena cava (SVC) syndrome and less commonly inferior vena cava (IVC). IVC stenting may provide symptomatic relief and can prevent secondary organ failure (renal or hepatic venous involvement).[14]

Hemorrhage can occur in up to 10% of patients with advanced cancer.[15] The role of interventional radiology in management of bleeding lies in embolization of a bleeding vessel, usually after active bleeding has been identified on computed tomography (CT) angiogram. This is performed most commonly via a femoral artery approach.[16]

Embolotherapy can be bland when agents that cause vessel occlusion alone are employed (Gelfoam, polyvinyl alcohol particles, microspheres, coils).[14,17] Chemoembolization combines chemotherapeutic agents with an embolic agent and is delivered directly to the target tumor by selective cannulation of the feeding artery. This method facilitates increased chemotherapy dose to the tumor.[17,18]

Radioembolization or selective internal radiation therapy (SIRT) enables delivery of high-dose brachytherapy (BT) to hepatic malignancies by the selective injection of yttrium-90 microspheres, used in the setting of hepatocellular carcinoma (HCC) and colorectal liver metastasis (CRLM).[17,19] This treatment exploits the finding that arterial supply to liver tumors is different to normal liver tissue, which is supplied by the portal vein system.[19] There is low penetration of the beta particles from yttrium-90 (approximately 2.5 mm in human tissues), so necrotizing effects are localized.[17]

Thermal ablation techniques involve placement of a specially designed probe/electrode into the center of a lesion, usually under ultrasound (US) +/− CT guidance. The device is connected to an energy source able to generate extremes of temperature to cause irreversible tumor necrosis, ranging from microwave or radiofrequency ablation (RFA) in excess of 60°C to cryotherapy using argon gas under pressure to create subfreezing temperatures.[17,19,20] Chemical ablation has also been described using absolute alcohol and phenol, although thermal ablation is more commonly performed.[20] A 0.5–1.0-cm zone of coagulation necrosis around the lesion is required to enable a tumor-free margin. Because RFA relies on electrical current flow, effective tissue/tumor heating is reduced by adjacent blood vessels >3 mm due to heat sink effect.[20] Microwave ablation can include larger treatment volumes (up to 8 cm diameter), provides optimal heating of cystic masses, causes less pain, and has less heat sink effect than RFA.[17]

Overall, thermal ablative therapies (primarily RFA and microwave) are the preferred treatment option for small lesions, with chemoembolization therapy preferred for larger lesions.

Esophagus

Esophageal carcinoma is the eighth most common cancer worldwide and sixth most common cause of cancer death.[21,22] Despite recent improvements in treatment and modest survival gains, overall 5-year survival for esophageal cancer remains disappointing at around 17%. Patients with inoperable local disease fare even worse with less than 3% of patients surviving 5 years.[23] The majority of symptoms from advanced esophageal cancer can now be palliated with nonsurgical techniques and, as such, palliative surgery in the form of resection or bypass is rarely performed.[23]

The most troublesome symptoms of incurable esophageal cancer, namely, dysphagia and bleeding, can be alleviated using less invasive methods. Esophageal self-expanding stents (SES), BT, external beam radiotherapy, and endoscopic recannulation techniques are highly effective as unimodal or multimodal therapy and are well tolerated by patients.[23] A 2014 Cochrane Review confirmed that the combination of BT with self-expanding metal stent insertion or radiotherapy should be used as the preferred options for palliative management of dysphagia.[24] Meta-analysis has shown that metallic stents are superior to plastic stents.[24] Patients have been reported to do badly with tumors requiring stents more than 12 cm in length.[23]

BT provides a less instant relief of dysphagia than SES but is associated with a better quality of life (QOL) and survival. The optimal dose is unknown but 8–20 Gy in single or double doses is common. SES can be placed endoscopically often without the need for esophageal dilatation.[25]

Malnutrition is common with advanced esophageal cancer due to malignant dysphagia and the catabolic state. Percutaneous gastrostomies (PEG) and radiologically inserted gastrostomies (RIG) can be placed and permit bolus feeding. The author prefers placement of a PEG tube at the time of esophageal stenting. Occasionally if the esophageal lumen is completely occluded, a surgical gastrostomy or feeding jejunostomy may be required. This can be placed via laparotomy or laparoscopy.[23]

Stomach

Gastric carcinoma represents the second leading cause of cancer-related death worldwide. Despite improvements in overall survival, the majority (60%–70%) of patients diagnosed with gastric cancer present with advanced stages. Bleeding is the most important adverse event caused by locally advanced gastric cancer. Other major complications are gastric outlet obstruction (GOO) and malnutrition.[26]

Hemorrhage and obstruction may often be controlled by endoscopic intervention or with radiotherapy, perforation almost always requires surgical intervention.[26] The effect of palliative surgery in patients with advanced gastric cancer on QOL is unknown. Currently two prospective randomized multicenter trials (RENAISSANCE/FLOT5, SURGIGAST) are assessing the role of combined chemotherapy and surgery for patients suffering from stage IV gastric cancer.[27]

Complications due to peritoneal carcinomatosis, i.e., stenosis, bleeding, or perforation, have to be treated considering tumor mass, distribution and localization, performance status, nutritional status, and overall prognosis. Potential surgical therapeutic approaches include small bowel resection, stoma formation, bypass surgery, or PEG placement to drain gastric and small bowel fluid.[26]

If bleeding is significant and cannot be controlled by endoscopic intervention, or if bleeding recurs more than once following endoscopic treatment, the following options remain:

- Angiography and selective embolization of the bleeding vessel (angiography is only capable to visualize bleedings of 1 mL/min or more; the stomach is perfused via five different arteries limiting the chances of successful embolization)
- Palliative gastrectomy
- Palliative radiation

In a meta-analysis comparing endoscopic stenting to gastroenterostomy, stenting was found to be associated with higher clinical success, a shorter time to starting oral intake, reduced morbidity, a lower incidence of delayed gastric emptying, and a shorter hospital stay, while there was no significant difference between the two methods for severe complications or 30-day mortality.[28] Surgical gastroenterostomy, however, appears to allow for longer symptom-free survival.[26]

In some patients, insertion of a jejunal feeding tube (percutaneous endoscopic jejunostomy, PEJ) is the only option to maintain enteral nutrition. In patients with an otherwise untreatable GOO, palliative placement of a PEG is indicated to drain gastric fluid (venting PEG). Palliative (partial) gastrectomy may prolong survival by as much as 3 months when compared with a bypass procedure. This comes with a significant risk of morbidity and mortality and should therefore only be performed in selected cases.[29]

Although gastrectomy remains a successful intervention for GOO related to gastric cancer, endoscopic stenting might be a preferable option for patients with limited life expectancy or where surgery is not possible. There are, however, no data on QOL outcomes postendoscopic stenting and the technology of duodenal stenting seems to lag behind that of biliary stents, and thus laparoscopic or open gastric bypass remains an important consideration.[26]

Radiation has been associated with good palliation in gastric cancer causing obstruction with symptom control rates of 80% in a small series and has the advantage of also controlling bleeding.[30]

Pancreas

Approximately 80% of newly diagnosed patients with pancreatic adenocarcinoma cannot benefit from a curative strategy. When the diagnosis of unresectable disease is made, nonsurgical endoscopic approaches should be prioritized in order to keep hospital stay as short as possible without delaying systemic chemotherapy. If an unresectable disease is diagnosed at laparotomy, an appropriate palliative surgical treatment should be considered to prevent biliary and enteral obstruction, as well as pain exacerbation due to tumor invasion. A more aggressive approach toward palliative resection can be justified only in specific circumstances. Hepatic metastases constitute a contraindication for resection of pancreatic adenocarcinoma. With treatment, median survival for locally advanced inoperable disease approaches 12 months in contemporary clinical trials and 6–8 months for metastatic disease.[31]

The assessment of life expectancy in pancreatic cancer is difficult. Jamal et al.[32] developed a symptom-based score (McGill-Brisbane Symptom Score, MBSS), which can be assessed during the first interview. They reported four symptoms independently predicting poor survival and weighted them regarding their influence on survival:

- Weight loss >10% (8 points)
- Pain (5 points)
- Jaundice (4 points)
- Smoking (4 points)

A low score (0–9 points) predicted an overall median survival of 14.6 months versus 6.3 months in the patient group with a high score (12–21 points).[32]

Patients with an estimated survival of less than 6 months benefit more from interventional stent placement in terms of morbidity and length of hospital stay. Patients with a life expectancy exceeding 6 months may benefit from a more lasting solution with a decreased need for reinterventions over time. In these patients, a surgical bypass procedure should be performed, especially if the diagnosis of unresectable disease is made at laparotomy.[31] These patients will benefit from double bypass procedures as this approach can reduce the incidence of GOO and obstructive jaundice.[33] The double bypass procedure including gastrojejunostomy does not increase postoperative morbidity compared with biliary bypass alone.[33] The retrocolic gastrojejunostomy is associated with a lower rate of postoperative delayed gastric emptying.[34] Some authors reported 20% morbidity and 4% mortality rates after palliative biliary bypass surgery.[31,35]

A Cochrane Review published in 2014 addressed the question whether resection of the pancreas with involved vessels (locally advanced pancreatic cancer) provides better outcome than palliative treatment alone.[36] This review identified some evidence that pancreatic resection increases survival and decreases costs compared with palliative treatment for selected patients (40% survival in resection group vs. 0% in palliative treatment group at 3 years follow up).[36]

At diagnosis, approximately one-third of pancreatic cancer patients complain of pain and 90% of them experience severe pain at end-stage disease. Therefore any good palliation must focus on pain management in order to improve QOL. Percutaneous and/or intraoperative neurolysis should always be attempted for pain relief.[31]

Biliary Tract/Liver

Most liver resections should be undertaken with curative intent. In the palliative setting, they are undertaken with two main aims, either to prolong survival or for symptom control.[37] Cholangiocarcinomas are the main indication for surgical palliation, in the form of a biliary-enteric bypass. Neuroendocrine tumors (NETs) are the predominant indication for palliative liver resection. Cytoreductive liver resections for NETs can be associated with enhanced survival and can relieve symptoms caused by the mechanical effects of the tumor and hormone secretion.[37]

The alleviation of biliary obstruction is preferable prior to instituting systemic therapy, if possible. Stenting endoscopically or percutaneously is an effective and less invasive option than surgical bypass, having been shown to have fewer short-term complications, although a higher reocclusion rate.[37]

Studies have failed to demonstrate any significant difference in overall survival between patients with hilar cholangiocarcinomas who undergo surgical and nonsurgical procedures to relieve biliary obstruction, and percutaneous, endoscopic, and combined biliary stents should be regarded as first-line palliative treatment.[38] The most common surgical approach for the palliation of hilar cholangiocarcinoma is a biliary-enteric bypass to segment III. For those patients in whom a segment III bypass is not feasible, a right-sided cholangiojejunostomy may be undertaken.[37] The preferred procedure to achieve surgical palliation for patients with distal cholangiocarcinoma depends on the exact site of the tumor but is either a hepaticojejunostomy or choledochojejunostomy. It has long been recognized that these bypasses yield superior results compared with those involving the gall bladder or duodenum. Concomitant gastrojejunostomy as a prophylactic measure to avoid GOO is now recommended by most authors.[39]

Unresectable gall bladder cancer is associated with a dismal survival of approximately 2–5 months, and nonsurgical methods of palliation should therefore be chosen in the vast majority of patients.[37]

More than 80% of patients with liver metastases from NETs cannot undergo curative resection. The management of these patients remains controversial. The main aims of palliative liver resections for NETs are to improve symptoms (and associated QOL) and facilitate the effect of nonoperative treatments. Palliative resections for neuroendocrine liver metastases (NELM) can also confer a survival benefit. Most authors advocate cytoreductive hepatic surgery when at least 90% of the bulk of the tumor can be resected, which is very likely to yield a successful outcome.[40] The current literature, however, does not provide evidence from randomized trials in order to definitely assess the role of cytoreductive surgery in these patients.[41]

Small and Large Bowel and Rectum

Less than 3% of gastrointestinal malignancies arise from the small bowel.[42] Malignant small bowel obstruction carries a poor prognosis, and usually survival is not expected to exceed 1 year.[43,44] Within the multitude of disease processes that can lead to malignant small bowel obstruction, patients with primary colorectal cancer appear to have better survival and palliation when treated with surgical intervention.[45] In the palliative setting, intestinal bypass or stoma formation needs to be considered. A high-output stoma carries significant risks for the patient and an intestinal bypass should always be preferred for the treatment of a nonresectable malignant small bowel obstruction.[2]

The estimated median survival of patients with inoperable malignant bowel obstruction (MBO) is 1 month with a 6-month survival of less than 8%.[46] A patient fit for surgery should only have a short trial of conservative management followed by surgery. Surgery should result in a definitive diagnosis, radical resection of the obstructing lesion, or bypass formation.[2]

Considering overall data of invasive measures in metastatic colorectal cancer, there are no statistically significant differences between median survival of patients treated with resection surgery (11–22 months) and of patients treated with intervention without tumor resection (7–22 months). The median survival of patients receiving only best supportive care does not exceed 2–3 months.[47] Studies involving a series of surgical cases of MBO have shown a 30-day mortality of 25% (9%–40%), postsurgical morbidity of 50% (9%–90%), a rate of reobstruction of 48% (39%–57%), and a median survival of 7 months (2–12 months).[45,46,48–50] Age, advanced disease, malnutrition, and poor performance status are considered factors for poor prognosis even in cases where surgery may technically be possible.[49,51]

Malignant colonic obstruction in a patient not suitable for surgery can often be managed effectively with a self-expanding colonic stent, under fluoroscopic guidance.[52,53] With this method, stents can be inserted into the rectum and distal sigmoid but with combined colonoscopic guidance stents can also be placed into the proximal colon.[52] Colonic stenting has a high success rate (80%–100%) with good symptomatic relief and improved QOL.[52] There is no difference in mortality and morbidity rates compared with surgery, but the advantage of stenting is a shorter hospital stay with shorter procedure time and less blood loss.[53] The most common complications of this technique are immediate or delayed perforation (4.5%), migration (11%), and obstruction (12%).[54]

Palliative medical treatment of inoperable MBO is multimodal and based on the combined use of glucocorticoids, antiemetics, antisecretors, and potent analgesic opioids. Due to their antiemetic action and reduction of mucosal edema, glucocorticoids are indicated in the initial phases of this complication and may increase the rate of spontaneous resolution. Antiemetics of choice are neuroleptics (haloperidol). Antagonists of 5-HT_3 receptors are effective for controlling emesis in the treatment of MBO, even in cases where the patient's response to other antiemetics is insufficient.[55]

There is considerable debate regarding the risks and benefits of elective resection of the primary tumor in asymptomatic patients with clearly incurable disease. The rationale for this approach is threefold. First, it may prevent development of acute complications during the lifetime of the patient, which is now significantly longer. In patients with metastatic colorectal cancer where the primary tumor remains in situ and there are no symptoms, only 11%–14% experience morbidity related to the primary tumor that may require surgical or nonsurgical intervention such as stenting or radiotherapy.[56] Second, primary tumor resection may prevent treatment complications such as hemorrhage or perforation that arise due to the use of the anti–vascular endothelial growth factor (VEGF) agent bevacizumab.[57] Third, primary resection may improve the efficacy of systemic treatment and prolong survival. There are, however, conflicting data on the survival benefit of primary tumor resection and no prospective randomized trials, although recent retrospective studies have suggested a survival benefit.[58] It is likely that carefully selected patients benefit from primary tumor resection followed by systemic therapy. Nonetheless, until the results of ongoing randomized trials are published, this patient population remains undefined.[59]

Abnormal volume of fluid in the peritoneal cavity as a result of cancer is termed malignant ascites and develops in up to 50% of cases.[19] Common underlying neoplasms include breast, ovarian, gastric, pancreas, and colon cancer, with up to 20% of unknown primary.[19,60] Associated life expectancy is short (less than 4 months); only in breast and ovarian cancer is survival usually longer.[19] Single drainage of ascites with nontunneled catheters is effective but if left in place long term these can cause complications, such as infection (35%), accidental removal, leakage (20%), and occlusion (30%). As a result, tunneled catheters are preferred for longer-term management of malignant ascites.[19,60]

Brain and Vertebral Column

Modern neurosurgery is much less invasive than even two decades ago, and it is much easier to tip the balance in favor of intervention for symptom reduction.[61] Autopsy studies suggest that 20%–25% of cancer patients have brain metastases.[62] Eight to ten percent of adults with cancer will develop symptomatic brain metastases.[63] There is some evidence supporting the treatment of up to three metastases, and for palliation of raised intracranial pressure or neurologic deficit, a large metastasis may be removed even if the magnetic resonance imaging (MRI) reveals other smaller asymptomatic lesions.[64]

While there is still debate regarding the influence of surgery on survival of glioblastoma, it can be very useful for palliation of symptoms, including headache and neurologic deficit.[61,65,66] Surgery will usually provide better palliation for accessible tumors in noneloquent areas, but radiosurgery (linear accelerator, Gamma knife) can be very useful for treating deep-seated tumors or those in eloquent areas.[61]

Ventriculoperitoneal shunting can provide dramatic palliation of symptoms of raised intracranial pressure with minimal morbidity.[15] In some cases, where there are malignant cells in the cerebrospinal fluid (CSF), there is a risk of peritoneal seeding as well as shunt blockage. In this situation, endoscopic third ventriculostomy is a minimally invasive procedure that can provide similar palliation.[61]

Epidural spinal cord or cauda equina compression from metastatic disease can have a significant negative effect on QOL. Treatment by posterior laminectomy often fails. Minimally invasive surgery (MIS) techniques provide a compromise better suited to palliation of pain and neurologic deficit. Using a combination of neuronavigation and MIS techniques, tumors can often be decompressed through the pedicle, and fixation can then be inserted percutaneously.[61]

Head and Neck

The complexity of care in the terminal period of life with head and neck cancer (HNC) results in the admission of many patients. A recent study reported that more than 50% of patients were hospitalized in their last month of life due to bleeding (17%), pain (9%), breathing difficulties (9%), swallowing difficulties (9%), inability to cope (6%), and fracture (3%).[67]

Cancer of the head and neck often requires treatment to provide patients with adequate voice use and the ability to swallow. Endoluminal debulking of pharyngeal and laryngeal lesions can provide good palliation, avoiding the need for a tracheostomy and allowing patients to undergo palliative chemotherapy or radiotherapy, or to buy time for definitive palliative surgery. The use of laser allows clean, hemostatic tumor removal or debulking.[68]

Weight loss and malnutrition are major problems in patients with advanced HNC, with more than half having significant weight loss and cachexia, and approximately 20% of all cancer-related deaths caused by cachexia.[69,70] Cancer cachexia is different from starvation and is associated with preferential loss of muscle over adipose tissue, increased proteolysis and lipolysis, increased metabolic activity of the liver, and increased production of acute-phase proteins.[71]

Pleura, Chest Wall, Lung, and Mediastinum

The main indications for thoracic surgical palliation in primary and secondary thoracic malignancies are:

- Cardiorespiratory compromise secondary to a malignant pleural effusion and/or pericardial effusion
- Pulmonary metastases from extrathoracic primary malignancy
- Pain resulting from chest wall tumors
- Sepsis resulting from obstructive bronchogenic malignancy[72]

Malignant pleural mesothelioma is an almost-always fatal tumor, and palliative platinum-based chemotherapy is the standard of care.[73] A recent Cochrane Review addressed the question whether the use of radical multimodality therapy with extrapleural pneumonectomy would provide better survival. This review does not support the use of radical multimodality therapy over routine clinical care.[73] In patients with malignant pleural mesothelioma it is therefore recommended that videoscopic talc pleurodesis and insertion of a tunneled indwelling pleural catheter are the most appropriate forms of palliation.[72]

Overwhelmingly, malignant pleural effusion is the main indication for surgical palliation in thoracic malignancy. It is generally accepted that pleurodesis should not be attempted if the predicted survival of the patients is less than 3 months.[72]

If, on postdrainage plain chest x-ray, the lung reexpands completely, full pleural apposition can be achieved and any intervention to affect a pleurodesis will have a high likelihood of success. If the lung fails to reexpand fully, this indicates entrapment by a malignant pleural rind and any attempt to achieve a pleurodesis will have a high failure rate.[72]

The most effective surgical treatment option for malignant pleural effusion is that of a videoscopic talc pleurodesis. This procedure requires general anesthesia, double-lumen endotracheal intubation, and positioning of the patient in the lateral decubitus position. Sterile talc is insufflated to effectively cover all areas of the visceral and parietal pleura. The standard dose is 5–10 g. A chest drain is inserted and should be removed when less than 150 mL of pleural fluid is produced over a period of 24 h. This usually occurs at 48–72 h postsurgery. The success rate of a talc pleurodesis has been reported to be greater than 75%.[74]

Talc slurry (talc mixed with normal saline 5 g talc: 50–100 mL sterile normal saline), instilled via an intercostal catheter, is a useful technique for achieving pleurodesis in patients not fit for or declining surgical intervention. This technique can be performed on the ward. The talc slurry is instilled via the intercostal catheter and the tube clamped. The patient is then positioned on each side in the supine position for approximately 20 min and then in the upright position, leaning left and right for a further 20 min. The procedure results in acute pleuritis and can be quite painful. Adequate analgesia should be provided to the patient. The author prefers to add local anesthetic agents to the talc slurry. Thoracoscopic talc pleurodesis has a significantly higher success rate than talc slurry (80% vs. 60%).[74] The effectiveness of talc slurry compared with a permanent indwelling pleural catheter is comparable.

For patients with failed videoscopic pleurodesis where significant symptomatic benefit is achieved by pleural drainage, a permanent indwelling tunneled pleural catheter may be the most effective option.[74]

Malignant pericardial effusions can be effectively managed in the acute setting by percutaneous drainage via an ultrasound-guided catheter introduced using Seldinger technique. For long-term management a pericardial window can be formed videoscopically on the left or right side.[74]

Breast

Women with metastatic breast cancer face remote disease as their dominant cause of death, but many will have concurrent locoregional relapse.[75] Often a standard mastectomy technique with carefully planned skin excision can remove a symptomatic, ulcerating cancer with primary closure of the skin and subcutaneous tissues.[76] Vacuum-assisted closure (VAC) dressings are the currently preferred dressing for split-skin grafting postmastectomy.[77] Latissimus dorsi (LD) myocutaneous flaps are the simplest option for new skin and soft tissue. They can be mobilized and rotated into a postmastectomy defect with relatively little surgical morbidity. An LD flap provides robust skin and muscle coverage, which allows postsurgical radiotherapy to be performed.[77]

In many cases axillary dissection to level III of the axilla can be a very important palliative surgical procedure. In the era of sentinel lymph node biopsy as standard therapy for early breast cancer, palliative completion axillary dissection is an important surgical tool.[78] The contraindications to resection of axillary disease are involvement of the axillary artery and brachial plexus.[77]

Patients often survive for considerable periods with stage IV breast cancer. In these patients, the majority of the tumor burden will often be the primary cancer in the breast or axilla. Retrospective studies have suggested improved survival for patients who have the primary malignancy resected in the presence of confirmed metastatic disease.[79] This view, however, is not entirely supported by a recent Cochrane Review.[80] Tosello et al.[80] did not identify evidence from randomized trials to make definitive conclusions on the benefits and risks of breast surgery associated with systemic treatment for women diagnosed with metastatic breast cancer.

The bone is the most common site for breast cancer metastases. Low-volume, bone-only disease is relatively common and often responds well to systemic therapy, particularly endocrine agents. Indications for surgery are lack of response to therapy, local pain, fracture, or high potential of fracture in weight-bearing long bones.[77]

Thyroid Gland

Anaplastic thyroid carcinoma (ATC) is one of the most aggressive solid neoplasms with a median survival of 6 months after diagnosis. It most commonly presents as a large, firm thyroid mass causing hoarseness, vocal cord paralysis, dysphagia, cervical pain, and dyspnea. Most cancer-related deaths are due to rapid locoregional growth; therefore therapeutic efforts should be concentrated here. These patients are often best managed by multimodal therapy, including surgery and external beam radiation therapy (EBRT) ± chemotherapy. Due to its poor prognosis, aggressive approaches in metastatic ATC should be used sparingly.[81] In cases of inoperability, neoadjuvant EBRT and/or chemotherapy should be considered, possibly rendering the tumor suitable for surgery. As there is a high risk of relapse after response to EBRT ± chemotherapy, surgery should be performed when feasible in these cases. There is no indication for tumor debulking with gross positive margins.[81]

Tracheostomy for airway compromise is technically challenging and has a high rate of healing complications, which can delay EBRT. It should be considered in cases of impending airway obstruction, not as a prophylaxis. Most patients requiring a tracheostomy have aggressive disease with a poor prognosis. It may relieve airway distress but provides minimal prolongation of life.[81]

Adrenal Gland

Adrenal incidentalomas may be found in 4%–7% of abdominal CT scans. Up to 5% of these will be adrenocortical carcinomas (ACC), and 2.5% will be metastatic cancers.[82] An endocrine syndrome can be found in 60% of ACC, most commonly Cushing syndrome (50%), virilization (<10%), or a combination of both (25%).[83] ACC are very rare malignant tumors (1–2 per million per year). In the presence of metastatic lesions, the 5-year survival drops from approximately 60% to below 20%, and survival is usually less than 13 months.[84] Debulking mainly serves to control tumor-related endocrine syndromes.

To diagnose a malignant pheochromocytoma (PCC), the presence of local invasion and distant metastasis is needed, and such lesions are not curable. Up to 25% are part of a hereditary syndrome, most commonly multiple endocrine neoplasia and von Hippel-Lindau. Treatment options for malignant PCC include surgery (the mainstay of treatment), metaiodobenzylguanidine (MIBG) radiotherapy, and systemic antineoplastic therapy. There are no randomized controlled trials to determine which nonsurgical treatment is more effective. If the PCC is not resectable, tumor debulking is considered a mainstay of treatment, palliating the hypersecretory state. However, its role is unclear in asymptomatic, low-secreting tumors.[85]

Urology

The most commonly performed palliative urologic procedures are ureteric stenting and fulguration of bleeding bladder and prostate tumors.[86] As cystectomy carries greater morbidity than radiotherapy, it should be considered only if there are no other options of palliative diversion (nephrostomy, ileal conduit).[87] Ureteric stents may not always be able to overcome the compressive forces, and nephrostomy tubes may be the only palliative option.[84]

Up to one-third of cases with renal cell carcinoma (RCC) will present with synchronous metastatic disease.[83] Cytoreductive nephrectomy has potential QOL benefits as it may reduce bleeding, pain from clot colic, as well as paraneoplastic symptoms. Patients who underwent cytoreductive nephrectomy also have better survival.[84]

The gold standard treatment for organ-confined ureteric or renal pelvis transitional cell carcinoma (TCC) is nephroureterectomy. Patients with synchronous or metachronous metastatic disease have poor outcomes.[84] For metastatic bladder TCC, the current standard of care involves a transvesical debulking of the bladder tumor with adjuvant chemotherapy and radiotherapy. However, palliative cystoprostatectomy (men) or anterior pelvic exenteration (women) remains an option for patients with significant local symptoms such as uncontrollable hemorrhage.[84]

Most patients with lymph node-positive prostate cancer will ultimately fail treatment.[88] While many urologists are reluctant to perform radical prostatectomy (RP) in patients who are lymph node-positive, there is evidence of improved cancer-specific and overall survival in those who undergo RP.[89] Thus RP is an important component of multimodal strategies of lymph node-positive prostate cancer.[88]

Gynecology

Epithelial ovarian cancer, which accounts for >90% of all ovarian malignancies, is advanced at diagnosis in approximately 70% of cases. Primary cytoreductive surgery is still the mainstay of therapy for its assumed benefit in three main areas:

- Physiological benefits of removing bulky tumor masses, particularly ovarian and omental disease, improving gut function and decreasing ascites.
- Improved tumor perfusion and increased growth fraction increasing the likelihood of response to chemotherapy and decreasing the potential for developing drug resistance.
- Immunologic benefits as large tumor masses appear to have an immunosuppressive function.[86]

There also appears to be a role for repeat surgical cytoreduction in patients with recurrent disease.[90]

The incidence of bowel obstruction in patients with ovarian cancer is 25%–50%, and the life expectancy of patients with bowel obstruction in ovarian cancer is 4 months. There are no definite prognostic factors to predict the outcome of surgery in patients with MBO, and the management of these patients remains controversial.[86] Kucukmetin et al.[91] confirmed in a Cochrane Review that there is evidence in support of palliative surgical management to prolong survival in patients suffering from bowel obstruction due to ovarian cancer.

Cancer of the cervix is the most common gynecologic cancer worldwide, with the incidence being much higher in third world countries without a screening program. Locally advanced or metastatic cervical cancer is usually primarily treated with chemoradiation rather than radical hysterectomy. When cervical cancer recurs centrally in a radiated field, pelvic exenteration may offer the only hope of cure. However, there may also be a role for palliative exenteration in certain cases of cervical cancer complicated by vesico- or colovaginal fistulae.[86] A Cochrane Review published in 2014, however, did not find evidence from which to determine whether exenterative surgery is better, equivalent to, or worse than nonsurgical treatment in women with recurrent gynecologic cancers (excluding recurrent ovarian cancer).[92] Recurrent cervical cancer may also present with ureteric obstruction. Retrograde stenting is often appropriate, but if this is not technically feasible, strong consideration must be given to the appropriateness of percutaneous nephrostomy in patients whose poor prognosis or symptoms from pelvic tumor may make a less traumatic demise from renal failure a kinder option.[86]

Large ovarian tumors, either primary or secondary from other sites (particularly gastrointestinal tract and breast), may cause local pressure effects resulting in pain, bloating, abdominal distension, and problems with gut function. Even if the removal of the ovarian tumor does not prolong survival, there is a role to debulk them to improve the patient's QOL for the time they have left.[86]

Recurrent ascites is a common complication in patients with advanced gynecologic malignancies, especially recurrent ovarian cancer. Repeated paracentesis may be required, and this can be a great inconvenience to patients. A tunneled peritoneal catheter drainage system (radiologic or surgical insertion is possible) can be used for repeated drainage of ascitic fluid in the community setting.[86]

Orthopedics

The aim of palliative orthopedic treatment is to alleviate pain and restore mobility and dignity to patients suffering with terminal cancer.[93]

The majority of metastatic bone lesions encountered are lytic in nature. Lysis is not due to direct tumor destruction. It occurs via the release of cytokines, causing recruitment of osteoclasts. This is thought to occur as part of the metastatic cell binding.[93]

Treatment for patients with metastatic bone disease (MBD) is primarily palliative, with the goals of limiting pain and rapidly restoring function. Renal and thyroid carcinoma lesions may be highly vascular. Embolization is advisable to decrease the risk of bleeding. This should be performed even if closed techniques such as intramedullary nailing are to be employed.[93]

Typically, clinicians have a tendency to underestimate the patients' life expectancy. The following features of MBD are associated with a better prognosis:

- Primary tumor breast, prostate, myeloma, or lymphoma
- Solitary skeletal metastasis
- Absence of visceral metastasis
- Absence of pathological fracture[93]

In the lower-limb intramedullary nailing is the treatment of choice. In the femur the use of long cephalomedullary nails is recommended. These maximize the amount of bone protected and reduce the need for reoperation. Controversy exists in the surgical management of diaphyseal lesions in the humerus. The surgical options are either intramedullary nailing or plate stabilization. There is no consensus within the literature, and surgeons should use the technique they feel most comfortable with.[93]

The femur and specifically the hip are disproportionately overrepresented in the frequency of long bone MBD locations. Up to 75% of all surgery for MBD is performed in the hip. In the proximal femur, lesions that cross the intertrochanteric line proximally should be treated with arthroplasty.[93]

Conclusions

Palliative surgery remains a challenging area of surgery with limited evidence to support therapeutic decision-making. Significant symptom relief can be achieved through close cooperation between different care providers and surgical (sub-) specialists. Early postoperative morbidity and mortality are high and this needs discussion with patients, family, and other members of the care team. Less traumatizing and minimal invasive approaches should always be preferred to reduce time spent in hospital and to avoid delays of palliative radio- and/or chemotherapy. Every decision in this area of surgery needs to be made with profound and humble respect for the person who is dying and their family.

Key Points

- Every surgeon should have a good understanding of the options and limitations of palliative surgery.
- 30-day mortality in palliative surgery is as high as 30%.
- Treatment decisions should be made in an MDT setting.
- Brain metastases, Karnofsky index less than 50%, severe pain, dyspnea, high LDH, and leukocytosis are indicators of a poor prognosis.
- Endoscopic stenting +/− BT is the preferred option for management of malignant dysphagia.
- Palliative gastrectomy for stage IV gastric cancer is currently under investigation.
- Complications of unresectable pancreatic cancer should be managed with nonsurgical endoscopic/radiologic approaches.
- If unresectable pancreatic cancer is found at surgery a double bypass procedure should be performed.
- Locally advanced pancreatic cancer is best palliated with resection.
- Endoscopic, percutaneous, and combined stents are the first line of palliative treatment for malignant biliary obstruction.
- Malignant small and/or large bowel obstruction should be managed surgically (bypass/stoma/resection) in a patient fit for surgery.
- Malignant colonic obstruction in patients not fit for surgery is best managed with a colonic stent.
- Asymptomatic patients with stage IV colorectal cancer benefit from primary tumor resection followed by systemic therapy.
- Malignant ascites indicates a life expectancy of less than 4 months (excluding breast and ovarian cancer).
- Tunneled catheters are optimal for management of malignant ascites and malignant pleural effusion (if pleurodesis fails).
- Palliative resection of up to three brain metastases is justified.
- Radiosurgery (Gamma knife, linear accelerator) is suitable for deep-seated tumors or those in eloquent areas.
- Videoscopic talc pleurodesis is the most effective treatment for malignant pleural effusions.
- Radical multimodality therapy of malignant pleural mesothelioma is not superior to palliative platinum-based chemotherapy plus pleurodesis.
- Primary cytoreductive surgery is the mainstay of therapy for advanced ovarian cancer.
- Palliative surgery for bowel obstruction due to ovarian cancer prolongs patient survival.

References

1. Dunn GP. Surgical palliative care: recent trends and developments. *Surg Clin North Am.* 2011;91(2):277–292.
2. Wichmann MW. Small bowel. In: Wichmann MW, Maddern G, eds. *Palliative Surgery*. Springer-Verlag; 2014:189–194.
3. Currow DC, Cartmill J. Surgery and palliative care: is there common ground or simply a clash of cultures. In: Wichmann MW, Maddern G, eds. *Palliative Surgery*. Springer-Verlag; 2014:3–7.
4. Tseng WH, Yang X, Wang H, et al. Nomogram to predict risk of 30-day morbidity and mortality for patients with disseminated malignancy undergoing surgical intervention. *Ann Surg.* 2011;254(2):333–338.
5. Miner TJ, Brennan MF, Jaques DP. A prospective, symptom related, outcomes analysis of 1022 palliative procedures for advanced cancer. *Ann Surg.* 2004;240(4):719–726.
6. McCahill LE, Smith DD, Bornemann T, et al. A prospective evaluation of palliative outcomes for surgery for advanced malignancies. *Ann Surg Oncol.* 2003;10(6):654–663.
7. Merrill RM, Hunter BD. Conditional survival among cancer patients in the United States. *Oncologist.* 2010;15(8):873–882.
8. Yu XQ, Baade PD, O'Connell DL. Conditional survival of cancer patients: an Australian perspective. *BMC Cancer.* 2012;12(1):460.
9. Wang SJ, Emery R, Fuller CD, Kim JS, Sittig DF, Thomas CR. Conditional survival in gastric cancer: a SEER database analysis. *Gastric Cancer.* 2007;10(3):153–158.
10. Gwilliam B, Keeley V, Todd C, et al. Prognosticating in patients with advanced cancer - observational study comparing the accuracy of clinicians' and patients' estimates of survival. *Ann Oncol.* 2013;24(2):482–488.
11. Workgroup SPC. Office of promoting excellence in end-of-life care: Surgeon's Palliative Care Workgroup report from the field. *J Am Coll Surg.* 2003;197(4):661–686.
12. Badgwell B, Krouse R, Cormier J, Guevara C, Klimberg VS, Ferrell B. Frequent and early death limits quality of life assessment in patients with advanced malignancies evaluated for palliative surgical intervention. *Ann Surg Oncol.* 2012;19(12):3651–3658.
13. Gripp S, Moeller S, Boelke E, et al. Survival prediction in terminally ill cancer patients by clinical estimates, laboratory tests, and self-rated anxiety and depression. *J Clin Oncol.* 2007;25(22):3313–3320.
14. Desai KR, Chen RI. Endovascular therapy for palliative care of cancer patients. *Semin Intervent Radiol.* 2007;24:382–390.
15. Gonda DD, Kim TE, Warnke PC, Kasper EM, Carter BS, Chen CC. Ventriculoperitoneal shunting versus endoscopic third ventriculostomy in the treatment of patients with hydrocephalus related to metastasis. *Surg Neurol Int.* 2012;3:97.
16. Pereira J, Phan T. Managment of bleeding in patients with advanced cancer. *Oncologist.* 2004;9:561–570.
17. O'Neill SB, O'Connor OJ, Ryan MF, Maher MM. Interventional radiology and the care of the oncology patient. *Radiol Res Pract.* 2011;2011:160867. doi:10.1155/2011/160867.
18. Lewandowski RJ, Geschwind JF, Liapi E, Salem R. Transcatheter intraarterial therapies: rationale and overview. *Radiology.* 2011;259(3):641–657.
19. Requarth J. Image-guided palliative care procedures. *Surg Clin North Am.* 2011;91:367–402.
20. Ahmed M, Brace CL, Lee Jr FT, Goldberg SN. Principles of and advances in percutaneous ablation. *Radiology.* 2011;258(2):351–369.
21. Melhado R, Alderson D, Tucker O. The changing face of oesophageal cancer. *Cancers (Basel).* 2010;2(3):1379–1404.
22. Ferlay J, Shin HR, Bray F, Forman D, Mathers CD. GLOBCAN. Cancer incidence and mortality worldwide. *Int J Cancer.* 2010;127(12):2893–2917.
23. Knight BC, Jamieson GG. Oesophagus. In: Wichmann MW, Maddern G, eds. *Palliative Surgery*. Springer-Verlag; 2014:125–144.
24. Dai Y, Li C, Xie Y, et al. Interventions for dysphagia in oesophageal cancer. *Cochrane Database Syst Rev.* 2014;30(10): CD005048.
25. O'Donnell CA, Fullarton GM, Watt E, Lennon K, Murray GD, Moss JG. Randomized clinical trial comparing self-expanding metallic stents with plastic endoprotheses in the palliation of oesophageal cancer. *Br J Surg.* 2002;89(8):985–992.
26. Albertsmeier M, Jauch KW, Angele MK. Stomach. In: Wichmann MW, Maddern G, eds. *Palliative Surgery*. Springer-Verlag; 2014:145–152.
27. Monig S, van Hootegem S, Chevallay M, Wijnhoven BPL. The role of surgery in advanced disease for esophageal and junctional cancer. *Best Pract Res Clin Gastroenterol.* 2018;36(37):91–96.
28. Hosono S, Ohtani H, Arimoto Y, Kanamiya Y. Endoscopic stenting versus surgical gastroenterostomy for palliation of malignant gastroduodenal obstruction: a meta-analysis. *J Gastroenterol.* 2007;42(4):283–290.
29. Yang K, Liu K, Zhang WH, et al. The value of palliative gastrectomy for gastric cancer patients with intraoperatively proven peritoneal seeding. *Medicine (Baltimore).* 2015;94:e1051.
30. Tey J, Back MF, Shakespeare TP, et al. The role of palliative radiation therapy in symptomatic locally advanced gastric cancer. *Int J Radiat Oncol Biol Phys.* 2007;1(67):385–388.
31. Wirsching A, Lesurtel M, Clavien PA. Pancreas. In: Wichmann MW, Maddern G, eds. *Palliative Surgery*: Springer-Verlag; 2014:153.
32. Jamal MH, Doi SA, Simoneau E, et al. Unresectable pancreatic adenocarcinoma: do we know who survives? *HPB (Oxford).* 2010;12(8):561–566.
33. Lesurtel M, Dehni N, Tiret E, Parc R, Paye F. Palliative surgery for unresectable pancreatic and periampullary cancer: a reappraisal. *J Gastrointest Surg.* 2006;10(2):286–291.
34. House MG, Choti MA. Palliative therapy for pancreatic/biliary cancer. *Surg Clin North Am.* 2005;85(2):359–371.
35. Distler M, Kersting S, Rueckert F, et al. Palliative treatment of obstructive jaundice in patients with carcinoma of the pancreatic head or distal biliary tree. Endoscopic stent placement vs. hepaticojejunostomy. *JOP.* 2010;11(6):568–574.
36. Gurusamy KS, Kumar S, Davidson BR, Fusai G. Resection versus other treatments for locally advanced pancreatic cancer. *Cochrane Database Syst Rev.* 2014(2):CD010244.
37. Thomasset S, Dennison A. Biliary Tract and Liver. In: Wichmann MW, Maddern G, eds. *Palliative Surgery*: Springer-Verlag; 2014: 171–187.
38. Witzigmann H, Lang H, Lauer H. Guidelines for palliative surgery of cholangiocarcinoma. *HPB (Oxford).* 2008;10(3): 154–160.
39. Mann CD, Thomasset SC, Johnson NA, et al. Combined biliary and gastric bypass procedures as effective palliation for unresectable malignant disease. *ANZ J Surg.* 2009;79(6):471–475.
40. Pavel M, Baudin E, Couvelard A, et al. ENETS Consensus Guidelines for the management of patients with liver and other distant metastases from neuroendocrine neoplasms of foregut, midgut, hindgut, and unknown primary. *Neuroendocrinology.* 2012;95(2):157–176.

41. Gurusamy KS, Pamecha V, Sharma D, Davidson BR. Palliative cytoreductive surgery versus other palliative treatments in patients with unresectable liver metastases from gastro-entero-pancreatic neuroendocrine tumours. *Cochrane Database Syst Rev.* 2009(1): CD007118.
42. Bojesen RD, Andersson M, Riis LB, Nielsen OH, Jess T. Incidence of, phenotypes of and survival from small bowel cancer in Denmark, 1994–2010: a population-based study. *J Gastroenterol.* 2016;51(9):891–899.
43. Verwaal VJ, van Ruth S, de Bree E, et al. Randomized trial of cytoreduction and hyperthermic intraperitoneal chemotherapy versus systemic chemotherapy and palliative surgery in patients with peritoneal carcinomatosis of colorectal cancer. *J Clin Oncol.* 2003;21(20):3737–3743.
44. Piso P, Arnold D. Multimodal treatment approaches for peritoneal carcinosis in colorectal cancer. *Dt Aerztbl International.* 2011;108(47):802–808.
45. de Boer NL, Hagemans JAW, Schultze BTA, et al. Acute malignant obstruction in patients with peritoneal carcinomatosis: the role of palliative surgery. *Eur J Surg Oncol.* 2019;45(3):389–393.
46. Tuca A, Guell E, Martinez-Losada E, Codorniu N. Malignant bowel obstruction in advanced cancer patients: epidemiology, managment, and factors influencing spontaneous resolution. *Cancer Manag Res.* 2012;4:159–169.
47. Ahmed S, Shahid RK, Leis A, et al. Should noncurative resection of the primary tumour be performed in patients with stage IV colorectal cancer? A systematic review and meta-analysis. *Curr Oncol.* 2013;20(5):e420–e441.
48. Miller G, Boman J, Shrier I, Gordon PH. Small-bowel obstruction secondary to malignant disease: an 11-year audit. *Can J Surg.* 2000;43(5):353–358.
49. Schwenter F, Morel P, Gervaz P. Management of obstructive and perforated colorectal cancer. *Expert Rev Anticancer Ther.* 2010;10(10):1613–1619.
50. Cauley CE, Panizales MT, Reznor G, et al. Outcomes after emergency abdominal surgery in patients with advanced cancer: opportunities to reduce complications and improve palliative care. *J Trauma Acute Care Surg.* 2015;79(3):399–406.
51. Roses RE, Folkert IW, Krouse RS. Malignant bowel obstruction: reappraising the value of surgerh. *Surg Oncol Clin N Am.* 2018;27(4):705–715.
52. Sato KT, Takehana C. Palliative nonvascular interventions. *Semin Intervent Radiol.* 2019;24:391–397.
53. Sagar J. Colorectal stents for the management of malignant colonic obstructions. *Cochrane Database Syst Rev.* 2011:1–CD007378.
54. Park YE, Park Y, Park SJ, Cheon JH, Kim WH, Kim TI. Outcomes of stent insertion and mortality in obstructive stage IV colorectal cancer patients through 10 year duration. *Surg Endosc.* 2019;33(4):1225–1234.
55. Tuca A. Large bowel and rectum. In: Wichmann MW, Maddern G, eds. *Palliative Surgery*: Springer-Verlag; 2014:195–208.
56. Scheer MGW, Sloots CEJ, van der Wilt GJ, Ruers TJM. Management of patients with asymptomatic colorectal cancer and synchronous irresectable metastases. *Ann Oncol.* 2008;19(11):1829–1835.
57. Hapani S, Chu D, Wu S. Risk of gastrointestinal perforation in patients with cancer treated with bevacizumab: a meta-analysis. *Lancet Oncol.* 2009;10(6):559–568.
58. Savas PS, Price TJ. Medical Oncology. In: Wichmann MW, Maddern G, eds. *Palliative Surgery.* Springer-Verlag; 2014:71–82.
59. van Rooijen KL, Shi Q, Goey KKH, et al. Prognostic value of primary tumour resection in synchronous metastatic colorectal cancer: individual patient data analysis of first-line randomised trials from the ARCAD database. *Eur J Cancer.* 2018;91:99–106.
60. Stokes LS. Percutaneous management of malignant fluid collections. *Semin Intervent Radiol.* 2007;24:398–408.
61. Jones N. Brain and vertebral column. In: Wichmann MW, Maddern G, eds. *Palliative Surgery.* Springer-Verlag; 2014:209–215.
62. Aizer AA, Lee EQ. Brain metastases. *Neurol Clin.* 2018;36(3): 557–577.
63. Tabouret E, Chinot O, Metellus P, Tallet A, Viens P, Goncalves A. Recent trends in epidemiology of brain metastases: an overview. *Anticancer Res.* 2012;32(11):4655–4662.
64. Salvati M, Tropeano MP, Maiola V, et al. Multiple brain metastases: a surgical series and neurosurgical perspective. *Neruol Sci.* 2018;39(4):671–677.
65. Vogelbaum MA. Does extent of resection of a glioblastoma matter? *Clin Neurosurg.* 2012;59:79–81.
66. Li XZ, Li YB, Cao Y, et al. Prognostic implications of resection extent for patients with glioblastoma multiforme: a meta-analysis. *J Neurosurg Sci.* 2017;61(6):631–639.
67. Cocks H, Ah-See K, Capel M, Taylor P. Palliative and supportive care in head and neck cancer: United Kingdom National Multidisciplinary Guidelines. *J Laryngol Otol.* 2016;130(S2):S198–S207.
68. Semdaie D, Haroun F, Casiraghi O, et al. Laser debulking or tracheotomy in airway management prior to total laryngectomy for T4a laryngeal cancer. *Eur Arch Otorhinolaryngol.* 2018;275(7):1869–1875.
69. Jager-Wittenaar H, Dijkstra PU, Dijkstra G, et al. High prevalence of cachexia in newly diagnosed head and neck cancer patients: an exploratory study. *Nutrition.* 2017;35:114–118.
70. Zaorsky NG, Churilla TM, Egleston BL, et al. Causes of death among cancer patients. *Ann Oncol.* 2017;28(2):400–407.
71. Tisdale MJ. Cachexia in cancer patients. *Nat Rev Cancer.* 2002;2(11):862–871.
72. Jurisevic CA. Pleura, chest wall, lung, and mediastinum. In: Wichmann MW, Maddern G, eds. *Palliative Surgery.* Springer-Verlag; 2014:239–244.
73. Abdel-Rahman O, Elsayed Z, Mohamed H, Eltobgy M. Radical multimodality therapy for malignant pleural mesothelioma. *Cochrane Database Syst Rev.* 2018(1):CD012605.
74. Stefani A, Natali P, Casali C, Morandi U. Talc poudrage versus talk slurry in the treatment of malignant pleural effusion. A prospective comparative study. *Eur J Cardiothorac Surg.* 2006;30(6):827–832.
75. Redig AJ, McAllister SS. Breast cancer as a systemic disease: a view of metastasis. *N Engl J Med.* 2013;367:256–265.
76. Alvarado M, Ewing CA, Elyassnia D, Foster RD, Shelley Hwang E. Surgery for palliation and treatment of advanced breast cancer. *Surg Oncol.* 2007;16(4):249–257.
77. Walsh DCA. Breast. In: Wichmann MW, Maddern G, eds. *Palliative Surgery.* Springer-Verlag; 2014:245–251.
78. Tryfonidis K, Senkus E, Cardoso MJ, Cardoso F. Management of locally advanced breast cancer-perspectives and future directions. *Nat Rev Clin Oncol.* 2015;12(3):147–162.
79. Petrelli F, Barni S. Surgery of primary tumors in stage IV breast cancer: an updated meta-analysis of published studies meta-regression. *Med Oncol.* 2012;29(5):3282–3290.
80. Tosello G, Torloni MR, Mota BS, Neeman T, Riera R. Breast surgery for metastatic breast cancer. *Cochrane Database Syst Rev.* 2018(3):CD011276.

81. Caron NR, Simard L. Thyroid and parathyroid. In: Wichmann MW, Maddern G, eds. *Palliative Surgery*. Springer-Verlag; 2014:253–261.
82. Young Jr WF. The incidentally discovered adrenal mass. *N Engl J Med*. 2007;356:601–610.
83. Wiechno P, Kucharz J, Sadowska M, et al. Contemporary treatment of metastatic renal cell carcinoma. *Med Oncol*. 2018;35(12):156.
84. Spernat D. Urology. In: Wichmann MW, Maddern G, eds. *Palliative Surgery*. Springer-Verlag; 2014:269–274.
85. Scholz T, Eisenhofer G, Pacak K, Dralle H, Lehnert H. Clinical review: current treatment of malignant pheochromocytoma. *J Clin Endocrinol Metab*. 2007;92:1217–1225.
86. Miller J. Gynaecology. In: Wichmann MW, Maddern G, eds. *Palliative Surgery*. Springer-Verlag; 2014:275–281.
87. Stenzl A, Cowan NC, De Santis M, et al. Treatment of muscle-invasive and metastatic bladder cancer: update of the EAU guidelines. *Eur Urol*. 2011;59(6):1009–1018.
88. Litwin MS, Tan HJ. The diagnosis and treatment of prostate cancer; a review. *JAMA*. 2017;317(24):2532–2542.
89. Heidenreich A, Bastian PJ, Bellmunt J, et al. EAU guidelines on prostate cancer. Part II: Treatment of advanced, relapsing, and castration-resistant prostate cancer. *Eur Urol*. 2014;65(2):467–479.
90. Suh DH, Kim HS, Chang SJ, Bristow RE. Surgical management of recurrent ovarian cancer. *Gynecol Oncol*. 2016;142(2):357–367.
91. Kucukmetin A, Naik R, Galaal K, Bryant A, Dickinson HO. Palliative surgery versus medical management for bowel obstruction in ovarian cancer. *Cochrane Database Syst Rev*. 2010(7):CD007792.
92. Ang C, Bryant A, Barton DPJ, Pomel C, Naik R. Exenterative surgery for recurrent gynaecological malignancies. *Cochrane Database Syst Rev*. 2014(2):CD010449.
93. Young S, Zellweger R. Orthopaedics. In: Wichmann MW, Maddern G, eds. *Palliative Surgery*. Springer-Verlag; 2014:283–297.

35

Frailty in the Perioperative Setting for Cancer Patients

HUI-SHAN LIN, NATASHA REID, AND RUTH E. HUBBARD

Introduction

The world's population is aging at an unprecedented rate with the number of older people growing at a faster rate than all other age groups. By 2050, one in six people will be over the age of 65 (16%), accounting for 1.6 billion worldwide.[1] The global population aged 80 years and over is expected to more than triple between 2015 and 2050, growing from 126.5 million to 446.6 million.[1]

As the population ages, there will be increasing numbers of older people with cancer. Age is the most important risk factor for developing cancer, and age is also associated with the poorest cancer survival. Sixty percent of all cancers and 70% of cancer mortality occur in people above 65 years of age. In addition, those above 65 years have an 11-fold increase in cancer incidence and a 16-fold increase in cancer mortality compared with their younger counterparts.[2] In the UK, between 2014 and 2016, more than half (53%) of all new cancer cases were in adults aged between 50 and 74 years while more than a third (36%) were in those aged 75 years and over. Furthermore, cancer incidence rates are the highest in the 85–89 years age group regardless of sex (see Fig. 35.1).[3] Despite its growth, the aging cancer population remains under-represented in clinical trials.

Surgery is an important treatment modality of cancer; oncologists and surgeons will see a growing population of older cancer patients undergoing surgery. Given that older cancer patients are such a heterogeneous group with varying degrees of frailty, decisions regarding the most beneficial oncology treatment are complex. Understanding the role of frailty in older cancer patients is paramount in making individualized treatment decisions and to minimize adverse outcomes.

This chapter will explore the concept of frailty, how it is measured, its prevalence in cancer patients, and its relevance in cancer care. It will then discuss geriatric syndromes, consider the importance of nutrition, and conclude with the principles of providing individualized care for older cancer patients in the perioperative period. Different models and pathways of perioperative care for older patients undergoing cancer surgery will be covered in another chapter.

Frailty in Cancer Patients

Chronologic age alone is a poor guide to tolerance of cancer treatment. An 80-year-old person who runs marathons and who is fully independent with his activities of daily living is likely to be a better candidate for cancer surgery than a 70-year-old person who is malnourished, cognitively impaired, has difficulty walking for more than 10 m, and who needs assistance for personal hygiene cares. The concept of frailty, in addition to age, has become an increasingly popular tool for assessing whether an older person has the reserve and resilience to benefit from aggressive therapies and surgery. Frailty is typically associated with advancing age; however, young people can also become frail.

Definition, Conceptualization, and Prevalence of Frailty

Frailty is a state of increased vulnerability leading to adverse health outcomes. It describes a diminished physiologic reserve that results in reduced resilience and adaptive capacity to respond to stressors and maintain homeostasis. Frailty is the result of a complex interplay between aging-related physiologic changes (such as inflammation and immune activation, sarcopenia, decrease in sex hormones, higher levels of cortisol, and vitamin D deficiency), genetic and epigenetic factors, environmental and lifestyle stressors, as well as acute and chronic diseases. Frailty is distinct from disability and chronic diseases although they overlap and share similarities.

Adverse health consequences can be viewed as a balance between frailty status or reserve and external insults to the body, such as a new disease, infection, cancer, or a change in medication. A fit individual with large physiologic reserves will require a major insult such as major surgery or intensive

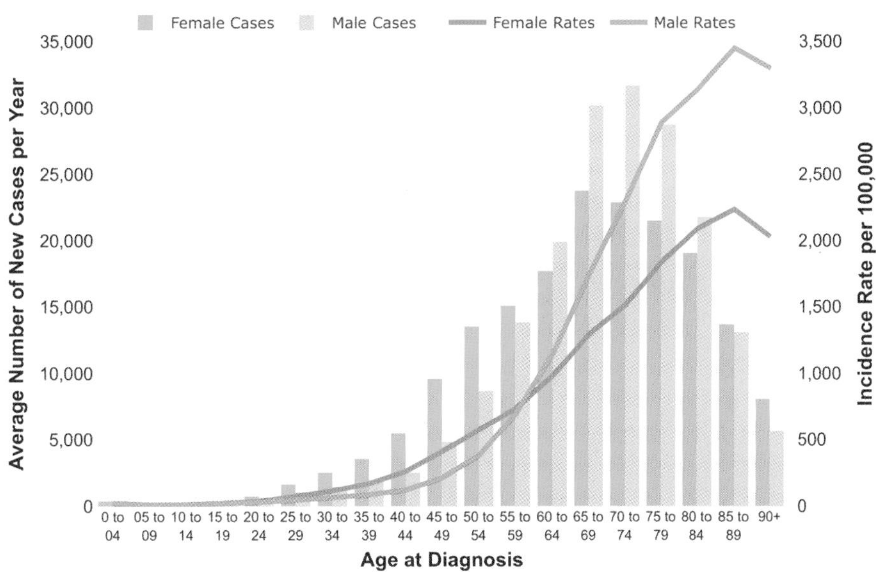

• **Fig. 35.1** All cancers, average number of new cases per year and age-specific incidence rates per 100,000 population, UK, 2014–2016. From Cancer Research UK.

care admission to render them functionally dependent. However, a frail individual with little reserves may suffer significant decline in their physical and functional abilities after even minor insults, such as a urinary tract infection or a medication change.[4] It is also important to remember that chronologic age still has a critical role. Consider a 75-year-old frail man: he will have a greater risk of adverse outcomes than a 75-year-old man with lower frailty but will have lower risks of adverse outcomes than a 95-year-old man with the same frailty status. Whether health assets (such as a positive health attitude and supportive caregivers) can mitigate the effect of frailty is an area of ongoing research. Fig. 35.2 depicts our current conceptualization of frailty, incorporating the impact of age, health assets, health deficits, and a health insult on three distinct types of people: (A) a healthy younger person with high assets and low deficits; (B) a healthy older person with high assets and low deficits; and (C) an older person with low assets and high deficits.

Although the prevalence of frailty in the general community-dwelling older population is estimated to be 10%,[5] in a systematic review of 20 studies the median prevalence of frailty in older adults with cancer was up to 42%.[6] The prevalence of prefrail older adults with cancer is reported to be 43%, with the minority being fit.[6] In older people with cancer, both the disease process and its intense treatment are important contributors to the high prevalence of frailty, making these patients particularly susceptible to adverse outcomes.

Sex Differences in Frailty

Previous cross-sectional evidence has proposed a male-female health-survival paradox, whereby females are found to be frailer yet live longer. To this effect, a recent meta-analysis confirmed a consistent relationship between sex, frailty, and mortality. The review synthesized seven studies using frailty index to assess frailty and found that in every age group, females had higher frailty than males yet tolerated this frailty better, evidenced by a lower mortality rate.[7]

A number of biological, behavioral, and psychosocial factors in the pathophysiology of sex differences in frailty, morbidity, and mortality have been proposed.[8,9] Perhaps most interestingly is the influence of chronic inflammation, which has been identified as a key driver of the development of frailty. It has been suggested that male-female variation in diet, the gut microbiome, and central adiposity all contribute to the more critical role of inflammation in the development of frailty in females compared to males.[8] In addition, estrogen and testosterone may contribute to sex differences in frailty by modulating inflammation,[10] as well as having direct effects on other tissues.

While females tend to be frailer than males, they may also cultivate more health assets to help them maintain function and independence for longer. To date, no studies have investigated the association of sex with frailty in cancer patients. It is an important area for future research given the emerging evidence showing that sex influences the pathophysiology, clinical signs, treatment outcomes, and responses to cancer.[11]

Frailty in Predicting Cancer and Surgical Outcomes

Frailty in general medical and surgical patients is associated with increased mortality and morbidity, and this is also observed in older cancer patients. Over the past decade, there has been a surge of research and publications evaluating the impact of frailty on adverse outcomes in cancer patients. In a meta-analysis by Handforth et al. frailty increased the risk of all-cause mortality at 5, 7, and 10 years of follow up by 1.8-, 2.3-, and 1.7-fold, respectively.[6] Multiple studies have also confirmed that frailty is predictive of chemotherapy,

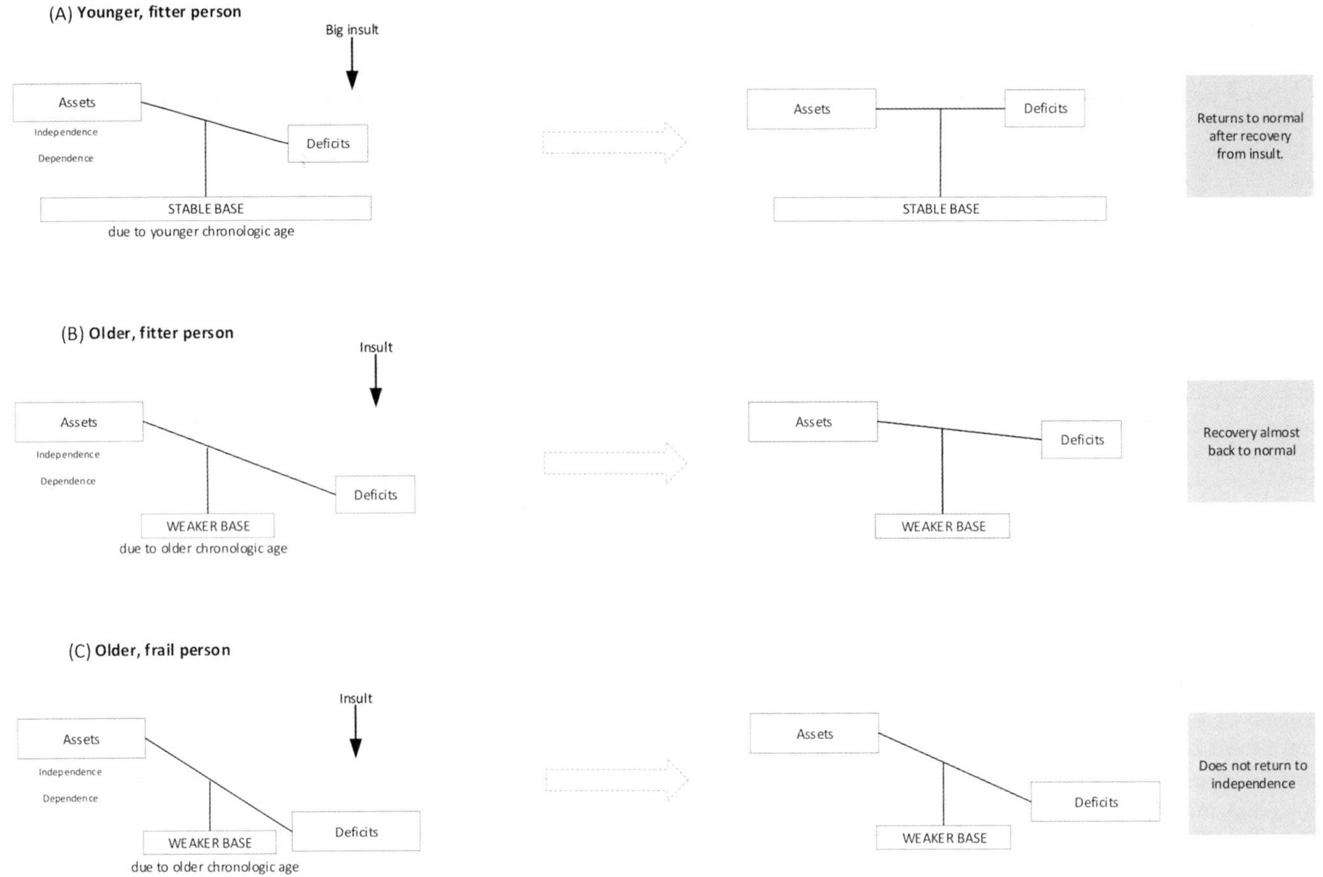

• **Fig. 35.2** Conceptualization of frailty.

toxicity, and intolerance.[12] Similarly, in cancer patients who have undergone surgery, frailty is associated with increased postoperative major complications (Clavien-Dindo grade ≥II), non-home discharge, increased hospital cost, and higher 30-day mortality and hospital readmission.[12] Table 35.1 summarizes the adverse outcomes associated with frailty in cancer surgery in key papers published since 2010. The most frequently assessed adverse outcome in these 44 studies was major postoperative complications: frailty was a significant predictor in all 29 studies that evaluated this outcome, regardless of the types of cancer surgery and tools of frailty measurement. Short-term mortality, including in-hospital mortality, was the next frequently assessed adverse outcome linked to frailty. Several studies found that frailty was a superior predictor of mortality and morbidity than chronologic age and American Society of Anaesthesiology (ASA) classification.[13–15]

As frailty is a strong predictor of poor outcomes in older cancer patients, frailty assessment is important for risk stratification before surgery and chemoradiotherapy. Detecting frail patients preoperatively has the potential to inform risk of postoperative complications and adverse outcomes, thus enabling treatment planning, prompting early detection of complications, and enhancing communication with family and patients regarding expected treatment outcome. Although there is no current consensus on how to incorporate frailty assessment into cancer treatment planning or perioperative care, screening for frailty may be a good starting point for detecting those who are the most vulnerable.

Principles of Frailty and Geriatric Syndromes

Geriatric syndromes contribute to frailty, and frailty also increases the risk of developing geriatric syndromes. Frailty screening may facilitate the detection of geriatric syndromes that can be optimized in cancer patients to prevent adverse outcomes. The mean number of geriatric syndromes per community-dwelling person above the age of 65 years has been found to be 2.9.[16] In the oncology population, the prevalence of geriatric syndromes is as high as 78%, and 43% have suffered three or more geriatric syndromes.[17] The presence of geriatric syndromes makes cancer treatment complex; cancer itself and the treatment required can also precipitate or exacerbate geriatric syndromes. Managing geriatric syndromes is important in cancer patients undergoing surgery because they are associated with increased complications, in-hospital mortality, prolonged hospital stay, high health care cost, and increased functional dependence on discharge from hospital.[18] Geriatric syndromes negatively impact on a cancer

TABLE 35.1 Adverse Outcomes Associated With Frailty in Oncologic Surgery

		Adverse Outcomes Associated With Frailty						
Cancer Type	Author; Sample Size	Long-Term Mortality[a]	Short-Term Mortality[b]	Postop Complications	Prolonged Hospital Stay	Readmission	Institutionalization	Postop Functional Status
Breast	Clough-Gorr 2012; **660** [52]	√						
	Mandelblatt 2017; **1280** [53]	√						
Colorectal	Chen 2018; **1928** [31]			√				
	Kristjansson 2010; **178** [54]			√				
	Kristjansson 2012; **176** [55]		√	√				
	Neuman 2013; **12,979** [56]	√	√					
	Ommundsen 2014; **178** [57]	√						
	Reisinger 2015; **310** [58]		√					
	Robinson 2011; **60** [59]					√ (30 days)	√	
	Rønning 2014; **93** [60]							X (non sig)
	Souwer 2018; **139** [35]		√	√	√	√ (30 days)		
	Tan 2012; **83** [61]			√				
Gastric	Choe 2017; **223** [62]					√ (1 year)		
	Lu 2017; **165** [63]	√		√				
	Tegels 2014; **180** [64]		√					
Gastrointestinal	Bateni 2018; **1928** [65]		√	√				
	Buettner 2016; **1326** [66]	√						
	Kenig 2015; **75** [67]			√				
	Vermillion 2017; **41,455** [68]		√	√	√			
Glioblastoma	Cloney 2016; **243** [29]			√	√			
Gynaecologic	Courtney-Brooks 2012; **37** [69]			√				
	Driver 2017; **88** [70]	√						
	George 2016; **66,105** [71]		√	√				
	Uppal 2015; **6551** [30]		√	√				
Head and neck	Abt 2016; **1193** [27]			√				
	Adams 2013; **6727** [13]		√	√				
	Nieman 2017; **159,301** [72]		√	√	√			
	Goldstein 2019; **274** [37]			√	√			

Continued

TABLE 35.1 Adverse Outcomes Associated with Frailty in Oncologic Surgery—*cont'd*

		Adverse Outcomes Associated With Frailty						
Cancer Type	**Author; Sample Size**	**Long-Term Mortality[a]**	**Short-Term Mortality[b]**	**Postop Complications**	**Prolonged Hospital Stay**	**Readmission**	**Institutionalization**	**Postop Functional Status**
Intra-cranial neoplasm	Youngerman 2018; **9149** [32]		√	√	√		√	
Liver	Gani 2017; **2714** [73]		√	√	√			
Ovarian	Ferrero 2017; **78** [74]			√				
	Kaibori 2016; **71**[75]			√				
	Kumar 2017; **535** [25]		√	√				
	Yao 2019; **535** [26]						√	
Pancreas	Mogal 2017; **9986** [76]			√				
	Dale 2014; **76** [36]			√	√	√		
Renal	Hoffen 2016; **11,755** [77]			√				
	Silvestri 2018; **162** [78]			√				
Urologic	Burg 2019; **123** [23]			√				
	Chappidi 2016; **2679** [79]		√	√				
	Lascano 2015; **41,681** [80]		√					
	Matsushita 2018; **41** [81]			√				
Various	Brown 2015; **416** [82]	√						
	Lascano 2015; **41,681** [80]		√					
	Shahrokni 2019; **1137** [83]	√			√			

[a]Worse survival on long-term follow up.
[b]Died within 6 months of surgery.

patient's fitness for surgery and their recovery from surgery. Comprehensive geriatric assessment (CGA) is the best way to identify and manage geriatric syndromes.

Dementia and Delirium

Dementia is a neurodegenerative condition that causes multidomain decline in cognitive function, which may manifest as memory loss, disorientation, impaired judgment and insight, impaired planning, impaired visual spatial awareness, impaired language, personality change, or behavioral disturbances. The biggest risk factor for dementia is age. Delirium is an acute onset fluctuating course of altered level of consciousness and inattention, usually precipitated by a medical illness or a change of environment. Dementia is a risk factor for delirium, and delirium is associated with high mortality and morbidity. Dementia is more prevalent in older cancer patients compared with their younger counterparts simply due to age. Cognitive impairment has implications for cancer treatments.

Cognitive impairment may affect a person's ability to understand in full the consequences of cancer treatments and the ability to weigh up benefits and risks when embarking on intensive therapies; hence the capacity to provide informed consent to a complex treatment regimen may be impaired. Dementia and delirium are associated with functional impairments and the need for prompting and supervision to carry out activities of daily living, such as driving, remember appointments, and taking regular medications. This means that cancer patients with cognitive impairment will likely need more help to adhere to medication regimes, frequent blood tests required when undergoing chemotherapy, and help with transportion to and from health appointments.

Falls

Falls are common in the older population and their causes are often multifactorial. Falls may be intrinsic in nature, for example, secondary to postural hypotension, dehydration, infections, blood dyscrasia, cardiac arrhythmias, seizures, strokes, Parkinson's disease, dyspraxia from dementia, sciatica, peripheral neuropathy, or lower limb muscle weakness due to frailty. Falls may also be extrinsic in nature, secondary to an external trigger; for example, wet floors, loose-fitting footwear, uneven walking surfaces, or loose carpet edges. The consequences of falls range from mild, such as soft tissue injury, to severe, such as intracranial bleed and fractures, or even death. In addition, the psychologic sequelae from falls can pathologically heighten anxiety level with a fear of falls, leading to fear of mobilizing and immobility.

Screening for falls in older cancer patients is important as falls may trigger investigations for underlying causes leading to treatment of previously undiagnosed medical problems, optimization of medications, a review of a person's home environment to prevent future falls, and physiotherapy to improve gait and balance. Falls may be an indicator of a person's underlying frailty, hence affecting the tolerability of intensive cancer treatments.

Depression and Anxiety

Older adults are particularly at risk of mood and anxiety disorders. Many psychosocial precipitants to depression and anxiety are associated with aging: functional impairments leading to increased dependence on their spouse, children, friends, or carers; sensory impairments affecting quality of life; physical slowing and falls; symptoms from medical comorbidities; social isolation due to being outside of the workforce; and loneliness as their peers and friends pass away from advancing age. Some older adults may experience existential crisis, losing the meaning of life and feeling they have lived longer than they wished. Depression in older people can present atypically where self-reported low mood may be absent, but psychomotor retardation, apathy, and reduced appetite are also prominent features that should not be overlooked. Reduced appetite from low mood can compound the malnutrition associated with cancer.

Cancer patients are particularly susceptible to depression and anxiety, not only due to physical symptoms that cancers cause, for example pain, nausea, general lethargy, and weakness, but also due to the uncertainty of future, in terms of survival, treatment plans, and potential side effects from cancer treatment. Depression and anxiety significantly impact on quality of life and are risk factors for adverse health outcomes as apathy can lead to functional decline and poor self-care.

Polypharmacy

Polypharmacy is commonly defined as taking five or more regular medications; however, other definitions exist, including taking unnecessary medications. Polypharmacy is common in older adults due to their multiple comorbidities and chronic pain from degenerative joint diseases. Cancer and chemotherapy treatment can also add to pill burden. For example, a patient undergoing chemotherapy can suddenly have five extra medications to take for pain, constipation, and nausea. Increased number of medications in a patient is associated with greater risks of drug interactions and side effects. In addition, psychotropic medications, such as benzodiazepines, antipsychotics, and antidepressants, increase the anticholinergic load in the body, predisposing an older adult to falls and cognitive impairment.

Malnutrition

Malnutrition is another syndrome common in the older population and overlaps with cancer cachexia. Malnutrition will be explored in more detail in a later section entitled Nutrition and How It Impacts on Surgical Journey.

Comprehensive Geriatric Assessment

Comprehensive geriatric assessment (CGA) is a way of identifying and managing geriatric syndromes. It is usually conducted by a multidisciplinary team with a geriatrician and/or a gerontology nurse taking the main roles. CGA gives a holistic view of an older person's physiologic and functional status and assesses multiple domains of health, including medical comorbidities, medications, nutrition, cognition, activities of daily living, continence, mobility, psychologic status, and social support. A CGA typically involves administering some or all of the following tools: a scale for personal and instrumental activities of daily living (such as Barthel's index or the Nottingham Extended Activities of Daily Living Scale), Mini-Nutritional Assessment (MNA), the Mini-Mental Status Exam (MMSE), or the Mini-Cog and Geriatric Depression Scale (GDS), a social support scale, each with set cutoff points to denote abnormality. A CGA also includes a review of comorbidities, medications, and physical-based tests, such as grip strength, Timed Up and Go Test, and balance test. CGA is versatile and the number of items can be modified to as few as three components depending on the size of the multidisciplinary team and time constraint. Abbreviated-CGA (aCGA) is a validated tool using shortened forms of GDS, MMSE, and number of impaired activities of daily living items.[19]

Frailty Screening and Measurement Tools

Having established that frailty predicts adverse outcomes, we need to consider how it can be detected, whether screening for frailty is sufficient, and if frailty should be quantified to guide management. There are a multitude of tools developed for measuring frailty in general medical and surgical patients; many of these have been applied in cancer patients. There is currently no consensus on which tool is the best for use in routine practice. Each tool has its own strengths and weaknesses, and the tools vary in the time taken to perform, training required, and their predictability of adverse outcomes. Some clinicians argue that each oncology and surgical unit needs to find the tools that are practical and applicable for their patient population, as different tools may be more suited for different surgical settings (acute versus elective) and different cancer types. On the other hand, the use of multiple instruments limits the ability of specialists to communicate risks across different cancer types and precludes the development of definitive Clinical Practice Guidelines.

Traditionally, frailty was diagnosed and detected using the "eye-ball" method. However, for clinicians without geriatric knowledge and training, the "eye-ball" method can be subjective and unreliable. Systematic geriatric assessment using validated measurement tools is superior to the oncologist's opinion in detecting frailty and prognosticating survival.[20]

Most frailty measurement tools evaluate the various domains of CGA discussed above and include a combination of self-reported measures and performance-based measures. However, some studies use single tests as markers of frailty, such as gait speed, grip strength, Timed Up and Go, albumin, or C-reactive protein (CRP) alone. The sensitivity and specificity of a more comprehensive tool need to be balanced with its feasibility and practicality, as the time taken to detect frailty will be longer than for single markers of frailty. CGA is considered the gold standard for identifying frail patients; however, each assessment can take up to 60 min and requires a specialist geriatrician and a gerontology nurse. The goal of CGA is to detect geriatric syndromes for which interventions may be offered, while brief frailty screening tools such as G8 and VES-13 aim to select patients who are vulnerable and who may benefit from the entire CGA, making more efficient use of resources.

In the next section, we will discuss in more detail six frailty measurement tools that have been validated in two or more studies evaluating older patients undergoing cancer surgery. Table 35.2 shows the different components of the six frailty measurement tools, and Table 35.3 summarizes the clinical utility of these tools. For more information on all frailty measurement tools trialed in cancer patients and their sensitivity and specificity, refer to a systematic review by Hamaker et al.[21]

TABLE 35.2 Frailty Screening Tools in Older Cancer Patients

Domains Assessed	G8	VES-13	Fried Criteria	mFI	FI
Age	✓	✓			
Weight/ nutrition	✓		✓		✓
ADLs		✓		✓	✓
Mobility/ slowness	✓	✓	✓		✓
Weakness			✓		✓
Exhaustion			✓		
Low physical activities			✓		✓
Cognitive impairment	✓				✓
Impaired sensorium				✓	
Self-rated health	✓	✓			✓
Depression					✓
Social support					✓
Comorbidities				✓[a]	✓
Medications	✓				✓

ADL, Activities of daily living; *FI*, Frailty Index; *G8*, Geriatric 8; *mFI*, modified Frailty Index; *VES-13*, Vulnerable Elders Scale.

[a]Specific comorbidities include COPD or recent pneumonia, congestive heart failure, myocardial infarction, PCI, PCS or angina, diabetes mellitus, hypertension requiring medication, peripheral vascular disease or ischemic rest pain, TIA or CVA, and CVA with neurologic deficit.

Fried Criteria

The phenotypic model developed by Fried et al. in the Cardiovascular Health Study (CHS) views frailty as an observed physical decline characterized by slowness, weakness, weight loss, inactivity, and exhaustion.[22] The assessment of these five domains of frailty incorporates self-reported domains, as well as in-office physical assessments with specific scoring criteria for each domain. The cutoff values for frailty vary in different studies; however, a score of 3 or more is commonly defined as frail, a score of 1–2 is defined as pre-frail, while a score of 0 is defined as fit. The Fried Criteria have been validated in colorectal, bladder, and gynecologic cancer surgeries.[23] The Fried Criteria do not take into account cognitive impairment and have limited use in non-ambulatory patients.

Frailty Index

The Frailty Index (FI) was developed by Rockwood et al. from the Canadian Study of Health and Aging (CSHA) based on the cumulative deficit model of frailty.[24] In this model, frailty is viewed as an accumulation of "deficits" leading to vulnerability. When a certain threshold of deficits is reached beyond which the system can cope with, the system collapses. In the original study, 70 health deficits were assessed, capturing deficits from multiple domains, which include physical and functional impairments, chronic diseases, medications,

TABLE 35.3 Clinical Utility of Frailty Screening Tools

	G8	VES-13	Fried	mFI	FI
No. of items	8	13	5	11	30–70
Time to perform (min)	4.4	5.7	5–10	5	10–15
Training required	No	No	Yes	No	Yes
Includes performance-based tests	No	No	Yes	No	No
Expresses frailty as a categorical or continuous value	Categorical	Categorical	Categorical	Categorical & continuous	Categorical & continuous
No. of papers validating the tool in cancer populations	5	3	7	14	2
Sample sizes tool has been trialed on	41,79, 139, 162, 205,	76, 114, 274	37, 76, 83, 123, 176, 274, 416	Largest sample 41, 455	535, 555
Predicts mortality (no. of studies)	2	1	1	7	2
Predicts morbidity (no. of studies)	4	1	5	13	2

FI, Frailty Index; *G8*, Geriatric 8; *mFI*, modified Frailty Index; *VES-13*, Vulnerable Elders Scale.

psychosocial risk factors, and nutrition. FI is a number between 0 and 1, derived from the number of health deficits present in an individual divided by total number of deficits evaluated. A FI close to 0 indicates fitness and a higher FI indicates a higher degree of frailty. FI can be used as a continuum to indicate increasing degree of frailty or used as a dichotomous system with <0.25 being fit and ≥0.25 being frail. Studies have found that denominators as few as 30 items could maintain the validity of the FI, while making it more time efficient. FI has been validated in breast cancer and ovarian cancer patients.[25,26] FI is comprehensive and multidimensional; however, each assessment takes 15–20 min to administer, depending on the number of domains assessed. There are ongoing research efforts looking at incorporating domains of FI into the wider electronic medical system using routinely collected health information, in which case FIs can be automatically generated to increase time efficiency.

Modified Frailty Index

Modified Frailty Index (mFI) is a variation of FI, matching 11 deficits routinely collected in the American College of Surgeons National Surgical Quality Improvement Program (ACS NSQIP) database to the original 70 items in the CHSA study, covering domains of functional status, impaired sensorium, and a range of medical comorbidities. The presence of each item yields 1 point. The mFI is expressed differently in different studies, with some using a cutoff value of ≥5 to identify frailty and others using the number of deficits divided by 11, to generate a ratio between 0 and 1. The mFI has been evaluated extensively in retrospective studies using the ACS NSQIP database as a predictor of poor outcome in a variety of cancer surgeries[27–32]; however, it has not been validated in prospective studies as a bedside screening tool. Its strength is brevity and ability to be derived from an existing database; however, its weakness is its reliance on the NSQIP database that is not available in countries other than the United States. mFI also weighs heavily on medical comorbidities in detecting frailty and lacks evaluation of the cognitive and psychologic aspects of frailty.

Geriatric 8

Geriatric 8 (G8) is a screening tool developed specifically for cancer patients with the aim of identifying potentially frail patients who may benefit from further geriatric assessment. G8 is composed of eight items covering several domains of a CGA with an emphasis on nutrition. Out of eight items, seven are derived from the mini nutritional assessment questionnaire (MNA), namely appetite changes, weight loss, mobility, neuropsychologic problems, body mass index, medication, and self-reported health. One item is age. A score of zero is severe impairment, while 17 is no impairment. A score of ≤14 points indicates potential frailty. G8 is easy and fast to administer and has been found to have an 85% sensitivity and 64% specificity for detecting frailty compared with geriatric assessment.[33] G8 has been widely used in oncology and has been validated in a variety of solid cancers and hematologic malignancies.[34,35]

Vulnerable Elder Survey

The Vulnerable Elder Survey (VES-13) consists of 13 self-administered questions incorporating age, self-rated health, physical abilities, and functional abilities. It was originally designed for screening community-dwelling adults to identify older persons at risk of impending health deterioration. A score of 3 of more indicates frailty. It has been validated in pancreatic, colorectal, and head and neck cancer surgeries.[36–38] Its strengths are the brevity and non-reliance on physical performance; however, the low cutoff points for being frail means that a person 85 years or older would qualify to be frail without any other impairments or disabilities. In addition, it does not take into account cognitive impairment.

Nutrition and How It Impacts on Surgery

Nutrition plays an important role in the surgical journey of older cancer patients, with both preoperative nutritional status and the effects of surgery on nutrition being important factors to consider. Malnutrition is both a geriatric syndrome and a cancer syndrome. Appetite reduces with aging; however, the protein requirement for an older person is double that of a middle-aged person. Due to physical frailty or cognitive impairment, an older person may have reduced ability or motivation to make complex nutritious meals, instead resolving to eating cold salads or sandwiches, which are lower in protein content. Nutritional deficiencies in vitamins, such as B_{12}, D, and folate, can lead to muscle weakness, loss of balance, and peripheral neuropathy, leading to falls. In addition, malnutrition affects healing of surgical scars and predisposes to development of pressure injury in a person with reduced mobility.

Cancers of the head, neck, esophagus, stomach, intestines, pancreas, and liver are often associated with impaired nutrient intake, while surgery as a treatment for cancer is associated with an increased need for nutrients and energy to aid recovery. For cancer patients, particularly those who are frail, malnutrition is strongly associated with an increased risk of mortality. This section will discuss common consequences of impaired nutritional status in cancer patients, including anorexia, cancer cachexia, sarcopenia, and sarcopenic obesity, before finishing with a discussion of nutritional support opportunities prior to surgery.

Anorexia, Cancer Cachexia, and Sarcopenia

Cancer patients can experience one or all of anorexia, cachexia, and sarcopenia. Loss of appetite or desire to eat (anorexia) is common in cancer patients and may present early or later in the disease. The majority of people with advanced cancer will be anorexic. Patients may simultaneously have anorexia and a condition called cachexia, which refers to marked weakness, decreased weight, and fat and muscle loss.[39] Even in patients who are eating well, certain tumors may alter the way nutrients are absorbed and used, or inhibit the storage of fat and formation of muscle tissue, leading to cachexia. Importantly, cachexia cannot be fully reversed by conventional nutritional support.[40] Cancer cachexia is often classified into three stages: precachexia (early clinical and metabolic signs), cachexia, and refractory cachexia, where active treatment of weight loss is no longer possible, and life expectancy is less than 3 months.[39] Cachexia is a multiorgan syndrome and impacts health through numerous pathways. Finally, sarcopenia refers to the loss of muscle mass and function.[41] While both cachexia and sarcopenia are associated with higher risks of chemotherapy-related toxicities, reduced treatment response, poorer surgical outcomes, and lower survival rates, particular attention needs to be paid to a condition known as sarcopenic obesity.[40]

Sarcopenic Obesity and the Obesity Survival Paradox

People with cancer are unique in that their muscle mass is not strongly correlated with their body mass index, and they do not lose or gain fat and muscle in equal proportions.[42] Importantly, cancer patients can accumulate fat while simultaneously losing muscle, hence the term sarcopenic obesity.[43] Approximately 10% of patients with advanced cancer are considered sarcopenic obese, while approximately 25% of patients who are obese are also sarcopenic.[42] Sarcopenic obese cancer patients are at an increased risk of mortality and treatment-related complications, of which surgical problems can include infections, sepsis, and cardiovascular, pulmonary, neurologic, renal, or gastrointestinal complications.[44]

An interesting contradiction to the negative surgical and cancer-related consequences of obesity is known as the "obesity survival paradox." The paradox was proposed after studies observed a protective effect of obesity in cancer patients, including in colorectal cancer,[45] hematologic cancers,[46] and metastatic cancer.[47] Nevertheless, critics of this theory suggest that the paradox is only observed when body mass index is considered without accounting for body composition.[44]

Nutrition Support Before and After Cancer Surgery

Nutritional support prior to cancer surgery is beneficial for malnourished patients, so much so that the European Society for Clinical Nutrition and Metabolism (ESPEN) guidelines indicate that supplementation should be given for 10–14 days preoperatively, even if surgery must be delayed.[48] Supplements to consider include protein, vitamins, minerals, and long-chain fatty acids.

Similarly, nutritional support following surgery is important to lessen surgical stress, minimize catabolism, maintain nutritional status, reduce complications, and optimize recovery.[40] In all perioperative settings, including cancer surgery, Enhanced Recovery after Surgery (ERAS) programs have become an important focus for management and care.[40] These programs are designed to lessen complications due to major surgery and malnutrition by optimizing physiologic and psychologic responses. The principles of ERAS programs include preoperative counseling, preoperative nutrition, avoidance of perioperative fasting and carbohydrate loading up to 2 h preoperatively, standardized anesthetic and analgesic regimens (epidural and nonopioid analgesia), and early mobilization.[40]

Perioperative Care for Older Cancer Patients: Clinical Implications

As older people are heterogeneous in their frailty status, comorbidities, function, and social supports, treatments for cancer must have a tailored approach. Individualized care involves matching an older person's health status, goals of care, and physical strengths and limitations to the treatment. Geriatric assessment identifies frailty and previously undiagnosed impairments that can be optimized before cancer surgery; it also informs perioperative and postoperative risks of adverse outcomes. As discussed earlier in this chapter, frail patients are at increased risk of postoperative complications, mortality, functional decline, and being discharged to long-term institutional care. The benefit of cancer surgery needs to be balanced with the potential deterioration in quality of life, functional status, and cognition due to treatment toxicities or due to deconditioning during hospitalization for surgery. These decisions are often very complex to make.

When cancer specialists perform this risk and benefit analysis in an older patient, specialists need to consider each patient's wishes and life goals, what they consider to be the most important in their health and life. They need to evaluate whether the cancer is symptomatic or an incidental finding, and whether a patient's cancer symptoms can be alleviated by the treatment offered. They also need to evaluate what the likely trajectory of disease progression is and an individual's prognosis due to other comorbidities and frailty. Cancer treatment is usually only recommended if a patient will live long enough to suffer from symptoms of cancer progression.

Traditionally, oncologists use age and the Eastern Cooperative Oncology Group (ECOG) performance status to determine if a patient is fit for chemotherapy, radiotherapy, and surgery. More recently, the International Society of Geriatric Oncology (SIOG) recommended that geriatric assessment be routine in older patients with cancer at baseline before cancer treatment and also repeated at regular intervals throughout therapy.[49] Geriatric assessment enables individualization of treatment; however, its utilization is limited by resources, time, and availability of geriatricians in a particular center. Screening for frailty, using brief tools such as G8, can identify vulnerable patients who will benefit from a more comprehensive assessment. There is neither a unified way of screening frailty nor a standardized way of performing CGA; however, any form of screening and CGA is likely to be beneficial if practical and feasible.

According to the SIOG recommendations, geriatric assessment should at minimum include a review of comorbidities, medications, activities of daily living, mobility, falls, nutritional status, cognition, mood, and social support.[49] CGA is often administered by a multidisciplinary team, but selective components of the CGA can be used if only smaller teams or a single gerontology nurse are available. Once areas of impairment are discovered from CGA, geriatricians and relevant allied health members can provide interventions to optimize health status and prevent adverse outcomes. When results from CGA are presented to oncology

TABLE 35.4 Preoperative Optimization for Geriatric Oncology Surgery

Geriatric Syndrome	Possible Interventions
Malnutrition	Dietitian review—high protein, high energy diet Supplemental nutritional drinks Review of dentition and oral health
Polypharmacy	Pharmacist review—review indications for each medication De-prescribe medications no longer required Reduce anticholinergic load Dose administration aid such as Webster pack to improve compliance
Falls and mobility issues	Physiotherapy review Home-based exercises/center-based rehabilitation program Prehabilitation, rehabilitation Occupational therapy—review of home environment to remove hazards Falls education and prevention
Functional dependence	Arrange community home supports to assist with activities of daily living Arrange support for transport to appointments if no family members available
Depression/anxiety	Psychology input for psychotherapy Antidepressants, antianxiolytics Counseling
Cognitive impairment	Referral to Memory Clinics to assess for dementia Look for and treat reversible causes for delirium Future planning by formalizing an Enduring Power of Attorney, Advanced Health Directives, and Resuscitation Orders

multidisciplinary teams, there is often a shift towards less intensive treatment options.[50]

The geriatrician's role in cancer care has multiple facets. The geriatrician contributes by supporting a patient-focused vision within the multidisciplinary team uncovers and optimizes geriatric syndromes and medical comorbidities. The geriatrician helps to evaluate a patient's reserve and ability to withstand intensive treatment, estimate life expectancy with and without the cancer, and predict risk of treatment-related toxicity and complications. The geriatrician can also take time to discuss and elucidate patient preferences and priorities to achieve patient-centered shared decision-making.[50]

In the preoperative assessment of older cancer patients undergoing surgery, it is essential to screen for malnutrition, impaired ability to manage their personal activities of daily living, delirium, depression, falls, polypharmacy, and to gather details about their social support system. Screening for geriatric syndromes in addition to the routine assessment of cardiorespiratory systems highlights areas for optimization prior to surgery. Table 35.4 shows examples of interventions that can be considered for geriatric syndromes uncovered in a CGA, depending on local resources. There are several randomized trials currently underway evaluating the effectiveness of prehabilitation before cancer surgery in reducing adverse outcomes postsurgery.[51] Multimodal interventions targeting nutrition, physical exercise, and psychologic health have the potential to reduce the degree of frailty and to improve outcomes.

Conclusion

Older cancer patients are a heterogeneous group with varying degrees of frailty and susceptibility to adverse outcomes; hence frailty screening is important for predicting adverse outcomes and should be part of cancer care. Treatment decisions must be holistic, individualized, multidimensional, and multidisciplinary to match the needs of older people with their life goals. Geriatric assessment is recommended in preoperative assessment to detect geriatric syndromes in order to help stratify surgical risks, paying particular attention to malnutrition and its sequelae. Perioperative care during cancer surgery should include assessment of frailty and optimization of potentially modifiable geriatric syndromes to improve outcomes.

References

1. Department of Economic and Social Affairs, Population Division. World Population Prospects 2019: Highlights. 2019. Available at https://population.un.org/wpp/Publications/Files/WPP2019_10KeyFindings.pdf.
2. Yancik R, Ganz PA, Varricchio CG, Conley B. Perspectives on comorbidity and cancer in older patients: approaches to expand the knowledge base. *J Clin Oncol.* 2001;19(4):1147–1151.
3. Cancer Research UK. Cancer Incidence by Age. 2019. Available at https://www.cancerresearchuk.org/health-professional/cancer-statistics/incidence/age#heading-Zero.
4. Mudge AM, Hubbard RE. Management of frail older people with acute illness. *Intern Med J.* 2019;49(1):28–33.
5. Collard RM, Boter H, Schoevers RA. Oude Voshaar RC. Prevalence of frailty in community-dwelling older persons: a systematic review. *J Am Geriatr Soc.* 2012;60(8):1487–1492.
6. Handforth C, Clegg A, Young C, et al. The prevalence and outcomes of frailty in older cancer patients: a systematic review. *Ann Oncol.* 2015;26(6):1091–1101.
7. Gordon EH, Peel NM, Samanta M, Theou O, Howlett SE, Hubbard RE. Sex differences in frailty: a systematic review and meta-analysis. *Exp Gerontol.* 2017;89:30–40.
8. Gordon EH, Hubbard RE. Physiological basis for sex differences in frailty. *Curr Opin Physiol.* 2018;6:10–15.
9. Gordon EH, Hubbard RE. Do sex differences in chronic disease underpin the sex-frailty paradox? *Mech Ageing Dev.* 2019;179:44–50.
10. Horstman AM, Dillon EL, Urban RJ, Sheffield-Moore M. The role of androgens and estrogens on healthy aging and longevity. *J Gerontol A Biol Sci Med Sci.* 2012;67(11):1140–1152.
11. Kim HI, Lim H, Moon A. Sex differences in cancer: epidemiology, genetics and therapy. *Biomol Ther (Seoul).* 2018;26(4):335–342.
12. Ethun CG, Bilen MA, Jani AB, Maithel SK, Ogan K, Master VA. Frailty and cancer: implications for oncology surgery, medical oncology, and radiation oncology. *CA Cancer J Clin.* 2017;67(5):362–377.
13. Adams P, Ghanem T, Stachler R, Hall F, Velanovich V, Rubinfeld I. Frailty as a ipredictor of morbidity and mortality in inpatient head and neck surgery. *JAMA Otolaryngol Head Neck Surg.* 2013;139(8):783–789.
14. Farhat JS, Velanovich V, Falvo AJ, et al. Are the frail destined to fail? Frailty index as predictor of surgical morbidity and mortality in the elderly. *J Trauma Acute Care Surg.* 2012;72(6):1526–1530 discussion 1530–1521.
15. Joseph B, Zangbar B, Pandit V, et al. Emergency general surgery in the elderly: too old or too frail? *J Am Coll Surg.* 2016;222(5):805–813.
16. Tkacheva ON, Runikhina NK, Ostapenko VS, et al. Prevalence of geriatric syndromes among people aged 65 years and older at four community clinics in Moscow. *Clin Interv Aging.* 2018;13:251–259.
17. Schulkes KJ, Souwer ET, Hamaker ME, et al. The effect of a geriatric assessment on treatment decisions for patients with lung cancer. *Lung.* 2017;195(2):225–231.
18. Tan HJ, Saliba D, Kwan L, Moore AA, Litwin MS. Burden of geriatric events among older adults undergoing major cancer surgery. *J Clin Oncol.* 2016;34(11):1231–1238.
19. Overcash JA, Beckstead J, Extermann M, Cobb S. The abbreviated comprehensive geriatric assessment (aCGA): a retrospective analysis. *Crit Rev Oncol Hematol.* 2005;54(2):129–136.
20. Kirkhus L, Saltyte Benth J, Rostoft S, et al. Geriatric assessment is superior to oncologists' clinical judgement in identifying frailty. *Br J Cancer.* 2017;117(4):470–477.
21. Hamaker ME, Jonker JM, de Rooij SE, Vos AG, Smorenburg CH, van Munster BC. Frailty screening methods for predicting outcome of a comprehensive geriatric assessment in elderly patients with cancer: a systematic review. *Lancet Oncol.* 2012;13(10):e437–e444.
22. Fried LP, Tangen CM, Walston J, et al. Frailty in older adults: evidence for a phenotype. *J Gerontol A Biol Sci Med Sci.* 2001;56(3):M146–M156.

23. Burg ML, Clifford TG, Bazargani ST, et al. Frailty as a predictor of complications after radical cystectomy: A prospective study of various preoperative assessments. *Urol Oncol.* 2019;37(1):40–47.
24. Rockwood K, Mitnitski A. Frailty in relation to the accumulation of deficits. *J Gerontol A Biol Sci Med Sci.* 2007;62(7): 722–727.
25. Kumar A, Langstraat CL, DeJong SR, et al. Functional not chronologic age: Frailty index predicts outcomes in advanced ovarian cancer. *Gynecol Oncol.* 2017;147(1):104–109.
26. Yao T, DeJong SR, McGree ME, Weaver AL, Cliby WA, Kumar A. Frailty in ovarian cancer identified the need for increased postoperative care requirements following cytoreductive surgery. *Gynecol Oncol.* 2019;153(1):68–73.
27. Abt NB, Richmon JD, Koch WM, Eisele DW, Agrawal N. Assessment of the predictive value of the modified frailty index for Clavien-Dindo Grade IV critical care complications in major head and neck cancer operations. *JAMA Otolaryngol Head Neck Surg.* 2016;142(7):658–664.
28. Augustin T, Burstein MD, Schneider EB, et al. Frailty predicts risk of life-threatening complications and mortality after pancreatic resections. *Surgery.* 2016;160(4):987–996.
29. Cloney M, D'Amico R, Lebovic J, et al. Frailty in geriatric glioblastoma patients: a predictor of operative morbidity and outcome. *World Neurosurg.* 2016;89:362–367.
30. Uppal S, Igwe E, Rice LW, Spencer RJ, Rose SL. Frailty index predicts severe complications in gynecologic oncology patients. *Gynecol Oncol.* 2015;137(1):98–101.
31. Chen SY, Stem M, Cerullo M, et al. The effect of frailty index on early outcomes after combined colorectal and liver resections. *J Gastrointest Surg.* 2018;22(4):640–649.
32. Youngerman BE, Neugut AI, Yang J, Hershman DL, Wright JD, Bruce JN. The modified frailty index and 30-day adverse events in oncologic neurosurgery. *J Neurooncol.* 2018;136(1):197–206.
33. van Walree IC, Scheepers E, van Huis-Tanja LH, et al. A systematic review on the association of the G8 with geriatric assessment, prognosis and course of treatment in older patients with cancer. *J Geriatr Oncol.* 2019;10(6):847–858.
34. Denewet N, De Breucker S, Luce S, Kennes B, Higuet S, Pepersack T. Comprehensive geriatric assessment and comorbidities predict survival in geriatric oncology. *Acta Clin Belg.* 2016;71(4):206–213.
35. Souwer ETD, Verweij NM, van den Bos F, et al. Risk stratification for surgical outcomes in older colorectal cancer patients using ISAR-HP and G8 screening tools. *J Geriatr Oncol.* 2018;9(2):110–114.
36. Dale W, Hemmerich J, Kamm A, et al. Geriatric assessment improves prediction of surgical outcomes in older adults undergoing pancreaticoduodenectomy: a prospective cohort study. *Ann Surg.* 2014;259(5):960–965.
37. Goldstein DP, Sklar MC, de Almeida JR, et al. Frailty as a predictor of outcomes in patients undergoing head and neck cancer surgery. *Laryngoscope.* 2020;130(5):E340–E345.
38. Ommundsen N, Nesbakken A, Wyller TB, et al. Post-discharge complications in frail older patients after surgery for colorectal cancer. *Eur J Surg Oncol.* 2018;44(10):1542–1547.
39. Fearon K, Strasser F, Anker SD, et al. Definition and classification of cancer cachexia: an international consensus. *Lancet Oncol.* 2011;12(5):489–495.
40. de Las Penas R, Majem M, Perez-Altozano J, et al. SEOM clinical guidelines on nutrition in cancer patients (2018). *Clin Transl Oncol.* 2019;21(1):87–93.
41. Cruz-Jentoft AJ, Bahat G, Bauer J, et al. Sarcopenia: revised European consensus on definition and diagnosis. *Age Ageing.* 2019;48(1):16–31.
42. Baracos VE, Arribas L. Sarcopenic obesity: hidden muscle wasting and its impact for survival and complications of cancer therapy. *Ann Oncol.* 2018;29(Suppl 2):ii1–ii9.
43. Muscaritoli M, Anker SD, Argiles J, et al. Consensus definition of sarcopenia, cachexia and pre-cachexia: joint document elaborated by Special Interest Groups (SIG) "cachexia-anorexia in chronic wasting diseases" and "nutrition in geriatrics". *Clin Nutr.* 2010;29(2):154–159.
44. Carneiro IP, Mazurak VC, Prado CM. Clinical implications of sarcopenic obesity in cancer. *Curr Oncol Rep.* 2016;18(10): 62.
45. Schlesinger S, Siegert S, Koch M, et al. Postdiagnosis body mass index and risk of mortality in colorectal cancer survivors: a prospective study and meta-analysis. *Cancer Causes Control.* 2014;25(10):1407–1418.
46. Brunner AM, Sadrzadeh H, Feng Y, et al. Association between baseline body mass index and overall survival among patients over age 60 with acute myeloid leukemia. *Am J Hematol.* 2013;88(8):642–646.
47. Tsang NM, Pai PC, Chuang CC, et al. Overweight and obesity predict better overall survival rates in cancer patients with distant metastases. *Cancer Med.* 2016;5(4):665–675.
48. Arends J, Bachmann P, Baracos V, et al. ESPEN guidelines on nutrition in cancer patients. *Clin Nutr.* 2017;36(1):11–48.
49. Wildiers H, Heeren P, Puts M, et al. International Society of Geriatric Oncology consensus on geriatric assessment in older patients with cancer. *J Clin Oncol.* 2014;32(24):2595–2603.
50. Hamaker ME, van Huis-Tanja LH, Rostoft S. Optimizing the geriatrician's contribution to cancer care for older patients. *J Geriatr Oncol.* 2020;11(3):389–394.
51. van Rooijen S, Carli F, Dalton S, et al. Multimodal prehabilitation in colorectal cancer patients to improve functional capacity and reduce postoperative complications: the first international randomized controlled trial for multimodal prehabilitation. *BMC Cancer.* 2019;19(1):98.
52. Clough-Gorr KM, Thwin SS, Stuck AE, Silliman RA. Examining five- and ten-year survival in older women with breast cancer using cancer-specific geriatric assessment. *Eur J Cancer.* 2012;48(6):805–812.
53. Mandelblatt JS, Cai L, Luta G, et al. Frailty and long-term mortality of older breast cancer patients: CALGB 369901 (Alliance). *Breast Cancer Res Treat.* 2017;164(1):107–117.
54. Kristjansson SR, Nesbakken A, Jordhoy MS, et al. Comprehensive geriatric assessment can predict complications in elderly patients after elective surgery for colorectal cancer: a prospective observational cohort study. *Crit Rev Oncol Hematol.* 2010;76(3):208–217.
55. Kristjansson SR, Ronning B, Hurria A, et al. A comparison of two pre-operative frailty measures in older surgical cancer patients. *J Geriatr Oncol.* 2012;3(1):1–7.
56. Neuman HB, Weiss JM, Leverson G, et al. Predictors of short-term postoperative survival after elective colectomy in colon cancer patients >80 years of age. *Ann Surg Oncol.* 2013;20(5):1427–1435.
57. Ommundsen N, Wyller TB, Nesbakken A, et al. Frailty is an independent predictor of survival in older patients with colorectal cancer. *Oncologist.* 2014;19(12):1268–1275.
58. Reisinger KW, van Vugt JL, Tegels JJ, et al. Functional compromise reflected by sarcopenia, frailty, and nutritional depletion

predicts adverse postoperative outcome after colorectal cancer surgery. *Ann Surg*. 2015;261(2):345–352.
59. Robinson TN, Raeburn CD, Tran ZV, Brenner LA, Moss M. Motor subtypes of postoperative delirium in older adults. *Arch Surg*. 2011;146(3):295–300.
60. Rønning B, Wyller TB, Jordhøy MS, et al. Frailty indicators and functional status in older patients after colorectal cancer surgery. *J Geriatr Oncol*. 2014;5(1):26–32.
61. Tan K-Y, Kawamura YJ, Tokomitsu A, Tang T. Assessment for frailty is useful for predicting morbidity in elderly patients undergoing colorectal cancer resection whose comorbidities are already optimized. *Am J Surg*. 2012;204(2):139–143.
62. Choe YR, Joh JY, Kim YP. Association between frailty and readmission within one year after gastrectomy in older patients with gastric cancer. *J Geriatr Oncol*. 2017;8(3):185–189.
63. Lu J, Cao LL, Zheng CH, et al. The preoperative frailty versus inflammation-based prognostic score: which is better as an objective predictor for gastric cancer patients 80 years and older? *Ann Surg Oncol*. 2017;24(3):754–762.
64. Tegels JJ, de Maat MF, Hulsewe KW, Hoofwijk AG, Stoot JH. Value of geriatric frailty and nutritional status assessment in predicting postoperative mortality in gastric cancer surgery. *J Gastrointest Surg*. 2014;18(3):439–445; discussion 445–436.
65. Bateni SB, Bold RJ, Meyers FJ, Canter DJ, Canter RJ. Comparison of common risk stratification indices to predict outcomes among stage IV cancer patients with bowel obstruction undergoing surgery. *J Surg Oncol*. 2018;117(3):479–487.
66. Buettner S, Wagner D, Kim Y, et al. Inclusion of sarcopenia outperforms the modified frailty index in predicting 1-year mortality among 1,326 patients undergoing gastrointestinal surgery for a malignant indication. *J Am Coll Surg*. 2016;222(4):397–407.
67. Kenig J, Olszewska U, Zychiewicz B, Barczynski M, Mituś-Kenig M. Cumulative deficit model of geriatric assessment to predict the postoperative outcomes of older patient with solid abdominal cancer. *J Geriatr Oncol*. 2015;6(5):370–379.
68. Vermillion SA, Hsu FC, Dorrell RD, Shen P, Clark CJ. Modified frailty index predicts postoperative outcomes in older gastrointestinal cancer patients. *J. Surg. Oncol.* 2017;115(8): 997–1003.
69. Courtney-Brooks M, Tellawi AR, Scalici J, et al. Frailty: an outcome predictor for elderly gynecologic oncology patients. *Gynecol Oncol*. 2012;126(1):20–24.
70. Driver JA, Viswanathan AN. Frailty measure is more predictive of outcomes after curative therapy for endometrial cancer than traditional risk factors in women 60 and older. *J Surg Oncol*. 2017;145(3):526–530.
71. George EM, Burke WM, Hou JY, et al. Measurement and validation of frailty as a predictor of outcomes in women undergoing major gynaecological surgery. *BJOG*. 2016;123(3): 455–461.
72. Nieman CL, Pitman KT, Tufaro AP, Eisele DW, Frick KD, Gourin CG. The effect of frailty on short-term outcomes after head and neck cancer surgery. *Laryngoscope*. 2018;128(1): 102–110.
73. Gani F, Cerullo M, Amini N, et al. Frailty as a risk predictor of morbidity and mortality following liver surgery. *J Gastrointest Surg*. 2017;21(5):822–830.
74. Ferrero A, Fuso L, Tripodi E, et al. Ovarian cancer in elderly patients: patterns of care and treatment outcomes according to age and modified frailty index. *Int J Gynecol Cancer*. 2017;27(9):1863–1871.
75. Kaibori M, Ishizaki M, Matsui K, et al. Geriatric assessment as a predictor of postoperative complications in elderly patients with hepatocellular carcinoma. *Langenbecks Arch Surg*. 2016;401(2):205–214.
76. Mogal H, Vermilion SA, Dodson R, et al. Modified frailty index predicts morbidity and mortality after pancreaticoduodenectomy. *Ann Surg Oncol*. 2017;24(6):1714–1721.
77. Hoffen J, Fahey N, Wang C, Park S. Patient frailty predicts for serious complications after renal cancer surgery—analysis from NSQIP. *J Urol*. 2016;195(4Suppl S):E241.
78. Silvestri T, Pavan N, Boschian R, et al. MP59-03 A multicentre analysis of the role of the G8 screening tool in the assesement of peri-operative and functional outcome in elderly patients with kidney tumours. *J Urol*. 2018;199:e782.
79. Chappidi MR, Kates M, Patel HD, et al. Frailty as a marker of adverse outcomes in patients with bladder cancer undergoing radical cystectomy. *Urol Oncol*. 2016;34(6):e251–e256.
80. Lascano D, Pak JS, Small AC, et al. Simplified frailty index predicts adverse surgical outcomes and increased length of stay in radical prostatectomy patients: An analysis of the ACS-NSQIP database. *J Urol*. 2015;193(4):e151–e152.
81. Matsushita K, Sandhu J, Horie S, et al. MP16-04 The role of G8 screening tool in the assesement of surgical outcome of elderly patients (=75yo) with high-risk prostate cancer: a pilot study. *J Urol*. 2018;199:e198.
82. Brown JC, Harhay MO, Harhay MN. The prognostic importance of frailty in cancer survivors. *J Am Geriatr Soc*. 2015;63(12):2538–2543.
83. Shahrokni A, Tin A, Alexander K, et al. Development and evaluation of a new frailty index for older surgical patients with cancer. *JAMA Netw Open*. 2019;2(5):e193545.

36

Delivering Perioperative Care for Older Patients Undergoing Cancer Surgery

EMILY JASPER, JUGDEEP DHESI, AND JUDITH PARTRIDGE

Introduction

The surgical population is aging at a faster rate than the general population.[1] A significant proportion of this group will undergo cancer surgery; in 2030 it is estimated that more than 75% of cancer patients will be aged over 65 years.[2] While there are clear benefits in terms of morbidity and mortality, older people undergoing cancer surgery remain at higher risk than younger patients of adverse postoperative outcomes.[3,4] With increasing age, the rate of surgical complications remains fairly static, with the excess observed morbidity seen in older patients related to higher rates of medical complications.[5,6] This is particularly relevant in oncological surgery where 90% of older patients with cancer live with multimorbidity, 40% have polypharmacy, and 70% are functionally dependent.[2] Furthermore, the frequent exclusion of older people from cancer treatment studies has led to a paucity of evidence describing disease and treatment outcomes in this age cohort.[7] As a result, treatment decisions in the older population can be complex, with uncertainty among professionals regarding the gold standard of care. Traditionally, treatment decisions have been based on age alone, without consideration of multimorbidity, frailty, and functional capacity as superior prognostic indicators.[8] In response to these issues, guidelines from professional bodies outline surgical care standards for older patients including the recommendation to use a comprehensive, structured approach to assessment and management of older patients with cancer.[9,10]

Patient Assessment

Treatment decisions for patients with cancer are traditionally made at multidisciplinary meetings between oncologists, surgeons, and radiologists, with other specialties contributing as necessary. For over 50 years, oncologists have used the Eastern Cooperative Oncology Group (ECOG) performance status as a method to assess function and guide treatment decisions. While the benefits of this performance status include face validity and clinical feasibility, it can be less discriminatory in older people because it does not distinguish between functional impairment, specifically attributable to malignancy and therefore potentially reversible through oncological treatment, and preexisting impairment secondary to frailty, multimorbidity, or dementia.[11] An awareness of the limitation of this approach has led to the inclusion of Comprehensive Geriatric Assessment (CGA) and optimization in oncological assessment for older people. CGA is an established, evidenced-based methodology for multidomain assessment of medical, functional, psychological, and social issues using objective tools. The role of CGA in the medical setting is well established and there is an increasing evidence base for CGA in surgical and oncological cohorts.[11–15]

Cancer treatment involves traditional chemotherapy and radiotherapy, often used in combination with biologic treatment and surgery. CGA is used to assess and optimize prior to oncological treatment,[16] resulting in amended oncological treatment decisions in a quarter of cases (intensifying or reducing treatment intensity) and increased survival.[16,17] In surgical settings, CGA has resulted in a reduction in length of stay and postoperative morbidity and mortality in elective and emergency surgical patients across surgical subspecialties,[12,14,18,19] including colorectal cancer surgery.[20]

Identifying patients most likely to benefit from CGA is important. The International Society of Geriatric Oncology (SIOG) recommends screening older patients with cancer using validated tools to identify patients requiring further assessment and optimization.[21] Three of the most widely used tools include the G8, Vulnerable Elder Survey-13 (VES-13), and the abbreviated Comprehensive Geriatric Assessment (aCGA).[22] The G8 is an eight-item questionnaire that takes less than 10 min to complete by any clinician, with a score <14 identifying a patient who may benefit from CGA.[23] VES-13 is a self-administered 13-question survey that takes <10 min, with a score ≤3 suggesting an older person who may benefit from CGA.[24] The third tool, the aCGA, is a 15-question survey assessing four domains, including functional status (e.g., activities of daily living [ADL]), independent ADL, depression, and cognition, with individual domain cutoffs identifying a need for further assessment.[25] All three have been validated in the oncological setting but have not been studied in patients undergoing cancer surgery specifically.[23,24,26]

Core Components of Perioperative Care for Older Patients Undergoing Cancer Surgery

Models of perioperative care for older patients with cancer undergoing surgery vary. There are a number of core components appropriately tailored to the perioperative and oncological settings (Table 36.1).

TABLE 36.1 Core Components of Perioperative Care for Older People Undergoing Cancer Surgery

	Component	Detail
Preoperative	Assessment	- Assessment of physiological reserve - Assessment of known comorbidities - Diagnosis of new comorbidities - Identification of geriatric syndromes - Assessment of functional capacity - Assessment of mental capacity - Assessment of psychosocial factors - Assessment of social situation
	Optimization	- Optimization of medical comorbidities - Comprehensive medication review - Optimization of geriatric syndromes - Optimization of malnutrition and obesity - Optimization of psychosocial factors and modifiable lifestyle risk factors - Optimization of functional reserve - Optimization of social situation
	Shared decision-making (SDM)	- Understanding patient goals and expectations - Counseling on risks, benefits, and alternatives to treatment - Collaboration across specialties to address specific aspects of SDM in older people - Planning the perioperative period - Advanced care planning
Intraoperative	Intraoperative care	- Following anesthetic and surgical guidelines
Postoperative	Prevention and treatment of medical complications	- Prevention of postoperative medical complications - Prompt identification of postoperative medical complications - Standardized treatment of postoperative medical complications
	Management of multidisciplinary issues	- Early mobilization to prevent functional decline and falls - Optimizing nutrition including early feeding - Prompt removal of urinary catheters - Ensuring pressure area care
	Discharge planning	- Early identification of potential barriers to discharge - Collaboration across disciplines and specialties to facilitate prompt discharge - Timely liaison with community services to support transitions of care - Appropriate follow up plan, with communication to primary care team
Organizational	Education and collaboration across disciplines and specialties	- Upskilled workforce - Perioperative medicine curricula - Structured teaching program - Avoidance of silo working - Joint clinical reflection through interdisciplinary, multispecialty morbidity and mortality review, development of guidelines and audit meetings, etc.
	Research	- Structured quality improvement projects - Collaborative multispecialty research programs - Use of "big data" to examine perioperative outcomes and inform local quality improvement (e.g., national audit)

Preoperative Care for Older Patients Undergoing Cancer Surgery

Regardless of patient age, the preoperative period is an opportunity to identify and modify conditions that may adversely impact a patient's perioperative journey. Improving patient-reported and clinician-reported outcomes can be more challenging in older patients with cancer due to concurrent multimorbidity and geriatric syndromes requiring optimization in a short preoperative timeframe. In planned cancer surgery, the optimization period is often just 1 to 2 weeks (possibly longer if neoadjuvant treatment is being administered first) with a preoperative period <24 h in emergency cancer surgery (such as acute bowel obstruction secondary to a gastrointestinal malignancy).

Assessment of Frailty

This important component of assessment of older patients is addressed in the chapter on Frailty (see Chapter 15).

Assessment of Comorbidities

A comprehensive assessment begins with reviewing the patient's known preexisting medical conditions, which in the older cohort will often include a number of pathologies. Common examples include ischemic heart disease, essential hypertension, anemia, chronic obstructive pulmonary disease (COPD), and osteoarthritis. This assessment involves an evaluation of severity, past and present treatments, and current disease control for each comorbidity, allowing identification of areas for optimization. Targeted investigations may be required to further assess these underlying conditions.

Older patients with cancer should also be routinely screened for the presence of undiagnosed comorbidities using history, examination, and routine investigations. Routine investigations may include a full blood profile, renal and liver function tests, electrocardiograph (ECG), and spirometry. These investigations may lead to new diagnoses. Multimorbidity is an independent predictor of reduced quality of life, adverse surgical outcomes, and mortality rates.[27,28] CGA provides an underpinning methodology with which to manage multimorbidity, cognizant of the interplay between individual comorbidities, and the necessary treatments with an understanding of the potential impact on the patient during the perioperative period.

Assessment of Geriatric Syndromes

Geriatric syndromes are distinct conditions occurring in older patients that do not stem from identifiable diseases but rather occur due to the accumulation of impairments across multiple systems affecting multiple domains in patient function. The most common geriatric syndromes and proposed tools for assessment are listed in Table 36.2.

The presence of geriatric syndromes, in particular frailty, is associated with worse postoperative outcomes in older patients with cancer and should therefore inform shared decision-making (SDM).[29] Assessment of cognition is important to inform capacity assessment, appraise delirium risk, and facilitate SDM. There is no single cognitive assessment cutoff score that deems a patient to have "capacity" regarding the surgical decision. National legislation will inform the assessment of capacity and guide how decisions are made in patients deemed to lack capacity.[30]

TABLE 36.2 Assessment Methods for Common Geriatric Syndromes

Geriatric Syndrome	Example Assessment Tool
Frailty	Clinical Frailty Scale (CFS) Edmonton Frail Scale (EFS)
Cognitive impairment	Montreal Cognitive Assessment (MoCA)
Delirium	4AT Rapid Assessment Test (4AT)
Falls/reduced mobility	Timed up and go Gait velocity
Incontinence	Clinical assessment
Pressure ulcers	Waterlow Braden Scale

Assessment of Functional Capacity

Assessment of an older patient's functional status is essential to:

- Refine perioperative risk assessment
- Identify areas for preoperative optimization
- Inform SDM
- Inform the postoperative plan to minimize functional deterioration
- Facilitate proactive discharge planning

Functional status should be assessed using a multidisciplinary approach, often with the use of a validated tool such as the Nottingham Extended Activities of Daily Living (NEADL).[31] Functional reserve can be appraised through self-reported exercise tolerance, scores such as 6-Minute Walk Test (6MWT), or an objective physiological assessment such as cardiopulmonary exercise testing (CPET). Other widely used scores such as the Duke Activity Status Index (DASI) estimate functional capacity using both a combination of ADL and estimated functional reserve.[32]

Assessment of Psychological Factors and Social Situation

Appraising psychological and social domains using CGA is useful to identify areas that can be optimized and used to anticipate potential barriers to postoperative recovery. Mental health disorders, particularly anxiety, depression, and social isolation, can impact postoperative recovery, including timely discharge from hospital. Preoperative screening for these issues should be undertaken using validated tools such as the Hospital Anxiety and Depression Scale (HADS) to supplement a clinical history including detail of support networks and reliance on formal or informal carers. Finally, as part of assessing the psychological domain it is important to assess the patient's understanding of their condition and expectations for ongoing treatment, e.g., managing a colostomy.

Optimization

Optimization of Medical Comorbidities

Evidence-based approaches should be utilized but applied with an awareness of the interplay between coexisting conditions (both comorbidities and geriatric syndromes), and treatments in the individual patient scheduled to undergo cancer surgery. This process can be challenging in the context of multimorbidity, e.g., addressing uncontrolled hypertension in a patient with Parkinson's disease who also has significant symptomatic postural hypotension. The approach to optimization must therefore be nuanced with clear instruction regarding preoperative interventions and planning for longer-term interventions to be instigated in the postoperative period.

Comprehensive Medication Review

Medication review is an integral component of preoperative CGA. The full medication list should be reviewed to identify:

- Drugs lacking a valid indication
- Adverse drug effects
- Drug-drug interactions
- Opportunities to optimize comorbidities
- Drugs to be withheld perioperatively (e.g., anticoagulants, oral hypoglycemic agents)

Additionally, medication adherence and use of medication aids should be assessed. This is important to prevent harm from introducing new agents or increasing doses of existing medications in the setting of poor disease control due to nonadherence as opposed to resistant disease.

Optimizing Geriatric Syndromes

Frailty is a common condition occurring frequently in older patients with cancer. Potential frailty modifiers include nutritional supplementation, exercise interventions, and pharmacological treatments (angiotensin-converting inhibitors and vitamin D).[33–35] However, there are no studies to date examining these or other frailty modifiers in improving postoperative outcomes in cancer surgery.

Cognitive impairment can be difficult to assess and optimize in a single preoperative consultation. However, given the timelines from assessment to cancer surgery and the impact of cognitive impairment on delirium risk, capacity, and SDM, a systematic approach should be used. Following screening (using 4AT) and clinical history/examination, assessment should be completed using a brief multidomain tool. Optimization strategies include:

- Identification and management of comorbidities known to impact cognition (e.g., depression, electrolyte abnormalities, pain, etc.)
- Optimization of cerebrovascular risk (e.g., statins, antiplatelets)
- Clear verbal and written preoperative instructions for the patient and/or carer (e.g., regarding medicine cessation)
- Planning of the intraoperative period (e.g., depth of anesthesia, use of benzodiazepines)
- Planning of the patient journey (e.g., admission on day of surgery to avoid additional bed moves)
- Communication of delirium-prevention strategies preoperatively to patients, their families, and ward staff
- Modification of delirium risk using Hospital Elder Life Program (HELP)-type interventions (e.g., provision of sensory aids, cognitive stimulation, mobilization) to effectively reduce the incidence of delirium in hospitalized patients[36]
- Communication regarding potential delirium related distress for patients, carers, and staff[37]
- Signposting to long-term condition management (memory clinic assessment and follow-up)

Similarly, other geriatric syndromes such as falls and incontinence should be addressed and optimized using a multidisciplinary approach throughout the perioperative pathway.

Optimizing Malnutrition

Malnutrition affects more than 50% of older patients with cancer due to a catabolic state secondary to malignancy, and depression and reduced appetite secondary to the physical tumor burden or adverse treatment effects.[38] Malnutrition should be assessed using a validated tool cognizant of the overlap with cachexia. Contributing factors, such as poor dentition, poor oral health care, dysphagia, and access to food, require a multidisciplinary approach to assessment and optimization. Oral nutritional supplements are often adequate to address malnutrition; however, more invasive methods such as enteral or parenteral feeding may be required preoperatively particularly when the timeframe to cancer surgery is short. Enlisting the help of a dietician with oncology experience as part of the multidisciplinary team (MDT) can be helpful.

Optimizing Psychosocial Factors and Lifestyle Risk Factors

Addressing psychosocial issues to improve patient-reported outcomes after cancer surgery might involve a variety of interventions. These range from pharmacological management of untreated mental health issues, psychology/counseling referral to address cancer-related distress, or occupational therapy and social work input to improve social engagement, ensure home support, and address financial issues.

Modifiable lifestyle risk factors should also be addressed in the preoperative period. These include support with smoking cessation, alcohol consumption, weight management, and exercise. Such risk factor management is relevant for all ages, noting that the "teachable moment" is also relevant in the management of older people.

Optimizing Functional Reserve

As discussed in Chapter 35, there is emerging evidence that prehabilitation with exercise, nutrition, and psychological support may improve cancer surgery outcomes. Evidence in the older patient cohort, however, is limited and further research is needed with regard to acceptability, feasibility, and impact of exercise on short- and long-term postoperative outcomes.

Shared Decision-Making

SDM is a collaborative process between health care professionals, patients, and their families used to inform a health-related decision. The clinician's role in SDM is to provide insight regarding the diagnosis and potential risks and benefits of relevant treatment options. In the setting of cancer surgery, discussion of treatment options should include proceeding with surgery, alternative surgeries (less radical), alternative treatments (chemotherapy, radiotherapy), palliative management, or "do nothing" options. In older people, the risk of cancer progression should be considered in the context of prognosis from coexistent frailty or multimorbidity, which may convey a shorter life expectancy than the cancer for which surgical treatment is being considered.

Preoperative risk assessment is essential to inform SDM and a number of validated tools are available. Examples include the American Society of Anesthetists (ASA) physical status, the Portsmouth Physiological and Operative Severity Score for the enumeration of Mortality and Morbidity (P-POSSUM), and the Surgical Outcome Risk Tool (SORT). The limitations of these population-based measures should be acknowledged when used to inform the SDM process, but coupled with clinical assessment can provide a systematic approach to risk assessment and planning of the perioperative period (e.g., ensuring appropriate use of level 2 and 3 care).

Advanced Care Planning

Advanced care planning is a crucial component of SDM in cancer surgery in older people and should be routinely undertaken with patients and their families. Timely incorporation of this into the discussion empowers patients to outline their wishes for future care and treatments, including planning for situations where the patient may no longer have capacity to make independent decisions. Important points to address in this discussion include ceilings of treatment, including what interventions would be offered and would be acceptable to patients (e.g., levels of care, single-organ support) and resuscitation status. This discussion is particularly important in oncology patients where the intent of treatment may not be curative, and prognosis is often uncertain.

Postoperative Care for Older Patients Undergoing Cancer Surgery

While intraoperative care for the particular surgery falls under the jurisdiction of the anesthetist and surgeon, standardizing postoperative care to minimize the incidence and severity of common postoperative medical complications is essential to provide value both for individual patients and for health care services. In the case of emergency cancer presentations (e.g., bowel obstruction secondary to malignancy), the postoperative period may often afford the first point of contact with CGA-based services. In such circumstances there may be an increased reliance on collateral history to inform the clinical team regarding premorbid status.

Prevention and Treatment of Medical Complications

Postoperative medical complications that commonly affect older people and examples of methods to reduce the incidence or severity of these are presented in Table 36.3. These examples do not represent exhaustive management strategies. *)*

Optimization and Recovery to Functional Baseline

Optimal functional recovery relies on a multidisciplinary approach. The combination of surgery-associated inflammation and malignancy results in a catabolic state. Overcoming this through MDT intervention is essential for full recovery. Examples of such interventions include nutritional optimization when maintaining adequate caloric intake, which is vital for a patient's medical (e.g., wound healing) and functional recovery. Early mobilization strategies result in improved functional recovery, mortality, and fewer medical complications.[39] Other important postoperative interventions include early catheter removal, both to reduce the risk of postoperative urinary tract infection and promote mobility.

Realistic postoperative goal setting acknowledges that for some patients functional recovery will continue to occur long after hospital discharge (up to 6 months) or in other situations may not result in a full recovery. Goal setting is an MDT process following the same principles as preoperative SDM, where realistic medical and therapy outcomes are incorporated with the patient's views and beliefs in order to effect safe and timely discharge planning.

Discharge Planning

Discharge planning should begin as early as possible in the preoperative stage. This will allow maximal use of available time to anticipate postoperative needs (e.g., use of a wheelchair in a new amputee), modify the home environment (e.g., creation of single-level living in a two-storey house through providing a commode and moving the bed), and organize support for discharge (e.g., formal or informal carers).

Current Models of Perioperative Care for Older People Undergoing Cancer Surgery

Various models of perioperative care for older people undergoing cancer surgery have developed in recent years. The most frequently encountered models are discussed as follows.

Traditional Surgical Model

Traditional models of care for older patients undergoing cancer surgery involve collaboration between the oncologist and surgeon, leading to the decision that surgical treatment is required. This decision triggers a preoperative assessment that is often junior doctor- or nurse-delivered with a primary focus on anesthetic risk profile. Such an approach is well suited to younger patients without multimorbidity or to those who are undergoing low-risk surgery. While this model of care may incur minimal operational costs, it can lack the capacity to comprehensively assess and optimize more complex older patients with cancer. This may result in medical optimization being deferred to primary care or in referrals to multiple specialties or disciplines with the risk

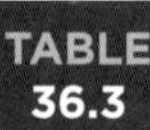

TABLE 36.3 **Prevention and Management Strategies for Common Postoperative Complications**

Condition	Prevention and Management Strategy
Delirium	• Patients at risk of delirium should be identified in the preoperative stage • Routine implementation of HELP-type prevention strategies • Prompt diagnosis of delirium using a recognized tool (e.g., 4AT) • Standardized management plan with clear emphasis on nonpharmacological management strategies and deescalation techniques (HELP) • Education regarding pharmacological management as a "last resort" treatment in the context of safety concerns for patient or staff • Patient follow up to evaluate for delirium resolution, cognitive impairment, and ongoing delirium-associated distress

Acute kidney injury (AKI)	• Patients at risk of AKI should be identified in the preoperative stage
	• Important components in reducing risk or severity of AKI include:
	  • Withhold medications that cause hypovolemia
	  • Withhold nephrotoxic agents (regular medications and other nephrotoxic insults, e.g., repeated contrast doses)
	  • Ensure adequate fluid balance
	  • Appropriate postoperative monitoring of renal function and fluid balance

Pulmonary complications	• Patients at risk of pulmonary complications should be identified in the preoperative stage • Prevention of postoperative respiratory complications (e.g., atelectasis, pneumonia) through early mobilization, time sitting out of bed, frequent deep-breathing exercises (self-initiated and physiotherapist-led), and ongoing use of regular inhalers • Prompt treatment of pneumonia with antibiotics and physiotherapy as required
Cardiac complications	• Patients at risk of cardiac complications should be identified in the preoperative stage • Continue appropriate secondary cardiac-prevention medications (e.g., beta blockers) • Monitor and optimize hemoglobin and mean arterial pressure to minimize risk of type II myocardial infarction • Ensure electrolytes in normal range to avoid arrhythmias
Pressure areas	• Patients at risk of pressure area damage should be identified in the preoperative stage • Encourage mobilization and pressure area-prevention strategies, including regular repositioning and use of pressure mattresses for high-risk patients • Optimize nutrition • Regular wound care for pressure ulcers

HELP, Hospital Elder Life Program.

of delay in the surgical pathway or a missed opportunity for joined-up, timely optimization. In this model, postoperative care is usually provided by the treating surgical team who may feel less confident in oncological, medical, and geriatric medicine issues, and in some settings can result in patients being moved to medical or rehabilitation teams for medical optimization and discharge planning.[40]

Enhanced Recovery After Surgery (ERAS) Programs

ERAS programs are now well established in both cancer- and noncancer-related surgery. An ERAS program aims to accelerate patient recovery through creating a structured approach with defined components of care at each perioperative stage (pre-, intra-, and post-). The content and supporting evidence for an ERAS program within the oncological setting is discussed in Chapter 56. Conclusive evidence for the benefits of ERAS programs in older patients is not yet established due to a lack of examination of adherence rates and impact on outcomes such as length of stay and readmission.[41]

Anesthetist-Led Model

With the advent of perioperative medicine as a subspecialty, predominantly led by anesthetic organizations, anesthetist-led perioperative services are increasingly being established. Within this model, a patient may be described as "high-risk" due to the complexity of the surgery or presence of anesthetic risk factors (e.g., known cardiorespiratory disease). This may prompt a "high-risk" patient to be referred to an anesthetist-led clinic, where expertise exists in quantifying risk to inform SDM. The assessment can result in a number of outcomes, including further targeted investigations, referrals to single-organ specialists, and/or referral back to primary care, for further optimization. In the postoperative period, anesthetists increasingly review their patients in the postsurgery period. The ownership of a patient's postoperative care may be shared by the MDT, including anesthesiological, surgical, oncological, and geriatric medicine team.

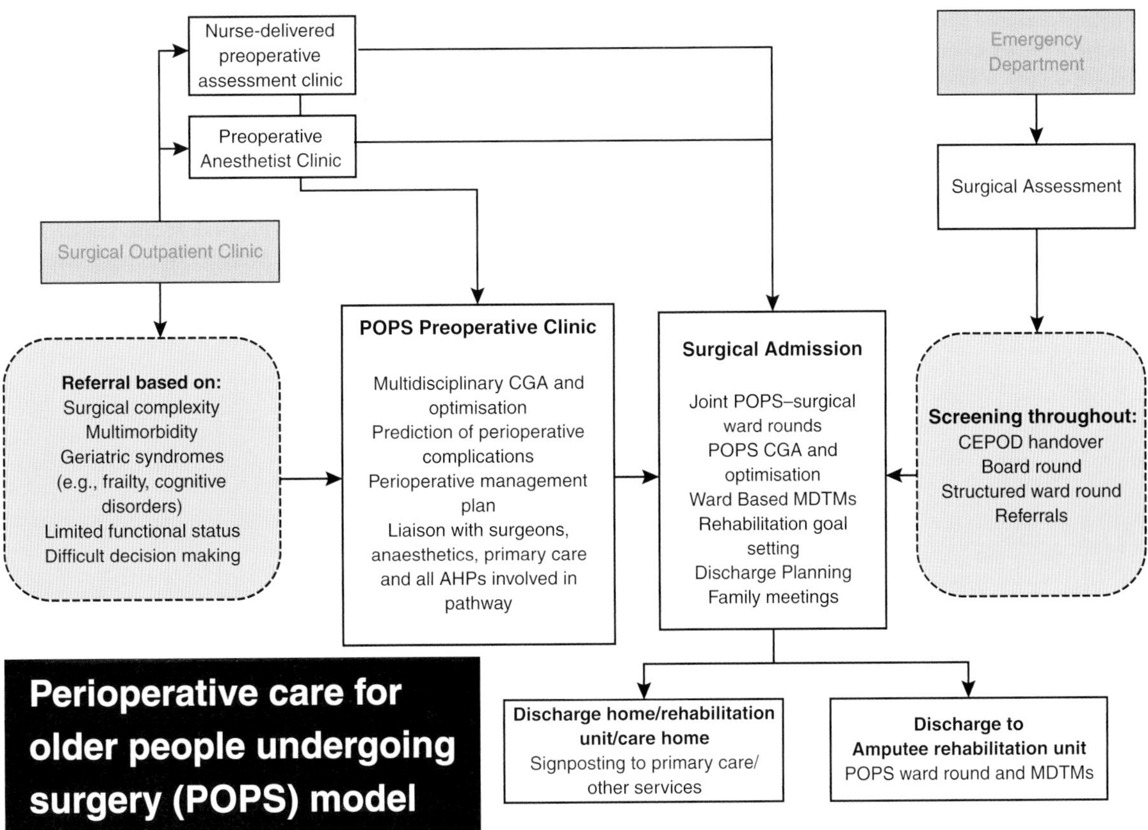

• **Fig. 36.1** Perioperative care for older people undergoing surgery (POPS) model. *CGA*, Comprehensive Geriatric Assessment.

Hospitalist-Led Model

The hospitalist model, most commonly seen in the United States, involves a physician-led service by a "generalist," who works in partnership with the surgeon. This model evolved due to the recognized need for increased medical expertise in the surgical pathway. This collaborative model has tentatively shown reductions in length of stay and improved postoperative outcomes when compared with a traditional care model.[42,43]

Geriatrician-Led Model

Geriatrician-led services encompass an MDT using CGA methodology to manage patients in the pre- and postoperative setting. This involves shared care with the surgical and anesthetic teams for both emergency and elective surgical patients. Evidence in support of this approach is emerging with studies showing decreased length of stay and reduced medical complications for elective and emergency surgical patients in a number of surgical specialties.[14,15,18,44] One example of such a service is given in Fig. 36.1.

Notable limitations of this model, however, include lack of dedicated perioperative subspecialty training within international geriatric medicine curricula and workforce shortages in geriatric medicine.

References

1. Fowler A, Abbott T, Prowle J, Pearse R. Age of patients undergoing surgery. *Br J Surg*. 2019;106(8):1012–1018.
2. Michel J, Beattie L, Martin F, Walston J. *Oxford Textbook of Geriatric Medicine*. Oxford University Press; 2017. 3rd ed.
3. St Louis E, Sudarshan M, Al-Habboubi M, et al. The outcomes of the elderly in acute care general surgery. *Eur J Trauma Emerg Surg*. 2016;42(1):107–113.
4. Lin H., Watts J., Peel N., Hubbard R. Frailty and post-operative outcomes in older surgical patients: a systematic review. *BMC Geriatrics*. 2016;16(1):157.
5. Patel S, Zenilman M. Outcomes in older people undergoing operative intervention for colorectal cancer. *J Am Geriatr Soc*. 2001;49(11):1561–1564.
6. Khuri S, Henderson W, DePalma R, et al. Determinants of long-term survival after major surgery and the adverse effect of postoperative complications. *Ann Surg*. 2005;242:326–341.
7. Simcock R, Lillis A, Cree A, Wright J, Reed M, Ugolini F. *Older People and Cancer*: Macmillan Cancer Support; 2018.
8. National Cancer Equality Initiative. *The Impact of Patient Age on Clinical Decision-making in Oncology*: Department of Health and Social Care; 2012.
9. Lees N, Peden C, Dhesi J, Quiney N, Lockwood S, Symons N. *The High-Risk General Surgical Patient: Raising the Standard*: Royal College of Surgeons; 2018.
10. Mohanty S., Rosenthal R., Russell M., Neuman M., Ko C., Esnaola N. Optimal Perioperative Management of the Geriatric

Patient - Best Practice Guideline: American College of Surgeons & American Geriatrics Society; 2016.
11. Whittle A, Kalsi T, Babic-Illman G, et al. A comprehensive geriatric assessment screening questionnaire (CGA-GOLD) for older people undergoing treatment for cancer. *Eur J Cancer Care*. 2017;26:e12509.
12. Eamer G, Taheri A, Chen S, et al. Comprehensive geriatric assessment for older people admitted to a surgical service. *Cochrane Database Syst Rev*. 2018;1:CD012485.
13. Kalsi T, Babic-Illman G, Ross P, et al. The impact of comprehensive geriatric assessment interventions on tolerance to chemotherapy in older people. *Br J Cancer*. 2015;112(9):1435–1444.
14. Partridge J, Harari D, Martin F, et al. Randomized clinical trial of comprehensive geriatric assessment and optimization in vascular surgery. *Br J Surg*. 2017;104(6):679–687.
15. Shipway D, Koizia L, Winterkorn N, Fertleman M, Ziprin P, Moorthy K. Embedded geriatric surgical liaison is associated with reduced inpatient length of stay in older patients admitted for gastrointestinal surgery. *Future Healthc J*. 2018;5(2):108–116.
16. Kenis C, Bron D, Libert Y, et al. Relevance of a systematic geriatric screening and assessment in older patients with cancer: results of a prospective multicentric study. *Ann Oncol*. 2013;24(5):1306–1312.
17. van de Water W, Bastiaannet E, Egan K, et al. Management of primary metastatic breast cancer in elderly patients–an international comparison of oncogeriatric versus standard care. *J Geriatr Oncol*. 2014;5(3):252–259.
18. Braude P, Goodman A, Elias TC, et al. Evaluation and establishment of a ward-based geriatric liaison service for older urological surgical patients: Proactive care of Older People undergoing Surgery (POPS)-Urology. *BJU Int*. 2017;1:123–129.
19. Vilches-Moraga A, Fox J. Geriatricians and the older emergency general surgical patient: proactive assessment and patient centred interventions - Salford-POP-GS. *Aging Clin Exp Res*. 2018;30(3):277–282.
20. Ommundsen T, Wyller T, Nesbakken A, et al. Preoperative geriatric assessment and tailored interventions in frail older patients with colorectal cancer: a randomized controlled trial. *Colorectal Dis*. 2018;20(1):16–25.
21. International Society of Geriatric Oncology. Comprehensive Geriatric Assessment (CGA) of the older patient with cancer. 2015. Available at https://www.siog.org/content/comprehensive-geriatric-assessment-cga-older-patient-cancer.
22. Korc-Grodzicki B, Holmes H, Shahrokni A. Geriatric assessment for oncologists. *Cancer Biol Med*. 2015;12(4):261–274.
23. Bellera C, Rainfray M, Mathoulin-Pelissier S, et al. Screening older cancer patients: first evaluation of the G-8 screening tool. *Ann Oncol*. 2012;23(8):2166–2172.
24. Soubeyran P, Bellera C, Goyard J, et al. Screening for vulnerability in older cancer patients: the ONCODAGE Prospective Multicenter Cohort Study. *PLoS One*. 2014;9(12):e115060.
25. Overcash J, Beckstead J, Moody L, Extermann M, Cobb S. The abbreviated comprehensive geriatric assessment (aCGA) for use in the older cancer patient as a pre-screen: scoring and interpretation. *Crit Rev Oncol Hematol*. 2006;59(3):205–210.
26. Kenig J, Zychiewicz B, O'lszewska U, Richter P. Screening for frailty among older patients with cancer that qualify for abdominal surgery. *J Geriatr Oncol*. 2015;6(1):52–59.
27. Jani B, Hanlon P, Nicholl B, et al. Relationship between multimorbidity, demographic factors and mortality: findings from the UK Biobank cohort. *BMC Med*. 2019;17(74). doi:10.1186/s12916-019-1305-x.
28. Lyons W. Approach to evaluating the multimorbid patient with cardiovascular disease undergoing noncardiac surgery. *Clin Geriatr Med*. 2016;32(2):347–358.
29. Souwer E, Verweij N, van den Bos F, et al. Risk stratification for surgical outcomes in older colorectal cancer patients using ISAR-HP and G8 screening tools. *J Geriatr Oncol*. 2019;9(2):110–114.
30. National Health Service England. Mental Capacity Act London: NHS England; 2019. Available at. https://www.nhs.uk/conditions/social-care-and-support-guide/making-decisions-for-someone-else/mental-capacity-act/.
31. Kristjansson S, Jordhoy M, Nesbakken A, et al. Which elements of a comprehensive geriatric assessment (CGA) predict post-operative complications and early mortality after colorectal cancer surgery? *J Geriatr Oncol*. 2010;1(2):57–65.
32. Wijeysundera D, Pearse R, Shulman M, et al. Assessment of functional capacity before major non-cardiac surgery: an international, prospective cohort study. *Lancet*. 2018;391:2631–2640.
33. Band M, Sumukadas D, Struthers A, Avenell A, et al. Leucine and ACE inhibitors as therapies for sarcopenia (LACE trial): study protocol for a randomised controlled trial. *Trials*. 2018;391:2631–2640.
34. Hubbard R, Fallah N, Searle S, Mitnitski A, Rockwood K. Impact of exercise in community-dwelling older adults. *PLoS One*. 2009;4(7):e6174.
35. Ju S, Lee J, Kim D. Low 25-hydroxyvitamin D levels and the risk of frailty syndrome: a systematic review and dose-response meta-analysis. *BMC Geriatr*. 2018;18(206). doi:10.1186/s12877-018-0904-2.
36. Hshieh T, Yang T, Gartaganis S, Yue J, Inouye S. Hospital elder life program: systematic review and meta-analysis of effectiveness. *Am J Geriatr Psychiatry*. 2018;26(10):1015–1033.
37. Partridge J, Crichton S, Biswell E, et al. Measuring the distress related to delirium in older surgical patients and their relatives. *Int J Geriatr Psychiatry*. 2019;34(7):1070–1077.
38. Van Den Broeke C, De Burghgraeve T, Ummels M, et al. Occurrence of malnutrition and associated factors in community-dwelling older adults: those with a recent diagnosis of cancer are at higher risk. *J Nutr Health Aging*. 2018;22(2):191–198.
39. Baer M, Neuhaus V, Pape H, Ciritsis B. Influence of mobilization and weight bearing on in-hospital outcome in geriatric patients with hip fractures. *SICOT-J*. 2019;5:4. doi:10.1051/sicotj/2019005.
40. Shipway D, Partridge J, Foxton C, et al. Do surgical trainees believe they are adequately trained to manage the ageing population? A UK survey of knowledge and beliefs in surgical trainees. *J Surg Educ*. 2015;72(4):641–647.
41. Fagard K, Wolthuis A, D'Hoore A, et al. A systematic review of the intervention components, adherence and outcomes of enhanced recovery programmes in older patients undergoing elective colorectal surgery. *BMC Geriatr*. 2019;19:157.
42. Auerbach A, Wachter R, Cheng H, et al. Comanagement of surgical patients between neurosurgeons and hospitalists. *Arch Intern Med*. 2010;170(22):2004–2010.
43. Wachter R, Goldman L. The hospitalist movement 5 years later. *JAMA*. 2002;287(4):487–494.
44. Harari D, Hopper A, Dhesi J, Babic-Illman G, Lockwood L, Martin F. Proactive care of older people undergoing surgery ('POPS'): designing, embedding, evaluating and funding a comprehensive geriatric assessment service for older elective surgical patients. *Age Ageing*. 2007;36(2):190–196.

SECTION 4

Acute Postoperative and Intensive Care of the Cancer Patient

37

Special Considerations in the Postoperative Care of the Cancer Patient

CELIA R. LEDET

According to the National Cancer Institute, an estimated 1.7 million new cases of cancer were diagnosed in the United States in 2018, and more than 600,000 people died from the disease. In fact, cancer is the leading cause of death in the United States. Cancer mortality is higher among men than women, and when comparing groups based on race/ethnicity and sex, cancer mortality is highest in African American men and the lowest in Asian/Pacific Islander women. There are an estimated 15.5 million cancer survivors in the United States, with this number expected to increase to 20.3 million by 2026.[1]

Because of the significant impact of cancer, there have been new advances in both diagnostic and therapeutic tools for cancer treatment that have allowed the number of patients living with cancer to increase. Intensive chemotherapy regimens and the use of new and more targeted therapeutic drugs have resulted in higher cancer cure rates. In addition, there are new, innovative clinical trials for treatments that may also prolong overall survival. Last, there are a number of drugs and surgical therapies that not only improve quality of life for patients but also extend overall survival. Although these treatments may increase the number of patients living with cancer, they also may lead to severe morbidity and mortality that increase the costs of cancer care. National expenditure for cancer care in the United States in 2017 was $147.3 billion, and in future years costs are likely to increase as the population ages and cancer prevalence increases. Costs are also likely to increase as new and often more expensive treatments are adopted as standards of care.[1,2]

Most cancer patients will have at least one surgical procedure during the continuum of their cancer care.[3] In patients with solid tumor malignancies, more than 75% of those patients will undergo a surgical procedure for cure, and almost 90% will have surgery for other reasons that include diagnostic or palliative procedures, brachytherapy, or surgery unrelated to cancer. The increasing age of patients with cancer, the increasing number of comorbid conditions, and the complexity of cancer care before surgery often affect their perioperative course.[4] Routine perioperative considerations in cancer patients do not differ from those in healthy patients. However, there are special considerations in the perioperative setting that should be considered in cancer patients who undergo surgical resection. These perioperative factors can influence postoperative outcomes. These factors include but are not limited to nutritional status, functional status of the patient, the complex issue of wound healing, and the effects of neoadjuvant and adjuvant therapies. In addition, postoperative factors, including postsurgical pain control and venothromboembolism prophylaxis, are also factors that need to be considered. In this chapter, we will specifically focus on unique considerations in postoperative care in the cancer patient.

Nutrition

Nutritional status is an important factor in cancer treatment and can greatly influence postoperative outcomes. Evolving evidence continues to demonstrate a relationship between nutritional status and various clinical outcomes, including quality of life, the ability to tolerate cancer treatment, and overall survival. Weight loss, which often occurs during the diagnosis and treatment of cancer, has been identified as a significant indicator of malnutrition and can portend a poor prognosis in postsurgical cancer patients. Specifically, malnutrition has been associated with poor performance status, increased frailty, and increased postoperative morbidity.[5–7] Weight loss alone has been associated with lower tolerance of chemotherapy resulting in shorter duration of treatment in patients with nonmetastatic breast cancer.[8] This correlates to higher recurrence and lower overall survival rates in this patient population.[9]

The stress of surgery increases protein utilization and creates a catabolic state. This can lead to the onset of protein calorie malnutrition that has been associated with delayed wound healing, postoperative pulmonary complications, increased incidence of anastomotic leak, and increased risk of postoperative wound infection.[10] All of the consequences of cancer-associated malnutrition can lead to prolonged hospital length of stay, need for rehabilitation, and increased cost of care.[11]

Perioperative cancer-related malnutrition is related to poor outcomes; therefore it is important to identify nutritional problems early. Historically, serum proteins, such as albumin and prealbumin, have been widely used to determine patients' nutritional status. However, in the oncologic setting, several nutritional screening tools have been validated and allow for early recognition of cancer patients at nutritional risk who are likely to benefit from dietary support. These tools include the Nutritional Risk Screening 2002 (NRS 2002), the Malnutrition Universal Screening Tool (MUST), the Malnutrition Screening Tool (MST), and the Mini Nutritional Assessment (MNA).[12] Most of these screening tools evaluate clinical and anthropometric data, including height, current and ideal weight, weight loss, rate of weight loss, and body mass index (BMI).[13] Other information, including current treatment regimens, planned nutritional intake, and gastrointestinal disorders, are also frequently assessed.

Preoperative patients at nutritional risk should be promptly identified and referred for comprehensive nutritional assessment prior to surgery. Nutritional intervention should be initiated if malnutrition is present at the time of preoperative evaluation or when nutritional intake is expected to be adequate for more than 7–10 days. For better postoperative outcomes, malnourished patients undergoing elective surgery should receive nutritional support for 10–14 days prior to surgery, even if surgery must be delayed. This nutritional support should be in the form of enteral nutrition, except in patients with poor swallowing function or parenteral nutrition in patients with compromised gastrointestinal (GI) function.[14,15]

Functional Status

For cancer patients, preoperative functional status greatly influences postoperative clinical outcomes. Functional status is a multidimensional concept defined as a patient-oriented health outcome that contains aspects of individual daily functioning, including physical, psychologic, and social factors. One measure of functional status is the Eastern Cooperative Oncology Group (ECOG) Performance Status, a score ranging from 0 ("fully active") through 3 ("capable of only limited self-care") to 5 ("dead").[16] The other scale often used is the Karnofsky scale. This scale ranges from 10 (moribund) to 100 (no limitations). An alternative measure of a patient's general health is the American Society of Anesthesiologists (ASA) score.[9] This measure of physical status ranges from 1 for a normal healthy patient to 5 for a moribund patient who is not expected to survive surgery.[17]

The postoperative period is associated with a 20%–40% reduction in functional and physiologic capacity.[18] In a study evaluating patients who underwent oncologic abdominal surgery postoperative pulmonary complications, specifically pneumonia, unplanned intubations and respiratory failure occurred most frequently in patients who underwent esophagectomy, with advanced ASA class and with partial and totally dependent functional status. These results underlie the importance of functional status on postoperative outcomes. It is essential in achieving and maintaining functional independence, a common prerequisite for hospital discharge and the ability to independently function.

Prehabilitation

Since we know that functional status can have a big impact on postoperative outcomes, determining methods to improve functional status before surgery is essential to improve postoperative recovery.[19] Prehabilitation has been defined as a strength-training program to increase functional capacity in preparation for stressful events such as a surgical procedure.[20] Prehabilitation was first documented in 1946 in the military, where physical medicine specialists trained men of "poor physique" who needed physical development or restoration. These military recruits were provided with nutrition, physical training, and education to help with the improvement of the patient's physical status.[21,22] In the past 20 years, most of the literature surrounding prehabilitation focuses on joint replacement and cardiac patients demonstrating improved functional status, decreased complications, and improved length of stay in various studies.[23,24]

Prehabilitation in cancer patients is an emerging field. It has become more common to treat solid tumor cancers (e.g., breast, gynecologic, pancreas, colorectal, and genitourinary) with neoadjuvant chemotherapy or radiation, or both, prior to surgical resection. Because of the risk of deconditioning and subsequent functional decline while receiving neoadjuvant treatment, the preoperative period is the prime time to intervene with a mobility program and structured exercise to circumvent and prevent some of the sequelae of treatment and improve postoperative outcomes.[25] Patients who do not receive prehabilitation have a risk for slower recovery of functional capacity after surgery as demonstrated in Fig. 37.1.

Wound Healing

Postsurgical wound healing in cancer patients is a complex process that can be influenced by myelosuppression; malignancy; and treatment-related immunosuppression, including steroids, neoadjuvant and adjuvant chemotherapy, and radiation. Normal wound healing requires an orderly progression of complex processes that result in restoration of the anatomic and functional integrity of tissues. This process involves a series of sequential and overlapping cellular activities, driven by growth factors and cytokines that promote the migration and recruitment of specific cells to the site of the tissue injury. Normal wound healing involves major cell types, including polymorphonuclear leukocytes (PMN), platelets, macrophages, keratinocytes, and fibroblasts.

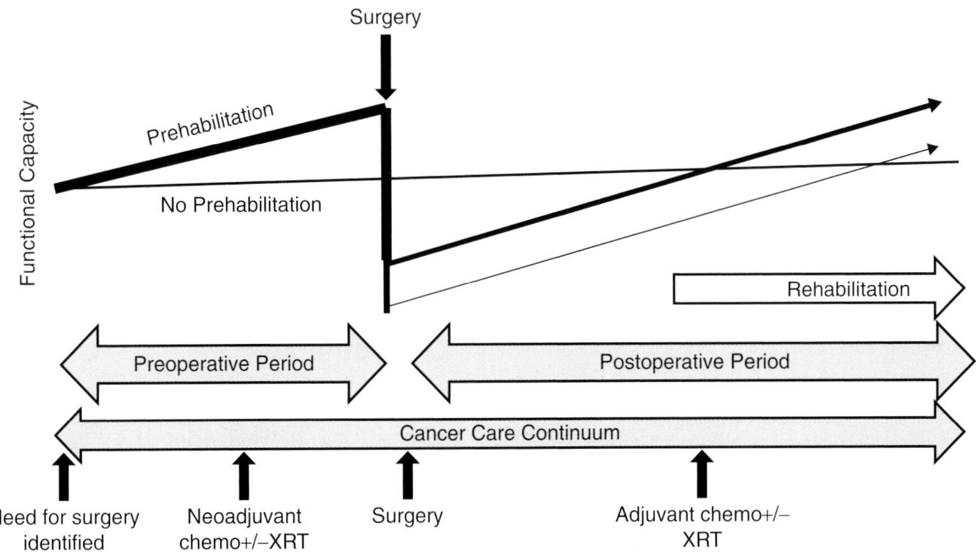

• **Fig. 37.1** Cancer continuum and prehabilitation.

Table 37.1 provides a summary of the phases of wound healing: inflammation, proliferation, and maturation.[26] The inflammatory phase lasts 4–6 days from surgery and is characterized by the cellular inflammatory processes. The proliferative phase lasts from 4–14 days after injury. Cytokines and growth factors secreted by platelets and macrophages from the inflammatory phase drive angiogenesis, fibroplasia, collagen synthesis, granulation tissue formation, and reepithelization. Maturation occurs from 8 days to 1 year postsurgery, and the focus is on collagen deposition and remodeling. At 1 year, the tensile strength of skin and fascial wounds is 80%–85% of unwounded tissue, essentially never attaining the same tensile strength as prior to surgery.[27–29] Along the same lines, GI wounds attain appropriately 65% of wounded tensile strength at 1 year.[28]

TABLE 37.1 Phases of Wound Healing

Phase of Wound Healing	Days Post Wound Healing	Major Cell Types	Major Growth Factors	Wound Healing Processes
Inflammatory phase	4–6 days	Platelets	Transforming growth factor β (TGF-β)	Homeostasis
			b-Fibroblast growth factor (bFGF),	Wound epithelization
		Macrophages	Epidermal growth factor receptor (EGFR)	
		T lymphocytes	Interleukin (IL)-2 (IL-2)	Tissue debridement
		Polymorphonuclear leukocytes (PMNs)	IL-1	Infection prevention
Proliferation	4–14 days	Platelets	IL-1	Angiogenesis
		Macrophages	IL-6	Granulation tissue formation
		Keratinocytes	Tumor necrosis factor-α (TNF-α)	Collagen synthesis
			Transforming growth factor α (TGF-α),	Organized collagen deposition
		Fibroblasts	Vascular endothelial growth factor (VEGF)	
Maturation	8 days to 1 year	Platelets	Fibroblast growth factor (bFGF)	Increased wound tensile strength
		Macrophages	Epidermal growth factor (EGF)	
		Keratinocytes		

Treatment of cancer patients often involves multiple modalities, all of which impact their ability to heal wounds. Within the spectrum of cancer treatment, surgery is often employed for curative purposes by eradication or tumor debulking in anticipation of further treatment. The timing of surgical intervention in relation to radio- or chemotherapy is fundamentally important in recovery and wound healing.

Adjuvant Therapy

Radiation Therapy

Radiation therapy is based on the ability of target tissues to absorb energy and can cause damage to vital structures, including cellular DNA. Wound healing complications are worsened by radiation exposure to skin, connective tissue, and underlying vasculature. Clinically, prior radiation exposure has been demonstrated to increase the incidence of flap failures, fistulas, wound necrosis, delayed or prolonged healing, and infection.[30,31] Of note, wound healing is most affected by ionizing radiation when surgery is performed 6 months or more after radiation therapy. During the intervening period, the irradiated tissue becomes hypoxic, and fibroblasts become dysfunctional, which can lead to increased wound-healing complications. Consequently, the timing of surgery in reference to proposed radiotherapy can have a significant impact on the outcome of wounds.[32–34]

Fewer wound complications have been demonstrated when radiation is given in the postoperative setting.[35] Because acute radiation exposure delays wound healing due to effects on the skin, connective tissue, and vasculature, it is logical to conclude that the effects on healing wounds can be minimized if the majority of wound healing has occurred prior to radiation treatment. Treatments should be initiated within 6 to 8 weeks postoperatively, as the benefits of radiotherapy may decrease if treatments are delayed further.[36]

Chemotherapy

Chemotherapy, alone or as a part of treatment regimen with surgery and radiation, is a fundamental treatment of cancer. Chemotherapy specifically targets proliferating cells by interfering with specific components of the cell cycle. Although chemotherapeutic agents preferentially target rapidly dividing cells, any tissue can be affected by these treatments. Macrophages and fibroblasts involved in wound healing are just as susceptible to these effects as cancer cells. Consequently, the timing of surgical intervention as well as the specific agents prescribed should be considered in wound healing in cancer patients.[32]

Typically, chemotherapy is delayed by 2 weeks postsurgery, and the optimal timing of perioperative treatment using various antineoplastic agents remains unknown. Individual cytotoxic agent classes and the potential adverse effects on wound healing are discussed in Table 37.2.

TABLE 37.2 Major Chemotherapy Drug Classes and Effects on Wound Healing

Agent Class	Common Chemotherapy Agent	Effect on Wound Healing
Antimetabolites	5-Flourouracil	Equivocal results on wound healing in human models
	Methotrexate	Neoadjuvant administration causes dose-dependent reduction of tensile strength
	Azathioprine, 6-mercaptopurine	Transient suppression of the proliferative phase of wound healing
	Gemcitabine	Effects on wound healing unknown
Alkylators	Cyclophosphamide, thiotepa, nitrogen mustard	Adjuvant administration of supratherapeutic doses causes reduction in wound tensile strength in animal models
	Cisplatin	Reduction in wound tensile strength up to 4 weeks postoperatively in animal models
Antitumor antibiotics	Bleomycin	Inhibition of skin fibroblasts resulting in delayed wound healing
	Doxorubicin	Macrophage dysfunction resulting in wound impairment during early phases of wound healing
Antimicrotubule agents	Paclitaxel, docetaxel, cabazitaxel, nab-paclitaxel	No impairment on wound healing
Hormonal therapies	Tamoxifen	No significant wound healing impairments. Increased risk of thromboembolism and possible flap loss in reconstructive surgery
	Letrozole	Impaired wound healing in animal models but not in human models
Corticosteroids	Glucocorticoids	Adverse effects on all phases of wound healing

Pain Management

Patients with cancer often require pain medication throughout their treatment course. As many as three-quarters of chronic pain syndromes result from a direct effect of the neoplasm; others are related to therapies administered to manage the disease or to disorders unrelated to the disease or its treatment.[37]

In surgical cancer patients, postoperative pain is both prevalent and undertreated, with 20%–30% of patients continuing to experience moderate-to-severe pain after surgery. High levels of postoperative pain are associated with an increased risk of pulmonary and cardiovascular complications and are the most common reason for delayed discharge or unexpected hospital admission after ambulatory surgery.[38] Those patients who chronically use opioid analgesics can be expected to have some degree of tolerance and may require dose escalation in the postoperative period to obtain adequate pain control.[39] Many patients who receive long-acting forms of opioids may have breakthrough pain and need conversion to short-acting forms of analgesia in the postoperative period.

Although the mainstay approach for the management of cancer pain is opioid-based medications, a range of potential strategies should be considered for each patient. The major pharmacologic approaches for pain management include opioids; nonopioid analgesics such as aspirin, acetaminophen, and nonsteroidal antiinflammatory drugs (NSAIDs); tramadol; and other adjuvant therapies such as antiepileptic drugs, including gabapentin and pregabalin, muscle relaxants, antidepressants, and topical analgesics.

Multimodal analgesia is recommended for the treatment of pain in postsurgical cancer patients.[37] Typically multimodal therapy uses combinations of drugs that target different metabolic pathways, which may result in improved analgesia and fewer side effects because lower doses of each drug can be used.

Multimodal Enhanced Recovery After Surgery (ERAS) is an integrated multidisciplinary approach to postsurgical care that can be used in patients with cancer. The goals of ERAS protocols include attenuating the surgical stress response and reducing end-organ dysfunction through integrated preoperative, intraoperative, and postoperative pathways. While each intervention has a small effect, all together they have a stronger synergistic impact.

Components of ERAS are demonstrated in Table 37.3. Preoperative elements include but are not limited to thromboprophylaxis, antibiotic prophylaxis, selection of bowel preparation, and fluid and carbohydrate loading. Intraoperative elements include avoidance of salt and water overload, use of short-acting anesthetic agents where appropriate, and the maintenance of normothermia. Postoperative components include initiation of early nutrition, early mobilization, prevention of nausea and emesis, early catheter removal, and the use of nonopioid oral analgesics and NSAIDs.[40]

In order to decrease the frequency of opioid use, regional anesthetics can be considered. In a nonrandomized study of laparoscopic colorectal surgery, local infiltration with a long-acting local anesthetic such as liposomal bupivacaine was associated with reduced opioid use, a shorter length of stay, and lower overall cost.[41] Examples of other regional techniques that cancer patients may receive in the perioperative period include scalp infiltrations and blocks for craniotomies, superficial cervical plexus blocks in head and neck surgeries, local blocks at flap harvest sites, transversus abdominis plain blocks, and mid- and low-thoracic epidurals utilized in abdominal, gynecologic, and urologic surgeries.[42–44] All of these adjunctive treatments help improve postoperative pain control and reduce the need for opioid analgesics.

TABLE 37.3 Components of The Enhanced Recovery After Surgery (ERAS) Program

Preoperative Management
Fluid/carbohydrate loading
No prolonged fasting
Antibiotic prophylaxis
Thromboprophylaxis
No selective bowel preparation
Intraoperative Management
Short-acting anesthetic agents
Mid-thoracic epidural anesthesia/analgesia
Avoidance of salt and water overload
Normothermia
Postoperative Management
Prevention of nausea and vomiting
Early removal of catheter
Early oral nutrition
Stimulation of gut mobility
Nonopioid oral analgesia/nonsteroidal antiinflammatory drugs (NSAIDs)
No nasogastric tubes

Postoperative Nausea and Vomiting Prevention

Postoperative nausea and vomiting (PONV) are two of the most frequent and distressing complications following surgical procedures, with as many as 80% of patients considered to be at risk. PONV can lead to aspiration, wound dehiscence, hematoma, dehydration, electrolyte imbalance, exhaustion, delayed mobilization, prolonged recovery, and an inability to begin oral medications.[45,46] PONV is one of the strongest predictors of prolonged hospital stay and unanticipated admission for outpatient cancer surgery patients, accounting for millions of dollars of health care costs annually. In gynecologic cancer operations alone, the rates of PONV can range from 60% to 85%.[47]

Surgery and the use of volatile anesthetics are responsible for causing nausea and vomiting in the postoperative period. From a surgical standpoint, abdominal distension and bowel manipulation stimulate peripherally and centrally located receptors that activate the central coordinating site for nausea and vomiting.[48] This "vomiting center" is not so much a discrete center of emetic activity as it is a "central pattern generator" (CPG) that sets off a specific sequence of neuronal activities throughout the medulla to result in vomiting.[49,50] A particularly important area is the chemoreceptor trigger zone, which is located outside the blood-brain barrier. Five distinct receptor mechanisms have been identified in the chemoreceptor trigger zone that are involved in nausea and vomiting. They are serotonergic-, dopaminergic-, histaminergic-, muscarinic-, and neurokinin-1-type receptors. A variety of different pharmacologic agents acting on one or more of the five major neurotransmitter categories are routinely used for the prophylaxis and/or treatment of PONV.[51] Frequently, serotonin antagonists such as ondansetron and dexamethasone are used to treat postoperative nausea. Antihistamines, phenothiazines, butyrophenones, and benzodiazepines can also be used but are generally avoided due to their sedating properties.

Thromboembolic Prophylaxis

The risk of venous thromboembolism (VTE), including deep venous thrombosis (DVT) and pulmonary embolism (PE), is increased fourfold in patients with cancer and increases sixfold in patients receiving chemotherapy.[52,53] The incidence of DVT following general surgery in patients with cancer is estimated to be almost 40%, in contrast to an estimated 20% in patients without cancer. Due to these increase risks, death associated with VTE in cancer patients is significantly higher than in the general population. In fact, the risk of fatal PE in patients with cancer undergoing surgery is threefold greater than in patients without cancer undergoing similar surgery.[54] Graduated compression stockings and intermittent pneumatic compression devices are recommended across surgical disciplines, with the timing of prophylactic chemoprophylaxis being variable. The initiation of VTE prophylaxis differs by surgical discipline.

Malignant brain tumors, hematologic malignancies, and adenocarcinomas of the pancreas, uterus, ovary, stomach, lungs, and kidneys are considered to carry the highest risk of VTE. Patients undergoing curative abdominal or pelvic surgery for cancer should receive Lovenox (enoxaparin) chemoprophylaxis within 1 h of incision and according the National Comprehensive Care Network (NCCN) guidelines and should be continued for 4 weeks postoperatively, which significantly lowers the incidence of VTE without a significant risk of bleeding.[54]

There are special circumstances for some postsurgical patients. For patients with malignant brain tumors, there are significant reservations in the initiation of chemical thromboembolic prophylaxis after craniotomy due to concerns of postoperative intracranial hemorrhage (ICH). The incidence of DVT and subsequent PE in patients undergoing neurosurgery has been reported to be as high as 25%, with a mortality rate from PE between 9% and 50%. Even with the use of mechanical prophylaxis such as pneumatic compression devices, the incidence of DVT has been reported to be greater than 30% in these patients, making prophylactic chemoprophylaxis desirable. Both unfractionated heparin and low-molecular-weight heparin have been shown to reduce the incidence of DVT consistently by 40%–50% in neurosurgical patients. The baseline rate for major ICH following craniotomy has been reported to be between 1% and 3.9%, but after initiation of heparin therapy, this rate has been found to be as high as 10.9%. Therefore neurosurgeons must balance the risk of PE against the increased risk of postoperative ICH from prophylactic heparin for DVT.[55]

Postoperative Quality of Life in Cancer Patients

There are special circumstances that must be considered in cancer patients with regard to the goals and intent of cancer surgery. Most patients who undergo oncologic surgery will fall into the category of patients undergoing surgery for curative intent. This is almost always disease driven, and the type or extent of resection is typically at the discretion of the surgeon. Most surgical reports have focused on preoperative risk factors and operative mortality along with long-term survival. Late functional disabilities and quality of life after surgical resection are not widely reported and are equally or more important to patients.

There are many tools available to measure quality of life. These can serve as outcome measures and may also be used to guide postsurgical patient counseling. One such tool, the Short-Form Health Survey (SF-36), was designed to be applicable in a wide range and severity of conditions. Its measures include behavioral functioning, perceived well being, social and role disability, and personal evaluations of general health. It aims to distinguish role changes attributable to physical limitations from those due to mental conditions.[56]

The utility of the SF-36 in longitudinal studies of patients undergoing non–small cell lung cancer surgery and thoracic aortic aneurysm repair has been reported. The SF-36 has been found to be a useful tool in the quantification of patient quality of life. It is brief and has gained general acceptance. At 6 and 12 months after surgery, lung cancer patients have reported significantly poorer levels of health perception, physical function, bodily pain, and vitality as compared with their preoperative assessment.[57]

Whereas surgeons often consider the probability of survival with regard to preoperative risk factors, patients may be more concerned with the possibility of needing home oxygen, poor exercise tolerance, and inability to perform activities of daily living. Information such as this should be reported in the literature and discussed during preoperative patient counseling. In the setting of surgical treatment for a chronic or potentially incurable disease, quality of life must be considered of prime concern and not forgotten.

Conclusion

In summary, there are multiple factors that influence postoperative outcomes in cancer patients. Understanding different dynamics that can influence wound healing, functional status, the effect of nutritional deficits, chronic pain issues, and higher risks of thromboembolism can all have a profound impact on postoperative outcomes in cancer patients. In addition, the timing of a surgical intervention in relation to adjuvant and neoadjuvant therapies is fundamentally important in optimizing surgical wound integrity and recovery.

Finally, surgical intent should be established in the preoperative period in order to better influence decision-making regarding disposition in the postoperative period. Diagnosis and treatment of cancer patients have many different important segments as demonstrated in Fig. 37.1. For cancer patients who need surgery, it is important to optimize patients for the stress of surgery and for close communication between all members of the cancer care team, including medical, surgical, and radiation oncologists, as well as anesthesiologists and surgical support staff to provide the best outcomes.

References

1. Institute NC. National Cancer Institute. Cancer Statistics. 2019. Available at https://www.cancer.gov/about-cancer/understanding/statistics.
2. American Cancer Society. Cancer Facts and Figures. 2018. Available at https://www.cancer.org/research/cancer-facts-statistics/all-cancer-facts-figures/cancer-facts-figures-2018.html.
3. Santos DA, Alseidi A, Shannon VR, et al. Management of surgical challenges in actively treated cancer patients. *Curr Probl Surg*. 2017;54(12):612–654.
4. Sahai SK, Zalpour A, Rozner MA. Preoperative evaluation of the oncology patient. *Med Clin North Am*. 2010;94(2):403–419.
5. Barao K, Abe Vicente Cavagnari M, Silva Fucuta P, Manoukian Forones N. Association between nutrition status and survival in elderly patients with colorectal cancer. *Nutr Clin Pract*. 2017;32(5):658–663.
6. Dewys WD, Begg C, Lavin PT, et al. Prognostic effect of weight loss prior to chemotherapy in cancer patients. Eastern Cooperative Oncology Group. *Am J Med*. 1980;69(4):491–497.
7. Nitenberg G, Raynard B. Nutritional support of the cancer patient: issues and dilemmas. *Crit Rev Oncol Hematol*. 2000;34(3):137–168.
8. Ross PJ, Ashley S, Norton A, et al. Do patients with weight loss have a worse outcome when undergoing chemotherapy for lung cancers? *Br J Cancer*. 2004;90(10):1905–1911.
9. Thivat E, Therondel S, Lapirot O, et al. Weight change during chemotherapy changes the prognosis in non metastatic breast cancer for the worse. *BMC Cancer*. 2010;10:648.
10. Carli F, Webster J, Ramachandra V, et al. Aspects of protein metabolism after elective surgery in patients receiving constant nutritional support. *Clin Sci (Lond)*. 1990;78(6):621–628.
11. Schricker T, Lattermann R. Strategies to attenuate the catabolic response to surgery and improve perioperative outcomes. *Can J Anaesth*. 2007;54(6):414–419.
12. Skipper A, Ferguson M, Thompson K, Castellanos VH, Porcari J. Nutrition screening tools: an analysis of the evidence. *J Parenter Enteral Nutr*. 2012;36(3):292–298.
13. Champetier S, Bataillard A, Lallemand Y, et al. Good clinical practice in the dietetic management of cancer patients. *Bull Cancer*. 2000;87(12):917–926.
14. Arends J, Bodoky G, Bozzetti F, et al. ESPEN guidelines on enteral nutrition: non-surgical oncology. *Clin Nutr*. 2006;25(2):245–259.
15. August DA, Huhmann MB. American Society for Parenteral and Enteral Nutrition (A.S.P.E.N.) Board of Directors. A.S.P.E.N. clinical guidelines: nutrition support therapy during adult anticancer treatment and in hematopoietic cell transplantation. *J Parenter Enteral Nutr*. 2009;33(5):472–500.
16. Sorensen JB, Klee M, Palshof T, Hansen HH. Performance status assessment in cancer patients. An inter-observer variability study. *Br J Cancer*. 1993;67(4):773–775.
17. Rades D, Bolm L, Kaesmann L, Bartscht T. Karnofsky performance score is predictive of survival after palliative irradiation of metastatic bile duct cancer. *Anticancer Res*. 2017;37(2):949–951.
18. Lawrence VA, Hazuda HP, Cornell JE, et al. Functional independence after major abdominal surgery in the elderly. *J Am Coll Surg*. 2004;199(5):762–772.
19. Mayo NE, Feldman L, Scott S, et al. Impact of preoperative change in physical function on postoperative recovery: argument supporting prehabilitation for colorectal surgery. *Surgery*. 2011;150(3):505–514.
20. Li C, Carli F, Lee L, et al. Impact of a trimodal prehabilitation program on functional recovery after colorectal cancer surgery: a pilot study. *Surg Endosc*. 2013;27(4):1072–1082.
21. PREHABILITATION, rehabilitation, and revocation in the Army. *Br Med J*. 1946;29: 1:192–197. PMID: 20989832.
22. Dobbins TA, Badgery-Parker T, Currow DC, Young JM. Assessing measures of comorbidity and functional status for risk adjustment to compare hospital performance for colorectal cancer surgery: a retrospective data-linkage study. *BMC Med Inform Decis Mak*. 2015;15:55.
23. Rooks DS, Huang J, Bierbaum BE, et al. Effect of preoperative exercise on measures of functional status in men and women undergoing total hip and knee arthroplasty. *Arthritis Rheum*. 2006;55(5):700–708.
24. Hulzebos EH, Smit Y, Helders PP, van Meeteren NL. Preoperative physical therapy for elective cardiac surgery patients. *Cochrane Database Syst Rev*. 2012;11:CD010118.
25. van Rooijen S, Carli F, Dalton S, et al. Multimodal prehabilitation in colorectal cancer patients to improve functional capacity and reduce postoperative complications: the first international randomized controlled trial for multimodal prehabilitation. *BMC Cancer*. 2019;19(1):98.
26. Schilling JA. Wound healing. *Surg Clin North Am*. 1976;56(4):859–874.
27. Broughton G. 2nd, Janis JE, Attinger CE. The basic science of wound healing. *Plast Reconstr Surg*. 2006;117(7 Suppl):12s–34s.
28. Diegelmann RF. Analysis of collagen synthesis. *Methods Mol Med*. 2003;78:349–358.
29. Peacock EE, Jr. Biology of wound repair. *Life Sci*. 1973;13(4):I–IX.
30. Luce EA. The irradiated wound. *Surg Clin North Am*. 1984;64(4):821–829.

31. Arnold PG, Lovich SF, Pairolero PC. Muscle flaps in irradiated wounds: an account of 100 consecutive cases. *Plast Reconstr Surg*. 1994;93(2):324–327 discussion 328–329.
32. Payne WG, Naidu DK, Wheeler CK, et al. Wound healing in patients with cancer. *Eplasty*. 2008;8:e9.
33. Marcial VA, Gelber R, Kramer S, Snow JB, Davis LW, Vallecillo LA. Does preoperative irradiation increase the rate of surgical complications in carcinoma of the head and neck? A Radiation Therapy Oncology Group Report. *Cancer*. 1982;49(6):1297–1301.
34. Snow Jr JB, Gelber RD, Kramer S, Davis LW, Marcial VA, Lowry LD. Randomized preoperative and postoperative radiation therapy for patients with carcinoma of the head and neck: preliminary report. *Laryngoscope*. 1980;90(6 Pt 1):930–945.
35. Bernstein EF, Sullivan FJ, Mitchell JB, Salomon GD, Glatstein E. Biology of chronic radiation effect on tissues and wound healing. *Clin Plast Surg*. 1993;20(3):435–453.
36. Vikram B. Importance of the time interval between surgery and postoperative radiation therapy in the combined management of head & neck cancer. *Int J Radiat Oncol Biol Phys*. 1979;5(10):1837–1840.
37. Carroll IR, Angst MS, Clark JD. Management of perioperative pain in patients chronically consuming opioids. *Reg Anesth Pain Med*. 2004;29(6):576–591.
38. Michel MZ, Sanders MK. Effectiveness of acute postoperative pain management. *Br J Anaesth*. 2003;91(3):448–449 author reply 449.
39. Dolin SJ, Cashman JN, Bland JM. Effectiveness of acute postoperative pain management: I. Evidence from published data. *Br J Anaesth*. 2002;89(3):409–423.
40. Scott MJ, Baldini G, Fearon KC, et al. Enhanced Recovery After Surgery (ERAS) for gastrointestinal surgery, part 1: pathophysiological considerations. *Acta Anaesthesiol Scand*. 2015;59(10):1212–1231.
41. Pricolo VE, Fei P, Crowley S, Camisa V, Bonvini M. A novel enhanced recovery protocol, combining multimodal analgesia with liposomal bupivacaine and pharmacologic intervention, reduces parenteral opioid use and hospital length of stay after colectomy: a cohort study. *Int J Surg Open*. 2018;13:24–28.
42. Azhar RA, Bochner B, Catto J, et al. Enhanced recovery after urological surgery: a contemporary systematic review of outcomes, key elements, and research needs. *Eur Urol*. 2016;70(1):176–187.
43. Gustafsson UO, Scott MJ, Schwenk W, et al. Guidelines for perioperative care in elective colonic surgery: Enhanced Recovery After Surgery (ERAS®) Society recommendations. *World J Surg*. 2013;37(2):259–284.
44. Nygren J, Thacker J, Carli F, et al. Guidelines for perioperative care in elective rectal/pelvic surgery: Enhanced Recovery After Surgery (ERAS®) Society recommendations. *Clin Nutr*. 2012;31(6):801–816.
45. Wesmiller SW, Sereika SM, Bender CM, et al. Exploring the multifactorial nature of postoperative nausea and vomiting in women following surgery for breast cancer. *Auton Neurosci*. 2017;202:102–107.
46. Miaskowski C. A review of the incidence, causes, consequences, and management of gastrointestinal effects associated with postoperative opioid administration. *J Perianesth Nurs*. 2009;24(4):222–228.
47. Janicki PK, Sugino S. Genetic factors associated with pharmacotherapy and background sensitivity to postoperative and chemotherapy-induced nausea and vomiting. *Exp Brain Res*. 2014;232(8):2613–2625.
48. Wang SC, Borison HL. The vomiting center; a critical experimental analysis. *Arch Neurol Psychiatry*. 1950;63(6):928–941.
49. Borison HL. Area postrema: chemoreceptor circumventricular organ of the medulla oblongata. *Prog Neurobiol*. 1989;32(5):351–390.
50. Watcha MF, White PF. Postoperative nausea and vomiting. Its etiology, treatment, and prevention. *Anesthesiology*. 1992;77(1):162–184.
51. Gan TJ, Diemunsch P, Habib AS, et al. Consensus guidelines for the management of postoperative nausea and vomiting. *Anesth Analg*. 2014;118(1):85–113.
52. Heit JA, Silverstein MD, Mohr DN, Petterson TM, O'Fallon WM, Melton 3rd LJ. Risk factors for deep vein thrombosis and pulmonary embolism: a population-based case-control study. *Arch Int Med*. 2000;160(6):809–815.
53. Lyman GH, Khorana AA, Falanga A, et al. American Society of Clinical Oncology guideline: recommendations for venous thromboembolism prophylaxis and treatment in patients with cancer. *J Clin Oncol*. 2007;25(34):5490–5505.
54. Gallus AS. Prevention of post-operative deep leg vein thrombosis in patients with cancer. *Thromb Haemost*. 1997;78(1):126–132.
55. Browd SR, Ragel BT, Davis GE, Scott AM, Skalabrin EJ, Couldwell WT. Prophylaxis for deep venous thrombosis in neurosurgery: a review of the literature. *Neurosurg Focus*. 2004;17(4):E1.
56. Treanor C, Donnelly M. A methodological review of the Short Form Health Survey 36 (SF-36) and its derivatives among breast cancer survivors. *Qual Life Res*. 2015;24(2):339–362.
57. Chen JC, Johnstone SA. Quality of life after lung cancer surgery: a forgotten outcome measure. *Chest*. 2002;122(1):4–5.

38

Early Warning and Rapid Response Systems

JOHN WILSON CROMMETT, JOSEPH L. NATES, DARYL JONES

Introduction

Rapid response teams arose out of the realization that inpatients are at risk for serious adverse events that were usually preceded by physiologic signs of instability that were not always recognized by ward staff.[1,2] These teams have evolved over time since the concept appeared in the medical literature in the 1990s. These teams of responders vary in composition, but most have critical care experience and training and were developed in an effort to reduce hospital mortality by responding to, or preventing, serious adverse events.[3]

Failure to rescue was originally defined as the death of a patient after developing a treatable condition, but has been refined to include these adverse events that could have been prevented or limited in severity by timely intervention or escalation of care.[4] This has become an important safety indicator that attempts to measure a hospital's ability to recognize and manage complications.[5] In 2008 the Joint Commission established Patient Safety Goal #16 to improve recognition and response to changes in a patient's condition. This has provided momentum to the international movement to develop and refine rapid response systems. Since their genesis, these teams have experienced a gradual transition from a primarily reactive response to a more proactive, early recognition model that utilizes early warning scoring systems, incorporating physiologic variables and trends to identify patients earlier in the process of deterioration.

The Rapid Response System

The term "rapid response system" describes the hospital-wide approach to recognition and treatment of a patient who is deteriorating. The major components are the afferent limb, the efferent limb, administrative (which oversees day-to-day function of the RRT), and audit and quality improvement.[6]

The **afferent limb** describes the triggering mechanism for the activation of the rapid response team. A wide range of criteria for activation currently exists worldwide, ranging from complex early warning scoring systems to vital sign trends, specific cutoff points for individual vital signs (single parameter systems), and the instincts of the bedside nurse that "something is not right" (staff worried criterion).[7–9] Experts feel that some objective criteria should be utilized, allowing standardization and education of staff, but that subjective reasons for escalating should not be deemphasized as this provides opportunities to intervene in patients for whom the objective criteria are unmet or not applicable.[10] There is no set of calling criteria considered all-inclusive, as patient populations vary in their baseline physiology. In addition, there may be a need to customize calling criteria because of the variability in the expertise of the responders and availability of intensive care unit (ICU) beds, as well as other systems and processes for clinical deterioration. Experts have proposed a set of clinical indicators that suggest the need for ICU admission, which can easily be adapted into a hospital's ICU admission criteria (see Table 38.1).[11]

Not all patients who demonstrate one or more of these indicators will require ICU admission, but at the very least, timely evaluation and intervention should be considered, and the patient should be closely monitored for further deterioration. For the afferent limb to be effective, this triggering mechanism should not only be utilized by the bedside nurse but also be available to other caregivers and even to family members who recognize deterioration.

The **efferent limb** refers to the responding team, including the members and the equipment they carry. As will be described, the composition of the team varies between institutions and situation but typically follows one of the following models (Table 38.2).[12] The response should be available and timely all hours of the day, and there should be no negative consequences for activations considered unnecessary by the responding team. These team members are typically experienced high-acuity providers with critical care experience. They should project calm reassurance and the ability to diagnose and initiate treatment, and possess the authority to transfer to a higher level of care as needed.[6]

Leadership and management of the rapid response system are essential to maintain an environment of patient safety. This key element should oversee team member

TABLE 38.1 Ten Clinical Indicators Suggesting the Need for ICU Admission

Clinical Indicator	Feature
Potentially threatened airway	Stridor, noisy breathing, airway swelling
Sustained tachypnea	Respiration rate >26 or increased work of breathing
Cyanosis/hypoxemia despite Fio_2 >0.4	Spo_2 <90%
Sustained tachycardia	Heart rate >120
Systolic blood pressure (SBP) <100 mmHg	Sustained SBP <100 or trend below baseline
Altered skin color	Cyanosis, mottling, cool periphery
Altered level of consciousness	Decreased Glasgow coma scale, new delirium, focal deficit
Frequent/prolonged seizures	Seizures recurrent or >5 min
Increasing creatinine	Rising creatinine level
Increasing lactate level	Serum lactate >3 mmol/L and rising

TABLE 38.2 Types of Response Team

Type	Leader	Focus	Function
Medical Emergency Team (MET)	Physician	Clinically important deterioration	Active interventions
Rapid Response Team (RRT)	Nurse	Abnormal vital signs, Ward staff concern	Assessment, triage, call in resources
Critical Care Outreach (CCO)	Nurse	Follow up ICU discharges, abnormal vital signs, pre-emptive review following ward nurse referral	Assessment, triage, call in resources
Code Blue Team	Varies	Responds to cardiac arrest	Cardiopulmonary resuscitation/ advanced cardiovascular life support (CPR/ACLS) protocol

selection and competency verification, sustained education of hospital staff, purchase and maintenance of equipment, collection and analysis of data from team activations, and communication of these data to hospital leadership to ensure patient safety and quality improvement.[13] Rapid response systems will be limited in their effectiveness or may even fail if these critical elements are not addressed in an ongoing way, and success is impossible to achieve without hospital leadership support.[14]

The **administrative and quality improvement** component is key in the collection and analysis of data, to allow feedback and appropriate allocation of resources. When coupled with hospital administrative support, this allows the team to improve function over time and to adapt to new challenges.[11]

Composition

In contrast to a typical code team, which is called emergently to the bedside in response to an acute life-threatening event such as cardiac or respiratory arrest, rapid response teams are often activated for trending abnormal vital signs, early signs of respiratory distress such as tachypnea or increasing oxygen requirements, or a decrease in level of consciousness. The composition of these teams varies according to the needs and resources of the institution.[13] Physician-led teams are conventionally titled medical emergency teams. Other teams may be led by advanced practice providers (nurse practitioners or physician's assistants), critical care nurses, or even respiratory therapists. These are often referred to as rapid response teams, though the terminology varies.[6] Critical care outreach services were initially deployed in the UK and led by nurses, with goals of avoiding admissions to the ICU, enabling discharges from the ICU, and educating ward staff.[15] Their roles have expanded since then, and they are being utilized in more countries. More recently, specialized teams have been constructed to provide rapidly deployable expertise for specific subgroups of patients such as sepsis response teams and pulmonary embolism response teams.[16,17] Many of these teams have also assumed a role in facilitating limitations of care discussions, particularly in the oncology patient population.[18]

Evidence

Due to the cost of implementing and maintaining rapid response systems, numerous trials have been performed to evaluate the effect on cardiopulmonary arrest events and

TABLE 38.3 Studies that Demonstrate Reduction in In-Hospital Cardiac Arrests[12,24,26–27]

Study	Risk Reduction (RR)
Solomon et al., 2016	RR, 0.62 (95% confidence interval [CI], 0.55–0.69) for adults
Maharaj et al., 2015	RR, 0.65 (95% CI, 0.61–0.70) for adults RR, 0.64 (95% CI, 0.55–0.74) for pediatrics
Winters et al., 2013	RR, 0.66 (95% CI, 0.54–0.80) for adults RR, 0.62 (95% CI, 0.46–0.84) for pediatrics
Chan et al., 2010	RR, 0.66 (95% CI, 0.54–0.80) for adults

in-hospital mortality in order to justify the cost. Earlier studies showed mixed results, with Chan et al., Shah et al., and Segon et al. failing to demonstrate the benefit of rapid response teams, while Lighthall et al. and Beitler et al. showed improved inpatient cardiac arrests and improved hospital-wide mortality.[19–23] The earlier studies were limited by some variables, including institutional acceptance of rapid response teams, low utilization of calling criteria, and newly developed teams without protocols to intervene effectively at the bedside of a deteriorating patient. An early systematic review and meta-analysis by Chan et al. concluded that "although RRTs have broad appeal, robust evidence to support their effectiveness in reducing hospital mortality is lacking."[24] The MERIT investigators enrolled 125,000 patients from 23 Australian hospitals in a randomized trial of medical emergency team implementation and found no difference in unexpected mortality, cardiac arrests, or unplanned ICU admissions.[25] These earlier studies and systematic reviews did not independently show reduction in hospital mortality or inpatient cardiac arrests but were able to show a significant impact when included in later meta-analyses. These later meta-analyses consistently show reduction in inpatient cardiac arrests. In a 2015 article, Maharaj et al. reviewed 29 eligible studies and showed that rapid response systems were associated with a reduction in hospital mortality and cardiopulmonary arrest. A meta-regression did not identify physician presence as a significant factor in this mortality reduction.[26] The review by Winters et al. published in 2013 demonstrated a reduction in cardiorespiratory arrest rates outside of the ICU in pediatric and adult patients with rapid response systems, but total hospital mortality was not reduced in adults. They noted that more recent studies were more likely to show positive results.[27] The currently available data support that rapid response teams reduce inpatient cardiac arrests (Table 38.3) and suggest that rapid response systems help to achieve the goals of identifying patients who would benefit from a higher level of care.

The ability to truly assess the impact of rapid response teams has become more difficult as these teams have evolved into accepted practice so that functional randomization is not possible. Before and after comparisons may still be made, particularly in the implementation of specialty rapid response teams; expanded roles and increased autonomy of existing teams; and refined calling criteria, including complex scoring systems and vital sign trends.

Oncology-Related Issues

The oncology patient population presents unique challenges to a rapid response system. They are typically complex patients with significant comorbidities and treatment-related complications, and the underlying physiology is often abnormal at their new "baseline," contributing to their high risk for rapid deterioration. In a large multinational study, So et al. associated a clinical frailty score with increased mortality, showing that clinical frailty has a significant influence on the outcome and trajectory for clinically deteriorating patients, which is highly relevant in the oncology population.[28] In addition to consideration of functional status, some treatment regimens may precipitate a specific set of physiologic stresses, such as acute neurotoxicity, cytokine release syndrome, capillary leak syndrome, or neurologic dysfunction that would require additional knowledge and training of rapid response members to recognize and react appropriately to a called event. Rapid response systems have unique roles in the perioperative care of high-risk cancer patients in understanding the patterns of deterioration in oncology patients and in end-of-life issues.

As the surgical management of cancer patients evolves, clinicians are encountering an increasing number of patients with advanced age and comorbidities undergoing surgical procedures for recurrent or secondary malignancies, or complications of chemotherapy or radiation therapy regimens. Up to 20% of surgeries performed in cancer patients have serious complications, which are related to the physiologic insult of the procedure superimposed upon the underlying disease processes and weakened immune systems. Such patients typically have decreased physiologic reserve and often experience more rapid clinical deterioration than other postoperative patients.[29]

Patients with malignancies account for approximately 13.5%–21.5% of all ICU admissions, and with recent progress in cancer treatment options coupled with studies that show that seriously ill cancer patients can benefit from ICU treatment, clinicians should expect more frequent rapid response team activations.[30–34] In 2013 Parmar et al. showed that rapid response team activations in patients with newly diagnosed acute myelogenous leukemia (AML) were 6.9 times more frequent than non-AML patients. The most common reasons for activation were respiratory distress and hemodynamic instability, with 73% of ICU admissions due to respiratory failure.[35] Oncology patients who require rapid response team activation have a significantly higher mortality rate, particularly if the patient requires ICU transfer.[36] In one US study, activation of the rapid response team was associated with high inpatient mortality in patients with solid tumors (43%) and hematologic malignancies (35%), as well as high 100-day mortality (78% and 55%, respectively).[37] The unanswered question regarding this increased mortality risk is which of these patients were exhibiting irreversible deterioration. For those in which the deterioration is considered potentially reversible, the activation triggers for the rapid response team should be reviewed and adjusted so that earlier interventions can be made in the future, potentially improving outcomes. For those in whom the deterioration is interpreted to be part of the dying process with misaligned goals of care, earlier awareness is also useful in promoting end-of-life discussions prior to the patient experiencing acute distress.[38] In any case, activation of rapid response in oncology patients can be interpreted as an indication to initiate or revisit discussion regarding goals of care and consideration of a palliative care mode.[37]

The role of the rapid response team in end-of-life care has been examined, and this evaluation extends beyond the realm of the oncology patient. Parr et al. showed that in 23% of medical emergency team activations over a 12-month period, a not for resuscitation (NFR) order would have been appropriate.[14] In a multicenter, prospective study, including hospitals in Australia, Sweden, and Canada, Jones et al. showed that issues around end-of-life care and limitations of medical therapy arose in approximately one-third of calls to the medical emergency team.[39] When appropriate, end-of-life discussions may result in less aggressive treatments and greater integration of palliative care interventions, which lead to improved quality of life closer to death.[40] In a retrospective study, a change in resuscitation status following rapid response team-led discussion was associated with reduced ICU transfers and increased access to palliative care services.[41] Interestingly, factors identified by patients, caregivers, and health care staff that negatively influence the quality of life closer to death include ICU admission and chemotherapy within the last 2 weeks of life.[42–44] The role of the rapid response team will continue to include assisting with end-of-life discussions and appropriateness of transfer to a higher level of care and should be able to utilize outcome-based data to assist patients and families with decision-making. Even when aggressive interventions are not indicated, assisting the bedside nurse with palliative interventions is within the scope of an rapid response team's responsibilities.

Future Directions

At many institutions rapid response teams are making a transition from a purely reactive service to a more proactive one that utilizes some component of early warning scoring systems, physiologic trends, and other potential identifiers of patients at risk for deterioration. In general, early warning scoring systems perform well when attempting to predict cardiac arrest or death within 48 h.[45] Uncertainty remains regarding which early warning scoring systems or physiologic variables are most useful and predictive. Numerous early warning scoring systems have been published in the literature, nearly all of which require the highly useful, but often inaccurate, respiratory rate measure. One study showed that the introduction of an early warning scoring system and a critical care outreach service improved the accuracy of recorded respiratory rates.[46] Fortunately, many devices that accurately measure this important physiologic parameter are in the development and evaluation phases.[47] In order to examine various predictors of patient deterioration, Green et al. compared the Between the Flags patient safety net system, which is a single-parameter track and trigger system developed in Australia in 2010, with the Modified Early Warning Score (MEWS), the National Early Warning Score (NEWS), and the electronic Cardiac Arrest Risk Triage (eCART) score. Results favored the eCART score as being more accurate than the other observation methods for predicting outcomes of in-hospital cardiac death, ICU transfer, and death within 24 h of observation.[48] This finding stimulates the idea that statistically derived algorithms that incorporate an array of variables, including vital signs, laboratory values, and demographics, can be more predictive than previously utilized methods, especially in the area of increasing functionality of electronic health records. As rapid response team leaders continue to strive for systems that predict deterioration even earlier, they must maintain awareness of the potential to overwhelm rapid response teams with frequent calls, limiting their effectiveness.

Summary

Since their inception, rapid response teams have been studied from various perspectives. The overriding principle that guides such teams, providing timely resources to patients who are experiencing clinical deterioration outside of a critical care environment, is without debate. The benefits of this service are not limited to decreasing in-hospital cardiac arrests and the potential for decreased mortality as they also include a role in end-of-life care and the bedside education of ward nurses, and may decrease intensive care bed utilization.[49] In order to optimize the impact of rapid response teams, future work should include (1) identification of at-risk patients using early warning scoring systems, (2) proactive rounding on such patients, along with (3) institutional culture change so that the entire hospital staff is working in unison to address failure to rescue.[50] To achieve success, these elements must be employed together and consistently. It would be ineffective, for example, to have a highly predictive scoring system with proactive rounding, but bedside clinicians who do not support the use of protocols for timely interventions. New technologies that alert staff of early deterioration may be met with disdain and mistrust instead of excitement and positive energy. As a result of these and other barriers, the rapid response team leadership must continually strive to demonstrate their value through quality improvement initiatives and to expose and overcome hospital-specific barriers in order to build interprofessional trust.[51]

References

1. Schein RM, Hazday N, Pena M, et al. Clinical antecedents to in-hospital cardiopulmonary arrest. *Chest.* 1990;98:1388–1392.

2. Franklin C, Mathew J. Developing strategies to prevent in-hospital cardiac arrest: analyzing responses of physicians and nurses in the hours before the event. *Crit Care Med*. 1994;22:244–247.
3. Brennan TA, Localio AR, Leape LL, et al. Identification of adverse events occurring during hospitalization; a cross-sectional study of litigation, quality assurance, and medical records at two teaching hospitals. *Ann Intern Med*. 1990;112(3):221–226.
4. Silber JH, Williams SV, Krakauer H, et al. Hospital and patient characteristics associated with death after surgery: a study of adverse occurrence and failure-to-rescue. *Med Care*. 1992;30:615–629.
5. Silber JH, Romano PS, Rosen AK, et al. Failure-to-rescue: comparing definitions to measure quality of care. *Med Care*. 2007;45:918–925.
6. Goldhill DR, Worthington L, Mulcahy A, et al. The patient at-risk team: identifying and managing seriously ill ward patients. *Anaesthesia*. 1999;54:853–860.
7. Smith GB, Prytherch DR, Jarvis S, et al. A comparison of the ability of the physiologic components of the medical emergency team criteria and the U.K. national early warning score to discriminate patients at risk of a range of adverse clinical outcomes. *Crit Care Med*. 2016;44(12):2171–2181.
8. Smith GB, Prytherch DR, Meredith P, et al. The ability of the national early warning score (NEWS) to discriminate patients at risk of early cardiac arrest, unanticipated intensive care unit admission, and death. *Resuscitation*. 2013;84:465–470.
9. DeVita MA, Hillman K. Potential sociological and political barriers to medical emergency team implementation. In: DeVita MA, Hillman K, Bellomo R, eds. *Medical Emergency Teams: Implementation and Outcome Measurement*: Springer Science and Business Media; 2006:91–103.
10. Jones D, DeVita M, Warrillow S. Ten clinical indicators suggesting the need for ICU admission after rapid response team review. *Intensive Care Med*. 2016;42:261–263.
11. Devita MA, Bellomo R, Hillman K, et al. Findings of the first consensus conference on medical emergency teams. *Crit Care Med*. 2006;34:2463.
12. Solomon RS, Corwin GS, Barclay DC, et al. Rapid response team meta-analysis. *J Hosp Med*. 2016;6:438–445.
13. Jones DA, Devita MA, Bellomo R. Rapid-response teams. *N Engl J Med*. 2011;365:139–146.
14. Parr MJ, Hadfield JH, Flabouris A, et al. The medical emergency team: 12 month analysis of reasons for activation, immediate outcome, and not-for-resuscitation orders. *Resuscitation*. 2001;50:39–44.
15. Gao H, Harrison DA, Parry GJ, et al. The impact of the introduction of critical care outreach services in England: a multicenter interrupted time-series analysis. *Crit Care*. 2007;11:R113.
16. Ju T, Al-Mashat M, Rivas L, et al. Sepsis rapid response teams. *Crit Care Clin*. 2018;34:253–258.
17. Kabrhel C, Rosovsky R, Channick R, et al. A multidisciplinary pulmonary embolism response team – initial 30-month experience with a novel approach to delivery of care to patients with submassive and massive pulmonary embolism. *Chest*. 2016;150(2):384–393.
18. Pattison N, O'Gara G, Wigmore T. Negotiating transitions: involvement of critical care outreach teams in end-of-life decision making. *Am J Crit Care*. 2015;24(3):232–240.
19. Chan PS, Khalid A, Longmore LS, et al. Hospital-wide code rates and mortality before and after implementation of a rapid response team. *JAMA*. 2008;300(21):2506–2513.
20. Shah SK, Cardenas VJ, Kuo YF, et al. Rapid response team in an academic institution: does it make a difference? *Chest*. 2011;139(6):1361–1367.
21. Segon A, Ahmad S, Segon Y, et al. Effect of a rapid response team on patient outcomes in a community-based teaching hospital. *J Grad Med Educ*. 2014;6(1):61–64.
22. Lighthall GK, Parast LM, Rapoport L, et al. Introduction of a rapid response system at a United States veterans affairs hospital reduced cardiac arrests. *Anesth Analg*. 2010;111(3):679–686.
23. Beitler JR, Link N, Bails DB, et al. Reduction in hospital-wide mortality after implementation of a rapid response team: a long-term cohort study. *Crit Care*. 2011;15(6):R269.
24. Chan PS, Jain R, Nallmothu BK, et al. Rapid response teams: a systematic review and meta-analysis. *Arch Intern Med*. 2010;170(1):18–26.
25. Hillman K, Chen J, Cretikos M, et al. Introduction of the medical emergency team (MET) system: a cluster-randomised controlled trial. *Lancet*. 2005;365:2091.
26. Maharaj R, Raffaele I, Wendon J. Rapid response systems: a systematic review and meta-analysis. *Critical Care*. 2015;19:254–269.
27. Winters BD, Weaver SJ, Pfoh ER, et al. Rapid-response systems as a patient safety strategy. *Ann Intern Med*. 2013;158:417–425.
28. So RKL, Bannard-Smith J, Subbe CP, et al. The association of clinical frailty with outcomes of patients reviewed by rapid response teams: an international prospective observational cohort study. *Crit Care*. 2018;22:227–235.
29. Story DA, Botz GH, Jones DA. The role of rapid response teams in the post-operative care of the high-risk cancer patient. *Curr Anesthesiol Rep*. 2015;5(3):340–345.
30. Shimabukuro-Vornhagen A, Boll B, Kochanek M, et al. Critical care of patients with cancer. *CA Cancer J Clin*. 2016;66:496–517.
31. Azoulay E, Thiery G, Chevret S, et al. The prognosis of acute respiratory failure in critically ill cancer patients. *Medicine (Baltimore)*. 2004;83:360–370.
32. Thiery G, Azoulay E, Darmon M, et al. Outcome of cancer patients considered for intensive care unit admission: a hospital-wide prospective study. *J Clin Oncol*. 2005;23:4406–4413.
33. Benoit DD, Depuydt PO. Outcome in critically ill cancer patients: past and present. *Rev Bras Ter Intensiva*. 2008;20:82–87.
34. Cherif H, Martling CR, Hansen J, et al. Predictors of short and long-term outcomes in patients with hematological disorders admitted to the intensive care unit for a life-threatening complication. *Support Care Cancer*. 2007;15:1393–1398.
35. Parmar A, Richardson H, McKinlay D, et al. Medical emergency team involvement in patients hospitalized with acute myeloid leukemia. *Leuk Lymphoma*. 2013;54(10):2236–2242.
36. Austin CA, Hanzaker C, Stafford R, et al. Utilization of rapid response resources and outcomes in a comprehensive cancer center. *Crit Care Med*. 2014;42(4):905–909.
37. Laothamatas KC, Bekker TD, Leiby BE, et al. Mortality outcomes in hospitalized oncology patients after rapid response team activation. *J Community Support Oncol*. 2018;16(6):e250–e255.
38. Jones DA, Dunbar NJ, Bellomo R. Clinical deterioration in hospital inpatients: the need for another paradigm shift. *Med J Aust*. 2012;196:97–100.
39. Jones DA, Bagshaw SM, Barrett J, et al. The role of the medical emergency team in end-of-life care: a multicenter, prospective, observational study. *Crit Care Med*. 2012;40(1):98–103.
40. Wright A, Zhang B, Ray A, et al. Associations between end-of-life discussions, patient mental health, medical care

near death, and caregiver bereavement adjustment. *JAMA*. 2008;300(14):1665–1673.

41. Tam B, Salib M, Fox-Robichaud. The effect of rapid response teams on end-of-life care: a retrospective chart review. *Can Respir J*. 2014;21(5):302–306.
42. Barbera L, Paszat L. Indicators of poor quality end-of-life cancer care in Ontario. *J Palliat Care*. 2006;22(1):12–17.
43. Earle C, Park E, Lai B, et al. Identifying potential indicators of the quality of end-of-life cancer care from administrative data. *J Clin Oncol*. 2003;21(6):1133–1138.
44. Miyashita M, Morita T, Sato K, et al. Factors contributing to evaluation of a good death from the bereaved family member's perspective. *Psycho Oncol*. 2008;17(6):61–620.
45. Smith ME, Chiovaro JC, O'Neil M, et al. Early warning system scores for clinical deterioration in hospitalized patients: a systematic review. *Ann Am Thor Soc*. 2014;11(9):1454–1465.
46. Odell M, Rechner IJ, Kapila A, et al. The effect of a critical care outreach service and an early warning scoring system on respiratory rate recording on the general wards. *Resuscitation*. 2007;74(3):470–475.
47. Massaroni C, Nicolo A, Lo Presti D, et al. Contact-based methods for measuring respiratory rate. *Sensors*. 2019;19(908): 1–47.
48. Green M, Lander H, Snyder A, et al. Comparison of the between the flags calling criteria to the MEWS, NEWS, and electronic cardiac arrest triage (eCART) score for the identification of deteriorating ward patients. *Resuscitation*. 2018;123:86–91.
49. Jones DA, Rubulotta F, Welch J. Rapid response teams improve outcomes: yes. *Intensive Care Med*. 2016;42:593–595.
50. Churpek MM, Edelson DP. In search of the optimal rapid response system bundle. *J Hosp Med*. 2015;10(6):411–413.
51. Olsen SL, Soreide E, Hillman K, et al. Succeeding with rapid response systems – a never-ending process: a systematic review of how health-care professionals perceive facilitators and barriers within the limbs of the RRS. *Resuscitation*. 2019;144: 75–90.

39

Intensive Care Considerations of the Cancer Patient

JOSHUA BOTDORF AND JOSEPH L. NATES

The Surgical Oncologic Patient

Burden of Disease

The International Agency for Research on Cancer reported that the incidence of cancer in 2018 was estimated at 18.1 million new cases and 9.6 million deaths. The cumulative risk for developing cancer is 22% in men and 18.3% for women; 12.7% of men and 8.7% of women will die from the disease.[1] Cancer incidence is predicted to continue to rise to 29.5% by 2040, and cancer deaths predicted to exceed 16 million by 2040[2]; however, cancer survival has improved significantly over time. Death rates from all cancers in the United States from 2000 to 2014 decreased by 1.8% per year among men and by 1.4% per year among women. Comparing the periods between 1975 and 1977 and 2006 and 2012, the 5-year relative survival for cancer in all sites improved from 50.3% to 66.4%.[3] The number of patients with malignancy admitted to the intensive care unit (ICU) ranges from 5% to 15%.[4–6] In Scotland, approximately 5% of patients with solid organ tumors will be admitted to an ICU during the first 2 years of diagnosis. Surgical admissions will comprise 84%, of which 63% will be elective. At MD Anderson, a comprehensive cancer center in the United States, surgical ICU admissions represent 60% of all ICU admissions. The utilization rate of surgical patients requiring ICU care is approximately 18.9%.[7] Head and neck surgery, and neurologic and gastrointestinal services represented 62% of the total ICU admissions.

Surgical Oncology Critical Care Outcomes

A large analysis of surgical ICU patients with cancer in West Scotland compared patients with and without cancer and found that surgical ICU patients with solid tumor diagnosis had an ICU mortality of 12.2% versus 16.8% ($P < 0.001$) in those without cancer. The hospital mortality for those with cancer was 22.9% versus 28.1% ($P < 0.001$). These patients were more likely to be admitted as a result of an elective admission to the ICU.[8] For those patients with cancer requiring organ support, the ICU mortality was 18.6%, and the hospital mortality of those admitted emergently was 39.5%. A review of the Dutch National Intensive Care Evaluation (NICE) registry found that the most frequent underlying malignancies included colorectal cancer (25.6%), lung cancer (18.5%), and tumors of the central nervous system (14.3%). Reasons for admission included need for mechanical ventilation (24.8%) and vasopressors (20.7%). In the surgical intensive care population, oncologic patients have a favorable ICU and hospital mortality rate of 1.4% and 4.7%, respectively, following admission after elective surgery.[9] Overall, those with cancer have comparable opportunity for recovery, and underlying malignancy should not disqualify acceptance to the surgical ICU. At MD Anderson, from 1994 to 2013 hospital mortality of surgical patients was 1.1% and 2.9% in the ICU.[7]

ICU Resource Allocation and Admission Prioritization

In 2017 a consensus group representing the fields of critical care in cancer patients was assembled from German and Austrian Societies and made recommendations with regard to those with cancer.[10] Three co-cohorts of patients were identified (Box 39.1). Surgical patients, especially those receiving elective procedures, would most likely be encompassed in the category of receiving full ICU management.

Intensive care admission criteria and resource allocation must be adapted at the institution level. Local resources often dictate the provision of critical care; therefore the threshold for ICU admission at lower acuity organizations may be much lower. The Society of Critical Care Medicine guidelines for ICU admission, discharge, and triage provide a sustained review of considerations for the development of institutional and departmental policies regarding the appropriate level of care of patients referred to the ICU.[11] Important concerns for making balanced decisions regarding patient assignment include patient interventions that can only be applied in the ICU, clinical expertise, patient condition, diagnosis, bed availability, evidence of stability, prognosis,

• Box 39.1 Types of Cancer Patients to Be Considered for Admission[10]

1. Full-code ICU management (without limitations of ICU resources) should be offered to all critically ill cancer patients if long-term survival may be compatible with the general prognosis of the underlying malignancy.
2. Patients with poor performance status not eligible for further anticancer therapy, dying patients, as well as those rejecting critical care treatment should not be admitted to the ICU in general.
3. For patients not in categories 1 or 2, a time-limited ICU trials or predefined do-not-escalate decisions (e.g., do-not-intubate or do-not-attempt-resuscitation) may be adequate options.

and potential benefit. Matching the needs of the patient to the interventions and level of care available at an institution is often a fluid process. The Society of Critical Care Medicine has developed two tools to aid leadership and the practitioner in the allocation of resources and prioritization to available units.[11] Table 39.1 provides a description of the components of care and how the level of care, patient needs, nursing-to-patient ratio, and potential interventions may align for the best interest of the patient.

Common Factors Affecting Patients Coming to the ICU

Patients arriving at the operating theater are likely to possess physiologic derangements secondary to their malignancy, or due to prior exposure to chemotherapy and newer targeted interventions including immuno- and biologic therapies. Frequently encountered factors complicating care include neutropenia and immunosuppression, thrombocytopenia, prothrombotic states, coagulopathic states, chemotherapeutic toxicities, malnutrition, and poor functional status.

Neutropenia and Immunosuppression

Neutropenia, defined as an absolute neutrophil count of less than 1500 cells per microliter, is a common complication of chemotherapy. Risk of infection increases with both severity and duration of neutropenia.[12,13] Among patients receiving myelosuppressive chemotherapy, the risk of developing neutropenic fever during the chemotherapy course is 13%–20%.[14,15] The Multinational Association of Supportive Care in Cancer (MASCC) index is a validated tool to identify a patient's risk for complications associated with febrile neutropenia. The assessment is based on age, history, outpatient or inpatient status, clinical signs, severity of fever and neutropenia, and presence of medical comorbidities.[16] Guidelines for prevention and treatment of neutropenic fever are outlined and supported by major societies.[17–19]

Thrombocytopenia

Thrombocytopenia is a common complication in oncologic patients. In solid tumor patients receiving chemotherapy, the 3-month risk of developing chemotherapy-induced thrombocytopenia is 13% (platelet count $<100 \times 10^9$/L), 4% with grade 3 (25 to $<50 \times 10^9$/L), and 2% with grade 4 ($<25 \times 10^9$/L).[20] Etiology of thrombocytopenia in cancer patients includes direct chemotherapy effects, splenomegaly, bone marrow infiltration, disseminated intravascular coagulation (DIC), thrombotic thrombocytopenic purpura, immune thrombocytopenia, infections, and medications.[21] Patients receiving gemcitabine or carboplatin-based chemotherapy regimens tend to have increased incidence of thrombocytopenia.[22] Several societies have recommended platelet count thresholds and targets for those patients undergoing elective surgery or invasive procedures (Table 39.2).[23] Preoperative consultation and

TABLE 39.1 ICU Levels of Care

Level of Care	Level of Monitoring	Nursing-to-Patient Ratio	Interventions
ICU	Continuous hemodynamic monitoring Invasive monitoring	1:1–1:2	External ventricular devices Mechanical ventilation Vasopressor support Continuous renal replacement Mechanical circulatory support Cardioversion/defibrillation Malingant or symptomatic arrhymia
Intermediate	Every 2–4 h monitoring Frequent laboratory monitoring	<1:3	Noninvasive ventilation
Telemetry	Continuous cardiac monitoring	<1:4	IV antiarrhythmic and vasodilator titration
Inpatient	Routine, every 4 h to every shift	<1:5	Additional evaluation Diagnostic studies IV medications IV chemotherapy

*Adapted from Nates JL, Nunnally M, Kleinpell R, et al. ICU admission, discharge, and triage guidelines: a framework to enhance clinical operations, development of institutional policies, and further research. *Crit Care Med.* 2016;44(8):1553–1602.

TABLE 39.2 Periprocedural Goal Platelet Count

Platelet Count	Planned Procedure
>100 × 10⁹/L	Surgery on the brain or posterior eye
>50 × 10⁹/L	Major nonneuroaxial surgery Therapeutic enteroscopy Liver, renal, or transbronchial biopsy
>20 × 10⁹/L	Central line placement Diagnostic enteroscopy Bronchoscopy with lavage
>10 × 10⁹/L	Prophylaxis against spontaneous bleeding

Modified from Nagrebetsky A, Al-Samkari H, Davis NM, Kuter DJ, Wiener-Kronish JP. Perioperative thrombocytopenia: evidence, evaluation, and emerging therapies. *Br J Anaesth*. 2019;122(1):19–31.

postoperative involvement of hematologic specialists are key for diagnostic evaluation and selecting appropriate interventions that may include platelet transfusions, procoagulants, antifibrinolytics, and thrombopoietin receptor agonists.[23,24]

Prothrombotic States

Cancer is a well-known prothrombotic state. Cancer patients have a 4 to 7-fold increased risk of venous thrombosis compared with the general population or patients without cancer.[25] Incidence rate of venous thrombosis amongst all patients with cancer is estimated at 13 per 1000 person-years.[26] Patients with cancer undergoing surgery are at increased risk of venous thromboembolism (VTE), the incidence of which is estimated at 1.3%–2.1% within 30 days with an annual prevalence of 4% following major cancer surgery.[27,28] Thrombotic events may manifest as VTE, arterial thrombosis, DIC, and thrombotic microangiopathy.[29] In addition to standard patient risk factors for thrombosis, cancer-associated risk factors include site of cancer, stage of cancer, histology, time after diagnosis, surgical interventions, hospitalization, chemotherapy, exposure to vascular endothelial growth factor inhibitors, and the presence of central venous catheters.[29] The American Society of Clinical Oncology (ASCO) updated guidelines for VTE in patients with cancer in 2019; these specifically address cancer patients undergoing surgery.[30] The recommended approach includes unfractionated heparin or low-molecular-weight heparin. Risks of active bleeding, high bleeding risk, or other contraindications must be weighed with potential benefit. All cancer patients should be offered pharmacologic thromboprophylaxis to be started preoperatively and continued for at least 7 to 10 days. In patients undergoing major open or laparoscopic abdominal or pelvic surgery for cancer who have restricted mobility, obesity, history of VTE, or who have risk factors for VTE, a 4-week course of prophylaxis is recommended.

• Box 39.2 Sources of Coagulopathy[31,32]

Antiangiogenic therapies
Pathogenic tumor endothelium
Drug related
Tumor-derived coagulation inhibitors
Treatment-related coagulation disorders
- Following radiation
- Chemotherapy related

Postoperative coagulation disorders
Fibrinolysis
A primary hyperfibrinolytic state associated with acute promyelocytic leukemia
Acquired hemophilia as is the case with factor VIII or
Acquired von Willebrand disease
Paraneoplastic hyperfibrinolysis

Coagulopathy

A state of hypocoagulopathy is less frequently encountered but can exist in the cancer patient. In addition to the more frequently encountered perioperative causes of coagulopathy, coagulation abnormalities secondary to hemorrhage, hemodilution, hemostatic factor consumption, exposure to anticoagulants and antiplatelet agents, renal disease, and liver disease, the oncologic patient may present with a variety of unique etiologies for the underlying cause of bleeding (Box 39.2).[31,32]

DIC in cancer generally presents as a subacute consumptive state or as acute DIC. Chronic DIC is typically seen in solid organ tumors of the lung, breast, prostate, colon, and rectum, which comprise the most frequent primary tumors. Approximately 7%–29% of solid organ malignancies experience DIC, of which bleeding occurs in 59%, while thrombosis occurs in 34%.[33,34] Acute DIC can be seen in 29%–32% of non APL acute leukemia.[35,36] DIC in acute leukemia predominantly presents with bleeding as opposed to thrombosis.[37] Management of DIC in cancer can require a complex and thoughtful approach and requires consideration of the thrombotic versus bleeding potential.[38] Involvement of a hematologist will be worthwhile. For those who are bleeding or need an invasive procedure, Box 39.3 outlines an approach.[38] Promyelocytic leukemia often presents with a particularly severe form of DIC associated with enhanced fibrinolysis.[39] Fifty-three percent of those with acute promyelocytic leukemia (APL) will present with some manifestation of bleeding: bruising, epistaxis, abnormal menstrual bleeding, hematuria, hemoptysis, hematochezia,

• Box 39.3 Approach to the Actively Bleeding Disseminated Intravascular Coagulation[38]

Platelet transfusion to keep platelet count >300–50 × 10⁹
Transfuse fresh frozen plasma or cryoprecipitate to maintain prothrombin time <3 s and fibrinogen >1.5 g/L
Vitamin K supplementation in case of deficiency
Antifibrinolytic treatment if excessive hyperfibrinolysis

• Box 39.4 Indicators of Malnutrition

Insufficient energy intake
Weight loss
Loss of muscle mass
Loss of subcutaneous fat
Localized or generalized fluid accumulation that may sometimes mask weight loss
Diminished functional status as measured by hand grip strengths

or melena. The coagulopathy associated with APL is particularly responsive to early induction therapy, thus mitigating bleeding risk.[40] White blood cell count at presentation is the most significant predictor of early hemorrhagic death and early thrombo-hemorrhagic death.[41] Use of recombinant thrombomodulin has been proposed as a rescue therapy for DIC.[42,43]

Malnutrition

Malnutrition is generally considered present by the American Society of Parenteral and Enteral Nutrition when at least two of six indicators are present (Box 39.4).[44] Generally, 26.6%–51% of oncologic patients will have nutritional impairment with 4.5%–9% overtly malnourished.[45,46] Malnutrition is consistently prevalent among hospitalized patients and present in approximately 40% of oncologic patients.[47,48] Given that the prevalence of malnutrition in hospitalized patients to admitted the ICU for more than 48 h is 70%, the burden of malnutrition in critically ill surgical oncology patients is likely to be substantial.[49]

Presence and degree of malnutrition can be affected by primary malignancy, metastases, prior and ongoing therapies, including chemotherapy and radiotherapy, prior surgeries, metabolic and mitochondrial derangements, procachexia cytokines and factors, homeostatic control in the central nervous system.[46,50] Severity of malnutrition was positively correlated with the stage of cancer.[45]

For those patients receiving cancer therapies, the routine administration of total parenteral nutrition (TPN) is not recommended by the American Society of Parenteral and Enteral Nutrition (ASPEN) to all patients undergoing major cancer operations.[51] These recommendations are due to the poor evidence to support the beneficial effects of parenteral and enteral nutrition in mortality and morbidity. In patients who are severely malnourished, there may be benefit with parenteral nutrition.[52,53] Additionally, there may be a role for nutrition support therapy beginning 7–14 days preoperatively in patients who have moderate and severe malnourishment.[51] Recommendations for those patients who are critically ill and in their perioperative phase are not well delineated in the literature. The 2016 SCCM/ASPEN Guidelines for Nutrition Support Therapy in the Adult Critically Ill Patient provide a framework for those patients in the ICU. No guideline, however, can replace the multidisciplinary dialogue between the surgeon, intensivist, and dietitian while taking into consideration the patient and operation performed. Key recommendations include initiation of enteral feeding within 24–48 h, interventions to reduce aspiration, application of feeding protocols, and avoidance of gastric residual measurements in assessing tolerance.[54]

Patients Requiring Monitoring

Neurologic

A common need for ICU admission following neurosurgery is the need for frequent neurologic monitoring and/or cerebral spinal fluid diversion via external ventricular drain. The level of intensive monitoring is considered necessary based on the rapidity of evolution of the physical exam and the need for rapid diagnostic evaluation and intervention required when a complication does arise. Challenges to the approach have occurred over time. Ziai et al. in 2003 retrospectively evaluated 158 consecutive patients having undergone brain tumor resection. Sixty-five (49%) patients required no interventions beyond postanesthetic care and frequent neurologic exams. Those who received ICU level interventions had the following: IV analgesics, IV anxiolytics, IV antihypertensives, hypertonic therapies, antiepileptics, treatment of bradycardias, mechanical ventilation, and vasopressors. Fifteen percent of patients required greater than 1 day of ICU stay after craniotomy for brain tumor resection.[55]

The best predictors of ICU stay greater than 1 day include postoperative intubation, tumor severity score based on radiologic findings, and a fluid score composed of estimated blood losses, combined with administration of crystalloid, colloid, blood products, and hypertonic saline. Other indicators included surgery lasting longer than 7 h, a new postsurgical hemiparesis or lower cranial nerve deficit, and intraoperative use of vasopressor therapy for hypotension.[55] The nursing skill set required for the management, as well as the concomitant diagnoses that preclude the need of an external ventricular device (EVD), will limit their use to the ICU at nearly all institutions. Methodical management with adherence to protocols and maintenance of procedural competencies can help to decrease the infectious complications associated with EVDs.[56] Bundles of care for EVD management may include hair removal and skin preparation prior to insertion, catheter selection, aseptic technique, appropriate dressing and frequency of dressing changes, standardized techniques of EVD maintenance, uniform cerebrospinal fluid sampling procedures, limiting duration of catheter placement, recurring competencies, and surveillance for infection and complications.[57] The Neurocritical Care Society 2016 evidence-based consensus statement regarding the insertion and management of external ventricular drains recommends a single dose of an antimicrobial at the time of EVD insertion for ventriculostomy-related infection prophylaxis and against the use of antimicrobials for the duration of EVD placement.[58]

• Box 39.5 Potential Complications Encountered Following Resection of Brain and Spinal Tumors

Potential Post Craniotomy Complications
Hematoma
Cerebral edema
Pneumocephalus
Stroke
Hydrocephalus
Cerebrospinal fluid leak
Seizures
Delirium secondary to steroids or other
Ethanol/drug withdrawal
Dysphagia/vocal cord paralysis
Corneal abrasion/exposure risk
Hyponatremia
Postoperative respiratory failure
Hemodynamic instability
Cardiac arrhythmia
Cardiac ischemia
Wound complication
Diabetes insipidus
Deep venous thrombus

• Box 39.6 Complications of Head and Neck Cancer Surgery

Superior laryngeal nerve injury
Recurrent laryngeal nerve injury
Bleeding
Hematoma formation
Acute hypocalcemia secondary to hypoparathyroidism
New tracheostomy associated bleeding, obstruction, and airway loss
Upper airway swelling and concern for compromised airway

Potential complications encountered following resection of brain and spinal tumors are outlined in Box 39.5.

ENT-Upper Airway

Medical morbidity and mortality from head and neck surgery are 5.65% and 2.98%, respectively.[59] Characteristics associated with increased risk of 30-day serious complications include American Society of Anesthesiologists (ASA) score ≥4 and operating room time >6 h. In patients ≥90 years of age, risk factors for increasing 90-day mortality included elevated Adult Comorbidity Evaluation-27 score, preoperative dysphagia, and large resections.[60] Complications unique to head and neck surgery that may require monitoring in the ICU are summarized in Box 39.6. Reasons for postoperative ICU admission of head and neck cancer patients can be categorized into complications related to respiratory, cardiac, and wounds.[61] Approximately 5% of head and neck cancer patients will have readmission within 30 days.

Factors associated with unplanned readmissions to the hospital include diabetes, preoperative dyspnea at rest and with moderate exertion, long-term use of corticosteroids, disseminated cancer, and a contaminated wound. The most frequent diagnoses to result in 30-day unplanned hospital readmission include superficial incisional surgical site infection, deep incisional surgical site infection, organ or space surgical site infection, wound disruption, pneumonia, deep vein thrombosis, pulmonary embolism, urinary tract infection, stroke, sepsis, and septic shock.[62]

Due to the high-risk nature of patients undergoing head and neck surgery, early elective tracheostomy is often incorporated into the primary surgery. Benefits of elective tracheostomy include decreased ventilator days, faster deescalation to floor status, decreased pneumonia, and decreased delirium.[63] Those patients with suspected at-risk airways due to surgical trauma, bleeding, swelling, edema, hematoma, vocal cord paralysis, and tracheomalacia who do not receive elective tracheostomy must be approached with caution. The Difficult Airway Society provides a schema for the planning, preparation, performance, and follow up of such high-risk patients.[64]

ICU utilization for head and neck surgery patients has dramatically evolved as clinical pathways of care have developed. Specialty specific floors with nurses specially educated in flap management, frequent vitals and flap checks, continuous oxygen saturation monitoring, and tracheostomy care have allowed for decreased ICU requirements.[65] Avoiding ICU admission has in turn allowed for a reduction in length of hospital stay and a decline in hospital costs.[66,67]

Postoperative delirium is common and is prevalent in approximately 17%–19% or patients undergoing head and neck cancer surgery.[68,69] Risk factors for delirium following head and neck cancer surgery include male sex, age >70 years, duration of surgery, history of hypertension, blood transfusions, tracheotomy, ASA physical status grade at least III, flap reconstruction, and neck dissection.[69] Postoperative delirium often is poorly recognized and managed.[70] The Society of Critical Care Medicine has incorporated a multifaceted approach in to their society guidelines (Box 39.7)[71]

Cardiac

The role of electrocardiographic monitoring is often incorrectly applied and utilization questioned. In fact the American Board of Internal Medicine Foundation's Choosing Wisely campaign highlighted the practice of continuous telemetry and recommended against the unnecessary use in the hospital.[72] It is estimated that 20% of patients may receive telemetry for noncardiac indications.[73] The clinical impact of telemetry in those deemed to have essential indications is in question as well. In the non-ICU, nonsurgical patient population physicians perceived cardiac telemetry helpful in only 12.6% of the patients and management decisions directly affected in only 7%.[74]

The 2017 Standards for Electrocardiographic Monitoring in Hospital Settings recommends against the routine

• Box 39.7 Management of Postoperative Delirium[71]

Assessment

Critically ill adults should be regularly assessed for delirium using a valid tool
CAM-ICU, ICDSC, and ICU-7

Avoidance of Modifiable Risks

Benzodiazepines and blood transfusions

Avoiding Pharmacologic Prevention

Haloperidol, dexmedetomidine, β-hydroxy β-methylglutaryl-coenzyme A (HMG-CoA) reductase inhibitor, and ketamine have not been shown to prevent delirium in all critically ill adults

Pharmacologic Treatment

Dexmedetomidine for delirium in mechanically ventilated adults where agitation is precluding weaning/extubation
Not routinely using haloperidol or an HMG-CoA reductase inhibitor to treat delirium

Nonpharmacologic Interventions

Reorientation, cognitive stimulation, use of clocks
Sleep hygiene and minimizing nocturnal light and noise
Reduce sedation and improve wakefulness
Increase mobility and early rehabilitation
Avoid sensory deprivation with the use of hearing aids or eyeglasses

use of arrhythmia monitoring after noncardiac surgery for asymptomatic patients.[75] Thoracic surgery and major vascular surgery patients represent two exceptions to this recommendation. Thoracic surgery patients are at increased risk for the development of atrial fibrillation, and for this reason 2–3 days of continuous electrographic monitoring is recommended. Atrial fibrillation rates can range from 3% to 30%, depending on the procedure performed.[76] Vascular surgery patients often have concomitant atherosclerosis that justifies postoperative monitoring. Indications and evidence for continuous electrographic monitoring are outlined in the guideline, and common postoperative indications are listed in Box 39.8.

Postoperative hemodynamic monitoring is generally not needed unless the patient has unstable hemodynamics, is at risk for unstable hemodynamics, or receiving vasopressors or inotropic agents. However, those requiring ongoing goal-directed resuscitation postoperatively will likely need hemodynamic monitoring.[77] An excellent example of the need for ongoing hemodynamic monitoring to aid resuscitation and continued Enhanced Recovery After Surgery (ERAS) is hyperthermic intraperitoneal chemotherapy (HIPEC), which is used for the treatment of peritoneal surface malignancies. HIPEC can result in significant hemodynamic instability and heightened inflammatory response.[78,79] Patients receiving HIPEC can have great individual intraoperative fluid therapy needs, highlighting the need for personalized resuscitation.[80] In a randomized controlled trial (RCT) of goal-directed versus standard fluid therapy, patients receiving hemodynamic-guided fluid therapy had reduced postoperative complications and hospital length of stay as compared with standard fluid therapy.[81]

• Box 39.8 Common Indications for Electrographic Monitoring[75]

Suspected coronary ischemia
Major cardiac interventions
Thoracic surgeries
Vascular surgeries
Those with mechanical circulatory support
New or recurrent ventricular tachycardia, nonsustained ventricular tachycardia
Acute atrial fibrillation
Chronic atrial fibrillation postoperatively
Symptomatic bradycardia or new bradycardia postoperatively
Atrioventricular block
Congenital or genetic arrhythmic syndromes
Intraoperative implantable cardioverter-defibrillator (ICD) shock
Acute decompensated heart failure
Infective endocarditis
Following stroke
Potassium and magnesium abnormalities

Plastics Flaps

A frequently encountered component in head and neck as well as plastic surgery procedures is the creation of a free flap. Free flaps require frequent monitoring for observed complications and specific perioperative management. Potential complications postoperatively include vascular compromise, hematoma, surgical site infection, and wound dehiscence.[82] Vascular compromise can be due to arterial thrombosis, venous thrombosis, hematoma, edema, recipient vessel disease, failure of anastomosis, and mechanical stress on the anastomosis.[83,84] In 990 consecutive free flaps, the overall thrombosis rate was 5.1%; 54% of thrombi occurred in the venous system, while 20% were arterial and 12% were combined artery and vein. In general, 80% of thrombi will occur within the first 48 h, highlighting the greatest yield for monitoring immediately postoperatively.[85]Various forms of invasive and noninvasive monitoring may take place (see Box 39.9) and those with the most supportive evidence include Cook-Swartz implantable Doppler, near-infrared spectroscopy, laser Doppler flowmetry, quantitative fluorimetry, and digital smartphone applications.[86]

Postoperative anticoagulation does not appear to have significant effect on free flap survival.[87,88] Fluid balance is of significant concern in the management of free flaps. Several studies have evaluated the role of fluids and outcomes with free flaps. Underlying principles are the maintenance of perfusion, avoiding hypotension, and avoiding fluid overload. Increased fluid administration is associated with increased graft failure and postoperative complications.[89,90] Conversely, perfusion and resuscitation may also place the patient at risk for flap failure. In a retrospective analyses

• Box 39.9 Free Flap Monitoring Techniques[86]

Implantable Doppler probe
Microdialysis
Pulse oximetry
Visible light spectroscopy
Multispectral spatial frequency domain imaging
Monitoring $SaCO_2$
Laser Doppler flowmetry
Temperature measurement
Glucose and lactate measurement
Smart phone applications
Photoplethysmography
Doppler ultrasound
Impedance plethysmography
Side stream dark field imaging
Hydrogen clearance

• Box 39.10 Sources of Perioperative Respiratory Failure

Respiratory infection/pneumonia
Respiratory failure
Pleural effusion
Atelectasis
Pneumothorax
Bronchospasm
Aspiration pneumonitis
Acute respiratory distress syndrome (ARDS)
Pulmonary embolism
Pulmonary edema
Transfusion-related acute lung injury (TRALI)
Abdominal compartment syndrome
Exacerbation of underlying lung disease (i.e., pulmonary fibrosis, chronic obstructive pulmonary disease [COPD], etc.)

of 682 patients, a below normal urine output and low rates of fluid resuscitation were associated with thrombotic events.[91] The Enhanced Recovery After Surgery Society has recommended an optimum fluid balance based on fluid responsiveness with use of cardiac output, stroke volume, or pulse pressure variation.[92] Vasopressor use has not shown to be associated with adverse flap events when studied retrospectively.[93-95] When epinephrine, norepinephrine, dobutamine, and dopexamine were studied in vitro using laser Doppler flowmetry to measure microcirculatory blood flow, norepinephrine was deemed suitable for preservation of flap blood flow in spite of its vasoconstrictor effect.[96]

Postoperative Respiratory Failure

Of cancer patients admitted to the ICU, respiratory failure and/or need for mechanical ventilatory support represents the most common indication for admission after cancer surgery. Respiratory failure is present in 25%–92% patients admitted to the ICU postsurgery.[8,9] These rates can be significantly impacted by the nature of the surgical intervention taking place, with head and neck surgeries being a significant contributor. Mortality rate from respiratory failure is dependent upon the surgical procedure, nature of respiratory failure, and underlying malignancy. In the case of cancer patients undergoing pneumonectomy that develop acute respiratory distress syndrome (ARDS), the mortality can be as high as 53%.[97]

Postoperative respiratory failure is defined in a variety of ways; definitions include ventilator dependence greater than 1 postoperative day, postoperative mechanical ventilation >48 h, unplanned reintubation within 30 days of surgery, reintubation within 3 days, postoperative acute lung injury, ARDS, mechanical ventilation within 7 days of surgery, and requiring noninvasive ventilation following surgery.[98] The European Society of Anesthesiology defines respiratory failure in the 2015 European Perioperative Clinical Outcome (EPCO) definitions as postoperative Pao_2 <8 kPa (60 mmHg) on room air, a Pao_2:Fio_2 ratio <40 kPa (300 mmHg) or arterial oxyhemoglobin saturation measured with pulse oximetry <90% and requiring oxygen therapy.[99]

In addition to the frequent causes of respiratory failure encountered in all surgical patients (Box 39.10),[99-101] cancer patients have also exposure to prior cancer therapy (e.g., immunotherapy, chemotherapy) and other complex underlying clinical conditions that may contribute (e.g., need for massive transfusion due to bleeding associated with vascularity of a tumor), if not the sole cause of postoperative respiratory failure (Table 39.3.)[102]

TABLE 39.3 Sources of Respiratory Failure Encountered in Cancer Patients

Central Neurologic	Peripheral Neurologic	Chest Wall	Pleura	Airways	Parenchymal
Primary tumors Metastatic tumors Leptomeningeal disease **Cerebellar degeneration**	**Myelopathy** Peripheral neuropathy Paraneoplastic syndromes Myasthenia gravis Guillain-Barré syndrome **Lambert-Eaton Myasthenic syndrome**	Chest wall tumors Pathologic rib fractures	Malignant pleural effusions Pleural tumors	Upper airway obstruction by tumor External compression by tumor Tracheoesophageal fistula Endobronchial metastases	Chemotherapy pneumonitis Radiation pneumonitis Periengraftment respiratory distress syndrome Diffuse alveolar hemorrhage Lymphangitic carcinomatosis Pulmonary leukostasis

Preoperative Risk Stratification

Several models assessing risk of developing postoperative pulmonary complications exist.[101,103–106] Risk stratification can aid in the assignment of level of care and preventative interventions postoperatively. Table 39.4 outlines many of the notable items associated with the development of postoperative pulmonary complications.[98] These factors consist of modifiable and nonmodifiable conditions and laboratory findings.

Prevention

Prevention strategies for postoperative pulmonary complications can be implemented in the preoperative, intraoperative, and postoperative phases. Preoperative interventions should start with a preoperative risk assessment to identify those at the highest risk.[107-109]

Preoperative physiotherapy has consistently reduced postoperative pulmonary complications.[108] Potential interventions include inspiratory muscle training, aerobic

TABLE 39.4 Risk Factors Associated with Postoperative Pulmonary Complications

Patient Factors	
Nonmodifiable	**Modifiable**
Age >60–65 years	Smoking
Sex: male	Chronic obstructive pulmonary disease
ASA ≥II	Asthma
Functional dependence (frailty)	Congestive heart failure
Acute respiratory infection (within 1 month)	Obstructive sleep apnea
Impaired cognition	BMI <18.5 or >40 kg/m^2
Impaired sensorium	BMI >27 kg/m^2
Cerebrovascular accident	Hypertension
Malignancy	Chronic liver disease
Weight loss >10% (within 6 months)	Renal failure
Long-term steroid use	Ascites
Prolonged hospitalization	Diabetes mellitus
	Alcohol use
	GERD
	Preoperative sepsis
	Preoperative shock
Procedural Factors	
Nonmodifiable	**Modifiable**
Type of surgery: upper abdominal, AAA, thoracic, neurosurgery, head and neck, vascular	Mechanical ventilation strategy
Emergency surgery	General anesthesia
Surgery >2 h	Long-acting NMBDs and TOF ratio <0.7 in PACU
Reoperation	Residual neuromuscular block
Multiple general anesthetics during admission	Intermediate-acting NMBDs with surgical time <2 h (not antagonized)
	Neostigmine
	Sugammadex with supraglottic airway
	Failure to use peripheral nerve stimulator
	Open abdominal surgery
	Perioperative nasogastric tube
	Intraoperative blood transfusion
Patient Physiologic and Laboratory Data	
BUN >45 mg/dL	
Creatinine >1.5	
Abnormal liver function tests	
Low preoperative oxygen saturation	
Positive cough test	
Abnormal preoperative CXR	
Preoperative anemia (<10 g/dL)	
Low albumin	
Predicted maximal oxygen uptake	
FEV_1:FVC <0.7 and FEV_1 <80% of predicted	

Modified from Miskovic, A. Lumb, A.B. Postoperative pulmonary complications. *Br J Anaesth.* 2017;118(3):317–334.

exercise, and breathing exercises. Smoking cessation is effective in reducing the risk of postoperative complications, though longer periods of cessation are more effective.[110]

Intraoperative Respiratory Failure Risk Reduction

Intraoperative interventions advocated for the prevention of postoperative respiratory failure include optimization of ventilation, avoidance of hyperoxia, avoidance of atelectotrauma and volumtrauma, and orotracheal tube management. Nonventilatory intervention measures include choice of anesthetic technique and restrictive fluid use strategies.[111]

Fio_2

When studied prospectively, adult patients undergoing noncardiothoracic surgery with tracheal intubation develop more major respiratory complications at 7 days in a dose-dependent manner in terms of intraoperative Fio_2. High median Fio_2 was also associated with 30-day mortality. Median Fio_2 for high- and low-oxygen groups was 0.79 (range, 0.64–1.00) and 0.31 (range, 0.16–0.34), respectively.[112]

Positive-End Expiratory Pressures

Avoidance of atelectotrauma is supported by studies evaluating the combination of increased positive end-expiratory pressure (PEEP) and low tidal volumes.[113–115] Target PEEP varies from 6 to 10 cmH_2O as compared to 0 cmH_2O for PEEP. A Cochrane review in 2013 reviewing available data concluded that there was insufficient evidence to draw conclusions whether intraoperative PEEP reduces the risk of postoperative mortality and respiratory complications.[116] It is possible that PEEP cannot be uncoupled from tidal volume in its association for reduced complications. In the IMPROVE study, patients undergoing abdominal surgery received recruitment maneuvers, tidal volumes of 6–8 mL/kg predicted body weight (PBW) and 6–8 cmH_2O PEEP versus 10–12 mL/kg PBW, zero PEEP, and no recruitment maneuvers. Patients receiving protective ventilation had significantly lower major pulmonary complications that included pneumonia, need for postoperative noninvasive positive pressure ventilation (NIPPV), and mechanical ventilation.[114] Idealized or personalized PEEP might provide a stronger indicator for improvement.[117]

Low Tidal Volume

Tidal volume size is associated with postoperative pulmonary complications in a dose-dependent fashion. Utilization of lung protective strategies using lower tidal volumes is widely endorsed with varying goals for PEEP in the reduction of postoperative pulmonary complications.[98,118] The patient's premorbid conditions and patient-specific factors will dictate how these strategies are implemented. However, in a meta-analysis involving 2127 patients undergoing general surgery, 8.7% developed postoperative pulmonary complications as compared with 14.7% with conventional ventilation. The analysis included 15 studies, the protective arm tidal volume ranged from 5 to 8 mL/kg predicted body weight, while the conventional tidal volume ranged from 6 to 12 mL/kg.[119]

Prevention of Postoperative Pneumonia

Preventing postoperative pneumonia will be of concern to the anesthesiologist and intensivist. Strategies are often bundled together in the ICU to prevent ventilator-associated pneumonias. The Infectious Diseases Society of America (IDSA) recommends the following in Box 39.11. Many of these items, while not studied specifically in the operating room, can easily be translated to intraoperative care and incorporated into the operating room practice.[120] These practices remain the standard of care for postoperative patients requiring mechanical ventilation (e.g., head of the bed elevation, deep vein thrombosis prophylaxis).

Fluid Administration

There exist mixed data with regard to intraoperative fluid management. Restrictive fluid strategies appear to have favorable respiratory complication outcomes as compared to liberal strategies in a number of studies.[121–123] However, a large-scale prospective study, including restrictive or liberal intravenous-fluid regimens in abdominal surgical patients, failed to show any differences between pneumonia, pulmonary edema, and duration of mechanical ventilation.[124]

Fluid management has emerged as a prominent element in the development of ERAS protocols. Typically goals of targeted euvolemia, cardiac output, and preservation of cellular function are aims in the intraoperative period.[125] Numerous outcomes improvements have been attributed to ERAS approaches, including the reduction of pneumonia and pulmonary complications in populations, including those receiving thoracotomy for lung cancer.[126] A large-scale comprehensive systematic review and meta-analysis of 95 RCTs demonstrated a reduction in the rates of respiratory failure, pneumonia, and prolonged mechanical ventilation in those patients receiving goal-directed therapy.[127]

Postoperative Considerations

High-Flow Nasal Cannula

High-flow nasal cannula (HFNC) use evaluated in the postoperative context has an unclear role with the prevention and treatment of postoperative respiratory failure. In a multicenter RCT in major abdominal surgery, receiving lung-protective ventilation intraoperatively, HFNC was used and compared to standard nasal cannula oxygen following extubation. There were no significant differences in postoperative hypoxemia or pulmonary complications.[128]

• Box 39.11 Postoperative Pneumonia Prevention Strategies

Use noninvasive positive pressure ventilation in selected populations
Manage patients without sedation whenever possible
Interrupt sedation daily
Assess readiness to extubate daily
Perform spontaneous breathing trials with sedatives turned off
Facilitate early mobility
Utilize endotracheal tubes with subglottic secretion drainage ports for patients expected to require greater than 48 or 72 h of mechanical ventilation
Change the ventilator circuit only if visibly soiled or malfunctioning
Elevate the head of the bed to 30–45 degrees
Selective oral or digestive decontamination
Regular oral care with chlorhexidine
Ultrathin polyurethane endotracheal tube cuffs
Automated control of endotracheal tube cuff pressure
Saline instillation before tracheal suctioning
Mechanical tooth brushing

By contrast, HFNC is essentially noninferior to noninvasive ventilation when evaluated in patients at increased risk for postoperative reintubation and postextubation respiratory failure, and it has shown lower rates in those receiving HFNC.[129] Authors have attempted to combine aggregate data in the form of meta-analyses, and HFNC ranged from being more favorable than conventional oxygen therapy (COT) or low-flow oxygen therapy to being noninferior to noninvasive ventilation and COT.[130,131]

Non-invasive Positive Pressure Ventilation

Noninvasive positive pressure ventilation is an accepted management modality in the postoperative management of respiratory failure and may have a role in prevention of respiratory failure. Noninvasive ventilation has proven to be successful in nonsurgical patients in the domains of chronic obstructive pulmonary disease, cardiogenic pulmonary edema, and obstructive sleep apnea.[132–134] The management of obstructive sleep apnea in the postoperative phase is well established, and formal recommendations encourage the use of positive airway pressure devices, when appropriate.[135] Noninvasive ventilation is recommended for postoperative respiratory failure by the European Respiratory Society and the America Thoracic Society.[136] In assorted surgical disciplines, noninvasive ventilation provides opportunities to reduce intubation and reintubation rates, mortality, and length of stay.[137–139] Noninvasive ventilation has not only reduced intubation rates with the attendant complications associated with mechanical ventilation, but has also reduced morbidity, hospital length of stay, and mortality in these patients.[140]

The use of noninvasive ventilation can be extremely problematic in the case of head and neck free flaps, hence the advantage of preemptive tracheostomy in proper candidates. Some authors have demonstrated safety in the use of noninvasive ventilation in this population.[141–143] However, a 2015 systematic review found insufficient evidence to endorse or refute its use in the postoperative period of esophagectomy patients.[144] The use of noninvasive ventilation in those with recent esophagectomy should be done in conjunction and careful consideration with the involved surgeons. Similar concerns are considered in the pneumonectomy and lung surgery patient. The post pneumonectomy has not been studied in great detail. A prospective randomized study of 24 patients revealed that noninvasive positive ventilation could be administered safely.[145] A 2019 Cochrane review evaluating noninvasive ventilation for the prevention of complications following pulmonary resection in lung cancer patients found that there was no additional benefit; however, the quality and quantity of evidence was low.[146] In abdominal surgery patients the use of noninvasive ventilation following extubation reduced the risk of reintubation as compared with standard oxygen therapy.[147] By contrast, a retrospective review of noninvasive ventilation in cardiothoracic patients did not significantly reduce reintubation rates.[148] When comparing noninvasive with HFNC the results are mixed, although high flow is likely noninferior to noninvasive ventilation in preventing reintubation and postextubation respiratory failure.[149,150]

References

1. Ferlay J, Ervik M, Lam F., et al. Global Cancer Observatory: Cancer Today. Lyon, France: International Agency for Research on Cancer. Accessed November 9, 2019. Available from: https://gco.iarc.fr/today.
2. International Agency for Research on Cancer. World Health Organization. Cancer Fact Sheets–All Cancer. Cancer Tomorrow. Available at http://gco.iarc.fr/tomorrow/home.
3. Jemal A, Ward EM, Johnson CJ, et al. Annual report to the nation on the status of cancer, 1975-2014, featuring survival. *J Natl Cancer Inst*. 2017;109(9):djx030.
4. Bos MM, de Keizer NF, Meynaar IA, Bakhshi-Raiez F, de Jonge E. Outcomes of cancer patients after unplanned admission to general intensive care units. *Acta Oncol*. 2012;51(7):897–905.
5. Puxty K, McLoone P, Quasim T, Sloan B, Kinsella J, Morrison DS. Risk of critical illness among patients with solid cancers: a population-based observational study. *JAMA Oncol*. 2015;1(8):1078–1085.
6. Taccone FS, Artigas AA, Sprung CL, Moreno R, Sakr Y, Vincent JL. Characteristics and outcomes of cancer patients in European ICUs. *Crit Care*. 2009;13(1):R15.
7. Wallace SK, Rathi NK, Waller DK, et al. Two decades of ICU utilization and hospital outcomes in a comprehensive cancer center. *Crit Care Med*. 2016;44(5):926–933.
8. Puxty K, McLoone P, Quasim T, Sloan B, Kinsella J, Morrison DS. Characteristics and outcomes of surgical patients with solid cancers admitted to the intensive care unit. *JAMA Surg*. 2018;153(9):834–840.
9. Bos MM, Bakhshi-Raiez F, Dekker JW, de Keizer NF, de Jonge E. Outcomes of intensive care unit admissions after elective cancer surgery. *Eur J Surg Oncol*. 2013;39(6):584–592.

10. Kiehl MG, Beutel G, Böll B, et al. Consensus statement for cancer patients requiring intensive care support. *Ann Hematol.* 2018;97(7):1271–1282.
11. Nates JL, Nunnally M, Kleinpell R, et al. ICU admission, discharge, and triage guidelines: a framework to enhance clinical operations, development of institutional policies, and further research. *Crit Care Med.* 2016;44(8):1553–1602.
12. Li Y, Klippel Z, Shih X, Reiner M, Wang H, Page JH. Relationship between severity and duration of chemotherapy-induced neutropenia and risk of infection among patients with nonmyeloid malignancies. *Support Care Cancer.* 2016;24(10):4377–4383.
13. Crawford J, Dale DC, Kuderer NM. Risk and timing of neutropenic events in adult cancer patients receiving chemotherapy: the results of a prospective nationwide study of oncology practice. *J Natl Compr Canc Netw.* 2008;6:109–118.
14. Weycker D, Barron R, Kartashov A, et al. Incidence, treatment, and consequences of chemotherapy-induced febrile neutropenia in the inpatient and outpatient settings. *J Oncol Pharm Practice.* 2014;20:190–198.
15. Weycker D, Li X, Edelsberg J, et al. Risk and consequences of chemotherapy-induced febrile neutropenia in patients with metastatic solid tumors. *J Oncol Pract.* 2015;11(1):47–54.
16. Klastersky J, Paesmans M. The Multinational Association for Supportive Care in Cancer (MASCC) risk index score: 10 years of use for identifying low-risk febrile neutropenic cancer patients. *Support Care Cancer.* 2013;21(5):1487–1495.
17. Taplitz RA, Kennedy EB, Bow EJ, et al. Antimicrobial prophylaxis for adult patients with cancer-related immunosuppression: ASCO and IDSA clinical practice guideline update. *J Clin Oncol.* 2018;36(30):3043–3054.
18. Freifeld AG, Bow EJ, Sepkowitz KA, et al. Infectious Diseases Society of America. Clinical practice guideline for the use of antimicrobial agents in neutropenic patients with cancer: 2010 update by the Infectious Diseases Society of America. *Clin Infect Dis.* 2011;52(4):e56–e93.
19. Klastersky J, de Naurois J, Rolston K, et al. ESMO Guidelines Committee. Management of febrile neutropaenia: ESMO Clinical Practice Guidelines. *Ann Oncol.* 2016;27(suppl 5):v111–v118.
20. Kilpatrick K, Marongiu A, Park J. Burden of thrombocytopenia in adult cancer patients receiving chemotherapy. *J Clin Oncol.* 2019;37(suppl15):1555.
21. Thrombocytopenia in cancer patients. *Thromb Res.* 2014;133(Suppl 2):S63–S69.
22. Weycker D, Hatfield M, Grossman A, et al. Risk and consequences of chemotherapy-induced thrombocytopenia in US clinical practice. *BMC Cancer.* 2019;19(1):151.
23. Nagrebetsky A, Al-Samkari H, Davis NM, Kuter DJ, Wiener-Kronish JP. Perioperative thrombocytopenia: evidence, evaluation, and emerging therapies. *Br J Anaesth.* 2019;122(1):19–31.
24. Pieri L. Management of thrombocytopenia in cancer. *Thromb Res.* 2018;164(Suppl 1):S89–S93.
25. Timp JF, Braekkan SK, Versteeg HH, Cannegieter SC. Epidemiology of cancer-associated venous thrombosis. *Blood.* 2013;122(10):1712–1723.
26. Horsted F, West J, Grainge MJ. Risk of venous thromboembolism in patients with cancer: a systematic review and meta-analysis. *PLoS Med.* 2012;9(7):e1001275.
27. Agnelli G, Bolis G, Capussotti L, et al. A clinical outcome-based prospective study on venous thromboembolism after cancer surgery: the @RISTOS project. *Ann Surg.* 2006;243(1):89–95.
28. Trinh VQ, Karakiewicz PI, Sammon J, et al. Venous thromboembolism after major cancer surgery: temporal trends and patterns of care. *JAMA Surg.* 2014;149(1):43–49.
29. Abdol Razak NB, Jones G, Bhandari M, Berndt MC, Metharom P. Cancer-associated thrombosis: an overview of mechanisms, risk factors, and treatment. *Cancers.* 2018;10(10):380.
30. Key NS, Khorana AA, Kuderer NM, et al. Venous thromboembolism prophylaxis and treatment in patients with cancer: ASCO Clinical Practice Guideline Update. *J Clin Oncol.* 2020;38(5):496–520.
31. Kvolik S, Jukic M, Matijevic M, Marjanovic K, Glavas-Obrovac L. An overview of coagulation disorders in cancer patients. *Surg Oncol.* 2010;19(1):e33–e46.
32. Mantha S. Bleeding disorders associated with cancer. In: Soff G, ed. *Thrombosis and Hemostasis in Cancer. Cancer Treatment and Research.* Springer; 2019.179.
33. Sallah S, Wan JY, Hguyen NP, et al. Disseminated intravascular coagulation in solid tumors: clinical and pathologic study. *Thromb Haemost.* 2001;86:828–833.
34. Nakagawa M, Tsuji H. Current trends in the diagnosis of disseminated intravascular coagulation in Japan: findings of questionnaire survey. *Rinsho Ketsueki.* 1999;40(5):362–364.
35. Yanada M, Matsushita T, Suzuki M, et al. Disseminated intravascular coagulation in acute leukemia: clinical and laboratory features at presentation. *Eur J Haematol.* 2006;77(4):282–287.
36. Uchiumi H, Matsushima T, Yamane A, et al. Prevalence and clinical characteristics of acute myeloid leukemia associated with disseminated intravascular coagulation. *Int J Hematol.* 2007;86(2):137–142.
37. Thachil J, Falanga A, Levi M, Liebman H, Di Nisio M. Scientific and Standardization Committee of the International Society on Thrombosis and Hemostasis. Management of cancer-associated disseminated intravascular coagulation: guidance from the SSC of the ISTH. *J Thromb Haemost.* 2015;13(4):671–675.
38. Levi M, Scully M. How I treat disseminated intravascular coagulation. *Blood.* 2018;131(8):845–854.
39. Asakura H. Classifying types of disseminated intravascular coagulation: clinical and animal models. *J Intensive Care.* 2014;2(1):20.
40. Chang H, Kuo MC, Shih LY, et al. Clinical bleeding events and laboratory coagulation profiles in acute promyelocytic leukemia. *Eur J Haematol.* 2012;88(4):321–328.
41. Mantha S, Tallman MS, Devlin SM, Soff GA. Predictive factors of fatal bleeding in acute promyelocytic leukemia. *Thromb Res.* 2018;164(Suppl 1):S98–S102.
42. Ikezoe T, Takeuchi A, Isaka M, et al. Recombinant human soluble thrombomodulin safely and effectively rescues acute promyelocytic leukemia patients from disseminated intravascular coagulation. *Leuk Res.* 2012;36(11):1398–1402.
43. Matsushita T, Watanabe J, Honda G, et al. Thrombomodulin alfa treatment in patients with acute promyelocytic leukemia and disseminated intravascular coagulation: a retrospective analysis of an open-label, multicenter, post-marketing surveillance study cohort. *Thromb Res.* 2014;133(5):772–781.
44. White JV, Guenter P, Jensen G, et al. Board of Directors. Consensus statement of the Academy of Nutrition and Dietetics/American Society for Parenteral and Enteral Nutrition: characteristics recommended for the identification and documentation of adult malnutrition. *J Acad Nutr Diet.* 2012;112(5):730–738.

45. Muscaritoli M, Lucia S, Farcomeni A, et al. PreMiO Study Group. Prevalence of malnutrition in patients at first medical oncology visit: the PreMiO study. *Oncotarget*. 2017;8(45):79884–79896.
46. Marshall KM, Loeliger J, Nolte L, Kelaart A, Kiss NK. Prevalence of malnutrition and impact on clinical outcomes in cancer services: a comparison of two time points. *Clin Nutr*. 2019;38(2):644–651.
47. Hébuterne X, Lemarié E, Michallet M, de Montreuil CB, Schneider SM, Goldwasser F. Prevalence of malnutrition and current use of nutrition support in patients with cancer. *J Parenter Enteral Nutr*. 2014;38(2):196–204.
48. Pressoir M, Desné S, Berchery D, et al. Prevalence, risk factors and clinical implications of malnutrition in French Comprehensive Cancer Centres. *Br J Cancer*. 2010;102(6):966–971.
49. Fontes D, Generoso Sde V, Toulson Davisson Correia MI. Subjective global assessment: a reliable nutritional assessment tool to predict outcomes in critically ill patients. *Clin Nutr*. 2014;33(2):291–295.
50. Baracos VE, Martin L, Korc M, Guttridge DC, Fearon KCH. Cancer-associated cachexia. *Nat Rev Dis Primers*. 2018;4:17105.
51. August DA, Huhmann MB. clinical guidelines: nutrition support therapy during adult anticancer treatment and in hematopoietic cell transplantation. *J Parenter Enteral Nutr*. 2009;33(5):472–500.
52. Bozzetti F, Gavazzi C, Miceli R, et al. Perioperative total parenteral nutrition in malnourished, gastrointestinal cancer patients: a randomized, clinical trial. *J Parenter Enteral Nutr*. 2000;24(1):7–14.
53. Wu GH, Liu ZH, Wu ZH, Wu ZG. Perioperative artificial nutrition in malnourished gastrointestinal cancer patients. *World J Gastroenterol*. 2006;12(15):2441–2444.
54. McClave SA, Taylor BE, Martindale RG. American Society for Parenteral and Enteral Nutrition. Guidelines for the Provision and Assessment of Nutrition Support Therapy in the Adult Critically Ill Patient: Society of Critical Care Medicine (SCCM) and American Society for Parenteral and Enteral Nutrition (A.S.P.E.N.). *J Parenter Enteral Nutr*. 2016;40(2):159–211.
55. Ziai WC, Varelas PN, Zeger SL, Mirski MA, Ulatowski JA. Neurologic intensive care resource use after brain tumor surgery: an analysis of indications and alternative strategies. *Crit Care Med*. 2003;31(12):2782–2787.
56. Champey J, Mourey C, Francony G, et al. Strategies to reduce external ventricular drain-related infections: a multicenter retrospective study. *J Neurosurg*. 2018;1:1–6.
57. Hepburn-Smith M, Dynkevich I, Spektor M, Lord A, Czeisler B, Lewis A. Establishment of an external ventricular drain best practice guideline: the quest for a comprehensive, universal standard for external ventricular drain care. *J Neurosci Nurs*. 2016;48(1):54–65.
58. Fried HI, Nathan BR, Rowe AS, et al. The insertion and management of external ventricular drains: an evidence-based consensus statement: a statement for healthcare professionals from the Neurocritical Care Society. *Neurocrit Care*. 2016;24(1):61–81.
59. Bhattacharyya N., Fried M.P. Benchmarks for mortality, morbidity, and length of stay for head and neck surgical procedures. *Arch Otolaryngol Head Neck Surg*. 2001;127(2):127–132.
60. L'Esperance HE, Kallogjeri D, Yousaf S, Piccirillo JF, Rich JT. Prediction of mortality and morbidity in head and neck cancer patients 80 years of age and older undergoing surgery. *Laryngoscope*. 2018;128(4):871–877.
61. Downey RJ, Friedlander P, Groeger J, et al. Critical care for the severely ill head and neck patient. *Crit Care Med*. 1999;27(1):95–97.
62. Bur AM, Brant JA, Mulvey CL, et al. Association of clinical risk factors and postoperative complications with unplanned hospital readmission after head and neck cancer surgery. *JAMA Otolaryngol Head Neck Surg*. 2016;142(12):1184–1190.
63. Meier J, Wunschel M, Angermann A, et al. Influence of early elective tracheostomy on the incidence of postoperative complications in patients undergoing head and neck surgery. *BMC Anesthesiol*. 2019;19(1):43.
64. Popat M, Mitchell V, Dravid R, Patel A, Swampillai C, Higgs A. Difficult Airway Society Extubation Guidelines Group. Difficult Airway Society Guidelines for the management of tracheal extubation. *Anaesthesia*. 2012;67(3):318–340.
65. Morse E, Henderson C, Carafeno T, et al. A clinical care pathway to reduce ICU usage in head and neck microvascular reconstruction. *Otolaryngol Head Neck Surg*. 2019;160(5):783–790.
66. Arshad H, Ozer HG, Thatcher A, et al. Intensive care unit versus non-intensive care unit postoperative management of head and neck free flaps: comparative effectiveness and cost comparisons. *Head Neck*. 2014;36(4):536–539.
67. Yetzer JG, Pirgousis P, Li Z, Fernandes R. Clinical pathway implementation improves efficiency of care in a maxillofacial head and neck surgery unit. *J Oral Maxillofac Surg*. 2017;75(1):190–196.
68. Booka E, Kamijo T, Matsumoto T, et al. Incidence and risk factors for postoperative delirium after major head and neck cancer surgery. *J Craniomaxillofac Surg*. 2016;44(7):890–894.
69. Zhu Y, Wang G, Liu S, et al. Risk factors for postoperative delirium in patients undergoing major head and neck cancer surgery: a meta-analysis. *Jpn J Clin Oncol*. 2017;47(6):505–511.
70. Montes DM. Postoperative delirium in head and neck cancer patients: a survey of oncologic oral and maxillofacial surgeon practices. *J Oral Maxillofac Surg*. 2014;72(12):2591–2600.
71. Devlin JW, Skrobik Y, Gélinas C, et al. Clinical practice guidelines for the prevention and management of pain, agitation, sedation, delirium, immobility, and sleep disruption in adult patients in the ICU. *Crit Care Med*. 2018;46(9):e825–e873.
72. Bulger J, Nickel W, Messler J, et al. Choosing wisely in adult hospital medicine: five opportunities for improved healthcare value. *J Hosp Med*. 2013;8(9):486–492.
73. Chen S, Palchaudhuri S, Johnson A, Trost J, Ponor I, Zakaria S. Does this patient need telemetry? An analysis of telemetry ordering practices at an academic medical center. *J Eval Clin Pract*. 2017;23(4):741–746.
74. Estrada CA, Rosman HS, Prasad NK, et al. Role of telemetry monitoring in the non-intensive care unit. *Am J Cardiol*. 1995;76(12):960–965.
75. Sandau KE, Funk M, Auerbach A, et al. Update to practice standards for electrocardiographic monitoring in hospital settings: a scientific statement from the American Heart Association. *Circulation*. 2017;136(19):e273–e344.
76. Vaporciyan AA, Correa AM, Rice DC, et al. Risk factors associated with atrial fibrillation after noncardiac thoracic surgery: analysis of 2588 patients. *J Thorac Cardiovasc Surg*. 2004;127(3):779–786.
77. Watson X, Cecconi M. Haemodynamic monitoring in the perioperative period: the past, the present and the future. *Anaesthesia*. 2017;72(Suppl 1):7–15.
78. Roth L, Eshmuminov D, Laminger F, et al. Systemic inflammatory response after hyperthermic intraperitoneal chemotherapy (HIPEC):

the perfusion protocol matters!. *Eur J Surg Oncol* 2019;45(9):1734–1739.

79. Coccolini F, Corbella D, Finazzi P, et al. Time course of cytokines, hemodynamic and metabolic parameters during hyperthermic intraperitoneal chemotherapy. *Minerva Anestesiol.* 2016;82(3):310–319.
80. Esteve-Pérez N, Ferrer-Robles A, Gómez-Romero G, et al. Goal-directed therapy in cytoreductive surgery with hyperthermic intraperitoneal chemotherapy: a prospective observational study. *Clin Transl Oncol.* 2019;21(4):451–458.
81. Colantonio L, Claroni C, Fabrizi L, et al. A randomized trial of goal directed vs. standard fluid therapy in cytoreductive surgery with hyperthermic intraperitoneal chemotherapy. *J Gastrointest Surg.* 2015;19(4):722–729.
82. Lahtinen S, Koivunen P, Ala-Kokko T, et al. Complications and outcome after free flap surgery for cancer of the head and neck. *Br J Oral Maxillofac Surg.* 2018;56(8):684–691.
83. Novakovic D, Patel RS, Goldstein DP, Gullane PJ. Salvage of failed free flaps used in head and neck reconstruction. *Head Neck Oncol.* 2009;1:33.
84. Chiu YH, Chang DH, Perng CK. Vascular complications and free flap salvage in head and neck reconstructive surgery: analysis of 150 cases of reexploration. *Ann Plast Surg.* 2017;78(3 Suppl 2):S83–S88.
85. Kroll SS, Schusterman MA, Reece GP, et al. Timing of pedicle thrombosis and flap loss after free-tissue transfer. *Plast Reconstr Surg.* 1996;98(7):1230–1233.
86. Chae MP, Rozen WM, Whitaker IS, et al. Current evidence for postoperative monitoring of microvascular free flaps: a systematic review. *Ann Plast Surg.* 2015;74(5):621–632.
87. Barton BM, Riley CA, Fitzpatrick JC, Hasney CP, Moore BA, McCoul ED. Postoperative anticoagulation after free flap reconstruction for head and neck cancer: a systematic review. *Laryngoscope.* 2018;128(2):412–421.
88. Lee KT, Mun GH. The efficacy of postoperative antithrombotics in free flap surgery: a systematic review and meta-analysis. *Plast Reconstr Surg.* 2015;135(4):1124–1139.
89. Ettinger KS, Arce K, Lohse CM, et al. Higher perioperative fluid administration is associated with increased rates of complications following head and neck microvascular reconstruction with fibular free flaps. *Microsurgery.* 2017;37(2):128–136.
90. Zhong T, Neinstein R, Massey C. Intravenous fluid infusion rate in microsurgical breath reconstruction: important lessons learned from 354 free flaps. *Plast Reconstr Surg.* 2011;128:1153–1160.
91. Nelson JA, Fischer JP, Grover R, et al. Intraoperative perfusion management impacts postoperative outcomes: an analysis of 682 autologous breast reconstruction patients. *J Plast Reconstr Aesthet Surg.* 2015;68(2):175–183.
92. Dort JC, Farwell DG, Findlay M, et al. Optimal perioperative care in major head and neck cancer surgery with free flap reconstruction: a consensus review and recommendations from the Enhanced Recovery After Surgery Society. *JAMA Otolaryngol Head Neck Surg.* 2017;143(3):292–303.
93. Kelly DA, Reynolds M, Crantford C, Pestana IA. Impact of intraoperative vasopressor use in free tissue transfer for head, neck, and extremity reconstruction. *Ann Plast Surg.* 2014; 72(6):S135–S138.
94. Chan JY, Chow VL, Liu LH. Safety of intra-operative vasopressor in free jejunal flap reconstruction. *Microsurgery.* 2013;33(5):358–361.
95. Knackstedt R, Gatherwright J, Gurunluoglu R. A literature review and meta-analysis of outcomes in microsurgical reconstruction using vasopressors. *Microsurgery.* 2019;39(3): 267–275.
96. Eley KA, Young JD, Watt-Smith SR. Power spectral analysis of the effects of epinephrine, norepinephrine, dobutamine and dopexamine on microcirculation following free tissue transfer. *Microsurgery.* 2013;33(4):275–281.
97. Blanc K, Dechartres A, Zaimi R, et al. Patients experiencing early acute respiratory failure have high postoperative mortality after pneumonectomy. *J Thorac Cardiovasc Surg.* 2018;156(6):2368–2376.
98. Miskovic AB. Lumb, postoperative pulmonary complications. *Br J Anaesth.* 2017;118(3):317–334.
99. Jammer I, Wickboldt N, Sander M, et al. Standards for definitions and use of outcome measures for clinical effectiveness research in perioperative medicine: European Perioperative Clinical Outcome (EPCO) definitions: a statement from the ESA-ESICM joint taskforce on perioperative outcome measures. *Eur J Anaesthesiol.* 2015;32(2):88–105.
100. Fernandez-Bustamante A, Frendl G, Sprung J, et al. Postoperative pulmonary complications, early mortality, and hospital stay following noncardiothoracic surgery: a multicenter study by the Perioperative Research Network Investigators. *JAMA Surg.* 2017;152(2):157–166.
101. Mazo V, Sabaté S, Canet J, et al. Prospective external validation of a predictive score for postoperative pulmonary complications. *Anesthesiology.* 2014;121(2):219–231.
102. Faiz S.A, Grosu H.B, Shannon V.R, et al. Pulmonary complications of cancer therapy. In Kantarjian H.M, Wolff R.A, eds. The MD Anderson Manual of Medical Oncology. McGraw-Hill; 2016. 3rd ed.
103. Canet J, Gallart L, Gomar C, et al. Prediction of postoperative pulmonary complications in a population-based surgical cohort. *Anesthesiology.* 2010;113(6):1338–1350.
104. Arozullah AM, Daley J, Henderson WG, Khuri SF. Multifactorial risk index for predicting postoperative respiratory failure in men after major noncardiac surgery. The National Veterans Administration Surgical Quality Improvement Program. *Ann Surg.* 2000;232(2):242–253.
105. Gupta H, Gupta PK, Fang X, et al. Development and validation of a risk calculator predicting postoperative respiratory failure. *Chest.* 2011;140(5):1207–1215.
106. Gupta H, Gupta PK, Schuller D, et al. Development and validation of a risk calculator for predicting postoperative pneumonia. *Mayo Clin Proc.* 2013;88(11):1241–1249.
107. Perelló-Díez M, Paz-Lourido B. Prevention of postoperative pulmonary complications through preoperative physiotherapy interventions in patients undergoing coronary artery bypass graft: literature review. *J Phys Ther Sci.* 2018;30(8):1034–1038.
108. Kendall F, Abreu P, Pinho P, Oliveira J, Bastos P. The role of physiotherapy in patients undergoing pulmonary surgery for lung cancer. A literature review. *Rev Port Pneumol* (2006). 2017;23(6):343–351.
109. Boden I, Skinner EH, Browning L, et al. Preoperative physiotherapy for the prevention of respiratory complications after upper abdominal surgery: pragmatic, double blinded, multicentre randomised controlled trial. *BMJ.* 2019;365: l1862.
110. Theadom A, Cropley M. Effects of preoperative smoking cessation on the incidence and risk of intraoperative and postoperative complications in adult smokers: a systematic review. *Tob Control.* 2006;15(5):352–358.

111. Canet J, Gallart L. Postoperative respiratory failure: pathogenesis, prediction, and prevention. *Curr Opin Crit Care.* 2014;20(1):56–62.
112. Staehr-Rye AK, Meyhoff CS, Scheffenbichler FT, et al. High intraoperative inspiratory oxygen fraction and risk of major respiratory complications. *Br J Anaesth.* 2017;119(1):140–149.
113. Severgnini P, Selmo G, Lanza C, et al. Protective mechanical ventilation during general anesthesia for open abdominal surgery improves postoperative pulmonary function. *Anesthesiology.* 2013;118(6):1307–1321.
114. Futier E, Constantin JM, Paugam-Burtz C, et al. A trial of intraoperative low-tidal-volume ventilation in abdominal surgery. *N Engl J Med.* 2013;369(5):428–437.
115. Hemmes SN, Serpa Neto A, Schultz MJ. Intraoperative ventilatory strategies to prevent postoperative pulmonary complications: a meta-analysis. *Curr Opin Anaesthesiol.* 2013;26(2):126–133.
116. Barbosa FT, Castro AA, de Sousa-Rodrigues CF. Positive end-expiratory pressure (PEEP) during anaesthesia for prevention of mortality and postoperative pulmonary complications. *Cochrane Database Syst Rev.* 2014(6):CD007922.
117. Pereira SM, Tucci MR, Morais CCA, et al. Individual positive end-expiratory pressure settings optimize intraoperative mechanical ventilation and reduce postoperative atelectasis. *Anesthesiology.* 2018;129(6):1070–1081.
118. Güldner A, Kiss T, Serpa Neto A, et al. Intraoperative protective mechanical ventilation for prevention of postoperative pulmonary complications: a comprehensive review of the role of tidal volume, positive end-expiratorypressure, and lung recruitment maneuvers. *Anesthesiology.* 2015;123(3):692–713.
119. Serpa Neto A, Hemmes SN, Barbas CS, et al. Protective versus conventional ventilation for surgery: a systematic review and individual patient data meta-analysis. *Anesthesiology.* 2015;123(1):66–78.
120. Stackhouse R.A, Beers R, Brown D, et al. Recommendations for Infection Control for the Practice of Anesthesiology (Third Edition). Available at http://www.asahq.org/For-Members/Standards-Guidelines-and-Statements.aspx#rec (refer to infection control section).
121. Shin CH, Long DR, McLean D, et al. Effects of intraoperative fluid management on postoperative outcomes: a Hospital Registry study. *Ann Surg.* 2018;267(6):1084–1092.
122. Corcoran T, Rhodes JE, Clarke S, Myles PS, Ho KM. Perioperative fluid management strategies in major surgery: a stratified meta-analysis. *Anesth Analg.* 2012;114(3):640–651.
123. Arslantas MK, Kara HV, Tuncer BB, et al. Effect of the amount of intraoperative fluid administration on postoperative pulmonary complications following anatomic lung resections. *J Thorac Cardiovasc Surg.* 2015;149(1):314–320 321.
124. Myles PS, Bellomo R, Corcoran T, et al. Restrictive versus liberal fluid therapy for major abdominal surgery. *N Engl J Med.* 2018;378(24):2263–2274.
125. Ljungqvist O, Scott M, Fearon KC. Enhanced recovery after surgery: a review. *JAMA Surg.* 2017;152(3):292–298. doi:10.1001/jamasurg.2016.
126. Van Haren RM, Mehran RJ, Mena GE, et al. Enhanced recovery decreases pulmonary and cardiac complications after thoracotomy for lung cancer. *Ann Thorac Surg.* 2018;106(1):272–279.
127. Chong MA, Wang Y, Berbenetz NM, McConachie I. Does goal-directed haemodynamic and fluid therapy improve perioperative outcomes? A systematic review and meta-analysis. *Eur J Anaesthesiol.* 2018;35(7):469–483.
128. Futier E, Paugam-Burtz C, Godet T, et al. Effect of early postextubation high-flow nasal cannula vs conventional oxygen therapy on hypoxaemia in patients after major abdominal surgery: a French multicentre randomised controlled trial (OPERA). *Intensive Care Med.* 2016;42(12):1888–1898.
129. Hernández G, Vaquero C, González P, et al. Effect of postextubation high-flow nasal cannula vs conventional oxygen therapy on reintubation in low-risk patients: a randomized clinical trial. *JAMA.* 2016;315(13):154–161.
130. Xu Z, Li Y, Zhou J, et al. High-flow nasal cannula in adults with acute respiratory failure and after extubation: a systematic review and meta-analysis. *Respir Res.* 2018;19(1):202.
131. Zhu Y, Yin H, Zhang R, et al. High-flow nasal cannula oxygen therapy versus conventional oxygen therapy in patients after planned extubation: a systematic review and meta-analysis. *Crit Care.* 2019;23:180.
132. Peter JV, Moran JL, Phillips-Hughes J, Graham P, Bersten AD. Effect of non-invasive positive pressure ventilation (NIPPV) on mortality in patients with acute cardiogenic pulmonary oedema: a meta-analysis. *Lancet.* 2006;367(9517):1155–1163.
133. Davidson AC, Banham S, Elliott M, et al. BTS/ICS guideline for the ventilatory management of acute hypercapnic respiratory failure in adults. *Thorax.* 2016;71(Suppl 2):ii1–ii35.
134. Berry RB, Chediak A, Brown LK, et al. Best clinical practices for the sleep center adjustment of noninvasive positive pressure ventilation (NPPV) in stable chronic alveolar hypoventilation syndromes. *J Clin Sleep Med.* 2010;6(5):491–509.
135. Chung F, Memtsoudis SG, Ramachandran SK, et al. Society of Anesthesia and Sleep Medicine Guidelines on preoperative screening and assessment of adult patients with obstructive sleep apnea. *Anesth Analg.* 2016;123(2):452–473.
136. Rochwerg B, Brochard L, Elliott MW, et al. Official ERS/ATS clinical practice guidelines: noninvasive ventilation for acute respiratory failure. *Eur Respir J.* 2017;50(2):1602426.
137. Jaber S, Chanques G, Jung B. Postoperative noninvasive ventilation. *Anesthesiology.* 2010;112(2):453–461.
138. Chiumello D, Chevallard G, Gregoretti C. Non-invasive ventilation in postoperative patients: a systematic review. *Intensive Care Med.* 2011;37(6):918–929.
139. Glossop AJ, Shephard N, Bryden DC, Mills GH. Non-invasive ventilation for weaning, avoiding reintubation after extubation and in the postoperative period: a meta-analysis. *Br J Anaesth.* 2012;109(3):305–314.
140. Ireland CJ, Chapman TM, Mathew SF, Herbison GP, Zacharias M. Continuous positive airway pressure (CPAP) during the postoperative period for prevention of postoperative morbidity and mortality following major abdominal surgery. *Cochrane Database Syst Rev.* 2014(8):CD008930.
141. Michelet P, D'Journo XB, Seinaye F, Forel JM, Papazian L, Thomas P. Non-invasive ventilation for treatment of postoperative respiratory failure after oesophagectomy. *Br J Surg.* 2009;96(1):54–60.
142. Yu KY, Zhao L, Chen Z, Yang M. Noninvasive positive pressure ventilation for the treatment of acute respiratory distress syndrome following esophagectomy for esophageal cancer: a clinical comparative study. *J Thorac Dis.* 2013;5(6):777–782.
143. Raman V, MacGlaflin CE, Erkmen CP. Noninvasive positive pressure ventilation following esophagectomy: safety demonstrated in a pig model. *Chest.* 2015;147(2):356–361.
144. Charlesworth M, Lawton T, Fletcher S. Noninvasive positive pressure ventilation for acute respiratory failure following oe-

sophagectomy: is it safe? A systematic review of the literature. *J Intensive Care Soc*. 2015;16(3):215–221.

145. Auriant I, Jallot A, Hervé P, et al. Noninvasive ventilation reduces mortality in acute respiratory failure following lung resection. *Am J Respir Crit Care Med*. 2001;164(7):1231–1235.
146. Torres MF, Porfírio GJ, Carvalho AP, Riera R. Non-invasive positive pressure ventilation for prevention of complications after pulmonary resection in lung cancer patients. *Cochrane Database Syst Rev*. 2019;3:CD010355.
147. Jaber S, Lescot T, Futier E, et al. Effect of noninvasive ventilation on tracheal reintubation among patients with hypoxemic respiratory failure following abdominal surgery: a randomized clinical trial. *JAMA*. 2016;315(13):1345–1353.
148. Melton N, Lazar JF, Childers WK, et al. Preventing respiratory failure after cardiac surgery using post-extubation bilevel positive airway pressure therapy. *Cureus*. 2019;11(3):e4236.
149. Hernández G, Vaquero C, Colinas L, et al. Effect of postextubation high-flow nasal cannula vs noninvasive ventilation on reintubation and postextubation respiratory failure in high-risk patients: a randomized clinical trial. *JAMA*. 2016;316(15):1565–1574.
150. Beng Leong L, Wei Ming N, Wei Feng L. High flow nasal cannula oxygen versus noninvasive ventilation in adult acute respiratory failure: a systematic review of randomized-controlled trials. *Eur J Emerg Med*. 2019;26(1):9–18.

40

The Challenges of Novel Therapies in the Care of the Critically Ill Cancer Patient

TIMOTHY WIGMORE, PHIL WARD

The global incidence of both hematologic and solid organ cancers continues to rise. This is due in part to the aging population and changes in socioeconomic-associated cancer risk factors such as tobacco and alcohol intake, as well as improved diagnostics and screening programs. The latter have also contributed to a simultaneous improvement in survival, where earlier diagnosis leads to greater chance of primary surgical resection. The advent of stem cell transplantation and a widening arsenal of systemic anticancer therapies (SACTs), including targeted therapies and immunotherapies, offer the possibility of remission even in refractory or advanced metastatic disease in select cancers.

Traditional reluctance to offer critical care therapies for patients with advanced cancers has been replaced with the concept of the "trial of therapy"[1,2] as evidence of improved survival has accumulated over the last 20 years.[3–8] This improved survival stems from a combination of progress in general critical care management and specific therapies (such as granulocyte-colony stimulating factor [G-CSF] and novel antibiotics) that have improved our ability to manage some of the common causes of acute illness in the oncologic population. However, the rapid development of novel therapies, which simultaneously offer hope in the most challenging cases but which often come with a raft of potential toxicities, some of which we are yet to fully elucidate, presents a new frontier in critical care. This new cohort of patients are often frail and deconditioned as a result of prolonged illness and serial courses of therapy, and may require high-level support for prolonged periods while allowing adequate time for presumptive treatment effects to occur.

The aim of this chapter is to review current novel anticancer treatments, the underlying immunology, their spectrum of activity, and the diagnosis and management of the associated complications.

Basic Sciences

Although a complete review of the current understanding of tumor cell biology and the immune response is outside the scope of this article, we will summarize key aspects relevant to the novel targeted agents and immunotherapies in current clinical practice.

Cell Proliferation

Cancer occurs as a result of mutations in the signaling pathways that regulate cell turnover, which is usually a tightly regulated process governed by complex interactions between the cell, the extracellular matrix, and circulating cytokines. The broad functional capabilities acquired by cancer cells include autonomous proliferative signaling, replicative immortality, resistance to apoptosis, and induction of angiogenesis.[9]

Cell survival, proliferation, and communication are triggered by ligand binding to cell membrane-bound receptors. Members of the receptor tyrosine kinase superfamily, such as epidermal growth factor receptors (EGFRs), anaplastic lymphoma kinase (ALK), and KIT, are implicitly involved, and are key targets for novel cancer agents. Once a ligand is bound, the intracellular kinase domain initiates effectors via second messenger systems, including the Ras-Raf-MEK-ERK, phosphoinositol-3-kinase (PI3K)/Akt/mTOR, and JAK/STAT pathways.[10] These in turn are regulated by negative feedback mechanisms, including PTEN phosphatase. Examples of mutations and dysregulation at each step have been identified in various cancer subtypes, including induction of growth factor secretion, increased expression of surface tyrosine kinase receptors, and constitutive activation of the intracellular cascade.

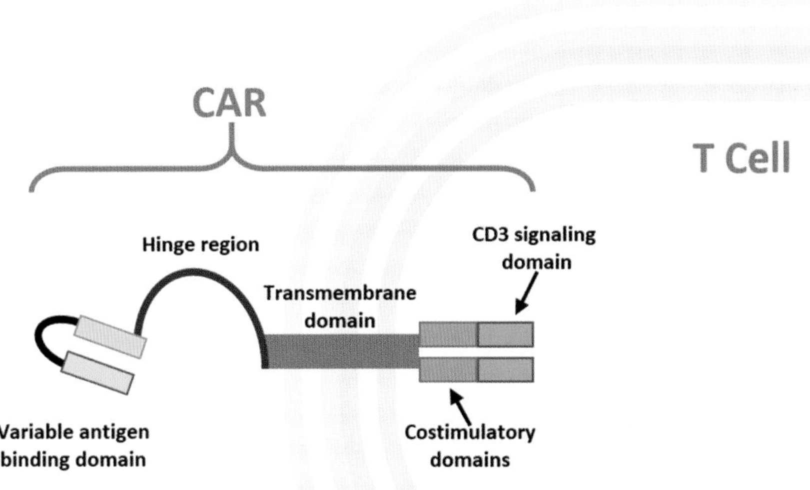

• **Fig. 40.1** Chimeric antigen receptor (CAR)-T cell structure.

Angiogenesis

Under normal conditions, angiogenesis is only transiently active in response to tissue damage and hypoxia. Activation of angiogenesis—the so-called "angiogenic switch"—is a characteristic of tumor growth and metastasis.[11] The key in vivo proangiogenic factor is vascular endothelial growth factor (VEGF), which exerts its effect via a further family of receptor bound tyrosine kinase receptors (VEGFRs).

The Immune Response

The effectors of both the innate and adaptive immune system are critical to tumor growth and suppression. Natural killer (NK) cells are able to induce cell death via apoptosis in the absence of antigen presentation, targeting cells with low expression of major histocompatibility complex (MHC).

The T-cell-mediated adaptive immune response requires priming by antigen presentation in the context of MHC. The T-cell receptor (TCR) has a CD3 domain and highly variable extracellular alpha/beta chains that are generated during T-cell maturation, enabling recognition of a diverse range of antigen. CD8+ T lymphocytes recognize antigen within MHC class I (present on all nucleated cells), whereas CD4+ T lymphocytes recognize antigen within MHC class II (expressed only by specialist antigen presenting cells). On antigen binding, activation is mediated via CD3-associated intracellular messenger systems, leading to cytokine release, and in the case of CD8+ cells, release of perforins.

In order to prevent autoimmunity, mechanisms exist to limit T-cell activation against self-antigens. Activation can only occur in the context of costimulation, regulated by immune checkpoint molecules, which include programmed cell death 1 (PD-1) and cytotoxic T lymphocyte-associated protein 4 (CTLA-4). These proteins, expressed on the surface of CD4+ and CD8+ T-cells, bind programmed cell death 1 ligand (PD-L1) and CD80/CD86 respectively and inhibit cell-mediated apoptosis. Through this mechanism, continued Tcell activation in response to chronic antigen exposure, as occurs with malignancy, leads to downregulation of the response and provides a further route by which tumor cells may escape apoptosis.

Adoptive Cell Transfer

Over the past decades, multiple strategies at adoptive cellular immunotherapy have been trialed. Tumor infiltrating lymphocytes (TILs) are CD8+ T cells that can be isolated from surgical specimens, expanded ex vivo and reinfused, leading to an effective antitumor response, particularly in melanoma.[12] However, TILs cannot be extracted from all tumor types, and as the native TCR requires MHC class I for activation, cytotoxicity can be downregulated or lost entirely when tumor cells do not express MHC class I.

The development of chimeric antigen receptor (CAR)-T cell technology overcomes this limitation. Here, T cells are acquired through peripheral blood culture and are genetically engineered with a CAR via retroviral transduction (Fig. 40.1). This CAR consists of an extracellular domain targeted to a specific tumor marker (e.g., CD19 in B-cell malignancy) linked via a transmembrane hinge protein to the intracellular components of CD3. Second- and third-generation therapies add costimulatory domains such as CD28/CD137 required for T-cell activation. After clonal expansion and reinfusion, CAR-T cells are able to target tumor cells independent of MHC, inciting a potent and persistent antitumor effect.[13–16]

Novel Cancer Therapies

SACTs may be used in isolation or as neoadjuvant or adjuvant treatment to surgical resection. SACTs traditionally involved only cytotoxic chemotherapy, which nonspecifically obtunds cell proliferation. Over the last 20 years, novel cancer therapies have been developed and licensed in specific malignancies. They can be classified as either:

Targeted therapies—where an agent (such as a monoclonal antibody) blocks or activates a specific receptor target on the tumor or cellular environment, inhibiting tumor growth;

Immunotherapy—involving modulation of the immune system response to tumor cells; this may include the administration of cytokines, viruses, vaccines, monoclonal antibodies, or cellular therapies in order to augment the immune response or to inhibit mechanisms by which tumor cells may evade destruction.

Examples of available novel agents and their current indications are summarized in Table 40.1, although ongoing trials will no doubt widen their range of use. The efficacy of many agents is dependent on the specific oncogenic phenotype of each patient's disease.

Targeted Therapies

The first targeted therapy to be licensed was imatinib, a tyrosine kinase inhibitor exerting activity against Bcr-Abl, a mutant constitutively active receptor expressed in Philadelphia chromosome t(9;22) chronic myeloid leukemia.[17] It has since been licensed in t(9;22)-positive acute lymphoblastic leukemia (ALL) and subtypes of gastrointestinal stromal tumors expressing c-Kit.

Other small molecule tyrosine kinase inhibitors have since been developed against a wide range of targets with varying degrees of selectivity. In metastatic non–small cell lung cancer (NSCLC), the first-generation selective EGFR inhibitor erlotinib improved median progression-free survival (PFS) from 5.5 to 11 months when compared against platinum-based chemotherapy.[18] NSCLC expressing anaplastic lymphoma kinase (ALK) fusion oncogene can be treated using ALK inhibitors such as alectinib, which in the ALEX trial, has shown a PFS approaching 3 years.[19] In metastatic clear cell renal cell cancer, the VEGF inhibitor sunitinib versus standard treatment with interferon-alpha was shown to enhance median PFS from 5 to 11 months.[20] On treatment resistance to tyrosine kinase inhibitors is common however, and disease will eventually progress during follow up. Here, second- and third-generation agents may be used (e.g., bosutinib and ponatinib in imatinib resistance, osimertinib in erlotinib resistance) which either exhibit a higher degree of specificity, target multiple proteins, or target a protein further down the intracellular signaling pathway.

Monoclonal antibodies against the membrane receptor tyrosine kinases and their ligands are also available, particularly in the treatment of NSCLC, clear cell renal cell carcinoma, and breast cancer. In the AVOREN trial, treatment with interferon-alfa plus bevacizumab (anti-VEGF) increased median PFS in metastatic clear-cell from 5.5 to 10.2 months when compared with a placebo.[21] Combination therapy with the VEGFR inhibitor ramucirumab, however, has shown only short increases in overall survival in gastric/gastroesophageal adenocarcinoma and

TABLE 40.1 Examples of Novel Targeted Agents and Immunotherapies, Their Targets, and Indications

Therapy	Target	Indications
Targeted Therapies		
Protein Kinase Inhibitors		
Imatinib Bosutinib Nilotinib Ponatinib	(BCR-) ABL c-Kit	CML ALL Ph+ve GIST (imatinib)
Afatinib Dacomitinib Erlotinib Gefitinib	EGFR	NSCLC Pancreatic (erlotinib)
Alectinib Brigatinib Ceritinib Crizotinib	ALK	NSCLC
Axitinib Pazopanib	VEGFR/c-KIT	Renal cell cancer GIST (sunitinib)
Lapatinib	EGFR/HER2	Breast cancer
Lenvatinib Sorafenib	VEGFR/RAF	Thyroid Renal cell cancer
Dabrafenib Vemurafenib	B-Raf	Melanoma
Idelalisib	PI3K	CLL Follicular lymphoma
Abemaciclib Palbociclib Ribociclib	CDK4/6	Breast cancer
Monoclonal Antibodies		
Bevacizumab	VEGF	Colorectal cancer Renal cell carcinoma NSCLC
Ramucirumab	VEGFR	Colorectal cancer Gastric/GOJ adenocarcinoma NSCLC
Cetuximab	EGFR	Colorectal cancer Head and neck SCC
Necitumumab	EGFR	Nonsquamous NSCLC
Panitumumab	EGFR	Colorectal cancer
Pertuzumab Trastuzumab	HER2/EGFR	Breast cancer

TABLE 40.1 Examples of Novel Targeted Agents and Immunotherapies, Their Targets, and Indications—cont'd

Therapy	Target	Indications
Monoclonal Antibody-Drug Conjugates		
Gemtuzumab	CD33	AML
Brentuximab	CD30	Hodgkin's lymphoma Cutaneous T-cell lymphoma Anaplastic large cell lymphoma
Inotuzumab	CD22	B-ALL
Immunotherapies		
Monoclonal Antibodies		
Rituximab Obinutuzumab	CD20	B-cell lymphoma CLL
Daratumumab	CD38	Myeloma
Bispecific T-Cell Engagers		
Blinatumomab	CD3/ CD19	B-ALL
Immune Checkpoint Inhibitors		
Nivolumab Pembrolizumab	PD-1	Melanoma NSCLC Renal cell carcinoma Hodgkin's lymphoma Head and neck SCC
Atezolizumab	PD-L1	NSCLC Urothelial carcinoma
Durvalumab	PD-L1	NSCLC
Ipilimumab	CTLA-4	Melanoma Renal cell carcinoma
CAR-T-Cell Adoptive Cell Transfer		
Tisagenlecleucel Axicabtagene-ciloleucel	CD19	B-ALL DLBCL

ALL, Acute lymphoblastic leukemia; *ALK*, anaplastic lymphoma kinase; *B-ALL*, B cell precursor ALL; *CLL*, chronic lymphocytic leukemia; *CML*, chronic myeloid leukemia; *CTLA-4*, cytotoxic T lymphocyte-associated protein 4; *DLBLC*, diffuse large B-cell lymphoma; *EFGR*, epidermal growth factor receptor; *GIST*, gastrointestinal stroma tumor; *GOJ*, gastro-esophageal junctional; *HER2*, human epidermal growth factor receptor 2; *PD-L1*, programmed cell death 1 ligand; *PI3K*, phosphoinositol-3-kinase; *NSCLC*, non–small cell lung cancer; *SCC*, squamous cell carcinoma; *VEGF*, vascular endothelial growth factor; *VEGFR*, vascular endothelial growth factor receptor.

NSCLC.[22,23] Combination treatments with trastuzumab, a monoclonal antibody against HER-2, a subtype of EGFR, improve overall survival in HER-2-positive breast cancer in both localized, surgically resected, and metastatic disease.[24]

Another use of monoclonal antibodies is in the treatment of hematologic malignancy through the targeted delivery of antimitotic agents. In CD33+ acute myeloid leukemia, combination therapy with gemtuzumab reduces relapse and overall 5-year survival.[25] Combination therapy with brentuximab increases median PFS in CD30+ anaplastic large cell lymphoma[26] and relapsed Hodgkin's lymphoma.[27]

Immunotherapies: Monoclonal Antibodies

The anti-CD20 monoclonal antibody rituximab, which induces B-cell death through antibody and complement-dependent cytotoxicity, has long been established as an adjunct to chemotherapy in diffuse large B-cell lymphoma and follicular lymphoma.[28] More recently, the bispecific T-cell engager blinatumomab has been licensed for treatment in Philadelphia-chromosome negative B-cell precursor ALL (B-ALL). It consists of a CD3- and CD19-specific antibody fragment linked together, which binds and bridges the CD19+ tumor cell directly to CD8+ T cells via the CD3 domain, inducing direct cytotoxicity independent of MHC class I.[14,29] In a multicenter, randomized controlled trial studying relapsed/refractory B-ALL (n=405), blinatumomab compared to standard chemotherapy increased median overall survival (4 vs. 7.7 months) and had higher rates of complete remission (34% vs. 16%).[30]

Immune Checkpoint Inhibitors

The efficacy of immune checkpoint inhibitors has been established throughout the phase III CheckMate and KEYNOTE trials, and they have largely superseded cytokine-based immunotherapy in renal cell carcinoma and melanoma.

In advanced treatment naive clear cell renal carcinoma, the CheckMate-214 trial (n=1096) showed higher response rate (42% vs. 27%) and overall survival favoring combination nivolumab (anti-PD-1) and ipilimumab (anti-CTLA-4) versus sunitinib.[31] KEYNOTE-426 (n=861) compared sunitinib with combination pembrolizumab (anti-PD-1) and axitinib (multitargeted small molecule tyrosine kinase) and reported improved overall and PFS.[32] However, with a median follow-up period of 25.2 and 12.8 months, respectively, longer-term data from both trials are eagerly awaited. In metastatic melanoma, the CheckMate-066 trial (n=405) compared nivolumab with standard care chemotherapy and reported a dramatic improvement in median overall survival (37.5 vs. 11.2 months),[33] outcomes which may be exceeded by combination therapy with ipilimumab, although with a significant increase in side effect profile.[34] KEYNOTE-006 compared pembrolizumab (administered up to 2 years) with ipilimumab and has demonstrated superior median overall PFS after 5 years of follow up.[35]

Checkpoint inhibitors are also established in the treatment of NSCLC. In KEYNOTE-407 (n=559) and KEYNOTE-189 (n=616) combination, pembrolizumab with platinum-based chemotherapy demonstrated superior median overall survival and PFS compared with chemotherapy alone in squamous and nonsquamous NSCLC, respectively, although better outcomes were seen in tumors with higher expression of PD-L1.[36,37] In CheckMate-227, nivolumab with ipilimumab also conferred longer median survival than standard chemotherapy, irrespective of PD-L1 expression.[38]

Cellular Immunotherapy

Two CD-19-targeted CAR-T cell therapies have shown dramatic efficacy in the treatment of refractory or relapsed B-ALL and diffuse large B-cell lymphoma (DLBCL); however, the evidence base currently consists of small phase II studies which are in the early stages of follow up. In the multicenter phase II ELIANA trial, tisagenlecleucel was administered to 75 patients with B-ALL, leading to complete remission at 3 months in 81%, although in responders the relapse free survival fell to 59% at 12 months.[39] In DLBCL, the ZUMA-1 and JULIET trials demonstrated complete response rates of 54% and 40% in patients treated with axicabtagene ciloleucel (n=101) and tisagenlecleucel (n=93), respectively.[40,41] CAR-T cells engineered to target myeloma and acute myeloid leukemia are under investigation, although trials in solid organ disease have yet to match the impressive response rates seen in hematologic disease.[14]

Novel Agent Toxicity

While these newer targeted agents and immunotherapies generally lack the constitutional side effects of the traditional cytotoxic chemotherapeutics, they are associated with life-threatening complications related to their specific biological target.[42] Severity may be classified using the five point Common Terminology Criteria for Adverse Events (CTCAE) scale, which provides a framework both to report and compare toxicity during trials and to guide the requirement for critical care in its management.[43]

Cardiovascular Sequelae of VEGF Inhibition

The direct or downstream signaling inhibition of the VEGF pathway through bevacizumab, ramucirumab, or tyrosine kinase inhibitors may be associated with hypertension, arterial and venous thromboembolism,[44] left ventricular dysfunction,[45] thrombotic microangiopathy,[46] and dysrhythmias through QT prolongation.[47] No specific treatment is indicated; initiation and withdrawal of the VEGF inhibitor in a patient with thromboembolic risk factors should be undertaken on an individual basis.[42]

Immune-Related Adverse Events

Checkpoint inhibitors are associated with a group of multisystemic complications termed immune-related adverse events (irAEs), where inflammation and autoimmunity occur due to the loss of immunologic tolerance mediated through PD-1/PD-L1 and CTLA-4. The most commonly recognized irAEs include dermatologic, gastrointestinal, pulmonary, hepatic, and endocrine syndromes, which again may be graded using the CTCAE system.

The incidence of severe irAEs (CTCAE grade ≥3) is approximately 0.5%–13%, varying widely between trials, treatment, and disease types. Toxicity appears to be greater and dose-dependent with ipilimumab or combination anti-CTLA-4/PD-1/PD-L1 therapy, compared with anti-PD-1/PD-L1 therapy alone.[35,48–51] Dermatologic (rash, mucositis) and gastrointestinal (diarrhea, gastrointestinal bleeding, enterocolitis) irAEs are most commonly encountered. Critical care admission may be required for fluid balance monitoring, electrolyte disturbance, or specialist dressings, or following surgery for perforation.

In one case series, pneumonitis complicated 5%–10% of checkpoint inhibitor treatments, with a median onset of 2.8 months (range, 9 days to 19.2 months). In contrast to other irAEs, pneumonitis appears to be more common with anti-PD-1/PD-L1 treatment, and appearances on high-resolution computerized tomography (HRCT) scan are nonpathognomonic. Twenty-seven percent classified as CTCAE grade 3 or above, and within this group (n=12), there were five deaths. Importantly, in the minority of patients who progressed despite corticosteroids, little response was seen on the addition of second-line immunosuppressants, conferring high mortality, principally due to opportunistic infection.[51–53]

In a recent meta-analysis, hypothyroidism was the most common endocrine irAE with an overall incidence of 6.6%, although the incidence of CTCAE grade 3 or above reactions was generally low (hypothyroidism, 0.12%; hypophysitis, 0.5%; primary adrenal insufficiency, 0.2%).[54] However, given the variable onset and often vague symptoms associated with this group of irAEs, a high index of suspicion should be maintained and prompt critical care admission and specialist endocrine input sought for all critically unwell patients presenting with possible thyrotoxic or hypoadrenal symptoms.

The American Society of Clinical Oncology (ASCO) has provided consensus guidelines on the management of irAEs.[55] Unfortunately, although there is ongoing research into markers of neutrophil activation such as CD177,[56] there is no clinically available biomarker to identify checkpoint inhibitor toxicity, and therefore the general approach is a systematic multidisciplinary clinical assessment and investigations to exclude other etiologies, principally infection and de novo idiopathic autoimmune disease.

Established irAEs are treated by temporary cessation of the checkpoint inhibitor and corticosteroid therapy (0.5–1 mg/kg for grade 2, 1–2 mg/kg for grade 3 reactions) alongside prophylaxis against opportunistic infection until clinical response is observed. An alternative immunosuppressant, such as infliximab, azathioprine, or mycophenolate mofetil, may be used in refractory irAEs. Once symptoms have resolved, patients

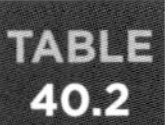
TABLE 40.2 **Stepwise Management of Cytokine Release Syndrome (CRS), According to CTCAE Grade[43]**

CRS Grade	Symptoms	Management
Grade 1	Mild reaction, fever with or without constitutional symptoms	Symptomatic management Antipyretics Antibiotics if neutropenic Consider tocilizumab 8 mg/kg (maximum 800 mg) 8-hourly if persistent fever for >3 days
Grade 2	Hypotension responding to fluids Hypoxia responding to <40% Fio_2	Fluid boluses If refractory hypotension, tocilizumab Consider siltuxumab 11 mg/kg if no response 6 h post 2 doses of tocilizumab Vasopressors if required (with ICU transfer) Consider dexamethasone 10 mg 6-hourly if hypotension persists
Grade 3	Hypotension managed with one pressor Hypoxia requiring ≥40% Fio_2	In addition to grade 2 management: Transfer to ICU Urgent echocardiogram Dexamethasone escalated to 20 mg 6-hourly if still refractory
Grade 4	Life-threatening consequences Pressor or ventilator support indicated	In addition to grade 3 management: High-dose methylprednisolone 1 g/day for 3 days, tapered rapidly over the next 6 days

may be rechallenged with the checkpoint inhibitor, although treatment is usually permanently discontinued for patients encountering grade 4 reactions.[55] Importantly, occurrence of an irAE, temporary treatment cessation, and immunosuppression does not appear to affect the efficacy of checkpoint inhibitor therapy.[57–59]

Cytokine Release Syndrome

As the name suggests, this is constellation of symptoms resulting from massive cytokine release secondary to the antigen recognition and T-cell activation, and as such tends to be greater when there is a higher tumor burden. It most commonly complicates CAR-T-cell therapy—77% of patients in the ELIANA trial suffered cytokine release syndrome (CRS)[39]—but it may also follow treatment with blinatumomab and monoclonal antibodies, such as rituximab and obinutuzumab. It is associated with high levels of interleukin (IL)-6, IL-10, IL-2, tumor necrosis factor (TNF), and interferon-alpha. It exhibits in a similar way to any major inflammatory response, with fever (often >40°C) as a minimum, tachycardia, hypotension, and hypoxemia, with potential for further progression to multiorgan failure. CRS timing is variable, but can be from a few hours postinfusion of CAR-T cells to more than a week.

Specific effects include:

- Cardiovascular effects: tachycardia, refractory hypotension, arrhythmias, prolonged QT; echocardiogram findings may include reduced left ventricular ejection fraction
- Respiratory: hypoxia, dyspnea, tachypnea secondary to pulmonary edema and/or pneumonitis
- Renal: acute kidney injury
- Gastrointestinal/hepatic: anorexia, nausea; colitis causing diarrhea; hyperbilirubinemia and transaminitis
- Hematologic: anemia, thrombocytopenia, clotting abnormalities

While a number of grading systems have previously been used, CRS was incorporated in CTCAE v5, providing a simple and comparable classification (Table 40.2).

The management of CRS is initially supportive, and as the syndrome evolves, the degree of that supportive therapy obviously escalates, with pressor support, ventilation, and renal replacement therapy, as indicated. However, for grade 2 CRS or above, tocilizumab, an IL-6 receptor antagonist, is recommended first-line treatment. Tocilizumab has been shown to reduce the severity of CRS, while not affecting the antitumor effect of CAR-T cells. Evidence for the optimum dosing regime and length of treatment is limited; however, our particular institutional algorithm is summarized in Table 40.2.

In patients with grade 3 CRS, steroids are introduced as adjunctive therapy. As T-cell suppressors, their action may impair the effect of CAR-T cells; therefore their use is reserved until this point. There is no evidence to support one steroid over another, but at our institution we use dexamethasone 10 mg IV every 6 h (increased to 20 mg every 6 h if there is no response) for grade 3 CRS, with pulsed high-dose methylprednisolone (1 g daily IV) for grade 4 CRS (following the recommendations of Neelapu et al.[60]); see Table 40.3.

Siltuximab is a chimeric anti-IL-6 monoclonal antibody utilized in the management of Castleman's disease. Its use in tocilizumab-refractory CRS has also been described, with the rationale being that it binds directly to IL-6, rather than to the receptors. It is also suggested as a potential first-line therapy in patients experiencing both CRS and immune effector cell-associated neurotoxicity syndrome (ICANS), because of the theoretical risk of elevated levels of IL-6 resulting from tozilizumab IL-6 receptor occupancy worsening ICANS.[61]

TABLE 40.3 Stepwise Management of Immune Effector Cell-Associated Neurotoxicity Syndrome (ICANS), According to CTCAE Grade[43]

Symptom/Sign	Grade 1	Grade 2	Grade 3	Grade 4
Level of consciousness	Mild drowsiness	Moderate	Obtundation	Unconscious/life-threatening
Confusion	Mild	Moderate	Severe	
Speech	Dysphasia not impairing communication	Moderate dysphasia, impaired communication	Severe	
Seizure	Brief partial seizure	Brief generalized seizure	Multiple seizures	Status epilepticus
Tremors	Mild	Moderate	Severe, limiting self-care	
Weakness	Mild, perceived by patient but not on objective exam	Symptomatic, evident on objective exam	Limiting self-care	
Cerebral edema				Life-threatening
Management	Neurology review	Critical care admission		
	Fundoscopy to assess for papilledema MRI brain plus MRI spine if focal peripheral neurologic deficits Diagnostic lumbar puncture Daily 30-min EEG until toxicity symptoms resolve Consider tocilizumab 8 mg/kg (maximum 800 mg dose) IV if associated concurrent CRS	If associated with concurrent CRS symptoms Tocilizumab Siltuximab if not associated with CRS Dexamethasone 10 mg IV every 6 h or Methylprednisolone 1 mg/kg IV every 12 h if refractory to IL-6 therapy	Tocilizumab/siltuximab if associated with concurrent CRS as per grade 2 and if not administered previously If not associated with CRS, siltuximab and if not administered previously Corticosteroids as above for worsening symptoms despite anti IL-6 therapy; continue corticosteroids until improvement to grade 1 and taper Treat stage 1 or 2 papilledema as per standard ICU management Repeat neuroimaging if persistent neurotoxicity[3] Grade 3 for more than 2–3 days	Ventilation for airway protection Tocilizumab/siltuximab and repeat neuroimaging as per grade 3 High-dose corticosteroids, e.g., methylprednisolone IV 1 g/day for 3 days followed by rapid taper at 250 mg every 12 h for 2 days; 125 mg every 12 h for 2 days and 60 mg every 12 h for 2 days. Continue steroids until improvement to grade 1 and then taper Stage 3, 4, or 5 papilledema, CSF opening pressure 20 mmHg[3] or cerebral edema, treat as per standard ICU management

CRS, Cytokine release syndrome; *CSF*, cerobrospinal fluid; *CTCAE*, Common Terminology Criteria for Adverse Events; *EEG*, electroencephalography; *IL*, interleukin; *MRI*, magnetic resonance imaging.

While the degree of CRS closely correlates with IL-6 levels,[62] the practicalities of obtaining a sufficiently rapid result preclude their use for anything but research purposes. C-reactive protein levels (CRP) also correlate but are nonspecific.

Immune Effector Cell-Associated Neurotoxicity Syndrome

ICANS is a blinatumomab or CAR-T treatment-related encephalopathy that ranges from confusion to seizures (with 10% of patients developing nonconvulsive status epilepticus and a smaller percentage convulsive status epilepticus) and cerebral edema. It manifests typically at the same time as CRS, but there can be a second phase (in approximately 10% of patients) that occurs following CRS resolution and which tends to be longer and of higher grade than that which occurs during CRS. In rare cases, this can result in severe (occasionally fatal) cerebral edema of rapid onset.[60]

Identification and monitoring of ICANS consists of a clinical scoring system, electroencephalography (EEG) monitoring, fundoscopy for papilledema, and MRI brain. The former is the CARTOX-10,[60] a 10-point neurologic scoring system. This consists of:

- Orientation to year, month, city, hospital, prime minister (5 points)
- Naming three objects (3 points)
- Writing a standard sentence (1 point)
- Counting backwards from 100 in 10 s (1 point)

EEG monitoring in ICANS may show frontal intermittent rhythmic activity, generalized periodic discharges, and slowing even in the absence of seizure activity. CT brain may be normal until very late in the progression of ICANS, but MRI may show T2/FLAIR hyperintensities involving the thalamus and brainstem with neurotoxicity greater than grade 2.[63]

The initial management of seizures follows standard practice, with benzodiazepines and antiepileptic medication. All patients exhibiting seizures should be admitted to ICU, as there may be rapid progression to status epilepticus and cerebral edema.

Specific medical management depends on whether ICANS is accompanied by CRS. If so, first-line therapy remains tocilizumab, unless the initial presentation is of both severe CRS and ICANS, in which case siltuximab may be preferred (because of the risk of transient increases of IL-6 with tocilizumab).

In the absence of CRS, specific therapy is corticosteroids (dexamethasone 10 mg IV every 6 h) for ICANS grade 2 or above with the addition of an antiepileptic (levetiracetam in our institution). In patients who fail to improve, or who deteriorate, the steroid dose can be increased with a switch to pulsed methylprednisolone.

The management and grading of ICANS are summarized in Table 40.3.

Hemophagocytic Lymphohistiocytosis

Hemophagocytic lymphohistiocytosis (HLH) occurs in roughly 1% of CAR-T recipients and has been reported with checkpoint inhibitor therapy. It is the result of the immune system, particularly macrophages, becoming overstimulated with resultant excessive inflammation and consequent tissue destruction. Activated macrophages are normally eliminated by NK cells and cytotoxic lymphocytes, and in HLH, this process does not occur, typically because of abnormalities in the proteins that are involved in perforins-dependent cytotoxicity. This results in a cytokine storm, which has similarities in presentation with CRS (i.e., fever, hypotension, and tachycardia) and can make diagnosis difficult in patients who have received CAR-T cells. This is of significance because HLH requires prompt treatment, initially with anti-IL-6 therapy and steroids as per CRS, but also with etoposide if there is no improvement within 48 h, repeated after 4–7 days if necessary.

Other features of HLH include splenomegaly, cytopenias, hepatitis, high ferritin, hypertriglyceridemia, hypofibrinogenemia, and hemophagocytosis (the engulfment of blood cells by macrophages, which can be visualized in the cytoplasm of macrophages). Diagnosis in the context of CAR-T-cell therapy is based upon a ferritin of >10,000 ng/mL together with two or more grade 3 organ toxicities and the presence of hemophagocytosis.

Conclusion

Novel therapies offer the hope of significant extension of life (and in some cases cure) for patients suffering from an expanding number of cancer subtypes. However, the pace at which they have been, and are, developing and subsequently entered clinical use has outstripped our knowledge of their toxicities, and a number of questions remain. While the immediate supportive management of organ failures is not dissimilar to that of stemming from other etiologies, that of the underlying immunoactivation is still empiric. In addition, we are unable to predict which patients will suffer more severe toxicities, and this compounds what is the potential issue of critical care resource use as the therapies become more widely utilized. As an exemplar, CAR-T-cell therapy is associated with ICU admissions rates of 15%–47%[64] and such high rates of ICU requirement carry implications for where therapy can, and should, be delivered and for the education of providers. We also need to be cognizant of the fact that in offering these treatments (and the critical care required to facilitate them) to patients who have exhausted other lines of therapy, there will inevitably be a subgroup for whom this will ultimately represent an extension of suffering, rather than cure or meaningful life extension. It will only be with larger trials and longer follow up that this cohort may be more readily identified.

References

1. Lecuyer L, Chevret S, Thiery G, et al. The ICU trial: a new admission policy for cancer patients requiring mechanical ventilation. *Crit Care Med.* 2077;35:808–814.
2. Carmona-Bayonas A, Gordo F, Beato C, et al. Intensive care in cancer patients in the age of immunotherapy and molecular therapies: commitment of the SEOM-SEMICYUC. *Med Intensiva.* 2018;42:363–369.
3. Ostermann M, Ferrando-Vivas P, Gore C, Power S, Harrison D. Characteristics and outcome of cancer patients admitted to the ICU in England, Wales, and Northern Ireland and national trends between 1997 and 2013. *Crit Care Med.* 2017;45:1668–1676.
4. Soubani AO. Critical care prognosis and outcomes in patients with cancer. *Clin Chest Med.* 2017;38:333–353.
5. Darmon M, Azoulay E. Critical care management of cancer patients: cause for optimism and need for objectivity. *Curr Opin Oncol.* 2009:21:318–326.
6. Hampshire PA, Welch CA, McCrossan LA, Francis K, Harrison DA. Admission factors associated with hospital mortality in patients with haematological malignancy admitted to UK adult, general critical care units: a secondary analysis of the ICNARC Case Mix Programme Database. *Crit Care.* 2009;13:R137.
7. Puxty K, McLoone P, Quasim T, Kinsella J, Morrison D. Survival in solid cancer patients following intensive care unit admission. *Intensive Care Med.* 2014;40:1409–1428.

8. Darmon M, et al. Changes in critically ill cancer patients' short-term outcome over the last decades: results of systematic review with meta-analysis on individual data. *Intensive Care Medicine.* 2019;45:977–987.
9. Hanahan D, Weinberg RA. Hallmarks of cancer: the next generation. *Cell.* 2011;144:646–674.
10. Asati V, Mahapatra DK, Bharti SK. PI3K/Akt/mTOR and Ras/Raf/MEK/ERK signaling pathways inhibitors as anticancer agents: structural and pharmacological perspectives. *Eur J Med Chem.* 2016;109:314–341.
11. Folkman J. Role of angiogenesis in tumor growth and metastasis. *Semin Oncol.* 2002;29:15–18.
12. Dudley ME, Rosenberg SA. Adoptive cell transfer therapy. *Semin Oncol.* 2007;34:524–531.
13. Sadelain M, Rivière I, Riddell S. Therapeutic T cell engineering. *Nature.* 2017;545:423–431.
14. Slaney CY, Wang P, Darcy PK, Kershaw MH. CARs versus biTEs: a comparison between T cell–redirection strategies for cancer treatment. *Cancer Discov.* 2018;8:924–934.
15. Yang Y, et al. CD4 CAR T cells mediate CD8-like cytotoxic anti-leukemic effects resulting in leukemic clearance and are less susceptible to attenuation by endogenous TCR activation than CD8 CAR T cells. *Blood.* 2015;126:100–100.
16. Vairy S, Garcia JL, Teira P, Bittencourt H. CTL019 (tisagenlecleucel): CAR-T therapy for relapsed and refractory B-cell acute lymphoblastic leukemia. *Drug Des Devel Ther.* 2018;12:3885–3898.
17. Druker BJ, et al. Efficacy and safety of a specific inhibitor of the BCR-ABL tyrosine kinase in chronic myeloid leukemia. *N Engl J Med.* 2001;344:1031–1037.
18. Wu Y-L, et al. First-line erlotinib versus gemcitabine/cisplatin in patients with advanced EGFR mutation-positive non-small-cell lung cancer: analyses from the phase III, randomized, open-label, ENSURE study. *Ann Oncol.* 2015;26:1883–1889.
19. Camidge DR, et al. Updated efficacy and safety data and impact of the EML4-ALK fusion variant on the efficacy of alectinib in untreated ALK-positive advanced non–small cell lung cancer in the global phase III ALEX study. *J Thorac Oncol.* 2019;14:1233–1243.
20. Motzer RJ, et al. Sunitinib versus interferon alfa in metastatic renal-cell carcinoma. *N Engl J Med.* 2007;356:115–124.
21. Escudier B, et al. Phase III trial of bevacizumab plus interferon alfa-2a in patients with metastatic renal cell carcinoma (AVOREN): final analysis of overall survival. *J Clin Oncol.* 2010;28:2144–2150.
22. Wilke H, et al. Ramucirumab plus paclitaxel versus placebo plus paclitaxel in patients with previously treated advanced gastric or gastro-oesophageal junction adenocarcinoma (RAINBOW): a double-blind, randomised phase 3 trial. *Lancet Oncol.* 2014;15:1224–1235.
23. Garon EB, et al. Ramucirumab plus docetaxel versus placebo plus docetaxel for second-line treatment of stage IV non-small-cell lung cancer after disease progression on platinum-based therapy (REVEL): a multicentre, double-blind, randomised phase 3 trial. *Lancet.* 2014;384:665–673.
24. Moja L, et al. Trastuzumab containing regimens for early breast cancer. *Cochrane Database Syst Rev.* 2012;(4):CD006243.
25. Hills RK, et al. Addition of gemtuzumab ozogamicin to induction chemotherapy in adult patients with acute myeloid leukaemia: a meta-analysis of individual patient data from randomised controlled trials. *Lancet Oncol.* 2014;15:986–996.
26. Horwitz S, et al. Brentuximab vedotin with chemotherapy for CD30-positive peripheral T-cell lymphoma (ECHELON-2): a global, double-blind, randomised, phase 3 trial. *Lancet.* 2019;393:229–240.
27. Chen R, Chen B. Brentuximab vedotin for relapsed or refractory Hodgkin's lymphoma. *Drug Des Devel Ther.* 2015;9:1729–1733.
28. Coiffier B, et al. CHOP chemotherapy plus rituximab compared with CHOP alone in elderly patients with diffuse large-B-cell lymphoma. *N Engl J Med.* 2002;346:235–242.
29. Klinger M, Benjamin J, Kischel R, Stienen S, Zugmaier G. Harnessing T cells to fight cancer with BiTE® antibody constructs–past developments and future directions. *Immunol Rev.* 2016;270:193–208.
30. Kantarjian H, et al. Blinatumomab versus chemotherapy for advanced acute lymphoblastic leukemia. *N Engl J Med.* 2017;376:836–847.
31. Motzer RJ, et al. Nivolumab plus ipilimumab versus sunitinib in advanced renal-cell carcinoma. *N Engl J Med.* 2018;378:1277–1290.
32. Rini BI, et al. Pembrolizumab plus axitinib versus sunitinib for advanced renal-cell carcinoma. *N Engl J Med.* 2019;380:1116–1127.
33. Ascierto PA, et al. Survival outcomes in patients with previously untreated BRAF wild-type advanced melanoma treated with nivolumab therapy: three-year follow-up of a randomized phase 3 trial. *JAMA Oncol.* 2019;5:187–194.
34. Wolchok JD, et al. Overall survival with combined nivolumab and ipilimumab in advanced melanoma. *N Engl J Med.* 2017;377:1345–1356.
35. Robert C, et al. Pembrolizumab versus ipilimumab in advanced melanoma (KEYNOTE-006): post-hoc 5-year results from an open-label, multicentre, randomised, controlled, phase 3 study. *Lancet Oncol.* 2019;20:1239–1251.
36. Gandhi L, et al. Pembrolizumab plus chemotherapy in metastatic non–small-cell lung cancer. *N Engl J Med.* 2018;378:2078–2092.
37. Paz-Ares L, et al. Pembrolizumab plus chemotherapy for squamous non–small-cell lung cancer. *N Engl J Med.* 2018;379:2040–2051.
38. Hellmann MD, et al. Nivolumab plus ipilimumab in advanced non–small-cell lung cancer. *N Engl J Med.* 2019;381:2020–2031. doi:10.1056/NEJMoa1910231.
39. Maude SL, et al. Tisagenlecleucel in children and young adults with B-cell lymphoblastic leukemia. N Engl J Med. 32018;78:439–448.
40. Neelapu SS, et al. Axicabtagene ciloleucel CAR T-cell therapy in refractory large B-cell lymphoma. *N Engl J Med.* 2017;377:2531–2544.
41. Schuster SJ, et al. Tisagenlecleucel in adult relapsed or refractory diffuse large B-cell lymphoma. *N Engl J Med.* 2019;380:45–56.
42. Kroschinsky F, et al. New drugs, new toxicities: severe side effects of modern targeted and immunotherapy of cancer and their management. *Crit Care.* 2017;21:89.
43. US Department of Health and Human Services. Common Terminology Criteria for Adverse Events (CTCAE) v5. 0. 2017. Available at: https://ctep.cancer.gov/protocolDevelopment/electronic_applications/ctc.htm#ctc_50.
44. Choueiri TK, Schutz FAB, Je Y, Rosenberg JE, Bellmunt J. Risk of arterial thromboembolic events with sunitinib and sorafenib: a systematic review and meta-analysis of clinical trials. *J Clin Oncol.* 2010;28:2280–2285.

45. Ghatalia P, et al. Congestive heart failure with vascular endothelial growth factor receptor tyrosine kinase inhibitors. *Crit Rev Oncol Hematol*. 2015;94:228–237.
46. Eremina V, et al. VEGF inhibition and renal thrombotic microangiopathy. *N Engl J Med*. 2008;358:1129–1136.
47. Bello CL, et al. Electrocardiographic characterization of the QTc interval in patients with advanced solid tumors: pharmacokinetic- pharmacodynamic evaluation of sunitinib. *Clin Cancer Res*. 2009;15:7045–7052.
48. Kumar V, et al. Current diagnosis and management of immune related adverse events (irAEs) induced by immune checkpoint inhibitor therapy. *Front Pharmacol*. 2017;8:49.
49. Hodi FS, et al. Improved survival with ipilimumab in patients with metastatic melanoma. *N Engl J Med*. 2010;363:711–723.
50. Naidoo J, et al. Toxicities of the anti-PD-1 and anti-PD-L1 immune checkpoint antibodies. *Ann Oncol*. 2015;26:2375–2391.
51. Naidoo J, et al. Pneumonitis in patients treated with anti-programmed death-1/programmed death ligand 1 therapy. *J Clin Oncol*. 2017;35:709–717.
52. Suresh K, Naidoo J, Lin CT, Danoff S. Immune checkpoint immunotherapy for non-small cell lung cancer: benefits and pulmonary toxicities. *Chest*. 2018;154:1416–1423.
53. Chuzi S, et al. Clinical features, diagnostic challenges, and management strategies in checkpoint inhibitor-related pneumonitis. *Cancer Manag Res*. 2017;9:207–213.
54. Barroso-Sousa R, et al. Incidence of endocrine dysfunction following the use of different immune checkpoint inhibitor regimens: a systematic review and meta-analysis. *JAMA Oncol*. 2018;4:173–182.
55. Brahmer JR, et al. Management of immune-related adverse events in patients treated with immune checkpoint inhibitor therapy: American Society of Clinical Oncology Clinical Practice Guideline. *J Clin Oncol*. 2018;36:1714–1768.
56. Shahabi V, et al. Gene expression profiling of whole blood in ipilimumab-treated patients for identification of potential biomarkers of immune-related gastrointestinal adverse events. *J Transl Med*. 2013;11:75.
57. Horvat TZ, et al. Immune-related adverse events, need for systemic immunosuppression, and effects on survival and time to treatment failure in patients with melanoma treated with ipilimumab at Memorial Sloan Kettering Cancer Center. *J Clin Oncol*. 2015;33:3193–3198.
58. Schadendorf D, et al. Efficacy and safety outcomes in patients with advanced melanoma who discontinued treatment with nivolumab and ipilimumab because of adverse events: a pooled analysis of randomized phase II and III trials. *J Clin Oncol*. 2017;35:3807–3814.
59. Weber JS, et al. Safety profile of nivolumab monotherapy: a pooled analysis of patients with advanced melanoma. *J Clin Oncol*. 2017;35:785–792.
60. Neelapu SS, et al. Chimeric antigen receptor T-cell therapy—assessment and management of toxicities. *Nature Rev Clin Oncol*. 2018;15:47–62.
61. Bonifant CL, Jackson HJ, Brentjens RJ, Curran KJ. Toxicity and management in CAR T-cell therapy. *Mol Ther Oncolytics*. 2016;3:16011.
62. Maude SL, et al. Chimeric antigen receptor T cells for sustained remissions in leukemia. *N Engl J Med*. 2014;371:1507–1517.
63. Santomasso BD, et al. Clinical and biological correlates of neurotoxicity associated with CAR T-cell therapy in patients with B-cell acute lymphoblastic leukemia. *Cancer Discov*. 2018;8:958–971.
64. Fitzgerald JC, et al. Cytokine release syndrome after chimeric antigen receptor T cell therapy for acute lymphoblastic leukemia. *Crit Care Med*. 2017;45:e124–e131.

SECTION 5

Pain and Palliative/ Integrative Medicine

41

Acute Postsurgical Pain Management in Patients With Cancer

VIKRAM B. PATEL AND BHAWNA JHA

Introduction

Postoperative pain management is an integral component of the perioperative management of patients requiring surgery. Perioperative management starts early, even before the patient is admitted to the hospital for surgical procedures. The perioperative care team's preoperative optimization of underlying comorbid diseases and associated medications ensures that optimal anesthesia and analgesic strategies are utilized. For example, patients with cardiac disease may have anticoagulants prescribed that need careful discontinuation when neuraxial analgesic modalities, such as epidural catheter placement, are considered.[1] Patients with brain metastases may have compromised neurologic function, which requires careful consideration of centrally acting analgesics. Similarly, patients with hepatic metastases may have impaired metabolic and synthetic liver function and therefore altered drug metabolism and coagulopathy, which may impact the choice of anesthetic and analgesic techniques.

Cancer is one of the leading causes of morbidity and mortality and is associated with a significant burden of pain. The World Health Organization (WHO) executive summary (2018) reported 18.1 million new cases and 9.6 million deaths related to cancer in 2018, with 70% of patients experiencing cancer-related pain while undergoing cancer-related treatment or during the terminal stages of illness.[2,3] A multidisciplinary approach to pain management in cancer patients is essential and should include pharmacologic, interventional, surgical, and psychologic approaches. Given that surgery remains a cornerstone of cancer care, an acute postoperative pain management strategy is essential. Perioperative pain management in patients with cancer poses distinct challenges that require a systematic, well-thought-out approach starting in the preoperative phase tailored to the individual patient's surgery, underlying comorbid disease, patient's previous experience, and outcomes.

Postoperative Pain Management in Cancer Patients

The perioperative team managing patients undergoing cancer-related surgery may experience specific challenges with regard to postoperative pain management. Some of these challenges include the following.

- Abnormal coagulation profile, particularly in patients with liver dysfunction. Impaired liver function and coagulation factors may be related to primary liver cancer, metastatic liver disease, chemotherapy, immunotherapy, or comorbid disease such as hepatitis C. Thrombocytopenia related to cancer treatment or bone marrow infiltration is another challenge that should be considered when considering neuraxial and regional blocks, for example, epidurals, spinal, plexus blocks, and so on. If a preintervention platelet transfusion is indicated, the risk-benefit profile of the planned intervention should be considered. Consideration should be given to preprocedural laboratory investigations, such as partial thromboplastin time (PTT), prothrombin time/international normalized ratio (PT/INR), and platelet count, to avoid hemorrhagic complications and other specialists (e.g., hematologists) consulted for complex clinical cases.
- Immune compromise, for example, neutropenia, may be seen in patients receiving chemotherapy, mandating regular blood counts to monitor their underlying immune state, and for early signs of infection.
- Preoperative analgesia requirements may be associated with opioid tolerance, a recognized side effect of opioid therapy that leads to dose escalation and higher opioid usage. A typical strategy would be to continue baseline long-acting opioids and add short-acting (prn, as required) opioid medications postoperatively.
- Other preoperative conditions that may affect postoperative analgesia requirements and the effectiveness of

interventions include neuropathic pain from radiation therapy, metastatic lesions in the spine or around the neural plexuses, inability to maintain steady posture, cognitive deficits due to cerebral metastasis, impaired drug metabolism, and clearance, such as metastatic liver disease and impaired renal function compromised by renal or pelvic cancers.

Various Analgesic Modalities

Successful postoperative pain management involves the application of multimodal analgesic modalities adapted to the surgical procedure and patient needs. Depending on the modality to be applied, specific precautions must be considered. Opioids are the most commonly used pharmacological agents for acute and chronic cancer-related pain. The WHO guidelines for the pharmacologic management of cancer pain in adults and adolescents are among the most commonly used and validated tools in clinical practice. Despite the availability of several rapid and short-acting opioid and nonopioid agents, a substantial number of patients reportedly have undertreated pain, which adversely affects their mood, activities of daily living (ADLs), and level of satisfaction. Some of the most common modalities for postoperative analgesia include the following.

Oral Analgesics

Oral analgesics play a limited role in postoperative analgesia after cancer surgery. Unless the surgical procedure is minor, most cancer-related surgeries require parenteral analgesics. Patients with cancer may receive preoperative oral analgesics (usually opioids) for chronic pain management. These medications should be considered as the patient's baseline analgesic requirement and then supplemented with other analgesic strategies as necessary.

Preoperative cessation of oral intake may necessitate conversion to parenteral analgesics during the perioperative phase, and the parenteral route continues until the patient can resume oral intake. Newer agents such as sufentanil sublingual tablet system (SSTS) are gaining attention as an option, notably for acute postoperative pain management. A meta-analysis reported that SSTS is a valuable option for managing moderate to severe postoperative pain control, with improved effectiveness and faster onset.[4]

Nonsteroidal antiinflammatory analgesics (NSAIDs) play an essential role in managing patients with bone metastases but should be weighed against the risk of bleeding in patients with gastrointestinal or hepatic disease.

Parenteral Analgesia

A historical article by Roe (1963) on the intravenous administration of morphine for postoperative pain control in adults and children reported that the IV route was significantly more effective than the conventional oral regimen, with a dose reduction from 50–100 mg to 4 mg.[5] Patient-controlled analgesia (PCA) with parenteral opioids is now one of the mainstays of postoperative analgesia after cancer surgery. Intravenous PCA can provide a baseline dosage (which may be equal to or greater than the preoperative opioid dosage), depending on the patient's needs and the demand dosage at a specified interval. A patient with intact cognitive function may properly administer programmed dosage on an as-needed basis.

Sechzer, the true pioneer of PCA, initially administered small IV doses given on patient demand but administered by a nurse, followed by the development of a pump-driven PCA in 1971.[6] PCA infusion pumps have since evolved in terms of technology, delivery system, flexibility offered to patients, safety features, and portability. A mechanical/electronic device providing PCA is considered superior to IV bolus analgesia.[7] Common opioids used for PCA include morphine and fentanyl, while other agents occasionally administered via PCA infusion pumps include hydromorphone, sufentanil, and rarely meperidine (if the patient is intolerant to other agents). Most modern PCA infusion pumps can be programmed in PCA mode or PCA plus continuous background infusion mode. There are three settings commonly considered when starting a patient on a PCA device: demand dose, background infusion, and lock-out intervals. The lock-out interval is programmed to avoid toxicity, and the demand dose should be closely monitored to avoid side effects.

Continuous infusion along with a patient-administered bolus may be required in patients with cancer undergoing surgical procedures that are on preoperative oral or transdermal forms of opioids. For these patients, the background analgesic requirement should be continued based on the preoperative opioid dosage of the patient.

Parent-controlled analgesia can be used for pediatric patients. This setup requires parents to understand the PCA mechanism and the potential of overdosing the patient by overly enthusiastic or concerned parents. A background dose may be programmed along with a demand bolus dose in patients with high preoperative opioid requirements. It is essential to monitor patients during parent-administered PCA and PCA programs that use a background dosage to prevent respiratory depression.

Nurse-administered intravenous analgesia is commonly observed in the immediate postoperative period in patients who have undergone routine surgery. Once the patient has recovered adequately and requires moderate amounts of opioids, transitioning to a PCA infusion pump is suitable for patients nursed on surgical wards. The nurse-administered route may continue to be required if a patient cannot operate the PCA equipment, for example, due to limitations such as cognitive impairment.

Neuraxial Modalities

Epidural Analgesia

Epidural analgesia is commonly used for postoperative analgesia following major cancer surgery. A well-placed functioning epidural infusion can provide near-complete analgesia without the sedating side effects of oral or intravenously administered analgesics. Epidural catheters are usually placed preoperatively before induction of anesthesia, as the placement of an epidural in the postoperative recovery phase is difficult in patients who are heavily sedated or in pain and thus not very cooperative. It is essential to consider the patient's coagulation profile, especially if hepatic metastases are present or if the patient has any blood dyscrasias. Once the epidural infusion catheter is placed, it is activated either intra- or postoperatively before the conclusion of anesthesia. A basal rate is usually programmed and may be sufficient for most patients.

The location of the epidural catheter tip is important and should be positioned close to the nerve route level of the dermatome of the surgical incision. For most abdominal surgeries, a catheter placed with the tip at the mid-abdominal dermatomes (e.g., T10) should provide sufficient abdominal coverage, hence thoracic epidurals are preferred to reach the desired dermatomal level. For thoracic surgery, a transcutaneous extrapleural catheter placed under direct videoscopic vision by the thoracic surgeon can be considered, which negates the need for preoperative placement of an epidural catheter. Thoracic epidural placement requires skill and proper training, as the interlaminar space in the thoracic spine is relatively narrow and difficult to access, especially without imaging such as fluoroscopy. For lower limb surgeries (such as amputations), a lumbar catheter should be considered.

Continuous epidural infusion with a set basal rate may be sufficient for most patients. The choice of agents to be infused is based on institution-specific standard protocols, often including a local anesthetic (e.g., bupivacaine or ropivacaine) combined with an opioid (fentanyl or hydromorphone) and occasionally with adjuncts (clonidine and adrenaline). The local anesthetic concentration is chosen to provide only a sensory blockade to allow early postoperative ambulation as part of enhanced recovery pathways. Lidocaine 0.5% or bupivacaine 0.25% provide sensory analgesia, but when combined with an opioid agent, the concentration required is significantly reduced to as little as bupivacaine 0.075%, which offsets the need for postoperative vasopressor support.

A patient-controlled epidural bolus may also be programmed to help a patient with the incidental increase in pain (patient-controlled epidural analgesia; PCEA). It is important to remember that the analgesic effect of a bolus may take several minutes, and it is advisable to educate the patient to use such boluses before any anticipated movements such as going to the bathroom. The duration of the epidural infusion is usually 2–3 days after surgery, before removal of the catheter to avoid infection. A bolus of long-acting, hydrophilic opioids, such as hydromorphone or morphine, should also be considered immediately before epidural catheter removal to extend the duration of analgesia. Catheters may be used for extended periods if the catheter is tunneled subcutaneously in the paraspinal area to minimize the risk of catheter infection.

Single bolus dosing of an epidural is not optimal unless conditions preclude the use of a catheter, such as difficulty in guiding the catheter in the epidural space. Single bolus dosing cannot provide long-term analgesia but may help during the immediate postoperative phase, for example, after lesser surgery, such as for debridement of tissue. A bolus dose that includes long-acting, hydrophilic opioids, for example, hydromorphone or morphine, would ideally suit such single-shot techniques.

Spinal Analgesia

Spinal analgesia is gaining increasing popularity, especially with minimally invasive surgery. Intrathecal opioids are also effective in open abdominal surgery and are accompanied by fewer postoperative complications that often accompany continuous infusions of epidural administered local anesthetic agents in the postoperative period. Intrathecal administration of opioids combined with local anesthetics has been in use for decades. A small amount of intrathecal opioid (e.g., 200 μg of morphine) and adjuncts such as clonidine (e.g., 20–30 μg) may enhance the analgesic effect and duration and help reduce the concentration of the local anesthetic, with dramatic sparing of systemic opioid requirements and reduced sedation in the first 24 h after surgery. Opioid requirements may increase slightly on the second postoperative day. Given the single-shot nature of this technique, the hemodynamic lability accompanying the sympatholytic effect of the local anesthetic agent is managed intraoperatively by the anesthesiologist and is resolved in the postoperative period, with less postoperative hypotension.

Regional Anesthesia

Regional anesthesia is a well-known method for intraoperative and postoperative analgesia. While it may avoid the need for general anesthesia entirely, it may also help reduce postoperative complications from general anesthesia and reduce the recovery time. In patients who are not suitable for neuraxial techniques, for example, due to poor coagulation profiles, spinal metastasis, and so on, a plexus blockade may be utilized with a lower risk of bleeding-related complications. The use of ultrasound has gradually replaced the need for a peripheral nerve stimulator. Ultrasound is considered a safer alternative as blood vessels are visualized and avoided.

Single-shot plexus blockade may be utilized for shorter surgeries, with analgesic effects lasting for several hours depending on the local anesthetic agent used. It is instrumental in ambulatory patients who are expected to be discharged from the recovery room. Continuous plexus blockade is a valuable modality for providing near-complete analgesia for several days. A continuous infusion catheter can remain in situ for 3–5 days. Catheter migration is one of the most common occurrences due to limb movement, hence a secure method such as suturing the catheter is recommended.

Side Effects and Complications

In addition to the type of modality, another critical aspect of postoperative analgesia is the choice of analgesic agent. Opioids are the most common agents used, but other agents, such as NSAIDs, antineuropathic drugs (e.g., gabapentin), and even muscle relaxants, can be used. It is crucial to appreciate the risk-benefit profile of each modality.

Opioids used via the PCA route have side effects similar to those of the oral administration route, including nausea, vomiting, pruritus, sedation, and respiratory depression. The most common side effects are nausea and vomiting, and the addition of antiemetic(s) is a common practice. Female sex, history of postoperative nausea and vomiting or motion sickness, nonsmoking status, younger age, general anesthesia with volatile anesthetics and nitrous oxide, postoperative opioids, duration of anesthesia, and type of surgery (cholecystectomy, laparoscopic, gynecologic) are recognized risk factors for postoperative nausea and vomiting.[8] The recommended pharmacologic agents for the prevention and management of postoperative nausea and vomiting include serotonin (5-HT3) receptor antagonists (ondansetron, dolasetron, granisetron, tropisetron, ramosetron, and palonosetron), neurokinin-1 (NK-1) receptor antagonists (aprepitant, casopitant, and rolapitant), corticosteroids (dexamethasone and methylprednisolone), butyrophenones (droperidol), antihistamines (diphenhydramine and meclizine), and anticholinergics (transdermal scopolamine). Current guidelines do not recommend prophylactic treatment in every patient, but only in the subset of at-risk patients.[8]

Pruritus occurs in about 2%–10% of patients treated with systemically administered opioids.[9] The risk is higher when the neuraxial route is utilized.[10] Opioid-induced pruritus is higher in obstetric patients, with the reported prevalence of opioid-induced pruritus ranging between 60% and 100%.[9] This high prevalence may be due to the interplay between estrogen receptors and opioid receptors.[10] Patients undergoing major orthopedic surgery had a 30%–60% prevalence after intrathecal opioid administration.[10] The type and dose of opioids used, and the method of drug administration, play a role in pruritus. Opioid agonists, such as morphine or methadone, excluding fentanyl or oxymorphone, cause local itching and a typical histamine weal and flare response.[11] However, after intrathecal or epidural administration of opioids, patients typically scratch the nose, perinasal area, and upper part of the face.[12] Facial itching may be explained by high concentrations of opioid receptors in the trigeminal spinal nucleus innervating facial areas.[9] Using lipid-soluble agents (fentanyl and sufentanil), the minimum effective dose and the addition of local anesthetic agents seem to decrease the prevalence and severity of itching.[9] Intrathecal agents such as morphine cause a longer duration of pruritus, which is also more difficult to manage. Medications used to manage pruritis include opioid antagonists such as naloxone and naltrexone, but are known to reduce the analgesic effects of opioids, particularly at higher doses.[8] Nalbuphine effectively prevented and treated opioid-induced pruritus without increasing pain. However, the treatment was associated with increased drowsiness,[13] whereas no reduction in pruritus was observed after subcutaneous injection of 400 μg of naloxone in patients who received intrathecal fentanyl and morphine.[11] Other medications to reduce pruritis include antihistamines (e.g., diphenhydramine and hydroxyzine).

Postoperative confusion may occur, particularly in older patients, due to delayed metabolism and accumulation of drugs, resulting in delirium. However, the treatment of pain may cause delirium. In a large population of patients undergoing noncardiac surgery, higher pain levels at rest correlated with the development of delirium, and the method of postoperative analgesia, type of opioid, and cumulative opioid dose were not associated with an increased risk of delirium.[7,14]

Epidural analgesia-related side effects include neuraxial hematoma and subsequent spinal cord compression, nerve injury, and infection that may lead to an epidural abscess and cord compression. Risk factors predisposing to neuraxial hematoma include low platelet count, anticoagulant use, and coagulation defects in patients with cancer. Rosero and Joshi reported that in more than 1.3 million nonobstetric epidural analgesic procedures the incidence of spinal hematoma and abscess was 1 per 5401 and 1 per 13,968 catheterizations, respectively.[15] Kupersztych-Hagege et al. reported one spinal hematoma and two spinal abscesses in 2907 patients who underwent lung surgery.

Patients should be monitored for any sign of cord compression or infection in the intraspinal space after placing (or attempting) a neuraxial block (spinal or epidural) or after removing an epidural catheter. Patients should be evaluated daily for any neurologic signs or symptoms that may arise from cord compression. An urgent MRI scan of the spine is essential if a hematoma or epidural abscess is suspected. A CT scan is limited in its ability to identify a collection of fluids. If a spinal hematoma or abscess is suspected, timely (within hours) surgical drainage is essential to avoid long-term neurologic complications. Regular postoperative laboratory investigations can help evaluate a possible infectious process and guide the removal of an infusion catheter.

Other complications include postoperative neurologic deficits, postdural puncture headache, and systemic local anesthetic toxicity.[16] Rare intracranial complications may also follow dural puncture, with the pathophysiology likely linked to intracranial hypotension with subsequent tearing of bridging veins.[17] Predisposing risk factors for a cranial hematoma in obstetric patients, including coagulation disorders, arteriovenous malformations, or multiple punctures, are present in a minority of patients. Close postoperative monitoring for a change in the nature of headaches from postural to nonpostural, prolonged, or onset of focal neurologic signs is recommended.[18]

Postoperative and Postdischarge Follow-up

During the immediate postoperative recovery phase after surgery, patients need to be carefully monitored for excessive sedation due to opioids prescribed for postoperative analgesia. Once intravenous PCA or epidural infusion is discontinued, it is essential to reassess patients to determine if their analgesic requirements are met. As the surgical pain gradually subsides, careful adjustment of the opioid dosage should be made to anticipate hospital discharge. In some patients who are on high doses of preoperative opioids, a reduction in postoperative dosing may occur after surgical resection of the painful part of the tumor or if a painful extremity is removed. This reduction should be titrated before hospital discharge.

Depending on the patient's pain, increased administration of analgesics may be required for a short period immediately after hospital discharge. A follow-up appointment with a pain physician in patients with significant pain at discharge can help manage long-term analgesic strategies. Some patients would also benefit from attending a transitional pain clinic to identify and manage acute and persistent pain to prevent chronic postsurgical and neuropathic pain.

Conclusion

In summary, considering that patients with cancer may already be on high doses of opioids preoperatively, careful choice of an analgesic modality should consider other comorbid diseases (including abnormal coagulation profile, spinal metastasis, decreased immunologic function, presence of neuropathic disease, and cognitive deficits). Careful choice of analgesic modality should aim to provide excellent postoperative analgesia with minimal or no side effects and related complications.

References

1. Horlocker TT, Vandermeulen E, Kopp SL, Gogarten W, Benzon HT, Leffert LR. Regional anesthesia in the patient receiving antithrombotic or thrombolytic therapy. American Society of Regional Anesthesia and Pain Medicine Evidence-Based Guidelines. *Reg Anesth Pain Med.* 2018;43(3):263–309.
2. Neufeld NJ, Elnahal SM, Alvarez RH. Cancer pain: a review of epidemiology, clinical quality and value impact. *Future Oncol.* 2017;13:833–841.
3. Chiu HY, Hsieh YJ, Tsai PS. Systematic review and meta-analysis of acupuncture to reduce cancer-related pain. *Eur J Cancer Care (Engl).* 2017;26:e12457.
4. Katz P, Takyar S, Palmer P, Leidgens H. Sublingual, transdermal and intravenous patient-controlled analgesia for acute postoperative pain: systematic literature review and mixed treatment comparison. *Curr Med Res Opin.* 2017;33(5):899–910.
5. Roe BB. Are postoperative narcotics necessary? *Arch Surg.* 1963;87:912–915.
6. Sechzer PH. Studies in pain with the analgesic-demand system. *Anesth Analg.* 1971;50:1–10.
7. McNicol ED, Ferguson MC, Hudcova J. Patient controlled opioid analgesia versus non-patient controlled opioid analgesia for postoperative pain. *Cochrane Database Syst Rev.* 2015;6:CD003348. doi:10.1002/14651858.CD003348.pub3.
8. Gan TJ, Diemunsch P, Habib A, et al. Consensus guidelines for the management of postoperative nausea and vomiting. *Anesth Analg.* 2003;97(1):85–113. (also: Anesth Analg. 2014;118:85–113). doi:10.1213/ANE.0000000000000002.
9. Reich A, Szepietowski JC. Opioid-induced pruritus: an update. *Clin Exp Dermatol.* 2010;35(1):2–6; doi:10.1111/j.1365-2230.2009.03463.x.
10. Szarvas S, Harmon D, Murphy D. Neuraxial opioid-induced pruritus pruritus: a review. *J Clin Anesth.* 2003;15(3):234–239; doi:10.1016/s0952-8180(02)00501-9.
11. Waxler B, Dadabhoy ZP, Stojiljkovic L, Rabito SF. Primer of postoperative pruritus for anesthesiologists. *Anesthesiology.* 2005;103:168–178.
12. Kyriakides K, Hussain SK, Hobbs GJ. Management of opioid-induced pruritus: a role for 5-HT3 antagonists? *Br J Anaesth.* 1999;82:439–441.
13. Lockington PF, Fa'aea P. Subcutaneous naloxone for the prevention of intrathecal morphine induced pruritus in elective Caesarean delivery. *Anaesthesia.* 2007;62:672–676.
14. Lynch EP, Lazor MA, Gellis JE, et al. The impact of postoperative pain on the development of postoperative delirium. *Anesth Analg.* 1998;86:781–785.
15. Rosero EB, Joshi GP. Nationwide incidence of serious complications of epidural analgesia in the United States. *Acta Anaesthesiol Scand.* 2016;60:810–820.
16. Kang XH, Bao FP, Xiong XX, et al. Major complications of epidural anesthesia: a prospective study of 5083 cases at a single hospital. *Acta Anaesthesiol Scand.* 2014;58:858–866.
17. Bos EME, Hollmann MW, Lirk P. Safety and efficacy of epidural analgesia. *Curr Opin Anaesthesiol.* 2017;30:736–742. doi:10.1097/ACO.0000000000000516.
18. Cuypers V, Van de Velde M, Devroe S. Intracranial subdural haematoma following neuraxial anaesthesia in the obstetric population: a literature review with analysis of 56 reported cases. *Int J Obstet Anesth.* 2016;25:58–65.

42 Chronic and Interventional Pain Management in Patients With Cancer

SABA JAVED AND SALAHADIN ABDI

Introduction

Pain is one of the most common symptoms reported in cancer patients.[1] This pain can be nociceptive (somatic or visceral) or neuropathic, or a combination of these. Chronic pain can arise secondary to the tumor burden itself or to cancer-related treatments, comprising radiation or chemotherapy that lead to radiation fibrosis and peripheral nerve damage, respectively.[2,3] This chapter will discuss the evaluation of patients with cancer who suffer from chronic pain, outline the assessment of cancer-related pain, and provide an overview of the pharmacologic and interventional treatment options available for managing chronic pain.

Evaluating the Patient With Cancer-Related Pain

Cancer pain can be nociceptive or neuropathic, or a combination of these two types of pain. Nociceptive pain can be either somatic or visceral (originating from internal organs mediated by the autonomic nervous system) and arises when receptors at the distal end of axons sense noxious mechanical, chemical, or thermal stimuli that subsequently produce electrical activity. By contrast, neuropathic pain is characterized by lesions or dysfunction of the pain-sensing nervous system.

Medical History and Physical Examination

Pain assessment for a patient with cancer-related pain begins with a thorough medical history. Specifically, the following information should be elicited in detail: location of the pain, the onset of pain, and whether the pain is constant or intermittent (essential to guide whether the patient may benefit from long-acting pain medication versus short-acting analgesics "as needed" [prn] pain medication), description of the pain in the patient's own words (i.e., sharp, dull, achy, gnawing, throbbing, etc.), factors that alleviate or aggravate the pain, and if there are any other systemic or autonomic symptoms associated with the pain. Most cancer pain is continuous, with some variation in intensity; the severity of pain is often worse at night. A thorough pain medication history should also be elicited. Specifically, an inquiry should elicit whether the patient is currently using or has used any pain medications in the past and whether this provided pain relief.

Information should also be gathered regarding the patients' cancer diagnosis, including documenting the cancer type, cancer stage, metastatic disease, and past and current cancer treatments (e.g., chemotherapy, radiation, immunotherapy, stem cell transplant).

An extensive physical examination should then follow history taking. For a new patient, the recommendation is to perform a complete multisystem examination. A more focused examination of the patient's pain complaint site could be considered for an established patient.

Radiologic and Electrophysiologic Studies

Radiologic studies are the mainstay tools for guiding cancer diagnosis, establishing disease progression or regression, or disease surveillance. Pertaining specifically to cancer diagnoses, x-ray images are used when there is a concern of fractures, bony spurs or overgrowth, or concern for bone metastases or disease involvement of the bone marrow. Computerized tomography (CT) and magnetic resonance imaging (MRI) are both high-resolution imaging modalities, with the latter proven to be more beneficial for disease in the soft tissue or spinal cord. In addition, nuclear imaging bone scans can help diagnose and localize pathologies affecting the skeletal bones.

In addition to diagnostic studies, several types of electrophysiologic study can further assist in diagnosing the etiology of pain. For example, a nerve conduction study (NCS) is a diagnostic test that can evaluate nerve function by assessing electrical conduction in both sensory and motor nerves. The NCS stimulates a specific nerve and records its ability to send impulses to the muscle. NCSs are usually performed along with electromyography (EMG), an electrodiagnostic modality for evaluating the electrical activity produced within skeletal muscles. Unlike NCSs, which typically test large fibers, quantitative sensory testing (QST) is a dependable way of assessing both large and small nerve fiber function. Quantitative sensory testing is a psychophysical test that tests the integrity of the entire sensory neuraxis; however, the results are subject to changes based on the patient's mental alertness.[4]

Pharmacologic Management of Cancer-Related Pain

The World Health Organization has developed a three-step ladder to treat cancer-related pain systematically.[5] While the three-step ladder is a treatment algorithm based on the severity of pain (mild, moderate, severe), the ultimate goal should be to assist with pain management while minimizing patient symptoms and maximizing their functionality. **Step 1** pertains to treating mild pain with aspirin, acetaminophen, and nonsteroidal antiinflammatory drugs (NSAIDs) along with "adjuvant" medications. Adjuvant medication is an umbrella term for nonopioid medicines used to assist with pain control and to minimize the use of opioids. Adjuvants can be antiinflammatories, muscle relaxants, anticonvulsants/antidepressants, local anesthetics, alpha-2 agonists, and many others. **Step 2** is geared toward treating patients experiencing moderate pain, using "weak opioids," such as codeine, hydrocodone, or oxycodone, along with other adjuvants. **Step 3** aims to manage patients' severe pain using strong opioids such as morphine, hydromorphone, methadone, or fentanyl, along with adjuvants. Unlike opioids, acetaminophen and NSAIDs have an analgesic ceiling effect and have no tolerance or addiction potential.

Acetaminophen

Although acetaminophen is widely used for its analgesic and antipyretic properties, its exact mechanism is unknown. Because of its antipyretic effect, acetaminophen is generally avoided in cancer patients who are actively undergoing chemotherapy, stem cell therapy, or immunotherapy to avoid masking fevers, thereby allowing early detection of neutropenic sepsis. In addition, acetaminophen should be used with caution in patients with liver dysfunction, as it may cause liver toxicity. The maximum dose is 4 g in a 24-h period.

Nonsteroidal Antiinflammatory Drugs(NSAIDs)

NSAIDs inhibit the cyclooxygenase (COX) enzyme, which can be found in either COX-1 (a constitutive form) or COX-2 (inducible under conditions of inflammation) analogs, and are responsible for the conversion of arachidonic acid to thromboxanes and prostaglandins. As such, NSAIDs help minimize the formation of inflammatory mediators that sensitize nerve endings.

The side effects of NSAIDs are associated with their mechanisms of action. Inhibition of the enzyme leads to inhibition of platelet aggregation and vasoconstriction, increasing the risk of gastric erosion and bleeding in the gastrointestinal tract and ischemic kidney injury. The risk of stomach ulcers and platelet inhibition is decreased with COX-2 specific medications. NSAIDs should be taken with food and used with caution in cancer patients with cachexia, reduced fluid intake, or dehydration.

Opioids

Opioids elicit their analgesic effects by binding to the central and peripheral mu-, kappa-, and delta-opioid receptors. Opioids can be full agonists, partial agonists, or mixed agonist-antagonists. However, to treat cancer-specific pain, we primarily focus on full agonists. Opioids can be administered via multiple routes, including oral, buccal, rectal, subcutaneous, transdermal, intravenous, epidural, and intraspinal, with a preference for the oral route due to ease of administration. Table 42.1 details the recommended doses for opioids.

Codeine

Codeine is a prodrug metabolized by CYP2D6 to its active form to achieve its analgesic effect. There are known variations in the CYP2D6 enzyme. Some variations have reduced enzymatic activity, with the formation of low levels of the active metabolite, providing insufficient pain relief in some patients. By contrast, some individuals are ultra-rapid metabolizers with overactivity of CYP2D6 and can experience symptoms of opioid overdose secondary to an overproduction of the active metabolite.[6] Due to the variability in the CYP2D6 enzyme, patients can often fail therapy, which requires switching to another opioid or alternate analgesic medication.

Tramadol

Tramadol is a weak opioid analgesic used to treat mild to moderate cancer-related pain. Tramadol binds to both mu- and kappa-opioid receptors. Furthermore, one benefit of tramadol is that it prevents the reuptake of norepinephrine and serotonin, which can serve as an effective analgesic for neuropathic pain.[7]

TABLE 42.1 Opioids: Typical Dosing

Drug	Dosage	Routes
Codeine	15–60 mg, Q4–Q6H, PRN	PO
Tramadol	50–300 mg, Q4–Q6H, PRN	PO
Tapentadol	50–100 mg, Q4–Q6H, PRN	PO
Morphine	Dose individualized 15–30 mg, Q4H, PRN 2.5–10 mg, Q2–Q6H, PRN 10–20 mg, Q4H, PRN 0.5–2.5 mg, IV-PCA, Q6–20 min, PRN	PO Subcutaneous/IM/IV Rectal IV-PCA
Oxycodone	Dose individualized, start 5–15 mg, Q4–Q6H, PRN	PO
Hydromorphone	Dose individualized = 2–3 mg immediate-release (IR), Q4–Q6H = 1–4 mg, Q3-Q6H, PRN	PO
	8 mg extended-release (ER), Q24H	
	3 mg, Q6-Q8H, PRN	IV/IM, subcutaneous
	0.05–0.4 mg, Q6–20 min, IV-PCA	IV-PCA
Methadone	2.5 mg, Q8–Q12H for moderate-severe pain	PO/subcutaneous/IM/IV
Fentanyl transdermal	12.5–100 µg/h	Transdermal

IV, Intravenous; *IM*, intramuscular; *PCA*, patient-controlled analgesia; *PO*, by mouth; *PRN*, as needed; *Q*, every.

Tapentadol

Tapentadol is a weak opioid involved with mu-agonism and norepinephrine reuptake inhibition, and minor serotonin reuptake inhibition. Tapentadol is more potent than tramadol, with no active metabolites. However, similar to tramadol, there is an increased risk of seizures, with a similar gastrointestinal side effect profile.[8]

Morphine

Morphine is a potent opioid that undergoes glucuronidation and is metabolized into two metabolites: morphine-3-glucuronide (M3G) and morphine-6-glucuronide (M6G). M6G has a high affinity for the mu receptors and provides analgesic relief; however, it also has the potential for respiratory depression.[9] On the other hand, M3G does not provide any analgesia and contributes to different adverse reactions, including seizures, myoclonus, allodynia, and hyperanalgesia.[10] Morphine can be administered via numerous routes, including oral,[11] intravenous,[12] epidural, and intrathecally.[13]

Oxycodone

Oxycodone is a semisynthetic opioid with high bioavailability and is prescribed in an extended-release or immediate-release form.[12] CYP2D6 metabolizes oxycodone into nor-oxycodone and oxymorphone; the latter is 14 times more potent than oxycodone.[14] Oxycodone is sold under different formulations in combination with aspirin or acetaminophen, which amplifies the synergistic properties. Again, caution must be exercised in patients undergoing active cancer treatment using formulations containing aspirin or acetaminophen, as these will mask fevers.

Hydromorphone

Hydromorphone is a strong opioid analgesic four times more potent than morphine, and it is metabolized into the inactive metabolite hydromorphone-3-glucuronide.[13] Due to its high affinity for the opioid receptor, hydromorphone is used for severe cancer pain that is not relieved by other methods. An extended-release formulation of hydromorphone is currently being formulated.

Methadone

Methadone is a mu- and delta-opioid agonist with *N*-methyl-D-aspartate (NMDA) antagonist properties. Methadone has been used as a drug of choice to treat opioid tolerance/addiction and heroin addiction. While the mechanism of action is not entirely understood, methadone also inhibits the reuptake of norepinephrine and serotonin, which, alongside its NMDA antagonist properties, makes it a good drug for treating neuropathic pain.[15]

Fentanyl

Transdermal patches have been shown to be effective for cancer-type pain, especially in patients who cannot take any oral medications.[16] Fentanyl patches come in different dosages, usually from 12.5 to 100 µg/h. On average, it takes approximately 4–6 h for fentanyl patches to start working, with maximum pain relief achieved after 12–24 h after application. Patches are usually changed every 3 days, and once removed, the medication half-life is approximately 17 h. Because of its slow onset of action, patients should be notified about using other narcotic medications, as opioid toxicity can occur hours later. In addition to the transdermal route, fentanyl can be administered via oral, buccal, and intravenous routes.

Anticonvulsants

Anticonvulsants, such as gabapentin, pregabalin, carbamazepine, valproic acid, and lamotrigine, are typically used as adjuvants along with opioids to manage neuropathic pain. These medications, listed in Table 42.2, have been shown to improve neuropathic pain resulting from trigeminal neuralgia, nerve root compression, diabetic neuropathy, and chemotherapy-induced peripheral neuropathy, among others.[17,18]

Antidepressants

Antidepressants, such as amitriptyline, nortriptyline, and desipramine, are a valuable class of drugs for treating neuropathic pain (Table 42.3). Antidepressants enhance the inhibitory modulation of nociceptive impulses in the dorsal horn. Unfortunately, anticholinergic side effects are commonly observed with antidepressants. Drugs that are selective serotonin and norepinephrine reuptake inhibitors, such as duloxetine and venlafaxine, have been used to treat chemotherapy-induced peripheral neuropathy and cancer-related neuropathic pain and have shown some positive outcomes; however, further studies are required.[19,20]

Corticosteroids

Corticosteroids can effectively manage cancer pain due to their antiinflammatory effects and improve patient well being through antiemetic, appetite stimulation, and mood improvement effects. Similar to NSAIDs, corticosteroids produce analgesic effects by reducing arachidonic acid release and subsequently decreasing prostaglandin formation. Side effects include hyperglycemia, myopathy, immunosuppression, infections, and psychosis, among others.[21]

Muscle Relaxants

Muscle relaxants, such as methocarbamol, cyclobenzaprine, or baclofen, can be used as adjuvants to pharmacologic therapy to alleviate cancer-related pain. Muscle relaxants can be particularly beneficial for myofascial-type pain or pain of musculoskeletal origin. Side effects include central nervous system depression, drowsiness, dizziness, weakness, fatigue, and impaired coordination.

Local Anesthetics

Local anesthetics, such as lidocaine or mexiletine, have been used as adjuvants to treat neuropathic pain.[22] Local anesthetic agents inhibit sodium channels and can be administered intravenously, orally, or topically. Common side effects include lightheadedness, tinnitus, nausea, vomiting, and topical skin rash, amongst others.

Alpha-2 Agonist

Alpha-2 agonists, such as clonidine or dexmedetomidine, can be used as adjuvants for both nociceptive and neuropathic pain[23]. Alpha-2 agonists act like opioids, except at different receptors. It is thought that alpha-2 agonists decrease sympathetic discharge, a characteristic intrinsic to neuropathic pain, thereby alleviating the quality of pain.[24]

TABLE 42.2 Anticonvulsants: Typical Doses

Carbamazepine	200–400 mg, BID	PO	Sodium channel blocker
Valproic acid	250–500 mg, BID	PO	Increasing GABA effects; may inhibit glutamate; NMDA excitation
Lamotrigine	100–200 mg, QD	PO	Sodium channel blocker
Phenytoin	300–400 mg/day	PO	Modulates sodium and calcium channels
Gabapentin	300–1200 mg, TID	PO	Blocks voltage-dependent calcium channels
Pregabalin	50–100 mg, BID	PO	Blocks voltage-dependent calcium channels

BID, Twice a day; *GABA*, gamma-aminobutyric acid; *NMDA*, *N*-methyl-D-aspartate; *PO*, by mouth; *QD*, once a day; *TID*, three times a day.

TABLE 42.3 Antidepressants: Typical Doses

Drug	Dosage	Routes	Mechanism of Action
Amitriptyline	25–100 mg, QHS	PO	Inhibits reuptake of norepinephrine and serotonin reuptake
Fluoxetine	20–50 mg, BID	PO	Selective inhibition of serotonin reuptake
Paroxetine	20–50 mg, QD	PO	Selective inhibition of serotonin reuptake
Sertraline	50–200 mg, QD	PO	Selective inhibition of serotonin reuptake

BID, Twice a day; *PO*, by mouth; *QD*, once a day; *QHS*, once at night.

However, side effects of alpha-2 agonists include hypotension, bradycardia, somnolence, fatigue, and dizziness. As such, this class of medications is typically not suited for cancer patients who are already experiencing hypotension, fatigue, nausea, and possibly are intravascularly depleted while undergoing cancer therapy.

NMDA Antagonists

NMDA receptor antagonists, such as ketamine, dextromethorphan, and methadone, may benefit patients with neuropathic pain, especially those resistant to high-dose opioids.[25] Intravenous ketamine infusions have been used for intractable pain; however, their efficacy has not been validated.[26,27] While the use of dextromethorphan and ketamine may be limited due to their side effects at higher doses, methadone seems to be well tolerated. However, adverse effects of methadone include QT prolongation, for which ECG monitoring is recommended for patients with long-term therapy.

Interventional Management of Cancer Pain

When noninvasive medical management of cancer pain provides suboptimal pain relief, interventional therapies, ranging from less invasive to more invasive, can be considered. These therapies include epidural steroidal injection, neurolytic procedures, vertebral augmentation, spinal cord stimulator, dorsal root ganglion stimulation, intrathecal drug delivery, and cordotomy. Each of these techniques is briefly discussed below.

Epidural Steroidal Injections

Epidural steroidal injections are the most frequently performed procedures by interventional pain physicians worldwide. Epidural steroidal injection is a minimally invasive procedure in which medication is focally deposited in the epidural space. Steroids aim to decrease inflammation of the spinal nerves and nerve roots due to spinal stenosis, disc herniation, facet arthropathy, degenerative disc disease, failed back surgery syndrome, extension of the disease into the epidural space, and so on. Two techniques commonly used to perform epidural steroidal injection are the interlaminar and transforaminal approaches, with systematic review articles not showing the superiority of one technique over the other.[28] Furthermore, recent studies have assessed the effectiveness of lumbar interlaminar epidural injections performed with or without steroids for chronic low back pain related to lumbar spinal stenosis. Interestingly, no significant difference was observed between the two groups at 3-, 6-, and 12-month follow up.[12,29]

Neurolytic Procedures

Neurolytic block of the sympathetic axis is effective in controlling visceral cancer pain. Examples of such blocks, including the celiac plexus, superior hypogastric plexus, and ganglion impar neurolytic blocks, are briefly discussed here.

The celiac plexus is located retroperitoneally at T12 and L1 vertebrae, anterior to the crura of the diaphragm, and comprises both sympathetic and parasympathetic fibers from greater, lesser, and least splanchnic nerves. A celiac plexus block is ideal for patients with pain in the upper abdominal region or pain originating from the liver, pancreas, gallbladder, stomach, spleen, kidneys, intestines, and adrenal glands.

The superior hypogastric plexus is located retroperitoneally from L5 to S1 vertebral body. A superior hypogastric plexus block is ideal for patients with pelvic pain originating from the uterus, ovaries, vagina, bladder, prostate, testes, and descending and sigmoid colon, secondary to cancer or noncancer-related etiology. This block is effective in patients with advanced pelvic cancer, suggesting that a significant visceral pain component is present.[30]

The ganglion impar is a retroperitoneal structure located at the level of the sacrococcygeal junction at the coccyx. A ganglion impar block is ideal for patients with pain in the perineum, rectum, anus, vagina, distal urethra, and vulva.

Vertebral Augmentation

Vertebral augmentation, which includes vertebroplasty and kyphoplasty, is an interventional technique that utilizes different acrylic- and nonacrylic-based cement polymers within the vertebral body to correct volume loss from a vertebral compression fracture. In the cancer population, for patients with compression fracture secondary to their disease state, this procedure may be an option when noninterventional treatments have failed. While multiple meta-analyses have shown superiority for vertebral augmentation compared to noninvasive surgical techniques,[31] others have found no benefit.[32]

Spinal Cord Stimulation and Dorsal Root Ganglion Stimulation

Spinal cord stimulation is a widely accepted pain treatment modality for failed back surgery, peripheral vascular disease causing claudication pain, complex regional pain syndrome, and more. Spinal cord stimulation works by placing electrodes in the epidural space overlying the dorsal column of the spinal cord and applying electrical currents, resulting in modulation of pain generation or processing by inhibiting the dorsal horn wide dynamic range (WDR) neuron excitability, increasing the release of neurotransmitters, such as gamma-aminobutyric acid (GABA), serotonin, and norepinephrine, and decreasing the release of glutamate.[33] Similarly, the dorsal root ganglion (DRG) is a sensory neural structure located within the intervertebral neural-foramen and comprises primary sensory neurons. The DRG acts as a T-junction, a signal modulation area for managing sensory information from peripheral and cell bodies to more central neural pathways.[34] The ACCURATE study, a prospective randomized controlled trial, was conducted to compare the safety and efficacy of spinal cord stimulation versus dorsal root ganglion stimulation in patients with complex regional pain syndrome. The study found DRG stimulation superior to tonic spinal cord stimulation when assessing pain reduction over a 3- and 12-month timeframe.[11] The pain associated with cancer can be focal peripheral nociceptive pain or neuropathic pain; both can be targeted and managed by dorsal root ganglion stimulation and spinal cord stimulation.

Intrathecal Drug Delivery System

An intrathecal drug delivery system (IDDS) is employed to achieve similar or superior therapeutic effects compared to oral medications, while minimizing typical dose-dependent side effects. Similar to dorsal root ganglion stimulation and spinal cord stimulation, a trial of therapy is first undertaken to evaluate improvement in pain. If this treatment trial is successful, a permanent implant is warranted. Although morphine, baclofen, clonidine, and ziconotide are currently approved by the Food and Drug Administration (FDA) for use in implantable IDDSs, various other medications are also used in clinical practice. In addition, the increasing incidence of cancer survivorship has shifted the treatment of cancer-related pain from short-term to long-term chronic pain management, including strategies that use IDDSs.[35]

Cordotomy

Cordotomy is an invasive procedure for the ablation of intractable, unilateral pain that is not controlled by conventional therapies. This procedure involves mechanical disruption of nociceptive pathways in the anterolateral column, specifically the spinothalamic and spinoreticular pathways, to relieve pain while preserving the fine touch and proprioceptive tracts. The plethora of analgesics available and advanced technologies has reduced the demand for cordotomy to manage intractable pain. However, some patients with pain unresponsive to medical and procedural management, particularly malignant pain, may benefit from this procedure. Thus it is a viable treatment option, especially for patients with a limited life expectancy whose severe, unilateral pain is unresponsive to analgesic medications.

Scrambler Therapy

Scrambler therapy is a novel neuromodulation therapy with noninvasive electrocutaneous stimulation of C-fiber surface receptors. It substitutes the pain information with synthetic "nonpain" information. The device produces different electrical currents that stimulate normal nerve action potentials. The impulses are transmitted via surface electrodes, which are placed around the area of pain. Scrambler therapy has proven to be a safe and effective alternative therapy for patients with refractory chronic neuropathic pain as well as chemotherapy-induced peripheral neuropathy.[36,37]

Conclusion

A cornerstone of cancer pain management starts with gathering a detailed history and performing a thorough physical examination to appropriately diagnose the pain and its etiology. Further radiographic and electrophysiologic studies can then be used for diagnostic confirmation. Finally, cancer pain can be treated by escalating pharmacologic therapy, interventional therapy, or both to help patients during their cancer treatment and improve quality of life in long-term cancer survivorship.

References

1. Portenoy RK, Thaler HT, Kornblith AB, et al. Symptom prevalence, characteristics and distress in a cancer population. *Qual Life Res*. 1994;3(3):183–189.
2. Hojan K, Milecki P. Opportunities for rehabilitation of patients with radiation fibrosis syndrome. *Rep Pract Oncol Radiother*. 2014;19(1):1–6.
3. Windebank AJ, Grisold W. Chemotherapy-induced neuropathy. *J Peripher Nerv Syst*. 2008;13(1):27–46.
4. Siao P, Cros DP. Quantitative sensory testing. *Phys Med Rehabil Clin N Am*. 2003;14(2):261–286.
5. World Health Organization. Cancer pain relief *With a Guide to Opioid Availability*. Geneva: World Health Organization; 1996. 2nd ed.
6. Dean L. Codeine therapy and CYP2D6 genotype. Medical Genetics Summaries. Bethesda, MD: National Center for Biotechnology Information; 2016.
7. Scott LJ, Perry CM. Tramadol: a review of its use in perioperative pain. *Drugs*. 2000;60(1):139–176.
8. Singh DR, Nag K, Shetti AN, Krishnaveni N. Tapentadol hydrochloride: A novel analgesic. *Saudi J Anaesth*. 2013;7(3):322–326.
9. Pasternak GW, Bodnar RJ, Clark JA, Inturrisi CE. Morphine-6-glucuronide, a potent mu agonist. *Life Sci*. 1987;41(26): 2845–2849.
10. Franken LG, Masman AD, de Winter BC, et al. Pharmacokinetics of morphine, morphine-3-glucuronide and morphine-6-glucuronide in terminally ill adult patients. *Clin Pharmacokinet*. 2016;55(6):697–709.
11. Deer TR, Levy RM, Kramer J, et al. Dorsal root ganglion stimulation yielded higher treatment success rate for complex regional pain syndrome and causalgia at 3 and 12 months: a randomized comparative trial. *Pain*. 2017;158(4):669–681.
12. Friedly JL, Comstock BA, Turner JA, et al. A randomized trial of epidural glucocorticoid injections for spinal stenosis. *N Engl J Med*. 2014;371(1):11–21.
13. Smith MT. Neuroexcitatory effects of morphine and hydromorphone: evidence implicating the 3-glucuronide metabolites. *Clin Exp Pharmacol Physiol*. 2000;27(7):524–528.
14. Tallgren M, Olkkola KT, Seppälä T, Höckerstedt K, Lindgren L. Pharmacokinetics and ventilatory effects of oxycodone before and after liver transplantation. *Clin Pharmacol Ther*. 1997;61(6):655–661.
15. Manfredi PL, Houde RW. Prescribing methadone, a unique analgesic. *J Support Oncol*. 2003;1(3):216–220.
16. Ibuki T. [Transdermal fentanyl patch for the treatment of chronic intractable pain]. *Masui*. 2013;62(7):784–790.
17. Backonja M, Beydoun A, Edwards KR, et al. Gabapentin for the symptomatic treatment of painful neuropathy in patients

with diabetes mellitus: a randomized controlled trial. *JAMA.* 1998;280(21):1831–1836.
18. Collins SL, Moore RA, McQuay HJ, Wiffen P. Antidepressants and anticonvulsants for diabetic neuropathy and postherpetic neuralgia: a quantitative systematic review. *J Pain Symptom Manag.* 2000;20(6):449–458.
19. Tasmuth T, Härtel B, Kalso E. Venlafaxine in neuropathic pain following treatment of breast cancer. *Eur J Pain.* 2002;6(1): 17–24.
20. Hou S, Huh B, Kim HK, Kim KH, Abdi S. Treatment of chemotherapy-induced peripheral neuropathy: systematic review and recommendations. *Pain Phys.* 2018;21(6):571–592.
21. Sørensen S, Helweg-Larsen S, Mouridsen H, Hansen HH. Effect of high-dose dexamethasone in carcinomatous metastatic spinal cord compression treated with radiotherapy: a randomised trial. *Eur J Cancer.* 1994;30A(1):22–27.
22. Galer BS, Harle J, Rowbotham MC. Response to intravenous lidocaine infusion predicts subsequent response to oral mexiletine: a prospective study. *J Pain Symptom Manage.* 1996;12(3):161–167.
23. Eisenach JC, Rauck RL, Buzzanell C, Lysak SZ. Epidural clonidine analgesia for intractable cancer pain: phase I. *Anesthesiology.* 1989;71(5):647–652.
24. Di Cesare Mannelli L, Micheli L, Crocetti L, Giovannoni MP, Vergelli C, Ghelardini C. Alpha2 adrenoceptor: a target for neuropathic pain treatment. *Mini Rev Med Chem.* 2017;17(2):95–107.
25. Nelson KA, Park KM, Robinovitz E, Tsigos C, Max MB. High-dose oral dextromethorphan versus placebo in painful diabetic neuropathy and postherpetic neuralgia. *Neurology.* 1997;48(5):1212–1218.
26. Maher DP, Chen L, Mao J. Intravenous ketamine infusions for neuropathic pain management: a promising therapy in need of optimization. *Anesth Analg.* 2017;124(2):661–674.
27. Moisset X, Clavelou P, Lauxerois M, Dallel R, Picard P. Ketamine infusion combined with magnesium as a therapy for intractable chronic cluster headache: report of two cases. *Headache.* 2017;57(8):1261–1264.
28. Chang-Chien GC, Knezevic NN, McCormick Z, Chu SK, Trescot AM, Candido KD. Transforaminal versus interlaminar approaches to epidural steroid injections: a systematic review of comparative studies for lumbosacral radicular pain. *Pain Phys.* 2014;17(4):E509–E524.
29. Manchikanti L, Cash KA, McManus CD, Damron KS, Pampati V, Falco FJ. A randomized, double-blind controlled trial of lumbar interlaminar epidural injections in central spinal stenosis: 2-year follow-up. *Pain Phys.* 2015;18(1):79–92.
30. de Leon-Casasola OA, Kent E, Lema MJ. Neurolytic superior hypogastric plexus block for chronic pelvic pain associated with cancer. *Pain.* 1993;54(2):145–151.
31. Beall D, Lorio MP, Yun BM, Runa MJ, Ong KL, Warner CB. Review of vertebral augmentation: an updated meta-analysis of the effectiveness. *Int J Spine Surg.* 2018;12(3):295–321.
32. Kallmes DF, Comstock BA, Heagerty PJ, et al. A randomized trial of vertebroplasty for osteoporotic spinal fractures. *N Engl J Med.* 2009;361(6):569–579.
33. Jensen MP, Brownstone RM. Mechanisms of spinal cord stimulation for the treatment of pain: still in the dark after 50 years. *Eur J Pain.* 2019;23(4):652–659.
34. Kent AR, Min X, Hogan QH, Kramer JM. Mechanisms of dorsal root ganglion stimulation in pain suppression: A computational modeling analysis. *Neuromodulation.* 2018;21(3):234–246.
35. Bruel BM, Burton AW. Intrathecal therapy for cancer-related pain. *Pain Med.* 2016;17(12):2404–2421.
36. Compagnone C, Tagliaferri FScrambler Therapy Group. Chronic pain treatment and scrambler therapy: a multicenter retrospective analysis. *Acta Biomed.* 2015;86(2):149–156.
37. Pachman DR, Weisbrod BL, Seisler DK, et al. Pilot evaluation of Scrambler therapy for the treatment of chemotherapy-induced peripheral neuropathy. *Support Care Cancer.* 2015;23(4):943–951.

43

Rehabilitation, Palliative Care, and Integrative Medicine Interventions in Cancer

NAVEEN SALINS, ARUNANGSHU GHOSHAL, AND KRITHIKA S. RAO

Rehabilitation Interventions in Patients With Cancer

Introduction

For patients with a broad range of serious life-threatening illness, loss of function and independence is a common struggle and a significant contributor to diminished quality of life. Among the factors that can contribute to loss of function are prolonged hospitalization, deconditioning, pain, fatigue, depression, malnutrition, organ failure, neurologic injury, and musculoskeletal problems. Patients with cancer can additionally experience sarcopenia from direct tumor effects and fatigue from cancer treatment.[1] Rehabilitation, even in the advanced phase of an illness, can help to maintain or restore function, permit patients to retain mobility and independence, and improve symptoms, all of which can contribute to a reduced burden on families and caregivers and improved quality of life.[2] The main rehabilitation modalities are physical therapy, occupational therapy, and speech/ swallowing rehabilitation. Regular and open communication with patients and their families regarding the goals of rehabilitation is critical in designing a rehabilitation plan so that realistic goals can be identified. The rehabilitation plan must also consider the patient's environment, existing functionality, and available resources. The measure of success of a palliative care rehabilitation program should not focus on length of survival but rather on enhancing quality of life, function/independence, and psychosocial well being. Patient condition and goals of care can shift dramatically while under palliative care, and therapists must maintain some flexibility, respecting patient choices and allowing for frequent interruptions in the rehabilitation treatment plan.[3]

Multi-disciplinary Assessment

A thorough patient assessment for rehabilitation potential involves gathering information on disease location and stage, previous and current therapies, estimated life expectancy, comorbidities, pain and nonpain symptoms, medications, cognition, mood, nutritional status, and physical function. A complete physical examination with special attention to the neurologic and musculoskeletal system is essential to evaluate motor strength, sensory deficits, joint flexibility, gait pattern, and fall risk. An evaluation of the home environment, the availability of community resources, and financial resources should also be carried out.[4] Using a systematized evaluation process will help to determine the patient's current level of disability, previous level of functioning, and potential to regain function, which are all important components of rehabilitation planning. Ideally, patient evaluation and planning for rehabilitation should be performed by an interdisciplinary team led by a physiatrist/ palliative care physician experienced in hospice and palliative medicine along with clinicians specializing in physical therapy, occupational therapy, speech therapy, nursing, nutrition, psychology, respiratory therapy, recreation therapy, and case management.[5] A variety of functional assessment tools may be utilized to assess function during the planning process for rehabilitation therapy and palliative care.[6]

Types of Rehabilitation

The type of rehabilitation depends on the patient's disease stage, function, and goals.[7,8] When applied to patients with life-limiting disease processes, it can be:

- Preventive rehabilitation: Begins after the diagnosis of the potentially life-limiting illness and attempts to mitigate functional morbidity caused by the disease or its treatment.
- Restorative rehabilitation: Attempts to return patients to their premorbid functional status when little or no long-term impairment is anticipated, and patients have remaining functional activity.
- Supportive rehabilitation: Attempts to maximize function by augmenting self care ability and mobility for patients

whose disease has been progressing, and whose functional impairments are increasing and may not be reversible.

- Palliative rehabilitation: Attempts to maintain the highest level of quality of life that is feasible in terminally ill patients by relieving symptoms (e.g., pain, dyspnea, edema) and preventing complications (e.g., contractures, decubitus ulcers). Aims to reduce dependence in mobility and self care activities in association with the provision of comfort and emotional support.

Indications and Benefit of Rehabilitation

Application of rehabilitation in hospice and palliative care settings is feasible and safe, and provides numerous benefits for both patients with cancer and noncancer illness. A systematic review of 13 studies (one randomized trial, three prospective single-armed studies of physical therapy interventions, and nine retrospective case series examining the utilization and benefits of physical therapy) examined the benefits of physical therapy interventions (mostly strengthening/therapeutic exercises, education, balance and fall-prevention training, and transfer training) in patients with a variety of life-threatening illnesses.[9] Benefits included a decrease in patient-rated musculoskeletal pain and improvements in function and performance of activities of daily living, mobility, endurance, mood, fatigue, and lymphedema.

All rehabilitation medicine's diagnostic and therapeutic effort is expended on enhancing or preserving patients' capacity for independent mobility, self care, communication, and cognition. Diseases, their treatments, and their symptoms are only relevant to the rehabilitation paradigm in the way they threaten or potentiate function. However, rehabilitation is underutilized in palliative care patients.[3] It is often thought that physical therapy and rehabilitation are not cost-effective, particularly for patients approaching the end-stage phase of their illness. However, limited evidence from randomized trials suggests that rehabilitation is cost-effective in patients with advanced cancer.[10] It is widely maintained that exercise and physical activity exacerbates fatigue although there is little evidence to support this assertion.

Current clinical practices in palliative care rehabilitation are largely based on the consensus statements for specific disease types (e.g., by the National Comprehensive Cancer Network), evidence derived from the early or acute stages of disease (e.g., aerobic conditioning during adjuvant chemotherapy), isolated case reports, and common sense. In areas where literature exists, such as acute rehabilitation of cancer patients, study cohorts are generally defined by diagnoses, rather than disease stage. Therefore uncertainty remains as to subjects' prospects for disease modification or cure and the proportion of their care delivered with palliative intent. As a result, limited inferences can be made as to the efficacy of rehabilitative interventions in far-advanced disease. At present, honest recognition of rehabilitation's incomplete evidence base in the palliative setting is the best means of preventing inappropriate adherence to therapies of equivocal benefit.

Palliative Care Interventions in Patients With Cancer

Introduction

Internationally, people often present late in their disease with limited treatment options. According to the Global Atlas of Palliative Care, it is estimated that 377 adults and 63 children out of every 100,000 of the population need palliative care. In the adult population, a cancer diagnosis constitutes one-third of the palliative care needs, while two-thirds are related to noncancer illness, such as cardiovascular disease, chronic kidney disease, dementia, HIV/AIDS, etc. In children, the major palliative care need is for noncancer conditions, with only 6% related to cancer. It is estimated that 78% of the adults and 98% of children in need of palliative care reside in low- and middle-income countries where access to palliative care is very limited.[11] The Lancet Commission report states that significant percentages of people are experiencing serious health-related suffering due to inequitable access to palliative care.[12] According to the International Association of Hospice and Palliative Care (IAHPC) 2018 definition, "Palliative care is the active holistic care of individuals across all ages with serious health-related suffering due to severe illness, and especially of those near the end of life. It aims to improve the quality of life of patients, their families and their caregivers." The 2002 World Health Organization (WHO) definition of palliative care was limited to people and their families with life-limiting illness. Therefore palliative care is not a passive approach toward illness. It is an active and holistic care that encompasses all domains of health care, that is, physical, emotional, social, and spiritual aspects of care. The aim is to improve serious health-related suffering in people with severe illness, and it is not restricted only to people with terminal illness or end-of-life care. The principal objective of palliative care provision is improvement in health-related quality of life. Moreover, the patients, their families, and caregivers are considered as a single unit and the care continues to the families and caregivers beyond the death of the patient.

Benefits of Palliative Care Referral in Patients With Cancer

A systematic review reported that palliative care in patients with advanced cancer attained improved quality of life, and that the effectiveness of palliative care intervention was more pronounced in patients when they were referred early.[13] An Italian study that assessed role of symptom control benefit of palliative care unit admission reported that the majority of symptoms were controlled within 7 days of palliative care intervention, with reduced pain, fatigue, nausea, anorexia, and breathlessness. Reduction in symptom prevalence and symptom intensity improved the quality of life.[14] Studies also showed that palliative care interventions in lung cancer improved emotional health (improved mood and reduced anxiety and depression) after 12 weeks of palliative care intervention. This effect was independent of antidepressant usage. In these studies, improvement in depressive symptoms was attributed to regular counseling and telephonic follow up that promoted adherence to antidepressants.[15,16]

There is empiric evidence to suggest that palliative care interventions influence treatment decision-making. A study in patients with non–small cell lung cancer showed that palliative care interventions positively influenced treatment decisions, and that these patients did not receive intravenous chemotherapy in the last few weeks before death.[17] Other studies demonstrate that palliative care interventions can increase prognostic awareness, end-of-life care awareness, and improving health-related communication.[18] Palliative care interventions can facilitate advance care planning, decreased intensive care unit admission and length of stay, and positively influence the course of illness and end-of-life care outcomes.[19,20] Palliative care intervention in hospitalized patients with advanced cancer also decreased intensive care unit readmission, decreased emergency room visits, and lowered health care costs. Palliative care intervention can reduce inpatient admission and inpatient deaths, decrease utilization of hospital resources, and promote death at home. Unrealistic expectations from the patients, families, or health care team can lead to unwarranted or unhelpful interventions, escalating the costs, and unnecessary utilization of limited resources and health facilities. Involving a palliative care team, discussing goals of care, and advance care planning can facilitate optimal resource utilization.[21,22] A study showed that in patients with metastatic non–small cell lung cancer, palliative care interventions led to stopping disease-modifying treatments in remaining weeks of life, transition to hospice care, hospice utilization, and provision of good end-of-life care.[17]

A study in non–small cell lung cancer showed that palliative care intervention also improved overall survival by 3 months. The improvement in survival was attributed to improvement in quality of life, better symptom control, knowledge of illness and understanding, and positive coping behaviors. In another study in patients with a mixed group of cancers, receiving palliative care intervention resulted in a survival benefit of 4 months.[23,24] Studies have shown that palliative care interventions significantly improve patient and family satisfaction of care.[25,26]

Delivery of Palliative Care

Inpatients who are either continuing to receive disease-modifying treatment or have completed disease-modifying treatment, have a good performance status, and are able to visit the outpatient department are offered ambulatory palliative care or outpatient palliative care service. Home-based palliative care is offered to patients who have poor performance status and are unable to visit outpatients, or prefer to remain at home, have stable symptoms, or wish to receive end-of-life care at home. The home-based palliative care intervention involves visit by a doctor or nurse either alone or together along with other members of the team on a needs basis. At home, patients receive medical consultation, palliative nursing interventions, including starting a syringe driver (e.g., analgesia) for patients in the terminal phase of illness, counseling, and support from volunteers. Hospice care is usually offered to patients with terminal illness, short prognosis, and where the goals of care are symptom control, comfort, and quality of life. The hospice is usually a standalone unit situated mostly outside the hospital setting where it has the infrastructure and environment to care for the dying. Inpatient palliative care is a specialized palliative care service for patients with poorly controlled symptoms or complications that require intensive management within the hospital setting. Inpatient palliative care involves rapid titration of medications either orally or parenterally for intractable symptoms, such as pain crisis, vomiting, breathlessness, delirium, and so on. It also involves managing complications like bowel obstruction, spinal cord compression, superior vena caval syndrome, etc. In the consultation liaison model, the patient is often admitted under other specialists, and palliative care providers provide consultation support for the management of physical symptoms, nursing care, or psychosocial interventions. In this integrated model of care, patients receive clinical input for disease-modifying therapies and for palliative care.

Pain Management in Patients With Advanced Cancer in a Palliative Care Setting

In a palliative care outpatient setting, the WHO analgesic step-ladder is used for cancer pain management. The WHO analgesic ladder is a simple treatment algorithm for pain management that is based on patient level of pain. Patients are treated using nonopioid analgesics such as nonsteroidal antiinflammatory drugs (NSAIDs) or paracetamol (acetaminophen) for mild pain. If the pain persists or worsens to moderate levels, a weak opioid analgesic is introduced alone or in combination with a nonopioid or adjuvant analgesic. If the pain persists or is severe, a strong opioid analgesic is introduced alone or in combination with a nonopioid or adjuvant analgesic.[27] Patients with poorly controlled cancer pain may require inpatient admission to an acute inpatient palliative care unit for rapid oral opioid titration along with adjuvants. An acute pain crisis is managed with intravenous opioid trial followed by maintenance opioid infusion. The infusions are converted to oral and transdermal preparations once stable pain relief is achieved. Patients with neuropathic pain crisis can benefit from intravenous lignocaine or ketamine bolus dosage followed by maintenance dosing until neuromodulation is achieved. Patients with cancer pain not achieving adequate pain relief with Step 3 of the WHO analgesic step-ladder may benefit from interventional pain management procedures.[28] Patients with cancer who are at end of life should have their pain assessed at least once a day. Their pain should be anticipated, and an anticipatory prescription should be provided to all patients admitted to a hospice or admitted for end-of-life care. Analgesics and doses of analgesics prescribed for pain management must be based on careful evaluation of patient pain. Doses of analgesics should be proportionate to patient pain, and response to treatment should be frequently reassessed. No attempt should be made to give a higher than required or inappropriate dose for patients who are in their end-of-life stage. As required (pro re nata [PRN], si opus sit [SOS]), orders should be prescribed to cover intermittent breakthrough pain. In the end-of-life setting, the PRN doses should be used liberally, and rapid readjustment of doses of background (round the clock) medication should occur. The administration route of analgesic delivery at end of life may also need to be changed to a subcutaneous or intravenous route, as some patients may not be able to take drugs via the oral route.[29]

Integrative Medicine Interventions in Patients With Cancer

Integrative oncology is defined as both a science and philosophy that focuses on the complexity of the health of cancer patients and proposes a multitude of approaches to accompany the conventional therapies of surgery, chemotherapy, molecular therapeutics, and radiotherapy to facilitate health.[30] Integrated oncology as a treatment model is tailor made for each patient based on their clinical history and treatments details, physical and psychologic adverse effects, spiritual belief, and family socio-economic status. CAM (Complementary and Alternative Medicine) modalities of care are integral components of integrative oncology and are terms that are commonly used to describe many kinds of products, practices, and systems that do not belong to or are not part of mainstream medicine. These CAM therapies are frequently sought out by patients and hence an understanding of these is essential for those practicing conventional medicine. It is important that clinicians explore which alternate therapies patients use to anticipate any negative or positive interactions with conventional cancer and symptom control therapies. Complementary often refers to therapies used alongside mainstream therapy and alternative refers to therapies used instead of proven medical treatment.

The four categories of CAM in health care are biochemical, lifestyle, biomechanical, and bioenergetics. According to CAM for cancer care (CAM-cancer), these therapies are classified as follows: [31,32]

1. Alternative medical systems (e.g., Ayurveda, Siddha, Unani, homeopathy, naturopathy, folk medicine)
2. Biologically based practices (e.g., naturopathy that uses food, vitamins, and herbs instead of drugs)
3. Energy medicine (e.g., Reiki, magnets, Qigong, healing touch)
4. Manipulative and body-based practices (e.g., massage, chiropractic care, osteopathy, reflexology, acupuncture, acupressure)
5. Mind-body medicine (e.g., yoga, spirituality, relaxation, art and music therapy, biofeedback, meditation, aromatherapy, deep breathing exercises, hypnosis, Tai Chi, progressive relaxation, guided imagery)

The exponential rise in cancer cases and the economic burden from out-of-pocket expenses toward cancer treatment and the late presentation with advanced stages of malignancy has prompted patients and families to look toward other modalities of treatment. A recent systematic review on CAM use in patients with cancer identified that CAM is perceived to influence cancer treatment (73.7%), treat cancer complications (62%), form part of holistic cancer treatment (57.8%), influence general health and well being (55.7%), give patients a sense of control over their therapy (45.9%), was tried by patients based on the recommendation of others (34.4%), or was tried by patients who had belief in CAM or were unsatisfied by conventional therapy (34.4%). A recent systematic review suggests that the use of CAM is increasing, with a prevalence rate of 51% in cancer patients, higher than that reported in two earlier systematic reviews, where average prevalence was 43% in 2012 and 31.4% in 1998.[33]

CAM therapies were used more often in patients with advanced cancer and those who had previously used CAM therapies. Other factors that influence CAM use include younger age, female sex, psychologic factors, higher education, and insurance coverage. Psychologic factors that associate with use of CAM therapies include anxiety, depression, increased symptom burden, poor quality of life, desire for control of treatment, and sense of trying all treatment options. The common reason cited by patients for using CAM therapy is to treat or cure their cancer, and it is perceived to fight the disease, enhance the immune response, and synergize or detoxify conventional treatment. These strategies are also commonly used as a method to reduce symptom burden and to improve quality of life during cancer disease-modifying therapy. Its noncurative benefits may include improvement in quality of life and well being, reduction of psychologic distress, addressing unmet emotional and spiritual needs, and boosting energy. Having positive illusionary beliefs about cure of cancer tends to be associated with CAM use as a positive coping and problem-solving mechanism for life-limiting illnesses. Spiritual faith and belief may influence the positive coping behavior or may indicate spiritual distress. Dissatisfaction with conventional therapy or care, poor quality of life, and patients under palliative care with progressive disease facing poor prognoses and a high symptom burden often seek health-care therapies and practitioners outside of mainstream medicine.[34]

References

1. Sakuma K, Aoi W, Yamaguchi A. Molecular mechanism of sarcopenia and cachexia: recent research advances. *Pflug Arch Eur J Physiol.* 2017;469(5–6):573–591.
2. Stanos S, Rivers W. *Physical Medicine and Rehabilitation. Elsevier.* 2014.
3. Barawid E, Covarrubias N, Tribuzio B, Liao S. The benefits of rehabilitation for palliative care patients. *Am J Hosp Palliat Care.* 2015;32(1):34–43.
4. Poduri KR. *Geriatric Rehabilitation: From Bedside to Curbside*: CRC Press; 2017.

5. McNeely ML, Dolgoy N, Al Onazi M, Suderman K. The interdisciplinary rehabilitation care team and the role of physical therapy in survivor exercise. *Clin J Oncol Nurs.* 2016;20(6):8.
6. Cohen ME, Marino RJ. The tools of disability outcomes research functional status measures. *Arch Phys Med Rehabil.* 2000;81:S21–SS9.
7. Kurtzman SH, Gardner B, Kellner WS. Rehabilitation of the cancer patient. *Am J Surg.* 1988;155(6):791–803.
8. Spence RR, Heesch KC, Brown WJ. Exercise and cancer rehabilitation: a systematic review. *Cancer Treat Rev.* 2010;36(2):185–194.
9. Putt K, Faville KA, Lewis D, McAllister K, Pietro M, Radwan A. Role of physical therapy intervention in patients with life-threatening illnesses: a systematic review. *Am J Hosp Palliat Care.* 2017;34(2):186–196.
10. Rexe K, Lammi B, von Zweck C. Occupational therapy: cost-effective solutions for changing health system needs. *Healthc Q.* 2013;16(1):69–75.
11. Connor S., Bermedo M.C. *Global Atlas of Palliative Care at the End of Life. Worldwide Palliative Care Alliance, World Health Organization*; 2014.
12. Knaul FM, Farmer PE, Krakauer EL, et al. Alleviating the access abyss in palliative care and pain relief—an imperative of universal health coverage: the Lancet Commission report. *Lancet.* 2018;391(10128):1391–1454.
13. Gaertner J, Siemens W, Meerpohl JJ, et al. Effect of specialist palliative care services on quality of life in adults with advanced incurable illness in hospital, hospice, or community settings: systematic review and meta-analysis. *Br Med J.* 2017;357:1–13.
14. Modonesi C, Scarpi E, Maltoni M, et al. Impact of palliative care unit admission on symptom control evaluated by the Edmonton Symptom Assessment System. *J Pain Symptom Manage.* 2005;30(4):367–373.
15. Jacobs JM, Greer J, El-Jawahri A, et al. The positive effects of early integrated palliative care on patient coping strategies, quality of life, and depression. *J Clin Oncol.* 2017;35(31_suppl):92.
16. Temel JS, Greer JA, Muzikansky A, et al. Early palliative care for patients with metastatic non–small-cell lung cancer. *New Eng J Med.* 2010;363(8):733–742.
17. Greer JA, Pirl WF, Jackson VA, et al. Effect of early palliative care on chemotherapy use and end-of-life care in patients with metastatic non–small-cell lung cancer. *J Clin Oncol.* 2011;30(4):394–400.
18. Jackson VA, Jacobsen J, Greer JA, Pirl WF, Temel JS, Back AL. The cultivation of prognostic awareness through the provision of early palliative care in the ambulatory setting: a communication guide. *J Palliat Med.* 2013;16(8):894–900.
19. Brinkman-Stoppelenburg A, Rietjens JA, van der Heide A. The effects of advance care planning on end-of-life care: a systematic review. *Palliat Med.* 2014;28(8):1000–1025.
20. Khandelwal N, Kross EK, Engelberg RA, Coe NB, Long AC, Curtis JR. Estimating the effect of palliative care interventions and advance care planning on ICU utilization: a systematic review. *Crit Care Med.* 2015;43(5):1102.
21. Alonso-Babarro A, Astray-Mochales J, Domínguez-Berjón F, et al. The association between in-patient death, utilization of hospital resources and availability of palliative home care for cancer patients. *Palliat Med.* 2013;27(1):68–75.
22. Gade G, Venohr I, Conner D, et al. Impact of an inpatient palliative care team: a randomized controlled trial. *Palliat Med.* 2008;11(2):180–190.
23. Bakitas MA, Tosteson TD, Li Z, et al. Early versus delayed initiation of concurrent palliative oncology care: patient outcomes in the ENABLE III randomized controlled trial. *J Clin Oncol.* 2015;33(13):1438.
24. Irwin KE, Greer JA, Khatib J, Temel JS, Pirl WF. Early palliative care and metastatic non-small cell lung cancer: potential mechanisms of prolonged survival. *Chron Respir Dis.* 2013;10(1):35–47.
25. Brumley R, Enguidanos S, Jamison P, et al. Increased satisfaction with care and lower costs: results of a randomized trial of in-home palliative care. *J Am Geriatr Soc.* 2007;55(7):993–1000.
26. Zimmermann C, Swami N, Krzyzanowska M, et al. Early palliative care for patients with advanced cancer: a cluster-randomised controlled trial. *Lancet.* 2014;383(9930):1721–1730.
27. Mercadante S, Fulfaro F. World Health Organization guidelines for cancer pain: a reappraisal. *Ann Oncol.* 2005;16(suppl_4):iv132–iv135.
28. Mercadante S, Villari P, Ferrera P, Mangione S, Casuccio A. The use of opioids for breakthrough pain in acute palliative care unit by using doses proportional to opioid basal regimen. *Clin J Pain.* 2010;26(4):306–309.
29. Qaseem A, Snow V, Shekelle P, Casey DE, Cross JT, Owens DK. Evidence-based interventions to improve the palliative care of pain, dyspnea, and depression at the end of life: a clinical practice guideline from the American College of Physicians. *Ann Intern Med.* 2008;148(2):141–146.
30. Sagar SM. Integrative oncology in North America. *J Soc Integr Oncol.* 2006;4(1):27–39.
31. Bhattacharyya P, Bishayee A. Ocimum sanctum Linn. (Tulsi): an ethnomedicinal plant for the prevention and treatment of cancer. *Anticancer Drugs.* 2013;24(7):659–666.
32. Rosenthal DS, Dean-Clower E. Integrative medicine in hematology/oncology: benefits, ethical considerations, and controversies. *Hematology Am Soc Hematol Educ Program.* 2005;2005(1):491–497.
33. Keene MR, Heslop IM, Sabesan SS, Glass BD. Complementary and alternative medicine use in cancer: A systematic review. *Complement Ther Clin Pract.* 2019;35:33–47.
34. Truant TL, Porcino AJ, Ross B, Wong M, Hilario C. Complementary and alternative medicine use in cancer: a systematic review. *J Support Oncol.* 2013;11(3):105–113.

44

Integrating Rehabilitative and Palliative Care Principles Within Acute Care Practice

SUSHMA BHATNAGAR AND SHVETA SETH

Introduction

From the time that we take our first breath, there is one thing that is inevitable and that is death. The journey from birth to death defines life, and how well it is spent defines its quality. To ensure good quality of life for our patients, we must understand palliative care and rehabilitative measures and that early integration of these measures could promote a better and complete recovery from an ailment or even a better quality of death.

Palliative Care

The World Health Organization (WHO) defines palliative care as "... an approach that improves the quality of life of patients and their families facing the problems associated with life-threatening illness, through the prevention and relief of suffering by means of early identification and impeccable assessment and treatment of pain and other problems, physical, psychosocial, and spiritual."[1]

Palliative Care in Acute Care Settings

The demand for palliative care is greater than ever before, largely driven by the increase in the aging global population and the accompanying increased burden of chronic disease, including stroke, ischemic heart disease, lung cancer, and other chronic progressive diseases—the leading causes of death globally.[2,3]

According to the *WHO Global Health Estimates,* more than 20 million people worldwide require palliative care at the end of their life every year, with the majority from the older population over 60 years of age. The major noncommunicable diseases that account for palliative care requirement are cardiovascular diseases, cancer, chronic obstructive pulmonary diseases, HIV/AIDS, and diabetes.[4] The increased burden of chronic disease that accompanies the aging population shows an alarming trend for increased palliative care requirements. This raises the question of where will all the people requiring palliative care be accommodated? Would it be at home, hospice, hospital, or communal establishment for the care of the sick? Are we future-ready to deliver these services?

Acute care hospital settings include more than one-third of inpatients who need palliative care services.[5] The requirement of such care in cancer patients is well recognized, but despite this, many cancer patients are missed by physicians[6] and die in hospitals without being identified as needing palliative care. Failure to recognize palliative needs could result in unnecessary interventions for the patient, and prolonged and inappropriate hospitalization, thereby increasing the financial stress on the patient and associated family members, thus impacting their quality of life.[7] There is a need to train health care professionals to identify patients who are facing their last stage of life and require palliative care.[8] Patients with chronic diseases often present to the hospital with acute exacerbations. At times, it becomes challenging for health care professionals to distinguish whether these deteriorations are treatable or require a palliative approach. Therefore it is very important to introduce the concepts of palliative care to all health care professionals to sensitize them to effectively deliver quality of care that embraces timely onset of palliative care when indicated.

Delivery of Palliative Care

Several models exist for the delivery of palliative care, including hospice care, care homes, community care, hospice programs in partnership with hospitals, or within acute care hospitals. Palliative care can be provided at three different levels: (a) *primary palliative care,* which refers to basic skills and knowledge acquired by all the physicians; (b) *secondary palliative care,* which refers to specialist clinicians providing consultation and specialty care; and (c) *tertiary palliative care,* which refers to an academic medical center where specialist care is provided along with academic research and the training of students and professionals.[9] The provision of secondary or tertiary levels of palliative care embraces a more comprehensive management for patients and their family members that incorporates control for physical symptoms, psychologic distress, and spiritual and financial issues during patient management.

Palliative care is conducted within the framework of interdisciplinary teamwork, which comprises physician, specialist clinician, nursing staff, social worker, physical and occupational therapist, dietitian, pharmacist, and spiritual counsellor.[10] They can provide their services on a consultative basis or be integrated within the hospital services.[11,12]

Goals of Palliative Care in the Acute Care Setting

As in other fields of medicine, palliative care clinicians aim to provide comfort to their patients, and patients and caregivers are at the center of their management plans. It is important to discuss the goals of care with patients, their family members, and caregivers. A clear communication of goals will improve patient satisfaction, avoid aggressive interventions, reduce hospitalization, and help patients deal with pending family issues or events, if any.[13] These factors contribute to better care through the end of life.

Transition or shift to palliative care also needs be addressed and studied carefully. Usually the patients are identified as palliative only a few months before death or at the final admission before death.[6] The timing and frequency of providing palliative care needs to be reviewed so that it is not seen as the last option of management. There is an urgent need to understand that if introduced early in the disease trajectory, palliative care will be more beneficial to patients.[14,15]

What Is Delivered Within a Palliative Care Pathway?

In an acute hospital environment, the intent of treatment is curative, and the majority of health care professionals are attuned to this approach of management. It is critical to integrate the knowledge of recognizing the palliative needs early in the trajectory of life-threatening diseases. Palliative care aims to manage physical symptoms, and the psychologic and spiritual needs of patients to provide maximum comfort to patients, their caregivers, and family members. Some of the most commonly experienced symptoms include pain, dyspnea, cough, nausea, vomiting, constipation, fever, anxiety, insomnia, and delirium,[16] and studies have shown better control of pain and other symptoms if the palliative approach begins along with the curative intent in the early course of disease.[17] The timing of providing palliative care is important; at the end stage of life, the focus of care should be linked with the physical symptoms and not with a specific diagnosis.[18] While managing patients with life-threatening conditions in an acute hospital setting, an early recognition of the palliative care needs of the patient is very critical. An early palliative care can help in maximizing the comfort of the patient and their caregivers.

Barriers to Palliative Care in the Acute Setting

Providing palliative care in an acute care setting, where needs of the patients are complex and varied, is challenging and many barriers may be encountered. These barriers may include the following.

The Hospital Environment

The acute hospital setting is typically an environment of curative intent, where nursing and medical staff are attuned to diagnostic tests, prescribing drugs, and therapeutic procedures, and is quite unlike hospice care.[19] The propensity to administer numerous procedures and medications, which are not actually required, places a barrier to effective palliative care. An acute setting often recognizes recovery as success and death as failure, thereby posing a hindrance to delivery of effective palliative care.

Reduced Awareness and Insufficient Knowledge

Although palliative care is gaining in much-deserved value, which is a need of the hour, there remains a dearth of awareness and knowledge amongst health care professionals. Specialist palliative care referrals are made in the hospital but are often limited to oncology patients, leaving a vast majority of noncancerous patients, especially in the older age group, requiring these specialized services.[20,21] It is important to educate nursing, allied health science, and medical students at the initial levels to sensitize them to the palliative requirements of the patient.[22,23] Working health care professionals also need to be updated regarding recent guidelines and practices for effective delivery of palliative services.[24,25]

Disease Trajectory

With the diagnosis of terminal illness patients may experience varied symptom levels up until death, as disease trajectory does not follow a straight path. There may be times when the patient deteriorates and needs hospitalization but with prompt management they can recover from an acute episode. Recovery from such acute episodes creates hope among the patients, family members, and caregivers.[26] Patients might experience such episodes repeatedly along the course of disease. Having seen patients recover from such acute episodes makes it difficult for the attending health care professionals, family members, and caregivers to recognize the terminal phase. It is important to identify transitions in the disease trajectory and to communicate this effectively to family members when the patient enters their terminal phase.[27] Knowledge in palliative care serves as a guide to making the right decision.

Lack of Advance Care Planning

A lack of advance care planning often results in situations where patients are not able to fulfill their wishes, especially their last wishes. For example, a patient may wish to spend the terminal days of life at home, or the patient may have unfinished family matters, or may be waiting to see a close relative or friend. There are many such issues that could be dealt with by having an effective advance plan of care. Patients must be encouraged to discuss their wishes with their family members so that they can attempt to fulfill these wishes. Respecting the patient's choice facilitates effective advanced planning, which is associated with more satisfied family members and caregivers.[104,105] The palliative care team must establish the goals of care and prepare in advance for the anticipated outcomes. The decision of withholding and withdrawal of treatments, consent for do not resuscitate (DNR) orders, role of parenteral feeding, diagnostic investigations, and intravenous antibiotic use are some of the points to be discussed.[106]

Rehabilitation

Palliative care is best delivered within a multidisciplinary framework that involves health care professionals from various fields, such as medicine, psychiatry, oncology, anesthesiology, neurology, and nursing, and allied health practitioners, e.g., dietitians and rehabilitation medicine specialists. The role of rehabilitation is crucial to achieving and maintaining the maximum functional capacity of the patients to help improve their quality of life.

What is Rehabilitation?

Rehabilitation is defined as "A set of measures that assist individuals, who experience or are likely to experience disability, to achieve and maintain optimum functioning in interaction with their environments."[28] Rehabilitation is provided in a variety of settings, including acute care hospitals, nursing homes, institutions, hospices, residential educational institutions, military settings, and single multiprofessional practices. Longer-term rehabilitation is also provided inside community settings and facilities, such as primary health care centers, rehabilitation centers, schools, workplaces, or homes.

Why Do We Need Rehabilitation in an Acute Care Setting?

Patients may need hospitalization due to an injury or acute illness, or an acute episode of exacerbation from a chronic illness. During the hospital stay, patients encounter reduced activity levels, decreased mobility status, and often prolonged bed rest. All these factors lead to a decrease in the patient's functional capacity, deconditioning of the body systems, and increased risk of disability. This is especially true for the patients with preexisting comorbidities or older age, and chronically ill or disabled patients.[29] The reason for hospitalization is often treated, but patients are in a worse situation due to decreased functional capacity. Given that increased levels of physical activity are associated with improved quality of life,[30,31] it therefore serves that early rehabilitation is important for a speedy and complete recovery from an acute illness or injury.

Goals of Early Rehabilitation

Rehabilitation should begin early in case of an acute illness. We must establish the goals of rehabilitation after a thorough assessment of the patient's musculoskeletal, neurologic, cardiovascular, psychologic, and functional status.[32,33] Their functional independence must be assessed, and they should be evaluated for the need of orthotic or prosthetic aids.

The goals of rehabilitation are to improve functioning, maximize recovery, achieve early mobility, minimize complications, and prevent long-term disabilities. Providing physical therapy in an acute setting can be challenging, in that therapists do not just treat a particular system or body part but rather manage the patient as a whole. The patient must be monitored for any fluctuations in their heart rate, blood pressures, oxygenation levels, pain levels, and other vital observations. After setting the goals for a prehabilitation program this must then be communicated to the treating physician, nursing staff, patients, and their family members.

Rehabilitation Interventions

To achieve the aforementioned goals of rehabilitation, the rehabilitation team or the physical therapist can make use of the following techniques/methods that consider the desired goals, patients' limitations, and abilities.

Therapeutic Exercises

Immobilization due to an acute illness can induce musculoskeletal deconditioning as a result of a decrease in the muscle mass and reduced recruitment levels.[34,35] Active exercises have been shown to improve muscle strength by increasing motor neuron recruitment and muscle mass.[36–38] Patients must be encouraged to actively move their joints and strengthen the muscles.[39] Therapeutic exercises are based on the needs of the patient and are outlined in Table 44.1. For example, if the patient has complete loss of muscle strength, passive range of motion exercises along with neuromuscular stimulation is the intervention of choice. If the patient is unable to initiate muscular contraction due to pain, neuromuscular electrical stimulation (NMES) can be used along with active-assisted exercises to prevent disuse atrophy of muscles.[40] NMES has been useful in many fields, including cardiovascular, orthopedic, neurologic, geriatric, and sports medicine and many more for improving muscle strength.[41,42] NMES is used extensively after total knee arthroplasty. Its early use in the postoperative phase has been shown to reduce the loss of quadriceps muscle strength and improve functional performance.[43]

Movement can also be promoted by using cycle ergometry either actively or passively. This enhances blood circulation and prevents bed rest complications. Studies pro-

TABLE 44.1 Types of Therapeutic Exercises

S. No.	Type of Exercise	Description of Exercise	Therapeutic Effects of Exercise
A.	**Active exercises**		
	Free Exercise	During these exercises the active muscle groups are subjected only to the force of gravity.	• Promotes relaxation • Improves neuromuscular coordination • Enhances cardiorespiratory endurance • Maintains and improves muscle power
	Assisted exercise	These exercises are assisted by an external force to compensate for inadequate muscle strength or coordination.	• Improves neuromuscular coordination • Used in early stages of neuromuscular reeducation • Helps to maintain joint mobility during painful conditions, e.g., rheumatoid arthritis
	Assisted-resisted exercise	During these exercises the active muscle groups are subjected to resistance only in a part of the range, as they are still not strong enough to endure resistance throughout the range.	• Improves neuromuscular coordination • Used in early stages of neuromuscular reeducation • Helps to maintain joint mobility during painful conditions, e.g., rheumatoid arthritis
	Resisted exercise	During these exercises the working groups of muscles are subjected to resistance systematically to develop power and endurance.	• Strengthens weak muscles • Enhances blood flow • Improves stability and coordinates
B.	**Passive Movements**		
	Relaxed passive movements	These movements are produced by an external force (by the therapist or an external device) during muscle inactivity or when the muscle strength is too low to permit active movements.	• Maintains and improves the extensibility of muscles and soft tissues • Prevents adhesion formation in the soft tissues • Stimulates kinesthetic sense hence helps to preserve memory of movement during absence of active muscle contraction • Assists in venous and lymphatic return • Promotes relaxation
	Mobilization of joints	Small repetitive oscillatory localized movements performed by the therapist.	• Improves joint play • Reduces pain • Reduces muscle spasm • Improves joint range of motion
	Manipulation of joints	These are small amplitude and high velocity movements performed by the therapist at the limit of the available range of motion of joint.	• Improves range of motion of joints • Stimulates joint receptors
	Controlled sustained stretching of tightened muscles	This involves passive stretching of the muscle and other soft tissue to increase the range of movement.	• Improves extensibility of soft tissues surrounding the joint • Reduces spasticity, e.g., after stroke

mote their early use to improve the functional status of the patient.[44,45]

Once the patient has mastered active exercises, they can be progressed by the addition of resistance. Resistance can be applied manually (by the therapist) or mechanically (using free weights, pulleys, springs, water, elastic tubing, etc.). Low-resistance strengthening exercises with high repetitions have been shown to improve muscle strength, force generation capacity, and overall physical function in patients with an acute illness or during an acute exacerbation of a chronic illness.[46,47]

When prescribing an exercise program the feasibility and safety of the exercises must also be considered. Berney et al. conducted a cohort study in which 74 patients admitted to the intensive care unit (ICU) received a protocolized rehabilitation program that began in the ICU and continued in the acute care ward for a further 8 weeks following hospital discharge to the outpatient program. The protocol included strength training, functional retraining, and cardiovascular exercises. These exercises were found to be safe and feasible for survivors of critical illness.[48]

Positioning

A comfortable position promotes the well being of the patient. Proper positioning should make the patient pain free, help to increase lung function, support the affected area or limb, and prevent bedsores.[49] Prone positioning is found to facilitate oxygenation, improve ventilation-perfusion mismatch, and enhance lung compliance and mobilization of secretions.[98,99] Positioning on the patient's side, with the affected lung on the upper side, helps to improve oxygenation of the affected lung.[100,101] Positioning can also be used in various neurologic conditions such as stroke, multiple sclerosis, and spinal cord injury to reduce abnormal tone, maintain skeletal alignment, and prevent contractures.[102,103]

Pulmonary Rehabilitation

Regular chest physiotherapy in an acute care setting helps in early recovery, reducing the dependency on mechanical ventilation and decreasing the days of hospitalization. It also helps in reducing the incidence of respiratory infection.[50] The goals of respiratory physiotherapy are to enhance lung function and lung capacities, promote secretion clearance, optimize oxygenation, and prevent ill effects of bed rest

TABLE 44.2 Pulmonary Rehabilitation Techniques

S. No.	Technique	Description	Therapeutic Effects
A.	Nonintubated Patients		
	Breathing Retraining		
	Diaphragmatic breathing	Controlled breathing with the optimal use of diaphragm and decreased used of accessory muscles.	• Decreases respiratory rate • Coordinates breathing pattern • Improves blood gases • Improves breathing efficiency • Decreases microatelectasis • Improves expansion of specific lung segments
	Pursed lip breathing	Involves controlled exhalation through lightly pursed lips.	
	Segmental breathing	Breathing exercise directed to expand specific segments of the lung.	
	Airway Clearance Techniques		
	Huffing	Frequent short expulsive bursts following a deep breath.	• Enhances removal of the secretions from airways
	Coughing	Involves deep breath followed by expiration against a closed glottis and an explosive release of air.	
	Chest percussion	Performed with cupped hands over the lung segment to be drained. Involves alternating repetitive flexion and extension at the wrist joint.	
	Vibrations	Performed by placing both the hands over the chest wall, then gently compressing and vibrating the chest wall. Applied only during the expiratory phase. Can also be done mechanically.	
	Postural drainage	Mobilizing secretions from various lung segments using postures where gravity assists in drainage.	
	Autogenic drainage	Involves mobilizing the secretions in smaller airways by breathing with low tidal volumes between the functional residual capacity and the residual volume. Followed by taking increasingly larger tidal volumes and forced expirations to transport mucus to the mouth.	

TABLE 44.2 Pulmonary Rehabilitation Techniques—cont'd

S. No.	Technique	Description	Therapeutic Effects
	Inspiratory Muscle Training		
	Inspiratory resistance exercise	Providing resistance training to inspiratory muscles using pressure or flow-based devices that resist the airflow.	• Improves endurance of respiratory muscles • Prevents alveolar collapse and atelectasis especially in postoperative patients
	Incentive spirometry	Utilizes a visual or auditory feedback to increase the inspiratory capacity by using a small handheld spirometer.	
	Reconditioning Exercises		
	Early mobilization		• Improves physical activity level • Improves cardiovascular endurance • Improves exercise tolerance • Enhances overall well being • Helps to overcome the deconditioning effects of bed rest due to acute exacerbations
	Aerobic exercises	Augmentation of energy utilization of the muscle by means of exercise program. A low intensity load at high frequency builds the aerobic capacity of muscles.	
	Strengthening exercises	A systematic procedure of a muscle or muscle group lifting, lowering or controlling loads for low number of repetitions or over a short period of time.	
	Stretching exercises	Increase extensibility of soft tissue, thereby improving range of motion and flexibility.	
B.	**Intubated Patient**		
	Manual hyperinflation (MHI)	I Involves delivering air above the baseline tidal volume using a manual resuscitation bag.	• Improves pulmonary compliance • Enhances removal of secretion • Reduces airways resistance • Promotes recruitment of collapsed segments
	Positioning	MHI and other pulmonary rehabilitation techniques are most frequently and effectively delivered with the patient in a side lying position with the affected lung uppermost.	• Facilitates oxygenation • Improves ventilation- perfusion mismatch • Enhances removal of secretions
	Manual techniques	Techniques such as chest percussion and vibrations are commonly employed.	• Enhances removal of the secretions from airways

such as atelectasis and infection.[51,52] There are various techniques utilized for pulmonary rehabilitation, and some are described in Table 44.2.

Intubated Patients

Intubated and mechanically ventilated patients are at increased risk of developing infections, barotrauma, and ventilator-associated pneumonia.[53,54] Regular pulmonary physiotherapy aims to prevent the aforesaid complications along with promoting early recovery and reduced length of hospitalization.[55] Different techniques are used in an acute care setting. Some of these include manual hyperinflation, suctioning, postural drainage, chest percussions, and vibrations. These techniques have been shown to enhance airway clearance and assist in lung inflation.[56–58]

Nonintubated Patients

Pulmonary physiotherapy in an acute setting for a nonintubated patient aims to improve lung expansion, enhance regional ventilation, reduce airway resistance, and improve pulmonary compliance. Various methods that have been used to enhance inspiratory volume include incentive spirometry, breathing exercises, inspiratory muscle training, and early mobilization.[59–62] In the acute phase, for example, the postoperative period, the techniques that enhance expiratory flow include huffing, coughing, autogenic drainage, positive pressure devices, and manually assisted coughing.[63–65] These techniques have been shown to be effective in removing secretions and improving pulmonary functions during acute exacerbations of chronic conditions like chronic bronchitis, cystic fibrosis, and other chronic obstructive pulmonary diseases. Their use is also recommended in the immediate postoperative phase to prevent pulmonary complications.[66–71]

Mobilization of the Patient

Early mobilization of the patient helps in preventing and reducing the negative effects of bed rest. It helps in improving ventilation, enhances central and peripheral perfusion levels, decreases the length of hospital stay, and reduces the risk of deep vein thrombosis by improving venous return. It also improves the overall activity and confidence level of the patient. This holds true for various orthopedic conditions, neurologic conditions, and the postoperative phase.[72–77]

We should mobilize the patient in a graded manner to prevent fall, injury, syncope, orthostatic hypotension, or a cardiovascular event. The vital signs of the patient must be monitored before, during, and after the mobilization session.[78,79]

We begin with passive or active movements within the bed, such as rolling/turning and sitting with the head end of the bed elevated, then progressing to sitting without support in the bed and sitting over the edge of the bed. As the condition improves, we progress to standing beside the bed with support and then without support. Further progression is made with chair exercises and walking.[80–83]

Speech and Swallowing Rehabilitation

In an acute phase many patients experience speech and swallowing difficulties due to the disease process itself or as a result of treatment side effects. Effective rehabilitation intervention from an early stage can prevent or lessen the adverse long-term effects.

Dysarthria is often seen in traumatic brain injury, parkinsonism, amyotrophic lateral sclerosis, multiple sclerosis, and other neurologic conditions.[87,88] The goal is to improve functional communication for the patient. We can use augmentative or alternative communication (AAC) systems that involve using techniques as simple as writing or a communication board to as complex as computer-based speech synthesis.[84–86] Consultation with other medical professionals, such as speech therapists, prosthodontists, and occupational therapists, is very often beneficial.

Patients with head and neck cancer often experience speech and swallowing difficulties.[89,90] For patients who undergo laryngectomy, esophageal speech or tracheal esophageal prosthesis are some of options for speaking after laryngectomy.[91,92] Dysphagia is common with cerebrovascular disease, traumatic brain injury, Parkinson's disease, Alzheimer's disease, and head and neck cancers.[93,95] Management of swallowing impairments include diet modification and changing the route of food intake (oral or nonoral), and the teaching of special postures, respiratory maneuvers, and therapeutic exercises.[94,96,97]

Conclusion

The role of palliative care and rehabilitative medicine must not be overlooked in an acute care setting. A timely integration of rehabilitation with the framework of acute medical management can bring major improvements in the treatment outcomes. The various rehabilitation modalities that can be utilized include therapeutic exercise, patient positioning, pulmonary rehabilitation, early mobilization, speech therapy, and occupational therapy, amongt others.

When designing a rehabilitation plan, it is crucial to consider the individualized need of every patient. Every patient is unique and the rehabilitation plan must be tailored as per their requirement. For successful rehabilitation, we must consider the patient as a whole and not focus solely on the affected system.

References

1. World Health Organization. WHO Definition of Palliative Care. Geneva: WHO. Available at http://www.who.int/cancer/palliative/definition/en
2. Bone AE, Gomes B, Etkind SN, et al. What is the impact of population ageing on the future provision of end-of-life care? Population-based projections of place of death. *Palliat Med.* 2018;32(2):329–336.
3. World Health Organization. World Health Organization fact sheet: the top 10 causes of death. Available at http://www.who.int/mediacentre/factsheets/fs310/en/index2.html. Published December 9, 2020. Accessed January 23, 2021.
4. World Health Organization. Global Health Estimates - Causes of Death 2000-2011. 2013. Available at www.who.int/healthinfo/global_burden_disease/en
5. Gardiner C, Gott M, Ingleton C, et al. Extent of palliative care need in the acute hospital setting: a survey of two acute hospitals in the UK. *Palliat Med.* 2013;27(1):76–83.
6. Tung J, Chadder J, Dudgeon D, et al. Palliative care for cancer patients near end of life in acute-care hospitals across Canada: a look at the inpatient palliative care code. *Curr Oncol.* 2019;26(1):43.
7. Detering KM, Hancock AD, Reade MC, Silvester W. The impact of advance care planning on end of life care in elderly patients: randomized controlled trial. *Br Med J.* 2010;340:c1345.
8. Gomes B, Calanzani N, Higginson IJ. Reversal of the British trends in place of death: time series analysis 2004–2010. *Palliat Med.* 2012;26(2):102–107.

9. Von Gunten CF. Secondary and tertiary palliative care in US hospitals. *JAMA*. 2002;287(7):875–881.
10. Bowen L. The multidisciplinary team in palliative care: A case reflection. *Indian J Palliat Care*. 2014;20(2):142.
11. Rosenberg M, Rosenberg L. Integrated model of palliative care in the emergency department. *West J Emerg Med*. 2013;14(6):633.
12. Mercadante S, Gregoretti C, Cortegiani A. Palliative care in intensive care units: why, where, what, who, when, how. *BMC Anesthesiol*. 2018;18(1):106.
13. Fallowfield LJ, Jenkins VA, Beveridge HA. Truth may hurt but deceit hurts more: communication in palliative care. *Palliat Med*. 2002;16(4):297–303.
14. Ferris F, Balfour H, Bowen K., et al. *A Model to Guide Hospice Palliative Care*: Ottawa: Canadian Hospice Palliative Care Association; 2013. Second Printing: June 2004. URL Updates: August 2005, Revision: September 2013.
15. Murray SA, Kendall M, Mitchell G, Moine S, Amblàs-Novellas J, Boyd K. Palliative care from diagnosis to death. *Br Med J*. 2017;356:j878.
16. Blinderman CD, Billings JA. Comfort care for patients dying in the hospital. *N Engl J Med*. 2015;373(26):2549–2561.
17. Bandieri E, Sichetti D, Romero M, et al. Impact of early access to a palliative/supportive care intervention on pain management in patients with cancer. *Ann Oncol*. 2012;23(8):2016–2020.
18. Sandgren A, Strang P. Palliative care needs in hospitalized cancer patients: a 5-year follow-up study. *Support Care Cancer*. 2018;26(1):181–186.
19. Chuah PF, Lim ML, Choo SL, et al. A qualitative study on oncology nurses' experiences of providing palliative care in the acute care setting. *Proc Singapore Healthc*. 2017;26(1):17–25.
20. Gardiner C, Cobb M, Gott M, Ingleton C. Barriers to providing palliative care for older people in acute hospitals. *Age Ageing*. 2011;40(2):233–238.
21. Dalgaard KM, Thorsell G, Delmar C. Identifying transitions in terminal illness trajectories: a critical factor in hospital-based palliative care. *Int J Palliat Nurs*. 2010;16(2):87–92.
22. Coyne P, Paice JA, Ferrell BR, Malloy P. Oncology end-of-life nursing education consortium training program: improving palliative care in cancer. *Oncol Nurs Forum*. 2007;34(4):801.
23. Robinson K, Sutton S, Gunten CF, et al. Assessment of the education for physicians on end-of-life care (EPEC™) project. *J Palliat Med*. 2004;7(5):637–645.
24. Glaetzer K, McHugh A, Parish K, Grbich C, Hegarty M, Hammond L. Dying for attention: palliative care in the acute setting. *Aust J Adv Nurs*. 2006;24(2):21.
25. Noble C, Grealish L, Teodorczuk A, et al. How can end of life care excellence be normalized in hospitals? Lessons from a qualitative framework study. *BMC Palliat Care*. 2018;17(1):100.
26. Middlewood S, Gardner G, Gardner A. Dying in hospital: medical failure or natural outcome? *J Pain Symptom Manage*. 2001;22(6):1035–1041.
27. Gott M, Ingleton C, Bennett MI, Gardiner C. Transitions to palliative care in acute hospitals in England: qualitative study. *Br Med J*. 2011;342:d1773.
28. World Health Organization. *World Report on Disability*. https://www.who.int/disabilities/world_report/2011/report.pdf. Published 2011. Accessed September 23, 2019.
29. Palmer RM. Acute hospital care of the elderly: minimizing the risk of functional decline. *Cleve Clin J Med*. 1995;62(2):117–1128.
30. Lowe SS, Watanabe SM, Baracos VE, Courneya KS. Associations between physical activity and quality of life in cancer patients receiving palliative care: a pilot survey. *J Pain Symptom Manage*. 2009;38(5):785–796.
31. Roach KE, Ally D, Finnerty B, et al. The relationship between duration of physical therapy services in the acute care setting and change in functional status in patients with lower-extremity orthopedic problems. *Phys Ther*. 1998;78(1):19–24.
32. Jette DU, Brown R, Collette N, Friant W, Graves L. Physical therapists' management of patients in the acute care setting: an observational study. *Phys Ther*. 2009;89(11):1158–1181.
33. Stucki G, Stier-Jarmer M, Grill E, Melvin J. Rationale and principles of early rehabilitation care after an acute injury or illness. *Disabil Rehabil*. 2005;27(7-8):353–359.
34. Kawahara K, Suzuki T, Yasaka T, et al. Evaluation of the site specificity of acute disuse muscle atrophy developed during a relatively short period in critically ill patients according to the activities of daily living level: a prospective observational study. *Aust Crit Care*. 2017;30(1):29–36.
35. Chambers MA, Moylan JS, Reid MB. Physical inactivity and muscle weakness in the critically ill. *Criti Care Med*. 2009;37(10):S337–S346.
36. Gabriel DA, Kamen G, Frost G. Neural adaptations to resistive exercise. *Sports Med*. 2006;36(2):133–149.
37. Keeler LK, Finkelstein LH, Miller W, Fernhall BO. Early-phase adaptations of traditional-speed vs. super slow resistance training on strength and aerobic capacity in sedentary individuals. *J Strength Cond Res*. 2001;15(3):309–314.
38. Griffin L, Cafarelli E. Resistance training: cortical, spinal, and motor unit adaptations. *Can J Appl Physiol*. 2005;30(3):328–340.
39. Troosters T, Probst VS, Crul T, et al. Resistance training prevents deterioration in quadriceps muscle function during acute exacerbations of chronic obstructive pulmonary disease. *Am J Respir Crit Care Med*. 2010;181(10):1072–1077.
40. Maffiuletti NA. Physiological and methodological considerations for the use of neuromuscular electrical stimulation. *Eur J App Physiol*. 2010;110(2):223–234.
41. Needham DM, Truong AD, Fan E. Technology to enhance physical rehabilitation of critically ill patients. *Crit Care Med*. 2009;37(10):S436–S441.
42. Zanotti E, Felicetti G, Maini M, Fracchia C. Peripheral muscle strength training in bed-bound patients with COPD receiving mechanical ventilation: effect of electrical stimulation. *Chest*. 2003;124(1):292–296.
43. Stevens-Lapsley JE, Balter JE, Wolfe P, Eckhoff DG, Kohrt WM. Early neuromuscular electrical stimulation to improve quadriceps muscle strength after total knee arthroplasty: a randomized controlled trial. *Phys Ther*. 2012;92(2):210–226.
44. Ballaz L, Fusco N, Crétual A, Langella B, Brissot R. Acute peripheral blood flow response induced by passive leg cycle exercise in people with spinal cord injury. *Arch Phys Med Rehabil*. 2007;88(4):471–476.
45. Burtin C, Clerckx B, Robbeets C, et al. Early exercise in critically ill patients enhances short-term functional recovery. *Crit Care Med*. 2009;37(9):2499–2505.
46. Heyland DK, Stapleton RD, Mourtzakis M, et al. Combining nutrition and exercise to optimize survival and recovery from critical illness: conceptual and methodological issues. *Clin Nutr*. 2016;35(5):1196–1206.
47. Troosters T, Probst VS, Crul T, et al. Resistance training prevents deterioration in quadriceps muscle function during acute exacerbations of chronic obstructive pulmonary disease. *Am J Respir Crit Care Med*. 2010;181:1072–1077.

48. Berney S, Haines K, Skinner EH, Denehy L. Safety and feasibility of an exercise prescription approach to rehabilitation across the continuum of care for survivors of critical illness. *Phys Ther.* 2012;92(12):1524–1535.
49. Johnson KL, Meyenburg T. Physiological rationale and current evidence for therapeutic positioning of critically ill patients. *Adv Crit Care.* 2009;20(3):228–240.
50. Castro AA, Calil SR, Freitas SA, Oliveira AB, Porto EF. Chest physiotherapy effectiveness to reduce hospitalization and mechanical ventilation length of stay, pulmonary infection rate and mortality in ICU patients. *Resp Med.* 2013;107(1):68–74.
51. Knight J, Nigam Y, Jones A. Effects of bedrest 1: cardiovascular, respiratory and haematological systems. *Nurs Times.* 2009;105(21):16–20.
52. Andrews J, Sathe NA, Krishnaswami S, McPheeters ML. Nonpharmacologic airway clearance techniques in hospitalized patients: a systematic review. *Resp Care.* 2013;58(12):2160–2186.
53. Anzueto A, Frutos–Vivar F, Esteban A, et al. Incidence, risk factors and outcome of barotrauma in mechanically ventilated patients. *Intensive Care Med.* 2004;30(4):612–619.
54. Konrad F, Schreiber T, Brecht-Kraus D, Georgieff M. Mucociliary transport in ICU patients. *Chest.* 1994;105(1):237–241.
55. Castro AA, Calil SR, Freitas SA, Oliveira AB, Porto EF. Chest physiotherapy effectiveness to reduce hospitalization and mechanical ventilation length of stay, pulmonary infection rate and mortality in ICU patients. *Respir Med.* 2013;107(1):68–74.
56. Denehy L, Berney S. Physiotherapy in the intensive care unit. *Phys Ther Rev.* 2006;11(1):49–56.
57. Berney S, Denehy L, Pretto J. Head-down tilt and manual hyperinflation enhance sputum clearance in patients who are intubated and ventilated. *Aust J Physiother.* 2004;50(1):9–14.
58. Pattanshetty RB, Gaude GS. Effect of multimodality chest physiotherapy in prevention of ventilator-associated pneumonia: a randomized clinical trial. *Indian J Crit Care Med.* 2010;14(2):70.
59. Westwood K, Griffin M, Roberts K, Williams M, Yoong K, Digger T. Incentive spirometry decreases respiratory complications following major abdominal surgery. *Surgeon.* 2007;5(6):339–342.
60. Possa SS, Amador CB, Costa AM, et al. Implementation of a guideline for physical therapy in the postoperative period of upper abdominal surgery reduces the incidence of atelectasis and length of hospital stay. *Rev Port Pneumol.* 2014;20(2):69–77.
61. Hulzebos EH, Helders PJ, Favié NJ, De Bie RA, de la Riviere AB, Van Meeteren NL. Preoperative intensive inspiratory muscle training to prevent postoperative pulmonary complications in high-risk patients undergoing CABG surgery: a randomized clinical trial. *JAMA.* 2006;296(15):1851–1857.
62. Holland AE, Hill CJ, Jones AY, McDonald CF. Breathing exercises for chronic obstructive pulmonary disease. *Cochrane Database Syst Rev.* 2012;10:CD008250.
63. Fink JB. *Forced expiratory technique, directed cough, and autogenic drainage. Respir Care.* 2007;52(9):1210–1223.
64. Olsén MF, Lannefors L, Westerdahl E. Positive expiratory pressure–common clinical applications and physiological effects. *Respir Med.* 2015;109(3):297–307.
65. Chatwin M, Ross E, Hart N, Nickol AH, Polkey MI, Siamonds AK. Cough augmentation with mechanical insufflation/exsufflation in patients with neuromuscular weakness. *Eur Respir J.* 2003;21(3):502–508.
66. Bellone A, Lascioli R, Raschi S, Guzzi L, Adone R. Chest physical therapy in patients with acute exacerbation of chronic bronchitis: effectiveness of three methods. *Arch Phys Med Rehab.* 2000;81(5):558–560.
67. Van der Schans CP, Prasad A, Main E. Chest physiotherapy compared to no chest physiotherapy for cystic fibrosis. *Cochrane Database Syst Rev.* 2000;2:CD001401.
68. Tang CY, Taylor NF, Blackstock FC. Chest physiotherapy for patients admitted to hospital with an acute exacerbation of chronic obstructive pulmonary disease (COPD): a systematic review. *Physiotherapy.* 2010;96(1):1–3.
69. Westerdahl E. Optimal technique for deep breathing exercises after cardiac surgery. *Minerva Anestesiol.* 2015;81(6):678–683.
70. Hanan Gaber M, Ragab EI, Bary MA, Elshazly M, Latif AFA, Beshay M. The impact of chest physiotherapy technique (CPT) on respiration, pain and quality of life post thoracic wall fixation surgery among flail chest patients (FC). *Am J Nurs Res.* 2018;6(6):471–483. doi:10.12691/ajnr-6-6-15.
71. Boden I, Skinner EH, Browning L, et al. Preoperative physiotherapy for the prevention of respiratory complications after upper abdominal surgery: pragmatic, double blinded, multicentre randomised controlled trial. *Br Med J.* 2018;360:j5916.
72. Pearse EO, Caldwell BF, Lockwood RJ, Hollard J. Early mobilisation after conventional knee replacement may reduce the risk of postoperative venous thromboembolism. *J Bone Joint Surg Am.* 2007;89(3):316–322.
73. Santos PM, Ricci NA, Suster ÉA, Paisani DM, Chiavegato LD. Effects of early mobilization in patients after cardiac surgery: a systematic review. *Physiotherapy.* 2017;103(1):1–2.
74. O'Connor ED, Walsham J. Should we mobilize critically ill patients? A review. *Crit Care Resusc.* 2009;11(4):290.
75. McWilliams DJ, Pantelides KP. Does physiotherapy led early mobilization affect length of stay on ICU. *Respir Care J.* 2008;40:5–11.
76. Stiller K, Phillips A, Lambert P. The safety of mobilization and its effect on haemodynamic and respiratory status of intensive care patients. *Physiother Theory Pract.* 2004;20(3):175–185.
77. Schaller SJ, Anstey M, Blobner M, et al. Early, goal-directed mobilisation in the surgical intensive care unit: a randomized controlled trial. *Lancet.* 2016;388(10052):1377–1388.
78. Hodgson CL, Stiller K, Needham DM, et al. Expert consensus and recommendations on safety criteria for active mobilization of mechanically ventilated critically ill adults. *Crit Care.* 2014;18(6):658.
79. Stiller K. Safety issues that should be considered when mobilizing critically ill patients. *Crit Care Clin.* 2007;23(1):35–53.
80. Cameron S, Ball I, Cepinskas G, et al. Early mobilization in the critical care unit: A review of adult and pediatric literature. *J Crit Care.* 2015;30(4):664–672.
81. Bourdin G, Barbier J, Burlem JF, et al. The feasibility of early physical activity in intensive care unit patients: a prospective observational one-center study. *Respir Care.* 2010;55(4):400–407.
82. Collings N, Cusack R. A repeated measure, randomized crossover trial, comparing the acute exercise response between passive and active sitting in critically ill patients. *BMC Anesthesiol.* 2015;15(1):1.
83. Schaller SJ, Anstey M, Blobner M, et al. Early, goal-directed mobilisation in the surgical intensive care unit: a randomised controlled trial. *Lancet.* 2016;388(10052):1377–1388.
84. Bramanti P. Augmentative and alternative communication improves quality of life in the early stages of amyotrophic lateral sclerosis. *Funct Neurol.* 2019;34(1):35–43.
85. Mackenzie C, Lowit A. Behavioural intervention effects in dysarthria following stroke: communication effectiveness, intelligibility and dysarthria impact. *Int J Lang Commun Disord.* 2007;42(2):131–153.

86. Mahler LA, Ramig LO. Intensive treatment of dysarthria secondary to stroke. *Clin Linguist Phon*. 2012;26(8):681–694.
87. Tomik B, Guiloff RJ. Dysarthria in amyotrophic lateral sclerosis: a review. *Amyotrophic Lateral Sclerosis*. 2010;11(1–2):4–15.
88. Wang YT, Kent RD, Duffy JR, Thomas JE. Dysarthria associated with traumatic brain injury: Speaking rate and emphatic stress. *J Commun Disord*. 2005;38(3):231–260.
89. Erikka Baehring BS. Postoperative complications in head and neck cancer. *Clin J Oncol Nurs*. 2012;16(6):E203.
90. Radford K, Woods H, Lowe D, Rogers SN. A UK multi-centre pilot study of speech and swallowing outcomes following head and neck cancer. *Clin Otolaryngol Allied Sci*. 2004;29(4):376–381.
91. Robertson SM, Yeo JC, Dunnet C, Young D, MacKenzie K. Voice, swallowing, and quality of life after total laryngectomy—results of the west of Scotland laryngectomy audit. *Head Neck*. 2012;34(1):59–65.
92. Finizia C, Bergman B. Health-related quality of life in patients with laryngeal cancer: a post-treatment comparison of different modes of communication. *Laryngoscope*. 2001;111(5):918–923.
93. Martino R, Foley N, Bhogal S, Diamant N, Speechley M, Teasell R. Dysphagia after stroke: incidence, diagnosis, and pulmonary complications. *Stroke*. 2005;36(12):2756–2763.
94. Cook AM, Peppard A, Magnuson B. Nutrition considerations in traumatic brain injury. *Nutr Clin Pract*. 2008;23(6):608–620.
95. Takizawa C, Gemmell E, Kenworthy J, Speyer R. A systematic review of the prevalence of oropharyngeal dysphagia in stroke, Parkinson's disease, Alzheimer's disease, head injury, and pneumonia. *Dysphagia*. 2016;31(3):434–441.
96. Logemann JA. Oropharyngeal dysphagia and nutritional management. *Curr Opin Clin Nutr Metab Care*. 2007;10(5):611–614.
97. Kulbersh BD, Rosenthal EL, McGrew BM, et al. Pretreatment, preoperative swallowing exercises may improve dysphagia quality of life. *Laryngoscope*. 2006;116(6):883–886.
98. Dirkes S, Dickinson S, Havey R, O'Brien D. Prone positioning: is it safe and effective? *Crit Care Nurs Q*. 2012;35(1):64–75.
99. Rossetti HB, Machado FR, Valiatti JL, Amaral JL. Effects of prone position on the oxygenation of patients with acute respiratory distress syndrome. *Sao Paulo Med J*. 2006;124(1):15–20.
100. Dennis DM, Jacob WJ, Samuel FD. A survey of the use of ventilator hyperinflation in Australian tertiary intensive care units. *Crit Care Resusc*. 2010;12(4):262.
101. Berney S, Denehy L, Pretto J. Head-down tilt and manual hyperinflation enhance sputum clearance in patients who are intubated and ventilated. *Aust J Physiother*. 2004;50(1):9–14.
102. Fleuren JF, Nederhand MJ, Hermens HJ. Influence of posture and muscle length on stretch reflex activity in post stroke patients with spasticity. *Arch Phys Med Rehabil*. 2006;87(7):981–988.
103. Ada L, Goddard E, McCully J, Stavrinos T, Bampton J. Thirty minutes of positioning reduces the development of shoulder external rotation contracture after stroke: a randomized controlled trial. *Arch Phys Med Rehabil*. 2005;86(2):230–234.
104. Seal M. Patient advocacy and advance care planning in the acute hospital setting. *Aust J Adv Nurs*. 2007;24(4):29.
105. Jethwa KD, Onalaja O. Advance care planning and palliative medicine in advanced dementia: a literature review. *Br J Psych Bulletin*. 2015;39(2):74–78.
106. You JJ, Fowler RA, Heyland DK. Just ask: discussing goals of care with patients in hospital with serious illness. *CMAJ*. 2014;186(6):425–432.

SECTION 6

Perioperative/Periprocedural Care of the Pediatric Patients With Cancer

45

Overview of Pediatric Cancers

SANA MOHIUDDIN, WAFIK ZAKY, AND JOSE CORTES

Introduction

The incidence of childhood cancer has been steadily increasing over the last few decades, from approximately 13 per 100,000 in 1975 to over 17 per 100,000 in 2005. While pediatric malignancies account for only 1% of all cancers diagnosed each year, cancer is the leading cause of death by disease in children aged 1–19 years. In the United States alone, each year an estimated 15,780 children and adolescents are diagnosed with cancer, and more than 40,000 children require cancer treatment.[1] Despite the improvement in the cure rate, approximately 12% of children diagnosed with cancer do not survive, and cancer remains responsible for more deaths (57%) than all other diseases combined in children.[2]

The incidence rate of cancer in children varies between races, with Caucasians followed by Hispanics having the highest incidence, while African Americans have the lowest incidence.[1] Incidence rates also vary between high- and low-income countries. Countries with the lowest income have fewer medical resources, lack advanced diagnostic tools, and have limited access to cancer therapy. In addition, these countries have higher environmental exposures such as secondhand tobacco exposure, carcinogens in air pollution such as asbestos and silica dust, and unpurified water containing traces of carcinogens. The incidence of cancer in children also varies according to age and sex. Overall, leukemia is the most common cancer among children and adolescents, while neuroblastoma, Wilms tumor, and retinoblastoma predominate in infancy.[2] Pediatric cancers, except for Wilms tumor, are slightly predominant in males.[3] Fig. 45.1 shows rhe common pediatric malignancies and their incidence.

The majority of pediatric cancers have no known cause or risk factor, and only 10% can be linked to a familial or genetic factor.[4] Specific prenatal and postnatal exposures have also been implicated in some childhood cancers.[5] While a wide range of environmental agents has been thought to be oncogenic, thus far, only prior chemotherapy and high-dose radiation have been proven to be causal.[3] Certain genetic and inherited conditions, such as Downs syndrome, Li Fraumeni syndrome, Beckwith-Wiedmann syndrome, neurofibromatosis, and cancer predisposition syndromes, have a higher risk of particular malignancies, requiring these patients to be screened for these malignancies periodically (Fig. 45.1).[4]

The survival rates of pediatric malignancies have improved significantly over the past 50 years, from less than 40% to as high as 80%. The mainstay of treatment for pediatric solid tumors (neural or nonneural) is chemotherapy for the overall reduction in tumor burden, along with a modality of local control. Local control is often achieved by surgical resection, radiation therapy, or a combination of both. The primary survival contributors have been early diagnosis and significant discoveries of new chemotherapeutic agents, which now constitute the standards of care for most of these malignancies.

Tables 45.1 and 45.2 summarize the classes of chemotherapy and radiotherapy for cancer treatment modalities, respectively.

The field of surgical oncology has also undergone significant advances over the last few decades, with a shift in focus to finding surgical procedures with maximal therapeutic impact while limiting late effects on quality of life, which has improved outcomes.[6] Unfortunately, many children who survive cancer still suffer from long-term sequelae of cancer treatments, with conditions such as mental disabilities, organ dysfunction, and secondary cancers. Developing more innovative and less damaging therapies is therefore crucial for pediatric malignancies. Cancers that are metastatic at diagnosis, those that do not respond to standard treatment, or progress/relapse despite appropriate treatment have poor survival rates (<20%).

Acute Lymphoblastic Leukemia

Acute lymphoblastic leukemia (ALL) is the most common cancer diagnosis in children. It accounts for 20% of all cancers diagnosed in children and young adults.[7] An estimated 3000 new cases of childhood ALL are diagnosed each year in the United States. After a peak incidence of 90 cases per million per year at the age of 2–3 years, ALL incidence rates decrease steadily into adolescence. Initial complete remission rates are achieved in 95% of patients. Survival in childhood ALL is approaching 90% through the application of reliable prognostic factors permitting risk-stratification-based treatment protocols.[8] Unfortunately, relapse occurs in approximately 20% of cases, with higher relapse rates in

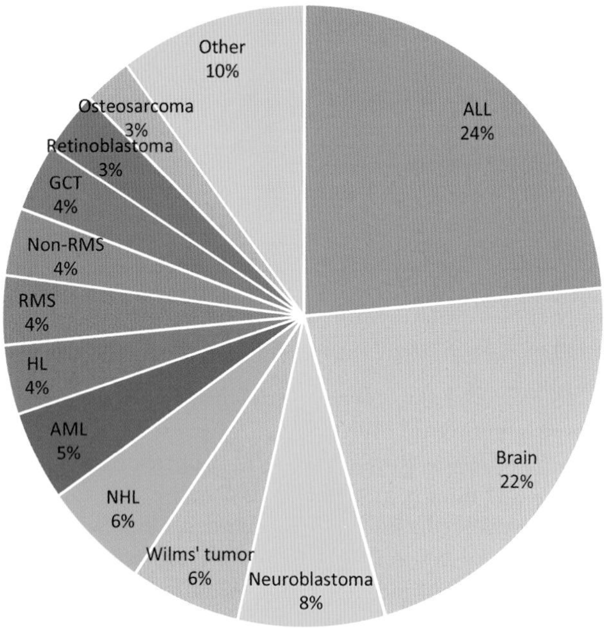

• **Fig 45.1** Pediatric malignancies, percentage distribution. *ALL*, Acute lymphoblastic leukemia; *AML*, acute myeloid leukemia; *GCT*, giant cell tumor; *HL*, Hodgkin's lymphoma; *NHL*, non-Hodgkin's lymphoma; *RMS*, rhabdomyosarcoma.

older patients and infants less than 1 year of age. The standard of care therapy for ALL is based on different phases and spans a total duration of 2–3 years of chemotherapeutic regimens. Traditionally, risk stratification is based on patient age, leukemic blast count at diagnosis, and high-risk genetic markers (e.g., BCR-ABL fusion or MLL rearrangement). Despite excellent outcomes overall, patients with relapsed ALL outnumber nearly all other childhood malignancies. With traditional intensive combination chemotherapy and allogeneic hematopoietic stem cell transplantation, 30%–40% of all children with relapsed ALL can be cured.[8]

Acute Myeloid Leukemia

Acute myeloid leukemia (AML) is the second most common type of leukemia in children, accounting for 15% of cases.[8] It has a bimodal pattern of incidence, with most patients either being diagnosed in the first 2 years of life or during teenage years. Unfortunately, survival is poorer than that for ALL, with approximately two-thirds of patients surviving for at least 5 years.[8] AML is associated with chromosomal abnormalities, including translocations (e.g., PML-RARA t15;17), gain or loss of chromosomes (chromosome 16), and other abnormalities (FLT3, MLL).[9] The disease is characterized by leukemic cells proliferating in the bone marrow, which then interferes with the production

TABLE 45.1 Classes of Chemotherapy Agents Used in Treatment of Childhood Cancers and Mechanisms of Action

Chemotherapy Class	Drug	Mechanism of Action
Antimetabolites		
Antifolates	Methotrexate	Inhibition of dihydrofolate reductase (DHFR)
Purine antagonists	Cytarabine, 5-fluorouracil, gemcitabine	Addition of faulty purine analogs between DNA base pairs
Pyrimidine antagonists	Fludarabine	Addition of faulty pyrimidine analogs between DNA base pairs
Purine analog	6-Mercaptopurine	Inhibition of DNA polymerase leading to DNA breaks
Tubular interactive agents		
Vinca alkaloids	Vincristine, vinblastine	Destruction of tubulin in microtubules leading to mitotic arrest
Alkylating agents		
Oxazaphosphorines	Cyclophosphamide, ifosfamide	Intercalate DNA double strand
Nitrogen mustards	Busulfan, melphalan	Intercalate DNA double strand
Platinum complexes	Cisplatin, carboplatin	Intercalate DNA double strand
Topoisomerase inhibitors		
Topoisomerase I inhibitors	Topotecan, irinotecan	Single-strand DNA breaks from inhibition of topoisomerase I
Topoisomerase II inhibitors	Etoposide	Double-strand DNA breaks from inhibition of topoisomerase II
Anthracyclines	Doxorubicin, daunorubicin	Formation of free radicals that lead to DNA breaks
Antibiotics	Bleomycin, actinomycin	
Enzymes	L-Asparaginase	Cleavage of amino acid L-asparagine
Tyrosine kinase inhibitors	Imatinib, dasatinib	Prevent activation and phosphorylation of tyrosine kinase

TABLE 45.2 Type of Radiation Therapy Used in Pediatric Cancers and Their Characteristics

Photon Therapy	Proton Therapy
X-ray, a source of energy without mass	Heavy part of the atom
Higher entrance and exit dose	Relatively low entrance dose, no exit dose
Scattered spillage beyond the tissue/region of interest	Ability to tailor peak intensity in target tissue, and minimal spillage beyond tissue of interest
Higher dose and gradual dose gradient in tissue	Lower dose and steep dose gradient in tissue
Heterogeneous dose within the tumor	Homogeneous dose within the tumor
Increased risk of second malignancies and late effect	Very sensitive to tumor motion regression
Lower cost	Much higher cost

of normal blood cells, leading to infections, bleeding, and other symptoms and complications. Similar to ALL, treatment risk grouping is based on molecular findings and the response to induction treatment. The relapse rate is high, with approximately 30% of children relapsing in the first 5 years. Treatment depends on the subtype and usually has a shorter duration but higher intensity than that of ALL. Most patients with relapsed disease are considered for stem cell transplantation.

Pediatric Lymphomas

Lymphomas are the third most common cancers in children. Hodgkin's lymphoma and non-Hodgkin's lymphoma are the main types of lymphoma in this age group. The most common presentation is painless lymphadenopathy with or without other symptoms such as fever, night sweats, and weight loss (known as B symptoms).

Hodgkin's lymphoma is the most common type of lymphoma in children and is the most common malignancy that affects adolescents between 15 and 19 years of age.[10] Non-Hodgkin's lymphoma in children is usually of high-grade nature, with Burkitt's lymphoma being an aggressive subtype. Both Hodgkin's lymphoma and non-Hodgkin's lymphoma can present as mediastinal masses. Lymphomas in the anterior mediastinum may risk significant respiratory or cardiovascular embarrassment (see Chapter 47). The role of surgery in the management of mediastinal masses depends on the primary diagnosis, the need for immediate decompression of vital organs, and the sensitivity of the tumor to chemotherapy or radiotherapy.

Bone Sarcomas

Osteosarcoma and Ewing sarcoma are the two most common malignant bone tumors in children and adolescents, with osteosarcoma being the most common. The peak incidence of osteosarcoma is around the growth spurt during adolescence and is rare before 5 years of age. Ewing sarcoma has a peak incidence in the preadolescent years. Both bone tumors present with pain and swelling. Diagnosis is usually delayed by 2–3 months, secondary to confusing it with sports-related injuries. The most common location for osteosarcoma is the metaphyseal region of the long bones, most commonly the femur. While the majority of Ewing sarcomas also arise from long bones, they mainly involve the diaphysis. Ewing sarcoma may also develop from the axial skeleton-like pelvis and chest wall, and very rarely from soft tissue.

Both tumors have different risk factors. Osteosarcoma is strongly associated with specific genetic syndromes, such as Li-Fraumeni syndrome, NF1, and Bloom syndrome. Ewing sarcoma has a strong racial predilection and is primarily seen in Caucasians, with almost none in children of African descent.

Bone cancer is diagnosed by biopsy. Open biopsy is preferred over core biopsy to obtain the highest chance of an accurate diagnosis. Magnetic resonance imaging (MRI) of the affected area may help determine the tumor size, the extent of local invasion into the soft tissue and neurovascular bed, and guide the surgeon during biopsy. Computed tomography (CT) of the chest is required to rule out metastatic pulmonary disease, and positron emission tomography (PET) helps diagnose distant metastasis. Ewing sarcoma can metastasize to the bone marrow; therefore bone marrow aspiration and biopsy are required for staging.[11]

The treatment of these sarcomas includes neoadjuvant chemotherapy followed by resection of the primary tumor and adjuvant chemotherapy, with or without radiation. Ewing sarcoma is more sensitive to radiation than osteosarcoma.

Historically, local control of bone cancer has been attempted by amputation of the affected extremities. However, with advancements in surgical approaches, innovation in prostheses, and better disease control with chemotherapy, the management of bone tumors has changed dramatically. Limb salvage surgery is the procedure of choice for most patients, along with endoprosthetic reconstructive surgery with allograft or autograft.[12] For adolescents who have not reached or are in their growth spurt, expandable prostheses are now available to avoid leg length discrepancy. Rotationplasty is another recent surgical technique for patients with above-the-knee amputation. It is an excellent option for patients aspiring to return to sports. In rotation-plasty, after above-the-knee amputation, the ankle joint is rotated 180 degrees and attached to function as a knee joint. A below-the-knee prosthesis is then applied to complete the restoration.

For Ewing sarcoma of the axial skeleton, the surgical approach for local control depends on the location, extent of disease, and presence of metastatic disease. Hemipelvectomy for pelvic tumors and rib resection for chest wall tumors are the standard therapeutic options. In patients with nonresectable tumors, radiation therapy is an effective option for Ewing sarcoma but is not indicated for osteosarcoma. Radiotherapy is only used for emergent situations such as cord compression or palliative treatment in patients with intractable pain.

Rhabdomyosarcoma

Rhabdomyosarcoma is the most common soft tissue sarcoma in the pediatric population, with a slight male predominance; it occurs more commonly in the first decade of life. Rhabdomyosarcoma accounts for 4.5% of all pediatric malignancies. Rhabdomyosarcoma is a heterogeneous tumor with distinct histologic subtypes that affects the prognosis of patients. Approximately half of rhabdomyosarcomas arise from skeletal muscle.

Any part of the body can be affected by rhabdomyosarcoma, including the orbit, head, neck, parameningeal space, and extremities. For extensive disease or metastatic spread at presentation, it is essential to discern the primary disease site to inform treatment decisions and prognosis. Patients are stratified into low, intermediate, and high risk based on histology, location of the primary tumor, extent of the disease, nodal involvement, and metastatic spread. In addition, four groups are formed based on how resectable the cancer is and the resection status of the tumor (residual disease postsurgical).

The overall survival rate for nonmetastatic disease is close to 70%. The treatment involves a combination of systemic chemotherapy and surgery, with or without radiation, for local control. For tumors that are considered resectable with negative margins, surgery is preferred before chemotherapy.[13] For large tumors surrounding vital or neurovascular structures, chemotherapy is preferred before surgery to reduce the disease mass and make it surgically resectable. After resection, all patients with any residual tumor, positive margins on resection, or suspicious lymph node involvement receive adjuvant radiation. For patients in whom complete resection was not achieved during the first surgery and radiation is not an option due to age or site of disease, a second-look surgery can be considered to achieve cure.[14]

Solid-Organ Tumors: Wilms Tumor and Hepatoblastoma

Wilms tumor is the most common primary malignant tumor of the kidney in children. The mean age at diagnosis is 3 years, and the prognosis is generally very good with current treatment modalities. The most common presentation is a painless abdominal mass palpated by a caregiver during bathing. Uncommonly, it also presents with hematuria and hypertension. The diagnosis is based on abdominal MRI, which provides information regarding tumor size, extent, proximity to surrounding structures, and the contralateral kidney's involvement.

Surgery is the mainstay of treatment. Biopsy of the tumor without resection is not recommended because of the upstaging of cancer secondary to local spread from capsule break. The most common surgical procedure performed for a unilateral Wilms tumor is radical nephrectomy, which includes the whole kidney, ureter, fatty pad around the kidney, and lymph node sampling. Postsurgical chemotherapy is administered to the majority of patients to reduce the risk of recurrence.[15]

In cases where the tumor has spilled from the renal capsule or the tumor is believed to be unresectable, preoperative chemotherapy is administered to control the local spread or shrinking the mass to improve resectability. Preoperative chemotherapy is used in bilateral Wilms tumors to salvage any functional kidney. When such a salvage procedure is not possible or fails, bilateral radical nephrectomy with renal transplant is the only option available.[15]

Hepatoblastoma is the most common liver malignancy in pediatric patients. This rare tumor is a disease of early childhood. Like Wilms tumor, hepatoblastoma has been associated with overgrowth syndromes such as Beckwith-Weidemann syndrome and familial adenomatous polyposis.[16] Most patients present with an asymptomatic abdominal mass. However, in some patients, anorexia and weight loss might be seen due to the mass effect of an enlarging tumor.[16] Although hepatoblastoma arises from the liver, elevated liver enzymes and liver dysfunction are rarely seen. Alpha-fetoprotein, a tumor marker, is elevated in most patients and can serve as a marker for disease persistence and treatment monitoring.[17] The use of imaging is standard for diagnosis; MRI of the abdomen is helpful to evaluate the disease extension, and CT of the chest is helpful to assess for metastatic pulmonary disease. Biopsy is usually indicated for diagnosis. If the tumor is thought to be resectable, attempts are made for complete resection. Historically, surgery with resection alone was the treatment for these tumors, but we now know that chemotherapy plays a significant role in curing hepatoblastoma, along with surgery.[18] For most tumors, a course of preoperative and postoperative chemotherapy is indicated.

Central Nervous System Tumors

Central nervous system tumors are the most common solid tumors in children. There have been significant advances in managing children with central nervous system tumors in the past few decades, but these are still associated with high morbidity and mortality rates. It is estimated that in the United States, 4700 new patients are diagnosed with central nervous system tumors annually, with the majority being malignant. Juvenile pilocytic astrocytoma is the most common central nervous system neoplasm, while medulloblastoma is the most common central nervous system malignant tumor.[19] The most common presentation is increased intracranial pressure, manifested by headache, vomiting, and altered mental status. Depending on the tumor location, patients may have motor weakness, sensory changes, seizures, or cranial nerve neuropathies. The incidence varies with age, with younger patients mostly having tumors of embryonal origin and older children having tumors of glial origin. However, overall survival has improved in the last few decades due to advances in chemotherapy, radiation therapy, and surgical techniques.

A gross total resection is performed whenever safe and feasible. Chemotherapy and radiation therapy are typically administered following surgery for malignant tumors, except for chemoresistant tumors such as ependymoma. Local spread, such as leptomeningeal disease, is seen in some tumors such as embryonal neoplasms (medulloblastoma), while metastatic spread outside the neuraxis is uncommon. For benign tumors such as low-grade gliomas, surgery is the standard of care if feasible, and chemotherapy is reserved for nonresectable or progressive tumors.[19] Radiation therapy is an effective adjuvant therapy for malignant central nervous system tumors and refractory central nervous system neoplasms. Some malignant central nervous system neoplasms with high neuraxis metastatic predilection also receive craniospinal radiation and focal radiation. The favored treatment modality is proton radiation, which is associated with fewer late effects in children younger than 10 years of age.[20]

Preoperative Care for the Pediatric Patient With Cancer

The advancement of new oncologic treatments, including chemotherapy, radiotherapy, immunotherapy, and targeted therapy, has brought more children to the operating/procedure room than ever before. Numerous procedures are performed in the operating/procedure room, including the following:

- Primary tumor resection of solid tumors.
- Secondary tumor resection (e.g., lung metastasis in Ewing sarcoma).
- Gastrostomy tube placement to facilitate enteral nutrition.
- Ventriculoperitoneal shunt placement for hydrocephalus in patients with central nervous system tumors.
- Central line placement for chemotherapy.
- Ommaya placement for interventricular chemotherapy delivery for central nervous system tumors and leukemia.
- Palliative procedures such as chordotomy in patients with severe pain related to their tumor or chest tube placement for malignant pleural effusion.

Prior to any procedure, the surgeon and the anesthesiologist need to be familiar with the pathophysiologic effects of cancer, side effects of chemotherapy, radiotherapy, immunotherapy, and their interactions with anesthetics. Chemotherapeutic agents affect every organ system but affect the gastrointestinal tract, bone marrow, and lymphoreticular system most severely.[21] The most common side effects of chemotherapeutic agents are nausea, vomiting, mucosal irritation, and bone marrow suppression (Table 45.1). The team involved in the care of these patients needs to understand the previous chemotherapeutic agents and doses administered to plan for any expected toxicity or side effect.[21] Radiation therapy also produces skin reactions that include inflammation, necrosis, and fibrosis that can compromise wound healing.

Every cancer patient should undergo a thorough assessment with a detailed medical history and a physical examination, emphasizing the patient's functional status before any procedure. The medical history should include the type and location of the cancer, prior medical treatment, total doses received, date of previous therapy, a list of all medications taken within the last 6 months, a history of glucocorticoid administration, and a history of all allergies. This assessment should have all the elements considered essential to ensure safety, as outlined by the American Society of Anesthesiologists (ASA) guidelines of preanesthetic evaluation of patients.[22] All patients should have basic laboratory testing. Patients with complex preexisting conditions should have a thorough preoperative laboratory workup and blood cross-matched.[23] A complete blood count should ideally have a platelet count of more than 50,000/mm^3 to prevent excessive bleeding and a hemoglobin concentration of more than 8.5 g/dL. The indication for transfusions should be based on expected surgical bleeding and patients' cardiorespiratory function. Coagulation studies should be performed as part of the screening for bleeding diathesis before invasive procedures. A full electrolyte panel should be obtained because electrolyte abnormalities and kidney dysfunction are common in pediatric oncology patients secondary to chemotherapy administration and dehydration. Patients who have received anthracyclines require a preoperative electrocardiogram (ECG) to rule out cardiac toxicity. Patients with ST-wave changes, decreased QRS voltage, or arrhythmias on their ECG should have an echocardiogram. Chest radiographs should be obtained, especially in patients with symptoms of cough, dyspnea, orthopnea, respiratory distress, and any patient with an abnormal physical examination and history of lung exposure to toxic chemotherapy such as bleomycin has a high likelihood of producing respiratory side effects.

The fasting (nil per os, NPO) guidelines for pediatric patients with cancer are the same as those for healthy pediatric patients (Table 45.3). However, investigators have found

TABLE 45.3 Fasting Guidelines for Pediatric Cancer Patients

Oral Intake	Time Prior to Procedure
Rich protein and fat meals	8 h
Formula, milk, or carbohydrate light meal	6 h
Breast milk	4 h
Clear liquids	2 h

that 1 h of fasting for clear liquids is sufficient for elective pediatric general anesthesia on the premise of no increased risk for pulmonary aspiration.[24,25] Most orally or intravenously administered medications are continued on the day of surgery, especially anticonvulsants, gastrointestinal reflux prophylaxis, and asthma medications. Anticoagulants should be withheld according to recommended guidelines before any procedure.[26] Age of the patient, grade ≥III ASA, history of prematurity, and break in fasting guidelines are independent risk factors to predict extended postoperative ICU admission and risk of mortality in pediatric patients.[27]

It is essential to make the need for a procedure or surgical operation a stress-free experience or at least decrease the anxiety to the minimum because most of the patients will require numerous other interventions in the future. It is essential to meet with the patient and family to explain the procedure in lay terms and answer their questions. The help of a child life specialist to bring information to the child at an age-appropriate level should be considered. The use of distraction techniques, music, electronic games, and videos are also good resources.[28] The use of sedatives prior to induction of anesthesia should be individualized to the child's previous experiences and parental expectations. The presence of a parent during induction of anesthesia is an alternative and an adjunct to premedication that works very well in decreasing patient anxiety. The presence of pain should be addressed using an analgesic prior to the induction of anesthesia. Gastrointestinal prophylaxis with an antihistamine-2 blocker should be considered in all patients who have received recent glucocorticoids for longer than 2 weeks. In addition, patients with recent steroid exposure should be supplemented with a stress dose of hydrocortisone to prevent potential adrenal insufficiency. If pharmacologic premedication is needed to induce anesthesia, midazolam, ketamine, or a combination of midazolam, ketamine, or dexmedetomidine are suggested.[29,30]

The Role of Pediatric Critical Care Unit in Preoperative Care

There are several specific situations in pediatric oncology that warrant admission to the pediatric critical care unit for preoperative stabilization and monitoring. Examples include:

- A pediatric patient with a mediastinal tumor is a candidate for monitoring in the pediatric intensive care unit. These patients may present with nonspecific symptoms such as fever, fatigue, dyspnea, cough, orthopnea, and respiratory distress that can be misdiagnosed as a common respiratory illness.[31] Evaluation for possible airway or vascular embarrassment is needed prior to any sedative administration for radiologic or surgical procedures (see Chapter 47).
- Patients with a primary or secondary brain tumor or patients with radiation-induced vasogenic edema and/or necrosis and elevated intracranial pressure should be monitored in an intensive care unit environment. CT scan or MRI with perfusion imaging scanning may help to differentiate radiation edema or necrosis from real progression.[32] In either case, patients may need management for raised intracranial pressure with high-dose steroids (e.g., dexamethasone 2 mg/kg loading dose) and hyperosmolar therapy with mannitol (1 mg/kg IV followed by 0.25–0.5 mg/kg every 6 h) or hypertonic saline (5 mL/kg IV followed by a continuous infusion of 0.1–1 mL/kg/h titrated to keep serum sodium between 150–155 mEq/L).[33] Mannitol has a blood viscosity reduction effect (an immediate effect that lasts up to 70 min) and an osmotic effect (onset of effect in 15–30 min that lasts up to 6 h). Mannitol should be discontinued if serum osmolality is >320 mOsm/L.[34] Hypertonic saline (3%–5%) has an osmotic effect on brain tissue. Hypertonic saline should be paused or discontinued if serum osmolality is >360 mOsm/L. Significant intraoperative blood loss and the need for mechanical intubation upon return to the pediatric intensive care unit are predictive of prolonged length of stay after craniotomy for tumor resection.[35]

References

1. Barbel P, Peterson K. Recognizing subtle signs and symptoms of pediatric cancer. *Nursing*. 2015;45(4):30–37 quiz 37–8.
2. Kaatsch P. Epidemiology of childhood cancer. *Cancer Treat Rev*. 2010;36(4):277–285.
3. Spector LG, Pankratz N, Marcotte EL. Genetic and nongenetic risk factors for childhood cancer. *Pediatr Clin North Am*. 2015;62(1):11–25.
4. Saletta F, Dalla Pozza L, Byrne JA. Genetic causes of cancer predisposition in children and adolescents. *Transl Pediatr*. 2015;4(2):67–75.
5. Sommelet D, Lacour B, Clavel J. Epidemiology of childhood cancer. *Bull Acad Natl Med*. 2003;187(4):711–737; discussion 738–41.
6. Veronesi U, Stafyla V. Grand challenges in surgical oncology. *Front Oncol*. 2012;2:127.
7. Siegel DA, Henley SJ, Li J, Pollack LA, Van Dyne EA, White A. Rates and trends of pediatric acute lymphoblastic leukemia—United States, 2001–2014. *MMWR Morb Mortal Wkly Rep*. 2017;66(36):950–954.
8. Cooper SL, Brown PA. Treatment of pediatric acute lymphoblastic leukemia. *Pediatr Clin North Am*. 2015;62(1):61–73.
9. Hageman IM, Peek AM, de Haas V, Damen-Korbijn CM, Kaspers GJ. Value of routine bone marrow examination in pediatric acute myeloid leukemia (AML): a study of the Dutch Childhood Oncology Group (DCOG). *Pediatr Blood Cancer*. 2012;59(7):1239–1244.
10. Allen CE, Kelly KM, Bollard CM. Pediatric lymphomas and histiocytic disorders of childhood. *Pediatr Clin North Am*. 2015;62(1):139–165.
11. Jackson TM, Bittman M, Granowetter L. Pediatric malignant bone tumors: a review and update on current challenges, and emerging drug targets. *Curr Probl Pediatr Adolesc Health Care*. 2016;46(7):213–228.
12. Bernstein M, Kovar H, Paulussen M, et al. Ewing's sarcoma family of tumors: current management. *Oncologist*. 2006;11(5):503–519.

13. Panda SP, Chinnaswamy G, Vora T, et al. Diagnosis and management of rhabdomyosarcoma in children and adolescents: ICMR consensus document. *Indian J Pediatr*. 2017;84(5):393–402.
14. Borinstein SC, Steppan D, Hayashi M, et al. Consensus and controversies regarding the treatment of rhabdomyosarcoma. *Pediatr Blood Cancer*. 2018;65(2).
15. Bhatnagar S. Management of Wilms' tumor: *NWTS vs SIOP*. *J Indian Assoc Pediatr Surg*. 2009;14(1):6–14.
16. Herzog CE, Andrassy RJ, Eftekhari F. Childhood cancers: hepatoblastoma. *Oncologist*. 2000;5(6):445–453.
17. Czauderna P, Lopez-Terrada D, Hiyama E, Häberle B, Malogolowkin MH, Meyers RL. Hepatoblastoma state of the art: pathology, genetics, risk stratification, and chemotherapy. *Curr Opin Pediatr*. 2014;26(1):19–28.
18. Hiyama E. Pediatric hepatoblastoma: diagnosis and treatment. *Transl Pediatr*. 2014;3(4):293–299.
19. Davidoff AM. Pediatric oncology. *Semin Pediatr Surg*. 2010; 19(3):225–233.
20. Knab B, Connell PP. Radiotherapy for pediatric brain tumors: when and how. *Expert Rev Anticancer Ther*. 2007;7(12 Suppl): S69–S77.
21. MacKenzie JR. Complications of treatment of paediatric malignancies. *Eur J Radiol*. 2001;37(2):109–119.
22. Apfelbaum JL, Connis RT, Nickinovich DG, et al. Committee on Standards and Practice Parameters; American Society of Anesthesiologists Task Force on Preanesthesia Evaluation. Practice advisory for preanesthesia evaluation: an updated report by the American Society of Anesthesiologists Task Force on Preanesthesia Evaluation. *Anesthesiology*. 2012;116(3):522–538.
23. Yang MM, Singhal A, Au N, Hengel AR. Impact of preoperative laboratory investigation and blood cross-match on clinical management of pediatric neurosurgical patients. *Childs Nerv Syst*. 2015;31(4):533–539.
24. Thomas M, Morrison C, Newton R, Schindler E. Consensus statement on clear fluids fasting for elective pediatric general anesthesia. *Paediatr Anaesth*. 2018;28(5):411–414.
25. Schmidt AR, Buehler P, Seglias L, et al. Gastric pH and residual volume after 1 and 2 h fasting time for clear fluids in children. *Br J Anaesth*. 2015;114(3):477–482.
26. Lerman J. Preoperative assessment and premedication in paediatrics. *Eur J Anaesthesiol*. 2013;30(11):645–650.
27. Lian C, Xie Z, Wang Z, et al. Pediatric preoperative risk factors to predict postoperative ICU admission and death from a multicenter retrospective study. *Paediatr Anaesth*. 2016;26(6):637–643.
28. Mainer JA. Nonpharmacological interventions for assisting the induction of anesthesia in children. *AORN J*. 2010;92(2): 209–210.
29. Kain ZN, MacLaren J, McClain BC, et al. Effects of age and emotionality on the effectiveness of midazolam administered preoperatively to children. *Anesthesiology*. 2007;107(4):545–552.
30. Funk W, Jakob W, Riedl T, Taeger K. Oral preanaesthetic medication for children: double-blind randomized study of a combination of midazolam and ketamine *vs* midazolam or ketamine alone. *Br J Anaesth*. 2000;84(3):335–340.
31. Singh AK, Sargar K, Restrepo CS. Pediatric mediastinal tumors and tumor-like lesions. *Semin Ultrasound CT MR*. 2016;37(3):223–237.
32. Brandes AA, Tosoni A, Spagnolli F, et al. Disease progression or pseudoprogression after concomitant radiochemotherapy treatment: pitfalls in neurooncology. *Neuro Oncol*. 2008;10(3):361–367.
33. Kim H, Lee JM, Park JS, et al. Dexamethasone coordinately regulates angiopoietin-1 and VEGF: a mechanism of glucocorticoid-induced stabilization of blood–brain barrier. *Biochem Biophys Res Commun*. 2008;372(1):243–248.
34. Mortazavi MM, Romeo AK, Deep A, et al. Hypertonic saline for treating raised intracranial pressure: literature review with meta-analysis. *J Neurosurg*. 2012;116(1):210–221.
35. Spentzas T, Escue JE, Patters AB, Varelas PN. Brain tumor resection in children: neurointensive care unit course and resource utilization. *Pediatr Crit Care Med*. 2010;11(6):718–722.

46

Preoperative Assessment of the Pediatric Patient With Cancer

RAVISH KAPOOR AND SHANNON M. POPOVICH

Introduction

Childhood cancers make up less than 1% of all newly diagnosed cancers each year.[1] However, with increasing survival rates, an increasing number of pediatric patients will present for surgery and/or procedures related to their cancer diagnosis. Many of these patients will require anesthesia, often multiple times, and thorough preoperative assessment and optimization is therefore essential to ensure successful outcomes from cancer surgery.

The preoperative assessment and optimization of a pediatric patient with cancer can be complex. The disease process itself along with associated cancer-related treatments can impact the preoperative physiologic reserve and the perioperative management of these patients. A comprehensive, multidisciplinary approach to evaluation and optimization needs to be undertaken for the best outcomes, including patient and parental satisfaction. However, since surgery or procedures related to a diagnosis of cancer are often not elective, a sense of urgency can sometimes preclude medical optimization.

Children with cancer are typically evaluated by their primary oncologist prior to being referred for procedures under anesthesia. As a result, details of their primary diagnosis, coexisting medical conditions, types of cancer-related treatment undergone, complications associated with those treatments, and the results of laboratory or diagnostic imaging procedures may be available for review. A preoperative clinic visit to evaluate patients prior to the day of surgery or procedure is ideal but not always feasible. This chapter will focus on the important aspects of preoperative evaluation and optimization as they specifically relate to the pediatric patient with cancer.

Neurologic Evaluation

An altered neurologic status may be secondary to tumor progression or related to cancer therapy. Platinum agents, L-asparaginase, ifosfamide, methotrexate, cytarabine, etoposide, vincristine, cyclosporine A, and craniospinal irradiation have been associated with neurotoxic side effects.[2–6] Commonly associated acute complications include altered mental status, seizures, cerebral infarctions, encephalopathy, hearing loss, vision changes, and peripheral neuropathies. A comprehensive preoperative neurologic evaluation to document the baseline neurologic status, as well as to determine optimal perioperative management strategies, is encouraged.

Patients should continue their regular antiepileptic medications on the morning of surgery, and regular dosing should be reestablished as early as possible after surgery. When multiple doses are likely to be missed, antiepileptic drugs should be administered parenterally, if possible.[7]

Cardiac Evaluation

Some chemotherapeutic agents, particularly cytotoxic antibiotics of the anthracycline class (doxorubicin, daunorubicin, idarubicin, and epirubicin), are commonly associated with cardiotoxicity.[8] Other commonly used drugs in pediatric patients with cancer, for example methadone and the 5-HT3 antagonist ondansetron, may prolong the QT interval and potentially decrease the threshold for cardiac arrhythmias. Chest irradiation, with or without concurrent anthracycline treatment, can potentially lead to pericarditis, pericardial effusions, cardiomyopathy, endocardial fibrosis, valvular fibrosis, conduction abnormalities, and/or coronary artery disease.[9] Children receiving cardiotoxic cancer therapies should undergo periodic cardiac evaluations starting with baseline electrocardiography and echocardiography. In children, physical examination alone has been shown to miss the early signs of chemotherapy-related congestive heart failure in more than 50% of patients.[10] The stress of surgery can also unmask a subclinical cardiomyopathy. Therefore past cardiovascular physical examinations and laboratory studies should be thoroughly reviewed prior to induction of anesthesia.

Pulmonary Evaluation

Pulmonary dysfunction may be associated with the primary disease process or side effects of cancer therapies. A history of treatment with bleomycin, carmustine, lomustine, busulfan, cyclophosphamide, or chest irradiation should warrant an in-depth evaluation of pulmonary status.[11] Symptoms of chronic cough, dyspnea on exertion, and wheezing should be further examined by chest radiography and possibly pulmonary function tests. Pulmonary function tests in children play an important role in evaluating the child with known or suspected lung dysfunction, and they provide baseline measurements, especially prior to undergoing a surgical treatment, which could potentially alter respiratory mechanics. Additionally, pulmonary function tests, chest radiography, and oxygen saturation measurement may be indicated in patients with unexplained symptoms or abnormal findings on physical examination. Obstructive lesions, such as anterior mediastinal masses, neck masses, or oropharyngeal masses, should be evaluated by computed tomography or magnetic resonance imaging. Clinically symptomatic pleural effusions may benefit from therapeutic thoracentesis prior to surgery to enhance physiologic reserve.

Gastrointestinal Evaluation

Gastrointestinal symptoms, such as vomiting, gastroparesis, and obstruction, may occur in pediatric patients with cancer. These symptoms may place the child at risk for malnutrition, electrolyte and acid-base disturbances, and increase the risk for pulmonary aspiration during anesthesia. Chemotherapy-associated nausea and vomiting has been estimated to occur in up to 70% of the pediatric population.[12] The risk of postoperative vomiting has been shown to be higher in children than in adults. Factors that increase the risk of postoperative vomiting include age >3 years, girls who are postpubertal, a previous history of motion sickness, and those who have a personal or family history of postoperative vomiting.[13] A focused gastrointestinal assessment should be performed preoperatively, and any pertinent imaging should be reviewed in order to formulate the safest anesthetic plan and perioperative management.

Hepatic/Renal Evaluation

Chemotherapy, radiation, and hematopoietic stem cell transplant, with associated preconditioning regimens, may be associated with hepatotoxicity, nephrotoxicity, or both. The most common agents associated with hepatic dysfunction in children are methotrexate, actinomycin D, and 6-mercaptopurine.[14] Similar to patients with known liver dysfunction, impaired drug metabolism, hypoglycemia, and decreased coagulation factor production should be considered in children with potential hepatic impairment.

The most common nephrotoxic agents in children are alkylating agents, such as cisplatin, as well as ifosfamide, cyclophosphamide, and methotrexate.[15] Patients with a history of previous nephrotoxicity have the potential for decreased renal excretion of drugs, electrolyte and/or acid-base derangements, and hypertension. Nephrotoxicity can be further compounded by factors such as perioperative administration of nephrotoxic medications and sustained perioperative hypotension. Renal and liver function tests may therefore be clinically indicated prior to surgery.

Endocrine Evaluation

Endocrine and neuroendocrine dysfunction may be seen in pediatric patients with cancer. Adrenal insufficiency, primary or secondary, is an important perioperative consideration. While primary adrenal insufficiency is rare and involves dysfunctional adrenal glands, secondary adrenal insufficiency is more common and often due to exogenous corticosteroid usage.[16] Several chemotherapeutic protocols include glucocorticoids, which are not only used for their antitumor effects but also to treat side effects related to chemotherapy (e.g., nausea). A blunted stress response may persist for several months after exogenous corticosteroid use. The need for stress dose steroids is debated in the literature.[17] However, considering that the stress response is unpredictable in children and that significant harm has not been shown from perioperative stress-dose steroids,[18] the administration of hydrocortisone (1–2 mg/kg) preoperatively, plus every 6 h on the day of surgery for up to 72 h for more complicated surgeries, has been recommended if hypothalamic-pituitary axis suppression is suspected.[19] In the postoperative period, steroid doses can be tapered depending on the degree of surgical stress and replaced with the child's usual oral steroid dose when appropriate. Hydrocortisone is preferred in children because of its mineralocorticoid and antiinflammatory properties, ease of titration, shorter half-life, and fewer adverse effects when compared with more potent longer-acting glucocorticoids. The dosage, duration, and last dose of exogenous steroids should be verified in the preoperative interview to best determine appropriate coverage.

The primary or metastatic tumor, as well as treatment associated surgical/radiation therapies, can lead to central (neurogenic) diabetes insipidus with resulting vasopressin deficiency. Polyuria and polydipsia are typical clinical symptoms. These patients can present with severe dehydration and hypernatremia if there is inadequate free water intake, such as on the morning of surgery. Accordingly, surgery should be scheduled earlier in the day for these patients. Desmopressin (DDAVP), a vasopressin analogue, prevents water loss by helping the kidneys reabsorb water. For patients with preexisting diabetes insipidus, at home doses of oral/intranasal DDAVP should be verified and administered on the morning of surgery for minor procedures. However, for major surgical procedures, it should be withheld, and careful fluid management should take place intraoperatively. A vasopressin infusion can be titrated to effect intraoperatively or postoperatively, should intra/postoperative diabetes insipidus be suspected.[20]

Concerns of endocrine dysfunction that might require further workup, including those conditions previously listed, or others, such as uncontrolled diabetes mellitus, thyroid dysfunction, and/or secondary electrolyte abnormalities, should be discussed with the patient's primary physician or appropriate consultant prior to surgery.

Hematologic Evaluation

Radiation and chemotherapeutic agents may potentially cause myelosuppression. Neutropenia should prompt further workup for fever, sepsis, and immunosuppression. If anemia is present, its degree and duration should be considered in perioperative planning. The patient's condition, comorbidities, type, and urgency of the surgical procedure, and the risk for bleeding should also be weighed to determine whether a preoperative transfusion is necessary. In thrombocytopenic patients, the type of procedure is an important determining factor in whether preprocedural platelet transfusion is warranted. For certain minor procedures such as lumbar punctures, platelet counts as low as 20×10^9 per liter have been shown to be safe.[21] Conditions that can induce coagulopathy include sepsis, leukocytosis, vitamin K deficiency, L-asparaginase treatment, or a new diagnosis of leukemia. The hematology service should be consulted for difficult questions regarding existing or potential coagulopathies.

Pain Evaluation

Tumor- or metastases-related pain is common at the time of cancer diagnosis in children.[22] It can also stem directly or indirectly from chemo/radiation therapy. It is estimated that approximately 89% of children with advanced disease experience pain.[23] Pain in the pediatric cancer patient is often underestimated and undertreated due to inadequate pain assessment tools, as well as physician reluctance to prescribe opioids due to the fear of respiratory complications and/or addiction. Self-reported pain scales work best for children >6 years of age but numerous observational pain scales exist for younger children. The reliability of the observational tool depends on the clinical context and the quality of the validation criteria, guiding the caregiver in choosing the correct tool.[24]

Understanding the underlying etiology of a patient's pain, determining what medication regimens have worked well (i.e., optimal analgesia with the least side effects), along with the current analgesic regimen being used, is important during the preoperative assessment to devise an appropriate analgesic plan. Tolerance to opioids can often exist; therefore a multimodal approach should be employed, if possible. Regional anesthesia, which can be safely provided for children while under a general anesthetic,[25] should be incorporated when appropriate and discussed with the family and surgical team prior to the procedure.

Preoperative Laboratory Testing

Routine preoperative laboratory or radiologic testing is not recommended in pediatric oncology patients presenting for minor or noninvasive procedures but rather ordered on a case-by-case basis or if it is deemed that the results may influence the anesthetic management. A complete blood count should be considered in conditions that increase the likelihood of anemia such as newly diagnosed leukemia or lymphoma, recent chemoradiation, stem cell transplant, a recent episode of bleeding, or age less than 6 months. Additionally, it can be considered if there is a concern for thrombocytopenia, which is also possible with newly diagnosed leukemia, recent chemoradiation, or due to splenic sequestration.[26] On the other hand, baseline complete blood counts are considered routine in children presenting for major surgical procedures.

Coagulation studies are rarely necessary, but may be considered if there is a clinical history of bleeding despite normal platelet counts, if there is potential for clinically significant blood loss, or if the expected blood loss would be poorly tolerated.

An electrolyte panel should be ordered if there is a known or suspected derangement. Common conditions associated with electrolyte abnormalities include syndrome of inappropriate antidiuretic hormone (SIADH), hypercalcemia (can be associated with bone tumors and neuroblastomas), pituitary tumors, malnutrition, hyperalimentation, dehydration, renal dysfunction, or existing or recent tumor lysis syndrome (hyperkalemia, hyperphosphatemia, hyperuricemia, and hypocalcemia).[27]

Fasting Guidelines

Practice guidelines for preoperative fasting in children undergoing elective procedures are shown in Table 46.1.[28] There has been recent interest in liberalizing the guidelines to 1 h for clear liquids in accordance with guidelines and consensus statements offered by some European societies.[29–31] The argument for allowing clear liquids up to 1 h prior to anesthesia is that some studies have shown that there is complete gastric emptying at 1 h after ingestion of clear fluids; hence the practice would not increase the risk of pulmonary aspiration.

Since prolonged fasting in children increases irritability and the potential for physiologic and metabolic derangements, shorter fasting periods can improve patient comfort

TABLE 46.1 Preoperative Fasting Guidelines in Children

Clear liquids	2 h
Breast milk	4 h
Nonhuman milk, formula, light meal	6 h
Fried/fatty foods or meat	8 h

and increase patient compliance.[32] The risk of dehydration and hypoglycemia in pediatric patients with cancer may be secondary to disease-related malnutrition, the side effects of therapy, as well as the need to undergo repetitive procedures over a relatively prolonged period. Therefore allowing clear liquids up to 1 h prior to elective procedures in patients without the risk of gastroparesis or difficult airway could help mitigate these issues.

Parental Concerns

Anesthetic-Related Neurotoxicity

The preoperative assessment of younger children will primarily involve interviewing parents, legal guardians, or caregivers. Quickly establishing rapport and understanding family dynamics and social concerns will help the anesthesiologist navigate the interview process efficiently.

A pediatric-specific anesthesia concern for parents is the potential for anesthetic-induced long-term neurocognitive effects on their children. While some preclinical studies have shown an unfavorable association between anesthetic exposure and neurodevelopmental outcomes in children, evidence from human prospective randomized controlled trials suggests that a single exposure to anesthesia in otherwise healthy children may not be associated with cognitive or behavioral issues.[33] On the other hand, some human studies, albeit retrospective in nature, have suggested an increased risk of unfavorable neurocognitive effects with multiple exposures to anesthetics.[34] In pediatric patients with cancer, multiple anesthetics may be required for diagnostic or therapeutic procedures.

In accordance with the recommendations of the US Food and Drug Administration, discussion regarding risks versus benefits of anesthesia amongt parents and providers of children with cancer is highly encouraged.[35] Many health care institutions have implemented this discussion as part of their informed consent process. Distribution of educational materials to caregivers prior to the day of evaluation can provide a foundational framework for an educated conversation at the time of the preoperative evaluation.

Parental Presence During Induction

Parental accompaniment into the operating room is a controversial topic in pediatric anesthesia. Proponents for parental presence argue that it could help decrease the psychologic stress of surgery on the child, reduce parental anxiety, and even increase operating room efficiency,[36] hence providing for a smoother induction. Possible disadvantages of parental presence include the unpredictability of parental behavior, increased liability of having another person in the operating room who is not a staff member, and increased time to induction.[37] Current literature and practice appears to be split on this topic. Some centers rely more on preoperative anxiolytic administration, while some allow a caregiver to be present for anesthetic induction. Tools such as comic books, videos, and employing child life specialists can also help to decrease the anxiety associated with anesthesia and surgery.[38–39]

Special Considerations

The Difficult Airway

It is important to be cognizant about general anatomic differences between the pediatric and adult airway. The physical examination should focus on an abnormal breathing pattern, tongue size and its relationship to pharyngeal structures, restricted mouth opening, configuration of the palate and mandible, dentition, range of neck motion, and abnormal baseline oxygen saturation on room air. A child's global appearance can also help identify certain clinical conditions such as a symptomatic anterior mediastinal mass (see Chapter 47) or congenital disorders often associated with difficult airway management (Table 46.2). All available imaging should be reviewed prior to formulating a plan, and in certain situations, additional imaging may be warranted to help guide the approach. In the past lateral x-rays were shown to be useful in delineating anatomic aberrations although ultrasound, MRI, and CT imaging have since replaced this modality.[40] Preoperative endoscopic evaluation of the airway can also be considered in cooperative older children if a difficult airway is suspected. Availability of proper equipment and assistance should be incorporated into the contingency plan for any anticipated difficult airway.

Syndromes Related to Cancer

A predisposition to cancer has been identified not only with hereditary conditions but also with a multitude of syndromes. A cursory list of common syndromes with a predisposition to cancer in children, along with anesthetic considerations, are listed in Table 46.2.[41–44] When a patient with an identified syndrome presents for preoperative evaluation, every effort should be made to obtain prior records to review any recent laboratory values, imaging, and prior anesthetic and/or consult notes. Providers should familiarize themselves with the most common syndromes related to a cancer diagnosis to tailor the preoperative interview and formulate the most appropriate anesthetic plan for the patient.

Vascular Access

Many children will have vascular access in the form of vascular ports or peripherally inserted central catheter (PICC) lines placed for chemotherapy administration and to facilitate regular bloodwork. For serial procedures such as proton or radiation therapy, where anesthesia is required on multiple consecutive days, accessing these lines is ideal. If a port is present, eutectic mixture of local anesthetics (EMLA) cream can be useful in mitigating the pain and anxiety associated with accessing the port.[46] EMLA consists of 2.5% lidocaine and 2.5% prilocaine. One to two grams of the cream per 10 cm^2 of skin in infants and children 3 months of age or

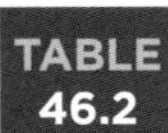

TABLE 46.2 Common Congenital Syndromes With a Predisposition to Cancer in Children

Gardner Syndrome (Subtype of Familial Adenomatous Polyposis)

APC gene mutation; features include multiple colonic polyps, dental anomalies, congenital retinal pigment epithelium hypertrophy, benign and malignant neoplasms including colon cancer, pancreatic cancer, papillary thyroid cancer, medulloblastoma, hepatoblastoma, desmoid tumors, and osteomas.

Preoperative Anesthetic Considerations:

Patients may require a prophylactic colectomy. Mouth opening and dentition should be carefully assessed. Patients may be on nonsteroidal antiinflammatory drugs as they have been shown to suppress the development of adenomatous polyps and can cause regression of existing polyps.

Beckwith-Wiedemann Syndrome

Genetic alterations of chromosomal region 11p15; features may include neonatal hypoglycemia, macrosomia, macroglossia, hemihyperplasia, omphalocele, visceromegaly, adrenocortical cytomegaly, renal abnormalities, ear anomalies, benign and malignant neoplasms such as Wilms tumor, hepatoblastoma, neuroblastoma, and rhabdomyosarcoma

Preoperative Anesthetic Considerations:

Macroglossia can cause upper airway obstruction and might make vocal cord visualization challenging during intubation. Visceromegaly can reduce functional residual capacity and possibly lead to hypoventilation under anesthesia. Blood glucose should be monitored perioperatively, as hypoglycemia can be severe. Intravenous access may be difficult.

Down Syndrome (Trisomy 21)

Chromosome 21 mutation, short stature, intellectual disability, congenital heart disease (primarily atrioventricular septal defects), hypothyroidism, hypotonia, and macroglossia can be present; predisposes to childhood acute lymphoblastic leukemia, transient myeloid neoplasms, and acute megakaryocytic leukemia.

Preoperative Anesthetic Considerations:

Intellectual disability or behavioral issues may affect anesthesia induction technique. Mask ventilation and intubation may be challenging. Increased frequency of obstructive sleep apnea and increased sensitivity to the respiratory depressant effects of opioids have been described. Atlantoaxial instability can occur after approximately 4 years of age but routine neck imaging is not warranted for patients without myelopathic symptoms. Intravenous access may be difficult.

Gorlin Syndrome (Basal Cell Nevus Syndrome)

Mutation of *SUFU* or *PTCH1*; features may include multiple jaw keratocysts, macrocephaly, frontal bossing, coarse face, facial milia, skeletal anomalies, and ectopic calcification of the falx; benign and malignant neoplasia including medulloblastomas, basal cell carcinomas, cardiac and ovarian fibromas, rhabdomyosarcomas, and ependymoma or rhabdomyomas.

Preoperative Anesthetic Considerations:

Dental abnormalities/dental caries may predispose to dental loss during laryngoscopy. It is recommended that teeth be inventoried before laryngoscopy. Extreme care should be used during positioning and laryngoscopy if cervical vertebral anomalies are present. Patients may have unrecognized hydrocephalus.

Neurofibromatosis 1 (Von Recklinghausen Disease)

Chromosome 17 mutation; features can include multiple café-au-lait spots, learning difficulties, scoliosis, vasculopathy, and other specific tumor-related issues; benign and malignant neoplasia including plexiform neurofibromas, low- and high-grade gliomas, malignant peripheral nerve sheath tumors, juvenile myelomonocytic leukemia, and other tumors.

Preoperative Anesthetic Considerations:

Mask ventilation and tracheal intubation may be challenging due to neck stiffness, facial bone deformities, macroglossia, or tumors of the airway. Kyphoscoliosis can cause restrictive lung disease as well as make supine positioning difficult. Mediastinal masses can exist. Hypertension is common in these patients and any unexpected intraoperative hypertension could be a potential pheochromocytoma. Imaging should be used to evaluate the spine/local area if neuraxial/regional anesthesia is being considered.

APC, Adenomatous polyposis coli.

older who weigh at least 5 kg should be utilized. Directions for proper application using an occlusive dressing over the cream for at least 45 min should be given to parents to make seamless accessing of the port more efficient. Sterile precautions should be taken prior to accessing any central line, especially in neutropenic children, and lines should be aspirated prior to use to withdraw any potential blood clot or heparin within the catheter. If central access is not available, ultrasound use is encouraged to obtain vascular access,[47] as veins can be fragile secondary to cancer therapies.

Conclusion

A multitude of challenges are faced by anesthesiologists providing care for children with cancer. The unique interplay amongst the direct effects of the tumor, complex pharmacologic management, and potentially extensive physiologic derangements mandates a firm knowledge of each of these components to best formulate an anesthetic plan that is appropriate for the individual patient and type of surgical procedure.

References

1. Siegel RL, Miller KD, Jemal A. Cancer statistics, 2019. *CA Cancer J Clin*. 2019;69(1):7–34.
2. Adamson PC, Balis FM, Berg S, et al. General principles of chemotherapy. In: Pizzo PA, Poplack DG, eds. *Principles and Practice of Pediatric Oncology*. 5th ed. Lippincott Williams & Wilkins; 2006:290.
3. Cordelli DM, Masetti R, Zama D, et al. Central nervous system complications in children receiving chemotherapy or hematopoietic stem cell transplantation. *Front Pediatr*. 2017;5:105.
4. Verstappen CC, Heimans JJ, Hoekman K, et al. Neurotoxic complications of chemotherapy in patients with cancer: clinical signs and optimal management. *Drugs*. 2003;63:1549–1563.
5. Hildebrand J. Neurological complications of cancer chemotherapy. *Curr Opin Oncol*. 2006;18:321–324.
6. Di Cataldo A, Astuto M, Rizzo G, et al. Neurotoxicity during ifosfamide treatment in children. *Med Sci Monit*. 2009;15:CS22–CS25.
7. Perks A, Cheema S, Mohanraj R. Anaesthesia and epilepsy. *Br J Anaesth*. 2012;108(4):562–571.
8. Bansal N, Amdani S, Lipshultz ER, et al. Chemotherapy-induced cardiotoxicity in children. *Expert Opin Drug Metab Toxicol*. 2017;13(8):817–832.
9. Bansal N, Amdani S, Hutchins KK, et al. Cardiovascular disease in survivors of childhood cancer. *Curr Opin Pediatr*. 2018;30(5):628–638.
10. Simbre VC, Duffy SA, Dadlani GH, et al. Cardiotoxicity of cancer chemotherapy: implications for children. *Paediatr Drugs*. 2005;7:187–202.
11. Huang TT, Hudson MM, Stokes DC, et al. Pulmonary outcomes in survivors of childhood cancer: a systematic review. *Chest*. 2011;140(4):881–901.
12. Dupuis LL, Sung L, Molassiotis A, et al. 2016 updated MASCC/ESMO consensus recommendations: Prevention of acute chemotherapy-induced nausea and vomiting in children. *Support Care Cancer*. 2017;25:323–331.
13. Hohne C. Postoperative nausea and vomiting in pediatric anesthesia. *Curr Opin Anesthesiol*. 2014;27(3):303–308.
14. King PD, Perry MC. Hepatotoxicity of chemotherapy. *Oncologist*. 2001;6:162–176.
15. Rossi R, Kleta R, Ehrich JH. Renal involvement in children with malignancies. *Pediatr Nephrol*. 1999;13:153–162.
16. Bowden SA, Henry R. Pediatric adrenal insufficiency: diagnosis, management, and new therapies. *Int J Pediatr*. 2018;1:1739831.
17. Liu MM, Reidy AB, Saatee S, et al. Perioperative steroid management: approaches based on current evidence. *Anesthesiology*. 2017;127(1):166–172.
18. Bornstein SR, Allolio B, Arlt W, et al. Diagnosis and treatment of primary adrenal insufficiency: an endocrine society clinical practice guideline. *J Clin Endocrinol Metab*. 2016;101:364–389.
19. Ghazal EA, Mason LJ, Cote CJ. Preoperative evaluation, premedication, and induction of anesthesia. In: Cote CJ, Lerman J, Todres ID, eds. *A Practice of Anesthesia for Infants and Children*. Saunders Elsevier; 2013:47 5th ed.
20. Maxwell LG, Goodwin SR, Mancuso TJ, et al. Systemic disorders. In: Davis PJ, Cladis FP, Motoyama EK, eds. *Smith's Anesthesia for Infants and Children*. 8th ed. Elsevier Mosby; 2011:1102–1103.
21. Schiffer CA, Bohlke K, Delaney M, et al. Platelet transfusion for patients with cancer: American society of clinical oncology clinical practice guideline update. *J Clin Oncol*. 2018;36:283–299.
22. Tutelman PR, Chambers CT, Stinson JN, et al. Pain in children with cancer: prevalence, characteristics, and parent management. *Clin J Pain*. 2018;34(3):198–206.
23. Hechler T, Ruhe AK, Schmidt P, et al. Inpatient-based intensive interdisciplinary pain treatment for highly impaired children with severe chronic pain: randomized controlled trial of efficacy and economic effects. *Pain*. 2014;155:118–128.
24. Beltramini A, Milojevic K, Pateron D. Pain assessment in newborns, infants, and children. *Pediatr Ann*. 2017;46(10):e387–e395.
25. Walker BJ, Long JB, Sathyamoorthy M, et al. Complications in pediatric regional anesthesia: an analysis of more than 100,000 blocks from the Pediatric Regional Anesthesia Network. *Anesthesiology*. 2018;129(4):721–732.
26. Latham GJ, Greenberg RS. Anesthetic considerations for the pediatric oncology patient—part 3: pain, cognitive dysfunction, and preoperative evaluation. *Pediatr Anaesth*. 2010;20(6):479–489.
27. Virk N, Senbruna B, Lerman J. Perioperative care of children with cancer. In: Astuto M, Ingelmo P, eds. *Perioperative Medicine in Pediatric Anesthesia. Anesthesia, Intensive Care and Pain in Neonates and Children*: Springer; 2016:245n.
28. Practice guidelines for preoperative fasting and the use of pharmacologic agents to reduce the risk of pulmonary aspiration: application to healthy patients undergoing elective procedures: an updated report by the American Society of Anesthesiologists Task Force on Preoperative Fasting and the use of pharmacologic agents to reduce the risk of pulmonary aspiration. *Anesthesiology*. 2017;126:376.
29. Smith I, Kranke P, Murat I, et al. Perioperative fasting in adults and children: guidelines from the European Society of Anaesthesiology. *Eur J Anaesthesiol*. 2011;28:556.
30. Thomas M, Morrison C, Newton R, et al. Consensus statement on clear fluids fasting for elective pediatric general anesthesia. *Paediatr Anaesth*. 2018;28:411.
31. Association of anaesthetists of Great Britain and Ireland. Preoperative Assessment and Patient Preparation. Available at: http://www.aagbi.org/sites/default/files/preop2010.pdf.
32. Dennhardt N, Beck C, Huber D, et al. Optimized preoperative fasting times decrease ketone body concentration and stabilize mean arterial blood pressure during induction of anesthesia in children younger than 36 months: a prospective observational cohort study. *Pediatr Anesth*. 2016;26:838–843.

33. McCann ME, de Graaff JC, Dorris L, et al. Neurodevelopmental outcome at 5 years of age after general anaesthesia or awake-regional anaesthesia in infancy (GAS): an international, multicentre, randomised, controlled equivalence trial. *Lancet*. 2019;393(10172):664–677.
34. Davidson AJ, Sun LS. Clinical evidence for any effect of anesthesia on the developing brain. *Anesthesiology*. 2018;128:840–853.
35. United States Food and Drug Administration. FDA Drug Safety Communication: FDA Review Results in New Warnings About Using General Anesthetics and Sedation Drugs in Young Children and Pregnant Women. Available at: https://www.fda.gov/Drugs/DrugSafety/ucm532356.htm.
36. Luehmann NC, Staubach ME, Akay B, et al. Benefits of a family-centered approach to pediatric induction of anesthesia. Benefits of a family-centered approach to pediatric induction of anesthesia. *J Pediatr Surg*. 2019;54(1):189–193.
37. Johnson YJ, Nickerson M, Quezado ZM. Case report: an unforeseen peril of parental presence during induction of anesthesia. *Anesth Analg*. 2012;115(6):1371–1372.
38. Kassai B, Rabilloud M, Dantony E, et al. Introduction of a paediatric anaesthesia comic information leaflet reduced preoperative anxiety in children. *Br J Anaesth*. 2016;117(1):95–102.
39. Scott MT, Todd KE, Oakley H, et al. Reducing anesthesia and health care cost through utilization of child life specialists in pediatric radiation oncology. *Int J Radiat Oncol Biol Phys*. 2016;96(2):401–405 1.
40. Litman RS, Fiadjoe JE, Stricker PA, Cote CJ. The Pediatric Airway. In: Cote CJ, Lerman J, Todres ID, eds. *A Practice of Anesthesia for Infants and Children*. : Saunders Elsevier; 2013:259. 5th ed.
41. Ripperger T, Bielack SS, Borkhardt A, et al. Childhood cancer predisposition syndromes—a concise review and recommendations by the Cancer Predisposition Working Group of the Society for Pediatric Oncology and Hematology. *Am J Med Genet*. 2017;173:1017–1037.
42. Baum VC, O'Flaherty JE, eds. Anesthesia for Genetic, Metabolic, and Dysmorphic Syndromes of Childhood, 3rd ed. Lippincott, Williams & Wilkins; 2015:52–53, 56–57, 121–123, 169–170, 319–321.
43. Koh JL, Harrison D, Myers R, et al. A randomized, double-blind comparison study of EMLA and ELA-Max for topical anesthesia in children undergoing intravenous insertion. *Paediatr Anaesth*. 2004;14:977.
44. Schindler E, Schears GJ, Hall SR, et al. Ultrasound for vascular access in pediatric patients. *Paediatr Anaesth*. 2012;22(10):1002–1007.

47

Intraoperative Management: Considerations for Specific Procedures in Children With Cancer

PASCAL OWUSU-AGYEMANG

Anesthetic Management of the Child With an Anterior Mediastinal Mass

Mediastinal masses may arise from structures normally located in the mediastinum, from those that pass through the mediastinum during development, or from metastatic disease that arises from tumors elsewhere in the body.[1] In children, mediastinal masses tend to be more prevalent in males than in females.[1,2] The majority are caused by lymphomas, followed by bronchial cysts, teratomas, vascular malformations, and neurogenic tumors.[3]

Mediastinal masses may present with nonspecific respiratory or cardiovascular symptoms, such as coughing, or present with more severe symptoms, such as superior vena cava syndrome, pulmonary artery obstruction, or culminate in superior mediastinal syndrome (airway compression/tracheal obstruction, vascular compression).[3]

The presence of an anterior mediastinal mass should be regarded as a clinical emergency. Early diagnosis and management are crucial for providing the best chance for a favorable outcome. The latter undoubtedly adds to the challenge of the anesthetic management of these patients, since symptoms such as respiratory or cardiovascular compromise may not be optimized before anesthesia.

General anesthesia confers considerable risk, since the effects of mediastinal masses on airway and vascular structures can impede gas exchange or reduce cardiac output. The symptoms at presentation are essential to developing an anesthetic plan and have been shown to be predictive of anesthetic-related morbidity. In a retrospective review of 118 pediatric patients who presented with mediastinal masses, four preoperative features were significantly associated with anesthetic complications: main-stem bronchus compression, great vessel compression, orthopnea, and upper body edema.[4] The presence of pleural or pericardial effusions, ventricular dysfunction, tracheal compression (cross-sectional area <50%), and stridor are also associated with anesthetic related morbidity.[3]

Anesthetic Management

The anesthetic management begins with a careful review of the child's history, symptoms, clinical signs, and radiographic images (computed tomography and/or chest x-ray). In general, patients without orthopnea or cardiovascular symptoms and minimal radiographic evidence of airway obstruction may likely be anesthetized safely. However, physical signs and radiographic evidence have not been consistently shown to be predictive of potential complications; therefore general anesthesia or deep sedation should be avoided whenever possible, and when required, it is essential that the anesthesiologist establishes communication with the surgeon, has a set plan for sedation or anesthesia, and has a plan for rescue in the event of cardiopulmonary compromise. These include repositioning the patient (lateral or prone), the ability to perform rigid bronchoscopy to relieve tracheal compression, and the ability to perform a sternotomy and provide cardiopulmonary bypass or extracorporeal membrane oxygenation (ECMO).[5]

Patients with signs of orthopnea, stridor, dyspnea at rest, and/or a >70% reduction in tracheal cross-sectional area are deemed high-risk, and general anesthesia should be avoided unless absolutely necessary.[5] In older children, tissue diagnosis under local anesthesia has been associated with lower risk of anesthetic complications and has been successfully accomplished in several series.[2,3] Distraction techniques such as counting, listening to music, and nonprocedure-related talk have been shown to be effective.[6] However, younger children and those undergoing surgical resection of large mediastinal masses may require a general anesthetic.

In this instance, an anesthetic plan that ensures spontaneous respiration is generally preferable. Spontaneous ventilation typically preserves the patency of the intrathoracic airways. On the other hand, positive pressure ventilation may worsen airway compression (e.g., through neuromuscular blockade and/or deep anesthesia reducing support of the surrounding tracheobronchial musculature) and also reduce cardiac output by reducing venous return.

The airway may be managed by mask ventilation only, with a laryngeal mask airway, or with endotracheal intubation. Several methods have been described for the maintenance of anesthesia, including a mixture of sevoflurane in oxygen and halothane in heliox, and low-dose infusions of propofol, dexmedetomidine, and ketamine.[7–9] The ability of dexmedetomidine and ketamine to provide sedation with minimal respiratory depression has proven beneficial in anesthetizing children with anterior mediastinal masses.

It is noteworthy that several authors have reported cases where intubation has been successfully performed in children with mediastinal masses.[10,11] In the event that an endotracheal intubation is necessary, advancement of the endotracheal tube past the segment of obstruction, typically through external compression, may have to be performed.[10] Regardless of the choice of airway management, neuromuscular blockade is generally not recommended because the relaxation of supporting tracheobronchial musculature may contribute to further worsening of airway compromise.[3] However, if neuromuscular blockade is deemed necessary, it is imperative to establish the ability to adequately ventilate the patient before administering muscle relaxants.

Summary

The management of the child with an anterior mediastinal mass poses a significant challenge to anesthesiologists. Potential respiratory and cardiovascular complications may be exacerbated under anesthesia, and plans to manage potential complications should be communicated to the entire team before initiation of care. Where possible, diagnostic procedures are best performed with local anesthesia with minimal-to-no sedation. Where deep sedation or general anesthesia is required, maintenance of spontaneous ventilation with or without an endotracheal tube is preferable. Neuromuscular blockade should be avoided whenever possible.

Anesthesia for Pediatric Radiotherapy

Unlike adults and older children, most children under 2 years of age require anesthesia or sedation for the successful completion of a course of radiotherapy treatments. This is mainly because complete immobilization, which is required for safe and effective radiotherapy, cannot be reliably accomplished in very young children without sedation or anesthesia.

This, in and of itself, presents several challenges. Perhaps most concerning is the fact that younger children may have to be exposed to multiple anesthetics over a relatively short period of time. The inherent risks associated with anesthetizing a very young child and the exposure to the side effects of anesthetic agents used are therefore amplified. In this regard, the safety profile of the chosen anesthetic technique gains further significance. Furthermore, to ensure that there is no interference with the radiotherapy plan from changes in airway management or patient positioning, it is important that the chosen method of anesthesia remains unchanged over the period of treatment and that it is easily replicable. Other challenges include choosing an anesthetic that may facilitate rapid awakening and rapid discharge, since most radiotherapy facilities treat multiple patients or may not have a designated postoperative recovery area.

Airway Management

Several studies have demonstrated that anesthesia in children undergoing radiation therapy may be safely performed by spontaneous ventilation and an unprotected airway. In a large series of 340 children who had undergone 9328 radiotherapy procedures under anesthesia, supplemental oxygen was provided with a face mask or nasal cannula.[12] In another large series describing the anesthetic management of 177 children who had undergone 3833 radiotherapy procedures, supplemental oxygen was provided by face mask in both the supine and prone positions. The placement of an oral airway or laryngeal mask airway was required in rare cases.[13]

General Anesthesia Versus Conscious Sedation

In a meta-analysis of anesthesia complications of pediatric radiation therapy, general anesthesia was shown to be superior to conscious sedation with regard to maintaining satisfactory procedural sedation while maintaining low respiratory and cardiovascular complication rates.[14]

Medications

Several medications and anesthetic agents have been used for the successful completion of daily recurrent anesthesia. These include intravenous propofol,[13] inhalational volatile anesthetics,[15] ketamine,[15,17] midazolam,[18] chloral hydrate,[19] and dexmedetomidine.[20,21]

Propofol

The rapid onset and quick recovery from propofol has made it the anesthetic of choice in several centers where daily recurrent anesthesia is performed.[13,15] In a retrospective study of 3833 pediatric radiotherapy/simulation procedures performed under propofol-based total intravenous anesthesia, Anghelescu et al. reported a very low rate of complications (1.3%). In this study, the authors described their technique of administering 1 mg/kg boluses of propofol until loss of consciousness, followed by 100–250 µg/kg/min (6–15 mg/kg/h). Additional boluses of 1 mg/kg were administered if the child responded to stimulation.[13] Furthermore, in a survey of anesthesia practices at proton radiotherapy centers worldwide, propofol was the maintenance anesthetic of choice in the majority of centers.[15] The reduction of recovery time by propofol has been consistently observed when propofol is used as a sole agent in children undergoing procedural sedation. The mean weighted difference in recovery time reduction has been estimated to be approximately 10 min.[22]

Volatile Anesthetics

The slower onset and recovery from volatile anesthetics pose a significant challenge during their use for multiple repeated anesthetics. That said, several institutions safely administer volatile anesthetics for daily repeated procedures. For example, in the aforementioned survey of anesthesia practices for proton radiotherapy, 36% of the respondents indicated that they used volatile anesthesia with a laryngeal mask airway.[15] This may be because treatment sessions during proton radiotherapy could be considerably longer than conventional radiotherapy, making differences in recovery times between volatile anesthetics and propofol less significant. Another factor may be the need to transport patients to recovery rooms that are located at a considerable distance from the treatment location, making rapid recovery less desirable.

Dexmedetomidine

Dexmedetomidine is a selective alpha-2-adrenoceptor agonist with anxiolytic and analgesic properties, and minimal respiratory depressant effects. The latter property makes it attractive as a sedative in remote settings where help from additional personnel may be difficult to obtain. In their description of two case reports, Kim et al. used dexmedetomidine to provide sedation for over 20 sessions of radiotherapy in two young children.[20] The authors administered a loading dose of 1.5–2.0 μg/kg of intravenous dexmedetomidine over 10 min, followed by a maintenance dose of 0.5–2 μg/kg/h. An increase in dexmedetomidine requirements was observed with subsequent treatment sessions. In another publication, Shukry et al. described the use of dexmedetomidine as the primary sedative agent in a 21-month-old child undergoing brain radiotherapy.[21] In this case report, the authors administered a loading dose of 1 μg/kg over 10 min, followed by an infusion at 10 μg/kg/h. A heart rate lower than 90 beats/min was treated with 10–20 μg/kg of atropine.

Ketamine

Ketamine is a dissociative agent with excellent amnestic and analgesic properties. However, its side effects, including increased secretions, involuntary movements, hallucinations, nightmares, and a slow recovery profile, make it less desirable as an agent for daily repeated anesthesia.[23] In a meta-analysis of anesthesia complications of pediatric radiation therapy, the complication rates associated with the use of ketamine were as high as 24%.[14] However, some authors have described its use in pediatric patients undergoing daily radiotherapy sessions.[16,17] In a single-blind prospective study, Sanusi et al. described the safe intravenous administration of a combination of ketamine (2 mg/kg) and atropine (10 μg/kg) to 33 children who were undergoing daily radiotherapy treatments. In that study, the investigators observed a progressive decrease in recovery times from a mean of 13.7 min at initiation of treatment to a mean of 7.7 min at the last treatment.[16] In another publication, Soyannwo et al. described the safe repeated intramuscular administration of ketamine at a dose of 5–13 mg/kg on 280 occasions to 15 children. In that study, involuntary movements were observed in more than half of the study population but resulted in interruption of treatment in only 2% of patients. Time to complete recovery varied and ranged from 15 to 90 min.[17]

Midazolam

Midazolam has been used in combination with ketamine for the successful completion of radiotherapy in children. This combination of drugs takes advantage of the anxiolytic properties of midazolam and the dissociative anesthesia offered by ketamine. Furthermore, the minimal respiratory depressant effects of lower doses of each of these drugs may be advantageous. In a retrospective study, describing the use of midazolam and ketamine for sedation for diagnostic and therapeutic procedures in children, Parker et al. described the intravenous administration of 0.05–0.1 mg/kg midazolam, followed by a 0.5–1 mg/kg dose of ketamine. Additional doses of ketamine 0.5–1 mg/kg were administered during lengthy procedures.[18] In that study, two patients experienced emergence agitation. Another two patients were reported to have sleep disturbances (nightmares). However, both of these patients received ketamine with subsequent procedures at a reduced dose without a repetition of the sleep disturbances. The incidence of vomiting was relatively high (2.9%), and recovery times ranged from 15 to 120 min. Compared to propofol, the use of midazolam for repeated sedations in children undergoing radiotherapy has been associated with lower odds of a successful outcome.[19]

Chloral Hydrate

The use of chloral hydrate for procedural sedation has been associated with a significant risk of complications and treatment failure. In a prospective observational study of repeated sedations for the radiotherapy in children with cancer, the use of chloral hydrate was associated with a 23% incidence rate of complications.[19] Furthermore, treatment was considered unsatisfactory in 40% of the patients, and in another 20%, treatment could not be initiated. As a result of these findings, the authors concluded that chloral hydrate was not the most suitable drug for children undergoing radiotherapy under anesthesia.[19]

Complications

Complication rates in children undergoing repetitive anesthesia for radiotherapy are generally low. In a series of 177 children who had undergone 3833 radiotherapy procedures under anesthesia, Anghelescu et al. reported an overall complication rate of 1.3%.[13] In their study, procedure duration;

total propofol dose; the use of use of adjuncts, such as opioids, benzodiazepines, and barbiturates, in addition to propofol; and anesthesia for simulation (vs. radiotherapy) were associated with an increased risk of complications. In another retrospective study of 130 children who had undergone 1376 radiation treatment sessions under anesthesia, Yildirim et al. reported an overall complication rate of 2.6%.[24] Similar to the findings of Anghelescu et al., the total propofol dose was associated with a risk of complications. However, unlike the study by Anghelescu et al., the use of adjuncts in addition to propofol was associated with a lower complication rate. This difference may be explained by the type of adjuncts used. Unlike the study by Yildirim et al. where ketamine and midazolam were used as adjuncts, opioids were used in the study by Anghelescu et al. and may have accounted for a higher rate of complications.

In a meta-analysis of anesthesia complications of pediatric radiation therapy, the most common complications were respiratory in nature (e.g., airway obstruction, broncho/laryngospasm, desaturation, apnea), followed by those that were cardiovascular in nature (e.g., tachycardia, bradycardia, arrhythmias, hypotension) and nausea/vomiting. Other complications included those associated with vascular access devices, such as infection, breakage, or extravasation, which was observed in up to 25% of patients.[14] Thus attention to sterility during daily access of venous devices is essential.

Neurotoxicity of Anesthetic Agents

Concerns regarding the possible neurotoxic effects of repetitive anesthesia continue to be raised by parents. To date there have been no studies examining the neurotoxic effects of repetitive anesthesia in children undergoing radiotherapy. However, in a recent cohort study of 212 survivors of childhood acute lymphoblastic leukemia who underwent 5699 exposures to general anesthesia, higher cumulative doses of anesthetics and longer anesthesia duration significantly contributed to neurocognitive impairment and neuroimaging abnormalities observed at a median of 7.52 years after diagnosis.[25] This timeframe was well beyond the expected neurotoxic effects of chemotherapy. The confounding neurotoxic effects of cranial irradiation make this challenging to study in children undergoing radiotherapy.

By contrast, Oba and Türk presented the case of a 9-year-old child who received 80 separate anesthetics over a period of 6 years in order to facilitate treatment for corrosive esophagitis. The anesthetic agents used included propofol, fentanyl, rocuronium, and sevoflurane. After the last anesthetic, cognitive function was measured using the Wechsler Intelligence Scale for Children-Revised. A total score of 97 (corresponding to normal intelligence) was obtained. The Child Behavior Checklist was completed by his mother. The questionnaire detected no abnormalities except for minor attention problems. In this particular case, there were no permanent adverse effects due to multiple anesthesia.[26] However, studies investigating the potential neurotoxic effects of repetitive anesthesia in children undergoing radiotherapy are warranted.

Summary

The anesthetic management of children undergoing repetitive anesthesia for radiotherapy presents unique challenges. The ability to replicate the anesthetic management with minimal to no interruption of the radiation plan is essential. To date, continuous propofol infusions with supplemental oxygen delivered by face mask or nasal cannula is preferred by most centers. There is still a lack of studies investigating the neurotoxic effects of repetitive anesthesia in children undergoing radiotherapy.

Cytoreductive Surgery With Hyperthermic Intraperitoneal Chemotherapy

Cytoreductive surgery with hyperthermic intraperitoneal chemotherapy (CRS-HIPEC) is an extensive surgical procedure that offers a chance for cure, or more frequently, palliative control of peritoneal spread of malignancies.[27] In children, this procedure can be performed in patients with peritoneal spread of tumors, such as desmoplastic round cell tumor, rhabdomyosarcoma, mesothelioma, and colorectal cancer.[28] Complete cytoreduction is critical to achieving prolonged survival in this group of patients.[29] The procedure may involve the removal of several hundred tumor nodules; thus aggressive cytoreduction is typically performed, with procedures typically lasting up to 12 h and blood loss estimates of up to 175 mL/kg.[30] This is then followed by the instillation of heated (40.5°C–41.0°C) chemotherapy (e.g., cisplatin) into the peritoneal cavity for up to 90 min.

Appropriate anesthetic management is essential for the success of this procedure. A preanesthetic evaluation is usually performed 1 to 2 weeks before the procedure. During this visit, aspects of care, including the possible preoperative transfusion of blood and blood products, and pain management options (epidural analgesia vs. patient controlled analgesia) are discussed. It is notable that children presenting for cytoreductive surgery with hyperthermic intraperitoneal chemotherapy may be anemic or coagulopathic from extensive disease or the side effects of neoadjuvant chemotherapy, thus necessitating possible correction of those factors before surgery. For the most part, children are admitted the day before surgery for preoperative hydration and mechanical bowel preparation. This presents an opportunity for correction of any hematologic or electrolyte abnormalities before surgery.

A general anesthetic with volatile agents, opioids, and epidural analgesia is typically performed. There has also been some limited experience with total intravenous anesthesia.[31] Adequate large bore venous access must be ensured and an arterial line is necessary. Although central lines are not always required during the intraoperative period, they are often used for the correction of potassium and calcium in the postoperative period or for hemodynamic support, for example, norepinephrine infusion.

Intraoperative analgesia typically consists of a combination of epidural analgesia (e.g., bupivacaine 0.075% with hydromorphone 2–5 µg/mL) and a balanced general anesthesia with a continuous infusion of opioids (fentanyl or sufentanil) and supplemental intravenous acetaminophen. Intraoperative opioid administration of up to 5.8 morphine equivalents per kilogram has been reported.[31] In general, total intravenous anesthesia with propofol, dexmedetomidine, and ketamine in combination with epidural analgesia has resulted in lower intraoperative opioid administration. However, this reduced opioid administration has not been associated with lower postoperative opioid consumption.

The nephrotoxic side effects of some of the intraperitoneal chemotherapeutic agents, for example cisplatin, make fluid management a critical component of the anesthetic management. In addition to preoperative hydration with crystalloid infusions at 1.5 times the maintenance rate, intraoperative fluids are given to maintain a urine output ≥2 mL/kg/h.[32] Respective intraoperative crystalloid and colloid transfusions of up to 208 mL/kg and 104 mL/kg have been reported.[30]

Packed red blood cells are transfused to maintain a hemoglobin value ≥100 mg/L (>10 g/dL), and blood products are transfused to keep values within normal limits. Red blood cell transfusion rates of up to 80% with an average transfusion volume of 39 mL/kg were reported by one retrospective study.[30] Children with either a lower preoperative hemoglobin value, lower body mass index, or higher American Society of Anesthesiologists physical status score were more likely to receive blood transfusions.

In the absence of any contraindications, the majority of children may be extubated in the operating room and transferred to the intensive care unit for further postoperative monitoring.

Conclusion

CRS-HIPEC in children is an extensive surgical procedure that requires careful attention to fluid management and may necessitate the transfusion of blood and blood products and hemodynamic lability in the postoperative period. Collaboration between the surgical, anesthesia, and critical care management teams is essential for the successful perioperative management of children undergoing this procedure.

References

1. Liu T, Al-Kzayer LFY, Xie X, et al. Mediastinal lesions across the age spectrum: a clinicopathological comparison between pediatric and adult patients. *Oncotarget*. 2017;8(35):59845–59853.
2. Gun F, Erginel B, Unuvar A, et al. Mediastinal masses in children: experience with 120 cases. *Pediatr Hematol Oncol*. 2012;29(2):141–147.
3. Malik R, Mullassery D, Kleine-Brueggeney M, et al. Anterior mediastinal masses: a multidisciplinary pathway for safe diagnostic procedures. *J Pediatr Surg*. 2019;54(2):251–254.
4. Anghelescu DL, Burgoyne LL, Liu T, et al. Clinical and diagnostic imaging findings predict anesthetic complications in children presenting with malignant mediastinal masses. *Paediatr Anaesth*. 2007;17(11):1090–1098.
5. Brenn BR, Hughes AK. The anesthetic management of anterior mediastinal masses in children: a review. *Int Anesthesiol Clin*. 2019;57(4):e24–e41.
6. Adler AC, Schwartz ER, Waters JM, et al. Anesthetizing a child for a large compressive mediastinal mass with distraction techniques and music therapies as the sole agents. *J Clin Anesth*. 2016;35:392–397.
7. Tutuncu AC, Kendigelen P, Kaya G. Anaesthetic management of a child with a massive mediastinal mass. *Turk J Anaesthesiol Reanim*. 2017;45:374–376.
8. Corridore M, Phillips A, Rabe AJ, et al. Dexmedetomidine-ketamine sedation in a child with a mediastinal mass. *World J Pediatr Congenit Heart Surg*. 2012;3(1):142–146.
9. Abdelmalak B, Marcanthony N, Abdelmalak J, et al. Dexmedetomidine for anesthetic management of anterior mediastinal mass. *J Anesth*. 2010;24(4):607–610.
10. Frost I, Ross-Russell R, Bass S, et al. A rapidly advancing mediastinal mass–overcoming tracheobronchial obstruction. *Paediatr Anaesth*. 2007;17(9):893–896.
11. Komura M, Kanamori Y, Sugiyama M, et al. A pediatric case of life-threatening airway obstruction caused by a cervicomediastinal thymic cyst. *Pediatr Radiol*. 2010;40(9):1569–1571.
12. Owusu-Agyemang P, Grosshans D, Arunkumar R, et al. Non-invasive anesthesia for children undergoing proton radiation therapy. *Radiother Oncol*. 2014;111(1):30–34.
13. Anghelescu DL, Burgoyne LL, Liu W, et al. Safe anesthesia for radiotherapy in pediatric oncology: St. Jude Children's Research Hospital experience, 2004–2006. *Int J Radiat Oncol Biol Phys*. 2008;71(2):491–497.
14. Verma V, Beethe AB, LeRiger M, et al. Anesthesia complications of pediatric radiation therapy. *Pract Radiat Oncol*. 2016;6(3):143–154.
15. Owusu-Agyemang P, Popovich SM, Zavala AM, et al. A multi-institutional pilot survey of anesthesia practices during proton radiation therapy. *Pract Radiat Oncol*. 2016;6(3):155–159.
16. Yalçın Çok O, Evren Eker H, Arıboğan A. Ketamine dosing for sedation during repeated radiotherapy sessions in children. *Turk J Med Sci*. 2018;48(4):851–855.
17. Soyannwo OA, Amanor-Boadu SD, Adenipekun A, et al. Ketamine anaesthesia for young children undergoing radiotherapy. *West Afr J Med*. 2001;20(2):136–139.
18. Parker RI, Mahan RA, Giugliano D, et al. Efficacy and safety of intravenous midazolam and ketamine as sedation for therapeutic and diagnostic procedures in children. *Pediatrics*. 1997;99(3):427–431.
19. Seiler G, De Vol E, Khafaga Y, et al. Evaluation of the safety and efficacy of repeated sedations for the radiotherapy of young children with cancer: a prospective study of 1033 consecutive sedations. *Int J Radiat Oncol Biol Phys*. 2001;49(3): 771–783.
20. Kim SK, Song MH, Lee IJ, et al. Dexmedetomidine for sedation in pediatric patients who received more than 20 sessions of radiation therapy: two cases report. *Korean J Anesthesiol*. 2016;69(6):627–631.
21. Shukry M, Ramadhyani U. Dexmedetomidine as the primary sedative agent for brain radiation therapy in a 21-month old child. *Paediatr Anaesth*. 2005;15(3):241–242.
22. Kim S, Hahn S, Jang MJ, et al. Evaluation of the safety of using propofol for paediatric procedural sedation: a systematic review and meta-analysis. *Sci Rep*. 2019;9(1):12245.
23. Slovis TL. Sedation and anesthesia issues in pediatric imaging. *Pediatr Radiol*. 2011;41(Suppl 2):514–516.

24. Yıldırım I, Çelik AI, Bay SB, et al. Propofol-based balanced anesthesia is safer in pediatric radiotherapy. *J Oncol Pharm Pract.* 2019;25(8):1891–1896.
25. Banerjee P, Rossi MG, Anghelescu DL, et al. Association between anesthesia exposure and neurocognitive and neuroimaging outcomes in long-term survivors of childhood acute lymphoblastic leukemia. *JAMA Oncol.* 2019;5(10):1456–1463.
26. Oba S, Türk HŞ. A case report of multiple anesthesia for pediatric surgery: 80 anesthesia applications in a period of 6 years. *BMC Anesthesiol.* 2018;18(1):175.
27. Sugarbaker PH. Peritonectomy procedures. *Ann Surg.* 1995;221(1):29–42.
28. Hayes-Jordan A, Green H, Lin H, et al. Cytoreductive surgery and hyperthermic intraperitoneal chemotherapy (HIPEC) for children, adolescents, and young adults: the first 50 cases. *Ann Surg Oncol.* 2015;22(5):1726–1732.
29. Huh WW, Fitzgerald NE, Mahajan A, et al. Peritoneal sarcomatosis in pediatric malignancies. *Pediatr Blood Cancer.* 2013;60(1):12–17.
30. Owusu-Agyemang P, Williams U, Van Meter A, et al. Investigating the association between perioperative blood transfusions and outcomes in children undergoing cytoreductive surgery with hyperthermic intraperitoneal chemotherapy. *Vox Sang.* 2017;112(1):40–46.
31. Owusu-Agyemang P, Hayes-Jordan A, Van Meter A, et al. Assessing the survival impact of perioperative opioid consumption in children and adolescents undergoing cytoreductive surgery with hyperthermic intraperitoneal chemotherapy. *Pediatr Anesth.* 2017;27(6):648–656.
32. Owusu-Agyemang P, Arunkumar R, Green H, et al. Anesthetic management and renal function in pediatric patients undergoing cytoreductive surgery with continuous hyperthermic intraperitoneal chemotherapy (HIPEC) with cisplatin. *Ann Surg Oncol.* 2012;19(8):2652–2656.

48

General Principles for Intensive Care Management of Pediatric Patients With Cancer

LINETTE EWING, SHEHLA RAZVI, AND RODRIGO MEJIA

Introduction/Overview

The most common cancers in the pediatric population are acute leukemia, central nervous system (CNS) tumors, nephroblastoma, neuroblastoma, lymphoma, and sarcoma (see Chapter 45). The most common surgeries performed in pediatric patients with cancer are for central access for treatment (port or central line placement) and tumor resections. Caring for these children in the postoperative period requires knowledge of their cancer and previous therapies. Commonly, patients are often immunocompromised and may have single or multiple organ dysfunction or damage resulting from the disease or treatment-related effects. This may include cardiac dysfunction, radiation-induced tissue damage, acute or acute-on-chronic kidney injury, electrolyte imbalances, adrenal insufficiency, or malnutrition.

A systematic preoperative evaluation of the patient is vital for successful postoperative management. Discussion between the intensive care unit and anesthesia clinicians before surgery may help mitigate problems in the postoperative period. Postoperative planning includes the timing of extubation, the optimal location for immediate recovery from anesthesia, and the anticipation of pain control issues. These decisions should be communicated ahead of time with staff in the postanesthesia care unit (PACU), intensive care unit, and pediatric ward. In addition, a complete and thorough handoff should be provided between teams. An example of a handoff form is shown in Table 48.1.[1]

Airway

The timing of extubation should be planned before the surgery begins. Extubation may occur immediately after surgery or be delayed for days in the intensive care unit due to airway risk (e.g., postoperative swelling), pulmonary edema, or hemodynamic instability. Patients who have undergone neurosurgery, oral-maxillary-facial surgery, or cardiac or thoracic surgery may benefit from postoperative mechanical ventilation for monitoring and management of tissue edema compromising the airway, or for hemodynamic and ventilatory optimization. Other considerations unique to pediatric patients with cancer include painful mucositis, restricted mouth opening (trismus), or a history of radiation to the neck requiring a well-planned process, given the potential for critical airway complications. Mucositis causes moderate to severe pain, friable oral tissue, edema, and bleeding. Restricted mouth opening may be seen in several pediatric conditions, including mandibular/temporomandibular joint radiation, Pierre Robin syndrome, Carpenter syndrome, Goldenhar syndrome, Crouzon disease, Freeman-Sheldon syndrome, Treacher-Collins syndrome, Klippel-Feil syndrome, ankylosing spondylitis, and rheumatoid arthritis (see Chapter 46). Macroglossia is associated with specific syndromes, including trisomy 21, Hurler syndrome, and Beckwith-Wiedemann syndrome, and can challenge reintubation or maintaining an oral airway.[2] Radiation to the neck can cause tracheal stenosis, affecting the airway, and may require fiberoptic intubation and a smaller than average endotracheal tube size, especially if the need for reintubation arises. Neurosurgical procedures, especially those involving the posterior or infratentorial fossa, may affect cranial nerve function and lead to a neurologic pathology affecting breathing and swallowing.

Residual anesthesia effects may lead to upper airway obstruction due to the loss of pharyngeal airway tone. The tongue falls back against the posterior pharynx and obstructs the gas flow. Vocal cord swelling or subglottic edema that may occur with intubation can also cause upper airway obstruction and stridor. Cool mist, sedation, pain medications, racemic epinephrine nebulizer treatments, and intravenous dexamethasone are treatment options for airway edema causing stridor. In patients who have undergone thyroid, parathyroid, or aortic surgery, damage to the recurrent laryngeal nerve is possible. This may cause vocal cord paresis or paralysis, resulting in stridor or voice hoarseness. Patients undergoing neurosurgery of the posterior or infratentorial fossa may also have paresis or paralysis of the vocal cords, leading to vocal cord dysfunction and difficulty

TABLE 48.1 PACU Handoff Checklist

Patient Identification (Name Band Check)	
Duration/length of procedure	Hours, minutes
Allergies	NKDA
Surgical procedure and reason for surgery	
Type of anesthesia (GA, TIVA, regional)	
Surgical or anesthetic complications	
Past medical history	
Preoperative vital signs	T, HR, BP, RR, O_2 sat
Position of the patient (if other than supine)	
Intubation conditions (grade of view, airway, quality of bag-mask ventilation)	
Circulation/need for vasoactive medications	Stable/unstable
Lines/catheters/drains	
Fluid management (fluids in, estimated blood loss, urine output)	IVF/UOP
Analgesia plan during case, postoperative orders	
Antiemetics administered	
Medications due for administration during PACU (antibiotics, etc.)	
Other intraoperative medications (steroids, antihypertensives)	
Family updated	Yes/No

BP, Blood pressure; *GA,* general anesthesia; *HR,* heart rate; *IVF,* intravenous fluid; *NKDA,* no known drug allergies; *O2 sat,* oxygen saturation; *PACU,* postanesthesia care unit; *RR,* respiratory rate; *T,* temperature; *TIVA,* total intravenous anesthesia; *UOP,* urine output.

in breathing. In addition, cranial nerve deficits may also impair swallowing and weaken cough, leading to pooling and aspiration of secretions.

Breathing

Mechanical Ventilation

Residual anesthesia is the most common cause of respiratory failure after surgery.[2] Volatile agents used for anesthesia, benzodiazepines used to decrease anxiety, or opioids used to manage surgical pain may cause prolonged sedation and respiratory depression. Lung protective ventilation strategies should be used in patients needing continued mechanical ventilation postoperatively. Inspiratory volumes up to 8–10 mL/kg, positive end-expiratory pressure (PEEP) of 5–8 cmH_2O, and an age-appropriate respiratory rate should be used in patients with compliant lungs. In diseased lungs, acute lung injury, or respiratory distress syndrome, the mechanical ventilator volumes should be set to 4–8 mL/kg while maintaining plateau pressures of less than 30 cmH_2O and allowing for permissive hypercapnia.[2]

Pediatric oncology patients may experience lung injury before surgery due to direct pulmonary toxicity from chemotherapy or radiation. Bleomycin, busulfan, cyclophosphamide, and nitrosoureas are chemotherapeutic agents known to cause rales, fever, and dyspnea at therapeutic levels. Methotrexate, cytarabine, ifosfamide, cyclophosphamide, interleukin (IL)-2, all-*trans* retinoic acid, and bleomycin may cause endothelial injury and vascular leakage, which can lead to noncardiac pulmonary edema. Dose-dependent radiation damage can present with cough, dyspnea, and pink sputum up to 3 months after treatment. One to two years after treatment, radiation damage can cause fibrosis, increased oxygen requirement, and decreased pulmonary function.[3] Reviewing previous cancer therapies, current symptoms, chest imaging, and previous pulmonary function testing can provide helpful knowledge regarding lung damage.

Noninvasive Ventilation

Discontinuing mechanical ventilation immediately postoperatively decreases the risk of iatrogenic lung injury. The use of noninvasive positive pressure ventilation (NIV), continuous positive airway pressure (CPAP), or bilevel positive airway pressure (BiPAP) provides respiratory support when patients are recovering from anesthesia. These strategies provide respiratory support by preventing alveolar collapse in patients who are spontaneously breathing. Contraindications for NIV use include the following:

- Patient's inability to protect their airway
- Glasgow coma scale <8
- High risk of cardiac arrest
- Hemodynamic instability
- Rapidly progressive neuromuscular weakness
- Unable to correctly fit the face mask (facial tumors, facial surgery)
- Untreated pneumothorax
- Vomiting or risk of aspiration
- Skin breakdown that may be exacerbated by tight-fitting mask

High-Flow Nasal Cannula Therapy

High-flow nasal cannula (HFNC) therapy delivers heated and humidified oxygen via nasal prongs at recommended flow rates of 2–8 L/min for neonates and 4–70 L/min for children. An air-oxygen blender allows the percentage of oxygen delivered to the patient to be adjusted. HFNC is well tolerated in pediatric patients, from neonates through adolescence, and works to improve alveolar oxygen delivery through the generation of PEEP and dead space carbon dioxide washout.[4] The heated and humidified flow prevents airway dryness, which preserves mucociliary function and enhances secretion clearance. Ideally, HFNC decreases the work of breathing and the need to escalate respiratory support to either CPAP or BiPAP and is often better tolerated than positive pressure ventilation with CPAP or BiPAP. HFNC may provide some positive pressure at sufficiently high flows, but this is limited due to multiple variables affecting the transmission of flow to the patient. The ability of HFNC to prevent the need for mechanical ventilation or to prevent mortality has been inconsistently supported in previous studies.[5–7]

Pulmonary Hygiene

Pulmonary hygiene techniques, including traditional chest physical therapy, use postural drainage, percussion, chest wall vibration, and coughing to assist with airway clearance and maintenance. Postural drainage utilizes gravity to facilitate the movement of secretions from the peripheral airways to the larger bronchi. Percussion loosens secretions from the bronchial walls and can be performed in different positions, supporting postural drainage. Chest wall vibrations loosen or move bronchial secretions similar to percussion, but the clinician's hand or device does not lose contact with the chest wall. Most sessions last 15–20 min and are scheduled 4–6 times per day. For acutely ill patients, pulmonary hygiene helps combat the hypoxemic effects of atelectasis, ventilation/perfusion mismatch, bronchospasm, or hypoventilation.[4] Contraindications to pulmonary hygiene include increased intracranial pressure (>20 mmHg), spinal injury, active hemoptysis, hemodynamic instability, pulmonary embolism, pulmonary edema with congestive heart failure, or an open wound over the area where chest physiotherapy would be applied.

Circulation

Physical examination may miss up to half of the patients with early chemotherapy-induced heart failure, primarily due to limitations of echocardiography in diagnosing diastolic dysfunction and right heart failure. Echocardiography is a generally accepted form of evaluating cardiac function, but is better suited for assessing left heart failure. Children at risk for cardiac disease from chemotherapy, especially those previously treated with anthracycline therapy (doxorubicin, daunorubicin, idarubicin, and epirubicin), should have a documented echocardiogram before surgery.[8] Early toxicity can occur within days or weeks of the initial dose of anthracycline.

Pericardial and Pleural Effusions

Cardiac dysfunction from pericardial effusion can progress to cardiac tamponade if left untreated. Pediatric oncology patients at the highest risk for pericardial effusion are those with Hodgkin's lymphoma or those who have received a hematopoietic stem cell transplant. The reported incidences in these patient populations are 5% to 25% and 0.2% to 16.9%, respectively.[9] Pericardial effusion may occur due to graft versus host disease, infection, or immune suppression.[10] Symptoms include tachycardia, S3, friction rub, narrow pulse pressure, dyspnea, cough, chest pain, electrocardiogram (ECG) changes (low voltage, electrical alternans, ST-segment elevation, or PR depression), pulsus paradoxus, Kussmaul sign (elevated jugular venous pressure with inspiration), and abdominal pain.[11] The majority of pericardial effusions seen in patients with Hodgkin's lymphoma are clinically silent and resolve with treatment of the underlying malignancy. Monitoring for the progression of pericardial effusion is performed using serial echocardiograms. Moderate to large effusions, as seen with hematopoietic stem cell transplantation, have a greater risk of life-threatening cardiac tamponade and require urgent pericardiocentesis.[9,11] Maintaining an appropriate fluid balance is essential for the management of pericardial and pleural effusions. A reduced preload due to under resuscitation could lead to cardiovascular collapse. By contrast, excessive administration of intravascular volume may worsen effusions.

Systemic Inflammatory Response Syndrome

Systemic inflammatory response syndrome (SIRS) is a stress response associated with hyperthermia, hypothermia, leukocytosis, leukopenia, tachycardia, and tachypnea. It is a systemic activation of the innate immune system triggered by infection, trauma, surgery, or other stressors. The degree of inflammation and the severity of the SIRS vary depending on the patient's situation.[12] The pediatric oncology population, especially hematopoietic stem cell transplant patients, may experience a SIRS after routine surgery.[3]

Fluid Management

Postoperative fluid management should consider the type and length of surgery, estimated fluid deficit, ongoing fluid loss, and maintenance fluid requirements. Preoperative dehydration or inadequate intraoperative fluids may manifest as tachycardia, diastolic hypotension, or concentrated urine. Postoperatively, endothelial dysfunction results in capillary leak and may increase the risk of acute renal injury and the accumulation of pleural effusions and ascites. Normal saline solutions, PlasmaLyte, lactated Ringer's solution, albumin, and blood products may be used for intravascular volume expansion. Although still controversial, albumin and fresh frozen plasma may have added benefits over large crystalloid volume infusion, protecting and repairing vascular endothelium.[13,14]

Postoperative laboratory studies should include a complete blood count, electrolyte levels, albumin, and coagulation studies to determine which fluid would provide the greatest benefit. Once euvolemia is established, intravenous maintenance fluids should be isotonic with appropriate amounts of sodium chloride, potassium chloride, and dextrose to help prevent hyponatremia, hypokalemia, and hypoglycemia.[15] The use of hypotonic fluids in the postoperative period should be restricted to patients with sizeable free water losses, such as neonates and children with diabetes insipidus. In addition, surgical patients are prone to developing the syndrome of inappropriate antidiuretic hormone, leading to hyponatremia and fluid retention. Serum sodium levels should therefore be checked regularly after surgery and corrected appropriately in any patient with a seizure or decreased level of consciousness.[2]

Inotropic Support

Postoperative hypotension should be treated with intravenous fluids or blood products until euvolemia is established. Early inotropic support should be considered in patients at risk of fluid overload and diastolic dysfunction. Hematopoietic stem cell transplant patients with endothelial damage are prone to a systemic inflammatory response after surgery, and fluid overload is detrimental to their overall survival. These patients may benefit from the inotropic, vasodilator, and lusitropic effects to improve cardiac output. Patients with preexisting preoperative or newly discovered postoperative heart dysfunction on echocardiography may benefit from milrinone's inotropic and afterload reducing properties. Low-dose epinephrine in combination with milrinone can be used in hypotensive patients with poor contractility. Vasopressin can be used as a vasopressor to elevate systemic vascular resistance and improve organ perfusion. Norepinephrine can be used in patients with cytokine release syndrome or septic shock. Calcium infusions may also be used as inotropic agents in young children.[3,16]

Pain Management

Postoperative agitation is common and may be due to the residual effects of anesthetics, hypoxia, hypercapnia, bladder distention, delirium, or pain. Many children with cancer have been exposed to opioids and narcotics earlier in their treatment plans and may experience pain before their surgical procedures. Pain is often related to anticancer therapies; however, the most painful events are medical procedures or surgery. A patient-specific multimodal pain management plan can be beneficial for patients with pain that is difficult to control before medical procedures or surgery. Both pharmacologic and nonpharmacologic modalities can provide effective and safe pain control. Epidural and regional anesthesia, patient-controlled analgesia (PCA), opioids, ketamine, dexmedetomidine infusions, acetaminophen, nonsteroidal antiinflammatory drugs (NSAIDs) gabapentin, and supplemental therapies are often used to provide a holistic approach to pain control.[17]

Epidural/Regional Analgesia

In the past decade, an emerging concept in cancer surgery was the opioid-sparing analgesic approach with multimodal use of regional analgesia/anesthesia, acetaminophen, NSAIDs, gabapentin, and low-dose ketamine. The growing success of regional anesthesia has led to a decrease in the need for and length of opioid infusions. For example, in one large children's hospital, local anesthetic infusions via peripheral nerve catheters increased 10-fold over 10 years. In addition, the need for PCA for narcotic delivery has decreased dramatically.[18]

Continuous peripheral nerve blocks are increasingly used in children for postoperative pain control, especially after orthopedic cancer surgeries or extensive tumor resections. These nerve blocks are generally used for a few days, while swelling and pain are the most problematic. Nerve blocks may also be used to relieve intractable pain during end-of-life care.[19] Thoracic surgeries for oncology patients are particularly painful. Nerve blocks have been reported to reduce pain scores, nausea, vomiting, pulmonary complications, and associated stress response markers.[20] In a study involving 204 pediatric patients undergoing minimally invasive surgery, children undergoing thoracic surgery had significantly higher pain scores than those who underwent gastrointestinal surgery. These patients were treated with epidural analgesia and a combination of acetaminophen, morphine, ketorolac, tramadol, and ibuprofen.[21]

Patient-Controlled Analgesia

PCA is an effective method for intravenous administration of opioids after surgery. The benefit is derived from the lack of a lag time between the demand for medication and its delivery. Most hospitals have protocols for using PCAs with options for continuous infusions, bolus infusions, and nurse and proxy (parent) administration. For example, in a Boston children's hospital study, 32,338 PCAs were used over a 22-year period with an extremely low (1%) rate of adverse events. In this study, there were only five incidents where patients could administer larger bolus doses of opioids themselves.[18]

Opioids

Opioids (e.g., morphine, hydromorphone, fentanyl) are the primary medications used to treat postoperative pain. Experimental research in cancer cells and in vivo animal models of cancer suggest that opioids facilitate cancer cell proliferation. However, other studies have demonstrated the opposite effect, reporting an inhibitory effect on cancer cells. Given the problems associated with opioid-related adverse events (ORADEs) opioid-sparing anesthesia (OSA) is gaining popularity in contemporary practice. OSA is administered, using dexmedetomidine, propofol, ketamine, and lidocaine infusions as appropriate; along with non-opioid adjuncts for analgesia utilizing acetaminophen, NSAIDs, gabapentinoids, and regional anesthesia in the absence of contraindications.[22]

Ketamine and Dexmedetomidine

Dexmedetomidine infusions are often used postoperatively in the pediatric intensive care unit to manage pain and anxiety because the drug does not suppress the respiratory drive. The side effects of dexmedetomidine commonly include bradycardia and hypotension. Additionally, ketamine infusion provides sedation and pain control. One study in adults showed that low-dose continuous infusion of ketamine in mechanically ventilated patients was associated with a significant decrease in opioid use without adversely affecting hemodynamic stability.[23]

Nerve Pain

Nerve pain is prominent in pediatric patients who have undergone leg amputation for osteosarcoma, Ewing sarcoma, or in patients with chemotherapy-induced peripheral neuropathy. Patients often complain of a burning, gnawing, or stabbing sensation of the limbs. Phantom nerve pain typically occurs within the first week following surgery and is present in up to 92% of pediatric patients in the first year.[24] Phantom nerve pain is often treated with narcotics, gabapentin, tricyclic antidepressants, opiates, nerve blocks, and epidural catheters. In addition, mirror therapy, psychotherapy, and acupuncture have been successfully used to treat phantom nerve pain.[25,26] In a prospective, double-blind, randomized controlled trial, preoperative administration of gabapentin was associated with reduced pain scores in the postoperative period. Adding opioids postoperatively further reduces postoperative pain levels.[26] Nerve pain is often challenging to treat. The benefits of a combination of therapies were demonstrated in a case study of a patient with significant preoperative opioid use undergoing a hemipelvectomy and hip disarticulation, where phantom pain was managed with a multimodal strategy of opioids, ketamine, gabapentin, clonidine, epidural, psychologic, and cognitive behavioral therapy, with a reduction in immediate postoperative pain that completely resolved over 2 years.[24]

References

1. Lane-Fall MB, Beidas RS, Pascual JL, et al. andoffs and transitions in critical care (HATRICC): protocol for a mixed methods study of operating room to intensive care unit handoffs. *BMC Surg.* 2014;14:96.
2. Stockwell J, Kutko M. *Comprehensive Critical Care: Pediatric.* 2nd ed. Mount Prospect, IL: Society of Critical Care Medicine; 2016.
3. Duncan C, Talano JA, McArthur J. *Critical Care of the Pediatric Immunocompromised Hematology/Oncology Patient.* Switzerland: Springer International Publishing; 2019.
4. Walsh BK, Smallwood CD. Pediatric oxygen therapy: a review and update. *Respir Care.* 2017;62(6):645–661.
5. Sklar MC, Mohammed A, Orchanian-Cheff A, Del Sorbo L, Mehta S, Munshi L. The impact of high-flow nasal oxygen in the immunocompromised critically ill: a systematic review and meta-analysis. *Respir Care.* 2018;63(12):1555–1566.
6. Cortegiani A, Crimi C, Sanfilippo F, et al. High flow nasal therapy in immunocompromised patients with acute respiratory failure: a systematic review and meta-analysis. *J Crit Care.* 2019;50:250–256.
7. De Jong A, Calvet L, Lemiale V, et al. The challenge of avoiding intubation in immunocompromised patients with acute respiratory failure. *Expert Rev Respir Med.* 2018;12(10):867–880.
8. Latham GJ, Greenberg RS. Anesthetic considerations for the pediatric oncology patient–part 2: systems-based approach to anesthesia. *Paediatr Anaesth.* 2010;20(5):396–420.
9. Marks LJ, McCarten KM, Pei Q, Friedman DL, Schwartz C, Kelly KM. Pericardial effusion in Hodgkin lymphoma: a report from the Children's Oncology Group AHOD0031 protocol. *Blood.* 2018;132(11):1208–1211.
10. Versluys AB, Grotenhuis HB, Boelens MJJ, Mavinkurve-Groothuis AMC, Breur JMPJ. Predictors and outcome of pericardial effusion after hematopoietic stem cell transplantation in children. *Pediatr Cardiol.* 2018;39(2):236–244.
11. Cully M, Buckley JR, Pifko E, Titus OM. Presenting signs and symptoms of pericardial effusions in the pediatric emergency department. *Pediatr Emerg Care.* 2019;35(4):286–289.
12. Chawla BK, Teitelbaum DH. Profound systemic inflammatory response syndrome following non-emergent intestinal surgery in children. *J Pediatr Surg.* 2013;48(9):1936–1940.
13. Straat M, Muller MC, Meijers J, et al. Effect of transfusion of fresh frozen plasma on parameters of endothelial condition and inflammatory status in non-bleeding critically ill patients: a prospective substudy of a randomized trial. *Crit Care.* 2015;19:163.
14. Jacob M, Bruegger D, Rehm M, Welsch U, Conzen P, Becker B. Contrasting effects of colloid and crystalloid resuscitation fluids on cardiac vascular permeability. *Anesthesiology.* 2006;104(6):1223–1231.
15. Feld LG, Neuspiel DR, Foster BA, et al. Clinical practice guideline: maintenance intravenous fluids in children. *Pediatrics.* 2018;142(6):e20183083.
16. Rowan CM, Nitu ME, Rigby MR. Inconsistencies in care of the pediatric hematopoietic stem cell transplant recipient with respiratory failure: opportunity for standardization and improved outcome. *Pediatr Transplant.* 2014;18(2):230–235.
17. Latham GJ, Greenberg RS. Anesthetic considerations for the pediatric oncology patient—part 3: pain, cognitive dysfunction, and preoperative evaluation. *Paediatr Anaesth.* 2010;20(6):479–489.
18. Donado C, Solodiuk J, Rangel S, et al. Patient- and nurse-controlled analgesia: 22-year experience in a pediatric hospital. *Hosp Pediatr.* 2019;9(2):129–133.
19. Anghelescu DL, Harris B, Faughnan L, et al. Risk of catheter-associated infection in young hematology/oncology patients receiving long-term peripheral nerve blocks. *Paediatr Anaesth.* 2012;22(11):1110–1116.
20. Semmelmann A, Kaltofen H, Loop T. Anesthesia of thoracic surgery in children. *Paediatr Anaesth.* 2018;28(4):326–331.
21. Molinaro F, Krasniqi P, Scolletta S, et al. Considerations regarding pain management and anesthesiological aspects in pediatric patients undergoing minimally invasive surgery: robotic *vs* laparoscopic-thoracoscopic approach. *J Robot Surg.* 2020;14(3):423–430.
22. Forget P, Aguirre J, Bencic I, et al. How anesthetic, analgesic and other non-surgical techniques during cancer surgery might affect postoperative oncologic outcomes: a summary of current state of evidence. *Cancers.* 2019;11(5):592.
23. Buchheit JL, Yeh DD, Eikermann M, Lin H. Impact of low-dose ketamine on the usage of continuous opioid infusion for the treatment of pain in adult mechanically ventilated patients in surgical intensive care units. *J Intensive Care Med.* 2019;34(8):646–651.
24. Grap SM, Fox E, Freeman M, Blackall G, Dalal P. Acute postoperative pain management after major limb amputation in a pediatric patient: a case report. *J Perianesth Nurs.* 2019;34(4):801–809.
25. DeMoss P, Ramsey LH, Karlson CW. Phantom limb pain in pediatric oncology. *Front Neurol.* 2018;9:219.
26. Wang X, Yi Y, Tang D, et al. Gabapentin as an adjuvant therapy for prevention of acute phantom-limb pain in pediatric patients undergoing amputation for malignant bone tumors: a prospective double-blind randomized controlled trial. *J Pain Symptom Manag.* 2018;55(3):721–727.

49

Anesthesia for Procedures Outside of the Operating Room

JESON R. DOCTOR AND MADHAVI D. DESAI

Introduction

Nonoperating room anesthesia (NORA) and anesthesia in the nontheatre environment (ANTE), as the names suggest, provide anesthesia services at locations outside of the safe confines of the operating room. Anesthesia services are being requested at a multitude of locations as diagnostic modalities become more complex and as interventional and therapeutic modalities provide less invasive treatment options. These locations have their own unique challenges, and guidelines have been proposed by various societies, such as the American Society of Anesthesiologists. (ASA) and the Royal College of Anaesthetists (RCoA),[1] for providing anesthesia care in nontheatre environments.

Not surprisingly, children form the largest group of patients in the NORA environment.[2] In addition, children with suspected or diagnosed malignancy may present with associated complications of their disease (severe anemia, hyperkalemia, tumor lysis syndrome, respiratory distress, infections, pleural/pericardial effusions, etc.), which present additional challenges to anesthesia for the pediatric population. This chapter discusses the management of ANTE in children with its specific challenges and problems.

Locations Requiring NORA

The various locations external to the operating room environment that require NORA include but are not limited to:

- Diagnostic and Interventional Radiology Suite: Diagnostic and interventional procedures performed in the computerized tomography (CT), digital subtraction angiography (DSA), magnetic resonance imaging (MRI), fluoroscopic, and ultrasound suites
- Radiation therapy units
- Endoscopy suite
- Positron emission tomography (PET) suite

Other nononcologic areas may include:

- Catheterization laboratory for cardiac and neurologic procedures
- Dental department
- Psychiatry unit for electroconvulsive therapy (ECT)
- Emergency department (ED), trauma units, intensive care units (ICU)

Challenges Associated With NORA

Patient Factors

A significant proportion of children scheduled for procedures in the NORA environment may be outpatients awaiting a diagnosis and may not have been clinically stabilized or medically optimized.[3–5] The functional and physiologic status of the same child may also continuously change during the course of the disease and following treatment with chemotherapy or radiotherapy. The same child may also require anesthesia at multiple times and different locations for various diagnostic and therapeutic procedures. Therefore the risk-benefit ratio of anesthesia needs to be assessed each time the child is scheduled for a procedure under anesthesia.

Children may be inadequately fasting in the absence of clear instructions or may experience dehydration and hypoglycemia from prolonged fasting.[6–8] The recommendations for preoperative fasting are provided in Table 49.1. Patients may present with an upper respiratory tract infection with a runny nose, may have mediastinal masses with dyspnea awaiting biopsy, or may be malnourished due to cancer cachexia. The child may have received chemotherapy in the past few weeks and may be neutropenic undergoing imaging to assess for response to therapy. Repeated chemotherapy in the absence of a vascular port, peripherally inserted central catheter (PICC), or a Hickman's catheter may make intravenous access increasingly difficult. Oral contrast may have been administered if the imaging involves the gastrointestinal tract, thereby increasing the risk of aspiration under anesthesia.

TABLE 49.1 Preoperative Fasting for Elective Procedures in Children[6–8]

	Hours	Examples
Light meal and nonhuman milk	6	Formula milk, cow/buffalo milk, bread without butter, fruit juice, biscuits
Breast milk	4	
Clear fluids up to 3 mL/kg	1	Water, sugar water, coconut water, clear liquids, oral rehydration solution, clear apple juice

Fatty meals require a longer time for fasting of at least 8 h due to the delayed gastric emptying of fats

Environment, Equipment, and Staffing Factors

Environmental Concerns

NORA locations are usually in remote areas of the hospital such as basements where obtaining extra help could prove difficult.[3] Access to patients may be challenging and bulky equipment may contribute to space constraints.[1] Children may need to be monitored and managed from a distance or remotely, thus increasing the dead space for venous access and limiting immediate access to the patient's airway (Fig. 49.1). Electric connections and cables may pose a safety hazard, and the hazards of radiation exposure and ferromagnetic fields in MRI warrant particular attention.

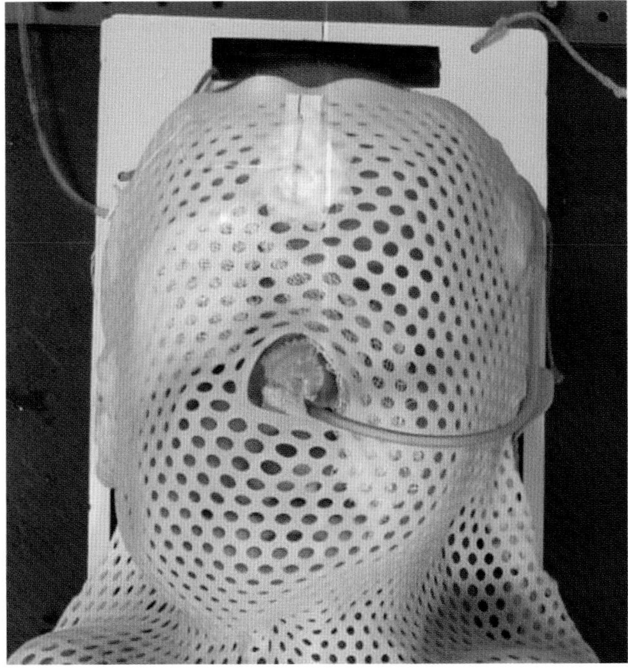

• **Fig. 49.1** Radiation oncology masks for immobilization and precision delivery of radiotherapy beams making the airway less accessible.

Equipment Concerns

It is essential that anesthesia and resuscitation equipment are available, checked, and well maintained.[9] A list of equipment that may be necessary for the provision of anesthesia service within NORA locations is provided in Table 49.2.

Staffing Concerns

It is essential for anesthesia staff to familiarize themselves with a particular NORA environment and its associated challenges before delivery of care. The remoteness of these locations makes calling for help in emergencies difficult. Identifying a fellow practitioner who could be called upon for emergencies could prove beneficial.

Procedural Factors

The anesthesiologist should be familiar with the nature of the procedure to be performed. The approach, position, and need for special equipment for the procedure should be discussed before the child is anesthetized. Adequate analgesia for the procedure, estimated duration, blood loss, blood product availability, and anticipated problems and complications should be discussed prior to beginning the

TABLE 49.2 ASA Standards for Equipment at NORA Locations[9]

1	Oxygen source with central pipeline and backup E-cylinder
2	Working suction
3	Scavenging system if inhalational agents are used
4	Anesthesia equipment • Appropriate sizes of self-inflating bags with reservoir • Anesthetic drugs • Operating room equivalent anesthesia machine
5	Adequate monitoring equipment as per ASA standards for basic monitoring Stethoscope, electrocardiogram, pulse oximeter, noninvasive blood pressure monitor and capnometer
6	Electrical outlets for anesthesia machine and monitors
7	Adequate illumination for patient, workstation, and monitoring equipment
8	Sufficient space to accommodate personnel and equipment
9	Defibrillator, emergency drugs, cardiopulmonary resuscitation equipment readily available
10	Adequately trained staff to assist the anesthesiologist
11	Emergency call list for facility should be available
12	Postanesthesia care monitoring with adequately trained staff including necessary equipment for transporting the patient to the intensive care unit.

procedure. Pediatric patients in these locations often require deep sedation or general anesthesia.[2,4]

Who Should be Administering Sedation and Anesthesia?

The Roles, Responsibilities, and Training Requirements for Anesthesiologists and Assistants

Societies, such as the ASA, offer clear guidelines on the roles, responsibilities, and minimum training requirements for professionals administering sedation and anesthesia.[10,11] Recommendations have also been proposed for pediatric procedural sedation outside the operating room.[12] The roles, responsibilities, and skill requirements for providing sedation and anesthesia outside the operating room are described in Table 49.3. Similarly, the RCoA provides guidelines defining the roles and training requirements for administering sedation and/or anesthesia.[1]

Patient Evaluation, Preparation, and Preprocedure Checklist

The ASA has recommended a checklist for the equipment necessary for providing sedation or anesthesia services within NORA locations (see Table 49.2). The mnemonic called SOAPME (Suction, Oxygen, Airway equipment, Pharmacy, Monitors, and Equipment) is useful in the anesthesia setup of NORA locations.[13]

A detailed medical history of the patient with an emphasis on the presenting symptoms and past medical history should be elicited. The last dose of chemotherapy, radiotherapy, or surgery should be documented. The anesthesiologist should be aware of the various implications of chemotherapeutic drugs on various body organ systems. A detailed physical examination, including an airway exam, should be performed.[14] The fasting status, WHO surgical safety checklist, and parental consent or child's assent should also be confirmed. For a complete evaluation of the pediatric patient for NORA, see Table 49.4. A frequent challenge is the management of the child presenting with a runny nose.

Infants and preschool children may have 6–8 episodes of an upper respiratory tract infection (URI) in any given year. Typically, the airway remains hyperactive for 3–6 weeks after an URI, increasing the risk of laryngospasm and other respiratory complications.[15] In the event of a suspected malignancy, diagnostic procedures or treatment may not always be delayed for possible medical optimization. This, in and of itself, presents a significant challenge to anesthesiologists, especially at NORA locations. An approach towards a child with an upper respiratory tract infection for a procedure under anesthesia is described in Figure 49.2.

Minimum Monitoring Standards

The ASA has recommended minimum monitoring standards for anesthesia, sedation, and monitored anesthesia care.[10,16]

1. Monitoring oxygenation:
   - Peripheral pulse oximetry (to detect alveolar hypoxemia early)
   - Fraction of inspired oxygen

TABLE 49.3 Staffing Requirements and Specific Additional Skills Requirement for Providing Sedation and Anesthesia to Children Outside the Operating Room[10,11]

Personnel	Skills and Training Required
Anesthesiologist Should be a licensed and board-certified physician	Preanesthesia assessment of children
	Pediatric airway management
	Use of equipment and medications
	Cardiopulmonary resuscitation
	Dedicated towards continuous monitoring and patient care
Nonanesthesia staff assisting anesthesiologist	Familiar with procedure and equipment
	Positioning for patients under anesthesia
	Basic life support
	Postprocedure monitoring
Sedation performed by nonanesthesiologist	Ability to assess the depth of sedation
	Pediatric advanced life support: techniques needed to open the airway and provide bag mask ventilation
	Should comply with hospital sedation policy
	Should be responsible for continuous monitoring and patient care during sedation with no other responsibilities

TABLE 49.4 Preoperative Evaluation of a Pediatric Patient for NORA

Demographics: age, sex, and weight of the child.
Current illness presenting complaints.
History of URTI/mediastinal mass with dyspnea at rest or in supine position. Functional status of the child with daily medications.
Past history
Birth and immunization history
Any comorbidities with hospital admissions
Allergies
Previous procedure and anesthetic history
The last dose of chemotherapy and radiotherapy; implications on various body organ systems
Personal and family history
Nature of procedure to be performed with position, risks and bleeding
Assessing the need for blood and blood products
Assessing the need for postprocedure hospital or ICU admission
Fasting status to be confirmed
Examination
General examination with ease of securing IV access
Airway examination
Systemic examination
Investigation review
Consent for the procedure from parent and child explaining the risks
WHO surgical safety checklist with site and side of procedure
Correct size of equipment and medication doses checklist with anesthetic plan

URTI, upper respiratory tract infection; *WHO*; World Health Organization.

2. Monitoring ventilation:
   - Capnography (to detect alveolar hypoventilation early). Capnography should be used in all cases requiring sedation.[17–19]
   - Ventilator disconnection alarms should be active.
3. Monitoring circulation: should be continuously monitored and recorded every 5 min
   - Electrocardiogram
   - Blood pressure (noninvasive or invasive)
4. Temperature monitoring: should be performed for all patients undergoing anesthesia.

In the event where there is no direct access to the patient, such as during radiotherapy and MRI, remote monitoring from a console is mandatory.

Anesthesia Techniques

Anesthetic options at NORA locations are similar to the operating room environment and include monitored anesthesia care (MAC), sedation, and general anaesthesia.[20] The definitions for general anesthesia and levels of sedation are described in Table 49.5. The presence of an upper respiratory tract infection, a history of obstructive sleep apnea, snoring, obesity, ASA class III, and older age are associated with an increased probability of failed sedation.[21] Neonates and infants may undergo NORA procedures with nonnutritive sucking, swaddling, and rocking.[22] Older children may undergo a diagnostic procedure which is not likely to be painful under MAC or sedation but younger children usually need general anesthesia.[2,4] Depending on the preference and skill of the

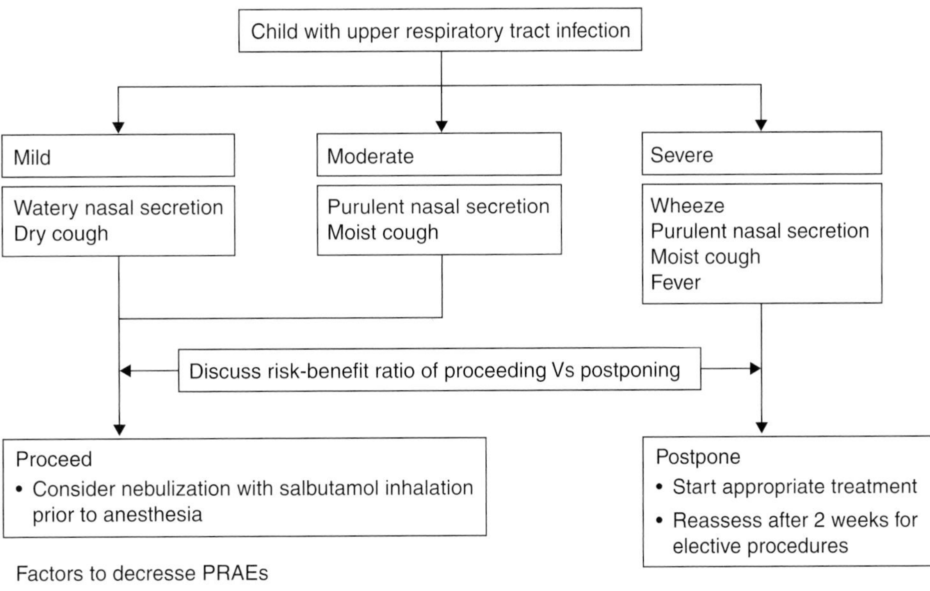

• **Fig. 49.2** Approach to a child with a upper respiratory tract infection

TABLE 49.5 ASA Definition of General Anesthesia and Levels of Sedation/Analgesia (as per ASA 2002 Practice Guidelines for Sedation and Analgesia by Nonanesthesiologists)[10-13]

	Minimal Sedation	Moderate Sedation	Deep Sedation	General Anesthesia
Responsiveness	Normal response to verbal stimulation	Purposeful response to verbal/tactile stimulus	Purposeful response on repeated or painful stimulus	Unarousable even with painful stimulus
Airway	Unaffected	No intervention required	Intervention may be required	Intervention often required
Breathing	Unaffected	Adequate	Spontaneous breathing may be inadequate	Spontaneous breathing frequently inadequate
Circulation	Unaffected	Usually unaffected	Usually maintained	May be impaired

anesthesiologist, the patient's condition and the availability of equipment, either an inhalational induction technique or an intravenous induction technique may be used. There are advantages and disadvantages of each technique. Securing intravenous access in a crying and combative child is a difficult task, and injection of propofol may cause a burning sensation and restlessness in a child.[23] However, there are also some advantages of intravenous over inhalational induction and maintenance, with lesser incidence of postoperative nausea and vomiting and emergence delirium.[23]

Inhalational Technique

Inhalational induction with sevoflurane may be used at NORA locations. Once the child is adequately anesthetized, intravenous access may be obtained after attaching appropriate monitoring devices. The airway may be secured with a supraglottic device or endotracheal tube, depending on the nature of the procedure. Children may be managed with spontaneous ventilation or controlled ventilation, depending on the nature of the procedure to be performed. A report from the Pediatric Sedation Research Consortium indicated that there was a very low prevalence of serious adverse events during nitrous oxide administration in children outside of the operating room. The incidence of vomiting increased when concomitant opioids were administered, and clear fluid intake was less than 2 h prior to the induction of anesthesia.[24]

Total Intravenous Anesthesia

Total intravenous anesthesia (TIVA) may be performed with or without target controlled infusions (TCI) of propofol. In addition to parental presence, a variety of distraction techniques, such as toys, books, balloons, puppets, bubbles, movies, games, videos, and smart phones, have been used for securing IV access.[22] Local anesthetic creams containing a mixture of lidocaine with prilocaine or tetracaine may also aid in reducing the pain associated with vascular access.[25] The various drugs used for sedation and anesthesia and their doses and routes of administration are described in Table 49.6.[26] Of these, propofol and dexmedetomidine have been associated with a very low risk of serious adverse events when used to facilitate anesthesia at NORA locations.[27,28]

The need for correct positioning and safety belts to prevent accidental falls and injuries should be borne in mind. Children should be adequately covered, and warm blankets or forced air warmers may be used to prevent hypothermia. Adequate analgesia and fluids should be given depending on the procedure involved and the duration for which the child has been fasting.

Complications

Complications at NORA locations can be disastrous due to the remoteness of the location and the nonavailability of trained help and equipment. The most frequent causes of adverse events are due to inadequate oxygenation and ventilation.[29] Other complications include, but are not limited to, anaphylactic shock, hypothermia, difficult airway maintenance, aspiration, hemodynamic instability, nausea and vomiting, falls, and trauma.[4,30–33] In addition, bleeding and equipment malfunction may be encountered during procedures at these remote locations. Anesthesia outside the operating room requires careful monitoring to avoid side effects, education of nonanesthetists, and improvement in the protocols and checklists to make anesthesia in these locations safer.[34] The presence of a dedicated, trained, and vigilant anesthesiologist is the best way of preventing adverse events and cannot be overemphasized. Providers must ensure proper monitoring of patients, and NORA locations need to maintain the same standard of care as the main operating room.[32] The various nonoperating room locations have their own specific sets of procedures, problems, and complications, and these are discussed briefly in Table 49.7.

Postprocedural Care

Recovery from anesthesia or sedation should be managed in a dedicated postoperative recovery area. The designated area for postoperative recovery should include a trained nurse, resuscitation equipment, oxygen source, monitoring,

TABLE 49.6 Medications Used, Their Routes of Administration, and Doses[28]

Drug	Route	Dose	Onset of Action	Desired Effect
Midazolam	Oral	0.5–1 mg/kg	15–20 min	Anxiolysis, sedation
	Intravenous	0.05–0.15 mg/kg	Immediate	Anxiolysis, sedation
	Intranasal	0.2–0.3 mg/kg	15–20 min	Anxiolysis, sedation
Fentanyl	Intravenous	0.5–2 µg/kg		Sedation, analgesia
	Intranasal	0.5–2 µg/kg	7–10 min	Sedation, analgesia
Ketamine	Oral	5 mg/kg	10–15 min	Sedation, analgesia
	Intranasal	3 mg/kg	10–15 min	Sedation, analgesia
	Intravenous	0.25–0.5 mg/kg	Immediate	Sedation, analgesia
	Intravenous	1–2 mg/kg	Immediate	Anesthesia
Propofol	Intravenous	25–100 µg/kg/min infusion		Sedation
		2–3 mg/kg	Immediate	Anesthesia
Dexmedetomidine	Intravenous	Bolus: 0.5–1 µg/kg over 10 min Maintenance: 0.2–0.6 µg/kg/h		Anxiolysis, sedation, analgesia
	Intranasal	1–2 µg/kg/min	25–30 min	Anxiolysis, sedation, analgesia
Chloral hydrate	Oral	40–100 mg/kg (maximum 2 g)	10–15 min	Anxiolysis, sedation,

Intramuscular injections are not widely practiced in pediatric oncology due to the risk associated with neutropenia and thrombocytopenia.

TABLE 49.7 Area-Specific Concerns for NORA

Location	Specific Problems Related to Location	Common Procedures Performed in Pediatric Oncology	Common Diseases	Associated Problems to be Checked	Complications Related to Procedures
Computed tomography (CT scan)	Radiation exposure to patient and personnel • Precautions: dosimeters • Protective gear (lead aprons, thyroid shields, etc.) Contrast allergy, anaphylaxis (iodinated nonionic contrast agents are safer than ionic contrasts)	CECT CT-guided biopsy of lesion CT-guided biopsy of mediastinal mass Angiography for bleeders	Suprarenal mass: Wilms tumor, neuroblastomas, pheochromocytoma. Abdominal mass: Hepatoblastoma, Burkitt's lymphoma Anterior mediastinum: NHL, ALL, germ cell tumors Posterior mediastinum: Neuroblastoma, PNET Neural crest tumors Miscellaneous: Chest wall tumors, pleuropulmonary blastomas	Suprarenal mass, hypertension Mediastinal mass, respiratory distress on crying or exertion	Contrast allergy Anaphylaxis Bleeding

Continued

TABLE 49.7 Area-Specific Concerns for NORA—cont'd

Location	Specific Problems Related to Location	Common Procedures Performed in Pediatric Oncology	Common Diseases	Associated Problems to be Checked	Complications Related to Procedures
Interventional radiology		Ophthalmic artery chemoembolization (OAC) Portal vein embolization Angioembolization of big/ vascular tumors/bleeders Radiofrequency ablation (RFA) Percutaneous transhepatic biliary drainage SOS with stenting	Retinoblastoma Hepatoblastoma Liver, lung, soft tissue lesion		Vagal response and hypotension during intraarterial chemotherapy drug injection during OAC Hypothermia Bleeding
Endoscopy suite	Radiation exposure in procedures such as ERCP Bulky equipment and space constraints	Esophagogastroduodenoscopy with or without endoscopic ultrasound Sigmoidoscopy Colonoscopy Endoscopic retrograde Cholangio pancreatography (ERCP)	Usual indications are bleeding in hematologic malignancies	Coagulopathy and hemodynamic instability	Aspiration risk especially for upper GI endoscopy Bowel perforation Bleeding Shared airway in upper GI endoscopy Airway obstruction due to upper GI scope in toddlers and infants
Bronchoscopy suite, operating room, ICU		Bronchoscopy Endobronchial biopsy Bronchoalveolar lavage (BAL) Endobronchial stenting	Febrile neutropenic child with consolidation for BAL Often palliative stenting in critically compromised intrathoracic airway for symptomatic relief	Respiratory distress	Often needs HFNC during procedure Postop HFNC/ NIV/ ETT and ICU in view of respiratory distress
Magnetic resonance imaging (MRI)[36]	Most of the chemo ports are MR safe Implantable cardioverter-defibrillators and cochlear implants are usually contraindicated Safety of the implanted device can be checked on the website www.MRIsafety.com Screening for ferromagnetic material with child and parent Needs MR conditional/safe equipment for anesthesia	MRI brain with spine MRI with spectroscopy and perfusion scan MRI soft tissue, abdomen	Ependymoma Pineal tumors Glial cell tumors Soft tissue sarcomas	Glasgow Coma Scale modified for children Raised intracranial pressure Lower cranial nerve function with bulbar palsy	Aspiration Hypothermia with cold environment (may need 40–120 min) Remote access to the patient with dead space for intravenous access and ventilator tubing Ferromagnetic field Remote monitoring may have a time lag to detect changes/ problems

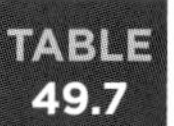

TABLE 49.7 **Area-Specific Concerns for NORA—cont'd**

Location	Specific Problems Related to Location	Common Procedures Performed in Pediatric Oncology	Common Diseases	Associated Problems to be Checked	Complications Related to Procedures
	Need to shift patient out of the MRI scanner room for resuscitation with designated space outside the MRI room Noise: acoustics exceeding 80 dB require ear protection for child Child needs to be monitored from console with MRI-compatible camera suited for dim light and slave monitor				
Radiotherapy Brachytherapy	No personnel/parent can accompany due to radiation hazard Monitoring exclusively through a camera in console and slave monitor or camera screen Radiotherapy includes daily treatment for 3–10 min for 3–7 weeks. Treatment requires immobilization with special immobilization mask (see Fig 49.1) with limited access to the airway unless removed		Ependymoma PNET Soft tissue sarcomas	Airway Difficult IV access due to repeated procedure	Aspiration Late detection of problem through camera Difficult intravenous access because of daily treatment
Bone marrow procedure room, operating room, ICU		Bone marrow aspiration and biopsy Lumbar puncture (CSF study, intrathecal chemotherapy)	Hematolymphoid malignancies Solid tumors (retinoblastoma, neuroblastoma for staging)	Cervical and mediastinal lymph node enlargements in hematolymphoid malignancies causing narrowing of upper or intrathoracic respiratory tract. Low platelets, severe anemia, coagulation disorders.	

ALL, Acute lymphocytic leukemia; *CECT*, contrast enhanced computed tomography; *CSF*, cerebrospinal fluid; *ERCP*, endoscopic retrograde cholangiopancreatography; *ETT*, endotracheal tube; *HFNC*, high frequency nasal cannula; *NHL*, non-Hodgkin's lymphoma; *NIV*, noninvasive ventilation; *PNET*, primitive neuroectodermal tumor.

suction, and all emergency medications. The patient's extremity should be splinted to prevent loss of intravenous access. Parental presence may be helpful in calming the child. The child should be monitored at all times to prevent sudden violent movements during emergence.

The nurse who is in charge of postoperative recovery should be trained in recognizing common postoperative problems and request assistance while starting resuscitation when needed. Common postoperative problems include pain, emergence delirium, postoperative nausea and vomiting, shivering, coughing, agitated behavior, and excessive crying.

Children should be given something to drink as soon as they meet the criteria.[35] Recovery and discharge criteria such as those suggested by ASA for procedural sedation and anesthesia should be followed before discharge from the recovery area.[10] Plans for transfer to the intensive care unit or operating room with transport monitors, ventilators, resuscitation drugs, and infusion pumps should be in place in case the need arises.

Conclusion and Key Messages

- Children are typically unable to cooperate with lengthy imaging procedures or painful treatments and are thus the largest group of patients requiring NORA.
- Societies, such as the ASA, have issued guidelines on the roles, responsibilities, and minimum training requirements for persons administering sedation and anesthesia.
- The ASA has recommended a checklist for the equipment necessary for providing sedation or anesthesia services at nonoperating room locations. The ASA has also recommended certain minimum monitoring standards for anesthesia, sedation, and monitored anesthesia care.
- The preoperative evaluation of the child should take into account the airway, any upper respiratory tract infection, dyspnea, and the anesthetic implications of chemotherapy or radiotherapy.
- The anesthesia technique for the child may be inhalational or intravenous depending on the nature of the procedure.
- The most frequent causes of adverse events at these locations are those related to inadequate oxygenation and ventilation.
- The designated area for postoperative recovery should have a trained nurse, resuscitation equipment, oxygen source, monitoring, suction and emergency medications.
- Each NORA location has its own set of unique problems that the health care provider needs to be aware of.

References

1. *Guidelines for the Provision of Anaesthesia Services in the Non-Theatre Environment Chapter 7*: Royal College of Anaesthetists; 2019.
2. Bell C, Sequeira PM. Nonoperating room anesthesia for children. *Curr Opin Anaesthesiol.* 2005;18(3):271–276.
3. Chang B, Urman RD. Non-operating room anesthesia: the principles of patient assessment and preparation. *Anesthesiol Clin.* 2016;34(1):223–240.
4. Youn AM, Ko YK, Kim YH. Anesthesia and sedation outside of the operating room. *Korean J Anesthesiol.* 2015;68(4):323–331.
5. Maddirala S, Theagrajan A. Non-operating room anaesthesia in children. *Indian J Anaesth.* 2019;63:754–762.
6. Practice guidelines for preoperative fasting and the use of pharmacologic agents to reduce the risk of pulmonary aspiration: application to healthy patients undergoing elective procedures: an updated report by the American Society of Anesthesiologists Task Force on Preoperative Fasting and the Use of Pharmacologic Agents to Reduce the Risk of Pulmonary Aspiration. *Anesthesiology.* 2017;126(3):376–393.
7. Smith I, Kranke P, Murat I, et al. Perioperative fasting in adults and children: guidelines from the European Society of Anaesthesiology. *Eur J Anaesthesiol.* 2011;28:556–569.
8. Thomas M, Morrison C, Newton R, Schindler E. Consensus statement on clear fluids fasting for elective pediatric general anesthesia. *Paediatr Anaesth.* 2018;28(5):411–414.
9. American Society of Anesthesiologists. Statement on Nonoperating Room Anesthetizing Locations. 2013. Available at http://www.asahq.org/quality-and-practicemanagement/standards-and-guidelines#
10. Practice Guidelines for Moderate Procedural Sedation and Analgesia. A Report by the American Society of Anesthesiologists Task Force on Moderate Procedural Sedation and Analgesia, the American Association of Oral and Maxillofacial Surgeons, American College of Radiology, American Dental Association, American Society of Dentist Anesthesiologists, and Society of Interventional Radiology. *Anesthesiology.* 2018;128(3):437–479.
11. American Society of Anesthesiologists Task Force on Sedation and Analgesia by Non-Anesthesiologists. Practice guidelines for sedation and analgesia by non-anesthesiologists. *Anesthesiology.* 2002;96(4):1004–1017.
12. Patino M, Samuels P, Mahmoud M. Pediatric sedation outside the operating room. *Int Anesthesiol Clin.* 2013;51(2):127–146.
13. Ramaiah R, Bhananker S. Pediatric procedural sedation and analgesia outside the operating room: anticipating, avoiding and managing complications. *Expert Rev Neurother.* 2011;11(5):755–763.
14. Tobias JD. Sedation of infants and children outside of the operating room. *Curr Opin Anaesthesiol.* 2015;28(4):478–485.
15. Becke K. Anesthesia in children with a cold. *Curr Opin Anaesthesiol.* 2012;25(3):333–339.
16. American Society of Anesthesiologists. Standards for Basic Anesthetic Monitoring. Last updated December 13, 2020. Available at http://www.asahq.org/quality-and-practice-management/standards-and-guidelines#.
17. Gozal D, Gozal Y. Pediatric sedation/anesthesia outside the operating room. *Curr Opin Anaesthesiol.* 2008;21(4):494–498.
18. Srinivasa V, Kodali BS. Capnometry in the spontaneously breathing patient. *Curr Opin Anaesthesiol.* 2004;17(6):517–520.
19. Whitaker DK, Benson JP. Capnography standards for outside the operating room. *Curr Opin Anaesthesiol.* 2016;29(4):485–492.
20. Sohn HM, Ryu JH. Monitored anesthesia care in and outside the operating room. *Korean J Anesthesiol.* 2016;69(4):319–326.
21. Grunwell JR, McCracken C, Fortenberry J, Stockwell J, Kamat P. Risk factors leading to failed procedural sedation in children outside the operating room. *Pediatr Emerg Care.* 2014;30(6):381–387.

22. Pillai Riddell RR, Racine NM, Gennis HG, et al. Non-pharmacological management of infant and young child procedural pain. *Cochrane Database Syst Rev*. 2015;1:CD006275.
23. Michel Foehn ER. Adult and pediatric anesthesia/sedation for gastrointestinal procedures outside of the operating room. *Curr Opin Anaesthesiol*. 2015;28(4):469–477.
24. Tsze DS, Mallory MD, Cravero JP. Practice Patterns and adverse events of nitrous oxide sedation and analgesia: a report from the Pediatric Sedation Research Consortium. *J Pediatr*. 2016;169:260–265 e2.
25. Manner T, Kanto J, Iisalo E, Lindberg R, Viinamäki O, Scheinin M. Reduction of pain at venous cannulation in children with a eutectic mixture of lidocaine and prilocaine (EMLA cream): comparison with placebo cream and no local premedication. *Acta Anaesthesiol Scand*. 1987;31(8):735–739.
26. Khurmi N, Patel P, Kraus M, Trentman T. Pharmacologic considerations for pediatric sedation and anesthesia outside the operating room: a review for anesthesia and non-anesthesia providers. *Paediatr Drugs*. 2017;19(5):435–446.
27. Cravero JP, Beach ML, Blike GT, Gallagher SM, Hertzog JH. Pediatric Sedation Research Consortium. The incidence and nature of adverse events during pediatric sedation/anesthesia with propofol for procedures outside the operating room: a report from the Pediatric Sedation Research Consortium. *Anesth Analg*. 2009;108(3):795–804.
28. Sulton C, McCracken C, Simon HK, et al. Pediatric procedural sedation using dexmedetomidine: a report from the Pediatric Sedation Research Consortium. *Hosp Pediatr*. 2016;6(9):536–544.
29. Robbertze R, Posner KL, Domino KB. Closed claims review of anesthesia for procedures outside the operating room. *Curr Opin Anaesthesiol*. 2006;19(4):436–442.
30. Melloni C. Morbidity and mortality related to anesthesia outside the operating room. *Minerva Anestesiol*. 2005;71(6):325–334.
31. Campbell K, Torres L, Stayer S. Anesthesia and sedation outside the operating room. *Anesthesiol Clin*. 2014;32(1):25–43.
32. Chang B, Kaye AD, Diaz JH, Westlake B, Dutton RP, Urman RD. Interventional procedures outside of the operating room: results from the National Anesthesia Clinical Outcomes Registry. *J Patient Saf*. 2018;14(1):9–16.
33. Beach ML, Cohen DM, Gallagher SM, Cravero JP. Major adverse events and relationship to nil per os status in pediatric sedation/anesthesia outside the operating room: a report of the Pediatric Sedation Research Consortium. *Anesthesiology*. 2016;124(1):80–88.
34. Garnier M, Bonnet F. Management of anesthetic emergencies and complications outside the operating room. *Curr Opin Anaesthesiol*. 2014;27(4):437–441.
35. Sümpelmann R, Becke K, Brenner S, et al. Perioperative intravenous fluid therapy in children: guidelines from the Association of the Scientific Medical Societies in Germany. *Paediatr Anaesth*. 2017;27(1):10–18.
36. Wilson SR, Shinde S, Appleby I, et al. Guidelines for the safe provision of anaesthesia in magnetic resonance units 2019: Guidelines from the Association of Anaesthetists and the Neuro Anaesthesia and Critical Care Society of Great Britain and Ireland. *Anaesthesia*. 2019;74(5):638–650.

50

Do Not Resuscitate and the Terminally Ill Child

NELDA ITZEP, KAREN MOODY, AND REGINA OKHUYSEN-CAWLEY

Introduction

Cancer is the leading cause of disease-related death in children in the United States.[1] Despite the numerous advances in pediatric oncology, some children are diagnosed with terminal malignancies and many others will become terminal later in their cancer trajectory. A child may die as a result of direct cancer progression or complications of treatment. For instance, uncontrolled invasion of cancer into major organs and bone marrow leads to a terminal prognosis. Additionally, the side effects of chemotherapy, including myelosuppression, cardiac toxicity, liver or renal toxicity, can also lead to death. At other times, the total body burden of cancer leads to cachexia, profound weakness, and eventual death. Reaching this stage in the cancer journey is a very difficult time in a child's and family's lives. Great care must be taken to provide compassionate care and support to families and children in this stage. This can begin by eliciting and then honoring their wishes and values.

Decision-Making in Pediatrics

Throughout the cancer journey parents and their child will have to make many decisions regarding their care, starting at diagnosis. Conversations about what is important to them early in their journey are necessary for developing a strong provider-parent relationship and will help establish goals of care.

Goals of Care

Ideally, conversations regarding goals of care start early in the cancer journey and are revisited periodically as the treatment and disease course progresses, and goals of care change. This is important all throughout the journey but is particularly crucial as the patient becomes terminal. These conversations must elicit the child's/parents' values, hopes, dreams, and fears, as well as assess their physical and emotional suffering. By carefully weighing the expected results of treatment and side effects against the child's/parents' values and goals, a picture begins to emerge that will help families make decisions regarding their care and help the physician to understand the family's decisions and to align the treatment with their goals.

Goals of care can be different for different families and children, and they will also change over time, depending on prognosis. Initially, the goal is most often for cure and thus treatment will be disease-directed and cure-oriented. Treatment regimens may be intense with the potential for high toxicity. As the disease advances, the goal may change to slowing the cancer progression to prolong life and increase quality of life (QoL). At this point the treatment will still be disease-directed, but it may be limited to treatments that allow for a good QoL and do not cause significant toxicity. Once a child enters a terminal stage, the goal may shift to providing comfort and minimizing suffering. Treatments, if desired, would ideally have little to no toxicity and allow for maximum comfort and QoL.

There are a few common goals that arise as children approach the end of life: minimizing physical and emotional suffering, enhancing QoL, dying peacefully, and leaving a legacy.[2] Palliative care physicians can help families achieve these goals, as well as align any remaining medical treatment with these goals. Table 50.1 shows a list of possible questions that may facilitate these difficult conversations.

Concurrent Care

Unique to pediatrics is the concept of concurrent care; this type of care allows children to continue receiving cancer treatment while enrolled in a hospice near the end of life. This is not the case for adults; they must stop all disease-directed treatment and even stop seeing their primary oncologist once they enroll in a hospice. Concurrent care allows for a gentle transition between the oncology treatment team and the palliative care/hospice team. Palliative care, which is an integrated, interdisciplinary team-based, holistic approach to address symptoms in seriously ill children, can also help to facilitate complex medical decision-making with patients, their families, and their primary medical teams. Patients can continue to see their oncologist until

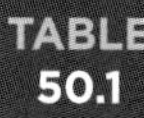

TABLE 50.1 Questions Used to Identify Goals

Is it ok to talk about some of the experiences of other families I have cared for?
Some children/families worry about what may happen if treatments don't work, is that something you worry about?
Can you tell us your understanding of the situation?
What are your concerns at this time and for the future?
I worry that [child's name] will not tolerate more chemotherapy. Can we talk about that?
I understand your primary hope is cure; what else do you hope for?
In light of what we have discussed, what is most important to you now?
How do you feel about your treatments?
What symptoms are the most bothersome?
What are the things that bring you joy/comfort?
What activities bring you peace or comfort?
How and where do you want to live the rest of your life?

they are no longer physically able. This may be very helpful to families, as there is often a strong bond with the physician who has been on this journey with them. Concurrent care allows time for the hospice/palliative care team to integrate themselves and build a rapport with families before having to discuss very difficult topics such as "do not resuscitate" (DNR) and end of life. Palliative care is ideally integrated early in the disease process so that the full benefits, including impeccable symptom control, truly partnered medical decision-making, advance care planning, and optimal end-of-life care. Furthermore, opportunities for legacy building and bereavement support are viewed as a thread of continuity from the time of initial contact to the present, rather than as the sudden introduction of a team of strangers at the end of an illness.

Although palliative care services are available in most academic children's hospitals in the United States, primary (basic symptom management and communication skills) and secondary (advanced symptom management, facilitation of complex medical decision-making, and management of complicated family dynamics) services are available to only a fraction of the 21 million children worldwide with serious diseases. Thus it is important that all physicians develop primary palliative care skills to care for terminal children and their families.

Communication

Honest, clear, and compassionate communication is critical for shared decision-making and subsequently advanced care planning. Two categories of communication needs have been described in the medical literature: cognitive and affective. The cognitive needs generally include the need to know medical facts, such as the diagnosis, treatment options, side effects, and prognosis. The affective needs in communication encompass the need to express oneself and to be understood, validated, and supported.[3] To meet both of these needs, the physician must have knowledge of the family and child and their preferences for receiving and delivering information, such as who will be present when important news is delivered and how much detail should be given. Eliciting preferences for information is an important step to take prior to family meetings.

Family Meetings

Family meetings are an important procedure for giving and receiving sensitive information with families. They must be planned with great thought given as to who will be present, who will lead, and what will be discussed. The presence of the interdisciplinary team may be helpful to encompass all aspects of the child and family's care but this must be weighed against the potential to overwhelm families with too many people in the room. Before the meeting, the medical team should meet first to discuss the medical aspects of the discussion, including prognosis, proposed treatment options, and palliative measures, to ensure everyone agrees and minimize opposing views in front of the family. The meeting should take place in a quiet, private place with care given to minimize distractions and interruptions. One person should be designated to lead. Someone from the team should review with the family their communication preferences, informational needs, whom they want present, and any other questions to be added to the agenda. Often parents and providers are unsure whether to include the child in these meetings. The answer to this will depend on the parents' wishes, the developmental age of the child, and sometimes the child's wishes. While honesty is always recommended, communication with children must be carried out delicately and in a developmentally appropriate way. When parents choose not to include the child in the team discussion, they can be encouraged to share the information later either by themselves or with the help of a trusted member of the care team. This allows time for parents to process the information first before sharing it with their child. Last, these difficult conversations will be performed all at once, albeit rarely. In many cases the conversation will be spread over several sessions to allow time for grieving and processing.

Tools for the Providers

Medical decision-making has become more complex as medicine has evolved, particularly since the introduction of life-sustaining technology in the 1950s. Difficult conversations can be challenging for providers. Training in such specialized communication skills has not traditionally been part of the medical training curriculum although this has changed in the last few years. Many tools exist to help medical providers as they navigate these conversations with families. One tool is NURSE, which is a helpful mnemonic that stands for Name, Understand, Respect, Support, and Explore and can help providers respond to the patient's or family's emotions.[4] These words refer to types of statements that can be used to respond to emotions. For example, the medical provider can name the emotion they are witnessing that demonstrates that the provider is paying attention to the emotion. Another option is for the provider to make a statement relating to how difficult, scary, or frustrating a situation is. Statements of respect refer to acknowledgments of the excellent care that a parent has provided for his or her child. Support statements can help foster trust in the patient/family-physician relationship and reassure families that they will not be abandoned. Last, the medical provider can simply explore the family's/patient's concerns or goals especially as disease or treatment progresses. Reflective listening and offering a silent ear are additional valuable communication tools that help families to feel heard, listened to, and supported. Other helpful resources include Vital Talk (www.vitaltalk.org), a communication skills course for medical providers for delivering serious news and the accompanying application for smartphones (Vital Tips), and the Courageous Parents Network (www.courageousparentsnetwork.org), an organization founded by parents to empower and equip parents and providers caring for children with serious illness.

Advanced Care Planning

Advanced care planning is now commonplace in the adult health care system; however, it is not standard practice in pediatrics. Data in the adult literature support advanced care planning, as it helps avoid aggressive yet futile interventions, and therefore minimizes suffering at the end of life. Advanced care planning improves concordance between care delivered and the patient's preferences for care.[5] This same benefit should be extended to children and adolescents approaching end of life. In fact, some literature already supports the use of advanced care planning in pediatrics, as well as the need for further research in this area.[6,7] Many tools for advanced care planning have been developed for adults but probably the most widely used tool is a legal advanced directive called *Five Wishes*, which takes into account medical, spiritual, emotional, and personal concerns. There are also pediatric versions, such as "My Wishes" or "Voicing My Choices," which take into account the developmental age of this special population.[8] Although these documents are not legally binding for pediatric patients they can help initiate these difficult conversations, as well as allow the child and parents to express their wishes. There are different aspects of advanced care planning but commonly it includes assigning a proxy medical decision-maker, preferences for end-of-life care, whether to attempt cardiopulmonary resuscitation (CPR) at end of life, the use of life-sustaining medical therapies, preferred location of death, and legacy planning.

Code Status

CPR was originally developed in the 1960s to reverse unexpected cessation of cardiopulmonary function in previously healthy individuals undergoing operations using anesthesia and with the expectation of recovery. However, blanket application of this intervention is not appropriate for all patients. By the mid-1970s, concerned clinicians created the first institutional policies seeking to protect patients who asserted their right to die without CPR in situations where it was known to be ineffective.[9] It is well known that chronically ill children tend to do poorly with CPR, even when witnessed arrest occurs in hospitals in well-resourced countries. Although cardiorespiratory activity may return with CPR, functional recovery is typically very poor; these children rarely return to their already-compromised baseline.

CPR is also, unfortunately, sometimes attempted for patients whose disease trajectory is well known to the clinical team and who are simply in the process of dying. Patients and families may be unable to accept the medical facts and continue to hold unrealistic expectations. Some clinicians may have formed strong bonds with patients and their families over the years and feel compelled to offer CPR as the child deteriorates, even when death is the expected outcome.

Palliative care providers can help patients and families reach decisions regarding whether or not their child should undergo CPR when arrest ensues. Most patients and families are able to agree with recommendations to forgo potentially harmful interventions when given the historical context of CPR, the dismal outcomes in debilitated patients, and an understanding of the beneficial interventions that can be implemented at end of life to ensure comfort. Families can usually understand the real risks of pain and prolonged suffering CPR may cause if implemented.

Presently, fully informed, joint decisions can be made by the patient or surrogate medical decision-maker and the attending physician to accept or forgo CPR, and this is documented as the "code status." A patient's code status is an important designation within the health care system. It can range from "full code" (all resuscitative and life-sustaining measures are provided) to "do not resuscitate" or DNR (no CPR is provided). At end of life, treatment can be personalized based on the patient's or family's wishes. The components of the code status encompass chest compressions, intubation, mechanical ventilation, defibrillation, and medications used during resuscitations.

The decision to withhold life-prolonging medical therapies and CPR at the end of life (DNR) is an important decision for families. Every attempt to honor this decision should be made and there may be legal consequences if it is not. Without these interventions, the disease course will progress and the child will reach the end of their natural life. Comfort measures should be in place for the child to ensure that the child does not suffer.

Palliative Procedures

Indications for surgical and other invasive procedures may arise in children with severe underlying medical conditions who have advanced directives, including a DNR already in place. A child may develop a problem that requires a surgical or interventional procedure under anesthesia that may be completely unrelated to the child's underlying process. One example would be a child with metastatic osteosarcoma who develops acute appendicitis. Other children may develop complications of treatment for their underlying condition; a fairly common example would be that of a child with refractory leukemia who develops neutropenic enterocolitis with perforation and septic shock, and in whom surgical intervention is considered. Some children may experience worsening of a symptom as their disease progresses that may be improved with an invasive intervention. Common examples are malignant effusions causing pain and respiratory distress, malignant ascites, and malignant bowel obstruction unresponsive to medical therapy.[10]

The decision to pursue an invasive procedure is always very difficult, especially as risks increase and significant moral distress can occur in providers trying to discern the best course of action. Multidisciplinary consultation may facilitate truly informed and empowered medical decision-making. Ethics committees can help individual clinicians, the entire health care team, and the patient and family members to comprehend the overall clinical situation, properly weigh the relative risks and benefits of specific proposed procedures, and may reassure clinicians, most often surgeons and interventional radiologists, who may be wary of performing the procedures. In some cases surgical intervention is not the right choice and the family may choose to spend the child's last days with an integrated palliative approach, which includes appropriate pharmacologic therapy (inclusive of palliative sedation, if indicated), nonpharmacologic adjuncts, and comprehensive psychosocial support, which certainly minimizes the existential pain even very young children may experience (see Table 50.2). Such an approach may help minimize decisional regret in parents, families, and clinicians, and may improve the overall family satisfaction with care, reduce costs, and mitigate the bereavement process after the child dies.

Perioperative DNR Orders

There has been an increased interest in the topic of perioperative DNR orders in the last few years.[11] During surgical interventions, even palliative ones, most institutional policies dictate that the DNR status must be temporarily suspended to allow for stabilizing measures in the operating room. The medical team must ensure that this is explained clearly to families and allow families to voice their concerns. Notably, position statements by the American Society of Anesthesiologists, the American College of Surgeons, the American Association of Nurse Anesthetists, and the Association of Perioperative Registered Nurses have cautioned against "blanket" revocation of DNR orders when surgical interventions are considered for patients who have life-limiting, life-threatening disorders, and in whom automatic perioperative revocation may impinge on the individual's right to self-determination. However, revocation of these orders generally does occur for many reasons, some of which are shown in Table 50.3.

In an effort to combat some of the challenges involved in maintaining a DNR in the perioperative setting, one model to consider is the "touchpoints" model (Table 50.4). This model focuses on specific opportunities for dialog regarding the previously agreed-upon plan for providing or withholding interventions in different clinical scenarios. The time points for discussion are analogous to the World Health Organization's "5 Moments for Hand Hygiene" schematic (1, before patient contact; 2, before aseptic task; 3, after body exposure risk; 4, after patient contact; and 5, after contact with surroundings). One benefit is that this model is familiar to clinicians throughout the world. In this model, documentation is provided at these time points so that all care providers are up to date with the current code status and intervention plans.[10]

TABLE 50.2 Examples of Palliative Procedures

Neurologic	Ventriculoperitoneal or other shunting procedures to relieve symptomatic hydrocephalus; deep brain stimulation for intractable movement disorders.
Otolaryngology	Airway dilations, laser-based and operative tracheostomy for obstruction or severe dyspnea in patients intolerant of noninvasive ventilation.
Thoracic	Thoracentesis/pericardiocentesis, airway stent placement.
Gastrointestinal	Gastrostomy, ileostomy, colostomy.
Musculoskeletal	Operative or minimally invasive fixation of fractures; debulking resections, palliative amputation for refractory pain.
Pain	Neuromodulation, ablation, deep brain stimulation, nerve blocks, epidurals.
Miscellaneous	Palliative radiation, central venous access devices, other drains.

Care at End of Life

As a child approaches end of life, more focus should be directed to comfort. The need for interventions, such as medication administration and laboratory assessments, should be reevaluated for their utility and discontinued if burden exceeds benefit. Decisions regarding antibiotics, transfusions, and fluid and nutritional therapies should be discussed with families based on prognosis, expected benefits, and the values/wishes of the family. Priority should be given to offering painless and comforting interventions, such as supplemental oxygen, pain medications, anxiolytics, and other integrative therapies.

TABLE 50.3 Reasons to Revoke Do Not Resuscitate (DNR) in the Perioperative Setting

General Reason	Context/Detail
Anesthesia risks	Anesthesia can lead to hemodynamic instability, respiratory compromise, and/or hypervolemia, which may require implementation of resuscitation efforts to reverse in the perioperative setting.
Unclear goals of care	In order to make educated decisions regarding DNR orders, providers and decision-makers must discuss in detail benefits and burdens of interventions for a myriad of complications and these decisions can be difficult, emotionally taxing, and time-consuming. This problem may be exacerbated when language and cultural differences exist between providers and families or when the primary team is unavailable.[12,13]
Hand-offs	Multiple physicians may care for a patient in tandem, further making clear communication in highly nuanced clinical scenarios very challenging.
Surgical culture	The culture of the operating room staff, including surgeons, nurses, and ancillary team members, is one that centers on execution of high-intensity interventions to reverse disease and complications. These teams may be wholly unprepared to deal with an intraoperative death, as all discharges to the recovery area are expected to be alive and stable.
Logistical challenges	Problems cited revolve around the precise time DNR orders are revoked and reinstituted, and determining the types of interventions that will or will not be performed (use of artificial airways, fluid boluses, transfusion, or vasoactive agents) if the patient becomes hypoxic or hypotensive, and whether more invasive measures (chest compressions/defibrillation) will be applied in the event of bradycardia or asystolic arrest.

Table 50.5 lists common symptoms at end of life and medications used to treat them, if appropriate or desired. As a patient approaches end of life, their wakefulness and ability to participate will decrease, and thus the medical team should be mindful of changing interventions to those that do not require patient participation. For example, for a child who is no longer awake or having difficulty swallowing, medications should be changed to sublingual, transdermal, rectal, or intravenous (IV). Subcutaneous routes are avoided unless urgent (e.g., lack of IV access and all other routes failing to control pain).

Withdrawal of life-sustaining treatments should be discussed with families as their child reaches end of life. This may include extubation or discontinuation of cardiac medications and will result in death of the child. The process should be carefully and gently explained to families, so that they can make an informed decision. This period can be very difficult and support services should be offered.

Anticipatory guidance should also be offered to families regarding children entering the active dying phase. Although predictions about remaining life span are notoriously inaccurate there are known symptoms and signs of the actively dying phase, such as excessive fatigue, increased sleeping hours, and decreased activity. Dying children may not have energy to engage with visitors or even with family members. Pain may also increase and pain medications will need to be titrated for effectiveness. Respiratory symptoms including pooling of oral secretions and irregular respiratory rate may also occur at end of life. Anorexia is also expected towards end of life, and iatrogenic feeds via nasogastric or gastric feeding tubes may not be tolerated. In the final hours a parent may

TABLE 50.4 Perioperative "Touchpoints" for the Care of Patients With Preoperative Do Not Resuscitate (DNR) Orders

Perioperative "Touchpoint"	Action
Planning stage	Clear, transparent, and inclusive discussion of anticipated benefits and potential risks of procedure. Patient, surrogate medical decision-maker, supportive family members, and clinicians should have the opportunity to participate in developing the contingency plans.
Immediate preoperative	"Huddle" with clinicians, with operating room staff, and specific discussion of contingency plans during or immediately after "time out" and before induction begins.
Intraoperative	Adherence to previously articulated contingency plans, including management of the airway, vasoactive infusions, elements of cardiopulmonary resuscitation to be implemented, management plan if patient unable to separate from ventilator, or in the very rare event of intraoperative death; timely communication with family members.
Immediate postoperative	Adherence to contingency plan in the postanesthesia care unit, intensive care unit, or acute care floor during the initial 24-h period after completion of procedure.
Duration of admission	Revision of "DNR" advance directive status: whether it should be continued or revoked, depending on clinical evolution and overall goals of care until live discharge or death during current hospitalization.

TABLE 50.5 Common Symptoms at End of Life

Symptom	Possible Therapy
Fatigue	Nonpharmacologic interventions, light therapy, steroids, stimulants, address any sleep disruptions.
Nausea/vomiting	5-HT3 antagonists, steroids, antihistamines, anticholinergics, benzodiazepines, neuroleptics, cannabinoids, NK1-receptor antagonists.
Anorexia	Megestrol acetate, cannabinoids, steroids, liquid meal replacements.
Dyspnea	Supplemental oxygen via nasal cannula, opioids, fan, raise head of bed, consider imaging for treatable etiology.
Constipation	Stimulant laxative (senna) plus osmotic agent (lactulose or polyethylene glycol), peripheral opioid receptor antagonist.
Pain	Opioids (see Chapter 51).
Delirium	Address day/night confusion, remove offending agents (benzodiazepines, anticholinergics); treat distressing symptoms with neuroleptics.

also notice evidence of multiorgan failure such as decreased mentation, decrease urine output, skin pallor and mottling, cool extremities, and agonal breathing (gasping) with inability to swallow secretions. These outward symptoms can be very distressing to families but they should be reassured that the child is not suffering and this is part of the dying process. At the time of death a child will stop breathing and heart function will cease. A medical provider will come to assess the child and pronounce the time of death.

The end of a child's life is very difficult for a family, but the medical team can provide some comfort at this time, if the family wishes. The medical staff can arrange for privacy during the initial grieving process, provide emotional support, offer memory making, facilitate holding or lying with the child, facilitate bathing or dressing the child, and help honor religious rituals. These seemingly small gestures can have monumental impacts on the manner in which the family grieves and ultimately remembers the end of their child's life.

References

1. Siegel RL, Miller KD, Jemal A. Cancer Statistics, 2017. *CA Cancer J Clin.* 2017;67(1):7–30.
2. Moody K, Siegel L, Scharbach K, Cunningham L, Cantor RM. Pediatric palliative care. *Prim Care.* 2011;38(2):327–361, ix.
3. Levetown M. American Academy of Pediatrics Committee on Bioethics. Communicating with children and families: from everyday interactions to skill in conveying distressing information. *Pediatrics.* 2008;121(5):e1441–e1460.
4. Back AL, Arnold RM, Baile WF, Tulsky JA, Fryer-Edwards K. Approaching difficult communication tasks in oncology. *CA Cancer J Clin.* 2005;55(3):164–177.
5. Houben CHM, Spruit MA, Groenen MTJ, Wouters EFM, Janssen DJA. Efficacy of advance care planning: a systematic review and meta-analysis. *J Am Med Dir Assoc.* 2014;15(7):477–489.
6. Lotz JD, Jox RJ, Borasio GD, Führer M. Pediatric advance care planning: a systematic review. *Pediatrics.* 2013;131(3):e873–e880.
7. Heckford E, Beringer AJ. Advance care planning: challenges and approaches for pediatricians. *J Palliat Med.* 2014;17(9):1049–1053.
8. Wiener L, Zadeh S, Battles H, et al. Allowing adolescents and young adults to plan their end-of-life care. *Pediatrics.* 2012;130(5):897–905.
9. Burns JP, Truog RD. The DNR order after 40 years. *N Engl J Med.* 2016;375(6):504–506.
10. Glass NL. Pediatric palliative care in the perioperative period. *Curr Anesthesiol Rep.* 2019;9(3):333–339.
11. Baumann LM, Williams K, Abdullah F, Hendrickson RJ, Oyetunji TA. Do-not-resuscitate orders and high-risk pediatric surgery: professional nuisance or medical necessity? *J Surg Res.* 2017;217:213–216.
12. Chandrakantan A, Saunders T. Perioperative ethical issues. *Anesthesiol Clin.* 2016;34(1):35–42.
13. Sanderson AD, Zurakowski D, Wolfe J. Clinician perspectives regarding the do-not-resuscitate order. *JAMA Pediatr.* 2013;167(10):954–958.

51

Chronic Pain and Palliative Care in the Pediatric Patient

NELDA ITZEP, KEVIN MADDEN, AND KAREN MOODY

Introduction

Pain is a common and troubling symptom among pediatric cancer patients in both the inpatient and outpatient settings.[1,2] In this chapter we will provide a comprehensive overview of chronic pain and its management in pediatric cancer patients. We will also discuss pediatric palliative care and how it can be of great benefit to this vulnerable population.

Pain Presentations

Pain is a complex entity that can manifest in many ways even within the same patient. It can present as acute or chronic pain. Acute pain is typically related to a specific insult and is self-limited, lasting no more than 3–6 months. Specifically, in cancer, it is usually related to tumor invasion or invasive interventions such as procedures or surgery. Acute pain occurs when the body sends signals to the brain to indicate injury, and it also occurs during the processes of preservation and repair. Treatment of acute pain is aimed at minimizing the pain perception while primarily treating the underlying etiology. Chronic pain can develop from long-standing tumor expansion, compression, or destruction of surrounding structures or their treatment. Chronic pain is generally defined as lasting for greater than 6 months and the treatment goals are markedly different, as often the underlying etiology cannot be reversed. While acute pain focuses on alleviating pain and treating the root cause, management of chronic pain focuses on maintaining function, while decreasing pain to a tolerable level.[3] There is also an acute on chronic pain presentation that is unique to chronic conditions such as malignancy. Also called breakthrough pain, acute on chronic pain presents as an episodic, significant increase in pain above the patient's baseline chronic pain. It is usually exacerbated by a specific event such as a surgical intervention, side effect of treatment, or progression of disease. The treatment for this type of pain is similar to that of acute pain, in which decreasing pain to baseline is the goal. In this chapter we will focus on chronic pain presentations, as these are common in the pediatric cancer population.

Types of Pain

Nociceptive pain is subdivided into somatic and visceral types and is caused by direct injury to anatomic structures, including internal organs (visceral pain) or connective tissues, muscles, and bone (somatic pain). Patients, who experience nociceptive visceral pain describe it as achy, crampy, and poorly localized. Examples of visceral pain are pancreatitis secondary to chemotherapy or bowel obstruction from tumor growth. Nociceptive somatic pain is described as sharp, stabbing, throbbing, or a pressure sensation and can be seen with bone metastases or leukemic skin infiltration. Neuropathic pain is characterized as sharp, electrical, shooting, tingling, or numbness and is the result of damage to the central and/or peripheral nervous system by direct tumor invasion, surgical trauma to nerves, or medication-induced neurotoxicity that leads to abnormal processing of somatosensory stimuli.

It is important to note that there are other types of pain, such as spiritual, psychologic, and social, that may manifest or be interpreted as physical pain by the child or their caregivers. Dame Cicely Saunders, the founder of modern hospice and palliative care, described a holistic concept of total pain in which pain affects different aspects of quality of life (physical well being and functioning, psychologic well being, social well being, and spiritual well being), and these aspects, in turn, affect the perception and presentation of pain.[4] This is well established in the literature, and other authors have built on this work.[5] A consequence of undertreated, nonphysical pain is usually an increase in the expression of physical pain. Early assessment and treatment of nonphysical pain may be helpful in minimizing confounding factors during the management of physical pain.

Chronic Pain Etiologies

Chronic pain can be the result of the malignancy or the treatment of the malignancy. Tumor extension can cause pain, as it puts pressure on solid organs or adjacent nerves. Direct infiltration into connective tissues, bone marrow, bones, or muscles can also produce long-standing pain, especially in patients with refractory, metastatic, or inoperable disease. Blockage of blood flow or lymphatics can lead to accumulation of fluid in the form of peripheral edema, ascites, or pleural effusions, which can also cause pain. Chronic neuropathic pain can also present after surgical interventions such as limb amputation (phantom limb), limb salvage, hemipelvectomies, or thoracotomies.

Pathologic fractures secondary to tumor invasion can produce chronic pain. Multimodal cancer therapy with a combination of chemotherapy, radiation, and/or surgery can be a source of great pain burden for patients. Chemotherapy can have painful side effects. For example, vincristine or paclitaxel can cause peripheral neuropathy that can lead to chronic pain. Osteopenia or osteoporosis secondary to chronic steroid use can result in vertebral body fractures, which in turn leads to chronic back pain. Radiation can produce many painful side effects, such as dermatitis and mucositis, which can be significant and prolonged. Iatrogenic procedures, such as indwelling catheters for pleural or ascitic fluid drainage or G-tubes for venting/feeding, can also be sources of chronic pain for patients. Central lines, which are commonplace for cancer treatment, can lead to thrombus or nerve damage.

Chronic Pain Evaluation

Chronic pain management requires not only a thorough physical and historical evaluation of the pain trajectory but also an understanding of both the physical and emotional burden on the patient and their family. Parents, as well as the patient, may experience significant distress that can impact their perception of pain. An example would be parent catastrophizing of a child's pain. This is when parents hold certain thoughts or beliefs that magnify the threat value of pain, and this has been found to be a significant predictor of adolescent somatic symptoms.[6] Wilson et al. described that parental catastrophizing increases the likelihood that adolescents will also catastrophize their pain, which in turns leads to more disability.[6] Additionally, it will be helpful to understand the status of the patient's primary malignancy, as this can greatly affect pain presentation, goals of care, and ultimately, management.

Pain assessment tools can be helpful in obtaining a subjective measurement of a patient's pain experience if the patient is able to self-report. For very young children, this may be impossible or very difficult, thus one has to rely on parent-proxy reports. The setting in which the pain evaluation takes place is also important. Depending on the developmental stage of a child, they may experience significant stranger anxiety and an accurate assessment of pain will be difficult by a medical provider that is unfamiliar to the child. In these situations the best strategy is to evaluate the child while they are held by a parent or simply by observing the child.

Many different pediatric pain scales exist for various chronologic and developmental age groups. For example, infant pain can be assessed through observations of the baby crying, grimacing, body stiffening, and withdrawal from painful stimuli. Several scales exist for neonatal pain assessment; for example, the Neonatal Pain, Agitation, and Sedation Scale (N-PASS)[7] or the Neonatal Infant Pain Scale (NIPS) can be used for neonates,[8] while the Premature Infant Pain Profile (PIPP) can be used for premature infants.[9] For toddlers, parent-proxy reports will still be the most helpful, and tools, such as the Faces, Legs, Activity, Cry, and Consolability Scale (FLACC), can be helpful.[10] Preschool children can have limited self-reporting abilities, and these should still be supplemented with parent's reports of pain or limitations. For children in this age group, the Wong-Baker FACES[11] or Oucher[12] pain rating scales can be used reliably. Most children aged 9 years and older can use the numerical (0–10) pain rating scale.

Although these pain scales are used primarily for assessment of acute pain, they may still be useful for periodic assessment of chronic pain. It is important that medical providers are aware that many of the typical pain signs and symptoms may be attenuated or absent in the chronic pain setting. For instance, children with chronic pain may not exhibit changes in vital signs or crying. They may have adapted to function with pain, and thus their functional status, emotional demeanor, and vital signs will not reflect their true level of pain.

Chronic Pain Management

Chronic pain management differs from that of acute pain in that the goal is to decrease pain to a tolerable level, not to alleviate it completely. Reducing pain allows increases in daily function and improvements in quality of life. It is very important to converse with parents and the child to set realistic expectations and establish goals. Goals should be life-centered and personalized to each patient.

General Strategy

The general strategy for management of chronic cancer pain in children is to use a minimum number of medications at the lowest effective dose in order to reduce pain and increase function. Treatment should be multimodal and include pharmacologic as well as nonpharmacologic interventions.

Nonpharmacologic Management

Nonpharmacologic therapies play a key role in the management of chronic pain. Physical and occupational therapies can offer patients exercises and stretches that can help decrease pain and improve mobility and function. Not only can these be performed with a skilled professional in the inpatient or outpatient setting but the therapist can also teach the patient and their caregivers exercises for the child to do on their own. This can be very helpful for children, as it gives them another method to control their pain. In a patient with advanced cancer that may have limited mobility, these therapies can also help prevent or alleviate painful contractures. Integrative medicine therapies, such as yoga, meditation, aromatherapy, acupuncture, massage, and guided imagery, are additional tools to help decrease pain without the use of medications.

Children with terminal cancer can suffer from severe pain and palliative surgical measures may provide adequate benefit to justify their use. For example, pleural, pericardial, or peritoneal effusion-related pain can be improved with catheter drain placement and improve respiratory status. Similarly, percutaneous gastrostomies for venting may be helpful in gastrointestinal obstructions secondary to tumor invasion. A more invasive but inarguably palliative measure is surgical debulking or stabilization of bones in the setting of terminal cancer. Refractory disease may be very painful due to direct tumor invasion into bones, body cavities, or solid organs. This progression can cause bowel obstruction or gross tumor burden that can perforate bowel or even skin. It is important to be mindful of the risks associated with surgery when planning these palliative interventions. Poor wound healing, infection, and significant pain among others may outweigh the benefits of the surgery. Radiation therapy can often also provide pain relief by decreasing tumor burden or growth rate without significant side effects or toxicity and often using less than five fractions.

Pharmacologic Management

Management of chronic pain will frequently require administration of pain-relieving medications. As is the general rule in pediatrics, medications should be dosed by weight and should not exceed maximal starting adult doses in opioid-naive patients. Oral medications should be the first choice but this can be transitioned to other routes, such as intravenous, transdermal, sublingual, subcutaneous, or even rectal, if the patient is unable to tolerate oral intake. Intravenous may be the route of choice in the case of severe, excruciating pain that requires immediate relief. Often, more than one medication may be needed to achieve adequate pain relief. Combination regimens, which may include both opioids and nonopioid medications, may be helpful for opioid-sparing effects but can also lead to polypharmacy, which can have numerous complications such as nephrotoxicity, hepatotoxicity, and oversedation among others. The decision to use combination pain regimens should be made by physicians with experience with these medications, their side effects, and possible interactions with other medications. Consultation with a palliative care physician or pain specialist is recommended. Finally, the pain medication choice and dose will, in part, depend on the patient's age, as this will affect their ability to take certain formulations. Liquid formulations or medication compounding may be necessary in children requiring small doses or unable to swallow pills.

The World Health Organization proposed a pain management plan that starts with nonopioid medications and escalates to stronger opioids.[13] This pain ladder can serve as a guide to initiate a pain regimen and then it can be titrated to effect. The correct dose of opioid will provide adequate analgesic effect with minimal toxicity. Common opioid toxicities include nausea, pruritus, and constipation. Less often and usually with larger doses, toxicities may include sedation, respiratory depression, myoclonus, and hallucinations. When toxicity outweighs the analgesic benefit, the provider may consider changing to a different opioid, also known as opioid rotation. Because the body becomes tolerant to opioids due to constant effect at its specific receptor, the analgesic effect may decrease over time while the side effect profile may increase. Changing to a different opioid that will affect a different receptor will increase the analgesic benefit and may decrease the side effect burden. Of note, opioid rotation requires conversion of the opioid dose to the new opioid dose using standardized tables and a 20%–30% dose reduction, as tolerance to the new opioid is generally incomplete (incomplete cross-tolerance).

Chronic cancer pain that is present on most days will require long-acting, in combination with short-acting, pain medications. The long-acting pain medication will provide a baseline level of pain relief and should be taken on a scheduled basis. The long-acting pain medication doses should be titrated to provide pain relief to a tolerable level. In addition, a short-acting pain medication will be necessary for breakthrough pain. This medication should be taken as needed only. The dose should be titrated to decrease pain to the baseline level. In the hospital setting, this combination of long- and short-acting pain medication can be delivered via a patient-controlled analgesia (PCA) pump. This method provides a continuous or basal dose of an opioid at a low rate, while allowing the patient to administer an additional dose for breakthrough pain at set intervals. The benefits of this method include faster pain medication delivery.

In general, opioids are the mainstay of cancer pain treatment; however, nonopioid medications also play a strategic role, as they can help spare opioid use. For mild pain, acetaminophen or nonsteroidal antiinflammatory medications should be the drugs of choice if no contraindications are present. For neuropathic pain, antiepileptic medications such gabapentin, serotonin-norepinephrine reuptake inhibitors (SNRIs) such as duloxetine, and low-dose methadone may be helpful. Methadone is particularly effective in relieving chronic cancer pain with minimal side effects; however, dosing is complicated and should be performed by an experienced provider or in consultation with a palliative care or pain physician. Other medications, such as topical lidocaine for mucosal pain, may be indicated depending on the child's pain or other comorbidities.

As mentioned earlier, opioids can be an important component of chronic cancer pain management and should be used with great care in order to avoid toxicity or disordered use. See Tables 51.1, 51.2, and 51.3 for opioids, neuropathic agents, and other adjuvant therapies used in pediatric cancer patients.

Procedural Anesthesia/Analgesia

Advances in pain control for pediatric cancer patients have brought about different procedural options. Local nerve blocks performed by experienced anesthesiologists can provide immediate and long-lasting pain relief for children

TABLE 51.1 Pain Medications Used in Pediatric Cancer Patients

Drug	Route	Initial Short-Acting Dose in an Opioid-Naive Patient	Onset (min)	Peak Effect (h)	Duration (h)	Initial Scheduled Dosing Frequency in Opioid-Naive Patients	Available Oral Dose Formulations	Notes
Acetaminophen	PO, IV, rectal	15 mg/kg/dose IV or PO q6 h (max 75 mg/kg/day or 4000 mg/day)						Use with caution in patients with liver disease.
Tramadol	PO	1–2 mg/kg/dose (max single dose 100 mg; max daily dose 400 mg)	30–60	1.5	3–7	Short-acting: every 4–6 h. Long-acting: every 12 h	Short-acting: 50 mg tablets Long-acting: 100, 200, 300 mg tablets	Not approved for children less than 18 years of age. May lower seizure threshold.
Hydrocodone	PO	0.1–0.2 mg/kg/dose (max 5–10 mg)	10–20	1–3	4–8	Short-acting: every 6 h	Short-acting in combination with acetaminophen: 5, 7.5, 10 mg tablets; 2.5 mg/5 mL liquid	Hydrocodone used for pain is only available in combination with acetaminophen or ibuprofen.
Morphine	PO	0.2–0.5 mg/kg/dose (max 15–20 mg)	30	0.5–1	3–6	Short-acting: PO: every 4 h. Long-acting: every 12 h	Short-acting: 15, 30 mg tablets; 10 mg/5 mL, 20 mg/5 mL, 20 mg/1 mL liquid. Long-acting: 15, 30, 60, 100, 200 mg tablets	Short-acting preparation can be compounded into very concentrate SL drops (20 mg/mL). Long-acting morphine for opioid-tolerant patients only.
	IV/SC	0.05–0.1 mg/kg/dose (max 2–3 mg)	5–10	None	None	every 4 h	None	
Oxycodone	PO	0.1–0.2 mg/kg/dose (max 5–10 mg)	10–15	0.5–1	3–6	Short-acting: every 4 h. Long-acting: every 12 h	Short-acting: 5, 15, 30 mg tablets; 5 mg/5 mL, 20 mg/mL liquid. Long-acting: 10, 15, 20, 30, 40, 60, 80 mg tablets	Available alone or in combination with acetaminophen. Long-acting form for opioid-tolerant patients only.
Hydromorphone	PO	0.03–0.08 mg/kg/dose (max 1–3 mg)	15–30	0.5–1	3–5	Short-acting: every 4 h; Long-acting: once daily	Short-acting: 2, 4, 8 mg tablets; 1 mg/mL liquid Long-acting: 8, 12, 16, 32 mg tablets	Long-acting form is for opioid-tolerant patients only.
	IV/SC	0.01–0.015 mg/kg/dose (max 0.5–1.5 mg)	15–30	None	4–5	every 4 h	None	
Methadone	PO/SC/IV	0.04 mg/kg/dose BID and titrated weekly to effect	30 min (PO)	3–5 days	Increases with repeater doses up to 60 h		Tablet, liquid	Consult expert provider. May prolong QTc; check baseline ECG.

BID, twice per day; *ECG*, electrocardiogram; *IV*, intravenous; *PO*, oral; *SC*, subcutaneous; *SL*, sublingual; *QTc*, corrected QT interval.

TABLE 51.2 Agents for Neuropathic Pain

Drug	Dose	Notes
Gabapentin	Day 1: 5 mg/kg/dose (max 300 mg/dose) PO at bedtime. Day 2: 5 mg/kg/dose (max 300 mg/dose) PO BID. Day 3: 5 mg/kg/dose (max 300 mg/dose) PO TID. Dose may be further titrated to a maximum dose of 35 mg/kg/day (max dose 3600 mg/day).	Comes in a liquid. May cause drowsiness, dizziness, and peripheral edema. Adjust dose for renal impairment.
Pregabalin	75 mg BID; can titrate up to 300 BID max.	Initial adult dose.
Clonidine	Oral: immediate release: initial: 2 µg/kg/dose every 4 to 6 h; increase incrementally over several days; range: 2 to 4 µg/kg/dose every 4 to 6 h. Topical: transdermal patch: may be switched to the transdermal delivery system after oral therapy is titrated to an optimal and stable dose; there is some variation in absorption between oral and transdermal routes.	Limited data available for pain in children and adolescents. Helps with opioid withdrawal, sleep, and dysautonomia pain. Can lower BP.
Topiramate	6–12 years (weight greater than or equal to 20 kg): 15 mg PO daily for 7 days, then 15 mg PO BID. ≥12 years: 25 mg PO at bedtime for 7 days, then 25 mg PO BID and titrate up to 50 mg PO BID. Maximum daily dose 200 mg.	May cause acidosis, drowsiness, dizziness, and nausea. Adjust dose for renal impairment and hepatic dysfunction.
Amitriptyline	0.1 mg/kg PO at bedtime. Titrate as tolerated over 3 weeks to 0.5–2 mg/kg at bedtime. Maximum: 25 mg/dose.	Consider for continuous and shooting neuropathic pain. May cause sedation, arrhythmias, dry mouth, orthostasis, and urinary retention. Caution use in patients with seizures and arrhythmias; avoid MAOIs, other SSRIs, or SNRIs due to potential for serotonin syndrome.
Duloxetine	Start with 30 mg capsule at bedtime and can titrate up to 60 mg qHS.	Approved for anxiety in children >7 years. Antidepressants can increase suicidal thinking in pediatric patients with major depressive disorder. Duloxetine may increase the risk of bleeding events. Concomitant use of aspirin, nonsteroidal antiinflammatory drugs, warfarin, and other anticoagulants may add to this risk. Taper slowly.

BID, Twice daily; *BP*, blood pressure; *MAOI*, monoamine oxidase inhibitor; *PO*, oral; *qHS*, nightly at bedtime: *SSRI*, selective serotonin reuptake inhibitor; *SNRI*, serotonin-norepinephrine reuptake inhibitor; *TID*, three times daily.

suffering from regional pain. Epidural anesthesia can be used to help manage acute pain related to surgical interventions or terminal pain that is localized below the thoracic cavity. One emerging therapy is a cordotomy, which is a procedure where the afferent nerve fibers are severed, effectively blocking incoming pain signals to the brain. This can be particularly helpful for patients who are approaching end of life and have significant tumor burden.

Chronic Pain Sequelae

Chronic pain can place additional strain on children already suffering from cancer. Sleep disorders are common among children suffering from cancer,[14,15] and these disturbances are worsened by pain. Sleep disorders can include difficulty falling asleep, difficulty staying asleep, achieving restful sleep, and daytime sleepiness. Treating pain will help alleviate some difficulty sleeping and can therefore lead to improved participation in daytime activity. Not only does the persistent experience of pain affect a child's physical health, it can also have a significant impact on their mental health. Depression and anxiety can be worsened by chronic pain. It is important to be mindful of the burdens of depression and anxiety on our pediatric patients and refer them early for mental health services and interventions. In addition to the child's suffering, family and caregivers who bear constant witness to their loved one's chronic pain also suffer. Familial distress is high during times of uncontrolled pain and treatment of pain can have widespread effects not only on the child but the entire family unit.

Palliative Care

Palliative care came from the necessity to care for some of the most vulnerable populations—those suffering from chronic or terminal illnesses. Great strides have been made in adult palliative care since its beginning in the second half of the 20th century as part of the hospice movement. However,

TABLE 51.3 Adjuvant Therapies

Drug	Indication	Dose	Notes
Dexamethasone	Inflammation, nerve compression	1 mg/kg/d IV or PO in divided doses every 6 h. Maximum: 16 mg/day. Use lowest effective dose.	May cause impaired healing, infection, thrush, hyperglycemia, weight gain, myopathy, stomach upset, psychosis, emotional instability.
Diazepam	Muscle spasms	Oral: children: 0.12 to 0.8 mg/kg/day in divided doses every 6 to 8 h.	
Tizanidine	Muscle spasms	Children 2 to <10 years: oral: 1 mg at bedtime, titrate as needed. Children ≥10 years and adolescents: oral: 2 mg at bedtime, titrate as needed.	Oral: titrate initial dose upward to reported effective range of: 0.3 to 0.5 mg/kg/day in three to four divided doses; maximum daily dose: 24 mg/day.
Cyclobenzaprine	Muscle spasms	≥15 years old: 5 mg PO three times daily Maximum 30 mg/day.	
Dicyclomine	Abdominal cramping	Infants ≥6 months and children <2 years: oral: 5 to 10 mg three to four times daily administered 15 min before feeding. Children ≥2 years oral: 10 mg three to four times daily. Adolescents: oral: 10 to 20 mg three to four times daily. If efficacy not achieved in 2 weeks, therapy should be discontinued.	
5% lidocaine patch	Nociceptive or neuropathic pain	1–3 patches applied daily (depending on size) up to 12 h per day.	Can be cut to fit.
OTC creams	Nociceptive or neuropathic pain	Apply topically to localized areas of neuropathic pain BID-TID.	
Prescription creams: diclofenac cream; compounded neuropathic agents	Nociceptive or neuropathic pain	Apply topically to localized areas of neuropathic pain BID-TID.	
Ice, heat	Nociceptive or neuropathic pain		

BID, twice daily; *IV*, intravenous; *OTC*, over the counter; *PO*, oral; *TID*, three times daily.

pediatric palliative care has lagged behind significantly. Fortunately, in the last few decades, several leading health organizations around the world have called attention to and provided resources for the advancement of pediatric palliative care.

Palliative care encompasses four main areas: pain and symptom management, psychosocial support, guidance in decision-making, and end-of-life care. The overarching goal of pediatric palliative care is to decrease suffering and improve quality of life. The palliative care team should be composed of multidisciplinary members in order to assist the child and family with all aspects of their cancer-related experience. For example, a team might include a physician, nurse, social worker, chaplain, and child life specialist.

Ideally, the palliative care team meets with the family early on in the cancer trajectory in order to build rapport prior to a medical emergency or when a difficult conversation is needed. The palliative care physician should meet with the child and their caregivers periodically to assess symptom burden and other areas where support can be offered to the entire family unit. Palliative care experts are highly skilled in pain and symptom management, communication skills, and care coordination. Their involvement in the care of pediatric cancer patients provides those patients and families with extra psychosocial support with keen attention to quality of life and suffering. These teams often have time for lengthy conversations about goals and values to assist in setting care goals. These functions can also be of enormous value to the primary oncology team.

As discussed earlier, cancer carries a very heavy symptom burden either from the disease itself or its treatment. See Chapter 50 on DNR and the terminally ill child for a table of symptoms and possible treatments. Decision-making, goals of care, and end of life are also discussed further in that chapter.

Palliative medicine can play an important role in a child's cancer experience. At its core, this specialty is focused on alleviating suffering and improving quality of life. The primary medical team should consider early referral in order to enhance the care of this vulnerable population.

References

1. Tutelman PR, Chambers CT, Stinson JN, et al. Pain in children with cancer: prevalence, characteristics, and parent management. *Clin J Pain*. 2018;34(3): 198–206.
2. Goodlev ER, Discala S, Darnall BD, Hanson M, Petok A, Silverman M. Managing cancer pain, monitoring for cancer recurrence, and mitigating risk of opioid use disorders: a team-based, interdisciplinary approach to cancer survivorship. *J Palliat Med*. 2019;22(11):1308–1317.
3. Grichnik KP, Ferrante FM. The difference between acute and chronic pain. *Mt Sinai J Med*. 1991;58(3):217–220.
4. Richmond C. Dame Cicely Saunders: Founder of the modern hospic movement—Obituary. *Br Med J*. 2005;331(7510):238.
5. Ferrell B, Grant M, Padilla G, Vemuri S, Rhiner M. The experience of pain and perceptions of quality of life: validation of a conceptual model. *Hosp J*. 1991;7(3):9–24.
6. Wilson AC, Moss A, Palermo TM, Fales JL. Parent pain and catastrophizing are associated with pain, somatic symptoms, and pain-related disability among early adolescents. *J Pediatr Psychol*. 2014;39(4):418–426.
7. Hillman BA, Tabrizi MN, Gauda EB, Carson KA, Aucott SW. The Neonatal Pain, Agitation and Sedation Scale and the bedside nurse's assessment of neonates. *J Perinatol*. 2015;35(2):128–131.
8. Lawrence J, Alcock D, McGrath P, Kay J, MacMurray SB, Dulberg C. The development of a tool to assess neonatal pain. *Neonatal Netw*. 1993;12(6):59–66.
9. Ballantyne M, Stevens B, McAllister M, Dionne K, Jack A. Validation of the premature infant pain profile in the clinical setting. *Clin J Pain*. 1999;15(4):297–303.
10. Manworren RC, Hynan LS. Clinical validation of FLACC: preverbal patient pain scale. *Pediatr Nurs*. 2003;29(2):140–146.
11. Garra G, Singer AJ, Taira BR, et al. Validation of the Wong-Baker FACES Pain Rating Scale in pediatric emergency department patients. *Acad Emerg Med*. 2010;17(1):50–54.
12. Beyer JE, Denyes MJ, Villarruel AM. The creation, validation, and continuing development of the Oucher: a measure of pain intensity in children. *J Pediatr Nurs*. 1992;7(5):335–346.
13. WHO. WHO Guidelines on the Pharmacological Treatment of Persisting Pain in Children With Medical Illnesses. Geneva: World Health Organization; 2012.
14. Ince D, Demirag B, Karapinar TH, et al. Assessment of sleep in pediatric cancer patients. *Turk J Pediatr*. 2017;59(4):379–386.
15. Lee S, Narendran G, Tomfohr-Madsen L, Schulte F. A systematic review of sleep in hospitalized pediatric cancer patients. *Psychooncology*. 2017;26(8):1059–1069.

52 Special Considerations for Intensive Care Management of Pediatric Patients With Cancer

KRISTIN P. CROSBY AND JAMES S. KILLINGER

Pediatric patients undergoing treatment for cancer may require intensive care at any time during their diagnostic and treatment courses. Caring for pediatric cancer patients in the intensive care unit requires skilled, specially trained members of the medical team to provide around the clock care for this distinct patient population. This chapter will focus on critical care issues of pediatric cancer patients, including the need for intensive monitoring following procedural or oncologic treatments, as well as perioperative and postoperative management following tumor resection.

Neurologic Diagnoses in the Pediatric Oncologic Critical Care Patient

Children are commonly admitted to the pediatric intensive care unit (PICU) after neurologic surgery for brain tumor resection. For both primary and metastatic disease, children are monitored postoperatively for acute neurologic changes, acute hemorrhage, and acute neurohormonal changes, such as central diabetes insipidus (CDI) and the syndrome of inappropriate antidiuretic hormone (SIADH) secretion. Furthermore, depending on the risk of increased intracranial pressure (ICP) following surgery, some patients will have an externalized ventricular drain (EVD) or lumbar drain (LD) for cerebral spinal fluid (CSF) diversion in place postoperatively, which demands close monitoring, typically only available in the PICU. In addition to the postoperative state, children with brain tumors may be admitted to the PICU preoperatively if they are at risk of acute increase in ICP, or if they need placement of an EVD for treatment of increased ICP.

In this section, two common circumstances that warrant PICU monitoring will be examined in greater detail: sodium balance and posterior reversible encephalopathy syndrome (PRES). Additionally, a relatively new surgical approach used for tumor-directed therapy convection-enhanced delivery (CED) will be discussed for its use in the treatment of pontine gliomas.

Disorders of Sodium Homeostasis Following Neurosurgery

Due to the location of many pituitary and suprasellar tumors, neurosurgery in these areas may lead to postoperative disorders under hormonal control from the pituitary stalk.[1] These common disorders can occur in isolation or in combination.[2,3]

Central Diabetes Insipidus

CDI can occur in more than 50% of patients after transsphenoidal surgery (TSS) to resect intrasellar or suprasellar tumors.[4] The diagnosis of CDI is made on the basis of both clinical and biochemical findings.[1] Polyuria (>4 mL/kg/h of urine output) and polydipsia, in combination with increased serum osmolality (>300 mOsm/L) and decreased urine osmolality with a urine/plasma osmolality ratio <1, is the hallmark of CDI in the postoperative period. Patients with an intact thirst mechanism and free access to oral fluids may not develop symptoms or hypernatremia. However, patients who are unable to maintain normal plasma osmolality and serum sodium levels need immediate intervention or they will develop symptoms of CDI, such as acute dehydration, nausea and vomiting, and alterations in mental status.

Monitoring of CDI includes following hourly urine output, hourly fluid intake, as well as measurements of serum and urine osmolality, serum electrolytes, and blood glucose levels every 6–8 h in the immediate postoperative period.[1]

For patients who show laboratory and/or clinical evidence of CDI, management will depend on the patients' thirst mechanism and access to oral fluids. For patients without an intact thirst mechanism or without free access to oral fluids, supplemental intravenous (IV) fluids are necessary. Institutional guidelines are very helpful in these circumstances, as a multidisciplinary approach to monitoring and treatment is warranted for consistency.[5] A reasonable approach to IV fluids with either normal saline or ½ normal saline with dextrose at one-third of maintenance needs or 400 mL/m^2/h, plus urine output replacement mL:mL with

½ normal saline or other balanced solution. If this fluid replacement method of CDI treatment is not successful, an alternative approach is to administer oral 1-desamino-8-D-arginine vasopressin (DDAVP) or vasopressin infusion for the hormonal replacement of endogenous vasopressin, which is often due to transient direct surgical injury or localized edema at the site of surgery.[5] The course of CDI most typically lasts up to 48 h from the immediate postoperative period[1,4,5] but may undergo what is termed a triphasic pattern of immediate postoperative CDI, followed by a period of SIADH for 5–7 days, followed once again by CDI, which may persist after discharge.[3,6] This triphasic pattern persists in more than 3% of patients undergoing TSS, and approximately 1% of patients experience the biphasic pattern of immediate postoperative CDI followed by SIADH.[3,6]

Syndrome of Inappropriate Antidiuretic Hormone

SIADH can occur in the immediate postoperative phase following TSS, either in isolation or as part of the triphasic pattern discussed earlier. SIADH occurs in isolation following TSS in up to 20% of patients.[7,8] The mechanism is likely the uncontrolled release of ADH from either degenerating posterior pituitary or from magnocellular neurons with damaged axons.[1] With this release of ADH, urine output decreases, and the patient remains in either a euvolemic or hypervolemic state with a subsequent drop in serum osmolality <270 mOsm/L.[9] The most important therapeutic intervention is fluid restriction and cessation of IV fluids, as soon as the patient is able to drink. Sodium replacement is only required for prolonged SIADH or in cases of severe hyponatremia. Symptoms of severe hyponatremia from SIADH include visual changes, focal neurologic changes, respiratory depression, and seizures. These symptoms are consistent with cerebral edema and can be treated carefully with hypertonic saline until symptoms resolve.[10,11]

Cerebral Salt Wasting

Cerebral salt wasting (CSW), characterized by polyuria and natriuresis, occurs in about 4% of children following neurosurgery.[1] CSW is thought to be due to a tubular defect in sodium transport, leading to extracellular volume depletion. CSW and SIADH can be present in both surgical and nonsurgical settings. Making a distinction between the two is important, as the treatment of CSW is different from that of SIADH. The treatment of CSW involves water and sodium repletion. The fundamental difference between these two syndromes is the presence of polyuria, which leads to dehydration in CSW. Replacement of both free water and sodium is therefore necessary because of the significant urine sodium losses and high urine output.[12,13] Depending on the severity, sodium replacement needs can be met with oral sodium, or CSW may require aggressive fluid and sodium replacement in the PICU with central venous pressure monitoring of intravascular volume status. In severe CSW, the mineralocorticoid fludrocortisone may be used,[13] although CSW typically resolves within a month of onset.[1]

Posterior Reversible Encephalopathy Syndrome

PRES is a clinical syndrome consisting of headache, impaired consciousness, seizures, visual disturbances, nausea and vomiting, and occasionally focal seizures.[14–16] These clinical features in the setting of specific cofactors often lead to its diagnosis. Cofactors, such as acute hypertension,[14,17–20] preeclampsia or eclampsia,[21–23] chemotherapeutic agents,[15,24–26] posttransplant immunosuppression,[27–33] and other diseases of inflammation,[15,16,18,34] have been associated with the development of PRES.

The best understanding of the etiology of PRES is that it is a disturbance in cerebral autoregulation, often in the face of severe hypertension, generating vasogenic edema.[35] Clinical diagnosis is often confirmed by magnetic resonance imaging (MRI). Classically, PRES affects the parieto-occipital region of the brain,[15,19–22] although it can also be located in the temporal and frontal lobes and posterior fossa.[19,36] On T2 and fluid-attenuated inversion recovery MRI, white matter intensities are demonstrated in the affected areas, confirming the diagnosis (Fig. 52.1).[18,19]

Treatment of encephalopathy, headache, and other neurologic findings surrounds the treatment of the underlying cause, and removing the offending medicines that are related to the PRES.[15,19,20,25,27] Hypertension requires timely intervention, including admission to a PICU, initiation of antihypertensive therapy, and close invasive blood pressure monitoring. Calcium-channel blockers or beta blocker infusions have been used in the acute treatment of hypertensive emergencies in children.[37–41] Treatment of PRES-associated seizures with valproic acid has been advocated for its favorable mechanism of action.[15,42]

Last, the removal of medications that are thought to contribute to the development of PRES should be strongly considered. Patients in whom the chemotherapy used to treat their underlying cancer diagnosis is thought to be the offending agent present difficult challenges to oncologists. The same is true for transplant physicians in managing immunosuppression following an episode of PRES, as cyclosporine and tacrolimus have both been implicated in the development of PRES and are staples of posttransplant immunosuppression.[27,29,31–33]

Convection-Enhanced Delivery

The delivery of chemotherapy to malignant gliomas has proven challenging. Systemic chemotherapy[43] and more direct methods such as chemotherapy-infused wafers and intrathecal administration of chemotherapy[44] have been ineffective at delivering tumor-directed therapy to deep gliomas. Developed in the 1990s, CED utilizes a syringe pump to generate a pressure gradient at the interstitium to enhance delivery of the therapy to the desired target.[45]

Diffuse intrinsic pontine glioma (DIPG) is a rare but lethal brain tumor seen in children. DIPG accounts for 15%–20%

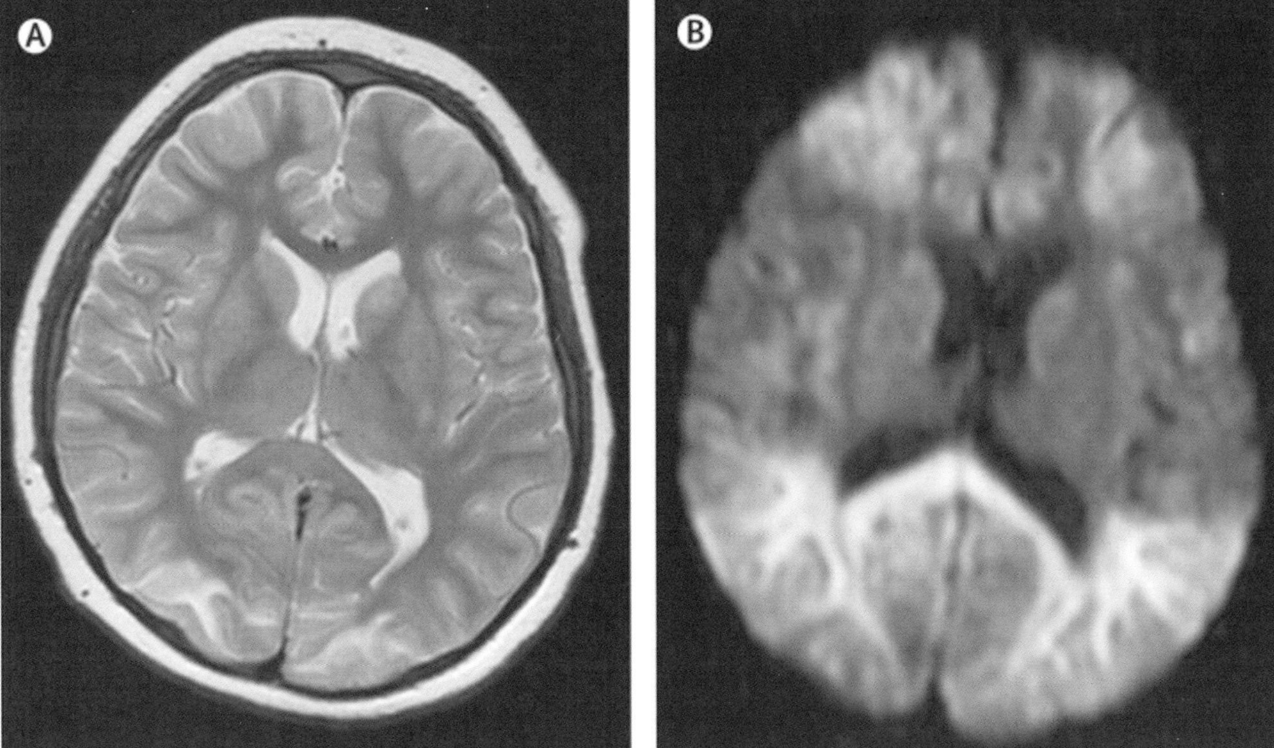

• **Fig. 52.1** MRI abnormalities in posterior reversible encephalopathy syndrome are mainly posterior. (A) T2-weighted image of a child who became hypersensitive on treatment with steroids for juvenile rheumatoid arthritis; high signal is seen posteriorly. (B) Diffusion-weighted abnormalities are more widespread, involving both frontal and posterior regions.
From Sharma, Madhu, Kupferman, Juan C, MD, et. al., The effects of hypertension on the paediatric brain: a justifiable concern, *The Lancet Neurology, Volume 9, Issues 9. Pages 933–940. © 2010.*

of all CNS tumors in children, and more than 90% will die within 2 years of diagnosis, with conventional fractionated radiation as the primary means of treatment.[46–49] In recent years, pediatric neurosurgeons have explored the use of CED in the delivery of tumor-directed therapy to children with DIPG (Fig. 52.2).

In phase I, dose-escalation trial using the radiolabeled antibody monoclonal ^{124}I-8H9, the first 16 subjects received the entire infusion under general anesthesia in the operating room, while the remaining 12 subjects were observed while receiving the infusion in the PICU after cessation of anesthesia for more complete neurologic monitoring.[48] In this cohort, the most common adverse event was the development of a transient facial palsy, which occurred in 9 of the 28 subjects. There was one grade 4 adverse reaction (respiratory failure requiring reintubation after the completion of the infusion) in the cohort. In a second phase I trial exploring the use of CED in the treatment of DIPG, investigators used the recombinant chimera of human interleukin 13 (IL-13) and the enzymatically active portion of *Pseudomonas* exotoxin A, which effectively targeted glioma cells in preclinical studies.[49] In this cohort, all subjects received the infusion (up to 13 h) in the operating room under general anesthesia. Similarly, the adverse reaction profile was acceptable, suggesting that further studies are warranted to study clinical effectiveness, including the use of liposomal doxorubicin via CED in DIPG.[50]

In all cases, admission to the PICU is necessary if patients are transferred from the operating room. Even small volumes delivered to the pons may cause acute neurologic changes that warrant close monitoring.[48]

Anterior Mediastinal Masses

The anesthetic approach to mediastinal masses is described in detail in Chapter 47. Tumors located in the thoracic cavity can pose challenges to patients, as they can compress or obstruct vital structures. Anterior mediastinal masses in pediatric patients are primarily caused by lymphoma (Hodgkin's and non-Hodgkin's) with other causes, including leukemia, thymoma, histiocytosis, and neuroblastoma.[51–53] Due to the wide range of possible etiologies, obtaining a tissue biopsy is needed to confirm the exact diagnosis, yet several risks are associated with obtaining such biopsies. The most significant risks include cardiovascular collapse and respiratory compromise; however, bleeding and other complications may also occur.

As described in Chapter 47, large anterior mediastinal masses can compress vital structures within the mediastinum,

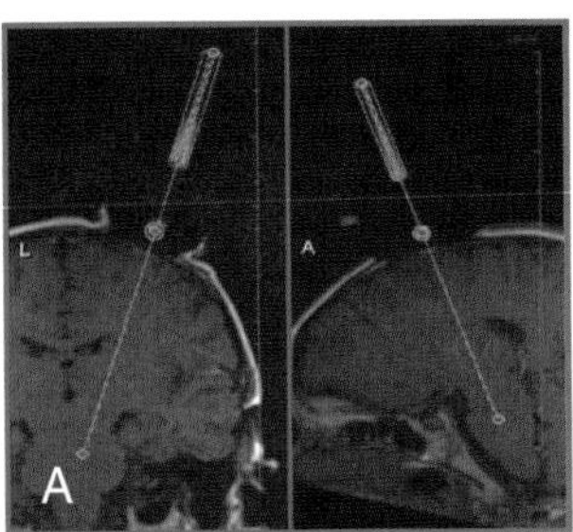

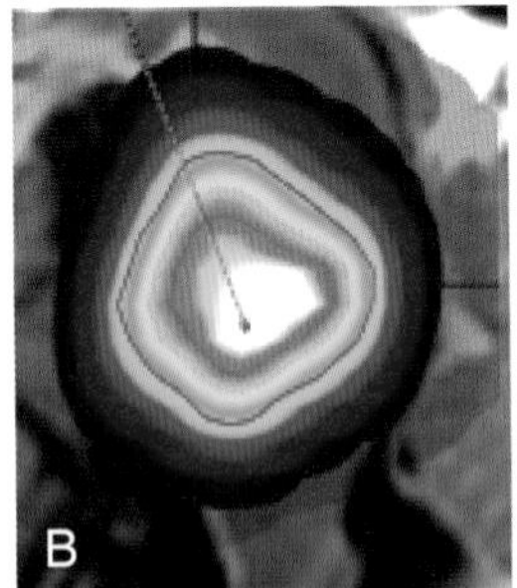

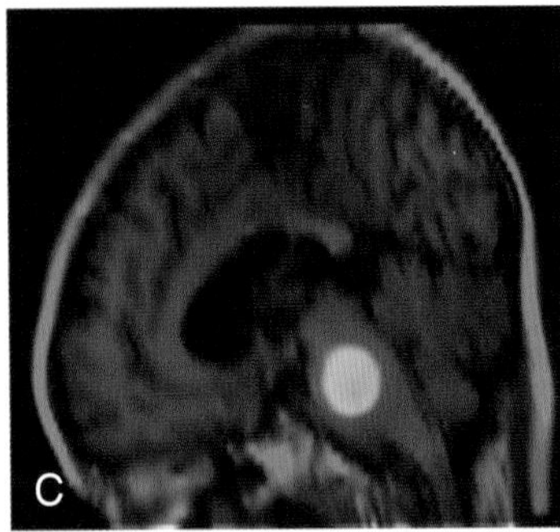

• **Fig. 52.2** (A) Stereotactic placement of the infusion catheter via supratentorial (transfrontal) route with fully MR-compatible navigational interface (ClearPoint, MRI Interventions, Irvine, CA, USA). (B) Radiolabeled ^{124}I-8H9 on infusion to the desired tumor site. (C) Radiolabeled ^{124}I-8H9 at completion of the infusion.

particularly affecting thin-walled structures, such as the right atrium, superior vena cava, and pulmonary artery. Preparing individualized plans for each patient's unique case addresses the needs and potential risks associated with surgical biopsies and anesthesia. Prior to sedation, patients should have a thorough workup, including computed tomography (CT) and echocardiogram at the minimum.[54] Patients with anterior mediastinal masses can be broadly classified into three categories defining the risk level associated with anesthesia (Table 52.1).[54]

Preoperative management of pediatric patients with anterior mediastinal masses should be performed in an intensive care unit or unit in which close airway monitoring can be maintained. Should patients develop inadequate ventilation or oxygenation, immediate attention and intervention are needed. Escalation of noninvasive respiratory support, including the use of high-flow nasal cannula, continuous positive airway pressure (CPAP), or bilevel positive airway pressure (BIPAP) ventilation, can be useful in this patient population. BIPAP devices allow the delivery of adjustable levels of continuous positive pressure during inspiration and expiration. Inspiratory positive airway pressure helps to

TABLE 52.1 Anesthesia Categories for Patients With Anterior Mediastinal Mass[54]

Risk Level	Symptoms	Percent Tracheal Compression
Low risk	None or mild	No radiographic evidence of compression
Intermediate risk	Mild-to-moderate postural symptoms	Less than 50%
High risk	Severe postural symptoms: orthopnea, stridor, cyanosis	50% or more

overcome upper airway resistance in cases of partial obstruction. However, CPAP alone provides expiratory positive airway pressure to open the upper airway, thereby preventing alveolar collapse.[55]

A helium/oxygen mixture or heliox can be used in these patients, as helium is less dense than oxygen, thus enhancing laminar flow through a compressed airway. Heliox must be delivered as a mixed gas. It is imperative to use the lowest oxygen content (i.e., FiO_2), thereby the highest concentration of helium in order to achieve the most beneficial clinical effects.[56]

Corticosteroids can be used in cases of severe airway or cardiovascular compromise. With its use, patients are at risk of tumor lysis syndrome, and additional monitoring is needed. Corticosteroid use prior to tumor biopsy does not necessarily interfere with making a diagnosis, as one small cohort had a 95% clear histologic diagnosis made in patients who had received corticosteroids.[57] Radiotherapy prior to diagnostic biopsy is uncommonly used in pediatric patients, as children may require anesthesia to tolerate the procedure.[57]

Finally, pediatric patients with the highest risk of cardiovascular collapse may be prophylactically placed on cardiopulmonary bypass prior to the procedure. Despite thorough planning and careful preparation, patients may need to be urgently placed on cardiopulmonary bypass should the need arise. This may be particularly true in adult populations, as they are less responsive to changes in positioning compared to pediatric patients.[58] In conclusion, advanced, experienced airway and critical care professionals should manage this high-risk patient cohort, having a variety of tools and cardiopulmonary support available.

Metastatic Lung Disease

Children with metastatic lung disease may require intensive care. One example of lung metastases in children is osteosarcoma, which is the most common bone tumor in children and young adults.[59] Metastatic lung disease can occur within the first year after diagnosis and more than 30% of patients with osteosarcoma relapse.[60] In order to maximize survival, complete metastatic tumor surgical resection is needed, as systemic antitumor therapies are not as reliable a treatment modality for improving survival.[61] Patients undergoing surgical resection of pulmonary metastases often need management and monitoring in the PICU before and following their surgery.

The surgical approach for patients with metastatic lung disease depends on several factors. The majority of patients have bilateral lung involvement but the literature shows that 24%–40% of patients may have unilateral disease.[60] The most common approach to surgical resection is thoracotomy; however, single-staged operations via median sternotomy are sometimes performed.

Pediatric patients who have undergone thoracotomy often recover in the PICU or a surgical step-down unit. Postoperative complications include bleeding, pain control, and respiratory failure. Anticipating these potential complications can mitigate harm and shorten the length of stay in the PICU. Monitoring for bleeding requires close monitoring of hemoglobin and platelet counts as well as coagulation factors, especially in patients who may have recently received chemotherapeutic agents, suppressing marrow production of blood cells. Pain control is the most common postoperative complication. The use of thoracic epidural patient-controlled analgesia (ePCA) has been proven to be safe and effective in controlling pain.[62,63] The use of ePCA can decrease the need for systemic analgesics, particularly opiates, in an effort to expedite mobility and reduce hospital length of stay. The care of patients with pulmonary metastatic disease requires a multidisciplinary team to achieve the best outcomes.

Intraabdominal Tumors

Pediatric tumors in the abdomen often require surgical management as a first-line or adjuvant therapy with antineoplastic medications.

Neuroblastoma

Neuroblastoma accounts for 8%–10% of all pediatric cancers and as high as 15% of all deaths in children with cancer,[64] prognosis of which depends on the stage of the tumor, determined using several tumor-specific and histologic factors. Patients with high-risk neuroblastoma often undergo complete surgical resection. Thoracoabdominal resections for neuroblastoma are tedious, long surgeries, during which blood loss, fluid shifts, and respiratory failure give rise to the need for intensive care monitoring. This unique patient population differs from other postsurgical patients in that some patients require additional exogenous catecholamines. This has been hypothesized to be caused by underlying neuroblastoma cells secreting catecholamines, which once removed may cause hemodynamic instability.[64]

Postoperative management of large thoracoabdominal resections in patients with neuroblastoma requires close attention from a team of providers, nurses, therapists, and other members of the care team. The development of a postoperative management protocol for patients undergoing any major surgical resection allows for a systematic approach, thereby ensuring that all aspects of care are met. Patients should have adequate blood pressures to ensure perfusion to all end organs, including adequate urine output (typically between 0.5 and 1 mL/kg/h for children), monitoring of central venous pressure, and trending of serum lactate. Administration of crystalloid fluid is recommended if any of these parameters are not met. The use of vasoactive medications, such as norepinephrine, should be considered if hypotension and hypoperfusion exist following fluid resuscitation or if there are signs of hypoperfusion in the setting of an elevated central venous pressure. The use of stress dose glucocorticoids should be considered if adrenal insufficiency is a concern.

Early extubation is the goal for postoperative patients in the PICU with stable hemodynamics, adequate ventilation and pulmonary compliance, and no major postoperative bleeding. Target respiratory goals include normal ventilation and oxygenation, while medical teams should anticipate the third spacing of fluid causing pulmonary edema, if large volumes of crystalloid or blood products are required perioperatively. Postoperative transfusion thresholds are discussed later. As with thoracotomies, ePCA is ideal for analgesia to minimize the systemic need for opiates or sedating medications. Maintenance of monitoring lines is imperative, including arterial lines and central venous catheters, along with assessing the daily need for any surgical drains, nasogastric tubes, and urinary catheters.

Immunotherapy for Neuroblastoma

Immunotherapy is a major component in the treatment of high-risk neuroblastoma. Several different antibodies target ganglioside GD2, which is expressed on the surface of neuroblastoma cells.[65] These immunotherapies require close monitoring during and after infusions because of their poor side effect profile. Commercially available dinutuximab is a chimeric human-murine antibody to GD2, and a similar monoclonal antibody, Hu3F8, is used at Memorial Sloan Kettering Cancer Center (MSKCC).

Intensivists and oncologists should be aware of the side effects of such antibodies and be prepared for treatment in the inpatient or intensive care setting. Pain is the most common adverse event, as GD2 is also expressed in peripheral nerve cells. High-dose opioids may be needed to control pain, which can in turn lead to respiratory depression. Continuous opioid infusions should be administered with caution when combined with other sedating medications. Opioids with dexmedetomidine, an alpha-2 agonist, can lead to hypotension and bradycardia, whereas ketamine infusions are generally well tolerated without respiratory compromise but may lead to dysphoria.[66,67]

Antibodies against GD2 can also cause anaphylactic-like hypersensitivity responses with symptoms, including bronchospasm, urticaria, hypotension, and capillary leak. Treatment with epinephrine, inhaled beta-2 agonists, fluid boluses, and antihistamines can improve many anaphylactic and anaphylactoid reactions. Hypertension can be a late side effect following immunotherapy infusion, and these patients should have close follow up as Hu3F8 has been associated with PRES as discussed earlier.[68] These patients with hypertension and any signs of symptoms of neurologic involvement should be treated with antihypertensives and require neuroimaging.

Wilms Tumor

Childhood kidney cancers account for approximately 7% of all pediatric cancers.[69] Wilms tumor is the primary type for all pediatric kidney cancers.[69] CT or MRI of the abdomen is imperative to assess disease burden. Approximately 11% of Wilms tumor patients have renal vein involvement and 4% present with inferior vena cava or atrial involvement.[69] Embolization of a caval thrombus to the pulmonary artery is a rare occurrence but can be fatal, necessitating precise surgical planning. Initial nephrectomy is recommended as the first-line treatment for stage I and II Wilms tumors by North American experts, and postoperative management often occurs in the intensive care unit or pediatric floor. Complications include the need for extensive resections, removal of addition organs, and intraoperative tumor contamination in stage III–V Wilms tumors.

Transfusion Medicine

Pediatric oncology patients are a special population who often require blood and platelet transfusions throughout their treatment course. There are limited evidence-based guidelines for transfusion thresholds for this population, yet recent experts have recommended restrictive transfusion strategies.[70] Current guidelines recommend transfusing for hemoglobin <7–8 g/dL, platelets $<10 \times 10^9$/L, and INR >2.5 with clinically significant bleeding.

Postoperative pediatric oncology patients pose an even more unique challenge with regard to the timing of transfusion. Current management of postoperative oncologic patients not only recommends a restrictive transfusion strategy for anemia but also a higher threshold for platelets, transfusion of platelets to maintain a count greater than 50×10^9/L. INR thresholds differ by clinician and surgeon in terms of when to transfuse plasma, most suggesting plasma transfusion if INR is prolonged and the patient has clinically significant bleeding. However, there is a lack of validated bleeding scales, and clinically relevant bleeding has not been universally defined.[70] Additional evidence-based studies and guidelines are needed to standardize transfusion practices that can be used in all critically ill patients.

Enhanced Recovery After Surgery

The goal of caring for pediatric oncologic patients following surgery is to provide high-quality medical care, optimize hospital resources, and expedite their discharge from the intensive care unit and hospital, while providing patient and parent support. Enhanced Recovery After Surgery (ERAS) programs are designed to achieve these goals (see Fig. 52.3). From presurgical counseling in an outpatient setting, to intraoperative pain control and conservative fluid management, to follow up after discharge, the ERAS program highlights the full spectrum of a surgical experience. Derived from adult ERAS programs, these concepts have been applied to pediatric patients and retrospectively studied in several common childhood surgeries.[71] Ideally, all elective surgeries would undergo screening for ERAS participation.

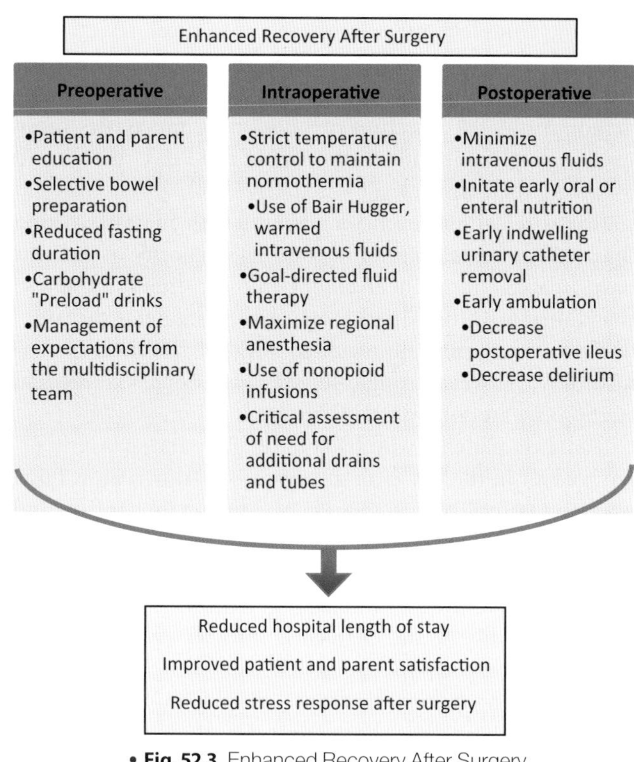

• **Fig. 52.3** Enhanced Recovery After Surgery.

The success of ERAS programs depends on active patient and family involvement, measurement of compliance and outcomes, and involvement of a multidisciplinary team. This comprehensive team approach involves members from hospital administration, nurses, advanced practice providers, primary providers in anesthesia, surgeons, and pediatricians, as well as physical and occupational therapists and child life specialists. To achieve a successful ERAS program, all representatives must be dedicated to achieving a unified goal. Ongoing research is being conducted to establish ERAS programs in the pediatric oncologic population.

References

1. Edate S, Albanese A. Management of electrolyte and fluid disorders after brain surgery for pituitary/suprasellar tumours. *Horm Res Paediatr*. 2015;83:293–301.
2. Kruis RWJ, Schouten-van Meeteren AYN, Finken MJJ, et al. Management and consequences of postoperative fluctuations in plasma sodium concentration after pediatric brain tumor surgery in the sellar region: a national cohort analysis. *Pituitary*. 2018;21:384–392.

3. Hensen J, Henig A, Fahlbusch R, Meyer M, Boehnert M, Buchfelder M. Prevalence, predictors and patterns of postoperative polyuria and hyponatraemia in the immediate course after transsphenoidal surgery for pituitary adenomas. *Clin Endocrinol (Oxf)*. 1999;50:431–439.
4. Cohen M, Guger S, Hamilton J. Long term sequelae of pediatric craniopharyngioma - literature review and 20 years of experience. *Front Endocrinol (Lausanne)*. 2011;2:81.
5. Pratheesh R, Swallow DM, Joseph M, et al. Evaluation of a protocol-based treatment strategy for postoperative diabetes insipidus in craniopharyngioma. *Neurol India*. 2015;63:712–717.
6. Hoorn EJ, Zietse R. Water balance disorders after neurosurgery: the triphasic response revisited. *NDT Plus*. 2010;3:42–44.
7. Olson BR, Gumowski J, Rubino D, Oldfield EH. Pathophysiology of hyponatremia after transsphenoidal pituitary surgery. *J Neurosurg*. 1997;87:499–507.
8. Olson BR, Rubino D, Gumowski J, Oldfield EH. Isolated hyponatremia after transsphenoidal pituitary surgery. *J Clin Endocrinol Metab*. 1995;80:85–91.
9. Sherlock M, O'Sullivan E, Agha A, et al. Incidence and pathophysiology of severe hyponatraemia in neurosurgical patients. *Postgrad Med J*. 2009;85:171–175.
10. Vaidya C, Ho W, Freda BJ. Management of hyponatremia: providing treatment and avoiding harm. *Cleve Clin J Med*. 2010;77:715–726.
11. Yeates KE, Singer M, Morton AR. Salt and water: a simple approach to hyponatremia. *CMAJ*. 2004;170:365–369.
12. Yee AH, Burns JD, Wijdicks EF. Cerebral salt wasting: pathophysiology, diagnosis, and treatment. *Neurosurg Clin N Am*. 2010;21:339–352.
13. Momi J, Tang CM, Abcar AC, Kujubu DA, Sim JJ. Hyponatremia—what is cerebral salt wasting? *Perm J*. 2010;14:62–65.
14. Hinduja A, Habetz K, Raina SK, Fitzgerald RT. Predictors of intensive care unit utilization in patients with posterior reversible encephalopathy syndrome. *Acta Neurol Belg*. 2017;117:201–206.
15. Ghali MGZ, Davanzo J, Leo M, Rizk E. Posterior reversible encephalopathy syndrome in pediatric patients: pathophysiology, diagnosis, and management. *Leuk Lymphoma*. 2019;60:2365–2372.
16. Fisler G, Monty MA, Kohn N, Assaad P, Trope R, Kessel A. Characteristics and outcomes of critically ill pediatric patients with posterior reversible encephalopathy syndrome. *Neurocritical Care*. 2020;32:145–151.
17. Raj S, Overby P, Erdfarb A, Ushay HM. Posterior reversible encephalopathy syndrome: incidence and associated factors in a pediatric critical care population. *Pediatr Neurol*. 2013;49:335–339.
18. Hinchey J, Chaves C, Appignani B, et al. A reversible posterior leukoencephalopathy syndrome. *N Engl J Med*. 1996;334:494–500.
19. Schwartz RB, Jones KM, Kalina P, et al. Hypertensive encephalopathy: findings on CT, MR imaging, and SPECT imaging in 14 cases. *AJR Am J Roentgenol*. 1992;159:379–383.
20. Hauser RA, Lacey DM, Knight MR. Hypertensive encephalopathy. Magnetic resonance imaging demonstration of reversible cortical and white matter lesions. *Arch Neurol*. 1988;45:1078–1083.
21. Ito T, Sakai T, Inagawa S, Utsu M, Bun T. MR angiography of cerebral vasospasm in preeclampsia. *AJNR Am J Neuroradiol*. 1995;16:1344–1346.
22. Schwaighofer BW, Hesselink JR, Healy ME. MR demonstration of reversible brain abnormalities in eclampsia. *J Comput Assist Tomogr*. 1989;13:310–312.
23. Trommer BL, Homer D, Mikhael MA. Cerebral vasospasm and eclampsia. *Stroke*. 1988;19:326–329.
24. Saad Aldin E, McNeely P, Menda Y. Posterior reversible encephalopathy syndrome on 18F-FDG PET/CT in a pediatric patient with Burkitt's lymphoma. *Clin Nucl Med*. 2018;43:195–198.
25. Navarro CE, Rodríguez PJ, Espitia OM. Fludarabine-induced posterior reversible encephalopathy syndrome in a pediatric patient with beta-thalassemia: case report and literature review. *Clin Neuropharmacol*. 2018;41:224–229.
26. Dicuonzo F, Salvati A, Palma M, et al. Posterior reversible encephalopathy syndrome associated with methotrexate neurotoxicity: conventional magnetic resonance and diffusion-weighted imaging findings. *J Child Neurol*. 2009;24:1013–1018.
27. Usta S, Karabulut K. A late complication occurring due to tacrolimus after liver transplant: posterior reversible encephalopathy syndrome. *Exp Clin Transplant*. 2018.
28. Chuk MK, Widemann BC, Minard CG, et al. A phase 1 study of cabozantinib in children and adolescents with recurrent or refractory solid tumors, including CNS tumors: trial ADVL1211, a report from the Children's Oncology Group. *Pediatr Blood Cancer*. 2018;65:e27077.
29. Shkalim-Zemer V, Konen O, Levinsky Y, et al. Calcineurin inhibitor-free strategies for prophylaxis and treatment of GVHD in children with posterior reversible encephalopathy syndrome after stem cell transplantation. *Pediatr Blood Cancer*. 2017;64:e26531. doi:10.1002/pbc.26531.
30. Cruz RJ Jr. DiMartini A, Akhavanheidari M, et al. Posterior reversible encephalopathy syndrome in liver transplant patients: clinical presentation, risk factors and initial management. *Am J Transplant*. 2012;12:2228–2236.
31. Siegal D, Keller A, Xu W, et al. Central nervous system complications after allogeneic hematopoietic stem cell transplantation: incidence, manifestations, and clinical significance. *Biol Blood Marrow Transplant*. 2007;13:1369–1379.
32. Kanekiyo T, Hara J, Matsuda-Hashii Y, et al. Tacrolimus-related encephalopathy following allogeneic stem cell transplantation in children. *Int J Hematol*. 2005;81:264–268.
33. Small SL, Fukui MB, Bramblett GT, Eidelman BH. Immunosuppression-induced leukoencephalopathy from tacrolimus (FK506). *Ann Neurol*. 1996;40:575–580.
34. Primavera A, Audenino D, Mavilio N, Cocito L. Reversible posterior leucoencephalopathy syndrome in systemic lupus and vasculitis. *Ann Rheum Dis*. 2001;60:534–537.
35. Bartynski WS. Posterior reversible encephalopathy syndrome, part 2: controversies surrounding pathophysiology of vasogenic edema. *AJNR Am J Neuroradiol*. 2008;29:1043–1049.
36. Shimizu Y, Tha KK, Iguchi A, et al. Isolated posterior fossa involvement in posterior reversible encephalopathy syndrome. *Neuroradiol J*. 2013;26:514–519.
37. Seeman T, Hamdani G, Mitsnefes M. Hypertensive crisis in children and adolescents. *Pediatr Nephrol*. 2019;34:2523–2537.
38. Saqan R, Thiabat H. Evaluation of the safety and efficacy of metoprolol infusion for children and adolescents with hypertensive crises: a retrospective case series. *Pediatr Nephrol*. 2017;32:2107–2113.
39. Stein DR, Ferguson MA. Evaluation and treatment of hypertensive crises in children. *Integr Blood Press Control*. 2016;9:49–58.
40. Baracco R, Mattoo TK. Pediatric hypertensive emergencies. *Curr Hypertens Rep*. 2014;16:456.
41. Sanford EF, Stein JC. Hypertensive encephalopathy presenting as status epilepticus in a three year old. *J Emerg Med*. 2012;42:e141–e145.
42. Bechstein WO. Neurotoxicity of calcineurin inhibitors: impact and clinical management. *Transpl Int*. 2000;13:313–326.

43. Papadakis V, Dunkel IJ, Cramer LD, et al. High-dose carmustine, thiotepa and etoposide followed by autologous bone marrow rescue for the treatment of high risk central nervous system tumors. *Bone Marrow Transplant*. 2000;26:153–160.
44. Portnow J, Badie B, Chen M, Liu A, Blanchard S, Synold TW. The neuropharmacokinetics of temozolomide in patients with resectable brain tumors: potential implications for the current approach to chemoradiation. *Clin Cancer Res*. 2009;15:7092–7098.
45. Shi M, Sanche L. Convection-enhanced delivery in malignant gliomas: a review of toxicity and efficacy. *J Oncol*. 2019;2019:9342796.
46. Baugh J, Bartels U, Leach J, et al. The international diffuse intrinsic pontine glioma registry: an infrastructure to accelerate collaborative research for an orphan disease. *J Neurooncol*. 2017;132:323–331.
47. Hargrave D, Bartels U, Bouffet E. Diffuse brainstem glioma in children: critical review of clinical trials. *Lancet Oncol*. 2006;7:241–248.
48. Souweidane MM, Kramer K, Pandit-Taskar N, et al. Convection-enhanced delivery for diffuse intrinsic pontine glioma: a single-centre, dose-escalation, phase 1 trial. *Lancet Oncol*. 2018;19:1040–1050.
49. Heiss JD, Jamshidi A, Shah S, et al. Phase I trial of convection-enhanced delivery of IL13-Pseudomonas toxin in children with diffuse intrinsic pontine glioma. *J Neurosurg Pediatr*. 2018;23:333–342.
50. Sewing ACP, Lagerweij T, van Vuurden DG, et al. Preclinical evaluation of convection-enhanced delivery of liposomal doxorubicin to treat pediatric diffuse intrinsic pontine glioma and thalamic high-grade glioma. *J Neurosurg Pediatr*. 2017;19:518–530.
51. Acker SN, Linton J, Tan GM, et al. A multidisciplinary approach to the management of anterior mediastinal masses in children. *J Pediatr Surg*. 2015;50:875–878.
52. Carter BW, Marom EM, Detterbeck FC. Approaching the patient with an anterior mediastinal mass: a guide for clinicians. *J Thorac Oncol*. 2014;9(9 Suppl 2):S102–S109.
53. Priola AM, Priola SM, Cardinale L, Cataldi A, Fava C. The anterior mediastinum: diseases. *Radiol Med*. 2006;111:312–342.
54. Shamberger RC, Holzman RS, Griscom NT, Tarbell NJ, Weinstein HJ. CT quantitation of tracheal cross-sectional area as a guide to the surgical and anesthetic management of children with anterior mediastinal masses. *J Pediatr Surg*. 1991;26:138–142.
55. Bassanezi BS, Oliveira-Filho AG, Miranda ML, Soares L, Aguiar SS. Use of BiPAP for safe anesthesia in a child with a large anterior mediastinal mass. *Paediatr Anaesthes*. 2011;21:985–987.
56. Polaner DM. The use of heliox and the laryngeal mask airway in a child with an anterior mediastinal mass. *Anesth Analg*. 1996;82:208–210.
57. Hack HA, Wright NB, Wynn RF. The anaesthetic management of children with anterior mediastinal masses. *Anaesthesia*. 2008;63:837–846.
58. Said SM, Telesz BJ, Makdisi G, et al. Awake cardiopulmonary bypass to prevent hemodynamic collapse and loss of airway in a severely symptomatic patient with a mediastinal mass. *Ann Thorac Surg*. 2014;98:e87–e90.
59. Dorfman HD, Czerniak B. Bone cancers. *Cancer*. 1995;75(Suppl 1):203–210.
60. Su WT, Chewning J, Abramson S, et al. Surgical management and outcome of osteosarcoma patients with unilateral pulmonary metastases. *J Pediatr Surg*. 2004;39:418–423. discussion 418.
61. Heaton TE, Hammond WJ, Farber BA, et al. A 20-year retrospective analysis of CT-based pre-operative identification of pulmonary metastases in patients with osteosarcoma: A single-center review. *J Pediatr Surg*. 2017;52:115–119.
62. Chou J, Chan CW, Chalkiadis GA. Post-thoracotomy pain in children and adolescence: a retrospective cross-sectional study. *Pain Med*. 2014;15:452–459.
63. Soliman IE, Apuya JS, Fertal KM, Simpson PM, Tobias JD. Intravenous versus epidural analgesia after surgical repair of pectus excavatum. *Am J Therapeut*. 2009;16:398–403.
64. Ross SL, Greenwald BM, Howell JD, et al. Outcomes following thoracoabdominal resection of neuroblastoma. *Pediatr Crit Care Med*. 2009;10:681–686.
65. Cheung NK, Kushner BH, Yeh SD, Larson SM. 3F8 monoclonal antibody treatment of patients with stage 4 neuroblastoma: a phase II study. *Int J Oncol*. 1998;12:1299–1306.
66. Bredlau AL, Thakur R, Korones DN, Dworkin RH. Ketamine for pain in adults and children with cancer: a systematic review and synthesis of the literature. *Pain Med*. 2013;14:1505–1517.
67. Zempsky WT, Loiselle KA, Corsi JM, Hagstrom JN. Use of low-dose ketamine infusion for pediatric patients with sickle cell disease-related pain: a case series. *Clin J Pain*. 2010;26:163–167.
68. Kushner BH, Modak S, Basu EM, Roberts SS, Kramer K, Cheung NK. Posterior reversible encephalopathy syndrome in neuroblastoma patients receiving anti-GD2 3F8 monoclonal antibody. *Cancer*. 2013;119:2789–2795.
69. National Cancer Institute. Wilms Tumor and Other Childhood Kidney Tumors Treatment (PDQ®): Health Professional Version. National Cancer Institute.
70. Nellis ME, Levasseur J, Stribling J, et al. Bleeding scales applicable to critically ill children: a systematic review. *Pediatr Crit Care Med*. 2019;20:603–607.
71. Grewal H, Sweat J, Vazquez WD. Laparoscopic appendectomy in children can be done as a fast-track or same-day surgery. *JSLS*. 2004;8:151–154.

SECTION 7

Value Proposition and Research in Perioperative Cancer Care

53

Value Proposition in Cancer Care: Quantifying Patient-Centered Value in a Comprehensive Cancer Care Center

THOMAS A. ALOIA

Radar Plots

A Comprehensive Value Equation for a Comprehensive Cancer Center

Over the past decade, many forms of the value equation have emerged from the original "Value = Outcomes/Cost" framework promulgated by Professors Michael Porter, Elizabeth Teisberg, and Robert Kaplan of the Harvard Business School.[1] Health care systems, hospital alliances, government health care funders, and even individual providers and health care administrators within the same institution have developed their own versions of the value equation. For example, many health systems have emphasized the concept of "high reliability," interpreting the value equation as "Value = Safety/Cost." However, by focusing the numerator only on harm, this form of the equation disregards the value of the positive outcomes that are sought from health care encounters. Alternative proposals have emphasized patient experience in the denominator, to the exclusion of either quality or safety. However, other versions combine these concepts:

"Value = (Quality + Outcomes)/Cost"

"Value = (Outcomes + Patient Experience)/(Direct + Indirect Cost)"

"Value = (Quality + Service)/Cost"

Each of the above variations of the value equation has fundamental flaws that prevent meaningful measurement of value. The major problem with each version is that the terms are nebulous, leaving too much room for interpretation when precision is needed. What is meant by safety? What is quality? Which costs should be included? Likewise, these equations do not always measure value from a patient's perspective. Frequently, the denominator of costs has been interpreted as institutional costs of provisioning care or third-party reimbursement when patient-centered value focuses only on out-of-pocket patient expenditures for health care, including copays and deductibles, but also on travel expenses and lost wages.

Adding to the already challenging task of developing measurement for a multidimensional equation is the complexity of cancer care and the heterogeneity of the patient population. Each type of cancer is not a single disease but a conglomerate of thousands of diseases with distinct characteristics that carry varying risks and require different treatments. Even within the same cancer disease type, there is variability in the genomic pathways that require individual considerations. Overlying the oncologic variability is variability in our patients' social determinants of health and their subjective outcome priorities. Faced with this compounded variability, our challenge was to develop a value equation that is inclusive of all the important domains while remaining scalable across a variety of diseases, perspectives, and priorities.

Defining Quality and Safety: Outcomes That Matter to Patients

To achieve this objective, we first expanded the terms in the numerator to contrast the outcome of "Quality" (defined as the achievement of a positive outcome) against the outcome of "Safety" (defined as the avoidance of a negative outcome). Here, "Safety" is mathematically equivalent to 1/"Harm." Although interrelated, the terms quality and safety are very different. Quality is the indication for the treatment, the *reason* we perform therapeutic intervention, while safety is *what* we do during the intervention to avoid harm. For almost every medical intervention (including drug therapies), at the time the intervention is initiated, the patient

A The relationship of Safety/Harm and Quality from Treatment Start

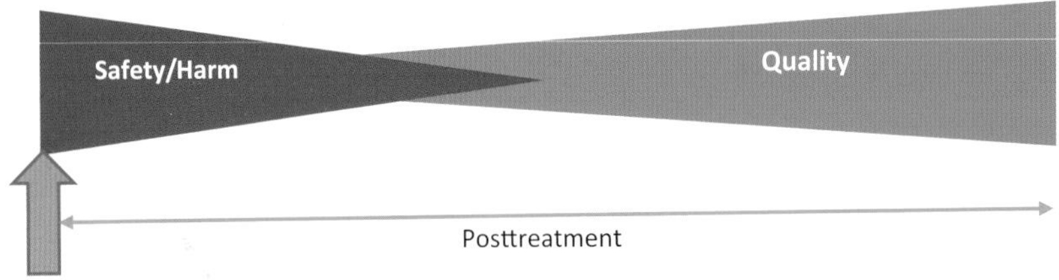

B High-Reliability Processes limit the Risk for Harm and allow Quality to emerge sooner and to a greater extent

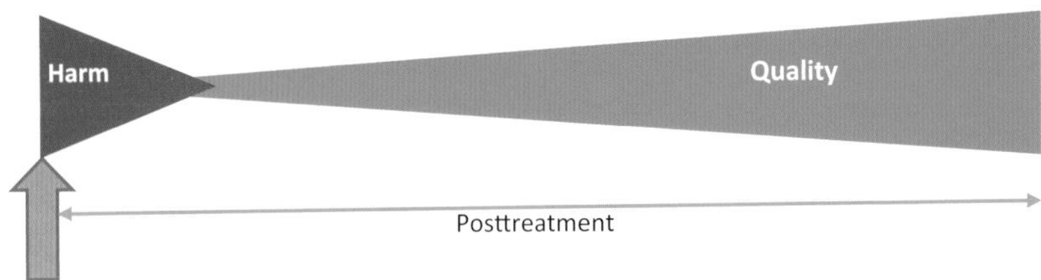

C Even one Harm Event can erase the possibility for patient and provider to experience the benefit of an intervention

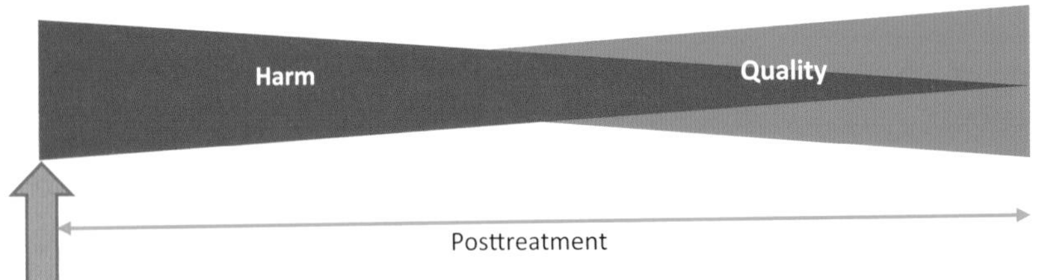

• **Fig. 53.1** (A) The relationship between safety/harm and quality from treatment start. (B) High-reliability processes limit the risk for harm and allow quality to emerge sooner and to a greater extent. (C) Even one harm event can erase the possibility of patients and providers experiencing the benefit of an intervention.

and provider cannot see the quality of the intervention (e.g., long-term survival after cancer surgery) (Fig. 53.1A). However, they are definitely exposed to the risk of harm (e.g., postoperative thromboembolism).

As previously discussed, a commonly derived transformation of the value equation has been tailored for high reliability, expressed as "Value = Safety/Cost." However, this version of the formula does not fully capture the impact of high reliability. The reason it is laudable to focus on a high-reliability environment is not only that it emphasizes the need to limit the risk for harm, but equally or more importantly, a narrowed risk for harm through high-reliability processes allows the patient and the provider to see the quality objective sooner and to a greater extent (Fig. 53.1B). In an error-prone, low-reliability environment, or in the case of chance complications, it is well understood that even one adverse event can completely erase the possibility of experiencing the intended quality of the intervention (Fig. 53.1C). The fact that 90% of "Quality measures" in health care are actually metrics describing harm, and we seldom measure and report on the positive quality outcomes of treatment, is a primary driver of provider burnout in medicine.[2] Based on these and other arguments, it is imperative that the value equation speak to both positive qualities and potential harm.

To account for both sides of this coin, we operationalized the numerator of the value equation as "Quality minus Harm." With these two domains defined, the patient can start to appreciate both the positive and negative attributes of the proposed intervention and to compare one therapy to another or one providing institution to another for the same therapy. This configuration likewise feels natural to providers, as it is the embodiment of the modern consent process, where we describe the benefits, risks, and alternatives of an intervention to the patient and their associated caregivers, allowing all parties to determine whether the balance favors (or not) the proposed procedure or treatment.

UTMDACC Value Equation featuring nine measured domains.

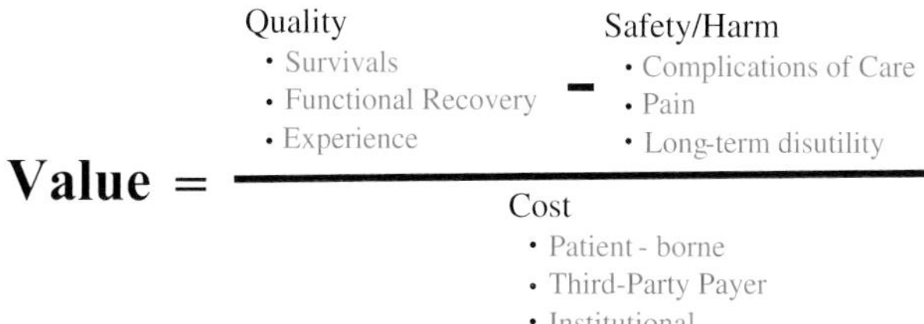

• **Fig. 53.2** UTMDACC value equation featuring nine measured domains.

The Full Value Equation

With the foundation of "Value = Quality minus Harm over Cost," we sought to define and measure the individual components of each of these three terms. To accomplish this, we interviewed patients, caregivers, and providers. We expected to find a vast array of qualities and harms that spoke to patients and providers alike. However, ultimately (and conveniently) all of the feedback we received could be folded under three primary qualities that patients seek from cancer care and three specific areas of harm that they seek to avoid (Fig. 53.2). In the next section, we define each of these subcategories of value.

Similar to the traditional basic form of the value equation, the University of Texas M.D. Anderson Cancer Center (UTMDACC) value equation is patient-centric, focusing on the value of care provided from the patient's perspective. However, unlike other forms of the value equation, this equation considers the factors that impact decisions from the perspective of all stakeholders, defines measurement for each component, and identifies their respective data sources to enable actual calculations and comparisons of care value. Additionally, the universality of the equation allows value calculations to easily transition between different cancers while still maintaining meaningful insights to inform decisions. The analyses are also easily dissectible to concentrate on specific patient populations, disease types, and outcome sets. The equation can be similarly utilized in noncancer-related care settings.

Defining the Value Equation

The Numerator: Quality

Based on our qualitative interviews and quantitative feedback, it is clear that patients seek three qualities from their cancer care: *survivals, functional recovery, and a positive experience (PE).*

• *Survivals*

Ninety percent of surveyed cancer providers reported that survival is the number one priority of our patients. Interestingly, only 50% of patients ranked survival as their first priority, as many more patients than might be expected were focused on returning to pressing life responsibilities that cancer had "interrupted" and/or maintaining their independence in the vein of "Quality of life over Quantity of life." Even patients who rank survival first, when pressed why their priority would be the achievement of a milestone birthday (e.g., So your first priority is to make it to 80 years old?). Most reply that the desire for longer survival is actually only driven by the observation that they "have more to do in life." **In other words, functional recovery from illness (discussed later) is clearly the primary goal of cancer care for the vast majority of our patients, and perhaps the most underaddressed value proposition in health care.** This having been said, cancer survival remains a crucial and highly measurable Quality metric. It can be calculated from when a patient is diagnosed or starts treatment for a specific cancer to the date of recurrence, progression, or death. Leveraging our Tumor Registry, which contains patient follow up data on over 1.5 million patients beginning in 1944, analyses are performed to determine long-term cancer survival after care at UTMDACC, which can then be benchmarked against equivalent populations in national datasets, as demonstrated in Fig. 53.3.

• *Functional Recovery*

Almost all patients come to medical care with some level of disease-induced disability. Patients with malignancy are no exception, as they are frequently diagnosed in a debilitated state with cachexia, malnutrition, infection, immunosuppression, anxiety, and cancer-related pain. Unfortunately, most cancer treatments further impair the patient's ability to perform desired activities by inducing symptoms and side effects. This sinister "double-hit" leaves patients with substantial levels of dysfunction. In part, this explains why functional recovery is the primary goal of cancer patients, as described earlier. It also implies that in addition to wearing badges that read "Surgical Oncology," "Medical Oncology," or "Radiation Oncology," all cancer providers are *also* rehabilitation specialists. **In fact, functional recovery is so preeminent in patient-centric value that a health care enterprise's ultimate true value could be summed to the degree to which it recovers patients from illness.** Rapid recovery also speaks to the value employers place on their employees rapidly returning to the workforce. Despite the preeminence of this value proposition, it is remarkable that functional recovery data are rarely found in our historical written medical records or our current electronic billing records (EHRs). This is because the only mechanism to assess functional recovery is to ask the patients how functional they are in their daily lives. Not only have we paternalistically never asked, we poorly recorded our own impressions of recovery via simple tools such as the Karnofsky status or Eastern Cooperative Oncology Group (ECOG) performance status.[3,4] Fortunately, we are evolving, and the field of patient-reported outcomes (PROs) has exploded into medical research and care, allowing patients to voice and numerically score their degree of recovery.[5,6] Only by using PRO surveys at strategic time points (e.g., preintervention and 14, 30, and 90 days postintervention) in clinical care can we measure our ability to achieve short-term functional recovery after interventions. Validated PRO instruments tend to be dominated by measures of symptom burden but the best tools for measurement of functional recovery contain measures of life interference from symptoms.[7] Our research shows that symptoms are variable, difficult to impact, and frequently affected by psychologic overtones. The goal of enhanced recovery

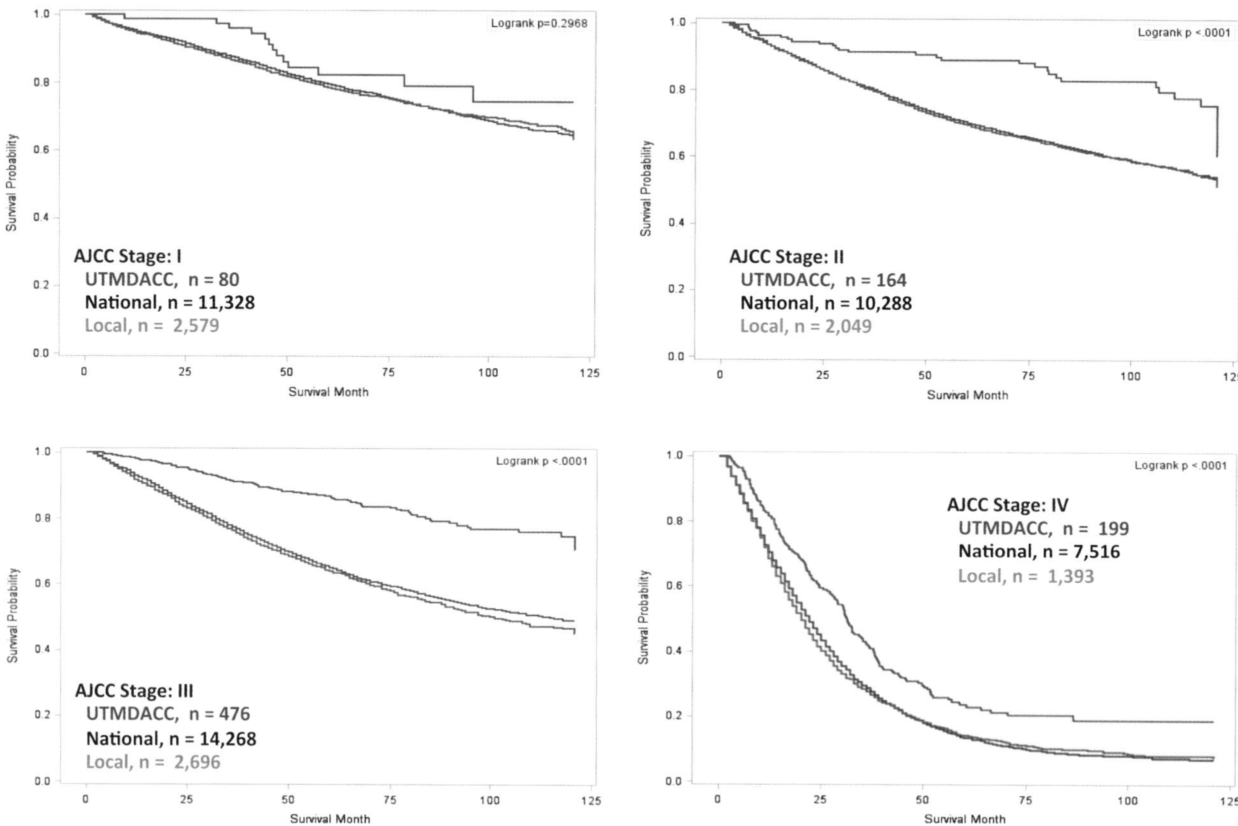

• **Fig. 53.3** Kaplan-Meier survival comparison for colorectal cancer by American Joint Commitee on Cancer (*AJCC*) Stage: 2005–2014 *Subsite: Rectum, Rectosigmoid.*

programs is to facilitate function with symptoms. Therefore PRO instruments that include questions about walking, work, ability to care for self, ability to care for others, and enjoyment of life serve as actionable dependent variables for hospitals to measure the value of their function recovery efforts. Armed with these measures of success, enhanced recovery programs have entered the cancer care environment with ubiquitous benefits that impact multiple areas of the value equation.

- *Patient Experience*

The third quality patients seek from cancer care is a positive experience (PE). PE is sometimes conflated with PROs, but symptoms and function are distinct from feelings of respect, courtesy, and open communication, as measured by patient experience and satisfaction surveys. An increasing number of institutions are collecting patient feedback through patient satisfaction reports, feedback surveys, and patient and family advisory councils.[8] These data points are assessed to rate an important part of the success of the service provided to patients along their cancer care journey.

The Numerator: Safety/Harm

Every cancer intervention has the potential to harm the patient before the benefits of treatment are ever realized. These unintended negative results, which may be preventable, include *acute complications of care, pain,* and *long-term disutility*. Both mathematically and qualitatively, if the harm encountered exceeds the quality, the numerator crosses into the negative and value is extinguished.

- *Complications of Care*

The medical profession is awash in short-term complication data that are produced locally, administratively, and even nationally by regulatory bodies. Surgeons, medical oncologists, radiation therapists, and all other care specialists collect and obsess over short-term harm data such as postoperative complications, toxicity grades, readmissions, and hospital-acquired infections. Ideally, these data are risk-adjusted for fair comparison, but frequently we have found even raw complication rate data to be actionable.[9] Despite the availability of these data, it has only recently been reported more transparently to patients and caregivers.

- *Pain*

Patient pain scores are ubiquitously collected throughout all facets of cancer care. Despite the availability of these data, substantial progress, and the development of medical specialties in pain management, pain continues to be a principle negative outcome for patients. More than 50% of patients receiving cancer treatment report severe pain during their continuum of care.[10] For this reason, we believe that pain warrants a unique place in the value equation and hope that calling it out will bring more attention to its profound impact on patients' quality of life. There is no doubt that intentional programs that successfully reduce pain to levels that permit function improve the value of cancer care.

- *Long-Term Disutility*

Much like short-term functional recovery, the measurement of long-term disutility from cancer care has been an underaddressed issue. As cancer treatments improve, patients live longer and rightfully demand durable functional recovery. Therefore the collection of long-term functional recovery data, again via PROs, has become a requisite to measure value. Urologic oncology providers who track long-term bowel, bladder, and sexual function after prostate surgery and radiation have demonstrated the feasibility of capturing these data and having them inform treatment decisions.[11] The widespread collection of these data will be a heavy lift for patients and providers but is required to completely factor the numerator of the value equation. To accomplish this, institutions are encouraged to form PRO Governance Committees to oversee the build of validated PROs into the EHR and to ensure that they take into consideration patient survey fatigue, changes to clinical workflow, and other factors that are critical to successful PRO implementation and data collection.

The Numerator: Accounting for All Three Tiers of Value

As originally proposed by Porter and Teisberg, value should be measured across time using the concept of three tiers of outcomes measures hierarchy.[1,12] Adhering to these principles, our detailed value formula incorporates the dimension of time by including short-term complications with long-term disutility, and both early and late survival with functional recovery.

Cost

Like the term "Outcomes," the value denominator term of "Cost" has been equally opaque. In one dimension, we must grapple with determining if we are describing charges, prices, collections, acquisition costs, costs of provisioning care, and/or amortization of indirect costs to overall costs. In another dimension, we are compelled to assume the perspective of the patient (who measures out-of-pocket payments and largely disregards third-party payer contributions or the institutional costs of provisioning care). At the same time, population-level value measurement requires the inclusion of third-party payor/society financial contributions and the institutions' expense side of the balance sheet. In a pure patient-driven value equation, we only concern ourselves with patient-borne cost, but holistically, we cannot effect positive change in the health care landscape without including the payor and provider perspectives. Given these seemingly conflicting priorities, we quarantined the denominator of our value equation to describe real dollars in the form of *collections from the patient (patient-borne cost) and third-party payors (including private, nonprofit, and governmental sources), as well as the institutional cost for the hospital system to provide care*. The institutional cost of care is optimally captured using time-driven activity-based costing (TDABC) methodologies but in the absence of this capability, financial data may also be acquired from traditional hospital costing systems. Importantly, charges are not included in any component of the equation, as these are not real dollars; they reflect inflated pricing of services and are subject to deep contractual discounts. The avoidance of the "monopoly money" of charges allows the Value equation to rigidly report on real dollars in the form of collections, and to subtract the institutional Cost to provision care yielding the margin. Deep knowledge of margin data is critically important for the future establishment of fair bundled payment pricing strategies.

- *Patient-Borne Cost*

Due to multiple factors, including the emergence of high-deductible insurance products and narrow network policies, the percentage and total amount of out-of-pocket health care costs that are being paid directly by patients are rising.[13] Although every state, demographic, and socioeconomic group has been impacted, the low- and middle-class wage earners have been disproportionately impacted by these trends, explaining the fact that medical costs account for over 60% of bankruptcies in the United States and multitudes of patients are avoiding necessary care in order to avoid financial toxicity.[13] Due to the complex nature of cancer, and extremely high-priced treatments (including robotic surgery, proton radiation therapy, and immunotherapy) financial toxicity for cancer patients is a serious concern. A portion of the patients' burden of out-of-pocket expenses can be determined by analyzing payments received directly from patients for care in the form of copays, deductibles, and/or coinsurance. However, travel costs and reduced income from lost work time cannot currently be factored into the equation. In the future, transparent disclosure of out-of-pocket estimates within the full framework of the value formula **prior** to the initiation of therapy is required to avoid catastrophic surprise billing and to allow for comprehensive shared decision-making. Previously, hospital systems have avoided these disclosures by hiding behind the perceived complexity of accurate determination of out-of-pocket cost estimates; however, with modern EHRs, this capability is now available ubiquitously. The time is now for every patient to know what out-of-pocket expenses they can anticipate from medical care.

- *Third-Party Payment Cost*

Reimbursement for care from third parties often involves complex contracts that outline discounts, plan maximums, stop-loss provisions, and nontransparent accounting. Given that most institutions accept a vast array of plans, the simplest method to calculate third-party payor contributions is to determine the actual payments received for care based on collections via the institutional accounting system. Modern systems can define these collections to the penny.

- *Institutional Cost*

Determining the actual cost of providing care to an individual patient has historically been elusive for all hospitals and remains a challenge. Fully loaded costs encompass goods, drugs, equipment, personnel, services, time, information technologies, capital purchases, and a multitude of indirect costs that require attribution and allocation. In the absence

TABLE 53.1 Specific Data Streams for Each Value Equation Component

Value Domain	Value Equation Component	Data Stream
Quality	Survivals	Tumor Registry
	Functional recovery	EHR-PRO builds
	Patient experience	External vendor PE data
Safety	Short-term complications	Registries and EHR data
	Pain	EHR data
	Long-term disutility	EHR-PRO builds
Costs	Patient-borne	Collections accounting
	Third party	Collections accounting
	Institutional	Traditional and TDABC cost accounting modules

EHR, Electronic health record; *PE*, positive experience; *PRO*, patient-reported outcome; *TDABC*, time-driven activity-based costing.

of a definitive strategy to accurately assess the true costs of medical care, many bodies, including quality reporters such as Vizient,[14] are forced to impute costs of care by applying a ratio of costs to charges based on each institution's Medicare Cost report. Although this methodology provides a rough surrogate estimate of resource utilization, it is an inaccurate way of representing the health care costs associated with cancer care because it neither factors in overhead costs associated with the facilities, administration, nonbillable items, and so on, nor considers the actual flow of expenses and revenue. TDABC is a more accurate accounting method for measuring the cost of care. It utilizes process maps to capture the resources actually attributable to patient care. Fully loaded cost, which accounts for direct and indirect costs of care, is then applied to each process to calculate the cost for the cycle of care. Although historically tedious to fully implement, electronic tools have substantially increased the pace and ability to accurately measure costs of care using the TDABC methodology.

The Value Equation: Summary

Fully realized, the Value equation is represented by three major domains as "Quality minus Harm over Costs." Each of the three main groups has three subcategories that are easily understood and measurable. The six numerator values account for all three tiers of outcome measures hierarchy, highlighting critically important factors for patients such as functional recovery and patient experience. Notably, two of the six factors (short-term functional recovery and long-term disutility) are dependent on PROs. For isolated patient-centric value, third-party payor contributions and institutional costs of care are dropped from the denominator, leaving seven total factors, as the denominator is limited only to the patient-borne expenses. When used for population health, payment reform, and institutional quality improvement is initiated, all nine factors are entered into the equation (Fig. 53.2).

Collecting Data

Many of the data sources for these nine elements are currently available in most health care systems (e.g., collections), whereas others require a build (e.g., PRO platforms). For the most part, the heavy institutional lift is simply the channeling of existing data streams to a central value group to assimilate them across patient types, diseases, stages, and interventions. The goal of this work is to integrate all of the data streams into the formula for transparent visualization at the patient encounter. Investing in and resourcing the QA capabilities for collecting and reporting these data can add expense, but has a tremendous return on investment (ROI). We predict that institutions that achieve this capability will have a substantial competitive advantage both in the ability to market their value proposition and negotiate premium reimbursement rates that reflect the full spectrum of the value they provide (Table 53.1).

Systems that enable real-time structured data entry before and during patient encounters promote automation of value measurement, accurate data reporting, and efficient use of data resources:

- Critical to survival analyses is the discreet documentation of the date of diagnosis, diagnosis, stage, previous treatment, toxicity, and vital status (these variables are referred to as the oncology data foundation or ODF). Electronically collecting this small set of significant fields permits the EHR, the Tumor Registry, and the financial systems to quickly identify the correct patient population for analyses and extract appropriate patient data across each domain of value.
- Ability to administer and collect PROs in the EHR.
- Accurate cost accounting system.

Patient Engagement

Data capture for two of the nine value equation components relies heavily on patient engagement—PROs for measurement of functional recovery and long-term disutility. The

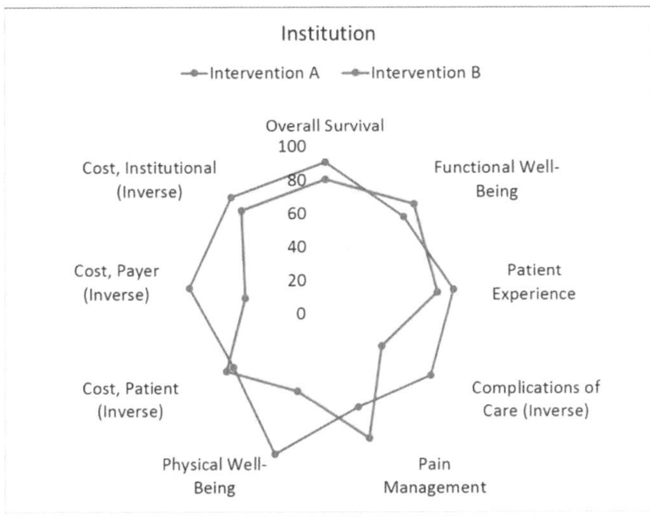

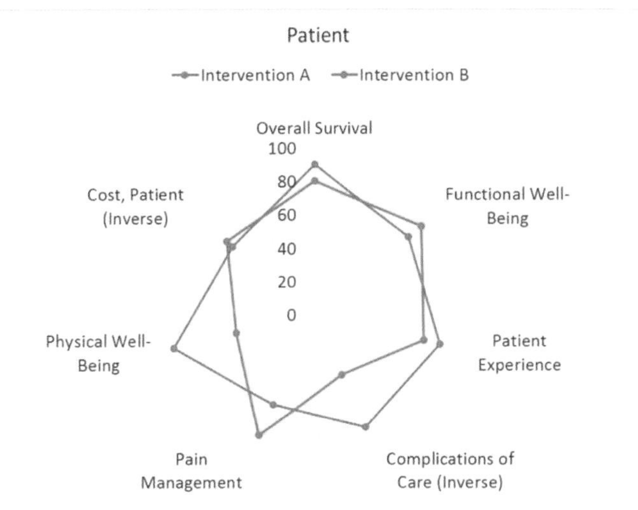

• **Fig. 53.4** The hypothetical values of nine measured domains are plotted on a radar graph with two resulting shapes symbolizing two comparable interventions.

engagement of patients starts with educating the patients on the purpose of answering surveys thoroughly and thoughtfully, and in a timely manner. Collected feedback from our Patient and Family Advisory Council has revealed that patients are willing to expend the time and effort to complete PROs as long as the providers review, acknowledge, and engage their responses. There are also opportunities to electronically tailor immediate feedback to symptoms and functional deficits based on patient inputs that motivate continued patient engagement with these surveys. Indeed, showing the patient an immediate personal ROI for survey completion creates long-term engagement.

Supportive Leadership

The success of accurately completing the value equation depends on the hospital, finance, and provider leadership support. Value measurement efforts benefit from executive leaders championing the collection of discreet data, providing resources to support PRO development and implementation, and emphasizing the importance of a holistic approach to value-based care to providers.

Visualizing and Comparing Value

Radar Value Plots

With so many individual components of the value equation, data visualization is crucial. We found that plotting the component values for the collected data on a radar chart facilitates both explanations to patients and comprehension by patients.[15] These charts arrange the data around a center point with a favorable value on each value axis plotted farthest from the center point. Connecting these points results in the formation of a geometric shape, where the internal area is a numeric summation of the total value of the treatment. The visualization tool has two main positive attributes. First, it enables quick comparisons between two treatment options at the same institution or for the same treatment option between the two providing institutions. Second, the individual values can be weighted differently by different stakeholders to visualize changes in value. For example, the institution may want to see the results of all nine elements; however, the patient may only want to know the factors that impact them, such as survival, complications, and patient-borne cost, with little need for including payor costs in their decision-making.

The Value Plot in Action

In Fig. 53.4, the hypothetical values of nine measured domains are plotted on a radar graph with two resulting shapes, symbolizing the value of two comparable interventions. The institution views all nine domains, while the patient views the seven domains they identified as priority. In the patient's narrower visualization, the two shapes are relatively close in the calculated area. Using this version, a discussion can ensue between providers and patients to determine how the patient's goals of care may weigh the factors in a different arrangement, allowing visualization (and even numerical calculation) of the optimal course of action for that patient. For example, a concert pianist may rate the long-term disutility of a neurotoxic drug far differently than another patient who may be most concerned with maximizing survival or eliminating the risk of loss of independence that may occur after major cancer surgery. The tailoring of treatment to individual patient-centered value is referred to as *goal-concordant care*.[16] Alternatively, the institution using the visualization with all the domains can make an informed decision to name Intervention A "standard of care" based on its greater all-domain value. Likewise, the institution can focus on specific improvements in the patient value domains while keeping the cost and reimbursement issues in view.

A Note About QALYs

Health care delivery researchers frequently attempt to represent value as a quality-adjusted life-year (QALY). This concept may be academically valuable, but it is challenging for providers and patients to bring to bear in medical decision-making. Furthermore, patients do not appreciate the academic community's arbitrary assumption that the reasonable value of one life-year is $50,000. We find that our version of the value equation is better accepted by patients and more easily described to them by providers. Further, if academic calculations with *P*-values are necessary for research, compared with QALYs, the area within the value radar plot serves as a more accurate, detailed, and objective measure of value-adjusted life-years (VALYs).

The Value Equation Payoff

Filling in the components of the value equation is not just a theoretical exercise. This detailed and expanded version of the equation is meant to be immediately implementable and actionable. The overarching goals of its implementation are to have **outcome data transparently available in real-time at patient encounters to facilitate shared decision-making and goal-concordant care**. These data must encompass quality, safety, and cost with attention to short-term complications, long-term disutility, and patient-borne costs so that **treatment plans can be formed around and evaluated based on patients' goals of care**. Institutions can then use these data to **inform workflows, pathways, and algorithms**. Furthermore, health systems should use this framework to **dashboard values across different components of their networks and systems**. Payors could partner to produce risk-adjusted scorecards that also **inform reimbursement models and patient choice**.

Institutional Value Improvement

The value equation helps define, measure, and analyze cancer care values. With these data, institutional improvement initiatives can be prioritized. Furthermore, specific areas could be targeted. For example, early sepsis detection algorithms can improve rescue and reduce the impact of early complications. Enhanced Recovery After Surgery programs can improve functional recovery with the added possibility of improving cancer-specific survival. In addition, Choosing Wisely campaigns can illuminate futile interventions, positively affecting multiple components of the value equation.[17]

Shared Decision-Making and Goal-Concordant Care Delivery

The ultimate goal of these efforts is to engage patients, caregivers, and providers with data to make informed decisions regarding their care. Cancer care can be physically taxing, emotionally draining, and financially toxic. By emphasizing patient-centered value-driven care, substantial improvements can be made to mitigate each of these hardships. Bringing the patient into the conversation about their care allows treatment to be reframed from the patient's perspective based on their life priorities.

References

1. Porter M, Teisberg E. *Redefining Health Care*. Boston, MA: Harvard Business School Publishing; 2006.
2. Aloia TA. Should zero harm be our goal? *Ann Surg*. 2020; 271(1):33.
3. Johnston BC, Patrick DL, Busse JW, Schünemann HJ, Agarwal A, Guyatt GH. Patient-reported outcomes in meta-analyses–part 1: assessing risk of bias and combining outcomes. *Health Qual Life Outcomes*. 2013;11:109.
4. Rahimi K, Malhotra A, Banning AP, Jenkinson C. Outcome selection and role of patient reported outcomes in contemporary cardiovascular trials: systematic review. *BMJ*. 2010; 341:c5707.
5. Day RW, Cleeland CS, Wang XS, et al. Patient-reported outcomes accurately measure the value of an Enhanced Recovery Program in liver surgery. *J Am Coll Surg*. 2015;221(6):1023.
6. Lillemoe HA, Marcus RK, Kim BJ, et al. Severe preoperative symptoms delay readiness to Return to Intended Oncologic Therapy (RIOT) after liver resection. *Ann Surg Oncol*. 2019;26(13): 4548.
7. Serlin RC, Mendoza TR, Nakamura Y, Edwards KR, Cleeland CS. When is cancer pain mild, moderate or severe? Grading pain severity by its interference with function. *Pain*. 1995;61(2):277.
8. Cunningham R, Walton MK. Partnering with patients to improve care: the value of patient and family advisory councils. *J Nurs Adm*. 2016;46(11):549.
9. Davis CH, Kao LS, Fleming JB, Aloia TA. Texas Alliance for Surgical Quality Collaborative. Multi-institution analysis of infection control practices identifies the subset associated with best surgical site infection performance: a Texas alliance for Surgical Quality Collaborative Project. *J Am Coll Surg*. 2017;225(4):455–464.
10. van den Beuken-van Everdingen MH, Hochstenbach LM, Joosten EA, Tjan-Heijnen VC, Janssen DJ. Update on prevalence of pain in patients with cancer: systematic review and meta-analysis. *J Pain Symptom Manage*. 2016;51(6):1070–1090.e9.
11. Resnick MJ, Koyama T, Fan KH, et al. Long-term functional outcomes after treatment for localized prostate cancer. *N Engl J Med*. 2013;368(5):436.
12. Porter M, Lee T. The strategy that will fix health care. *Harv Bus Rev*. 2013:10.
13. The US Health Care Cost Crisis: Gallup; 2019. Available from: https://news.gallup.com/file/poll/248081/The_US_Healthcare_Cost_Crisis.pdf. Accessed June 1, 2020.
14. Chatfield SC, Volpicelli FM, Adler NM, et al. Bending the cost curve: time series analysis of a value transformation programme at an academic medical centre. *BMJ Qual Saf*. 2019;28(6):449.
15. Thaker NG, Ali TN, Porter ME, Feeley TW, Kaplan RS, Frank SJ. Communicating value in health care using radar charts: a case study of prostate cancer. *J Oncol Pract*. 2016;12(9):813.
16. Sanders JJ, Curtis JR, Tulsky JA. Achieving goal-concordant care: a conceptual model and approach to measuring serious illness communication and its impact. *J Palliat Med*. 2018;21(S2):S17–S27.
17. Born KB, Levinson W. Choosing wisely campaigns globally: a shared approach to tackling the problem of overuse in healthcare. *J Gen Fam Med*. 2019;20(1):9.

54

Enhanced Surgical Recovery and Cancer

ANOUSHKA M. AFONSO AND VIJAYA N. R. GOTTUMUKKALA

Introduction

Globally, cancer is the second leading cause of death in the developed world.[1,2] It is estimated that up to 50% of inpatient admissions worldwide are for a diagnosis of cancer.[3] As cancer prevalence increases over time, an even larger number of cancer patients will need anesthesia services for perioperative and periprocedural care. Despite significant immunologic advances in cancer care, surgery will continue to be a mainstay strategy for reducing tumor burden, particularly for solid tumors. Frequently chemoradiation therapies are administered before surgical resection as neoadjuvant therapy, or after the surgical resection as adjuvant therapies, to minimize the risk of locoregional or distant metastasis and prolong diseasefree survival. In addition to routine presurgical evaluation and optimization, patients with cancer need special perioperative considerations. These relate to evaluating and optimizing the anatomic and physiologic effects of cancer on specific organ function, paraneoplastic effects of cancer, and the systemic effects of cancer therapies. Anesthesia providers should therefore be cognizant of immediate and long-term systemic effects of cancer therapies (organ toxicities) and the effects of chemoradiation on nutrition, fatigue, anemia, and physical deconditioning, all of which could influence the recovery profile after major surgery.

To optimize surgical care and enhance oncologic outcomes, multidisciplinary programs should be implemented in the entire perioperative care continuum to minimize symptom burden, enhance functional recovery, and minimize preventable postoperative complications. These coordinated multidisciplinary care pathways and principles of care aimed to enhance functional recovery of the surgical patient are the enhanced surgical recovery programs (ESRPs) (Fig. 54.1). An ESRP should focus on minimizing the neuroinflammatory signaling (stress) response to surgical trauma through minimal access surgery when indicated; utilize procedure-specific multimodal opioid sparing strategies; minimize periprocedural oxygen debt; and provide optimal anesthesia care with emphasis on rapid emergence, utilizing lung-protective ventilatory strategies, and ensuring complete reversal from neuro-muscular blockade. In addition, the postoperative phase demands a focused approach to safely implement early drinking, eating, and ambulating measures. An important postoperative component of enhanced recovery principles is procedure-specific pathway-based care, and institution of monitoring systems for rapid rescue from postoperative complications.[4] The enhanced recovery pathways therefore have specific elements of care in each of the preoperative, intraoperative, postoperative, and postdischarge phases of surgical practice. Adherence to the key elements in each of these phases of care is vital to improve outcomes for the surgical patients. In fact, Gustafsson et al. indicated a dose-response relationship with Enhanced Recovery After Surgery (ERAS) protocol adherence and clinical outcomes after major colorectal surgery.[5]

While earlier recovery to baseline function without major postoperative complications is important for any surgical patient population, this is particularly relevant for patients with cancer as frequently adjuvant therapies are part of the cancer care plan for many diseases. In pancreatic,[6] thoracic,[7] and breast cancer,[8] there is a correlation between postoperative complications and timely delivery of adjuvant therapies and survival. Delaying adjuvant therapies after a successful ablative surgery leads to worse prognosis. Frequently, common causes for delayed adjuvant therapies are postoperative complications, postoperative fatigue, and poor general physical condition (a general measure of recovery after major surgery). One of the major goals for surgical patients with cancer should therefore be faster recovery after surgery so that they can get back to their intended oncologic therapy. Thus every enhanced recovery protocol implemented for cancer patients should take into account the stage of the disease, overall prognosis, and appropriateness of care for maintaining quality of life (QoL), and ability to withstand the treatment plan, risks associated with therapies, and patient's wishes.

Preoperative Preparation

In addition to routine presurgical evaluation and medical optimization of comorbidities, surgical patients with cancer

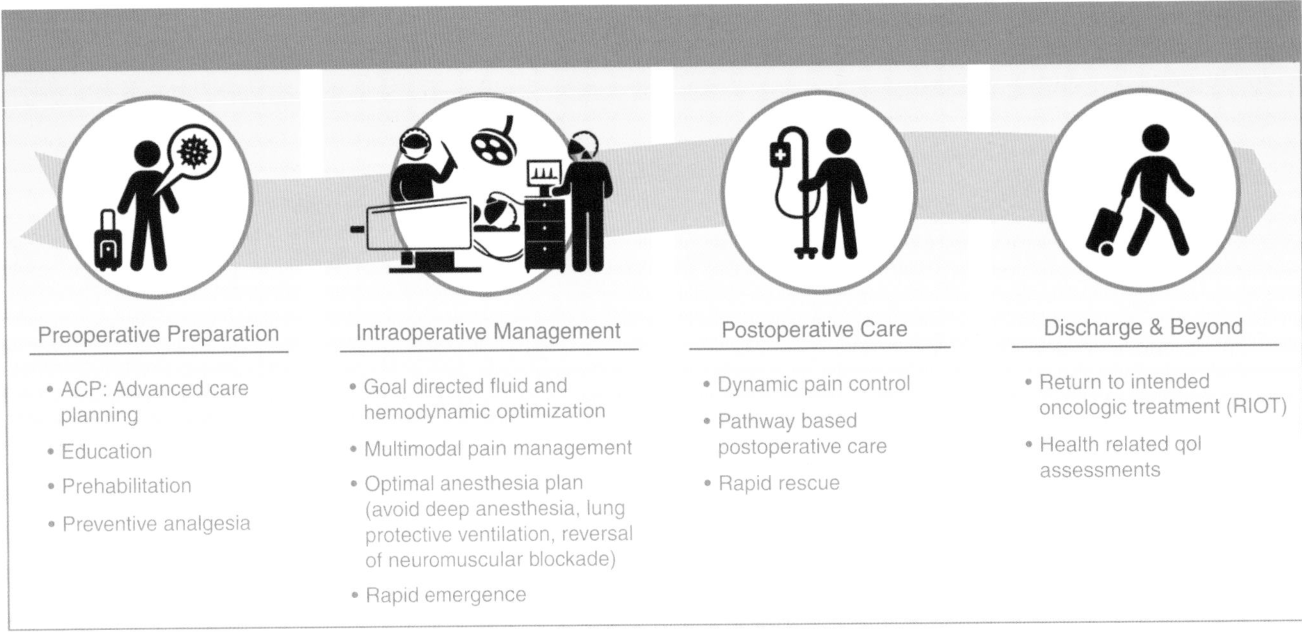

Preoperative Preparation
• ACP: Advanced care planning
• Education
• Prehabilitation
• Preventive analgesia
Intraoperative Management
• Goal directed fluid and hemodynamic optimization
• Multimodal pain management
• Optimal anesthesia plan (avoid deep anesthesia, lung protective ventilation, reversal of neuromuscular blockade)
• Rapid emergence
Postoperative Care
• Dynamic pain control
• Pathway based postoperative care
• Rapid rescue
Discharge & Beyond
• Return to intended oncologic treatment (RIOT)
• Health related qol assessments

• **Fig. 54.1** Enhanced recovery of cancer care.

have certain special considerations. The critical components that encompass preoperative care of patients with cancer are advanced care planning (ACP), patient education, prehabilitation, anemia management, and nutritional optimization.

Advanced Care Planning

In the United States, cancer treatments utilize an exorbitant amount of resources, particularly during advanced stage disease with little-to-no chance for cure, and often at the expense of offering meaningful QoL that meets patient's wishes. This is also true during end-of-life care, with increasing hospitalization rates, intensive care unit stays, several emergency department visits in the last month of life, and consistently high rates of terminal hospitalizations.[9] Approximately 25% to 30% of terminally ill cancer patients will die in hospital.[9] Additionally, terminally ill patients often receive more intensive care regimens than their stated preferences for treatment.[9]

Unlike noncancer conditions, functional decline is an innate characteristic of cancer's trajectory and thus is a distinct period in which patients can benefit from ACP and early introduction palliative care principles for symptom management and psychosocial behavior management.[9,10] Professional oncologic organizations such as the National Comprehensive Care Network (NCCN) and the American Society of Clinical Oncology (ASCO) have long emphasized the importance of ACP in providing optimal palliative care.[9,11] ACP should therefore be routinely discussed in all phases of cancer care plans, including surgery. Cognitive screening and frailty assessment in high-risk patients and the elderly cancer patient population is gaining momentum. In fact, Shahrokni et al. demonstrated that in oncogeriatric patients (age ≥75 years), the comprehensive geriatric assessment (CGA) deficits were strongly associated with 6-month mortality, whereas the ASA (American Society of Anaesthesiologists) classification was not.[12] Additionally, measuring frailty in older cancer patients can potentially identify those with increased risk of treatment-related complications. Data from 20 studies with over 2900 older cancer patients reported a prevalence rate of frailty as 42% (range 6%–86%). Frailty was independently associated with increased postoperative mortality (hazard ratio [HR], 2.67; 95% confidence interval [CI], 1.08–6.62) and increased treatment complications (odds ratio [OR], 4.86; 95%, CI 2.19–10.78).[13] Accurate evaluation of risk for perioperative complications, options available for treatment planning, and the prognosis after surgery with particular reference to QoL form the mainstay of informed choice, shared decision-making, and ACP, fulfilling patient's choices, expectations, and goals for care.

Education

A well-designed preoperative education program sets the stage for patient empowerment and improved outcomes through the oncologic perioperative journey. Usually, preoperative education begins in the surgical office, is continued through the preadmission clinic and testing, and emphasized at the preadmission phase when these patients and family come into the hospital. Understanding the risks and benefits of effective preoperative and psychologic preparation is the benefit of effective preoperative education. Additionally, it is important to provide patients and family with a detailed understanding of their surgical procedure so there are clear expectations of, and anticipation for, potential events that could happen in the perioperative period. Setting patient expectations in terms of pain management, ambulation, and resuming oral intake can pave the way for accelerated recovery. It has been demonstrated that perioperative education has been associated with decreased anxiety, better postoperative outcomes, and improved patient and family satisfaction.[4] While patient education is important during the perioperative process, physicians must familiarize themselves with the health literacy of their patients for effective engagement of patients and care givers. Providing patients with appropriate educational materials that they can read and instructions that are written in clear, simple language can also facilitate learning.[4] Pereira et al. showed in 104 patients that an empathic patient-centered approach can reduce preoperative anxiety, and increase surgical recovery and patient satisfaction.[14]

Prehabilitation

In addition to optimizing the nutritional status of the cancer patient, prehabilitation strategies should be implemented during the preoperative period to decrease the psychologic and physiologic stress associated with surgery.[15] Defining cancer prehabilitation is "a process on the continuum of care that occurs between the time of cancer diagnosis and the beginning of acute treatment, includes physical and psychological assessments that establish a baseline functional level, identifies impairments, and provides targeted interventions that improve a patient's health to reduce the incidence and the severity of current and future impairments."[16] Maintaining a high level of physical activity, in particular, can attenuate the perioperative risks associated with surgery.[15] Those that implement an exercise regimen prior to surgery have a faster return to baseline.[17] Preoperative exercise capacity serves as a strong marker for health status and is also related to decreased postoperative complications and mortality.[18] Because delays in cancer treatment can lead to poor outcomes, the timing of prehabilitation implementation as it relates to the anticipated date of surgery is critical to take into account when building an exercise regimen.[16] As little as 3 weeks prior to surgery may be sufficient time to build up a physiologic reserve, which can further improve surgical outcomes.[15] Additionally, the integration of neoadjuvant radiation therapy and chemotherapy expands the window in which exercise prehabilitation can be implemented.[4,15] Prehabilitation also provides psychologic benefit to cancer patients, as it gives them a sense of control over their state of health and thereby decreases anxiety.[17] Psychologic interventions should also be implemented in the prehabilitation landscape to address any psychiatric disturbances (i.e., depression, anxiety, etc.) and provide psychosocial support,[16] as a cancer diagnosis can be particularly burdensome both mentally and emotionally.

Cancer patients who undergo neoadjuvant chemotherapy often have a decline in overall physical fitness, which has been associated with worse outcome after surgery.[19] Preoperative exercise training may have an important benefit for surgical outcome and recovery after surgery in cancer patients. For those awaiting oncologic surgery, a preoperative exercise training program is a feasible option with regard to participation and adherence.[20] Licker et al. demonstrated that high-intensity interval training (HIIT) resulted in "significant improvement in aerobic performances, but failed to reduce early complications after lung cancer resection."[21] Objective measures of physical fitness, such as cardiopulmonary exercise testing (CPET), have been used to determine the association between postoperative morbidity and decreased exercise capacity.[22] The effect of exercise on cancer patients was evaluated by Loughney et al.[23] with acceptable feasibility adherence rates and safety in patients scheduled for neoadjuvant chemotherapy and surgery. The concept of the "dual hit" of neoadjuvant chemotherapy and surgery was explored in the context of preoperative exercise training. Larger randomized controlled trials are necessary to truly evaluate the effect of preoperative exercise programs in the different cancer populations. Wijeysundera et al.[24] performed an elegant multicenter international prospective trial comparing preoperative subjective assessment with alternative markers of fitness, such as cardiopulmonary exercise testing, serum N-terminal pro-B-type natriuretic peptide (NT pro-BNP), and Duke Activity Status Index (DASI) questionnaire scores, for predicting death or complications after major elective noncardiac surgery. They included 1404 patients in the study, with 28 (2%) having died or suffering a myocardial infarction within 30 days of surgery. Subjective assessment of preoperative functional capacity consistently performed poorly and did not predict postoperative myocardial complications, while the simple DASI questionnaire scores were associated with improved prediction.

Anemia Management

Optimization of an anemia management protocol is crucial to adapt and sustain best practices in enhanced recovery for the cancer patient. Preoperative anemia in cancer patients is prevalent and associated with higher perioperative morbidity and a transfusion risk factor.[25] The pathophysiology of anemia in the cancer patient who has nutritional deficiencies, chronic anemia, and concurrently on chemotherapeutic agents that affect red blood cell production is multifactorial. There is a need to reduce perioperative transfusions and its risks, and lessen the impact of postoperative anemia given the association with preoperative anemia and patient morbidity. Enhanced recovery from surgery in cancer patients can potentially be improved with an opportunity to intervene in the preoperative window in patients with treatable anemia. For example, Munoz et al.[26] describe a patient blood management strategy that involves a multidisciplinary multimodal individualized strategy for addressing perioperative anemia in the colorectal cancer patient. Treating anemia early and aggressively in colorectal patients allows for optimization of preoperative hemoglobin, which transforms transfusion risk from high to low and improves outcomes overall.[26] Iron therapy, erythropoiesis-stimulating agents under appropriate recommendations, restrictive transfusion protocols, and other measures to decrease blood loss should be undertaken. Follow up in these cancer patients is important as they often receive adjuvant chemotherapy and radiotherapy. For successful implementation across services and technology integration, patient and clinician educational programs are critical for both implementation and sustainability.

Nutrition

Nutritional optimization is important to increase anabolism and minimize the catabolic state in the postoperative period. Malnourished surgical patients benefit from perioperative nutrition. Klek et al. aimed to assess the clinical significance of route and type of nutritional support (enteral, parenteral, standard, or immunomodulating) in the perioperative setting of malnourished cancer patients with comparable results.[27] However, another prospective randomized trial that implemented the administration of a supplemented enteral formula during the perioperative period significantly reduced both postoperative infections and length of stay in cancer patients undergoing surgery.[28] Protein supplementation has also been used in prehabilitation programs. A double-blinded randomized controlled trial, which provided a more comprehensive prehabilitation program, with nutritional counseling, whey protein, exercise, and psychologic care, initiated 4 weeks prior for patients undergoing colorectal resection showed a clinical meaningful improvement in functional walking capacity.[29] Optimizing functional capacity and minimizing complications are the cornerstone of most enhanced recovery programs.

Optimizing the Nutritional Status of a Cancer Patient Prior to Surgery

In high-risk patients, objective perioperative nutritional screening should be used to assess a cancer patient's nutritional status.[18] Adequate tests that can be used to evaluate nutritional status prior to surgery include the Nutritional Risk Indicator (NRI), the Patient Generated-Subjective Global Assessment (PG-SGA), the Nutritional Risk Screening (NRS) tests, and Reilly's NRS.[4] Each of these tests provides a scoring system that categorizes the nutritional status of the patient, which can then be used as a guideline to triage and implement proper preoperative nutrition protocols. Malnutrition is a risk factor for increased mortality, complications, costs, and readmission,[4,30] reduced QoL, and decreased functional status.[9,31] Malnutrition and subsequent weight loss in cancer may be related to an amalgamation of factors including undernutrition, cancer catabolism, and inflammation, which can further lead to cachexia and sarcopenia.[30] Furthermore, there is an increased risk of gradual nutritional decline; thus it is imperative to decrease the deleterious metabolic effects of oncologic treatments by correcting for nutritional deficiencies.[30] When managing the nutritional status of a cancer patient prior to surgery, strategies should be implemented that avoid decrease insulin resistance, prevent negative protein balance, and modulate the immune system.[18] Additionally, when determining the proper nutritional intervention necessary for treating the cancer patient, it should be determined if a patient's cancer therapy is high risk or low risk with regard to its impact on the patient's nutritional status.[32] Utilizing both the patients' baseline nutritional status and the risk of nutritional deterioration associated with their treatment regimen, a nutritional intervention can be determined for those who fall below the threshold for adequate preoperative nutrition.[32]

For those who are deemed malnourished prior to surgery, nutritional supplementation should be implemented 5 to 7 days prior to surgery via enteral nutrition or total parenteral nutrition as an alternative, if needed.[4,18,33] However, total parenteral nutrition should be implemented 7 to 10 days prior to surgery.[33] Enteral feeding is preferred to total parental feeding; however, it has a decreased risk of complications and length of stay for patients who are critically ill.[18] In addition to properly correcting for any nutritional deficiencies before surgery, there are key steps that should be taken immediately prior to surgery to optimize recovery. Patients should receive liberal hydration with intake of clear liquids up to 2 h prior to scheduled arrival for surgery. Rather than fasting prior to surgery, patients should consume clear carbohydrate beverages to allow for the replication of normal metabolic responses and place the patient in a fed state prior to surgery.[4,33] This method can decrease the body's metabolic stress response to surgery, thereby decreasing the risk of postoperative complications.[4,33] Furthermore, a carbohydrate drink may decrease protein loss by placing patients in an anabolic state.[18] As cancer patients mostly have low immune function, the intention of immunesupplementation was to improve the immune status of these patients. However, guidelines that refer to specific immune nutrients (fish oils, glutamine) and vitamin C have not been adequately cited or studied. Given that there is cancer-related inflammation and cachexia in this patient population, investigation into antiinflammatory medications could be the next focus of research from a cancer standpoint.

One must also balance the heterogeneity in nutrition guidelines with their own cancer patients' nutritional needs. Zhao et al. demonstrated that the quality of the nutrition care procedure guidelines was highly variable for cancer patients.[34] Upon further analyses, heterogeneity was due to insufficient attention to nutrition risk screening, differences in nutritional assessment recommendations, immune nutrient support, and lack of high-quality research on energy and nitrogen demand.

Intraoperative Management

Postoperative Nausea and Vomiting Prophylaxis

As stated by Wesmiller et al., postoperative nausea and vomiting (PONV) has a large impact on the overall health of breast cancer patients and is related to significant morbidity (dehydration, wound dehiscence, pain, and immobility).[35] In women with breast cancer, PONV has a significant impact on both the well-being and health of these women.[36]

PONV should also be addressed vigilantly in the cancer patient population during the preoperative period to minimize its potential effects. After surgery, as many as 80% of women with early-stage breast cancer will experience PONV.[35,37] PONV prophylaxis prior to surgery is recommended rather than reactively treating PONV as it occurs.[4] A risk assessment of PONV can be conducted using the Apfel score.[4] The Apfel score evaluates the risk of PONV by using female sex, nonsmoking status, history of PONV, and administration of postoperative opioids as predictive measures.[4,37] Because prophylaxis for PONV is expensive, it is important to identify those who are at a higher risk and provide them with targeted prophylaxis.[38] Low-risk patients should not receive prophylaxis for PONV unless the surgery in which they are undergoing is emetogenic.[38] However, for those who are moderate- to high-risk for PONV, combination therapy that targets more than one type of receptor and pathway may be more effective than single therapy for prophylaxis.

For surgeries that are associated with a high risk for PONV, such as gynecologic, laparoscopic, HEENT (head, eyes, ears, nose, throat), intraabdominal, breast procedures, as well as those that are of longer duration, PONV prophylaxis should be administered regardless of Apfel score.[38] Preoperative psychologic factors can intensify the severity of PONV in patients with breast cancer.[35,39] Despite the use of multiple antiemetic agents, approximately 30% of women experience nausea after breast cancer surgery, with 10% having both nausea and vomiting.[35]

Fluid Management and Hemodynamic Optimization

Fluid management of the patient should be optimized throughout the perioperative period with the goal of a euvolemic, hydrated state prior to surgery.[40] For the cancer patient, preoperative radiation and chemotherapy can cause treatment-related diarrhea, which can lead to dehydration and fluid depletion.[41] Radiation can cause increased intestinal motility, while chemotherapy can cause damage to the intestinal mucosa leading to decreased absorption.[41] Prolonged fasting and bowel preparations should be avoided, as they may lead to dehydration prior to surgery.[40] Thus it is of pivotal importance to ensure that the surgical cancer patient is optimized throughout the perioperative period. Perioperative goal-directed fluid therapy (GDFT) is defined as "the concept of using indices of continuous blood flow and/or tissue oxygen saturation to optimize end-organ function."[4] Monitoring dynamic flow indices can be used to predict the hemodynamic effects of fluid administration to optimize oxygen delivery to tissues.[18] GDFT should be customized on the basis of patients' surgical risk, vascular access, monitoring needs, and the operating context to optimize hemodynamic stability.[4,40,42] During surgery, fluid administration should be carefully adjusted to reduce perioperative organ dysfunction and to restore tissue perfusion and cellular oxygenation.[4] Intraoperative fluid management should aim to maintain euvolemia and minimize excess salt and water through low-crystalloid therapy and fluid boluses (when necessary) to replace blood/fluid loss and maintain intravascular volume.[40] GDFT may decrease major complications and length of stay, and improve outcomes.[4,40] However, in a recent meta-analysis in noncardiac surgical patients, GDFT had questionable benefit over standard care as it relates to mortality postoperatively, length of ICU stay, and length of hospital stay overall.[43] However, incidence of all complications including wound infection, abdominal complications, and postoperative hypotension is reduced.[43] There is no evidence of benefit for the use of crystalloid or hydroxyethylstarch (HES) for colorectal cancer surgery for GDFT, despite a lower 24-h fluid balance with HES.[43,44] In addition, results from a pragmatic international trial showed that among patients at increased risk for complications during major abdominal surgery, a restrictive fluid group was not associated with a high rate of disability-free survival than a liberal fluid regimen but was associated with a higher rate of acute kidney injury (8.6% vs. 5.0%; $P <$ 0.001).[45] In a 2014 randomized trial of high-risk patients undergoing major gastrointestinal surgery,[46] use of cardiac output-guided hemodynamic therapy algorithm compared with usual care did not reduce the composite outcome of complications and 30-day mortality. We must take into consideration the results from both the above trials as we apply optimal fluid management for our cancer patients.

Salmasi et al.[47] showed that mean arterial pressures (MAPs) below absolute thresholds of 65 mmHg or relative thresholds of 20% were progressively related to both myocardial and kidney injury. At any given threshold, prolonged exposure to hypotension was associated with increased odds for both myocardial and kidney injury. Furthermore, there were no clinically important interactions between preoperative blood pressures and the relationship between hypotension and myocardial or kidney injury at intraoperative MAPs less than 65 mmHg. The authors concluded that anesthetic management can thus be based on intraoperative pressures without regard to preoperative pressure. A recent review on preoperative hypertension mentioned that most of the data regarding perioperative blood pressure management are based on epidemiologic data rather than randomized controlled trials; and hence that it may not be appropriate to defer anesthesia and surgery in a patient with mild or moderate hypertension. The anesthesiologist shares the responsibility to ensure that a patient with persistently elevated blood pressure during preassessment is referred for further management before or after surgery as appropriate.[48] In order to minimize oxygen debt, optimal management of fluid therapy, cardiac index (stroke volume), perfusion pressure, and anemia indices have to be considered collectively and not in isolation.

Multimodal Pain Management

Because pain can prolong recovery time and delay discharge, it is important to optimize the management of pain throughout the perioperative period.[49] Multimodal analgesia is a key element of the ERAS pathway that is defined as "the use of more than one modality of pain control to achieve effective analgesia while reducing opioid-related side effects."[49] The concept of a multimodal analgesic plan allows us to improve postoperative analgesia through different mechanisms and reduce the incidence of any opioid-related effects due to lower dosages. Multimodal pain management consists of the combinatory use of analgesics with different modes of action to minimize side effects and maximize analgesic effects.[50] Multiple agents that act at different receptors within the central and peripheral nervous system to improve pain control should be utilized intraoperatively and postoperatively. Nonopioid analgesics include nonsteroidal antiinflammatory drugs (NSAIDs), acetaminophen, paracetamol, alpha-2 agonists, ketamine, gabapentin-type drugs, dexamethasone, neuraxial/regional techniques using local anesthetics, hypnosis, and acupuncture. Ultimately, multimodal analgesia serves to minimize postsurgical length of stay, accelerate recovery, and improve outcomes.[49] Pain management strategies should be carefully planned, initiated prior to incision, tailored precisely to patient-specific considerations, and geared towards the surgical procedure in which the patient is undergoing. This careful selection of pain management can allow for the best outcomes for cancer patients.[2] Because pain secondary to cancer is a common occurrence due to both the pathophysiology of cancer and as a result of therapeutic interventions,[2] anesthesiologists must take cancer pain into account when planning an analgesic regimen for their cancer patients. Additionally, surgical interventions for cancer therapies are complex; adequate analgesia should be administered that allows for improved functionality to allow patients to return to chemotherapy and radiation therapy expeditiously.[2] Analgesic plans should aim for early mobilization, decreased perioperative complications, and the improvement of quality care, in addition to lowering pain in the cancer patient.[50] In addition, controversy exists around perioperative opioids and cancer recurrence. Currently, there is no level 1 evidence that opioids influence the perioperative period. A recent meta-analysis[51] showed no conclusive evidence for avoiding the use of opioids with the goal of reducing the risk of recurrence in colorectal cancer. Stress reduction and optimal pain control for our surgical cancer patients should be the goal, with opioids for rescue if needed.

Avoiding Hypothermia

Avoiding hypothermia is also part of the optimal anesthetic plan for cancer patients undergoing an enhanced recovery protocol. Enhanced recovery programs emphasize the need for maintenance of normothermia, as perioperative hypothermia is associated with poor outcomes that could be preventable. Perioperative hypothermia causes impaired pharmacodynamics, surgical site infections, blood loss and coagulopathy, transfusion requirements, thermal discomfort, prolonged recovery, and prolonged duration of hospitalization. Measurement of central core temperature, maintaining normothermia, and consequent warming of patients in the perioperative period are therefore essential.[52] In the National Institute for Health and Clinical Excellence (NICE) guidelines,[53] there is acceptable evidence showing significant dependence of a surgical wound infection and incidence of morbid cardiac events on the incidence of inadvertent perioperative hypothermia (IPH). In addition, complete reversal of neuromuscular blockade and lung protective ventilation strategies are strategies in an optimal anesthesia plan in ERAS for cancer patients.

Postoperative Care

Pain Management Maintenance

In the realm of postoperative care during the perioperative period, continued effective pain management, complication-free recovery, reduced symptom burden, and enhanced QoL should be emphasized for the cancer patient. Postsurgically, major physiologic changes can occur that can delay recovery.[4] Pain, in particular, can amplify these physiologic changes thereby increasing the time to restoration to baseline function.[54] Similar to intraoperative multimodal pain management strategies, this approach should be also utilized postoperatively.[49] Postoperative analgesia should focus on maximizing the pharmacologic benefits while minimizing side effects to allow for enhanced recovery and functional restoration to ultimately improve outcomes.[4,49]

Postsurgical Complications and Return to Intended Oncologic Therapies

The concept of return to intended oncologic therapies (RIOT) was introduced by Kim et al.[55] as a novel metric to measure and monitor how perioperative interventions impact functional recovery in cancer patients. RIOT has two components: whether the patient did or did not initiate intended oncologic therapies after surgery and the time between surgery and initiation of these therapies.[56] When RIOT was introduced into the enhanced recovery pathways, the team noted significant practice change management. For example, in colon cancer patients with metastases to the liver the identified RIOT rate was 75%. During the introduction of an enhanced recovery protocol in the liver surgery department, the RIOT rate increased to 95%.[57] Merkow et al. analyzed the American College of Surgeons National Surgical Quality Improvement Program and the National Cancer Database from 2006 to 2009 and showed that 61.8% of the patients who did not experience a complication after pancreatic resection for stages I–III adenocarcinoma received adjuvant chemotherapy.[58] The impact of postoperative complications and RIOT can be seen in the pancreatic surgical population. Patients with no complications had a median time of 52 days to adjuvant chemotherapy, as compared with patients with complications such as deep surgical-site infections, who had a median time of 70 days to adjuvant chemotherapy. Breast cancer overall survival

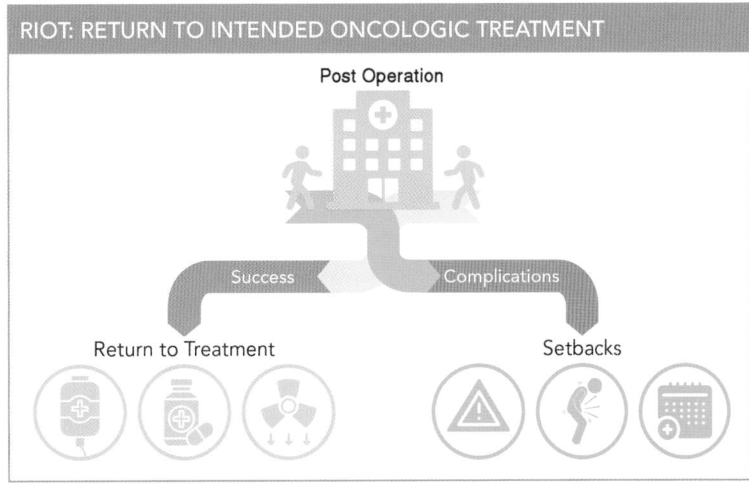

• **Fig. 54.2** Return to intended oncologic treatment (RIOT).

is dependent on both completion and amount of adjuvant chemotherapy. If there is a delay of more than 12 weeks, recurrentce-free survival and overall survival are adversely affected.[8] The rate of survival of cancer patients undergoing surgical procedures is highly dependent on the biology of the tumor, comorbidities associated with the cancer, effects of cancer and cancer therapies on QoL and functionality, and the impact of surgery on recovery.[56] Implementation of an enhanced recovery protocol was associated with receiving on-time adjuvant chemotherapy, defined as at ≤8 weeks postoperatively, in a cohort of 363 colorectal patients.[59] In the non–small cell lung cancer patient, enhanced recovery after thoracic surgery is associated with improved adjuvant chemotherapy completion.[60] Enhanced recovery pathways can potentially allow for a more rapid recovery and shortened time to patient oncologic therapy, which has a meaningful impact on survival (Fig. 54.2)

Health-Related Quality of Life Assessment

After discharge, patient recovery and health QoL measures are an increasingly valuable component in the landscape of ERAS.[4] While morbidity and mortality serve as markers for surgical outcomes, health-related QoL should be incorporated in the overall postoperative assessment of the cancer patient.[61] Health-related QoL assessments are subjective measures answered by the patient that are used to determine how the patient's health state affects their QoL through the evaluation of various health domains.[62] Additionally, health-related QoL is a multidimensional measure that encompasses psychologic, social, and physical well-being.[61] Each of these measures should be globally assessed in the cancer patient to allow for the optimization of treatment and overall well-being.[61] The assessment of QoL for cancer patients can serve to evaluate complications and side effects,[61] both of which can have deleterious effects on standards of living. Additionally, QoL assessments can help to determine the most appropriate surgical procedure[61] that incorporates the needs of the cancer patient and the goals of the surgical oncologist. In the case of palliative care, it is especially important to consider the impact that surgical procedures may have on a cancer patient's QoL. The treatment of cancer patients can be rather complex,[63] often utilizing chemotherapy or radiation therapy, in addition to surgery as treatment modalities. While this multifactorial approach may serve as curative treatment, the morbidities associated with these therapies can lead to a decreased QoL. The prospect of cure may render the toxicity associated with cancer treatment tolerable.[62] However, for cancer patients who have a decreased probability of cure, these adverse side effects may be less acceptable.[62] Thus, it is important to assess QoL measures to ensure that the patient has the best possible QoL in the postsurgical setting.

Conclusion

ERAS protocols for the cancer patient should encompass the risks associated with both oncologic pathologies and surgical procedures to allow for optimization of patient outcomes. Additionally, cancer patients who recover quickly after surgery can, in turn, return to their intended therapy expeditiously. This can further serve to improve the overall outcomes of cancer patients undergoing adjuvant oncologic treatment postoperatively. By adhering to ERAS protocols and tailoring treatment with specific regards for the clinical sequelae associated with cancer pathophysiology and cancer treatment regimens, physicians can improve the status of cancer patients in the perioperative setting and beyond.

References

1. Siegel RL, Miller KD, Jemal A. Cancer Statistics, 2017. *CA Cancer J Clin*. 2017;67(1):7–30.
2. Popat K, McQueen K, Feeley TW. The global burden of cancer. *Best Pract Res Clin Anaesthesiol*. 2013;27(4):399–408.
3. Rose J, Weiser TG, Hider P, Wilson L, Gruen RL, Bickler SW. Estimated need for surgery worldwide based on prevalence of

diseases: a modelling strategy for the WHO Global Health Estimate. *Lancet Glob Health*. 2015;3(Suppl 2):S13–S20.
4. Gan TJM, Thacker JK, Miller TM, Scott MJM, Holubar SDM. *Enhanced Recovery for Major Abdominopelvic Surgery*. Professional Communications, Inc.; 2016. 1st ed.
5. Gustafsson UO, Hausel J, Thorell A, et al. Adherence to the enhanced recovery after surgery protocol and outcomes after colorectal cancer surgery. *Arch Surg*. 2011;146(5):571–577.
6. Wu W, He J, Cameron JL, et al. The impact of postoperative complications on the administration of adjuvant therapy following pancreaticoduodenectomy for adenocarcinoma. *Ann Surg Oncol*. 2014;21(9):2873–2881.
7. Salazar MC, Rosen JE, Wang Z, et al. Association of delayed adjuvant chemotherapy with survival after lung cancer surgery. *JAMA Oncol*. 2017;3(5):610–619.
8. Lohrisch C, Paltiel C, Gelmon K, et al. Impact on survival of time from definitive surgery to initiation of adjuvant chemotherapy for early-stage breast cancer. *J Clin Oncol*. 2006;24(30):4888–4894.
9. Narang AK, Wright AA, Nicholas LH. Trends in advance care planning in patients with cancer: results from a national longitudinal survey. *JAMA Oncol*. 2015;1(5):601–608.
10. Teno JM, Weitzen S, Fennell ML, Mor V. Dying trajectory in the last year of life: does cancer trajectory fit other diseases? *J Palliat Med*. 2001;4(4):457–464.
11. Levy MH, Weinstein SM, Carducci MA, NCCN Palliative Care Practice Guidelines Panel. NCCN: Palliative care. *Cancer Control*. 2001;8(6 Suppl 2):66–71.
12. Shahrokni A, Vishnevsky BM, Jang B, et al. Geriatric assessment, not ASA physical status, is associated with 6-month postoperative survival in patients with cancer aged ≥75 years. *J Natl Compr Canc Netw*. 2019;17(6):687–694.
13. Handforth C, Clegg A, Young C, et al. The prevalence and outcomes of frailty in older cancer patients: a systematic review. *Ann Oncol*. 2015;26(6):1091–1101.
14. Pereira L, Figueiredo-Braga M, Carvalho IP. Preoperative anxiety in ambulatory surgery: the impact of an empathic patient-centered approach on psychological and clinical outcomes. *Patient Educ Couns*. 2016;99(5):733–738.
15. West MA, Wischmeyer PE, Grocott MPW. Prehabilitation and nutritional support to improve perioperative outcomes. *Curr Anesthesiol Rep*. 2017;7(4):340–349.
16. Silver JK, Baima J. Cancer prehabilitation: an opportunity to decrease treatment-related morbidity, increase cancer treatment options, and improve physical and psychological health outcomes. *Am J Phys Med Rehabil*. 2013;92(8):715–727.
17. Santa Mina D, Brahmbhatt P, Lopez C, et al. The case for prehabilitation prior to breast cancer treatment. *PM R*. 2017;9(9S2):S305–S316.
18. Ericksen LM, Miller TEMC, Mythen M, Gan TJM. Enhanced surgical recovery: from principles to standard of care. Washington, DC: *Annual Congress of Enhanced Recovery Perioperative Medicine*; 2017.
19. Lakoski SG, Eves ND, Douglas PS, Jones LW. Exercise rehabilitation in patients with cancer. *Nat Rev Clin Oncol*. 2012;9(5):288–296.
20. Valkenet K, Trappenburg JC, Schippers CC, et al. Feasibility of exercise training in cancer patients scheduled for elective gastrointestinal surgery. *Dig Surg*. 2016;33(5):439–447.
21. Licker M, Karenovics W, Diaper J, et al. Short-term preoperative high-intensity interval training in patients awaiting lung cancer surgery: a randomized controlled trial. *J Thorac Oncol*. 2017;12(2):323–333.
22. Jack S, West MA, Raw D, et al. The effect of neoadjuvant chemotherapy on physical fitness and survival in patients undergoing oesophagogastric cancer surgery. *Eur J Surg Oncol*. 2014;40(10):1313–1320.
23. Loughney L, West MA, Kemp GJ, Grocott MP, Jack S. Exercise intervention in people with cancer undergoing neoadjuvant cancer treatment and surgery: a systematic review. *Eur J Surg Oncol*. 2016;42(1):28–38.
24. Wijeysundera DN, Pearse RM, Shulman MA, et al. Assessment of functional capacity before major non-cardiac surgery: an international, prospective cohort study. *Lancet*. 2018;391(10140):2631–2640.
25. Diaz-Cambronero O, Matoses-Jaen S, Garcia-Claudio N, Garcia-Gregorio N, Molins-Espinosa J. Preoperative management of anemia in oncologic surgery. *Rev Esp Anestesiol Reanim*. 2015;62(Suppl 1):45–51.
26. Munoz M, Gomez-Ramirez S, Martin-Montanez E, Auerbach M. Perioperative anemia management in colorectal cancer patients: a pragmatic approach. *World J Gastroenterol*. 2014;20(8):1972–1985.
27. Klek S, Sierzega M, Szybinski P, et al. Perioperative nutrition in malnourished surgical cancer patients - a prospective, randomized, controlled clinical trial. *Clin Nutr*. 2011;30(6):708–713.
28. Braga M, Gianotti L, Radaelli G, et al. Perioperative immunonutrition in patients undergoing cancer surgery: results of a randomized double-blind phase 3 trial. *Arch Surg*. 1999;134(4):428–433.
29. Gillis C, Loiselle SE, Fiore Jr JF, et al. Prehabilitation with whey protein supplementation on perioperative functional exercise capacity in patients undergoing colorectal resection for cancer: a pilot double-blinded randomized placebo-controlled trial. *J Acad Nutr Diet*. 2016;116(5):802–812.
30. Sandrucci S, Beets G, Braga M, Dejong K, Demartines N. Perioperative nutrition and enhanced recovery after surgery in gastrointestinal cancer patients. A position paper by the ESSO task force in collaboration with the ERAS society (ERAS coalition). *Eur J Surg Oncol*. 2018 Apr;44(4):509–514.
31. Bozzetti F. Nutritional support of the oncology patient. *Crit Rev Oncol Hematol*. 2013;87(2):172–200.
32. Ottery FD. Definition of standardized nutritional assessment and interventional pathways in oncology. *Nutrition*. 1996;12(Suppl 1):S15–S19.
33. Gupta R, Gan TJ. Preoperative nutrition and prehabilitation. *Anesthesiol Clin*. 2016;34(1):143–153.
34. Zhao XH, Yang T, Ma XD, et al. Heterogeneity of nutrition care procedures in nutrition guidelines for cancer patients. *Clin Nutr*. 2019;39(6):1692–1704.
35. Wesmiller SW, Sereika SM, Bender CM, et al. Exploring the multifactorial nature of postoperative nausea and vomiting in women following surgery for breast cancer. *Auton Neurosci*. 2017;202:102–107.
36. Murphy MJ, Hooper VD, Sullivan E, Clifford T, Apfel CC. Identification of risk factors for postoperative nausea and vomiting in the perianesthesia adult patient. *J Perianesth Nurs*. 2006;21(6):377–384.
37. Gan TJ, Diemunsch P, Habib AS, et al. Consensus guidelines for the management of postoperative nausea and vomiting. *Anesth Analg*. 2014;118(1):85–113.

38. Habib AS, Gan TJ. Evidence-based management of postoperative nausea and vomiting: a review. *Can J Anaesth.* 2004;51(4):326–341.
39. Montgomery GH, Schnur JB, Erblich J, Diefenbach MA, Bovbjerg DH. Presurgery psychological factors predict pain, nausea, and fatigue one week after breast cancer surgery. *J Pain Symptom Manage.* 2010;39(6):1043–1052.
40. Miller TE, Roche AM, Mythen M. Fluid management and goal-directed therapy as an adjunct to Enhanced Recovery After Surgery (ERAS). *Can J Anaesth.* 2015;62(2):158–168.
41. Shaw C, Taylor L. Treatment-related diarrhea in patients with cancer. *Clin J Oncol Nurs.* 2012;16(4):413–417.
42. Colantonio L, Claroni C, Fabrizi L, et al. A randomized trial of goal directed vs. standard fluid therapy in cytoreductive surgery with hyperthermic intraperitoneal chemotherapy. *J Gastrointest Surg.* 2015;19(4):722–729.
43. Som A, Maitra S, Bhattacharjee S, Baidya DK. Goal directed fluid therapy decreases postoperative morbidity but not mortality in major non-cardiac surgery: a meta-analysis and trial sequential analysis of randomized controlled trials. *J Anesth.* 2017;31(1):66–81.
44. Yates DR, Davies SJ, Milner HE, Wilson RJ. Crystalloid or colloid for goal-directed fluid therapy in colorectal surgery. *Br J Anaesth.* 2014;112(2):281–289.
45. Myles PS, Bellomo R, Corcoran T, et al. Restrictive versus liberal fluid therapy for major abdominal surgery. *N Eng J Med.* 2018;378(24):2263–2274.
46. Pearse RM, Harrison DA, MacDonald N, et al. Effect of a perioperative, cardiac output-guided hemodynamic therapy algorithm on outcomes following major gastrointestinal surgery: a randomized clinical trial and systematic review. *JAMA.* 2014;311(21):2181–2190.
47. Salmasi V, Maheshwari K, Yang D, et al. Relationship between intraoperative hypotension, defined by either reduction from baseline or absolute thresholds, and acute kidney and myocardial injury after noncardiac surgery: a retrospective cohort analysis. *Anesthesiology.* 2017;126(1):47–65.
48. Howell SJ. Preoperative hypertension. *Curr Anesthesiol Rep.* 2018;8(1):25–31.
49. Tan M, Law LS, Gan TJ. Optimizing pain management to facilitate Enhanced Recovery After Surgery pathways. *Can J Anaesth.* 2015;62(2):203–218.
50. Jakobsson JG. Pain management in ambulatory surgery—a review. *Pharmaceuticals (Basel).* 2014;7(8):850–865.
51. Diaz-Cambronero O, Mazzinari G, Cata JP. Perioperative opioids and colorectal cancer recurrence: a systematic review of the literature. *Pain Manage.* 2018;8(5):353–361.
52. Ruetzler K, Kurz A. Consequences of perioperative hypothermia. *Handb Clin Neurol.* 2018;157:687–697.
53. National Collaborating Centre for Nursing and Supportive Care. National Institute for Health and Clinical Excellence: Guidance. *The Management of Inadvertent Perioperative Hypothermia in Adults*: Royal College of Nursing (UK). National Collaborating Centre for Nursing and Supportive Care; 2008.
54. Kehlet H. Multimodal approach to control postoperative pathophysiology and rehabilitation. *Br J Anaesth.* 1997;78(5):606–617.
55. Kim BJ, Caudle AS, Gottumukkala V, Aloia TA. The impact of postoperative complications on a timely return to intended oncologic therapy (RIOT): the role of enhanced recovery in the cancer journey. *Int Anesthesiol Clin.* 2016;54(4):e33–e46.
56. Aloia TA, Zimmitti G, Conrad C, Gottumukalla V, Kopetz S, Vauthey JN. Return to intended oncologic treatment (RIOT): a novel metric for evaluating the quality of oncosurgical therapy for malignancy. *J Surg Oncol.* 2014;110(2):107–114.
57. Day RW, Cleeland CS, Wang XS, et al. Patient-reported outcomes accurately measure the value of an enhanced recovery program in liver surgery. *J Am Coll Surg.* 2015;221(6):1023–1030 e1021–e1022.
58. Merkow RP, Bilimoria KY, Tomlinson JS, et al. Postoperative complications reduce adjuvant chemotherapy use in resectable pancreatic cancer. *Ann Surg.* 2014;260(2):372–377.
59. Hassinger TE, Mehaffey JH, Martin AN, et al. implementation of an enhanced recovery protocol is associated with on-time initiation of adjuvant chemotherapy in colorectal cancer. *Dis Colon Rectum.* 2019;62(11):1305–1315.
60. Nelson DB, Mehran RJ, Mitchell KG, et al. Enhanced recovery after thoracic surgery is associated with improved adjuvant chemotherapy completion for non-small cell lung cancer. *J Thorac Cardiovasc Surg.* 2019;158(1):279–286.
61. Langenhoff BS, Krabbe PF, Wobbes T, Ruers TJ. Quality of life as an outcome measure in surgical oncology. *Br J Surg.* 2001;88(5):643–652.
62. Darling GE. Quality of life in patients with esophageal cancer. *Thorac Surg Clin.* 2013;23(4):569–575.
63. Breeze J, Rennie A, Dawson D, et al. Patient-reported quality of life outcomes following treatment for oral cancer. *Int J Oral Maxillofac Surg.* 2018;47(3):296–301.

55

Symptom Assessment, Patient-Reported Outcomes, and Quality of Life Considerations in Perioperative Care for Patients With Cancer

XIN SHELLEY WANG AND QIULING SHI

Introduction

It is imperative that patients with cancer are followed closely, so as to maximize treatment benefit while minimizing complications;[1] thus monitoring the severity of symptoms and functional impairment is a critical component of patient care. Many stakeholder groups (e.g., clinicians, patients, patient advocates, those interested in quality assurance) have made a strong case for the inclusion of patient-reported outcomes (PROs) in routine oncology practice.[2,3] A PRO has been defined as "any report of the status of a patient's health condition that comes directly from the patient, without interpretation of the patient's response by a clinician or anyone else."[4] PRO assessments can detect worsening of symptoms (whether disease- or treatment-related) and decline in functioning, either before a clinic visit or between visits, when active symptom intervention is possible. Although PROs have been widely accepted in *clinical research*[5,6] and are endorsed by the US Food and Drug Administration (FDA) for use in *drug labeling-claim trials*,[7] the introduction of PROs in *perioperative patient care* has not been well established. PRO use has been limited mainly to tracking pain (and, more recently, fatigue and distress).

Recognition of the potential benefits of incorporating PROs into the trajectory of surgical care has been tempered somewhat by various practical difficulties with implementing PROs.[8] Nonetheless, significant progress has been made toward using PROs to support patient-centered care and recognizing the value of PROs in perioperative care. Studies show that PRO-based measures of symptom severity and functional impairment are sensitive to the posttreatment recovery trajectory when administered frequently and that PRO-based quality-of-life (QoL) measures can predict objective clinical outcomes, such as surgical complications.[8,9]

Patients with cancer who undergo major surgery experience an acute systemic inflammatory, neuroendocrine, and metabolic stress response to procedure-related tissue injury and the medications used during the perioperative period. Collectively, this response often encompasses a cluster of *systemic symptoms* (e.g., fatigue, poor appetite, drowsiness, disturbed sleep) and *organ-specific symptoms* (e.g., pain, abdominal bloating). Morbidity, including high symptom burden and other complications, may cause significant postoperative functional impairment, prolong the patient's convalescence and recovery trajectory, lead to unscheduled clinic or emergency department visits, and delay the return to intended cancer treatment.[10]

Insufficient empirical research has combined the patient's perspective (PROs) with clinical outcomes (risk for complications, length of hospital stay, return to planned treatment) in order to assess such issues as recovery to preoperative symptom levels or the effectiveness of Enhanced Recovery Programs (ERPs).[11,12] The knowledge gained from such research could be a clinically relevant and a critical component of routine surgical practice. Additionally, this kind of information is vital for clinicians, as it may help to determine the patient's ability to resume additional intended cancer therapies. Thus integrating PROs into standard postoperative care has multiple advantages for monitoring and evaluating recovery from cancer surgery.

Recent advances in data-gathering methods are facilitating the use of PROs in routine clinical practice.[5,9] In the past few years, a transition from earlier methods, such as paper-and-pencil assessment at clinic visits, to electronic data capture via telephone-computer interactive voice or web-based methods on computers or smartphones has enabled frequent PRO assessments to be obtained from patients at home. These newer methods increase the feasibility of tracking patients after discharge repeatedly and with relatively little patient burden, while making these data available to clinicians in real time.

Breakthrough projects are needed to establish (1) a workable *methodology* for using PRO measures to characterize postoperative recovery from the patient's perspective after complex procedures, focusing on symptom burden and functional impairment (especially once the patient is discharged from hospital), and (2) *knowledge* about barriers to adopting PROs in routine patient care. This chapter presents considerations for the development and use of PROs in perioperative care.

Defining PRO concepts

Ideal PRO Instruments

The ideal PRO instrument will satisfy the FDA requirements for certain development procedures that promote reliability, validity, and sensitivity (see later). Beyond such formal requirements, a good PRO instrument will also be brief, simple, and understandable by patients with diverse educational and cultural backgrounds. We find that a 0–10 numeric severity rating scale is ideal for obtaining reliable information directly from patients, because only the anchors have to be translated and adapted for different cultures, thereby minimizing possible misunderstanding. However, categorical responses (i.e., none, mild, moderate, severe) are used on many scales, including the PROMIS assessment method[13] and the PRO-based version of the Common Terminology Criteria for Adverse Events (PRO-CTCAE).[14] Finally, the ideal PRO instrument will have been validated for repeated use and will include specific symptoms related to the site, disease stage, and treatment to be studied—in other words it will be "fit for purpose"—and will allow acquisition of real-time data during recovery, which can be viewed as a continuous process.

PRO Instrument Development

In 2009 the FDA set forth guidance on how to develop PRO instruments that are acceptable to the FDA for supporting labeling claims in medical product development.[4] In accordance with this guidance, the development of procedure-specific PRO instruments for use in surgical settings must include both qualitative studies to establish content validity (i.e., which symptomatic outcomes might be expected) and psychometric validation studies to establish reliability, validity, and sensitivity. Besides reliability and validity, responsiveness (change in ratings when they are to be expected) also is important.[4] To acquire comparable clinical data across various patient populations, the impact of cultural and linguistic factors on patient-reported symptoms should be reviewed and minimized to support the use of these methods in other languages and cultures.[15]

Similarities and Differences Between Symptoms and QoL as Concepts

A long history of QoL research within clinical cancer research has focused on various dimensions of the patient's perspective. Wilson and Cleary[16] established a classic conceptual model of PROs that well defines the differences among the terms "symptom," "functional status," and "heath perception," as they relate to overall QoL. They noted that "Patient-reported symptoms not only cause patients to enter the medical system, they also may affect subsequent use and the costs of medical care." Their model indicates that how the individual evaluates his or her overall QoL depends on multiple levels of PROs; symptom status is one important determinant of functioning, whereas the physical, psychologic, social, and role functioning domains are indicative of health status. Wilson and Cleary conceived of overall QoL as "distinct from health, though related to it."[16]

Indeed, the similarity among these various health-related QoL domains (symptoms, functional status, health status, and overall QoL) is that all are measurable by PROs; the difference among them is that only one—symptom burden (symptoms and/or functional status)—has clinically relevant outcomes that could point to medically actionable targets for implementation in routine patient care.

Clinical Research on PRO Application in Perioperative Care

Ground Knowledge From PROs

To inform research, health care delivery, and policy, patient-centered outcomes research and comparative effectiveness research require that PRO data be captured appropriately.[17] PRO instrument validation processes and minimum measurement standards for specific diseases or procedures are rapidly being developed to promote the proper use of PROs.

Particularly in surgical oncology practice, where debilitating radical procedures and oncoplastic reconstruction after resection are common, the advent of ERP concepts and strategies[11,18] is challenging the conventional evaluation and definition of "postoperative recovery" after major cancer surgery. Undoubtedly, following ERAS guidelines has led to fewer complications, shortened hospital stays, fewer hospital readmissions, and decreased 30-day mortality.[19] Nonetheless, the time course and level of recovery associated with current standard care versus newer ERAS principles are still being characterized. Factors that might contribute to complications, such as advanced age, higher body mass index, the complexity and extent of resection, higher American Society of Anesthesiologists physical status classification score,[20] and existing medical comorbidities,[21] have been studied, but these concepts add little to our knowledge about the patient's experience during the post-discharge recovery period.[22]

Being free of symptoms (e.g., nausea, pain) and being independently mobile were identified by both patients and health care professionals as the most important goals of postsurgical recovery.[23] Indeed, functional recovery after major cancer surgery dictates whether adjuvant therapy will be delayed or cancelled, either of which can negatively affect long-term clinical outcomes.[24] Thus discussion regarding the design of PRO assessments has progressed from assessing one dimension of recovery, such as physiologic variables, to a multidimensional assessment of physical, emotive, functional, and cognitive performance.[6,8,23]

Establishing solutions that better serve key stakeholders (in particular, patients and clinicians) in tailoring and evaluating procedure-specific perioperative care after major surgery will require collaboration among investigators from surgery, symptom research, nursing, and anesthesiology. To incorporate PRO-based methods for defining major symptom burden, a research plan should include a validated PRO instrument that measures symptom burden and has been shown to be sensitive for detecting both acute and chronic treatment effects on symptoms and functioning in the patient population of interest (i.e., a fit-for-purpose measure). These methods can then be used to establish the utility of PROs as clinical outcomes in ERP practice, such as for defining functional interference and recovery during perioperative care and predicting poor recovery.

Further research is needed to investigate the challenges and barriers to adopting PROs in real-world perioperative care. Adding a measure of multisymptom and functional outcomes in care that provides the patient's perspective on their recovery trajectory would undoubtedly improve our understanding of the impact of surgery. Other than for pain, this is yet to be studied at any depth in surgical clinical research.

Challenges and Opportunities

Recognition of the potential benefits of incorporating PROs into the trajectory of care has been tempered somewhat by awareness of problems in implementing PROs.[8] Implementation requires not only sufficient research to provide PRO parameters that will be useful in routine patient care, but also the ability to transition from research to practice, which can take 10–20 years in a large population. A systematic review with a national focus on postacute care, which reported evidence from studies that used PROs during recovery after adult cardiac surgery,[25] encapsulates the challenges that are similarly faced by cancer researchers.[12] Multiple significant heterogeneity and methodological weaknesses were found, such as differing follow-up periods, lack of standardization in the frequency of measurement and the tools used to assess recovery, variations in the handling of missing data, limited domains that were assessed, and the fact that most were single-site studies without external validation. These weaknesses support concerns that the evidence base regarding postoperative patient-centered outcomes still needs to be strengthened to guide data-driven improvement in oncologic postoperative recovery.

For clinicians and nurses involved in perioperative care after cancer surgery, the feasibility of using PROs in this setting is influenced by difficulties with integrating PROs into clinical workflows and concerns that PRO assessment is a time-consuming effort that adds little in terms of clinical benefit.[3] The length of time needed for patients to complete a multi-item PRO instrument has been an issue for both patients and clinicians. Further, although validated PRO instruments are available, their utility and meaning within a defined clinical setting remain relatively unexplored. These challenges to PRO adoption might be met by providing empirically established methods for interpreting PRO measurements.

One result of time-related concerns related to multiitem PRO assessments is low temporal granularity in measurement. However, today's digital platforms may allow for high-frequency PRO measurements, as frequent as on a daily basis.[26] Leveraging such technology provides novel opportunities to obtain granular insights into the recovery process. The methods could enhance perioperative care, not only during hospitalization after surgery, when patients are highly symptomatic, but also after discharge during the functional recovery period.

The expansion of electronic data-capture systems to be deployable on home phones or computers, smartphones, and tablet computers makes it much more feasible to collect patient reports outside the clinic in real time.[9,27] This allows patient status to be followed frequently throughout active treatment and even after treatment has been discontinued. As the feasibility of adopting electronic PRO capture increases, the relationship between the patient's perspective and postoperative clinical outcomes as associated with different diseases and procedures should be further examined. Questions to be answered include: What symptom score presents a clinically meaningful trigger point that needs an intervention? What functional interference score should trigger action, so as to prevent further delay of adjuvant cancer therapy?

Clinical Research Outcomes

Despite the challenges inherent in PRO implementation, incorporating PROs as clinical research outcomes in perioperative care has numerous potential benefits.[8] When collected longitudinally, PROs can be used to quantify *perioperative symptom severity* and *functional status trajectories*, which should be interpretable for both clinical research and practice. The *definition of symptom recovery and functioning recovery* can be established either by using preoperative symptom and functional impairment levels in comparison with postsurgical and postdischarge levels, or by using mild-level symptom and interference severity cutoff points, below which patients can perform their daily activities without medical assistance. *Time to recovery*, which is the time needed to return to preoperative or no/mild symptom and interference levels, can inform comparisons between surgical techniques or between perioperative care strategies, for example, ERP versus standard care. It is worth mentioning that, because patients may report a PRO score below a predefined severity threshold at one time and above it at the next assessment, two consecutive below-threshold scores might better signify a recovery event; in this scenario, the time of the first assessment is considered as the time of recovery.

Methodologies for Applying PRO Measures in Perioperative Care

How can PROs inform and change real-world practice? We already have a widely used, acceptable PRO-based method for assessing *pain* in routine patient care: verbally asking patients to rate their pain on a 0–10 scale. This method is standard care across most health care systems and offers an excellent example of how PROs can be feasible and useful in real-world applications. Nonetheless, the transition from academic knowledge to good clinical utility for other PROs in perioperative practice is hindered by multiple factors, as represented by Rogers' classic *Diffusion of Innovation Theory*.[28] This theory provides an appropriate framework for understanding the challenges inherent in bringing a new process, characterized by Rogers as "hardware" and "software," to acceptance by users and, ultimately, successful adoption. Hardware is "the tool that embodies the technology in the form of a material or physical object"; in PRO implementation, it is the instrument itself, its method of delivery, and the real world clinical needs by cohort. Software is "the information base for the tool"; in PRO implementation, it is a set of clear and simple methods for how to use the instrument, its compatibility for patient-care clinicians implementing it as a new outcome measure (awareness, advice, concern), and its acceptability to patients (complexity of delivery). We are hopeful that the decision by various electronic medical record builders to include fit-for-purpose PROs in their foundational system for nationwide use will meet the software needs for most patient-care clinicians in a perioperative setting, as a part of an ERP.

The methods and procedures for using PROs in patient care include assessment tool selection, data collection and display, and data interpretation with clinically meaningful trigger points, algorithms, or pathway-of-action points, all of which must be carefully studied and supported by clinical research.

Considerations in Selecting Assessment Tools

Currently, PROs are used mainly in clinical research and are endorsed by the FDA for use in drug labeling-claim trials.[4] The PRO-CTCAE is mostly used in clinical trials.[29] Symptom tools are far more relevant to the disease and treatment process for everyday clinical care than are QoL measures, as symptom alleviation is the first critical step toward improving a patient's overall QoL, the final endpoint in Wilson's model.[16] Understanding this *theoretical* difference between symptom and functional interference measures versus more conceptually broad health-related QoL measures is challenging for most clinicians and is a major barrier to the adoption of PROs in practice, as is the *historical* use of health-related and overall QoL measures, rather than symptom-specific measures, in clinical trials and research (e.g., the 36-item Short Form Health Survey [SF-36], Functional Assessment of Cancer Therapy [FACT], and European Organization for Research and Treatment of Cancer core QoL questionnaire [EORTC-QLQ-C30]). In contrast, only pain and distress are typically assessed quantitatively in routine patient care.

Nonetheless, several validated multi-symptom assessment tools are available for focusing directly on symptom burden and its impact on functional status (e.g., the Edmonton Symptom Assessment System [ESAS],[30] MD Anderson Symptom Inventory [MDASI],[31] and the short form of Patient-Reported Outcomes Measurement Information System [PROMIS]).[32] Few symptom PRO measures have been adopted in perioperative care, even though they are already accepted in other areas of oncology research, academia, and patient care,[5] nor has the concept of PRO outcomes been broadly included in existing ERP-style programs or censuses.

Using PROs to assess symptom severity and its impact on daily functioning has proven to be a valid and sensitive approach to quantifying the patterns of change in perioperative symptoms and functioning over the course of recovery.[33] When used to longitudinally measure physical functioning status, PRO-measured interference with walking ability significantly correlated with an objective performance-measured outcome, the 6-min walk test. In a population with decreased physical functioning, the PRO measure generated less missing data than the 6-min walk test.[34]

The 2009 FDA guidance[4] suggests that it is preferable for patients to report their current or recent symptom and functional status with a short recall period. In the perioperative setting, especially in the first few days after surgery, symptoms and functional status change every day. Thus a recall period of 7 days may not capture the daily changes in a patient's status. Tools with a shorter recall periods (e.g., in the past 24 h, or currently) would be more suitable for this situation.

To successfully integrate PROs into patient care, an evidence-based subset of clinically meaningful symptoms that can be used to identify, triage, and treat patients at high risk for postoperative complications is needed. However, no symptom-specific PRO questionnaire has yet been adopted for evaluating relevant patient-reported symptom burden after patients are discharged from the hospital during postoperative recovery; this is a vital need, because an objective measure of functioning would not be feasible after

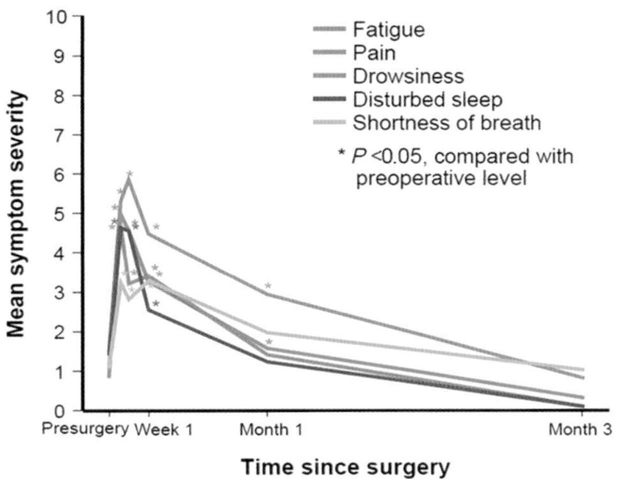

• **Fig. 55.1** Trajectories of fatigue, shortness of breath, disturbed sleep, drowsiness, and pain (the most severe symptoms after thoracic surgery) as assessed with the MD Anderson Symptom Inventory. From Fagundes CP, Shi Q, Vaporciyan AA, et al. Symptom recovery after thoracic surgery: measuring patient-reported outcomes with the MD Anderson Symptom Inventory. *J Thorac Cardiovasc Surg*. 2015;150(3):613–619. With permission from Elsevier.

discharge, when patients are at home. A recently published study demonstrated that critical PROs (such as the walking and general activity interference items on the MDASI) could quantify a patient's physical functioning that was verified by the Get up and Go test after gynecologic surgery.[35]

Assessment Schedules

PRO assessment schedules must match perioperative care needs and more importantly, align with expected changes in patient status. Further, the schedule should minimize the assessment burden for both patients and professionals. For example, PROs should be assessed more frequently during hospitalization (probably daily), but only weekly or twice weekly after discharge. Such a measurement schedule ensures timely capture of changes in symptoms and functional status, which should accurately describe the recovery trajectory and identify high-risk individuals in need of symptomatic intervention.

Cutoff Points as Thresholds to Trigger Intervention

A PRO measure should be easily understood and its scores must be interpretable, if it is to be of any clinical use. Although the use of continuous variables is statistically preferable to the use of categorical variables,[36] in practice, changing a PRO variable from continuous to categorical form by using empirically derived cutoff points may better inform treatment decision making for clinicians. The National Comprehensive Cancer Network (NCCN) Clinical Practice Guidelines in Oncology for Adult Cancer Pain[37] defined "mild," "moderate," and "severe" as clinically meaningful severity categories. These guidelines define a rating of 1–3 on a 0–10 numeric scale as mild, 4–5 as moderate, and 7–10 as severe, for the purposes of establishing alerts to inform clinical consequences or actions according to treatment algorithms and for defining high-risk complications. The NCCN used a similar approach to establish guidelines for fatigue and distress management.[38,39]

Although mild, moderate, and severe categories are discrete, a specific cutoff point for triggering clinical action still needs to be established for different symptom items. Cutoff points should be based on an anchor that is clinically interpretable (e.g., change in performance status or postdischarge complications to define the cutoff points for PRO-assessed physical functioning) and should be well correlated with the PRO measure.

Examples of Using PROs to Define Recovery After Thoracic Surgery

As an integral part of the development of the PRO outcomes for recovery from thoracic surgery in patients with early-stage non-small cell lung cancer (NSCLC), treatment-naive patients undergoing either standard open thoracotomy (n = 31) or video-assisted thoracoscopic surgery (VATS; n = 29)[33,40] used the MDASI, an extensively validated PRO measure of cancer-related symptom burden, to rate symptoms and their impact on daily functioning in the past 24 h. The MDASI asks patients to rate the severity of each symptom and functional interference item at its worst on a 0–10 numeric rating scale: for the symptom items, 0 represents "not present" (no symptom) and 10 represents "as bad as you can imagine"; for the interference items, 0 represents "did not interfere" and 10 represents "interfered completely." Fig. 55.1 shows MDASI trajectories for fatigue, shortness of breath, disturbed sleep, drowsiness, and pain, the most severe symptoms after thoracic surgery.[40] The MDASI was sensitive enough to detect differences in symptom and functional recovery between open surgery versus VATS.[33]

To define postsurgical recovery, the cutoff points for both symptom severity and inference were set at 3, 4 (0–3, no/mild symptom or interference; 4–10, moderate/severe symptom or interference).[40] Time to recovery of symptoms (i.e., return to mild level) was examined, with fatigue requiring the longest recovery time (median recovery time = 28 days postsurgery; Fig. 55.2). The recovery time for pain was significantly shorter for VATS lobectomy, compared with standard open thoracotomy (Fig. 55.3). The recovery of daily functioning (walking ability, relationship with others, mood, and enjoyment of life) to mild levels was significantly shorter for VATS than for open surgery.

Examples of Using PROs to Evaluate Pathway and Procedure-Specific Benefits After Gynecologic Surgery

PRO assessment of symptoms and inference was used to evaluate the effectiveness of an ERP pathway before and after its implementation in patients undergoing open

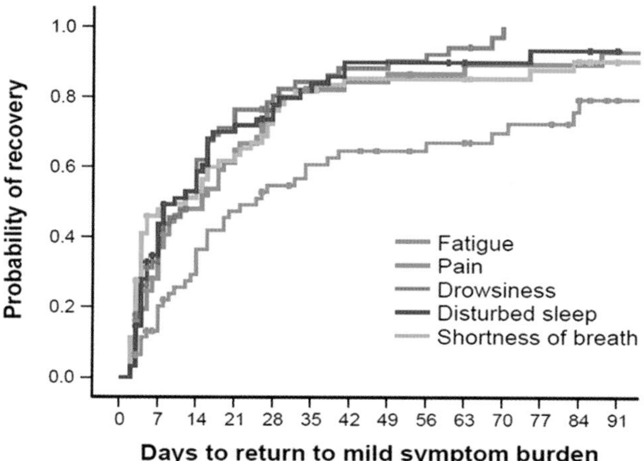

• **Fig. 55.2** Time to symptom recovery, by symptom. From Fagundes CP, Shi Q, Vaporciyan AA, et al. Symptom recovery after thoracic surgery: measuring patient-reported outcomes with the MD Anderson Symptom Inventory. *J Thorac Cardiovasc Surg.* 2015;150(3):613–619. With permission from Elsevier.

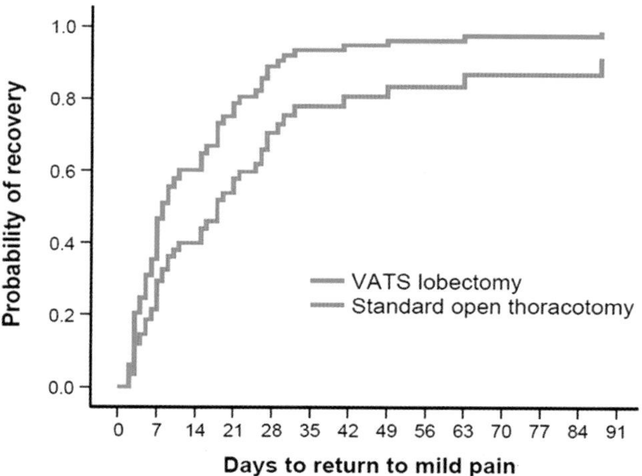

• **Fig. 55.3** Time to pain recovery, by procedure. From Fagundes CP, Shi Q, Vaporciyan AA, et al. Symptom recovery after thoracic surgery: measuring patient-reported outcomes with the MD Anderson Symptom Inventory. *J Thorac Cardiovasc Surg.* 2015;150(3):613–619. With permission from Elsevier.

surgery for gynecologic cancer.[41] A procedure-specific measure, the MDASI-Ovarian Cancer module, was developed in accordance with the 2009 FDA guidance.[42] The assessment schedule was set as presurgery, daily after surgery during hospitalization, on days 3 and 7 after discharge, then weekly for up to 6 weeks. Compared with patients who had standard perioperative care, the ERP patients had a shorter median times to return to no or mild fatigue (10 vs. 30 days) and to no or mild inference with walking (5 vs. 13 days).

In a tertiary cancer center with a standardized, systematic method of patient selection for primary cytoreductive surgery and a standardized ERP pathway, meaningful differences were observed in patient-reported symptom burden and symptom interference assessed with the MDASI-Ovarian Cancer module, by surgical complexity score.[43] Patients undergoing intermediate- or high-complexity surgery had more nausea, fatigue, and total interference than did patients undergoing low-complexity surgery.

Examples of Using PROs to Improve Postoperative Care

Cancer patients frequently report multiple severe symptoms for the first few weeks after tumor-removal surgery, which can prolong postoperative recovery, lead to unscheduled clinic or emergency department visits, delay the resumption of planned cancer treatment, and ultimately result in poorer QoL and shortened survival. Although the cost of clinician follow-up calls to patients could be high, the growing literature on randomized clinical trials indicates that computer-assisted electronic symptom monitoring (1) provides a symptom benefit, even without threshold alerts to clinicians,[43–45] (2) enhances patient-provider communications,[46] (3) increases patients' sense of control over their care,[47] and (4) may lower costs by identifying problems early enough for rapid intervention. The clinical utility and adoption of monitoring postdischarge PROs has not been well studied and could be considered an innovation.

In a nationwide study, more than half of patients with head and neck cancer were not yet receiving adjuvant therapy 6 weeks after surgery, the timeframe promoted in NCCN guidelines as optimal for functional recovery with fewer long-term clinical outcomes.[48,49] PRO-based strategies to address this concern, such as severe symptom alerts that trigger clinician response to reduce postoperative symptoms and to prevent delay in further treatment due to worsening complications, have not been well studied.

However, preliminary evidence with clinically significant data from symptom research in perioperative care supports the use of cutoff points to trigger triage and active care for symptoms in patients with lung cancer after thoracic surgery. Cleeland et al.[50] reported results from a randomized clinical trial showing that at-home symptom monitoring for 3 weeks postdischarge, plus feedback to clinicians when any symptom exceeded a predefined threshold, was feasible and contributed to more-effective postoperative symptom control (Fig. 55.4). Patients (n = 79) rated symptoms twice weekly on the MDASI via a computerized, telephone-based interactive voice response system. For the intervention arm, an email alert was sent to clinicians if ratings on the 0–10 scale reached a threshold of 5 for pain, distress, or disturbed sleep, or 3 for shortness of breath and constipation. The intervention group had a significant reduction in threshold events on those selected symptoms compared with the control group (19% vs. 8%).

This discussion of PRO application has illustrated the necessity of a standardized procedure that incorporates fit-for-purpose tool development, procedure-driven study design, and expert data analysis and interpretation. With such a procedure, PRO-defined perioperative outcomes can quantify the benefit obtained from implementing a new perioperative care pathway, such as an ERP, and provide tracking targets for routine perioperative care.

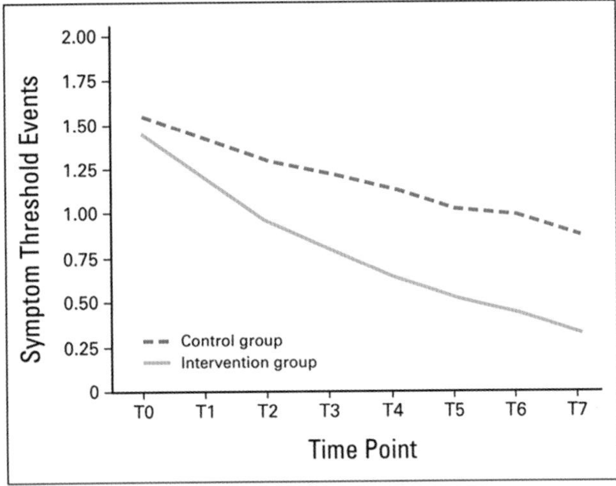

• **Fig. 55.4** Mean number of symptoms exceeding a predefined severity threshold as reported over time by patients using an automated, telephone-based monitoring system. From Cleeland CS, Wang XS, Shi Q, et al. Automated symptom alerts reduce postoperative symptom severity after cancer surgery: a randomized controlled clinical trial. *J Clin Oncol.* 2011;29(8):994–1000. With permission from ASCO.

Future Considerations Regarding the Use of PROs in Perioperative Care

The application of PROs in perioperative care depends on the purpose of the assessment within a specific context, as well as the burden on clinicians who must assess and interpret the scores. In research and quality-of-care assessments, one usually aims for optimal accuracy when using a screening measure such as the numeric rating scale. However, in daily practice, clinicians who screen for cancer-related symptoms in their patients generally aim to minimize the number of false-positive test results. In this context, symptom screening with a brief, easy-to-administer PRO questionnaire is usually followed by a more comprehensive symptom history to identify patients who actually experience clinically relevant burden. For instance, the NCCN guidelines suggest that symptoms such as pain, fatigue, and distress need additional clinical attention when rated ≥4.[37–39] However, a meta-analysis of papers published between September 2005 and January 2014 found that the prevalence of moderate to severe pain (≥5 on a 0–10 scale) in patients receiving anticancer treatment was 32%[51] but that symptom-specific clinical actions were taken for only one-third of those patients, even though an electronic PRO instrument was available for patients to complete at every clinic visit.[52] The contrast between the high rate of over-threshold scores and low response rates suggests that routine PRO assessment in practice generates a high potential burden for clinicians and other health care providers. To relieve this "alert burden," effective approaches (e.g., defining actionable thresholds according to both derived cutoff points and clinical feasibility) will be needed to promote PRO integration into surgical practice.

Conclusion

Timely symptom management is an essential component of effective patient care.[53] However, given the lack of studies showing that reducing symptom burden improves postsurgical clinical outcomes, the clinical utility of PRO monitoring in perioperative care has not yet been generally accepted or adopted by many surgical care professionals. Although the number of studies using PROs in research has increased, and although pain assessment on a 0–10 severity scale is routinely used as a screening tool in perioperative care, PROs remain a relatively new measurement in everyday patient care. For PROs to be acceptable as outcomes measures in routine practice, clinicians involved in multidisciplinary cancer care need precise, evidence-supported PRO-based monitoring pathways and guidance on when symptoms need immediate attention or may be predicting impending compromised clinical outcomes.

References

1. Amanam I, Gupta R, Mita A, Scher K, Massarelli E. Perspectives in head and neck medical oncology. *Cancer Treat Res.* 2018;174:163–185.
2. Basch E. Patient-reported outcomes - harnessing patients' voices to improve clinical care. *N Engl J Med.* 2017;376(2):105–108.
3. LeBlanc TW, Abernethy AP. Patient-reported outcomes in cancer care - hearing the patient voice at greater volume. *Nat Rev Clin Oncol.* 2017;14(12):763–772.
4. US Food and Drug Administration. Guidance for Industry. Patient-Reported Outcome Measures: Use in Medical Product Development to Support Labeling Claims. 2009. Available at http://www.fda.gov/downloads/Drugs/GuidanceCompliance-RegulatoryInformation/Guidances/UCM071975.pdf.
5. Basch E, Abernethy AP, Mullins CD, et al. Recommendations for incorporating patient-reported outcomes into clinical comparative effectiveness research in adult oncology. *J Clin Oncol.* 2012;30(34):4249–4255.
6. Cleeland CS. Symptom burden: multiple symptoms and their impact as patient-reported outcomes. *J Natl Cancer Inst Monogr.* 2007(37):16–21.
7. Eremenco S, Pease S, Mann S, Berry P. PRO Consortium's Process Subcommittee. Patient-Reported Outcome (PRO) Consortium translation process: consensus development of updated best practices. *J Patient Rep Outcomes.* 2017;2(1):12.
8. Bilimoria KY, Cella D, Butt Z. Current Challenges in using patient-reported outcomes for surgical care and performance measurement: everybody wants to hear from the patient, but are we ready to listen? *JAMA Surg.* 2014;149(6):505–506.
9. Bingener J, Sloan JA, Novotny PJ, Pockaj BA, Nelson H. Perioperative patient-reported outcomes predict serious postoperative complications: a secondary analysis of the COST trial. *J Gastrointest Surg.* 2015;19(1):65–71.
10. Lillemoe HA, Marcus RK, Kim BJ, et al. Severe preoperative symptoms delay readiness to return to intended oncologic therapy (RIOT) after liver resection. *Ann Surg Oncol.* 2019;26(13):4548–4555.
11. Nicholson A, Lowe MC, Parker J, Lewis SR, Alderson P, Smith AF. Systematic review and meta-analysis of enhanced recovery programmes in surgical patients. *Br J Surg.* 2014;101(3):172–188.

12. Avery KNL, Richards HS, Portal A, et al. Developing a real-time electronic symptom monitoring system for patients after discharge following cancer-related surgery. *BMC Cancer*. 2019;19(1):463.
13. Cella D, Yount S, Rothrock N, et al. The Patient-Reported Outcomes Measurement Information System (PROMIS): progress of an NIH Roadmap cooperative group during its first two years. *Med Care*. 2007;45(5):S3–S11.
14. US National Institutes of Health. Patient-Reported Outcomes Version of the Common Terminology Criteria for Adverse Events (PRO-CTCAE™) Item Library (Version 1.0). 2018. Available at https://healthcaredelivery.cancer.gov/pro-ctcae/item-library.pdf.
15. Wang XS, Cleeland CS, Mendoza TR, et al. Impact of cultural and linguistic factors on symptom reporting by patients with cancer. *J Natl Cancer Inst*. 2010;102(10):732–738.
16. Wilson IB, Cleary PD. Linking clinical variables with health-related quality of life. A conceptual model of patient outcomes. *JAMA*. 1995;273(1):59–65.
17. Reeve BB, Wyrwich KW, Wu AW, et al. ISOQOL recommends minimum standards for patient-reported outcome measures used in patient-centered outcomes and comparative effectiveness research. *Qual Life Res*. 2013;22(8):1889–1905.
18. de Groot JJ, van Es LE, Maessen JM, Dejong CH, Kruitwagen RF, Slangen BF. Diffusion of Enhanced Recovery principles in gynecologic oncology surgery: is active implementation still necessary? *Gynecol Oncol*. 2014;134(3):570–575.
19. Memtsoudis SG, Fiasconaro M, Soffin EM, et al. Enhanced recovery after surgery components and perioperative outcomes: a nationwide observational study. *Br J Anaesth*. 2020;124(5):638–647. doi:10.1016/j.bja.2020.01.017.
20. Owens WD, Felts JA, Spitznagel Jr EL. ASA physical status classifications: a study of consistency of ratings. *Anesthesiology*. 1978;49(4):239–243.
21. Reid BC, Alberg AJ, Klassen AC, Koch WM, Samet JM. The American Society of Anesthesiologists' class as a comorbidity index in a cohort of head and neck cancer surgical patients. *Head Neck*. 2001;23(11):985–994.
22. Blazeby JM. Systematic review of outcomes used to evaluate enhanced recovery after surgery. *Br J Surg*. 2014;101(3):159–170.
23. Aahlin EK, von Meyenfeldt M, Dejong CH, et al. Functional recovery is considered the most important target: a survey of dedicated professionals. *Perioper Med*. 2014;3:5.
24. Aloia TA, Zimmitti G, Conrad C, Gottumukalla V, Kopetz S, Vauthey J-N. Return to intended oncologic treatment (RIOT): a novel metric for evaluating the quality of oncosurgical therapy for malignancy. *J Surg Oncol*. 2014;110(2):107–114.
25. Mori M, Angraal S, Chaudhry SI, et al. Characterizing patient-centered postoperative recovery after adult cardiac surgery: a systematic review. *J Am Heart Assoc*. 2019;8(21):e013546.
26. Jaensson M, Dahlberg K, Eriksson M, Nilsson U. Evaluation of postoperative recovery in day surgery patients using a mobile phone application: a multicentre randomized trial. *Br J Anaesth*. 2017;119(5):1030–1038.
27. Gilbert A, Sebag-Montefiore D, Davidson S, Velikova G. Use of patient-reported outcomes to measure symptoms and health related quality of life in the clinic. *Gynecol Oncol*. 2015;136(3):429–439.
28. Rogers EM. Diffusion of Innovations. Free Press; 2003. 5th ed.
29. Dueck AC, Mendoza TR, Mitchell SA, et al. Validity and reliability of the US National Cancer Institute's Patient-Reported Outcomes Version of the Common Terminology Criteria for Adverse Events (PRO-CTCAE). *JAMA Oncol*. 2015;1(8):1051–1059.
30. Hui D, Bruera E. The Edmonton Symptom Assessment System 25 years later: past, present, and future developments. *J Pain Symptom Manage*. 2017;53(3):630–643.
31. Cleeland CS, Mendoza TR, Wang XS, et al. Assessing symptom distress in cancer patients: the M.D. Anderson Symptom Inventory. *Cancer*. 2000;89:1634–1646.
32. Cella D, Yount S, Rothrock N, Gershon R, Cook K, Reeve B, et al. The Patient-Reported Outcomes Measurement Information System (PROMIS): progress of an NIH Roadmap cooperative group during its first two years. *Med Care*. 2007;45(5 Suppl 1): S3–S11.
33. Shi Q, Wang XS, Vaporciyan AA, Rice DC, Popat KU, Cleeland CS. Patient-reported symptom interference as a measure of postsurgery functional recovery in lung cancer. *J Pain Symptom Manage*. 2016;52(6):822–831.
34. Shah N, Shi Q, Giralt S, et al. Utility of a patient-reported outcome in measuring functional impairment during autologous stem cell transplant in patients with multiple myeloma. *Qual Life Res*. 2018;27(4):979–985.
35. Wang XS, Kamal M, Chen TH, et al. Assessment of physical function by subjective and objective methods in patients undergoing open gynecologic surgery. *Gynecol Oncol*. 2021;161(1):83–88.
36. Royston P, Altman DG, Sauerbrei W. Dichotomizing continuous predictors in multiple regression: a bad idea. *Stat Med*. 2006;25(1):127–141.
37. National Comprehensive Cancer Network. NCCN Clinical Practice Guidelines in Oncology: Adult Cancer Pain - Version 3. 2019. Available at https://www.nccn.org/professionals/physician_gls/pdf/pain.pdf.
38. National Comprehensive Cancer Network. NCCN Clinical Practice Guidlines in Oncology: Cancer-Related Fatigue - Version 2. 2019. Available at https://www.nccn.org/professionals/physician_gls/pdf/fatigue.pdf.
39. National Comprehensive Cancer Network. NCCN Clinical Practice Guidlines in Oncology: Distress Management - Version 3. 2019. Available at https://www.nccn.org/professionals/physician_gls/pdf/distress.pdf.
40. Fagundes CP, Shi Q, Vaporciyan AA, et al. Symptom recovery after thoracic surgery: Measuring patient-reported outcomes with the MD Anderson Symptom Inventory. *J Thorac Cardiovasc Surg*. 2015;150(3):613–619.
41. Meyer LA, Lasala J, Iniesta MD, et al. Effect of an Enhanced Recovery After Surgery Program on opioid use and patient-reported outcomes. *Obstet Gynecol*. 2018;132(2):281–290.
42. Sailors MH, Bodurka DC, Gning I, et al. Validating the M. D. Anderson Symptom Inventory (MDASI) for use in patients with ovarian cancer. *Gynecol Oncol*. 2013;130(2):323–328.
43. Meyer LA, Shi Q, Lasala J, et al. Comparison of patient reported symptom burden on an enhanced recovery after surgery (ERAS) care pathway in patients with ovarian cancer undergoing primary vs. interval tumor reductive surgery. *Gynecol Oncol*. 2019;152(3):501–508.
44. Berry DL, Hong F, Halpenny B, et al. The electronic self report assessment and intervention for cancer: promoting patient verbal reporting of symptom and quality of life issues in a randomized controlled trial. *BMC Cancer*. 2014;14:513.
45. Avery AJ, Anderson C, Bond CM, et al. Evaluation of patient reporting of adverse drug reactions to the UK 'Yellow Card Scheme':

literature review, descriptive and qualitative analyses, and questionnaire surveys. *Health Tech Assess.* 2011;15(20): 1–234, iii-iv.

46. Berry DL, Blumenstein BA, Halpenny B, et al. Enhancing patient-provider communication with the electronic self-report assessment for cancer: a randomized trial. *J Clin Oncol.* 2011;29(8):1029–1035.
47. Velikova G, Booth L, Smith AB, et al. Measuring quality of life in routine oncology practice improves communication and patient well-being: a randomized controlled trial. *J Clin Oncol.* 2004;22(4):714–724.
48. Graboyes EM, Garrett-Mayer E, Sharma AK, Lentsch EJ, Day TA. Adherence to National Comprehensive Cancer Network guidelines for time to initiation of postoperative radiation therapy for patients with head and neck cancer. *Cancer.* 2017;123(14):2651–2660.
49. Lewis CM, Hessel AC, Roberts DB, et al. Prereferral head and neck cancer treatment: compliance with national comprehensive cancer network treatment guidelines. *Arch Otolaryngol Head Neck Surg.* 2010;136(12):1205–1211.
50. Cleeland CS, Wang XS, Shi Q, et al. Automated symptom alerts reduce postoperative symptom severity after cancer surgery: a randomized controlled clinical trial. *J Clin Oncol.* 2011;29(8):994–1000.
51. van den Beuken-van Everdingen MH, Hochstenbach LM, Joosten EA, Tjan-Heijnen VC, Janssen DJ. Update on prevalence of pain in patients with cancer: systematic review and meta-analysis. *J Pain Symptom Manage.* 2016;51(6): 1070–1090.
52. Seow H, Sussman J, Martelli-Reid L, Pond G, Bainbridge D. Do high symptom scores trigger clinical actions? An audit after implementing electronic symptom screening. *J Oncol Pract.* 2012;8(6):e142–e148.
53. Bernard H, Foss M. Patient experiences of enhanced recovery after surgery (ERAS). *Br J Nurs.* 2014;23(2):100–102, 104–106.

56

Shared Decision-Making and Advance Care Planning in the Cancer Care Journey

DAVID L. BROWN AND DEBRA LEUNG

Introduction

Shared decision-making (SDM) in cancer care seems to state the obvious. What other kinds of decision-making are ethical for oncologic patients, or in fact, any patient? Despite this self-evident truth, the widespread corporatization of health care across many countries and cultures forces the issue of SDM into this text and into daily clinical life in both primary and specialty cancer centers.

Although it is increasingly being recognized as crucial, there are a multitude of reasons that SDM is increasingly difficult to implement in our clinical practice. First, clinical production pressure experienced by patients and professionals often "nudges" care decisions for individuals into what is best for the health system (i.e., keeping the enterprise running smoothly), rather than what is best for varied and unique individuals. Overwhelmingly, the corporatization of medical care has drawn upon Frederick Taylor's assembly-line optimization[1] that focuses on knocking the variability out of processes. Although reducing variability is an admirable aim with regard to clinical practice outcomes, it can contribute to a lack of recognition of the individual behind the statistics. The quality improvement industry has embraced this limiting variability theme,[2] and it appears that this phenomenon is now impacting clinical decision-making.

Secondly, the rapid introduction and nature of electronic health records (EHRs) is an additional factor that pushes clinical decision-making toward the preeminence of health system autonomy in decisions. Contemporary EHRs do not contain an easily accessible, comprehensive, and true-to-life picture of patients as unique individuals with values that reflect this.[3] Rather, the records have become a compilation of drop-down menu facts that is more system-centric rather than focusing on our patients as unique individuals.

Finally, a third variable in patient care today that makes SDM difficult to implement is the increasing subspecialization of physicians caring for cancer patients. With this near hyper-specialization in many practices, the fragmentation of specialty care coupled with the time pressure of seeing more patients in a given appointment session makes it difficult to elicit unique individuals' goals. The time to listen is likely one of the features of modern health care, which is in the shortest supply. It takes time to get to "know" someone so that decision-making can truly be shared.

Advance care planning (ACP) is a disparate but related process that is integrally linked with SDM. ACP provides patients with the opportunity to document in their own voice the values and goals that they consider integral to the medical decision-making process. Therefore it is a part of and necessitates an informed SDM. Planning ahead cannot be effective in any fashion without the underpinnings of shared framing of the issues. Therefore we assume that SDM is the bedrock upon which effective ACP rests. Without true SDM about options, ACP can be too abstract and, hence, potentially of limited value.

What Is Shared Decision-Making?

Turning to a precise definition, and arguably a more academic and dry description, SDM is defined as an approach to medical decision-making where clinicians share the best available evidence, and where patients are supported to consider options, with the ultimate aim of achieving informed preferences.[4] In this chapter, we will also use the word individual, rather than patient, whenever practical. This is because adopting the role and attitudes of a patient almost always involves some loss of individuality and autonomy, which is necessary for truly shared and effective decision-making. Professional relationships need to be horizontal, rather than hierarchical, in decision-making. In essence, a partnership exists in the truest sense of the word.

Framing SDM in a slightly less dry fashion, in order for physicians to join with individuals in making shared decisions, a basic understanding of what is at the heart of medicine is required. The heart or center of medicine allows one to create a relationship with the individual (patient) so that they determine the type of care they want and need, using their values and goals for living to inform their choice. These care decisions are, of course, guided by physicians who define the range of appropriate treatment options that are deliverable within the capacity and expertise of their physician teams and the health systems that contain them. This philosophy embodies the concept of SDM as a dual expert model where both the physician and the patient are experts in disparate, but both equally important domains. The physician is the expert on the medical treatment options and the patient is the expert on what is important to them.

Many believe that this type of decision-making paradigm already occurs as a standard of care across the world, and indeed sometimes it does. The finest physicians practice SDM even if they may not be consciously aware of it. However, in today's busy clinical environment, operationalizing SDM is becoming increasingly challenging. In modern clinical practice, with its production pressure, time is in short supply. With time limitations, what is also limited is listening by our physician colleagues, as evidenced by a study that demonstrated an average time of 11 s before a physician interrupts a patient when in an exam room.[5] Without time to actively listen to an individual's values and goals, it is difficult to utilize them to truly make a shared decision.

Why Is Shared Decision-Making Needed?

1. Health care needs to be personalized and contextualized.

Physicians often view health care interactions as being based primarily on professionalism. There is little to argue about that insight, yet it is incomplete in scope. As individuals, health care must be personalized and impactful. Professionalism relating purely to clinical judgment and medical education is only a piece of it. The bridge between purely professional care and personalized care is the sacred commitment to put the individual's values and goals uppermost when determining an agreed-upon plan of care. This is especially true when decisions regarding cancer care are the focus of SDM.

Our focus on "evidenced-based medicine" can lead many to believe that there is only one singular correct treatment approach endorsed by the best available medical evidence for an individual condition. Of course, missing from this decision-making paradigm is the uniqueness of the individual in question. Does that individual have caregiving responsibilities that make some approaches to the proposed cancer treatment difficult? Do they have concurrent diseases that make a cardiac side effect of treatment problematic? Do they have certain treatments that they would be unwilling to accept? These examples of individual variables should also inform the SDM process.

The key to being able to keep the individual at the forefront is contextualization, which can be lost when care teams focus primarily on the clinical aspects of medical decision-making. Without contextualization, evidenced-based approaches can morph into an algorithmic approach to care that gets translated to the individual (patient), as "this is the way we approach your condition at our institution."

In spite of the availability of internet-based search engines that put a universe of information at an individual's fingertips, using that information effectively requires insight and experience. Experience that can only be provided by skilled and trained physicians. However, although physicians are in a position to understand the array of treatment options and accompanying medical evidence, it is the individual who is best able to contextualize those options into their choices for an approach forward. This is the essence of SDM.

2. Risk discussion is often performed suboptimally, and SDM encourages us to be comfortable and comprehensive in our approach.

What is often not shared with patients in early consultations is the plethora of side effects linked to the options for cancer treatment. When cancer survivorship is the focus of research, it deals almost exclusively with the lingering side effects of treatment, how the side effects can continue long past the treatment phase, and possible cure of the disease. Given that a key portion of the discussion leading to SDM involves disclosing the potential side effects of treatment, physicians need to be comfortable routinely covering these side effects and quality of life measures in our risk discussions with patients.

3. Patients feel disempowered due to the phenomenon of "hostage bargaining syndrome" and SDM may provide a means to overcome this.

One of the key reasons that SDM is needed is that individuals (patients), their families, and caregivers can become disempowered in the face of the multitude of challenges that accompany medical care. During our senior author's (DLB) experiences as a physician, and as a patient, he has often pondered why individuals, when they enter the health care environment, move from their typical, fiercely independent, and consumer-oriented mindset to a more submissive one than is characteristic in almost any other area of their lives. A recent Mayo Clinic Proceedings article provides a most interesting look at one of the reasons they postulate that this is occurring.

Berry and colleagues from the business school at Texas A&M University published the work: When Patients and Families Feel Like Hostages to Health Care.[6] In their manuscript, they defined in detail a concept they termed "hostage bargaining syndrome" (HBS). They assumed that it was HBS that was responsible for those submissive feelings and actions exhibited by patients in clinical interactions. They posit that when patients and families are in the presence of clinicians, they may behave like hostages, negotiating from a position of fear and confusion over their health decision-making. The authors outline that when HBS occurs there is a reluctance for patients and their families to challenge authority figures in the form of doctors, nurses, and other health care workers. These authority figures retain de facto control because of their attributes, such as expertise, prestige, and position. The authors hypothesize that this phenomenon exists because health care, especially that of a critical or life-threatening nature, is a "need" service, rather than a "want" service. This situation shifts the balance of power in favor of those in charge, rather than those consuming the service (i.e., the patient and/or patient's family).

Furthermore, the authors go on to frame the situation where HBS is allowed to persist and escalate to the extent that patients and their families may enter the second step along the HBS continuum—a state of learned helplessness. After the escalation of HBS into learned helplessness, the individuals involved begin to expect that future events will also be uncontrollable and thus have feelings of helplessness reinforced and amplified. Once this helpless mindset has been adopted, individuals become moldable to the system's standard operating practices. These standard operating practices are most often based on optimizing system functioning, rather than focusing decision-making on the unique human being facing a specific, and for them, distinctive health challenge.

Our senior author (DLB) spent several months chronically, and then critically ill, and as a result, he believes he understands some of these feelings. To him, what seems most often needed inside health systems to overcome and surmount this situation of learned helplessness is a focus on true "*informed choice*," rather than the standard practice of obtaining informed consent for procedures or treatment plans. By this, an individual (patient), or their family, if they are appointed as substitute decision-makers, is informed of all their options, and the potential impact of these options on their quality of life. This is in stark contrast to simply being asked to sign a form giving legal consent to a procedure and direction for care. This concept of informed choice amplifies true SDM, rather than a system-centric decision-making model. However, this takes time and heart, both of which are being "weaned out" of many health system interactions, due to perceived clinical production pressures.

At a personal level, our senior author (DLB) understands more today about what patients want from a health care interaction than he did before switching careers from academic leadership and clinical practice to advising others on health care decision-making. Providing background on his bona fides as a physician, he practiced across the United States in some elite institutions[a] that delivered wonderfully complex and high-tech medical care, viewed as some of the very best institutions in the United States. Again, he also knows what it is to be a patient, both with a critical illness and cancer, dependent on others for his life. Bearing these credentials in mind, he believes there are six things patients desire from their physicians and care team, even if they know their illness or injury cannot be "fixed" or "cured." If modeled by health care providers, these six things can empower patients and either prevent or lift them out of this state of "hostage" or learned helplessness. They are outlined below:

Value me as a unique human being—not special, but unique.

Truly care for me when coming into contact with me: I can tell.

Provide a value that is affordable to me and understandable.

Share with me your competence, not an insider's arrogance.

Give me a sense that I am at the center of this care encounter.

Do not abandon me: Provide me with communication and follow up.

4. SDM provides value in health care over and above traditional measures of value.

Unbeknownst to those not looking for it, the rhetoric of SDM is also present in all manner of texts. As the notable author, C.S. Lewis, stated many years ago, "the next best thing to being wise oneself is to live in a circle of those who are." SDM is about using physicians and health care resources as "wise friends" to inform decision-making. In this case, one of our wise friends is David W. Johnson. His book, *Market vs. Medicine*, is a "should read" for any of us seeking to heal health care decision-making and move toward true SDM and value in health care.[7] In his text, the concluding chapter is a timely reminder for all of us attempting to straddle a volume-based and value-based health delivery system. He cautions us that "the straddle" is failing US society, self-insured employers, and the larger health care system. In this concluding chapter he quotes John Maynard Keynes, who observed, "The difficulty lies not so much in developing new ideas as in escaping from old ones." Johnson encourages the health care industry to escape from its "revenue as the highest good" and move to providing measurable value to individuals, and secondarily to society. This is only possible through effective SDM.

Again, using our senior author's (DLB) experience as both a physician and a patient, it is evident that value discussions often take on a utilitarian societal view, and the individual's voice is muffled. Both voices are needed to deliver health care value through the SDM. Michael Porter constructed his health care value equation by placing "health outcomes that matter to patients" as the numerator and the costs of delivering those outcomes in the denominator. See Fig. 56.1 for a formula-derived overview of SDM.[8]

As an example of this, the literature surrounding this area tends to suggest that most individuals desire less care near

$$\text{Value} = \frac{\text{Health Outcomes that matter to Patients}}{\text{Cost of Delivering the Outcomes}}$$

• **Fig. 56.1** A formula-derived overview of shared decision-making.

[a]Virginia Mason, Seattle, Washington, Mayo Clinic, Rochester, Minnesota, University of Iowa, Iowa City, IA, UT-MD Anderson Cancer Center, Houston, TX, Cleveland Clinic, Cleveland, OH.

the end of life than is provided.[9] Ensuring that the individual's values and goals for life are driving decision-making is key in delivering just the right amount of care for that individual. When value, as defined by the individual, is the measure of success in health care, the constant pressure placed on clinicians by health care institutions with a volume-based (and arguably revenue-based) focus becomes less influential. However, the gap between volume and value remains an ever-present challenge for society.

What Elements Are Required to Make Shared Decision-Making Successful?

To make SDM successful, four factors must be present and accounted for. These are:

1. The ability to elicit an individual's values and goals for living.
2. Physician and multidisciplinary care teams with their expert knowledge of medical treatment options.
3. Time in an unhurried setting.
4. Communication skills training to enable physicians to comfortably and effectively carry out conversations about 1 and 2.

Another key in successful SDM that underpins all of the factors outlined above is mutual respect. Each party must believe the other has their best interest uppermost. It is this tenet that fosters trust between an individual and their physician. Again, turning to our senior author's (DLB) experience as a cancer patient, he believes that establishing trust is made possible by everyone on the health care team demonstrating empathy for the individual they are serving.

This is possible through the following steps:

Making eye contact upon greeting the individual
Taking the time to understand them as an individual, even if it means small talk
Opening your heart to their concerns, even if they seem trivial
Showing you care
Demonstrating real technical competence
Providing hope
Make sure they know that a follow up doesn't mean starting the process over.

These steps really just validate that they respect the patient as valuable, with unique characteristics and goals for care.

Building trust in the physician-patient relationship ensures that the phenomenon of "nudging" is not used to influence medical decision-making so that it favors the health system, rather than the needs of the individual. In brief, nudging, as described by popular authors Thaler and Sunstein, is "any aspect of the choice architecture that alters people's behavior in a predictable way without forbidding any options or significantly changing their economic incentives." To count as a mere nudge, the intervention must be easy and cheap to avoid. Nudges are not mandates. For example, placing fruit at eye level to encourage a healthy diet counts as a nudge. Banning junk food does not.[10]

If unfamiliar with "nudging in health care," the book, *Nudging Health: Health Law and Behavioral Economics*,[11] edited by three co-editors, Christopher T. Robertson, an associate dean and law-school professor at the University of Arizona; I. Glenn Cohen, professor at Harvard Law School and faculty director of the law school's Petrie-Flom Center; and Holly Fernandez Lynch, executive director of the Petrie-Flom Center, can be a guide. After the book's publication, the Wall Street Journal's Lisa Ward interviewed Professor Robertson, and it seems nudging is really the antithesis of SDM, as it subtly influences patient treatment choices.

Nudging in health care recalls the power imbalance present in the utilization of health care information. Without a balance in the relationship between a patient and their health care provider, nudging has the capacity to become coercive. If this nudging technique is widely and intentionally introduced into health care decision-making, it is likely that the impetus behind nudging may be designed around a public health policy framework. Ultimately, societal or government interests are primary and foregoing the best interests of the individual. This means that individual values and goals of the patient may not be the primary motivator for the designers of said nudge.[b] When public health policy issues are framed by utilitarian ethics, choices around the greater good seem clear, and yet utilitarian ethics are unsavory at the bedside, as they sacrifice the good of the individual in favor of the greater good. Nudging individual patients has the capacity to come perilously close to embracing utilitarianism at the bedside or in the clinic exam room. Nuances are often present in health care decision-making, and therefore as clinicians, we need to divest ourselves of biases that can inadvertently lead to nudging. In addition, we need to devote time to noncoercive framing of treatment options with our patients and their families.

Individual and Societal Advantages of Shared Decision-Making

1. Informed choice is more likely to be achieved

With respect to the advantages of SDM, the principle advantage is that when fully informed of their treatment options, the individual receives the care that achieves the outcomes most closely aligned with their stated values and beliefs. Primarily, being fully informed of options leads to the nuance between informed consent and informed choice, as discussed earlier in the chapter. When patients enter operating rooms, each day, across the world, a question is often asked: "where is the informed consent?" Far too often, the process of locating informed consent is as mechanical as the process of obtaining signed consent forms. Many involved in operating room care scurry around ensure there is a signature on the form. Far fewer are actually involved in ensuring

[b]Admittedly, Robertson and co-editors, included some chapters on the ethics of the nudge, and the lengthy forward by Cass Sunstein covers the ethical issue of nudging.

that the signed form reflects informed choice rather than simply consent.

Why has informed consent evolved to be so mechanical? In the early 20th century, court cases developed the principles that underpin informed consent.[12] Yet informed consent really came to the forefront of biomedical ethics following the Nuremberg trials after World War II.[12] Society, through the law, desired to recognize the basic right each of us has for self-determination over our own body. This is when a procedural quality became necessarily attached to informed consent. There was an explosion of innovative surgical and procedural techniques in the late 20th century that benefited many. However, as technical ability progressed, some of these procedures began to be associated with a good deal of futility. These individuals would have benefited from more robust informed choice discussions.

What individuals should expect from our health system and its physicians is more than a mechanical focus on informed consent. Rather, we should demand a more comprehensive understanding of our options, which builds upon the informed choice construct. In this setting, individuals learn all their options and what they might expect from acting on that range of options. Too often, clinicians do not want to slow the discussion in the exam room long enough to effectively elicit values and goals completely integrated into their decisions. However, our patients need to fully understand the choices available to them and what side effects accompany them. Truly understanding the frequency and impact of side effects associated with a procedure might produce quite different decisions for the individual.

Informed choice should be the foundation upon which the informed consent process exists and SDM is undertaken. Informed consent has a legalistic and often bureaucratic feel; informed choice produces understanding that is aligned with an individual's goals and values. This is the ideal for SDM.

2. Lower health care costs associated with end-of-life care

A further potential advantage of effective SDM is that health costs can be lowered for a society, especially at the end of life when delivery of nonbeneficial care can be prevented. Gibson and Singh have described this phenomenon effectively in their book, *The Treatment Trap*.[13] The team at Gundersen-Lutheran Health System in La Crosse, Wisconsin (USA) has shown that developing a means to obtain county-wide completion of advance directives to their local populous decreased health care costs by 25% during the last 2 years of life.[14,15] This decrease was possible with implementation of ACP countywide. One can further theorize that real-time informed SDM with patients and surrogate decision-makers might lower the cost saving even more. This must remain speculative at present.

We must also remain cognizant that although there is a correlation between ACP and lower health care costs, the key is that those patients with effective ACP receive the care they want, not more and not less.

How Does Advance Care Planning Fit Into Shared Decision-Making?

Incorporating ACP into SDM requires that individuals who will act as substitute decision-makers for an individual if decision-making capacity is lost are engaged in conversations about what that individual (patient) desires in approaches to their care at the end of life. It is clear that most individuals do not want intensive care as the end nears; rather, most want to die at home, or a home-like setting.

Effective ACP frames the contents of relevant documentation to reflect an individual's wishes. However, the single most important advance planning decision to be made is to designate the person who will serve as the substitute decision-maker, if you lack capacity at the end of life—even more crucially, that their elected substitute decision-maker understands the values and goals held by the individual that would guide medical decision-making. It is this person, in their role as a substitute decision-maker, who provides the much-needed context and interpretation of ACP documents. The substitute medical decision-maker in the United States is designated as an individual with durable power of attorney for health care. Since nuances in decision-making are difficult to capture with rapid advances in medicine, the selection of this substitute is important, since they alone may be able to incorporate their knowledge of the individual's wishes with facts that develop. They need to be able to reflect a model of SDM that mimics what the individual (patient) would have chosen had they maintained decision-making capacity.

Conclusion and Key Points

SDM has a sacred quality to its method. This is not new. Hippocrates reflected this when he said:

> It is more important to know what sort of a person has a disease than to know what sort of a disease a person has.[16]

Hippocrates was emphasizing a timeless truth that the individual needs to be the focus of decision-making in health care. This has not changed, yet the corporatization of health care (some frame it as the health care–industrial complex) has made keeping the individual uppermost more challenging. SDM requires each physician and health care professional to keep the patient fully informed about options, and to seek to fully understand and communicate the patient's values and goals to others caring for them to ensure that there is alignment in decision-making.

When we reflect on key points of SDM, we believe they are:

The individual's values and goals need to underpin medical decision-making, and a process needs to be established to record them accurately and meaningfully.

Informed choice, rather than informed consent, needs to be used in making decisions.

Time needs to be invested into SDM to make it effective.

Health system-centric nudging needs to be guarded against in decision-making.
Effective ACP is not possible outside the context of effective SDM.
SDM can be associated with lower costs at the end of life for care, but more importantly provides individuals with the opportunity to determine the end-of-life care that is most consistent with their values and goals.

References

1. Hartzband P, Groopman J. Medical Taylorism. *N Engl J Med.* 2016;374:106–108.
2. Orszag P. *Opportunities to increase efficiency in health care: Statement at the Health Reform Summit of the Committee on Finance, United States Senate.* Washington, D.C: Congressional Budget Office; 2008 June 16, 2008.
3. Sable-Smith B. Storytelling Helps Hospital Staff Discover the Person Within the Patient. 2019. Available at https://www.npr.org/sections/health-shots/2019/06/08/729351842/storytelling-helps-hospital-staff-discover-the-person-within-the-patient.
4. Elwyn G, Coulter A, Laitner S, Walker E, Watson P, Thomson R. Implementing shared decision making in the NHS. BMJ. 2010;341:c5146.
5. Singh Ospina N, Phillips KA, Rodriguez-Gutierrez R, et al. Eliciting the patient's agenda- secondary analysis of recorded clinical encounters. *J Gen Intern Med.* 2019;34:36–40.
6. Berry LL, Danaher TS, Beckham D, Awdish RLA, Mate KS. When patients and their families feel like hostages to health care. *Mayo Clin Proc.* 2017;92(9):1371–1381. https://www.mayoclinicproceedings.org/article/S0025-6196(17)30394-4/fulltext.
7. Johnson DW. *Market vs Medicine: America's Epic Fight for Better, Affordable Healthcare.* USA: Academy Press; 2016.
8. Porter ME, Teisberg EO. *Redefining Health Care: Creating Value-based Competition on Results.* Boston: Harvard Business School Press; 2016.
9. Committee on Approaching Death: Addressing Key End of Life Issues; Institute of Medicine. Dying in America: improving quality and honoring preferences near the end of life. Washington (DC): National Academies Press (US); March 19, 2015.
10. Thaler RH, Sunstein CR. *Nudge: Improving Decisions About Health, Wealth, and Happiness* 6. New Haven, CT: Yale University Press; 2008.
11. Cohen IG, Lynch HL, Robertson CT. *Nudging Health: Health Law and Behavioral Economics.* Baltimore: Johns Hopkins University Press; 2016.
12. Jonsen AR, Siegler M, Winslade WJ, *Clinical Ethics: A Practical Approach to Ethical Decisions in Clinical Medicine*, 8th ed: McGraw Hill; 2010. 50 [Schloendorff v Society of New York Hospital (NY 1914)].
13. Gibson R, Singh JP. *The Treatment Trap.* Chicago: Ivan R. Dee; 2010:185–195.
14. Hammes BJ, Rooney BL. Death and end of life planning in one Midwestern community. *Arch Int Med.* 1998;158:383–390.
15. MacGillis A. Debate Over End-of-Life Care Began in Small Midwestern Town. *Washington Post.* 2009. Available at http://www.washingtonpost.com/wp-dyn/content/article/2009/09/03/AR2009090303833.html?hpid=topnews&noredirect=on.
16. Hippocrates. It is more important to know what sort of person has a disease than to know what sort of disease a person has. Available at https://www.brainyquote.com/quotes/hippocrates_132701.

57

Ethics in Cancer Care Delivery—Do Not Resuscitate

MARIA ALMA RODRIGUEZ AND COLLEEN M. GALLAGHER

Introduction

The National Cancer Act, also known as the "War on Cancer" Act, was signed into law in 1971.[1] Thanks to the Act's support for ongoing cancer-related research, the number of cancer survivors in the United States has been progressively increasing. Today, nearly 70% of those diagnosed with cancer will be alive after 5 years. It is predicted that in 2026 there will be 20.3 million persons in the United States who have survived cancer.[2]

The cure rates for patients with localized cancer have steadily improved, and many patients with metastatic disease are now able to live for years with their malignancy as a chronic illness (e.g., prostate, breast, and colorectal cancers). Many unprecedented discoveries within the last few decades, most notably in the fields of molecular genetics, cancer cellular biology, and immunology, have led to the development of many novel anticancer therapeutic modalities, from molecular targeted agents to bioengineered cellular treatments. Due to these therapeutic advancements, cancer patients with advanced stage disease, once considered to be an imminently fatal diagnosis, are anticipated to have a longer life expectancy.

Thus for many patients, a diagnosis of cancer does not imply a prognosis of imminent death. Certain complex therapeutic interventions in cancer patients such as surgery, or rescue procedures such as cardiac resuscitation, are not necessarily futile or contraindicated under the appropriate circumstances. Evidence-based risk assessments, including anticipated prognosis of the malignancy, are therefore important considerations in treatment planning. To establish appropriate goals of care, these issues should be discussed with the patient and their family well in advance of acute care interventions.

In this chapter, we will review the evolving evidence on the outcomes of cardiac resuscitation as well as palliative surgery in cancer patients. We will also discuss the regulatory requirements for ensuring that patients' rights to do not resuscitate (DNR) decisions are safeguarded, and the ethical dilemmas that such decisions could generate for clinicians.

Cardiopulmonary Resuscitation

"Closed-chest cardiac massage" was introduced into medical practice in 1960 by Kowenhoven, Jude, and Knickerbocker when they published in the *Journal of the American Medical Association* a series of 20 selected patients who each had an in-hospital cardiac arrest (IHCA) event that was witnessed. Their cardiac arrest events were reversed through the application of a technique of external chest compressions, accompanied by external electrical shocks in some cases. Fourteen of the 20 patients survived and left the hospital, leading to their conclusion: "The use of this technique on 20 patients has given an over-all permanent survival rate of 70%. Anyone, anywhere, can now initiate cardiac resuscitative procedures. All that is needed are two hands."[3]

The application of this technique, which was renamed "cardiopulmonary resuscitation," or "CPR," quickly caught on, and began to be applied literally "anywhere," both within the setting of hospitals and in the community at large. Within a few years, outcomes in large series of cases were being published. One of the largest early in-hospital CPR case series included over 500 patients who had experienced an IHCA at the Royal Victoria Hospital in Montreal Canada.[4] Published in 1967, they defined resuscitation as successful if the patient survived 24 h or longer. By this definition, resuscitation was successful in 32% of the cases, but only half of these patients (15%) recovered completely and were discharged from the hospital. These results were vastly different from those of the original publication and, until recently, have remained remarkably constant across institutions and across time. In 1987, nearly 30 years after the original study, McGrath conducted an extensive literature review of published in-hospital CPR outcomes in studies that included at least 100 patients. Forty-two publications met his criteria and in total included 12,961 patients. The summary of results demonstrated essentially the same outcomes as the early Canadian series: on average, 15% of patients had long-term survival after in-hospital CPR.[5] An additional observation was that patients with coronary artery disease, who likely had developed an arrhythmia or asystole due to cardiac ischemia, were the group that most seemed to benefit from CPR.

Law, Regulations, and Guidelines

Rescuing patients from what previously had been fatal events, regardless that the numbers were relatively small, was considered clinically significant, and CPR became widely used. The results, however, were consistently showing that in the setting of a general hospital patient population, most patients with IHCA were not benefitting from CPR, and some who survived were left with late effects, including cognitive deficits and even in vegetative states of existence. Due to concern that CPR was not appropriate for all IHCA patients, the American Medical Association in 1974 issued a recommendation that patients be informed of risks/benefits of this procedure, and the patient's decision regarding their preferences for CPR (or "code status") be documented in the medical record. Nearly a decade later, in 1983, the President's Commission for the Study of Ethical Problems in Medicine published their opinion that consent for CPR be considered implicit, unless otherwise explicitly stated with an order issued to withhold CPR. This stemmed from a position of moral reasoning that a person would rationally want to be given an opportunity, even if small, that they would survive a cardiac arrest.[6] Cardiopulmonary resuscitation thus became the only intervention for which patient consent is required to NOT have the procedure, and an order must be written to NOT perform it.[7]

In 1988 the Joint Commission issued a standard that hospitals must have policies regarding CPR. The Patient Self-Determination Act of 1991 further required that hospitals receiving Medicare or Medicaid funds were to inform patients of their right to self-determination, including the right to refuse life support procedures such as CPR.[8] The American Society of Anesthesiologists (ASA), in alignment with the Patient Self-Determination Act, first published guidelines in 1993 stating that the practice of automatic perioperative suspension of DNR orders was in direct conflict with patients' rights to self-determination. This principle has been reiterated in more current updates to the ASA's guidelines, with support from the American College of Surgeons.

Intraoperative CPR Outcomes

Despite the time elapsed since the first publication of the ASA guidelines, there have been conflicting points of view with regard to the suspension of CPR intraoperatively, due to several considerations. First, some argue that because cardiopulmonary failure may be secondary to the processes of anesthesia itself, there is a responsibility to attempt to reverse this adverse effect. Second, the published outcomes of CPR in the intraoperative setting have been generally more successful than those in the hospital at large. An example of these outcomes is a published study by Keenan and Boyan in 1986 in which they focused on identifying anesthesia-related causes of cardiac arrest in over 100,000 anesthesia cases within a single institution in the United States.[9] They reported an incidence of 1.7 events/10,000 anesthesia cases. Among 27 anesthesia-related cardiac arrests, they identified that the most common cause of the arrests was failure to ventilate appropriately, followed by overdose of anesthetics, and third by hemodynamic instability. Forty-eight percent of the patients who had an intraoperative cardiac arrest were rescued and survived to hospital discharge.

Technological advances in intraoperative monitoring devices, newer anesthetics, and pain control agents, as well as checklists, have improved anesthesia-related safety in the operating room (OR) environment. Surgical procedures have also progressively moved to the ambulatory setting, making the hospital OR a selective environment in which the more complex and higher-risk surgical procedures are performed. Thus, the number and type of cardiac arrest events within the OR have also changed. A more recently published analysis of events in a Portuguese series of 122,289 anesthesia cases identified 62 cases of intraoperative cardiac arrests over a period of 7 years.[10] In this case series, the most common causes of the arrests were due to underlying comorbid conditions, and not the anesthesia itself. The incidence of anesthesia-specific related events was 0.74/10,000 anesthesia cases. The identified risk factors for a cardiac arrest were ASA PS score higher than 3, underlying cardiac disease, and use of vasopressors. Nine cases were attributable to the anesthesia process itself. All nine survived the arrest and left the hospital, while 43% of the 62 patients who had an intraoperative cardiac arrest survived to discharge. Thus the overall survival expectation from intraoperative CPR seems to be holding above 40%, and in this particular series all anesthesia related cardiac arrest events were reversible.

Outcomes of CPR in Cancer Patients

Until recently, very little was known about the outcomes of CPR in cancer patients who had experienced an IHCA, other than studies stating that the diagnosis of cancer portended a poor outcome, with a predominant focus on patients with advanced cancer. A recently published multi-institutional study compared survival outcomes post-CPR for IHCA in patients with a diagnosis of cancer that is not metastatic versus a propensity-matched cohort of patients without cancer.[11] The data source is the National Inpatient Sample dataset, compiled by the Agency for Healthcare Research and Quality (AHRQ). The data for this analysis is from 2003 to 2014, with a total of nearly 2 million hospitalizations complicated by an IHCA event. Of these, 112,926 occurred in patients with a history of cancer, not metastatic. Overall the CPR to discharge survival was better for the noncancer cohort (46%) compared to the nonmetastatic cancer patients (31%), even when controlling for general prognosis and comorbid conditions. Of note is that from 2003 to 2014 the overall survival to discharge improved for both the cancer patients and their matched cohort: from 23% to 31% in the cancer cohort and from 40% to 46% in the noncancer cohort. These survival to discharge rates for CPR are thus significantly higher than published in the latter decades of the 1900s.

Additionally, the study compared postarrest procedure utilization for each of these groups and determined that the cancer cohort statistically was less likely to receive postarrest procedures, such as coronary angiography, percutaneous coronary intervention, or targeted temperature management. The authors hypothesize that the less intense post event management of the cancer cohort contributed to the lower survival outcome and imply that biases may exist against implementing aggressive postarrest management in those with a cancer history, even though there was a potentially good cancer prognosis in most cases. They conclude: "Additional research is needed to clarify the role of patient-physician perceptions of cancer diagnosis and selective applications of post-resuscitation care."

A second recent study focused on the post-cardiac arrest CPR outcomes of patients with advanced (metastatic) cancer.[12] The data source for this analysis was similarly a large database, the Get With The Guidelines Resuscitation registry. The data encompassed the time period of April 2006 to June 2010, included 369 hospitals, and 47,157 adult patients with an IHCA. Of these, 6585 IHCA events occurred in patients with advanced cancer, and 1143 of these in turn occurred in cancer patients who were hospitalized for a surgical intervention (177 were cardiac surgeries). Independent of other risk factors, the survival to discharge for patients with advanced cancer was much lower than those without cancer (7.4% vs. 13.4%). The study did not report on the outcomes of the surgical subset of advanced stage cancer patients.

Similarly to the nonmetastatic cancer patients, the postarrest care for the metastatic cancer patient cohort was significantly less intense, with a higher rate of DNR orders within 48 h of the arrest compared to the noncancer patients. Of note, the authors of this study comment that despite the low rate of survival to hospital discharge for the advanced cancer patient group, in their opinion this rate is not so low as to be considered futile and merits discussion in setting goals of care for patients with advanced cancer. However, compared with patients with nonmetastatic cancer, and noncancer patients, the CPR to discharge survival rate for patients with disseminated cancer is clearly very low (Table 57.1).

Outcomes of Palliative and Rescue Surgery in Cancer Patients

For centuries, surgery has been the primary intervention for many types of malignancies. It continues to be a primary and potentially curative treatment modality for most solid tumor malignancies presenting with localized or limited stages of disease, whether as a single treatment strategy or in combination with chemotherapy and/or radiation. While the benefit of surgery in those circumstances is not questioned, the benefit of surgical interventions for patients with disseminated (metastatic) disease has been controversial. In many instances, surgery can have significant benefit in palliating symptoms, improving quality of life, and even prolonging survival in these patients. On the other hand, there are unique and higher risks of morbidity and mortality associated with surgery in patients with metastatic cancer, and therefore assessing risk/benefit is a critical element of treatment planning.

The National Surgical Quality Improvement Program database of the American College of Surgeons (ACS NSQIP) has made it possible to analyze outcomes in large cohorts of patients across multiple institutions. Thus, risk analysis nomograms have been published for many surgical procedures. Tseng et al. formulated a predictive nomogram of morbidity and mortality specifically for patients with disseminated cancers who undergo surgery.[13] The authors queried the ACS NSQIP database from 2005 to 2007 and identified 7447 patients with disseminated malignancy diagnoses who had undergone surgery. The overall morbidity and mortality in this cohort of patients were 28.3% and 8.9%, respectively. They analyzed in total 133 factors, including preoperative, intraoperative, demographic, postoperative, as well as surgical type factors for their significance in the risk of morbidity and mortality and identified 14 factors as significant for risk: DNR status prior to procedure, weight loss >10% of body weight, dyspnea at rest, functional dependence, the presence of ascites, chronic steroid use, active sepsis, elevated serum creatinine, low serum albumin, high white cell count, low hematocrit, surgical acuity (emergent procedures), type of procedure, and patients' age. These factors are ranked and are weighted by point scores in the nomogram, and when totaled for the individual patient, a percentage risk can be calculated for that unique individual. While it is complex given the number of risk factors that are taken into account, the nomogram can help assess relative risk for an individual patient in an objective manner, and support treatment decisions.

TABLE 57.1 CPR to Discharge Survival for Patients with Inpatient Hospital Cardiac Arrest (IHCA)

Location	Patients without Cancer	Patients with Disseminated Cancer	Patients with Nondisseminated Cancer
Hospital	15%–46%[5,11,12]	<10%[12]	31%[11]
Operating room	43%–48%[9,10]	-	-

A more recent outcomes analysis in a larger ACS NSQIP database cohort of 21,755 patients with disseminated malignancies, who had a surgical procedure from 2006 to 2010, noted that more than half of all the surgeries (54%) were either bowel resections or other type of gastrointestinal procedures, and an additional 10% were multivisceral resections.[14] The authors examined the trends of morbidity and mortality across the 5-year period of the analysis and identified improvements in the outcomes: morbidity decreased from 33.7% to 26.6%, and mortality decreased from 10.4% to 9.3%. They attributed the improvements to fewer emergency procedures, fewer patients with acute sepsis, as well as improvements in presurgery performance status and body weight.

Another situation to consider is that of patients who are undergoing chemotherapy that can lead to leukopenia and while under treatment, develop acute complications that require surgical rescue. A prior study looking at the risks of emergency surgery in 956 cancer patients (ACS NSQIP database, 2005–2008) who had received chemotherapy within 30 days of surgery showed an increased risk of morbidity and mortality for the cancer patients when compared to a matched noncancer cohort. The morbidity risks were 44% vs. 39%, and mortality risk 22.4% vs. 10.3%, respectively[15] (Table 57.2). Thus, unless surgery is absolutely emergent, medical management of neutropenic patients until counts are recovered should be considered. If surgery must be performed, the patients and their families or surrogates should be aware of the relatively high morbidity and mortality risk of such procedures.

Outcomes of Patients with DNR Orders

The presence of a DNR order prior to surgery is a recognized risk factor for less favorable outcomes in both cancer and noncancer patients. This has been documented across various surgical specialties, regardless of whether the surgical procedures are emergent or elective.[16–19] A speculative explanation is that this may be because the DNR status designates a very serious illness and thus is a surrogate marker for impending death. While this may be true for some patients, there is evidence in the literature of physician bias against aggressive treatment for patients with DNR status. Based on comparative outcomes analyses of matched clinical risk cohorts of elderly patients undergoing emergency surgery, comparing those "with" to those "without DNR" status, there is a demonstrated higher postsurgical failure to rescue the DNR patients (56.7%) versus those without DNR orders (41.4%).[16] Similar results were previously shown in a large cohort of more than 14,000 Medicare patients hospitalized for medical conditions. Despite adjusting for clinical risk factors, those with DNR status had a much higher mortality than those without DNR status (40% vs. 9%). The authors concluded at that time that further studies were needed to assess whether the patients' loss of "willingness to live" or the providers' withholding "aggressive care" were factors that could explain the differences.[20]

TABLE 57.2 Surgical Morbidity and Mortality in Cancer Patients: Palliative or Rescue Procedures

Type of Surgery	Overall Morbidity	Overall Mortality
Palliative Surgery		
Disseminated cancer[13]	28%	10%
Disseminated cancer[14]	27%	9%
Emergency Rescue Surgery		
Chemotherapy <30 days[15]	44%	22%
Noncancer cohort[15]	39%	10%

It is still not known whether the generally observed higher mortality in DNR status patients, despite adjusted risk factors, is driven by the patients' losing the will to live, or by providers shifting goals of treatment to comfort care. Failure to rescue could be due to providers' misunderstanding of DNR orders. A DNR order is not intended to withhold appropriate medical or surgical interventions for patients. A DNR order is active only when a person becomes unresponsive and has a cardiac arrest, at which time the order requires that CPR be withheld.[7] This order has no meaning or value in any condition other than in cardiac arrest. All other interventions require the same level of discussion and decision-making as would be applicable to any persons without a DNR order, taking all other relevant and appropriate clinical parameters into the decision process.

Potential biases can be further complicated in the cancer population by the assumption that a diagnosis of any cancer carries a dire prognosis. As reported in the recent analyses of post-IHCA care, nonmetastatic cancer patients receive statistically less diagnostic and supportive measures after a cardiac arrest compared to noncancer patients.[11] As we have previously noted, many cancer survivors, even some groups with metastatic disease, today have significantly longer life expectancy related to their cancer diagnosis, and thus goals of care discussions are necessary in each case. It is interesting, however, that in the two independent large cohort analyses of patients with disseminated malignancy performed by Tseng et al. and Bateni et al., only a very small percentage of patients had DNR status (3% and 2.4% respectively).[13,14] These numbers are not much different than those reported in noncancer cohorts from the ACS NSQIP database, in which DNR status reports have ranged from 0.5% to 4.2%.[16] This implies that despite having a serious illness, patients with disseminated cancer wish and hope for care that will prolong their life and relieve their suffering, and thus open discussions of risk/benefit of surgical interventions are needed so that patients can make an informed decision regarding the appropriateness of DNR status.

Ethical Considerations on Sustaining or Withholding DNR Status During Palliative Surgical Procedures

Patients who require surgical procedures for palliative purposes are looking to improve their quality of life. There is the underlying expectation that consenting to the procedure will enhance their life experience while they are dying. The controversy lies in the possibility of being able to provide a palliative benefit from surgical procedures when the patient refuses CPR, versus the professional obligation of sustaining the patient's life through surgery. Can a patient with the presumed capacity for understanding the risks and benefits of surgery make the autonomous decision of continuing their DNR status during a procedure? Does a perioperative DNR interfere with the ability of the surgeon and anesthesiologist to perform their professional duties to the best of their capabilities? What are the possibilities to find a consensus between the patient's wishes and the physicians' responsibilities?

Among the ethical principles to apply here are respect for persons, professional duty, and justice based on agreed upon expectations. Those that argue in favor of respecting the patient's DNR status generally allude to the patients' autonomy and the physicians' duty of beneficence. The physician has a duty to provide appropriate treatment options that have the possibility of benefiting the patient. The physician's views of physical and psychosocial benefits should be balanced with the patient's view of their own goals of care. This can be challenging in the palliative surgical setting. The sought-after benefit by the patient is quality of life, and not necessarily prolongation of life, even if this could be a byproduct of the surgical procedure. Thus respecting the patient's goals in seeking care means honoring their wish to remain in DNR status.

The argument on the side of not sustaining the DNR status has also been based on the principle of beneficence, meaning that if there is an intervention that will do "good" for the patient, then the physician should provide such a procedure. Some would say the basic nature of medicine is to preserve life at all cost, thus creating the duty of the physician to do resuscitation if needed during surgery. However, patients may refuse any treatment, even if it is part of standard medical practice and considered the "best" for the patient. Smith wrote that the right to refuse treatment is not diminished if the treatment is required to save the individual's life, and this right of refusal is essentially inalienable.[21] Thus if a patient refuses CPR, then CPR may not be given. He then equates performing a surgery on a patient with a DNR order the same as surgery for a Jehovah's Witness patient. One may die if a cardiac arrest occurs and the other may die if there is significant blood loss. "It is the patient who accepts the risks and it is the patient who suffers the consequences of the decision." Furthermore, he states that since operating on a Jehoore, he states that since operating on a Jehovah's Witness patient is a common and acceptable medical practice, then operating on a patient with a DNR order should also be commonplace and acceptable.

Those that argue in favor of withholding the DNR status also question the patients' understanding of intraoperative CPR and thus their ability to truly exercise an informed decision. They also raise their concerns for potential institutional, professional, and moral burdens on physicians for "allowing" perioperative deaths in patients with DNRs. Layon and Dirk suggest that patients and their surrogates must understand the nature of the possible risks and complications of both surgery and anesthesia.[22] They state that by doing so, and having the patient rescind the perioperative DNR, it will allow the medical team to access all modalities of therapy to preserve the patient's life. This arises from the concept that if a patient is requesting a procedure, their intention is not to die during the surgery. Then, it will be in the best interests of the patient to perform CPR in the case of a cardiac arrest, thus honoring the duty of beneficence. However, as Margolis et al. state, the decision to refuse intraoperative resuscitation does not necessarily exclude maximal therapeutic efforts for complications short of complete cardiac or respiratory arrest and could conceivably allow for therapies for surgical or anesthesia complications.[23] The goal then is to make sure that patient and physician have a conversation in which consent is truly informed and the expectations are agreed upon. It is possible to agree to not provide CPR if the patient understands the procedure's potential risks and benefits.

For more than 25 years, many authors have written in favor of sustaining perioperative DNRs. In 1993 the ASA formulated their "Ethical Guidelines for the Anesthesia Care of Patients and Do Not Resuscitate Orders or Other Directives that Limit Treatment." This guideline was approved in 2001, amended in 2013, and reaffirmed in 2018. The ASA guidelines respect informed suspension of DNR orders during the perioperative period if explicitly discussed with the patient or surrogate. The policy also allows airway management and other treatment options, including honoring perioperative DNR orders if the patient so states. Nonetheless, it is difficult for all parties involved when DNR patients undergo procedures, and careful documentation of advance care planning (ACP) discussions must be implemented in order to ensure that the physicians not suffer professional harm in the case of perioperative deaths.

Advance Care Planning—Communicating and Defining Goals of Care

ACP is often mistakenly viewed as equivalent to completing the advance directive documentation or that it is only about end-of-life care. While completing the documents may be part of the process for some patients, which we encourage, it is not the same. ACP is communication with the purpose of establishing what care is to be provided based on the medical possibilities and on the values, wishes, and goals of the patient related to their medical care. It is a conversation in which the physician explains current condition, what has changed, what is possible, risks and benefits for each possibility, and seeks to understand the patient's goals for their care. It is a conversation in which the patient expresses their goals, asks questions, and understands what the physician is able and not able to provide. In other words, it is defining the goals of care (Table 57.3).

TABLE 57.3 **Elements of Advance Care Planning (ACP) Discussions**

Major Components of ACP	Elements of the Discussion	When to Have Discussion
Clinical goals of care	Discuss with the patient and family the cancer stage, treatment options, risks and benefits of the treatments, and realistic outcome expectations. Clarify goals of care: potential for cure, or life prolongation (meaningful prolongation is when anticipated treatment benefit is in terms of months to years of life) versus symptom control and palliation.	At onset of treatment, and at any time that disease process changes. Document the discussions, and who was present.
ACP documents/ surrogate designation	Request copies of any documents the patient may already have, and upload to the health record; educate patient on ACP documents—Medical Power of Attorney, Advance Directives/Living Wills—and their benefit in clarifying for the medical team the patient's wishes, including surrogate designations.	At onset of treatment, and at any time that disease process changes; ask if any updates or changes to the documents have been made, and add new forms to the health record. Elicit surrogate designation with the simple question: "Who do you wish to speak on your behalf if you were not able to talk to your doctors?"
Personal values	Inquire about the patient's preferences (yes/no) for treatments that may prolong life but have low probability of restoring quality of life, particularly for patients with disseminated malignancy such as CPR, ICU ventilation support, or dialysis; discuss risks of morbidity and mortality.	At any time that high risk treatments with potential for mortality or impaired quality of life are anticipated, or if the patient's life expectancy from the malignancy or other underlying comorbid illness is anticipated to be a year or less.

ACP is not solely about end-of-life care. It should be performed each time the care of the patient needs to change because of their medical condition or a change in the patient's goals/wishes. This fluid discussion of goals of care facilitates a person-centered care allowing both physicians and surrogates to understand the patient's wishes.

In the case of cancer patients, the surgeon and anesthesiologist usually are not the first physicians to discuss a DNR order. If a patient has had that discussion with their primary physician or oncologist and determined that CPR does not fit their goals for medical care outside of surgery, then the surgeon and anesthesiologist need to discuss the goals of the procedure together with the patient and together determine if CPR fits the goals during the procedure. It would be of benefit for members of the surgery-anesthesia team to have a clinic consult with the patient dedicated to this conversation, allowing for nonpressurized goal/values discussions with ample time prior to the procedure. This coordinated care setting should provide the necessary information for a patient to make informed decisions regarding interventions of care, including intraoperative CPR (Fig. 57.1).

Bires et al. showed that patients preferred that their physicians initiate the conversation.[24] In general, physicians indicated a moderate-to-high self-assessment of knowledge, preparedness, and comfort discussing ACP or advance directives. However, there was an apparent gap between perceived abilities versus their actual clinical practices. Clinicians often shy away from the complex process of ACP. Nonetheless, it is within the physician's duty of beneficence toward their patients to initiate these conversations and provide the tools necessary for the patient to exercise truly autonomous decisions. Epstein et al. have developed a Person-Centered Oncologic Care and Choices (P-COCC) communication program, as a novel ACP intervention that combines a patient values interview with an informational care goals video. This approach assists cancer patients and their families to formulate questions for their physicians about disease prognosis, and also introduces information about advance directives and how patients can participate in informed decisions about their care.[25]

Burkle and colleagues surveyed 500 patients undergoing a surgical procedure, as well as 384 physicians (anesthesiologists, surgeons, and internists), regarding their attitudes about perioperative DNR orders being suspended or maintained.[26] A significant number of surgeons (38%) felt that DNR orders should be automatically suspended, while only a minority of anesthesiologists favored automatic suspension of DNR orders (18%). The results revealed, however, that the overwhelming majority (92%) of the patients who participated in the survey believed the physicians involved in the surgical procedure should have a discussion with the patient regarding DNR before suspending DNR orders. In addition, more than half of the patients (57%) were willing to suspend their DNR orders if the physicians discussed and explained why the orders should be suspended. The first step of ACP therefore is the clinicians' willingness to embrace the "necessary discomfort" of initiating important conversations with their patients, who are willing to listen, and expect their clinicians to initiate the conversations.

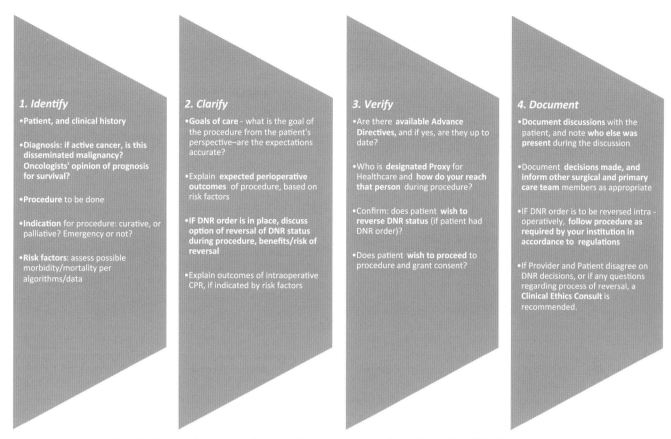

1. Identify
•Patient, and clinical history
•Diagnosis: if active cancer, is this disseminated malignancy? Oncologists' opinion of prognosis for survival?
•Procedure to be done
•Indication for procedure: curative, or palliative? Emergency or not?
•Risk factors: assess possible morbidity/mortality per algorithms/data
2. Clarify
•Goals of care - what is the goal of the procedure from the patient's perspective–are the expectations accurate?
•Explain expected perioperative outcomes of procedure, based on risk factors
•IF DNR order is in place, discuss option of reversal of DNR status during procedure, benefits/risk of reversal
•Explain outcomes of intraoperative CPR, if indicated by risk factors
3. Verify
•Are there available Advance Directives, and if yes, are they up to date?
•Who is designated Proxy for Healthcare and how do your reach that person during procedure?
•Confirm: does patient wish to reverse DNR status (if patient had DNR order)?
•Does patient wish to proceed to procedure and grant consent?
4. Document
•Document discussions with the patient, and note who else was present during the discussion
•Document decisions made, and inform other surgical and primary care team members as appropriate
•IF DNR order is to be reversed intra - operatively, follow procedure as required by your institution in accordance to regulations
•If Provider and Patient disagree on DNR decisions, or if any questions regarding process of reversal, a Clinical Ethics Consult is recommended.

• **Fig. 57.1** Process for perioperative care planning and goals of care discussion. *CPR*, Cardiopulmonary resuscitation; *DNR*, do not resuscitate.

There is certainly a need for further research to find the approaches that could aid both the physicians and patients in this process. However, it should not be overlooked that a deeply humanistic issue such as ACP requires a more humane than technical approach. In the end, the basic trust of the patient-physician relationship and compassionate communication are the key elements needed for a successfully fluid ACP process.

Conclusion

A diagnosis of cancer today does not necessarily portend a fatal illness. Nearly 70% of those diagnosed with cancer will be alive 5 years past their diagnosis. Thus decisions regarding appropriateness of interventions in cancer patients, such as surgery, or rescue interventions, such as CPR, should be considered with this information in mind. All patients, whether they have a diagnosis of cancer or not, have the right to self-determination under our laws. However, a patient's decision for a DNR status does not mean foregoing appropriate medical care. It simply means they do not wish to be resuscitated in the event of a cardiac arrest. All other care alternatives, outside of CPR, thus should be considered and applied, as appropriate. In the case of patients who have a DNR and need surgery, it is recommended that the patients and their families be fully informed of the surgical and anesthesia risks, and that they be made aware of the option of reversal of DNR in the intraoperative setting. The literature supports the reversal of the patient's DNR choice if the clinicians explain to them why it is appropriate, or will accept intermediate rescue procedures, such as cardiac medications or vasopressors. In the event that they do not wish to reverse their DNR choice, the ASA guidelines and ethical principles support honoring the patient's wishes. Clear and complete documentation of what was discussed and who witnessed the discussions is strongly recommended.

References

1. The National Cancer Act of 1971 [Public Law 92–218, 92ND Congress, S. 1828], Dec. 23, 1971. Available at Cancer.gov.
2. National Cancer Institute. Sureveillance Epidemiology, and End Results Program. Cancer Stat Facts. 2021. https://seer.cancer.gov>about-cancer>understanding> statistics. Viewed 10/26/2021.
3. Kowenhoven WB, Jude JR, Knickerbocker GG. Closed-chest cardiac massage. *JAMA*. 1960;173:1064–1067.
4. Johnson AL, Tanser PH, Ulan RA, Wood TE. Results of cardiac resuscitation in 552 patients. *Am J Cardiol*. 1967;20:831–835.
5. McGrath RB. In-house cardiopulmonary resuscitation—after a quarter of a century. *Ann Emerg Med*. 1987;16(12):1365–1368.

6. President's Commission for the Study of Ethical Problems in Medicine and Biomedical and Behavioral Research. *Deciding to Forego Life-Sustaining Treatment: Ethical, Medical, and Legal Issues in Treatment Decisions*: Government Printing Office; 1983.
7. Loertshcer L, Reed DA, Bannon MP, Mueller PS. Cardiopulmonary resuscitation and do-not-resuscitate orders: a guide for clinicians. *Am J Med.* 2010;123(1):4–9.
8. The Patient Self-Determination Act: Omnibus Budget Reconciliation Act of 1990. Title IV, Section 4206. *Congressional Record.* 1990;136:H12456–H124567 Oct. 26.
9. Keenan RL, Boyan CP. Cardiac Arrest due to anesthesia: a study of incidence and causes. *JAMA.* 1985;253(16):2373–2377.
10. Sobriera-Fernandes D, Teixeira L, Lemos TS, et al. Perioperative cardiac arrests—a subanalysis of the anesthesia-related cardiac arrests and associated mortality. *J Clin Anesth.* 2018; 50:78–90.
11. Guha A, Buck B, Biersmith M, et al. Contemporary impacts of a cancer diagnosis on survival following in-hospital cardiac arrest. *Resuscitation.* 2019;142:30–37.
12. Bruckel JT, Wong SL, Chang PS, Bradley SM, Nallamothu BK. Patterns of resuscitation care and survival after in-hospital cardiac arrest in patients with advanced cancer. *J Oncol Pract.* 2017;13(10):e821–e830.
13. Tseng WH, Yang X, Wang H, et al. Nomogram to predict risk of 30-day morbidity and mortality for patients with disseminated malignancy undergoing surgical intervention. *Ann Surg.* 2011;254:333–338.
14. Bateni SB, Meyers FJ, Bold RJ, Canter RJ. Current perioperative outcomes for patients with disseminated cancer. *J Surg Res.* 2015;197(1):118–125.
15. Sullivan M, Roman SA, Sosa JA. Does chemotherapy prior to emergency surgery affect patient outcomes? Examination of 1912 patients. *Ann Surg Oncol.* 2012;19(1):11–18.
16. Scarborough T, Pappas TN. The effect of do-not-resuscitate status of postoperative mortality in the elderly following emergency surgery. *Adv Surg.* 2013;47:213–225.
17. Jawa RS, Shapiro MJ, McCormack JE, Huang EC, Rutigliano DN, Vosswinkel JA. Preadmission Do Not Resuscitate advanced directive is associated with adverse outcomes following acute traumatic injury. *Am J Surg.* 2015;210:814–821.
18. Siracuse JJ, Jones DW, Meltzer EC, et al. Impact of "Do Not Resuscitate" status on the outcome of major vascular surgical procedures. *Ann Vasc Surg.* 2015;29(7):1339–1345.
19. Brovman EY, Walsh EC, Burton BN, et al. Postoperative outcomes in patients with a do-not-resuscitate (DNR) order undergoing elective procedures. *J Clin Anesth.* 2018;48:81–88.
20. Wenger NS, Pearson ML, Desmond KA, Brook RH, Kahn KL. outcomes of patients with do-not-resuscitate orders. *Arch Intern Med.* 1995;155:2063–2068.
21. Smith AL. DNR in the OR. *Clin Ethics Rep.* 1994;8(4):1–8.
22. Layon AJ, Dirk L. Resuscitation and DNR: ethical aspects for anaesthetists. *Can J Anaesth.* 1995;42(2):134–140.
23. Margolis JO, McGrath BJ, Kussin PS, Schwinn DA. Do Not Resuscitate (DNR) orders during surgery: ethical foundations for institutional policies in the United States. *Anesth Analg.* 1995;80:806–809.
24. Bires JL, Franklin EF, Nichols HM, Cagle JG. Advance care planning communication: oncology patients and providers voice their perspectives. *J Canc Educ.* 2018;33:1140–1147.
25. Epstein AS, O'Reilly EM, Shuk E, et al. A Randomized trial of acceptability and effects of values-based advance care planning in outpatient oncology: person-centered oncologic care and choices. *J Pain Symptom Manage.* 2018;56(2):169–177.
26. Burkle CM, Swetz KM, Armstrong MH, Keegan MT. Patient and doctor attitudes and beliefs concerning perioperative do not resuscitate orders: anesthesiologists' growing compliance with patient autonomy and self determination guidelines. *BMC Anesthesiol.* 2013;13:2.

58

Economics of Cancer Care Delivery: Opportunities and Challenges

RONALD S. WALTERS

Introduction

Cancer is an intensely emotional disease that places much of one's life in jeopardy.

The total cost of cancer care increased from $124 billion in 2010 to at least an estimated $206 billion in 2020.

Some articles quote at least 42% of cancer patients deplete their life savings within 2 years of a cancer diagnosis.

Cancer patients file for bankruptcy at least 2.6 times more frequently than those without cancer.

Financial toxicity correlates with a reduced life expectancy.

Economics of Cancer Care, 2019

Hearing the words "you have cancer" is extremely distressing and immediately raises a number of concerns about life expectancy, functional status, income and employment, family relationships, and the impact of treatments on each of these.[1] Multiple surveys have documented the classic response mechanisms of denial, anger, bargaining, and sadness, but immediate practical considerations, such as impact on job, income, bills, and quality of life, dominate early conversations. Increasingly, another serious consideration is coming to the forefront—that of the costs of care, especially the self-borne ones. This tends to arise once the treatment plan is formulated, as the direct line of association crystallizes between the diagnosis and the plan of action. It is also highly dependent on the presence or absence of insurance benefits, the details of those benefits, and how well they are understood by the patient. A continuous and rapid rise over the last few years of these patient-borne costs, which are projected to persist and increase over an indeterminate period of time, not only threatens one's ability to pay for treatment but also the access to such treatment.[2] As the article by Paul points out, once the words "you have cancer" are spoken, everything that contributes to a delay in getting to a treatment plan, or at least information about the diagnosis, becomes high priority for most individuals. In this article, at least one-third to one-half of patients in Sydney Australia reported treatment-phase dependent concerns about access to treatment, especially those of lower socioeconomic status, those who were younger, and those born outside of Australia. The same concerns are true in the United States, especially in rural areas, for which insurance coverage is a contributing factor.[3] In rural areas, Medicare is the predominant insurance for eligible individuals, and having no insurance has decreased slightly to approximately 15% to 25%. Initiation of the treatment itself, when disease is evaluable, provides a temporary emotional buffer to the costs of treatment, as it at least contributes subjective data about the imputed benefit-to-cost ratio. This is much more nebulous when the treatments are purposed to prevent recurrence, as the benefit/cost ratio is much more statistical in nature, rather than directly evaluable. Once treatment is concluded, as the proportion of survivors continues to increase (a positive outcome), long-term side effects of care will continue to escalate, leading to an increase in chronic noncancer but treatment-related financial and medical issues.[4,5] The Kline article proposed a risk-based model to optimize post-treatment care to the site most clinically appropriate for that care, and potentially delivered at a lower cost, such as the active incorporation of a primary care provider into the model. Future employment and insurability issues for those who have had cancer continue and are subject to local, regional, and federal regulatory changes. The looming threat of recurrence likely never disappears but certainly remains an emotional burden for a long time and is very disease dependent. Moreover, some treatments may actually predispose individuals to other cancers, further increasing long-term concerns. Adolescents who have survived cancer carry this burden for the rest of their lives. While this is shared with diseases such as diabetes, heart disease, chronic lung disease, and arthritis, the rapid increase in the costs associated with cancer has recently received much attention.

Cost of Treatments

Magnitude of the Issue

In any discussion about costs, one must decide whether the focus is on total societal costs of care (usually difficult to measure), payer costs (usually easiest to measure as the payments to providers and applicable to those patients with some sort of coverage), provider costs (extremely variable, unique to the provider, and usually estimated from charges to reimbursement), patient-borne costs (relevant to insured and uninsured patients), and those costs not captured by classical reimbursement systems, such as travel expenses and out-of-pocket expenditures (very difficult to capture). Nonetheless, when reported, and regardless of the above variable definitions, all have shown a significant increase in cancer costs, especially over the last decade,[6] from $124.57 billion in 2010 to between $186.59 billion and $206.59 billion estimated for 2020. These estimates are based on both incidence and survival trends. There is no evidence that the increase in costs will change in the near future, and most projections are that the rate of increase will also increase with the explosion of new technology and drugs. The cost associated with the initial year of treatment has grown by 19.4% in that time frame, while the cost in the last year of life has grown by 28.3%. The increasing role of continuing care (between the two endpoints) is shown by an increase of 31.6% over the same 10-year period. Not only is cancer being treated more effectively initially, it is increasingly a chronic disease with treatment extended over a longer period of time (similar to the diseases above). Furthermore, relapses that occur between the initial and last year of life have increasing options available to bring the disease back under control, contributing to longer survival after relapse. The average initial year of cancer treatment varies by disease from $5000 for most confined melanomas to $115,000 for brain tumors, ranging from a few hundred dollars a year to $11,000 for pancreatic cancer but these are averages and obviously very stage dependent. However, this group of costs is most likely to continue to increase as the periods of "maintenance" therapy expand for most cancers. The last year of life also varies by disease but ranges from $56,000 for melanoma to $135,000 for brain tumors. Much of this care is palliative in nature, some in intensive care units, and a majority in the hospital. Efforts to reduce these latter figures have thus far been unsuccessful, despite the increase in palliative care units and hospice locations. End-of-life care remains a considerable cultural issue and is relatively unique to the United States.[7]

Given the lag in tabulation, most of the cited data are either 5–10 years old or rely on projections based on newer treatments. In a recent study released by the American Association of Cancer Research (AACR), projections are for cancer costs of approximately $450 billion by 2030, worldwide.[8] Long-term data and even projections, by their very nature, are becoming subject to extreme variation and based on the utilization of current and newly released treatments, research developments and expectations of results, and population demographics. It is likely that even this projection will be refined long before that date to a much larger number. Medicare, Medicaid, and private payers provide some of the most recent expenditure data available and are generally searchable on the web pages of The National Cancer Institute and the American Cancer Society.

Medically Induced Bankruptcy

At an alarming rate, due to the cost of treatments and the distress caused by the rising cost of treatments, the number of people who file for a subsequent bankruptcy is increasing.[9,10] A recent article published in the *American Journal of Medicine* found that 42.5% of patients lost their entire life savings within 2 years of diagnosis.[9] Total financial insolvency extended to 38.2% over 4 years. Fifty-seven percent of the patients in the study were Medicare and 34% had private insurance. Medicaid accounted for only 2% of the population, for whom the results would be even more dramatic. Cancer patients are 2.65 times more likely to file for bankruptcy than those without cancer. Estimating expected costs before the initiation of treatment remains an imprecise art, based on the experience of others or on the averages of a population, and subject to unexpected events during treatment. Historically, physicians have not felt comfortable about having financial discussions with patients, mostly in fear that the perception would be that doctors were basing recommendations on costs. In most locations, this role has been delegated to financial advisors after a specific treatment recommendation has been offered. This makes it difficult for financial advisors to discuss other options on a comparative basis. The American Society of Clinical Oncology has been wrestling with this issue for over a decade and, at an annual meeting in 2018, noted the continuing barriers to a difficult situation. Frequently, costs become an issue long after anything can be done to reduce them or inform decision-making.

To compound the issue, financial insolvency has been shown to be a risk predictor for early mortality among patients with cancer[10] according to Ramsey, with a hazard ratio of 1.79. The endless circle of high costs, insolvency, inability to continue care, and worse outcomes is an unfortunate reality and story repeated over and over. It has become an all-to-frequent newspaper, magazine, or television article.

Besides the sheer cost of treatments, this is also a reflection of changing structures in the way cancer care is paid for. Cancer is not specifically treated any differently than other major medical illnesses; however, due to its escalating costs, it has drawn the attention of preexisting condition legislation, targeted preauthorization requirements, and coverage policies for newer treatments. Changing insurance plans with a history of cancer treatment or current treatment is difficult. With the very conscious effort to shift costs to the beneficiaries, regardless of plan, patients with cancer tend to be hit by coinsurance and out-of-pocket requirements very rapidly. As alluring as high-deductible plans can be with a lower premium, it is not always clear to purchasing patients how this affects cancer treatment access and costs. Delays in access and treatment have been reported in patients with breast cancer.[11] Cancer-specific insurance policies do exist but frequently have significant limitations and exclusions.[12] For those with Medicare, it is critical to have a supplemental plan, as out-of-pocket exposure can be unlimited.[13]

Financial Distress and Toxicity

Because of the above and across the board regardless of insured status or resources, the emotional and psychologic aspects of financial distress are increasing.[14] In that article they cite the effect on all age groups: young adults with generally fewer assets and savings are dramatically affected for life. Blending into the middle adult age group, there is a need for loans, debt, and an inability to pay for care. Minorities were especially affected, depending on their socioeconomic status. The intensity of treatment, which also increases in duration, is a major driver of certain diseases. Newer molecular therapies are increasingly expensive and a major contributor.[15] There are also data that it is either delaying care or discouraging care.[16] It has also been shown to correlate with increased pain, greater symptom burden, and poorer quality of life in a study by Lathan.[17] Methods of measurement for financial distress are evolving and will hopefully be applied as a routine part of assessment at more institutions, just as patient experience of care and patient-reported outcomes are currently.[18,19]

Current Strategies to Reduce Cost

The Ultimate Solution to Reduce Costs

Of course, to the extent it applies, which is not known to be true for all cancers, prevention and early detection are the optimal solutions. Risk factors for the most common diseases have been known for a long time, and while some risk reduction efforts have been successful, there is still much room for improvement. Many revolve around lifestyle changes, which have been adopted, would reduce cancer incidence. They are (1) a reduction in tobacco use, (2) adoption of a healthy diet, (3) maintenance of healthy weight, (4) physical activity, (5) protection from excessive sun exposure, (6) limitations of alcohol exposure, (7) vaccinations for relevant viruses, (8) regular medical care, and (9) avoiding risky behaviors. Estimates by the Harvard School of Public Health are that adoption of these could reduce preventable cancer deaths by up to 75%.[20] In the case of smoking, a 50% reduction in smoking (for smokers of more than 15 cigarettes per day) reduced the hazard ratio for future lung cancer to 0.73.[21] In addition, regular medical care with appropriate screening for selected cancers has been effective in detecting disease in earlier stages and has been shown to reduce the costs associated with more advanced disease. Depending on the criteria and population chosen for analysis, the results vary when applied to many cancers. Many of the comorbidities that are present in people who are cured of their cancer would also be reduced by such activities, such as smoking reduction. It is recognized that we do not know how to prevent all cancers from developing, but the effects on the most preventable ones, colorectal, lung, cervix, pancreas, bladder, breast, ovarian, melanoma, stomach, kidney, hepatocellular, uterine, and prostate, as well as the genetically linked inheritable ones, happen to overlap greatly with the most common cancers and therefore have the biggest effect.

Health Plan Efforts in Wellness

Unfortunately, benefits programs in virtually all plans have spent more dollars in treating illness than preventing illness. This is beginning to change for the first time since the implementation of health maintenance organizations (HMOs), with some benefits now being provided for free or at markedly reduced costs, such as screenings and vaccinations. Health coaches and wellness programs are becoming a common feature of plan offerings. A recent survey found that 86% of employers use their wellness programs.[22]

Strategies in Benefit Design to Lower Costs

Cost-sharing strategies take different forms, but the most common are increases in copays and coinsurance and tiering of pharmaceutical and imaging benefits. Structural strategies, including out-of-network obligations, narrow networks, annual or lifetime maximum benefit caps, and utilization management programs with financial implications for "nonpathway" treatments have been implemented by insurance plans and self-insured employers.

Changes in copay, coinsurance, and deductible requirements play a key role in the design of most plans. In fact, the increases in cost-sharing payments exceed wage growth over a 10-year period, thus becoming less affordable for the average patient with cancer.[23] In the study by Claxton et al. the average deductibles increased from $303 to more than $1200 between 2006 and 2016. Unfortunately, this contributes to prescription abandonment and delaying refills in order to postpone costs. In the study by Doshi et al.[24] the abandonment rate was 18% overall and highly correlated with the out-of-pocket cost, with a rate of 49.4% for out-of-pocket costs greater than $2000. Delayed initiation was prolonged in this group.

Pharmaceutical benefit tiering is another tactic for increasing sharing costs, particularly relevant to cancer. The article by Dubanski[25] discusses this issue with regard to oral anticancer drugs and Medicare Part D, noting that a 25%–33% coinsurance requirement is in place for drugs in the highest tier, which includes many cancer drugs. Almost all private insurance plans have similar structures. This trend has not abated and is not likely to do so in the current benefit structures.

As cancer costs increase, it is critical to know whether the provider is in-network or out-of-network. The difference in plan responsibility can vary from 0% (100% for you) to 100% (0% for you) of a very large number. As the 1-year costs of treatment (extremely disease- and stage-dependent) can vary from approximately $10,000 to well over $500,000, the implications are obvious. Unfortunately, not all geographic areas of the country have equal access to "high-quality" oncology providers, although most cancer care is available at a reasonable distance. Legislative efforts have been directed at ensuring access to high-quality care for all, but this is still not reality for most people with cancer. Geographic location has been shown to be one of the most important factors in cancer mortality, partly due to access and partly due to incidence.[26,27] Although health plans are required to have specialty coverage in the network as required by state laws, there continue to be opportunities for improvement.

Alternate Payment Models

In an attempt to deal with the rising costs, alternative payment models may be tested with various levels of one-side or two-side risk. Such programs include the oncology care model, centered on chemotherapy, a proposed radiation oncology model, and many examples of various bundled payment programs in both the private and public sectors. In most of these, payment is also tied to quality outcomes and the achievement of system efficiency. It is still too early to assess whether these types of programs will evolve into a primary payment model for cancer.[28]

The Uninsured

Those without insurance, especially if not well resourced, avoid these issues but are faced with the cost of care directly and immediately, unless public funding is available. Frequently, it forces one immediately to ask questions that nobody should have to ask: Is it worth it? Or, should I or my family go bankrupt? Financial distress has risen to the top of the chief concerns of people with few resources who are diagnosed with cancer. Unfortunately, there appears to be no immediate solution on the horizon to alleviate these concerns or questions.

Conclusion

The cost of cancer care, while achieving some rather remarkable results, is rapidly increasing and quickly becoming out of reach for all but the group with the most resources. It is of great significance to those without resources and is increasing, resulting in substandard care for individuals with even modest resources. Cost shifting to the patient has become a new norm, as is bankruptcy filings in cancer patients undergoing treatment. The emotional distress caused by this extremely frustrating situation affects the ability to receive quality care and affects long-term outlook. In 2019, there were no immediate or satisfying solutions.

References

1. National Cancer Institute. Feelings and Cancer. 2018 Aug 20. https://www.cancer.gov/about-cancer/coping/feelings.
2. Paul C, Carey M, Anderson A, et al. Cancer patients' concerns regarding access to cancer care: perceived impact of waiting times along the diagnosis and treatment journey. *Eur J Cancer Care*. 2012;21(3):321–329.
3. Charlton M, Schlichting J, Chioreso C, Ward M, Vikas P. Challenges of rural care in the United States. *Oncology*. 2015; 29(9):633–640.
4. Kline RM, Arora NK, Bradley CJ, et al. Long-term survivorship care after cancer treatment—summary of a 2017 National Cancer Policy Forum Workshop. *J Natl Cancer Inst*. 2018; 110(12):1300–1310.
5. Lorgelly PK, Neri M. Survivorship burden for individuals, households, and society: estimates and methodology. *J Cancer Policy*. 2018;15:113–117.
6. National Cancer Institute. Available at costprojections.cancer.gov.
7. Jha AK. End-of-life-care, not end-of-life-spending. *JAMA*. 2018;320(7):631–632.
8. No editor. *Managed Care*. 2015 Oct 24;10:65.
9. Gilligan AM, Alberts DS, Roe DJ, Skrepnek GH. Death or debt? National estimates of financial toxicity in persons with newly-diagnosed cancer. *Am J Med*. 2018;131(10): 1187–1199.e5.
10. Ramsey SD, Bansal A, Fedorenko CR, et al. Financial insolvency as a risk factor for early mortality among patients with cancer. *J Clin Oncol*. 2016;34(9):980–986.
11. Wharam JF, Zhang F, Lu CY, et al. Breast cancer diagnosis and treatment after high-deductible insurance enrollment. *J Clin Oncol*. 2018;36(11):1121–1127.
12. Alabama Department of Insurance.
13. Gurbikian G, Forbes Finance Council. Medicare Out-of-Pocket Costs for Cancer Treatment Every Retiree Should Know: November 18, 2019. Available at Forbes.com/sites/forbesfinancecouncil/2019/medicare-out-of-pocket-costs-for-treatment-every-retiree-should-know.
14. Snyder R, Chang G. Financial toxicity: a growing burden for cancer patients. *Bulletin of the American College of Surgeons*. Sep 1 2019.
15. Tran G, Zafar SY. Financial toxicity and implications for cancer care in the era of molecular and immune therapies. *Ann Transl Med*. 2018;6(9):166.
16. Highleyman L. Many people with cancer face serious financial hardship. Cancer Health. 2018 Sep;30.
17. Lathan C. How financial distress can affect cancer care. *J Clin Pathways*. 2016;2(7):24–27.
18. Witte J, Mehlis K, Surmann B, Lingnau R, Damm O, Greiner W, Winkler EC. Methods for measuring financial toxicity after cancer diagnosis and treatment: a systematic review and its implications. *Ann Oncol*. 2019;30(7):1061–1070.
19. Carrera PM, Kantarjian HM, Blinder VS. The financial burden and distress of patients with cancer: understanding and stepping-up action on the financial toxicity of cancer treatment. *CA Cancer J Clin*. 2018;68(2):153–165.
20. Health. harvard.edu.

21. Godtfredsen NS, Prescott E, Osler M. Effect of smoking reduction on lung cancer risk. *JAMA*. 2005;294(12):1505–1510.
22. Beaton T. 86% of Employers Use Financial Incentives in Wellness Programs. *Health Payer Intelligence*. 2018 May 7. Available at healthpayerintelligence.com.
23. Claxton G, Levitt L, Rae M, Sawyer B. Increases in Cost-Sharing Payments Continue to Outpace Wage Growth. Peterson-KFF Health System Tracker 2018 Jun 15. Available at https://www.healthsystemtracker.org/brief/increases-in-cost-sharing-payments-have-far-outpaced-wage-growth/.
24. Doshi J, Pengxiang L, Hairong H, Pettit A, Armstong K. Association of patient out-of-pocket costs with prescription abandonment and delay in fill of novel oral anticancer drugs. *J Clin Oncol*. 2017;36(4):476–482.
25. Cubanski J, Koma W, Neuman T. The Out-of-Pocket Cost Burden for Specialty Drugs in Medicare Part D in 2019. 2019. Available at https://www.kff.org/medicare/issue-brief/the-out-of-pocket-cost-burden-for-specialty-drugs-in-medicare-part-d-in-2019/.
26. Rolleri C. Cancer Care by ZIP Code: Examining Geographic Health Disparities in the United States. ASCO Connection 2019 Mar 7. Available at https://connection.asco.org/magazine/features/cancer-care-zip-code-examining-geographic-health-disparities-united-states.
27. Lin CC, Bruinooge SS, Kirkwood MK, et al. Association between geographic access to cancer care, insurance, and receipt of chemotherapy: geographic distribution of oncologists and travel distance. *J Clin Oncol*. 2015;33(28):3177–3185.
28. Aviki EM, Schleicher SM, Mullangi S, Matsoukas K, Korenstein D. Alternative payment and care-delivery models in oncology: a systematic review. *Cancer*. 2018;124(16):3293–3306.

59 The Costs of Postoperative Complications After Major Abdominal Surgery: Opportunities and Challenges

LAURENCE WEINBERG AND BERNHARD J. RIEDEL

Key Points

- Major abdominal surgery is associated with a high prevalence of complications.
- Postoperative complications are associated with increased hospital costs.
- Postoperative complications are associated with increased hospital length of stay.
- Minor complications (Clavien-Dindo grade I and II) are common and associated with a significant increase in costs.
- Preventing complications is a key target for cost containment.

Introduction

Cost-effective health care in the hospital setting is crucial for the sustainability of our health care system. With the rising costs of providing health care,[1] governments and health care institutions need to consider the composition of cost expenditure. Internationally, health care expenditure has increased at a faster annual rate than economy growth,[2] and now represents approximately 10% of global gross domestic product (GDP).[2] On a global perspective, $7.2 trillion is estimated to be spent on health care annually,[3] with 35%–40% of these costs attributed directly towards hospital costs.[4] In some countries, hospital expenditure has been reported to represent more than 38% of total health care expenditure.[1] Logically, hospital costs represent the single greatest economic target for reducing health care expenditure. Postoperative complications have been reported as being the strongest indicators of in-hospital costs.[5,6] While numerous mitigation strategies have aimed at reducing their occurrence, postoperative surgical complications remain common[5] and are associated with both poorer health and cost outcomes.[7]

In order to better understand opportunities for cost containment to reduce improvident spending, it is imperative to appreciate the hospital costs of complications following surgery. Given that major abdominal surgery is a commonly performed complex intervention of high acuity, with known risks of complications causing morbidity and mortality, we provide a contemporary overview of the drivers for hospital costs associated with major surgical procedures. Relevant to colonic, rectal, liver resection and pancreatic surgery, this chapter reviews (i) the costs of individual complications after surgery, (ii) the association of severity of complications and hospital costs, (iii) the costs associated with postoperative complications by surgical technique, (iv) the costs associated with postoperative complications by surgical urgency (emergency or elective), and (iv) the impact of complications on length of hospital stay and 30-day readmission rates.

A detailed search strategy was constructed based on the topic title and applied to EconLit MEDLINE, EMBASE, and The Cochrane Library. MeSH terms and free-text terms on costs, health economics, colonic, rectal, pancreatic and liver resections, and complications were used. Eligible studies had their data extracted into predetermined categories, which included study characteristics, procedure and surgical technique used, incidence of complications, their severity and mortality, length of stay, and 30-day readmission rates. All currencies were converted to a standardized form of $USD, taking into account inflation for the respective currency using a validated online application.

Rectal Resection Surgery

The incidence of complications ranged from 6.41%[8] to 64.71%,[9] with a consistent pattern that the presence of complications was associated with increased costs (Fig. 59.1).

Open surgery may have a smaller additional cost based on depth of infection as compared with a laparoscopic approach,[10,11] and laparoscopy for a low anterior resection was associated with a decrease in complication (anastomotic leak, surgical site infection [SSI], and bleeding) rates and therefore costs.[10] All studies[11–16] that reported length of stay demonstrated that where complications occurred, the length of stay increased. The presence of complications was also associated with a higher mortality. The highest mortality rate reported was 4.9%.[15] Only one study[17] reported 30-day readmissions.

Colonic Resection Surgery

Postoperative complication incidence varied greatly between the studies ranging from 6.0%[18] to 66.0%.[19] This variance can be attributed to the different definitions of complications adopted by the studies with some studies reporting the incidence of specific complications, while others reported the incidence of any complication. The use of different hospital resource utilization measures amongst the studies restricted the ability to directly compare the study outcomes. Postoperative complications resulted in a substantial increase in hospital costs (Fig. 59.2). The additional costs of complications varied from $2290[20] to $43,146[21]; this is in part due to the heterogeneous definitions of hospital costs adopted by the different studies, as well as the different complication types reported. Asgeirsson et al.[22] and Knechtle et al.[23] further demonstrate a positive correlation between the number of complications and the additional cost incurred by the hospital.

Asgeirsson et al.[22] and Fukuda et al.[11] demonstrated increasing hospital resource use with increasing SSI severity. The additional cost of SSI increased from $24,563 to $33,211 if an SSI was classified as deep.[22] Similarly, additional hospital charges for SSI in open colonic surgery increased from $995 for superficial SSI to $2155 and $2337 for deep and space/organ SSI, respectively.[11] Similar increases in additional charges were evident in laparoscopic

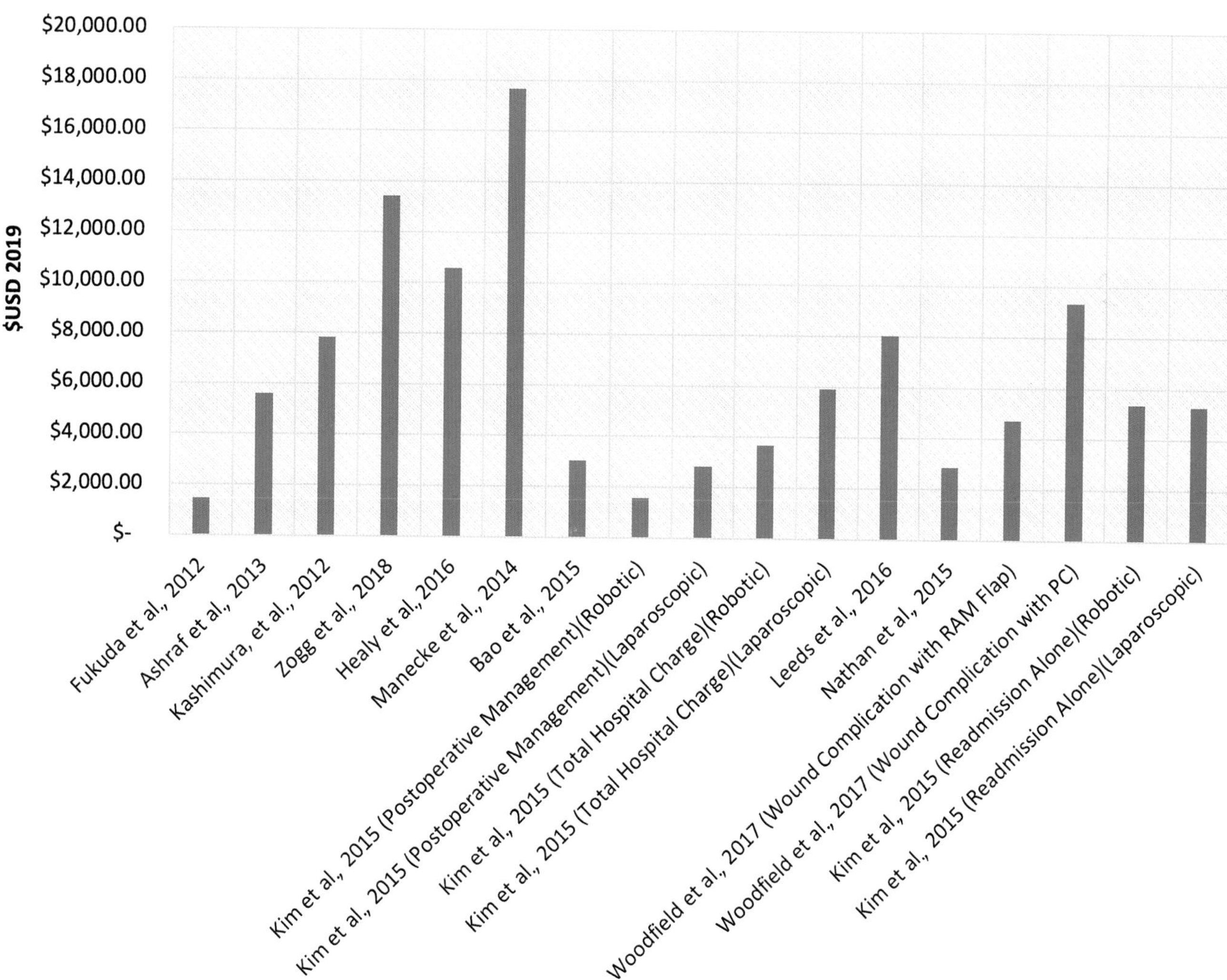

• **Fig. 59.1** Costs of complications after rectal surgery. Values reported as means.

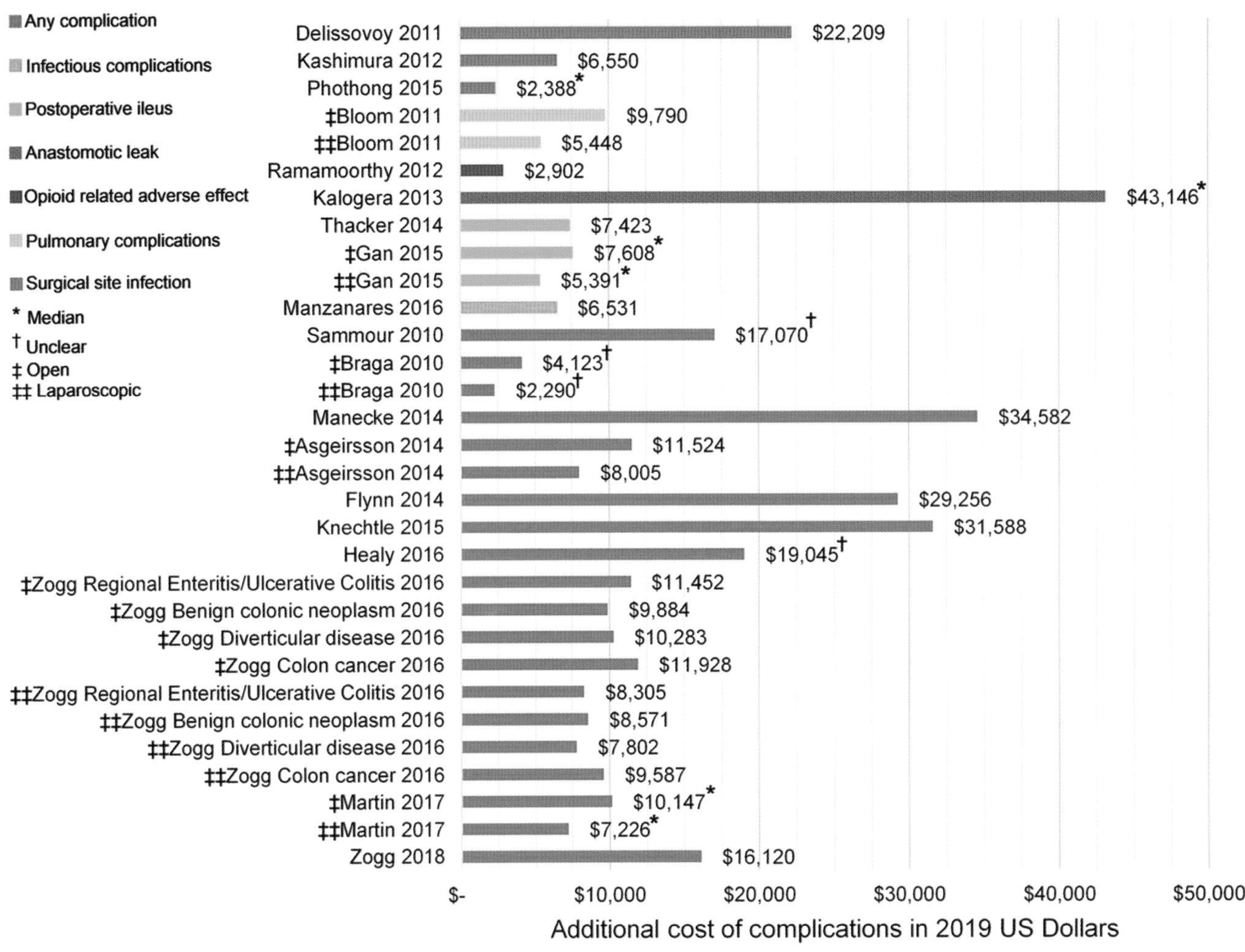

• **Fig. 59.2** Costs of complications after major colon resection. Values reported as means.

colonic surgery.[11] Widmar et al.[24] further explored the relationship between costs and complication severity by analyzing the impact of complication severity on Medicare reimbursements by utilizing the Clavien-Dindo classification. Thirty-day hospital reimbursements increased from $3756 for no complication to $5943 and $8119 for grade I and grade II complications, respectively.[24] Grade I and grade II complications occurred at a prevalence of 29% and 49%, respectively. This highlights the high prevalence of minor complications and emphasizes the significant health care burden of minor complications on total hospital costs. Notably, there was an exponential rise in reimbursements to $18,270 for grade ≥III complications.[24]

SSI and anastomotic leak were associated with the greatest financial burden amongst postoperative complications in colon resection surgery. The additional hospital cost of SSI varied greatly across studies from $2388[25] to $22,209,[26] whereas the hospital cost of postoperative ileus remained relatively consistent across studies ranging from NZD $5486[37] to $7608.[21] This significant variation in costs for SSI can be attributed to the geographic differences in health care system costs with the study by Phothong et al.[25] being completed in Thailand, whereas the studies by Asgeirsson et al.[22] and Delissovoy et al.[26] were completed in the United States. Asgeirsson et al.[22] was the only study directly comparing SSI with postoperative ileus demonstrating significantly higher additional costs in the presence of SSI $24,563 and deep SSI $33,211 than with postoperative ileus $5792. Anastomotic leak was shown to be associated with significant postoperative costs of $29,340[19] and $43,146.[21] One study compared the impact of SSI and anastomotic leak on diagnosis related group (DRG)-based cost coverage and demonstrated a 2.6-fold greater decrease in cost coverage for SSI, as compared with anastomotic leak $8026 versus $3128, respectively.[27] Postoperative complications in open surgery were shown to be associated with higher hospital costs than postoperative complications in laparoscopic surgery across all studies except Kashimura et al.[13] In addition to greater hospital costs, the incidence of complications was consistently higher in open surgery, as compared with laparoscopic surgery. Postoperative complications in open surgery were observed to be associated with greater additional hospital charges than postoperative complications in laparoscopic surgery[11,28]; however, the statistical significance of this association was not reported.

All studies demonstrated an increased hospital length of stay with postoperative complications, as compared with patients with an uncomplicated postoperative course. In addition, the greater the cumulative number of complications a patient experienced the greater their hospital length of stay.[29] Increasing SSI severity is also associated with increased hospital length of stay.[11] No study assessed the cost impact of length of stay. Three studies[15,30,31] reported increased mortality rates associated with incidence of postoperative complications. No study reported the cost impact of mortality.

Phothong et al.[25] demonstrated consistently higher costs with SSI, as compared with without SSI in all cost categories assessed except for anesthetic and instrument costs where the difference did not reach statistical significance. However, the greatest cost difference was in the combined cost of nursing, medication, laboratory, and radiology,[25] which can be explained by the increased length of stay associated with SSI in this study. Wick et al.[32] demonstrated consistently higher reimbursements with SSI, as compared with without SSI in inpatient, ambulatory, emergency department, home care, and pharmacy costs. The impact of surgical urgency on incidence and cost of complications is inconclusive across all studies. Fukuda et al.[11] reported no statistical association between surgical urgency and risk of SSI. However, Asgeirsson et al.[22] reported higher complication incidence and hospital costs with urgent/emergent admissions, as compared with elective admissions.

Liver Resection

The complication incidence across all studies varies between 7.6%[15] and 73.2%.[33] Despite variability in complication incidence, increasing costs with the occurrence of complications was a common finding across all studies[34] (Fig. 59.3). All four studies that graded complications[33,35–37] demonstrated that costs increased along with severity of complications. The increase in cost due to major complications varied between $3282[37] and $64,677.[35] The only exception was the group of patients experiencing minor complications following open resection in the study by Vanounou et al.,[36] where the cost was $1185 less than those without complications. Two studies[29,38] reported increasing costs with increasing number of complications, which supported the evidence across all studies of increasing costs with increasing complication incidence and severity.

Three studies reported the costs of mortality in addition to complications,[38–40] with a consistent finding of greatly increased costs associated with mortality. In high-volume hospitals, Gani et al.[39] reported a $30,102 increase in costs due to mortality compared with patients having complications and an increase of $70,633 compared with patients with an uncomplicated course. A similar finding was reported for low- and intermediate-volume hospitals. Lock et al.[40] found patients dying following liver resection cost $88,379 more

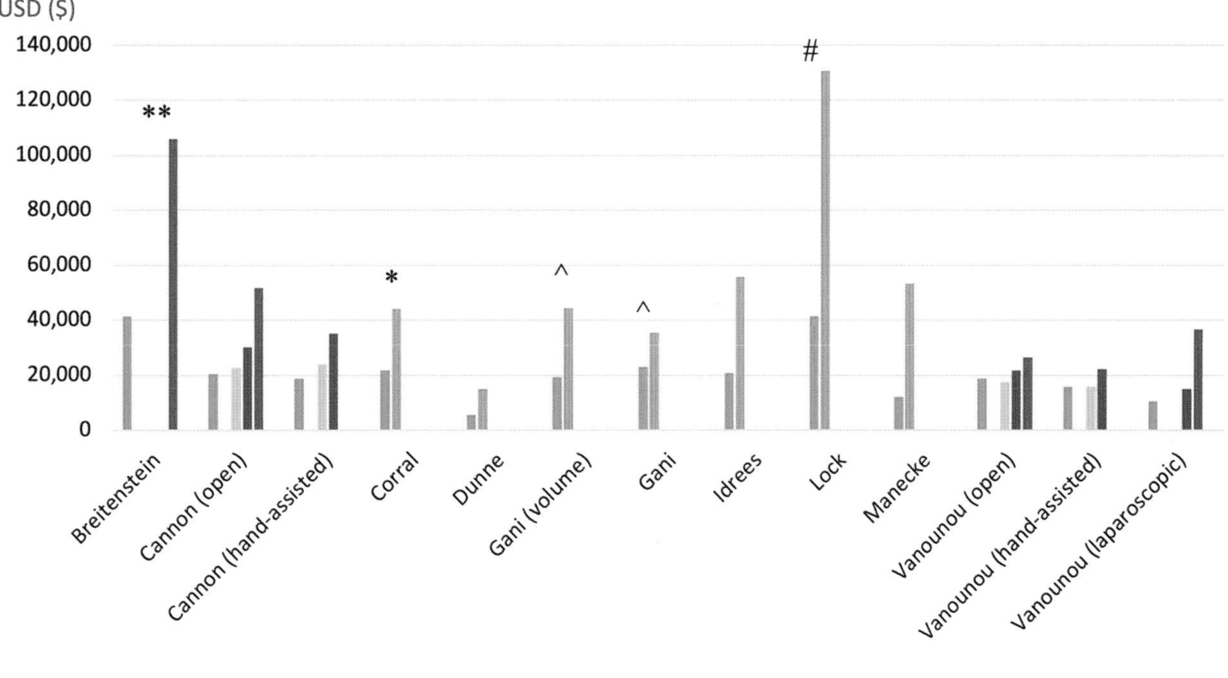

• **Fig. 59.3** Costs of complications for liver resection surgery. Data presented as means unless otherwise stated. ^Cost reported as median, *only assessed major bleeding, #only assessed postoperative liver failure, **no complications group includes Clavien-Dindo grade I/II, complications group includes Clavien-Dindo grade III/IV. To allow for comparison, the charges reported in Cannon et al.[33] were multiplied by a hospital specific cost-charge ratio[29] to obtain an estimate of costs.

than patients who recovered, corresponding to findings by Idrees et al.,[38] which found an increased cost of $88,337 for mortality compared with those without complications. Lock et al.[40] reported a $89,450 increase in costs as a result postoperative liver failure, which was the most expensive complication across the included studies. Additionally, 87.5% patients with postoperative liver failure died, highlighting the clinical cost of postoperative liver failure.

There was disagreement amongst the three studies reporting financial information by surgical technique. Cannon et al.[33] reported mixed results, finding the laparoscopic and open techniques were equivocal for all patients aside those experiencing major complications. As only the open resection group experienced major complications, which carried a higher cost, the overall cost was $11,902 less for the laparoscopic group. Vanounou et al.[36] supported this finding, reporting the overall cost for the laparoscopic group was $3198 less than the open group, and additionally laparoscopy without a hand-port was $3068 cheaper the hand-assisted technique. However, Fretland et al.[37] found the overall costs of laparoscopic and open resection to be equivocal.

The cause of the disagreement is likely attributable to the heterogeneity amongst studies. Vanounou et al.[36] and Fretland et al.[37] included only minor resections, while Cannon et al.[33] included both major and minor resections. Additionally, all three studies had varying selection criteria, and study design varied greatly between Fretland et al.,[37] a randomized controlled trial, and the two retrospective studies.[33,36]

Increased length of stay following the occurrence of complications was a consensus finding amongst the six studies[15,28,35,38,40,41] reporting the outcome. Additionally, Knechtle et al.[29] demonstrated that length of stay increased as the number of complications increased. Only Idrees et al.[38] described the financial impact associated with length of stay, reporting a mean incremental cost of $8929 (95% CI, $3321–14,536; $P < 0.001$) for patients exceeding a length of stay beyond 8 days. Fretland et al.[37] was the only study to report the cost of readmission and did so in the context of laparoscopic versus open resection, reporting that the two techniques were equivocal in terms of readmission costs: $1886 (4869) versus $2027 (7490), $P = 0.914$. Knechtle et al.[29] was the only study to report readmissions in terms of complications: rate of readmission increased from 5% for patients with no complications to 14.3% for patients with four or more complications.

Studies comparing the cost between major and minor resection showed an increased cost associated with major liver resection.[33,38] Only Idrees et al.[38] drew a direct comparison, reporting a mean incremental cost of $15,291 (95% CI, $5272–$25,310; $P < 0.001$) for hemi-hepatectomy, compared with a partial resection. Cannon et al.[33] reported an increased cost of $11,709 for the laparoscopic right hepatectomy subgroup, in comparison to the entire cohort, although found that open resection was $1536 cheaper for the right hepatectomy subgroup. No statistical analysis was included for this comparison. In the two studies,[36,37] including only minor resections, both had lower total cost than the major resection groups of Idrees et al.[38] and Cannon et al.[33] However, given the heterogeneity of different hospital and economic environments, comparison across studies was difficult.

Pancreatic Resection

The incidence of complications after pancreaticoduodenectomy has been previously reviewed[42] and ranged from 38%[43] to 77%.[44] The distribution of minor and moderate–major complications, defined as Clavien-Dindo I or II and Clavien-Dindo III or above, respectively, was heterogeneous among included studies. Notably deviant results include the studies by Topal et al.[45] and Santema et al.[46] These results can be explained by the utility of modified Clavien-Dindo systems. The incidence of postoperative pancreatic fistula (POPF) was similarly heterogeneous between cohorts, with overall incidence ranging from 7.9% to 36.8%. The incidence of delayed gastric emptying varied between studies. Brown et al.[43] reported an overall incidence of 14.6% in their cohort, while Eisenberg et al.[47] reported a 19.4% incidence of delayed gastric emptying. According to the International Study Group of Pancreatic Surgery criteria for delayed gastric emptying, 55.7% were grade A, 25.7% were grade B, and 18.6% were grade C. Santema et al.[46] found isolated delayed gastric emptying occurred at an incidence of 18%, compared with 12.2% in Eisenberg's primary delayed gastric emptying group.[47]

A consistent finding across all included studies is the substantial increase of hospital cost with complications, and when applicable, the severity of the complication. Costs were generally higher in North American and European studies compared with Asian studies.[42] Cost stratification according to Clavien-Dindo or similar systems was available in four studies.[45,46,48,49] The development of major complications (Clavien-Dindo grade III or above) led costs to more than double compared with uncomplicated patients in multiple studies.[45,46,48,50] Vanounou et al.[48] found that major deviations from the expected postoperative course after clinical pathway implementation cost $65,361 compared with $23,868 for uncomplicated patients. Similarly, Enestvedt et al.[50] found that patients with a major complication cost $64,898 compared with $33,518. Cecka et al.[49] was the only study reporting full cost data for each severity grade, and interestingly found only a small cost increase from no complications ($5147) to grade III complications ($8415), yet a substantial increase when a grade IV complication occurred ($39,464). This may reflect the relative costs of performing a procedure for a grade III complication compared with ICU stay with a grade IV complication.

Pancreatic fistula was the most commonly studied complication, with its impact on costs analyzed in eight studies.[42,44–46,51–54] The vast financial consequences of POPF have once again been shown in the included studies, with an incremental burden according to severity. Studies that analyzed hospital costs, not charges, of POPF are displayed

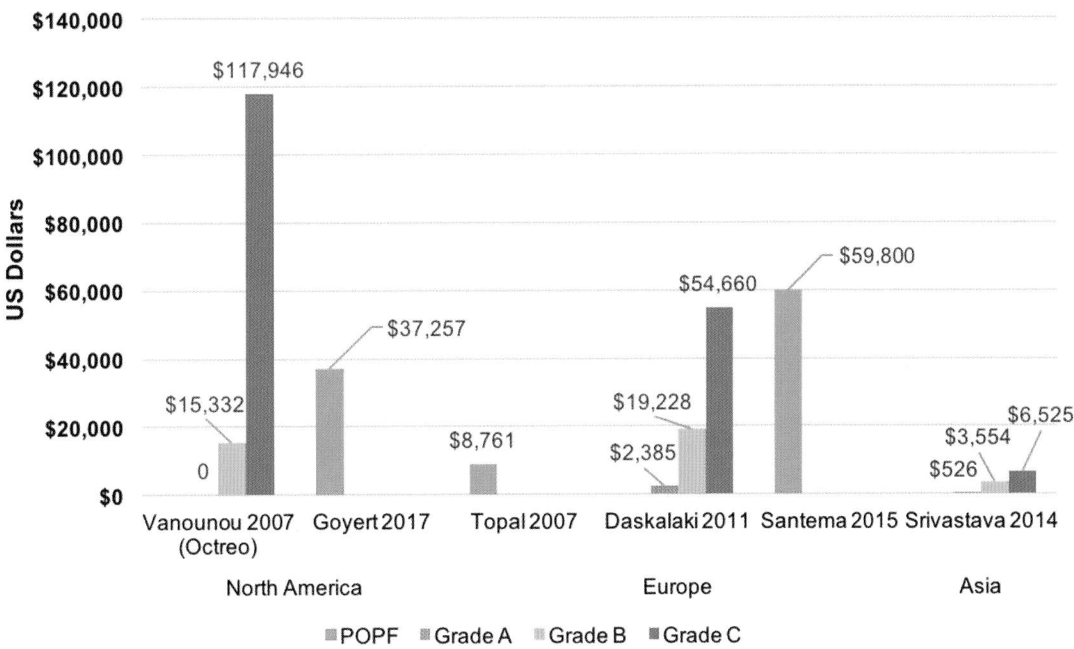

• **Fig. 59.4** Costs of postoperative pancreatic fistula (*POPF*) stratified by grades. Values reported as means.

in Fig. 59.4. Clinically insignificant fistulas, also known as "transient fistulas" and classified as grade A,[55] were found across our studies to contribute little to patients' hospital costs. Grade B and C fistulas, however, had significant clinical burden among the included articles. Daskalaki et al.[52] found that grade B and C fistulas had total hospital costs of $32,657 and $75,601, compared with patients without fistulas ($12,282). Similarly, Vanounou et al.[51] found patients with grade B and C fistulas had costs of $39,466 and $145,939 compared with $23,557 in patients without POPF. Huang et al.[53] found that patients with a clinically relevant POPF had a hospital charge of $14,077 compared with $10,601 in patients without. Goyert et al.[54] reported that patients with clinically relevant POPF cost $70,819 compared with $33,562 in patients without.

One study examined the cost of delayed gastric emptying specifically,[47] finding a $10,000 incremental increase in hospital charge per grade of delayed gastric emptying severity. In analyzing common complications following pancreaticoduodenectomy, Santema et al.[45] found that isolated delayed gastric emptying resulted in a cost differential of $8253 over uncomplicated patients—a 43% increase. The cost of delayed gastric emptying may be largely due to costs associated with length of stay, rather than medical intervention; however, when compared with a model of estimated charge for uncomplicated patients based on length of stay, delayed gastric emptying was found to be 7.2% less costly.[43]

Four studies examined the differences in hospital cost constituents, with an emphasis on the sources of cost variation due to complications. Topal et al.[45] found a statistically significant ($P \leq 0.05$) increase in the cost of hospitalization, laboratory work, medical staffing, and pharmacy work between patients with no complications, patients with complications other than POPF, and patients with POPF. Furthermore, they found that the contributions to hospital cost in all patients, in decreasing order, were hospitalization (33%), operation room (23%), medical staff (20%), pharmacy (14%), and others.[45] Daskalaki et al.[52] similarly found increasing costs of hospitalization and laboratory work across patients with increasing POPF grades. There were also added costs resulting from therapeutic interventions for POPF grades B and C, due to costs of antibiotics, parenteral/enteral nutrition, and in some cases, ICU stay and reoperation. Statistical significance for each cost center cannot be determined, however, as *P*-values were not individually reported.[14] Santema et al.[46] reported statistically significant ($P \leq 0.05$) cost increases in general diagnostics, imaging, clinical care, ICU, and surgery between patients with a grade II (Clavien-Dindo IIIb) complication and those with a grade I complication (Clavien-Dindo I, II, and IIIa). Interestingly, they found no significant differences in any cost categories between patients with postoperative hemorrhage and those with POPF. Enestvedt et al.[50] reported a greater than double increase in charges of blood bank, laboratory, imaging, ICU, pharmacy, and respiratory therapy between patients with major complications (Clavien-Dindo III and above) compared with those without.

Discussion

There is a considerable degree of heterogeneity in the reporting of complications between studies impeding direct comparisons of costs and outcomes. Further, there are important discrepancies in factors, such as study design, defining and reporting on complications, and methodology used to calculate "cost" and associated outcomes. Despite accounting for currency and inflation, the inherent differences in medical and financial structure of health care systems between countries limited the generalizability and comparison of cost outcome.

Despite these limitations, there is a high overall complication incidence arising from major abdominal surgical procedures with associated increased costs and greater resource utilization. Hospital readmissions are associated with significant financial burden, and postoperative complications are associated with greater incidence of hospital readmission. There is weaker evidence that postoperative SSIs and anastomotic leak for colon resections are associated with greater costs and resource utilization relative to other postoperative complications.

There are also significant shortcomings in defining and reporting of hospital resource utilization in economic studies of postoperative complications in surgery. First, the measure of hospital resource utilization adopted by numerous studies varied and was poorly defined. Second, the currency year was not reported in most of the studies, thus it was assumed to be the publication year. Third, reporting of costs using means and medians varied, impeding on direct comparison between studies.

Hospital costs, hospital charges, and hospital reimbursements are three resources which use measures that represent different financial aspects of health economics.[56,57] Hospital charges for a given service may differ greatly between hospitals and health care systems and are considered a poor representation of hospital costs.[58] Similarly, calculation of costs using cost-to-charge ratios is also considered an inaccurate method of calculating hospital costs.[50] Hospital reimbursement was the resource use measure adopted by many studies utilizing Medicare databases.[59–67] Reimbursement systems demonstrate significant geographical variation in their coding classification and payment value.[68] In the United States and many European countries, hospital reimbursements are predetermined and based on DRG codes, with greater reimbursements for patients with complications, as compared with those without complications.[68,69] This system in limited in that it does not account for cost variation within DRG codes, which acts as a source of uncertainty in estimating the financial burden of specific complications. As such, the most reliable measure of hospital costs involves recording actual resource consumption for each admission.[58] Secondary to this, studies should clearly define and report the utilized hospital resource use measure to enable accurate analysis of a study's results.

Poorly defined and inconsistent reporting of hospital resources acts as a barrier to accurate comparison of cost and clinical outcomes between studies. Hospital costs consist of fixed direct, variable direct, and indirect costs.[57] Inclusion or exclusion of specific hospital cost components resulted in variation in total financial burden of complications amongst the included studies. Furthermore, some studies did not specify the hospital resource use components included in their analysis, significantly weakening the clinical utility of their results. The reporting of health cost studies should adhere to a minimal standard of reporting including the definition of hospital cost components analyzed. In addition, cost currency and currency year should also be reported to allow accurate comparison of outcomes.

Adjusting for cost currency and currency year is essential in allowing comparison of cost data across years. Inaccurate inflation may form a source of error in interpreting a study's outcomes. Many studies fail to report the currency year. Complete reporting of costing studies should include the cost currency and the currency year, including any adjustments for inflation that the authors performed. In addition, skewed distributions are expected in medical costing data,[70] therefore it is recommended that both mean and median costs are reported to avoid misinterpretation of results.[70]

Most of the included studies reported the cost of a specific complication type or compared the cost of one complication type to another. Though specific complication data improve the clinical relevance of these studies, the inconsistency in complication definition limits the ability to compare complication types across studies. Many studies utilized local institutional definitions or the definitions of the national databases they analyzed. Few studies specified the use of the International Classification of Diseases, Ninth Revision, Clinical Modification (ICD-9-CM) codes to classify complications. Reporting on postsurgical complications should be aligned with established international standards for definitions and use of outcome measures, designed for clinical effectiveness research in perioperative medicine.[71]

Additionally, most studies failed to recognized complication severity as a significant factor in determining hospital resource use. There is a strong association of greater complication severity and increased costs. Complication severity is therefore an important factor to analyze and should be reported using internationally validated grading systems, such as the Clavien-Dindo classification system.[72]

There also is an inconsistency in the reporting of mortality. The reporting of mortality at 30 days may not provide an adequate measure of the clinical effectiveness of a treatment designed to improve patient-centered outcomes, as many patients who develop severe complications may survive to 30 days. Mortality should be reported to a minimum of 90 days after surgery and ideally at 1 year. By providing guidance on the choice of outcome measures and the optimal time frame for use, such standards will enable researches to develop high-quality cost research methodologies that meet an internationally agreed benchmark.

Hospital readmissions are a well-recognized and significant source of costs. Specifically, in the United States, the Hospital Readmissions Reduction Program was introduced which penalizes hospitals that demonstrate high 30-day readmission rates for specific conditions/procedures.[73] This initiative creates a significant financial incentive for hospitals to introduce measures that reduce readmissions. There is an increased readmission rate in patients who experience postoperative complications, highlighting the financial benefit of reducing postoperative complication rates. The reporting of readmissions should be standardized to at least 30 days postdischarge and should also be reported in all cost outcome studies.

Conclusion

There is a high rate and cost of complications arising from major abdominal surgery. High-quality prospective economic studies are still needed to evaluate the detailed cost of complications arising from surgery. Cost-effectiveness studies examining interventions that aim to reduce postoperative complications are also required to guide strategies designed to reduce costs and improve quality of practice, with the ultimate aim being cost-effective and sustainable surgical practice. Given that complications are a major contributor to total hospital costs, strategies aimed at reducing surgical complications postcolonic surgery should be an integral part of improving the cost-effectiveness of our health care systems. Multimodal stratagies include comprehensive prehabilitation initiatives to optimize physiological and psychological well being, intra- and postoperative Enhanced Recovery After Surgery multimodal treatment bundles to decrease the perioperative stress response to surgical trauma and reduce complication rates with surgery, and the establishment of early warning score systems and rapid response teams to minimize the frequency of unplanned intrahospital escalations and clinical deteriorations.

Further, it is imperative that costing studies of postoperative complications follow a detailed and consistent methodology and reporting standard. In addition, studies must report, as a minimum, the following variables: hospital cost definition, cost currency, cost year adjusted for inflation, complication definition, follow-up duration, and mean and median cost with confidence intervals and interquartile range. Accurate and consistent economic evaluations of complications are needed to inform cost-containment strategies, target interventions to reduce costs, and ultimately improve safety and the sustainability of our health care systems.

References

1. Australian Institute of Health and Welfare. *Health expenditure Australia 2016–17. Health and Welfare Expenditure Series no. 64. Cat. no. HWE 74*. Canberra: AIHW; 2018.
2. Xu K, Soucat A, Kutzin J, et al. *Public Spending on Health: A Closer Look at Global Trends*. Geneva: World Health Organization; 2018. (WHO/HIS/HGF/HFWorkingPaper/18.3). Licence: CC BY-NC-SA 3.0 IGO. Available at. http://www.who.int/iris/handle/10665/276728.
3. Global Health Observatory (GHO) Data World Health Organization. Global Health Observatory. 2015. Available at https://www.who.int/gho/health_financing/en/.
4. *Australian Institute of Health and Welfare. Health Expenditure Australia 2014–15*. Canberra: AIHW; 2016 Contract No.: HWE 67.
5. Vonlanthen R, Slankamenac K, Breitenstein S, et al. The impact of complications on costs of major surgical procedures: a cost analysis of 1200 patients. *Ann Surg*. 2011;254(6):907–913.
6. Patel AS, Bergman A, Moore BW, Haglund U. The economic burden of complications occurring in major surgical procedures: a systematic review. *Appl Health Econ Health Policy*. 2013;11(6):577–592.
7. Tevis SE, Kennedy GD. Postoperative complications and implications on patient-centered outcomes. *J Surg Res*. 2013;181(1):106–113. doi:10.1016/j.jss.2013.01.032.
8. Floodeen H, Hallbook O, Hagberg LA, Matthiessen P. Costs and resource use following defunctioning stoma in low anterior resection for cancer—a long-term analysis of a randomized multicenter trial. *Eur J Surg Oncol*. 2017;43(2):330–336. doi:10.1016/j.ejso.2016.12.003.
9. Woodfield J, Hulme-Moir M, Ly J. A comparison of the cost of primary closure or rectus abdominis myocutaneous flap closure of the perineum after abdominoperineal excision. *Colorectal Dis*. 2017;19(10):934–941. doi:10.1111/codi.13690.
10. Lim S, Chen BP, Marsh W, Ghosh W, Entwistle J, Goldstein LJ. Economic impact of laparoscopic vs open low anterior resection for rectal cancer surgery: a budget impact analysis. *Value Health*. 2018;21:S21–S22. doi:10.1016/j.jval.2018.04.131.
11. Fukuda H, Morikane K, Kuroki M, et al. Impact of surgical site infections after open and laparoscopic colon and rectal surgeries on postoperative resource consumption. *Infection*. 2012;40(6):649–659. doi:10.1007/s15010-012-0317-7.
12. Ashraf SQ, Burns EM, Jani A, et al. The economic impact of anastomotic leakage after anterior resections in English NHS hospitals: Are we adequately remunerating them? *Colorectal Dis*. 2013;15(4):e190–e198. doi:10.1111/codi.12125.
13. Kashimura N, Kusachi S, Konishi T, et al. Impact of surgical site infection after colorectal surgery on hospital stay and medical expenditure in Japan. *Surg Today*. 2012;42(7):639–645. doi:10.1007/s00595-012-0126-8.
14. Kim CW, Baik SH, Roh YH, et al. Cost-effectiveness of robotic surgery for rectal cancer focusing on short-term outcomes. *Medicine*. 2015;94(22):e823. doi:10.1097/MD.0000000000000823.
15. Manecke GR, Asemota A, Michard F. Tackling the economic burden of postsurgical complications: Would perioperative goal-directed fluid therapy help? *Crit Care*. 2014;18(5):566. doi:10.1186/s13054-014-0566-1.
16. Zogg CK, Ottesen TD, Kebaish KJ, et al. The cost of complications following major resection of malignant neoplasia. *J Gastrointest Surg*. 2018;22(11):1976–1986. doi:10.1007/s11605-018-3850-6.
17. Nathan H, Atoria CL, Bach PB, Elkin EB. Hospital volume, complications, and cost of cancer surgery in the elderly. *J Clin Oncol*. 2015;33(1):107–114. doi:10.1200/JCO.2014.57.7155.
18. Phothong N, Akaraviputh T, Chinswangwatanakul V, Methasate A, Trakarnsanga A. Cost-effective and potential benefits in three-port hand-assisted laparoscopic sigmoidectomy. *J Med Assoc Thai*. 2015;98(9):864–870.
19. Sammour T, Zargar-Shoshtari K, Bhat A, Kahokehr A, Hill AG. A programme of Enhanced Recovery After Surgery (ERAS) is a cost-effective intervention in elective colonic surgery. *N Z Med J*. 2010;123(1319):61–70.
20. Braga M, Frasson M, Zuliani W, Vignali A, Pecorelli N, Di Carlo V. Randomized clinical trial of laparoscopic versus open left colonic resection. *Br J Surg*. 2010;97(8):1180–1186.
21. Kalogera E, Haas L, Borah B, Dowdy S, Cliby W. A cost-analysis of anastomotic leak vs. prophylactic bowel diversion at the time of large bowel resection for primary ovarian cancer. *Gynecol Oncol*. 2013;130(1):e62.
22. Asgeirsson T, Jrebi N, Feo L, Kerwel T, Luchtefeld M, Senagore AJ. Incremental cost of complications in colectomy: a warranty guided approach to surgical quality improvement. *Am J Surg*. 2014;207(3):422–426; discussion 425–426.

23. Knechtle WS, Perez SD, Medbery RL, et al. The association between hospital finances and complications after complex abdominal surgery: deficiencies in the current health care reimbursement system and implications for the future. *Ann Surg*. 2015;262(2):273–279.
24. Widmar M, Strombom P, Keskin M, et al. Burden of surgical complications: contribution of long-term costs by Clavien-Dindo classification. *J Am Coll Surg*. 2016;223(4 Suppl 1):e90.
25. Phothong N, Akaraviputh T, Chinswangwatanakul V, Methasate A, Trakarnsanga A. Cost-effective and potential benefits in three-port hand-assisted laparoscopic sigmoidectomy. *J Med Assoc Thai*. 2015;98(9):864–870.
26. Delissovoy G, Pan F, Patkar AD, Edmiston CE, Peng S. Surgical site infection incidence and burden assessment using multi-institutional real-world data. *Value Health*. 2011;14(7):A271–A272.
27. Langelotz C, Hammerich R, Muller V, et al. Negative effects of surgical site infections after colonic resections on clinical course and costs are worse than anastomotic insufficiency. *Eur Surg Res*. 2017;58(Suppl 1):45–46.
28. Vaid S, Tucker J, Bell T, Grim R, Ahuja V. Cost analysis of laparoscopic versus open colectomy in patients with colon cancer: results from a large nationwide population database. *Am Surg*. 2012;78(6):635–641.
29. Knechtle WS, Perez SD, Medbery RL, et al. The association between hospital finances and complications after complex abdominal surgery: deficiencies in the current health care reimbursement system and implications for the future. *Ann Surg*. 2015;262(2):273–279.
30. Thacker J, Mountford W, Mythen M, Krukas M, Ernst F. An updated evaluation of postoperative ileus in colon surgery-associations and outcomes. *Dis Colon Rectum*. 2014;57(5):e306.
31. Zogg CK, Najjar P, Diaz AJ, et al. Rethinking priorities: cost of complications after elective colectomy. *Ann Surg*. 2016; 264(2):312–322.
32. Wick EC, Hirose K, Shore AD, et al. Surgical site infections and cost in obese patients undergoing colorectal surgery. *Arch Surg*. 2011;146(9):1068–1072.
33. Cannon RM, Scoggins CR, Callender GG, Quillo A, McMasters KM, Martin 2nd RC. Financial comparison of laparoscopic versus open hepatic resection using deviation-based cost modeling. *Ann Surg Oncol*. 2013;20(9):2887–2892.
34. Cosic L, Ma R, Churilov L, Nikfarjam M, Christophi C, Weinberg L. Health economic implications of postoperative complications following liver resection surgery: a systematic review. *ANZ J Surg*. 2019;89(12):1561–1566. doi:10.1111/ans.15213.
35. Breitenstein S, De Oliveira ML, Raptis DA, et al. Novel and simple preoperative score predicting complications after liver resection in noncirrhotic patients. *Ann Surg*. 2010;252(5): 726–734.
36. Vanounou T, Steel JL, Nguyen KT, et al. Comparing the clinical and economic impact of laparoscopic versus open liver resection. *Ann Surg Oncol*. 2010;17(4):998–1009.
37. Fretland AA, Dagenborg VJ, Bjornelv GMW, et al. Laparoscopic versus open resection for colorectal liver metastases: the OSLO-COMET randomized controlled trial. *Ann Surg*. 2018;267(2):199–207.
38. Idrees JJ, Johnston FM, Canner JK, et al. Cost of major complications after liver resection in the United States: are high-volume centers cost-effective? *Ann Surg*. 2017;11:11.
39. Gani F, Pawlik TM. Assessing the costs associated with volume-based referral for hepatic surgery. *J Gastrointest Surg*. 2016; 20(5):945–952.
40. Lock JF, Reinhold T, Malinowski M, Pratschke J, Neuhaus P, Stockmann M. The costs of postoperative liver failure and the economic impact of liver function capacity after extended liver resection–a single-center experience. *Langenbecks Arch Surg*. 2009; 394(6):1047–1056.
41. Corral M, Ferko N, Hollmann S, Broder MS, Chang E. Health and economic outcomes associated with uncontrolled surgical bleeding: a retrospective analysis of the premier perspectives database. *Clinicoecon Outcomes Res*. 2015;7:409–421.
42. Wang J, Ma R, Churilov L, Eleftheriou P, Nikfarjam M, Christophi C, Weinberg L. The cost of perioperative complications following pancreaticoduodenectomy: A systematic review. *Pancreatology*. 2018;18(2):208–220.
43. Brown EG, Yang A, Canter RJ, Bold RJ. Outcomes of pancreaticoduodenectomy: Where should we focus our efforts on improving outcomes? *JAMA Surg*. 2014;149:694–699.
44. Srivastava M, Kumaran V, Mehta N. The impact of a postoperative pancreatic fistula on clinical and economic outcomes following pancreaticoduodenectomy. *Curr Med Res Opin*. 2014;4:1–6.
45. Topal B, Peeters G, Vandeweyer H, Aerts R, Penninckx F. Hospital cost-categories of pancreaticoduodenectomy. *Acta Chir Belg*. 2007;107(4):373–377. doi:10.1080/00015458.2007.11680078.
46. Santema TB, Visser A, Busch OR, et al. Hospital costs of complications after a pancreatoduodenectomy. *HPB*. 2015;17:723–731.
47. Eisenberg JD, Rosato EL, Lavu H, Yeo CJ, Winter JM. Delayed gastric emptying after pancreaticoduodenectomy: an analysis of risk factors and cost. *J Gastrointest Surg*. 2015;19:1572–1580.
48. Vanounou T, Pratt W, Fischer JE, Vollmer Jr CM, Callery MP. Deviation-based cost modeling: a novel model to evaluate the clinical and economic impact of clinical pathways. *J Am Coll Surg*. 2007;204:570–579.
49. Cecka F, Jon B, Cermakova E, Subrt Z, Ferko A. Impact of post-operative complications on clinical and economic consequences in pancreatic surgery. *Ann Surg Treat Res*. 2016;90:21–28.
50. Enestvedt CK, Diggs BS, Cassera MA, Hammill C, Hansen PD, Wolf RF. Complications nearly double the cost of care after pancreaticoduodenectomy. *Am J Surg*. 2012;204:332–338.
51. Vanounou T, Pratt WB, Callery MP, Vollmer Jr CM. Selective administration of prophylactic octreotide during pancreaticoduodenectomy: a clinical and cost-benefit analysis in low- and high-risk glands. *J Am Coll Surg*. 2007;205:546–557.
52. Daskalaki D, Butturini G, Molinari E, Crippa S, Pederzoli P, Bassi C. A grading system can predict clinical and economic outcomes of pancreatic fistula after pancreaticoduodenectomy: results in 755 consecutive patients. *Langenbecks Arch Surg*. 2011; 396:91–98.
53. Huang R, Liu B, Chen H, Bai X, Kong R, Wang G, et al. Risk factors and medico-economic effect of pancreatic fistula after pancreaticoduodenectomy. *Gastroenterol Res Pract*. 2015; 2015: 917689.
54. Goyert N, Eeson G, Kagedan DJ, et al. Pasireotide for the prevention of pancreatic fistula following pancreaticoduodenectomy: a cost-effectiveness analysis. *Ann Surg*. 2017;265:2–10.
55. Bassi C, Dervenis C, Butturini G, et al. Postoperative pancreatic fistula: an international study group (ISGPF) definition. *Surgery*. 2005;138:8–13.
56. Arora V, Moriates C, Shah N. The challenge of understanding health care costs and charges. *AMA J Ethics*. 2015;17(11):1046–1052.
57. Rubin GD. Costing in radiology and health care: rationale, relativity, rudiments, and realities. *Radiology*. 2017;282(2):333–347.

58. Finkler SA. The distinction between cost and charges. *Ann Intern Med*. 1982;96(1):102–109.
59. Birkmeyer JD, Gust C, Dimick JB, Birkmeyer NJ, Skinner JS. Hospital quality and the cost of inpatient surgery in the United States. *Ann Surg*. 2012;255(1):1–5.
60. Etter K, Sutton N, Wei D, Yoo A. Impact of postcolectomy adhesion-related complications on healthcare utilization. *Clinicoecon Outcomes Res*. 2018;10:761–771.
61. Liu JB, Berian JR, Chen S, et al. Postoperative complications and hospital payment: implications for achieving value. *J Am Coll Surg*. 2017;224(5):779–786.
62. Nathan H, Atoria CL, Bach PB, Elkin EB. Hospital volume, complications, and cost of cancer surgery in the elderly. *J Clin Oncol*. 2015;33(1):107–114.
63. Regenbogen SE, Cain-Nielsen AH, Norton EC, Chen LM, Birkmeyer JD, Skinner JS. Costs and consequences of early hospital discharge after major inpatient surgery in older adults. *JAMA Surg*. 2017;152(5):e170123.
64. Wick EC, Hirose K, Shore AD, et al. Surgical site infections and cost in obese patients undergoing colorectal surgery. *Arch Surg*. 2011;146(9):1068–1072.
65. Birkmeyer JD, Gust C, Baser O, Dimick JB, Sutherland JM, Skinner JS. Medicare payments for common inpatient procedures: implications for episode-based payment bundling. *Health Serv Res*. 2010;45(6 Pt 1):1783–1795.
66. Regenbogen SE, Gust C, Birkmeyer JD. Hospital surgical volume and cost of inpatient surgery in the elderly. *J Am Coll Surg*. 2012;215(6):758–765.
67. Lawson EH, Hall BL, Louie R, et al. Association between occurrence of a postoperative complication and readmission: implications for quality improvement and cost savings. *Ann Surg*. 2013;258(1):10–18.
68. Busse R, Geissler A, Aaviksoo A, et al. Diagnosis related groups in Europe: moving towards transparency, efficiency, and quality in hospitals? *BMJ*. 7 Jun 2013;346:f3197. doi: 10.1136/bmj.f3197.
69. Quentin W, Scheller-Kreinsen D, Blumel M, Geissler A, Busse R. Hospital payment based on diagnosis-related groups differs in Europe and holds lessons for the United States. *Health Aff*. 2013;32(4):713–723.
70. Bang H, Zhao H. Cost-effectiveness analysis: a proposal of new reporting standards in statistical analysis. *J Biopharm Stat*. 2014;24(2):443–460.
71. Jammer I, Wickboldt N, Sander M, et al. Standards for definitions and use of outcome measures for clinical effectiveness research in perioperative medicine: European Perioperative Clinical Outcome (EPCO) definitions: a statement from the ESA-ESICM joint taskforce on perioperative outcome measures. *Eur J Anaesthesiol*. 2015;32(2):88–105.
72. Dindo D, Demartines N, Clavien PA. Classification of surgical complications: a new proposal with evaluation in a cohort of 6336 patients and results of a survey. *Ann Surg*. 2004;240(2):205–213.
73. *Readmissions Reduction Program [Internet]*. Maryland: Centers for Medicare and Medicaid Services; 2019. Available at https://www.cms.gov/Medicare/Medicare-Fee-for-Service-Payment/AcuteInpatientPPS/Readmissions-Reduction-Program.html.

60

Research in Perioperative Care of the Cancer Patient: Opportunities and Challenges

JUAN P. CATA, CARLOS E. GUERRA-LONDONO, AND GERMAN CORRALES

It is estimated that 30%–40% of men and women will be diagnosed with cancer in their lifetime.[1] In those patients, cancer will be a major cause of death. Therefore, it is anticipated that millions of patients will die of cancer every year worldwide. Several advances in diagnostic technologies have allowed an early stage diagnosis of cancer, where surgery plays a major role in the cure. Furthermore, if we consider the five most prevalent cancers in the adult patients (lung, breast, prostate, colorectal, and bladder), surgery is still the treatment of choice in nonmetastatic stages.[1] Due to the increased aging population, some of those cancers will be more prevalent in older patients, who will in turn become surgical candidates due to the improvements in perioperative care. Therefore the volume of surgical procedures to treat cancers will likely increase in the future.[2]

One of the basic questions in perioperative oncology medicine is whether surgery itself, anesthetics, analgesics, beta blockers, antiinflammatory drugs, and blood transfusions can promote or reduce cancer progression.[3,4] Although basic science research has proven that inflammation, immunosuppression, angiogenesis, and surgical stress (i.e., catecholamines) can promote a local and distant tumor microenvironment conducive for tumorigenesis and metastasis,[5–9] the clinical studies are inconclusive. A major drawback of the current clinical evidence is that only a few trials were designed to show causality between the exposure variable (i.e., anesthesia technique) and hard oncological outcomes (i.e., mortality).

In this chapter, we summarize the advantages, limitations, and challenges related to conducting perioperative oncology investigations with emphasis on clinical research.

Basic Science and Translational Studies

Since the early 1990s there has been a rapid increase in in vitro and in vivo animal investigations evaluating the effect of single or combined perioperative interventions on tumorigenesis and metastasis. Most of those preclinical studies indicate that surgical stress, volatile anesthetics, and opioids can mediate cancer progression by (1) acting on signaling mechanisms that promote cell survival, proliferation, epithelial-mesenchymal transition, and metastatic cell behaviors; (2) inducing inflammation and suppression of the immune response against cancer; (3) triggering angiogenesis; and (4) promoting cancer "stemness."[10,11] On the other hand, laboratory studies suggest that a reduction of the surgical stress and inflammatory response via regional anesthesia, infusions of the local anesthetic lidocaine, beta blockers, and antiinflammatory agents, such as nonsteroidal antiinflammatory drugs (NSAIDs), reduce the metastatic burden associated with surgery.[5–7,12–14]

Unfortunately, in the context of perioperative cancer medicine, the translation of experimental animal research into humans has largely failed. For instance, while studies in rodents indicate that minimally invasive surgery reduces cancer progression, well-conducted clinical studies have shown no benefits or the opposite effects in terms of benefits in survival.[15–18] In addition, significant advances in the areas of genomics, proteomics, and metabolomics have permitted clinicians and clinical researchers to reclassify and treat cancers based on their actionable targets instead of histological subtypes of disease.[19,20] However, it is still unknown how drugs with multiple potential receptor targets or epigenetic effects, such as anesthetics and some analgesics, can affect oncological outcomes in an era of "precision oncology."

Clinical Endpoints

When considering randomized controlled trials (RCTs) designed to test the efficacy of perioperative interventions in patients with cancer, improvements in overall survival and quality of life should be considered as the two most important endpoints.[21,22] While other survival endpoints, such as recurrence-free survival, disease-free survival, progression-free survival, or biochemical-free survival are also commonly used in clinical trials, they do not always correlate well with improvement in overall survival. In other words, when intervention A proves to significantly extend recurrence-free survival time in favor of intervention B, the actual impact on overall survival may not be clinically relevant.[21,22]

Furthermore, it has to be understood that most clinically available biological surrogate endpoints are poor indicators of the ultimate goal in the treatment of cancer, which is cure (long overall survival).[23] In other terms, a single biomarker or a combination of biomarkers that can be easily measured and/or modulated by perioperative interventions is not always highly predictive of overall survival. As an example, findings from randomized controlled studies in breast cancer patients suggesting that the use of paravertebral block anesthesia caused a significant reduction in biomarkers of inflammation and angiogenesis did not translate in a longer overall survival.[24–28]

Short- and long-term psychophysical and social recovery after surgery could be considered as endpoints of postoperative quality of life. From the patients' point of view, recovery is defined as return to "normality."[29,30] In the patient with cancer, the definition of recovery can be broadened to their ability to continue with the cancer treatments (adjuvant therapies), such as chemotherapy or radiotherapy. For some malignancies, such as breast cancer, early return to adjuvant therapies is associated with benefits in survival.[31] However, it must be considered that a disconnect between clinical indicators of recovery and patients' perception of recovery can exist before patients are able to return to their cancer journey, thus patients may still receive adjuvant therapies before achieve psychosocial recovery. We strongly believe that in all patients but specially in those with cancer, postoperative quality of life and recovery should be measured using patient-centered multidimensional tools, in addition to traditional and institutional measures of recovery, such as adequate pain controlled, minimum nausea and vomiting, ambulation, and return to basic physiological functions.[29,30]

In summary, it is of outmost importance to consider overall survival as the main endpoint in studies testing the efficacy of perioperative interventions in cancer outcomes.

Retrospective and Population Database Studies

Recent improvements in data capture, data integration from large registries, and the use of sophisticated statistical models permit clinical and translational investigators to evaluate associations between different perioperative interventions—in the so-called "real clinical practice"—and oncologic outcomes.[32] Thus it is not surprising that more than 30 retrospective studies have been conducted to evaluate the association between the use of different anesthetic or analgesic techniques with improvements in recurrence-free survival or overall survival.[33–36] While this type of research methodology can be seen as relatively inexpensive with results that are obtained in a relatively short period of time, it can require extensive technical support and personnel dedicated to "clean, mine, and combine" large databases that are not always created with investigational purposes.[37]

Retrospective studies and large registry databases have other disadvantages. First, missing information is a significant source of bias and a confounding factor.[38] In addition, most published studies do not report how missing data were analyzed. In our opinion, the use of multiple imputation analysis is generally accepted as a good strategy to handle missing information since the list-wise deletion or single imputation method can significantly reduce the sample size and or assign values incorrectly to missing variables; both of which are sources of bias.[39,40] Second, while sophisticated statistical analyses (i.e., propensity score matching) have been created to diminish imbalances in baseline demographic characteristics, the lack of randomization introduces selection bias.[37,41] Moreover, even when propensity scores analyses are designed to control for nonrandom treatment effects, retrospective studies tend to overestimate treatment effect. Another significant issue arising from the use of large database analysis can be the exaggerated interpretation of the findings based on traditional thresholds for type I error ($a = 0.05$). Researchers and clinicians demonstrating statistically significant differences not always or necessarily suggest a clinically relevant effect. Therefore, they use complementary approaches, such as the Bonferroni correction to obtain a more "strict" alpha error and thus avoid the presence of false positive findings, or the use of confidence intervals (*estimates of effect*) seems more prudent.[41] In line with this idea, *The New England Journal of Medicine* has recently adopted new guidelines for statistical reporting, emphasizing the importance of measures of estimates of effect over *P*-values for primary outcomes.[42] Last and perhaps most important, it is to remember that retrospective studies only evaluate an association and not cause-effect between an exposure variable and the studied outcome or outcomes. Hence findings and conclusions from retrospective studies should be considered hypothesis generating and their findings may require rigorous experimental testing by RCTs.

In summary, researchers will likely continue to use databases or large registries to evaluate associations between perioperative interventions and cancer-related survival or overall survival. However, in our opinion the results from such studies will be complementary to those obtained from RCTs. Last, the clinical significance of the findings generated from large registries and database studies can be limited by the lack of significant external (generalizability) and internal (bias) validity.[41]

Randomized Controlled Trials

Over the last two decades, there has been an increase in the number of RCTs designed to address causation between regional anesthesia, intravenous lidocaine, beta blockers, and cyclooxygenase inhibitors and longer survival. However, the results of only one of those trials was recently reported by Sessler et al. who tested the hypothesis that in comparison to opioid and volatile-based general anesthesia, paravertebral block anesthesia in combination with propofol sedation (or general anesthesia) would reduce cancer recurrence in women with no metastatic breast cancer having mastectomies without extensive breast reconstruction.[28] The authors found no clinically relevant differences in survival between the two treatment groups.[28]

Clinical decisions should be based on high-quality unbiased evidence.[43] In our opinion, RCTs are the best methodology to experimentally compare the efficacy of different perioperative interventions.[44] One of the main premises of any RCT is to reduce any potential selection bias by evenly distributing patient-related variables across treatment groups and assuming that prognostic factors of cancer progression do not interact with the intervention's (anesthetics or analgesic) specific effect. Taking into consideration our premise for RCTs as the standard for testing causation (cause-effect relationship) between anesthetic techniques and cancer outcomes, we should therefore assume that patients enrolled in comparative studies testing a perioperative intervention A versus B should have at the completion of the study similar demographics, tumor-related variables, neo- or adjuvant treatments, and neither of them will interfere with the potential effects of the allocated anesthesia or analgesia technique.

Large RCTs in perioperative medicine require extensive funding to institute a robust clinical research infrastructure and to support costs involved with screening and necessary diagnostic tests, follow-up programs for monitoring and evaluating needed interventions, data management, and research personnel.[48] Underfunded clinical research programs frequently result in RCTs that are not adequately powered for meaningful and clinically impactful endpoints. Another limitation is the lack of properly trained personnel dedicated to clinical research in perioperative medicine. Given the complexity of the perioperative period, and the multitude of factors that can affect clinical outcomes, poorly designed and conducted RCTs can lead to erroneous findings or conclusions. Poorly constructed RCTs are frequently limited by significant bias, and methodological flaws such as a lack of blinding or allocation concealment, lack of statistical power, and significant failures in follow-up.[45–48]

One of the major challenges of conducting and completing large RCTs in the areas of cancer and perioperative medicine research is related to difficulties in enrolling patients into studies. In general, less than 10% of subjects with cancer are recruited in clinical trials, which translates to several months or even years of patients' enrolment and study completion.[49–51] For instance, the results of a major RCT testing the efficacy of paravertebral block anesthesia to reduce breast cancer recurrence were released almost a decade after the study initiation.[28] Since new cancer treatment strategies can be discovered during follow-up periods, the translational value of those studies may be hampered. Thus after the completion of such RCTs the external generalizability of their results can be questioned. Alternatively, pragmatic clinical trials conducted in real-world settings, in which study drug(s) or intervention(s) are tested against usual care (rather than placebo), have been proposed to increase patients' eligibility and enrolment, enhance the generalizability of the results, and reduce costs.[52,53]

Conclusion

The field of perioperative oncology medicine is continuously evolving due to important strides in basic, translational, and clinical research. On the one hand, experimental laboratory research will help to answer mechanistic questions on how perioperative interventions can delay the growth of the so-called minimal residual disease. On the other hand, RCTs will be needed to rigorously answer the questions raised by preclinical and retrospective studies. While a single and short-term perioperative intervention (i.e., regional or general volatile anesthesia) is unlikely to reduce cancer recurrence or progression after oncologic surgery, it remains unknown whether the use combined therapies (i.e., beta blockers and NSAIDs) over a longer period of time that extends days before and after surgery can bring a much-needed benefit in the overall survival of patients with cancer.

Key Points

- Cancer trials currently have one of the lowest enrollment rates among all clinical trials.
- The future of perioperative cancer research will rely on improved collaboration, as well as conventional and novel study designs.
- The identification of super-responders and nonresponders to cancer therapies will bring light to design novel strategies.
- Basic and clinical researchers should take more responsibility to learn how to translate from bench to bedside and to design trials that address important clinical outcomes.

References

1. Siegel RL, Miller KD, Jemal A. Cancer statistics, 2017. *CA Cancer J Clin*. 2017;67:7–30.
2. Siegel R, DeSantis C, Virgo K, et al. Cancer treatment and survivorship statistics, 2012. *CA Cancer J Clin*. 2012;62:220–241.
3. Cata JP, Gottumukkala V, Sessler DI. How regional anesthesia might reduce postoperative cancer recurrence. *Eur J Pain Suppl*. 2012;5:345–355.
4. Buggy DJ, Borgeat A, Cata J, et al. Consensus statement from the BJA workshop on cancer and anaesthesia. *Br J Anaesth*. 2015;114:2–3.
5. Bar-Yosef S, Melamed R, Page GG, Shakhar G, Shakhar K, Ben-Eliyahu S. Attenuation of the tumor-promoting effect of surgery by spinal blockade in rats. *Anesthesiology*. 2001;94: 1066–1073.

6. Goldfarb Y, Sorski L, Benish M, Levi B, Melamed R, Ben-Eliyahu S. Improving postoperative immune status and resistance to cancer metastasis: a combined perioperative approach of immunostimulation and prevention of excessive surgical stress responses. *Ann Surg.* 2011;253:798–810.
7. Melamed R, Bar-Yosef S, Shakhar G, Shakhar K, Ben-Eliyahu S. Suppression of natural killer cell activity and promotion of tumor metastasis by ketamine, thiopental, and halothane, but not by propofol: mediating mechanisms and prophylactic measures. *Anesth Analg.* 2003;97:1331–1339.
8. Sloan EK, Priceman SJ, Cox BF, et al. The sympathetic nervous system induces a metastatic switch in primary breast cancer. *Cancer Res.* 2010;70:7042–7052.
9. Sood AK, Bhatty R, Kamat AA, et al. Stress hormone-mediated invasion of ovarian cancer cells. *Clin Cancer Res.* 2006;12: 369–375.
10. Seguin L, Desgrosellier JS, Weis SM, Cheresh DA. Integrins and cancer: regulators of cancer stemness, metastasis, and drug resistance. *Trends Cell Biol.* 2015;25:234–240.
11. Hiller JG, Perry NJ, Poulogiannis G, Riedel B, Sloan EK. Perioperative events influence cancer recurrence risk after surgery. *Nat Rev Clin Oncol.* 2018;15:205–218.
12. Melamed R, Rosenne E, Shakhar K, Schwartz Y, Abudarham N, Ben-Eliyahu S. Marginating pulmonary-NK activity and resistance to experimental tumor metastasis: suppression by surgery and the prophylactic use of a beta-adrenergic antagonist and a prostaglandin synthesis inhibitor. *Brain Behav Immun.* 2005;19:114–126.
13. Benish M, Bartal I, Goldfarb Y, Levi B, Avraham R, Raz A, Ben-Eliyahu S. Perioperative use of beta-blockers and COX-2 inhibitors may improve immune competence and reduce the risk of tumor metastasis. *Ann Surg Oncol.* 2008;15:2042–2052.
14. Glasner A, Avraham R, Rosenne E, et al. Improving survival rates in two models of spontaneous postoperative metastasis in mice by combined administration of a beta-adrenergic antagonist and a cyclooxygenase-2 inhibitor. *J Immunol.* 2010;184: 2449–2457.
15. Ramirez PT, Frumovitz M, Pareja R, et al. Minimally invasive versus abdominal radical hysterectomy for cervical cancer. *New Eng J Med.* 2018;379:1895–1904.
16. Da Costa ML, Redmond HP, Finnegan N, Flynn M, Bouchier-Hayes D. Laparotomy and laparoscopy differentially accelerate experimental flank tumour growth. *Br J Surg.* 1998;85: 1439–1442.
17. Da Costa ML, Redmond P, Bouchier-Hayes DJ. The effect of laparotomy and laparoscopy on the establishment of spontaneous tumor metastases. *Surgery.* 1998;124:516–525.
18. Jayne D, Pigazzi A, Marshall H, et al. Effect of robotic-assisted vs conventional laparoscopic surgery on risk of conversion to open laparotomy among patients undergoing resection for rectal cancer: the ROLARR randomized clinical trial. *JAMA.* 2017;318:1569–1580.
19. Schutte M, Ogilvie LA, Rieke DT, et al. Cancer Precision medicine: why more is more and DNA is not enough. *Public Health Genomics.* 2017;20:70–80.
20. Bogaerts J, Cardoso F, Buyse M, et al. Gene signature evaluation as a prognostic tool: challenges in the design of the MINDACT trial. *Nat Clin Pract Oncol.* 2006;3:540–551.
21. Nishikawa G, Prasad V. Diagnostic expansion in clinical trials: myocardial infarction, stroke, cancer recurrence, and metastases may not be the hard endpoints you thought they were. *Br Med J.* 2018;362:k3783.
22. Prasad V, Kim C, Burotto M, Vandross A. The strength of association between surrogate end points and survival in oncology: a systematic review of trial-level meta-analyses. *JAMA Intern Med.* 2015;175:1389–1398.
23. Kemp R, Prasad V. Surrogate endpoints in oncology: when are they acceptable for regulatory and clinical decisions, and are they currently overused? *BMC Med.* 2017;15:134.
24. Buckley A, McQuaid S, Johnson P, Buggy DJ. Effect of anaesthetic technique on the natural killer cell anti-tumour activity of serum from women undergoing breast cancer surgery: a pilot study. *Br J Anaesth.* 2014;113 Suppl 1:i56–i62.
25. Desmond F, McCormack J, Mulligan N, Stokes M, Buggy DJ. Effect of anaesthetic technique on immune cell infiltration in breast cancer: a follow-up pilot analysis of a prospective, randomised, investigator-masked study. *Anticancer Res.* 2015;35:1311–1319.
26. Looney M, Doran P, Buggy D. Effect of anesthetic technique on serum vascular endothelial growth factor C and transforming growth factor β in women undergoing anesthesia and surgery for breast cancer. *Anesthesiology.* 2010;113:1118–1125.
27. Sessler DI, Ben-Eliyahu S, Mascha EJ, Parat MO, Buggy DJ. Can regional analgesia reduce the risk of recurrence after breast cancer? Methodology of a multicenter randomized trial. *Contemp Clin Trials.* 2008;29:517–526.
28. Sessler DI, Pei L, Huang Y, et al. Recurrence of breast cancer after regional or general anaesthesia: a randomised controlled trial. *Lancet.* 2019;394:P1807–P1815.
29. Bowyer A, Royse C. The importance of postoperative quality of recovery: influences, assessment, and clinical and prognostic implications. *Can J Anaesth.* 2015;63:176–183.
30. Borrell-Vega J, Humeidan ML, Bergese SD. Defining quality of recovery—What is important to patients? *Best Pract Res Clin Anaesthesiol.* 2018;32:259–268.
31. Raphael MJ, Biagi JJ, Kong W, Mates M, Booth CM, Mackillop WJ. The relationship between time to initiation of adjuvant chemotherapy and survival in breast cancer: a systematic review and meta-analysis. *Breast Cancer Res Treat.* 2016;160:17–28.
32. Ramachandran SK, Kheterpal S. Outcomes research using quality improvement databases: evolving opportunities and challenges. *Anesthesiol Clin.* 2011;29:71–81.
33. Perez-Gonzalez O, Cuellar-Guzman LF, Soliz J, Cata JP. Impact of regional anesthesia on recurrence, metastasis, and immune response in breast cancer surgery: a systematic review of the literature. *Reg Anesth Pain Med.* 2017;42:751–756.
34. Perez-Gonzalez O, Cuellar-Guzman LF, Navarrete-Pacheco M, Ortiz-Martinez JJ, Williams WH, Cata JP. Impact of regional anesthesia on gastroesophageal cancer surgery outcomes: a systematic review of the literature. *Anesth Analg.* 2018;127:753–758.
35. Yap A, Lopez-Olivo MA, Dubowitz J, Hiller J, Riedel B. Anesthetic technique and cancer outcomes: a meta-analysis of total intravenous versus volatile anesthesia. *Can J Anaesth.* 2019;66:546–561.
36. Diaz-Cambronero O, Mazzinari G, Cata JP. Perioperative opioids and colorectal cancer recurrence: a systematic review of the literature. *Pain Manag.* 2018;8:353–361.
37. Porter G, Skibber J. Outcomes research in surgical oncology. *Ann Surg Oncol.* 2000;7:367–375.
38. Freundlich RE, Kheterpal S. Perioperative effectiveness research using large databases. *Best Pract Res Clin Anaesthesiol.* 2011;25:489–498.
39. White I, Royston P. Imputing missing covariate values for the Cox model. *Stat Med.* 2009;28:1982–1998.

40. Croy C, Novins D. Methods for addressing missing data in psychiatric and developmental research. *J Am Acad Child Adolesc Psychiatry*. 2005;44:1230–1240.
41. Nathan H, Pawlik T. Limitations of claims and registry data in surgical oncology research. *Ann Surg Oncol*. 2008;15:415–423.
42. Harrington D, D'Agostino RB, Gatsonis C, et al. New guidelines for statistical reporting in the journal. *N Eng J Med*. 2019;381:285–286.
43. Guyatt GH, Oxman AD, Kunz R, Vist GE, Falck-Ytter Y, Schunemann HJ. What is "quality of evidence" and why is it important to clinicians? *Br Med J*. 2008;336:995–998.
44. Jüni P, Altman D, Egger M. Systematic reviews in health care: assessing the quality of controlled clinical trials. *BMJ*. 2001;323:42–46.
45. Moher D, Pham B, Jones A, et al. Does quality of reports of randomised trials affect estimates of intervention efficacy reported in meta-analyses? *Lancet*. 1998;352:609–613.
46. Huwiler-Müntener K, Jüni P, Junker C, Egger M. Quality of reporting of randomized trials as a measure of methodologic quality. *JAMA*. 2002;287:2801–2804.
47. Lachin J. Introduction to sample size determination and power analysis for clinical trials. *Control Clin Trials*. 1981;2:93–113.
48. Stolberg H, Norman G, Trop I. Randomized controlled trials. *Am J Roentgenol*. 2004;183:1539–1544.
49. Curran W, Schiller J, Wolkin A, Comis R. Scientific Leadership Council in Lung Cancer of the Coalition of Cancer Cooperative Groups. Addressing the current challenges of non-small-cell lung cancer clinical trial accrual. *Clin Lung Cancer*. 2008;9:222–226.
50. Albrecht T, Eggly S, Gleason M, et al. Influence of clinical communication on patients' decision making on participation in clinical trials. *J Clin Oncol*. 2008;26:2666–2673.
51. Brawley O. The study of accrual to clinical trials: can we learn from studying who enters our studies? *J Clin Oncol*. 2004;22:2039–2040.
52. Haff N, Choudhry NK. The promise and pitfalls of pragmatic clinical trials for improving health care quality. *JAMA Netw Open*. 2018;1:e183376.
53. Sessler DI, Myles PS. Novel clinical trial designs to improve the efficiency of research. *Anesthesiology*. 2020;132:69–81.

61

Big Data, Advances in Computational Sciences, and Oncology Care

JOHN FRENZEL

As information technology has matured, organizations and industries embracing the use of data-driven analytics to guide services has profoundly changed the human experience. Just-in-time inventory, predictive pricing models and simple applications such as web searches have generated immense gains in productivity, efficiency, and reliability. The past 40 years have also seen a revolution in the use of data in health care. Within medicine there is an explosion of registries, such as the National Anesthesia Clinical Outcomes Registry (NACOR) from the Anesthesia Quality Institute, tracking clinical events and providing practice benchmarks and quality reporting for its members.[1] Requiring a mix of manual data entry and automated data extraction, these efforts attempt to build a data storehouse to help identify trends and understand practice. Within the wider scope of medicine, efforts are underway to incorporate information from many diverse sources, such as electronic health records (EHRs), genomic testing, claims, and public data sets. These advances will profoundly sculpt the face of health care from patient experience to patient outcomes. The impact of these forces cannot be underestimated.

Little Data to Big Data

Database technology is ubiquitous in our modern existence. Its roots trace back to the 1970s when computer systems were fairly novel. Commonly, the mainframe vendor engineered a closed software platform and was the sole source for the end-user applications. The hardware, operating system, and software were only available from one source. Since there were no competitors at the software layer, standards were internal and ad hoc. This issue created hardware vendor silos inhibiting third party developers. With no competition general product advancement was slow and development costly. Each application was a unique development effort and rarely leveraged work from other products. Due to this vertical integration, it was common for application designers to create and recreate ways to store, access, and aggregate data.

To overcome this, on the data side researchers at the IBM Corporation began to investigate how a layer of abstraction could be constructed between the application and the data. In creating this boundary, application programmers were no longer required to code their own data handling routines or other tools to manipulate the data cache. This break between data management and application programming was foundational. To support this, a standard interface was created to bridge this divide. In 1970, a team led by Dr. Edgar F. Codd at the Almaden Research Center published their work on building a standardized data query language called SEQUEL.[2] SEQUEL became the bridge and interface between data and application. Shortened to SQL over time, the language provided standard tools for programmers to manipulate data without regard to how it actually was stored or represented at the file level. In creating this split, the database management function (DBMS) became a separate service to the programmer, much like the screen display or the network. The SQL language was initially proprietary, but in 1979, a company named Relational created its own competitive and compatible database management software, having reverse engineered SQL. Relational would later be known by the corporate name of Oracle.

The database that Codd described in his publications and implemented in IBM software was known as a relational model. The main competing structure was called hierarchical and could be thought of as a tree with branches or nodes for different items. Relational databases organize data into tables. Tables can be stand alone, like a spreadsheet, or be linked together by keys. The use of keys traces a map of data, linking and defining how the data elements relate to each other. A SQL query leverages these relationships to pull data that conforms to both the constraints of the data model as well as the constraints of the SQL language. Given the standardization of database technology and explosion in data storage, relational databases became part of the fabric of computing. They enforced discipline on the data model through the syntax of the SQL language and ensured that in using a database engine (relational database management system; RMDBS) data could not be inadvertently corrupted through SQL-based manipulation. Designed in the 1970s, these structures worked well and delivered a robust and reliable performance. As computing, storage, and networking continued to evolve, however, the flood of data requiring processing and analysis expanded at an exponential rate. SQL was born in the primacy of the mainframe. In the world of the web, the Internet of Things (IoT), and digitization of whole new categories of daily artifacts, SQL and the relational database began to show its 50-year roots as challenged by the rise of the server.

NoSQL Technology

SQL-based technologies were hitting the performance wall. As the size of the database increased, it required more processing horsepower. While processors were accelerating in capacity, the rate of data generation outstripped their ability to scale. In the 1990s the World Wide Web (WWW) was beginning to grow by leaps and bounds. Architects in this environment scaled their web server performance using multiple compute cores spread across multiple servers to expand their ability to handle the increasing load. They were able to scale horizontally. The RDBMS vendors struggled to use this type of architecture. Mainframes where SQL was born were single processor devices. Due to the way the RDBMS interacted with data, it was technically difficult to make the application work when using multiple servers. It was constrained to scale only vertically, i.e., a single compute core that had to run faster to deliver improved performance. This pressure to create a more scalable and flexible model continued to build.

Driven by the large web utilities, Facebook, Google, LinkedIn, and others, internal research and development resources were tasked to explore alternative paths. The goals were to create a flexible framework that could handle a diverse set of data types (video, audio, text, discrete and binary) using racks of inexpensive hardware. Unlike the RDBMS/SQL solution with a standard interface, defined language and deterministic performance, the new framework, now known as NoSQL, was extremely heterogeneous and spawned a number of database management systems built to optimize specific classes of use cases. Over the past decade, work has gone into classifying data storage and retrieval challenges. From this work the specific task typically can be addressed using one of four categories of NoSQL topologies: Key-value, Column-oriented, Document-oriented, and Graph databases. Underlying these tools is the ability to replicate data across multiple servers, harness the power of numerous processors, and scale horizontally. These database management systems underpin the infrastructure of Facebook, Twitter, Verizon, and other large data consumers.

In health care, the data environment is still evolving. As the installed base of EHR continues to climb, volumes of granular data about and surrounding the management of each encounter are recorded in digital form. Dwarfing this is the volume of imaging data captured. Penetration of digital radiology workflows is substantial, and the images captured result in petabytes of data just within institutions. By 2013, more than 90% of US hospitals had installed digital imaging, and adoption of 3D image reconstruction in hospitals now exceeds 40%.[3] Technology is now transforming pathology workflow with digital whole slide image capture becoming more widely adopted. This is a massive data management exercise, as images contain terabytes each. Additionally, the slide images required to support a diagnosis would include scanning of the entire specimen at differing levels of magnification. For liquid slides, such as bone marrow of blood smears, this is increased due to the need to capture images at different focal planes also.

Within the operating room (OR) and critical care environments, streaming data is ubiquitous. The current generation of anesthesia machines, infusion pumps, noninvasive monitors, and ventilators emit a continuous river of information on a second by second basis. Physiologic and machine data from a large hospital can comprise hundreds of kilobits of discrete data per second 24 h a day. Buried in this data are clues warning of patient deterioration, sepsis, and intraoperative events. The tools necessary to find these signals must function on data that is streaming rather than at rest. While NoSQL technology can be used to store data, its value is manifest when it is also used to process data. In the example above, streaming data from different patients flow into a data processing engine and are segregated by patient. These individual patient data streams can be processed by algorithms colocated on the same server as the data. This combination of processing and storage on the same platform sets NoSQL apart from a performance standpoint. These algorithm/storage pipelines can continuously process data looking for predetermined signals. Compared to a traditional RDBMS, applications outside the database would be continuously making SQL calls for data to feed the analytics. This analytic SQL traffic would be competing against the SQL traffic driven by the data ingestion. Leveraging a NoSQL data structure that incorporates pipelines and the ability to process data locally enables analysis with low cost hardware and high throughput.

Medicine is in an age of information. Whether the application requires a SQL-type database or a NoSQL data processing engine to handle the ingestion and analysis of terabytes, the tools and technology to cope with this torrent of data are well developed and readily available.

Computational Advances

The first operational electronic computing machines were built during World War II to assist in code breaking of enemy message traffic. These were purpose-built machines and used the technology of the day: telephone relays, vacuum tubes, and paper tape. With the commercial advent of the transistor

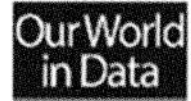

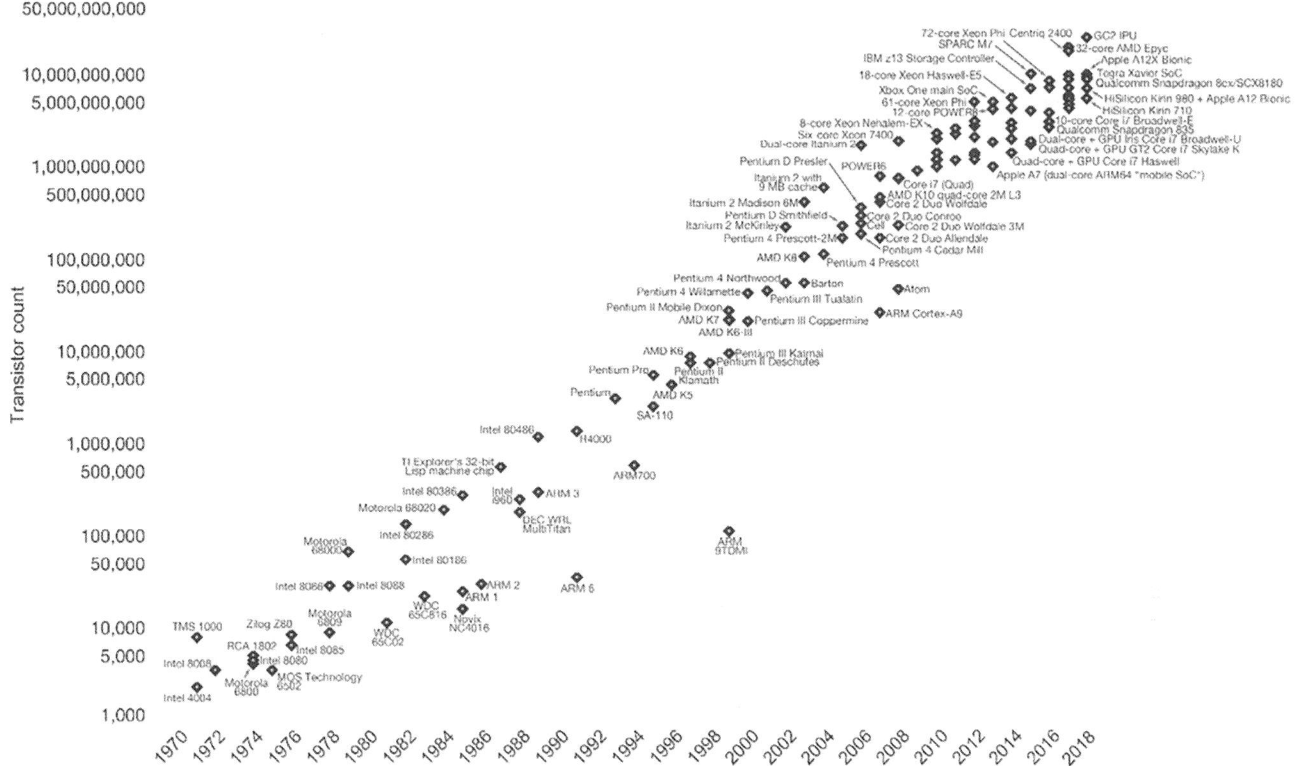

• **Fig. 61.1** From Max Roser. https://ourworldindata.org/uploads/2019/05/Transistor-Count-over-time-to-2018.png, CC BY-SA 4.0, https://commons.wikimedia.org/w/index.php?curid=79751151.

in the mid-1950s, an enormous change took place as vacuum tubes were replaced with integrated circuits.[4] Now, the function of a tube to switch from on to off, representing a logic one or zero went from the size of a baseball to that of a flea. By the early 1960s, designers were able to put more than one transistor in a package and in being able to connect multiple transistors together on a single piece of silicon they could create "chips" used as logic building blocks.[5]

During this era, Gordon Moore was director of Research and Development at Fairchild semiconductor, and through his observation of the technological trends within the industry, the underlying physical science, and the economic economies of scale, he formulated what has become to be known as Moore's Law. Dr. Moore stated, "The complexity for minimum component costs has increased at a rate of roughly a factor of two per year. Certainly over the short term, this rate can be expected to continue, if not to increase. Over the longer term, the rate of increase is a bit more uncertain, although there is no reason to believe it will not remain nearly constant for at least 10 years."[6] In this statement from 1965, he predicted a log-linear relationship that would hold true for over 50 years (see Fig. 61.1). Gordon Moore went on to found Intel Corporation.

The relentless advance of semiconductor technology has paved the way for smaller devices and increased computing capacity. Paired with this is the bountiful harvest of connected technologies benefiting from an increased understanding of materials science and physics. Storage technology, networking bandwidth, and video display all have similar cost-performance curves with incredible capabilities contained within inexpensive packages. Modeled after Moore's law and driven by some of the same economic pressures, Edholm's law[7] (data rates on wired and wireless networks, see Fig. 61.2) predicts the log-linear relationship of performance in these industries.

Cloud Computing

In the mid-2000s as predicted by Edholm's law, network bandwidth had increased to the point where connectivity was not usually a limiting factor in regard to application functionality. Previously, on-premise compute and storage using specialized data centers had been seen as the only choice to host business class applications. With many applications moving to the WWW, mobile platforms becoming more robust and the continually increasing server

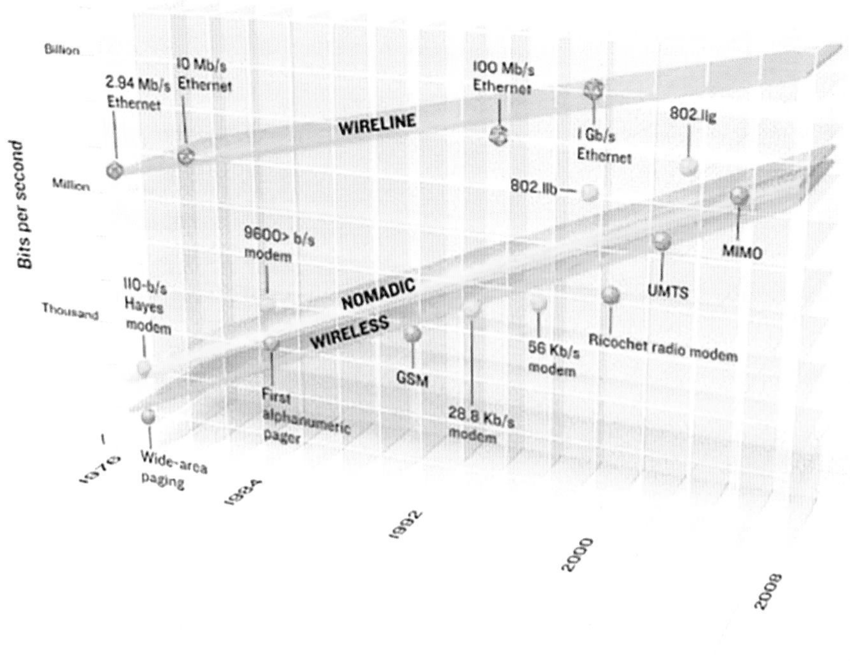

• **Fig. 61.2** From Cherry, S. Edholm's law of bandwidth. *IEEE Spectrum*. 2004;41(7):58–60. doi:10.1109/MSPEC.2004.1309810.

compute power, application owners were looking to outsource management of hardware.

Cloud computing refers to the use of shared resources (storage, compute, and processing) that are located oftentimes in IT infrastructure owned by a third party. Cloud has become widely adopted due to ease of use and low upfront capital costs. In July 2002 Amazon Corporation launched Amazon Web Services (AWS). Used until that point as an internal resource, Amazon began to open its platform to customers to run their applications. From the end-user perspective, items such as maintenance, upkeep, and security become contractual terms handled by the cloud provider, not tasks staffed by the customer. Eliminating this overhead enabled organizations to take advantage of an incremental approach to the technology with the ability to increase size or capability rapidly, needing only a contract amendment. For individual researchers using these services for analytics or machine learning applications, they are charged only for the resources they use, when they use them, lowering the bar to access technology of a world-class platform. Today Amazon (AWS), Microsoft (Azure), Google (Google Cloud Platform), VMWare, and IBM (IBM Cloud) are dominant forces within the industry.

Analytics and Visualization

Analytics is defined as "the discovery, interpretation, and communication of meaningful patterns in data. It also entails applying data patterns towards effective decision-making. In other words, analytics can be understood as the connective tissue between data and effective decision-making within an organization."[8] Society and industry have been transformed through the use of data. Early analytics tended to be static charts or tables, and the presentation of that data was left for the end user to process and understand the implications. Over time the discipline of data visualization began to mature. This field understood that presentation of data was half the job of a good visualization. The more important half was to guide the user to the correct interpretation of the data presented. Quality visualizations make understanding the implications of the data intuitive.

The price to pay for poor visualizations can be high. On the morning of January 28, 1986, the space shuttle Challenger was launched. Seventy-three seconds into the flight, the external fuel tank ruptured and the crew were lost. In the subsequent root cause analysis, it was discovered that rubber O-rings joining fuel sections together of the solid rocket boosters had failed. This came as a shock to the engineers who had been following the health of the O-rings closely each mission. Analytics used to understand previous nonfatal O-ring failures provided no real insight into a sporadic event. They had been plotted many ways including versus ambient temperature because the flight engineers understood that O-rings became less flexible as they cooled. In the visualization from the congressional report, O-ring failure is plotted by location and flight in sequential order with temperature noted individually. In constructing this

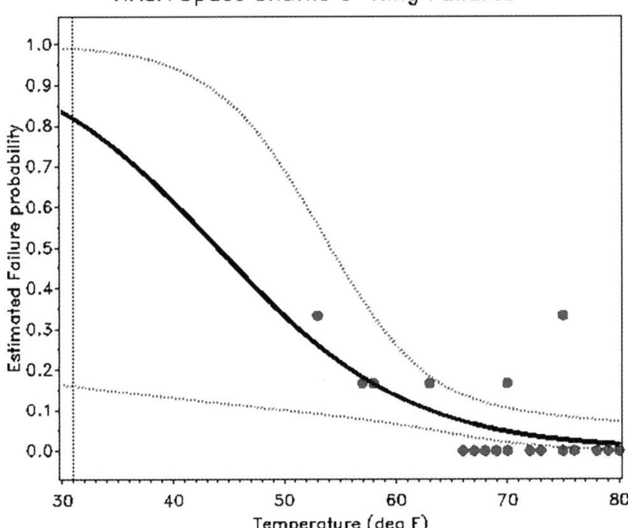

• **Fig. 61.3** Friendly, Michael (2001), Gallery of Data Visualization, Electronic document, http://www.datavis.ca/gallery/, Accessed: 09/23/2021.

analytic, the engineers made it difficult to extrapolate O-ring performance at launch temperatures more than 20°F cooler (32°F ambient at launch) than any other previous flight. When the elements are visualized appropriately, the dramatic effect of temperature on O-ring performance becomes intuitive (Fig. 61.3). Failure to grasp this insight by highly motivated, intelligent, and data rich engineers at NASA cost seven lives and the loss of over a billion dollars worth of hardware.

Visualization of medical data can be similarly high risk. As more clinical data moves onto electronic platforms such as EHRs, how that data is presented can influence how it is interpreted and acted upon. This comes not only from the representation of clinical data but the usability of the system interface. In the early stages of the nationwide push to install EHRs, focus rested squarely on end-user adoption. Moving from a paper and verbal-based system of patient management to one with a keyboard, mouse, and screen was difficult. The Office of the National Coordinator for Health Information Technology estimates that in 2017, 96% of all nonfederal acute care hospitals possessed certified health IT, nearly 9 in 10 (86%) of office-based physicians had adopted any EHR, and nearly 4 in 5 (80%) had adopted a certified EHR.[9] Humans become effective and efficient at performing tasks when their mental model, their internal representation of the problem space, closely matches and predicts reality. Building a good mental model requires time and repetition.

With EHRs now close to a decade in wide use, the next generation of providers has little experience with the paper chart. How the health provider interacts with the application and the way data is presented shape patient interactions. The user interface not only displays information but guides clinical interactions and potentially the interpretation of the data on the screen.

Augmented Decision Support

When understanding the potential return on dollars invested for health information technology, one of the most common cited was the promise that digital platforms would reduce waste and improve the quality of care delivered. On the current EHR platforms, the realization of these promises is mixed. The most common feature to be cited when discussing the improvement of quality is clinical decision support (CDS). While CDS has been widely adopted, it is seen as falling short of its full potential in clinical practice. As a rigid rule-based framework in an extremely fluid environment, many alerts are redundant, not germane, or simplistic. The highest impact has been around positive patient ID and in-patient medication/transfusion administration. To work in the current complex clinical environment, decision support must incorporate deeper knowledge of the process of care, goals of therapy, and the state of the patient. This requires moving from a rule-based framework to one with a more overarching "understanding" of the patient.

Machine Learning and Artificial Intelligence

From the advent of electronic computing machines, the idea to use them to emulate or augment the process of human decision-making has been ongoing. Early attempts began in the 1950s with chess-playing programs. Scientists' initial tendencies were to imagine the world and our interactions with it governed by a set of rules and associated supporting logic, ironically much like a chess board and the current EHR decision support framework. The assumption being that if all the rules and logic could be coded and captured, the computer would begin to mimic human thoughts. Progress was slow and early predictions of rapid success fell away as the problem space expanded and the limitations of computational power were reached. Over time, the field matured, and it became obvious that some problems, such as image recognition, were not tractable in a rule-based framework. During the 1980s and 1990s, the science progressed, and the term artificial intelligence (AI) became more generic. A spectrum of approaches began to emerge, including machine learning, deep learning, and classic rule-based AI. Over the next 20 years, machine-learning techniques took advantage of increasing computational power to create applications capable of addressing real-world problems.

Machine learning[10] and deep learning have become popular topics. Deep learning is a machine learning method based on understanding data representations rather than task-specific algorithms. Technologies supporting this sort of machine learning effort tend to be neural network-based and produce applications that are found in everyday life, such as speech recognition, natural language processing, and image processing. In this work, all these terms will be used interchangeably.

The impact of machine learning and deep learning is manifest today across society. In medicine, the most visible and common interaction that providers have with this type of technology is machine learning driven speech to text. Companies such as Nuance Communications and M*Modal have created the infrastructure to ingest dictation at the point of care, perform voice to text translation, and display the spoken word within the EHR in near real time.[11] Physicians and other health care providers had relied for decades on humans to transcribe recorded speech. The ability for health care organizations to deploy this technology without enormous training costs and end-user adoption problems has only occurred recently. This technology enables physicians to continue to work as they are accustomed while deriving benefit of rapid turnaround and low training cost.

But voice to text only impacts the user interface. The greater utility of the dictation exists when the concepts embedded in the text can be codified and shared as independent discrete concepts. Talking about an episode of sepsis is useful to others only after the document is opened and read. Being able to extract the concept of sepsis using machine learning enables this discrete information to become actionable in many places without the need to search for, find, read, and understand the base document. Automated concept extraction is a form of machine learning known as natural language processing (NLP).

NLP uses deep learning techniques to extract data and concepts from the written or spoken language. The utility of this capability is manifest within health care. While widespread EHR implementation has reduced the number of paper forms and other documents within the care ecosystem, there exists a legacy of scanned as well as physical documents that are poorly indexed and essentially inaccessible.

In our mobile society, records such as these are transferred from provider to provider commonly as physical documents that become invisible within the scanned/outside documents tab of the destination EHR. Using NLP, these documents could be mined for concepts and organized for search. The impact of this on clinical care would be substantial. The most expensive disease categories, those encompassing chronic conditions, represent an overwhelming percentage of cost. The ability to understand the longitudinal course of a disease and therapies that have succeeded as well as failed could have an outsized impact.

NLP is an area of intense innovation and research. The machine-based understanding of language and its meaning is extraordinarily complex. In medicine, accuracy and reliability are critically important. Current technology continues to evolve and within constrained universes accuracy is relatively good. The commercial product Nuance One is a relevant specific example. The Nuance One offering contains a component called Dragon Medical Advisor. Nuance One is a speech to text application with the capability for real-time medical concept extraction. Using the extracted concepts, Dragon Medical Advisor begins to create a profile of the patient. A knowledge engine built specifically for diagnosis and billing criteria then evaluates the concepts presented with facts from the specific text and the applicable coding criteria. It notifies the physician on the EHR screen of areas where additional language or finding specificity is needed. Within the context of billing codes and documentation completeness, the system is extremely accurate, unobtrusive, and easy to use. It is essentially a just-in-time learning system focused around coding and documentation. The promise of machine learning to help find, correlate, and display relevant information within the patient-physician interaction is appealing.

Neural Networks and Deep Learning

As opposed to machine learning, neural networks are often used for complex analysis of nontextual artifacts such as images. Applied to image data, neural networks use layers of interconnected nodes that focus and analyze small sections of an image. Working in parallel, they combine to judge whether the image contains the target. This parallel nature enables the neural network to be spread across multiple servers, increasing the speed of the application. Traditional programming languages are used to create the neural network environment. Once constructed, these networks are trained with large sets of data. This is different to how we normally think about software applications. Training occurs where multiple samples, such as images containing the desired feature (true positive), are ingested by the network.[12] This process causes the nodes to adjust their connections and create feedback loops. When presented, for example, with multiple images of chest x-rays known to be positive for tuberculosis (TB), the network begins to distinguish those features that are indicative for TB, similar to the method of training for residents in radiology. Shown a slightly different set of training images results in a neural network with different properties.

The training process causes the features to be recognized implicitly within the network, rather than explicitly programmed by a developer. In the example for TB, the application had a sensitivity (accurate identification of true positives) of 97% and a specificity (accurate identification of true negatives) of 100%. The impact of this technology on health care costs is evident. A deep learning application for automated image analysis has the potential to exceed the accuracy and reliability of human radiologists. While this is perceived as a controversial point and currently dismissed, automated image analysis has several compelling economic and quality advantages. Given the low impact of imaging procedures to the patient, it is a frequently used modality. For patients with chronic disease states, they accumulate numerous studies over time. While radiologists use previous images to compare and discern disease progression or discover new findings, there exists a functional limitation as to how far back and how many different modalities can be examined.

With a deep learning-based approach, this is only constrained by the available computing resources. Deep learning has the advantage of ingesting all the images within the Picture Archiving and Communication System (PACS) that are relevant to the analysis. Having the unlimited ability to ingest the longitudinal course of the disease could potentially bring insights into the subclinical evolution of the disease process. Second, improvements to the application can occur continuously and the most effective models instantly moved into operation, benefiting all subsequent studies. Radiologists accumulate knowledge and insight with experience over time. The resources for training and enabling a provider to become proficient are substantial and limited. This creates a scaling problem leading to multiple tiers of access to this resource gated by location, practice environment, and compensation resulting in variability of cost, quality, and availability.

Deep learning has the potential to feed forward information into the ordering cycle. Many organizations use a radiologist to protocol upcoming studies. This requires the radiologist to review the referring physician's order and the chart to ensure that the study ordered is going to actually help answer the clinical question. While ordering a CT scan of the head seems like the appropriate test for a patient with a metastatic lesion to the brain, the protocoling radiologist would correct that to CT of the head with and without contrast to enable evaluation of the perineural edema visible due to contrast enhancement. Missing in this workflow also is a comprehensive review of prior images. Coupled with natural language processing, this deep learning augmented activity could reduce inappropriate ordering and radiologist time and improve diagnostic efficiency. This is similarly applicable to other highly visually oriented specialties including pathology, ophthalmology, and dermatology.

The common conception is that deep learning applications must be associated with a keyboard, screen, and many racks of equipment behind the scenes. The level of semiconductor integration available today enables powerful applications to be constructed to fit in the palm of one's hand. Combining embedded deep learning models, commercially available image sensor, and the computing power found in a cell phone, DermaSensor has created a small handheld package that will image skin lesions (freckles, moles, etc.) and render a score of potential for malignancy. This type of technology could enable earlier detection of skin cancers for more people at a substantially lower cost. Current skin screenings are usually performed by dermatologists at a greater cost. With devices such as these, lower-skilled professionals would be able to deliver comparable results. This directly affects the economics of medicine through its impact on labor costs and potential curability of skin malignancies.

The impact of deep learning, machine learning, and the other technologies discussed will have a profound impact on the cost, quality, and availability of healthcare. The use cases cited above exist and are in clinical practice. This sort of technology has the potential to cause extreme disruption in the structure of medicine. As in most other industries, technology has caused displacement and upheaval. The travel industry is a clear example with the role of the travel agent dramatically shifting. Uber and Lyft have completely disrupted the cab industry, resulting in wage compression, bankruptcy, and suicides.[13–15] Technology and innovation are a double-edged sword, and their impact in medicine is not to be underestimated.

Genomic Data

Following the discovery of the nature of DNA by Watson and Crick in the mid-1950s, scientific attention turned to methods to understand and sequence the molecule. In 1973 Fred Sanger and his collaborators successfully created the first process to sequence segments of DNA.[16] These efforts gave rise to a diversity of approaches and technologies. Slowly the science matured and larger sequences of base pairs were able to be more rapidly decoded. By the late 1980s, the state of the industry was beginning to create commercial products and viable companies. Government funding supported much of this work and it was clear that sequencing the complete human genome was a realistic goal. Launched in 1990 and coordinated by the National Institutes of Health, the Human Genome Project was singularly focused on accomplishing this task. It was successfully concluded in 2003 at a cost of $3 billion.[17]

With the realization of the potential for this technology, genomic sequencing became a multibillion-dollar industry. Current sequencing using the "Ion Torrent" methodology uses specially formed micro wells on a semiconductor chip. Since this methodology leverages the same forces as Moore's law, similar cost performance curves can be expected. In 2003 Robert Carlson formalized this with an eponymous law calling out the log-linear relationship emerging in sequencing cost over time. In practice this is borne out with sequencing costs actually declining faster than predicted over some time periods (Fig. 61.4). Today viral and bacterial sequencing is routine. For patients with HIV, their therapeutic regimen is driven by recurring sequencing of their virus. Understanding what mutations the virus has undergone guides drugs used. Likewise, genome sequencing for cancer is expanding and for breast disease

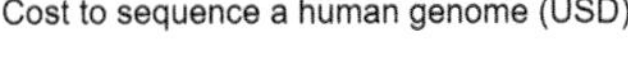

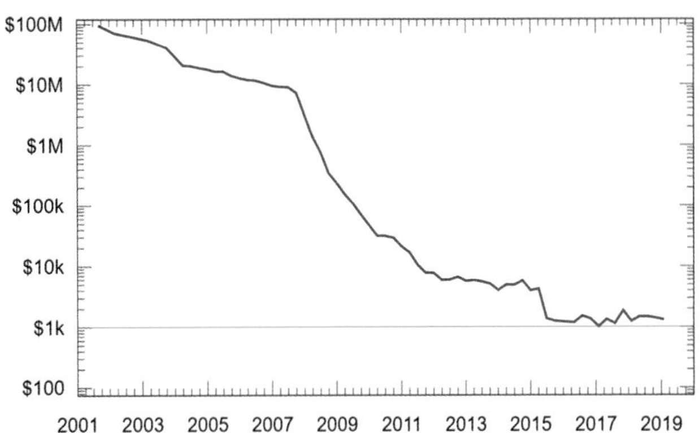

• **Fig. 61.4** Courtesy: National Human Genome Research Institute, http://www.genome.gov/about-genomics/fact-sheets/Sequencing-Human-Genome-cost.

the use of specific genetic markers such as HER2 (Human Epidermal Growth Factor 2) and BRCA1 (BReast CAncer type 1 susceptibility protein) is best practice. The revolution to enable these advances included biochemistry, physics, and information technology.

Sequencing begins with sample DNA enzymatically sliced into millions of overlapping fragments because current technology is limited to strand lengths numbering in the hundreds of base pairs. Once the sequence information of all the slices is obtained, complex algorithms and computing resources map and reassemble the overlapping segments, recreating the original strand. Depending on the organism, these can stretch to tens of billions of base pairs. The human genome contains 46 chromosomes with 50 million to 300 million base pairs in each.

While the raw sequence information is foundational, the understanding of what specific genes are present or other regions these base pairs represent is the critical information at the point of care. Translating sequence information to actual functional maps is complex. This translation step is known as alignment. In the work of the Human Genome Project, as sequences were read, existing protein data were explored to help match the sequence to an expressed protein.

There exist many unique changes in each person's DNA. Replicated sequences of genes can amplify their cumulative expression, whereas deletions can make a trait disappear. Sequences exist that act as promoters and switches, modifying the expression of adjacent encoded elements. Many of these regions are not used to produce proteins at all. Our understanding of what DNA sequences actually represent continues to evolve at a rapid pace, and previous understanding is clarified, with new discoveries incorporated. As more is understood as to what specific segments of DNA actually do, these maps change, so alignment done with one map can be altered significantly if aligned using an older or newer map. It is from the alignment information that individual genes can be isolated and variants analyzed. These findings are the distilled information that comes back to the provider in the genetic analysis.

Incorporation of genetic findings into point-of-care clinical decision-making remains a difficult problem. Unlike other laboratory test data, the clinical implications of genomic findings can be obscure, many times lacking a one-to-one relationship with a clinical impact. Mapping billions of base pairs onto tens of thousands of genes results in a useful abstraction from the underlying genetic mechanics, but continues to be a visualization and decision support problem. There are a few tests that produce the familiar cause and effect relationship of classic laboratory data. Many of these examples are in the field of pharmacogenomics, where genomic characteristics affect how the body responds to pharmaceutical compounds. Several genes have been recognized to have specific effects (sensitivity, side effect profile, or duration of action), CYP2D6 (tamoxifen, tramadol, venlafaxine and several others), HLA-B1502 (carbamazepine), CYP2C19 (clopidogrel, citalopram), and SLCO1B1 (simvastatin).

The clinical implications and management of various cellular mutations, replications, and deletions are unclear, as there exists great interplay between the various components. It is clear, however, that when we do begin to understand, what results will not be a one-to-one relationship. The ability for a provider to understand and anticipate the interactions of these various elements is extremely complex. With the rapid advance of the state of the science and continually evolving understanding of cellular mechanics, it seems to be clear that the use of machine learning to augment human decision support is where the future lies.

Population Health

Use of data to assess health impacts on populations has traditionally been within the province of public health. Understanding the social fabric within communities and its impact of health-related behavior has served as the basis for formulation of health policy and subsequent governmental spending. This type of analysis was typically performed from an economic and regulatory perspective. Information driving these analyses was commonly derived from publically available data sets, such as US government census, local property tax records, and crime reporting statistics. Lacking in this picture, however, was any sort of clinical information or personally identifiable data.

Since 2009, following the passage of the Affordable Care Act (ACA), the environment of care has continued to rapidly evolve. One of the goals of this transformation was to enable data collection and aggregation on patients. To support this data gathering, two barriers had to be addressed. The first was the paper-based workflow. Information had to exist in native digital form and moving providers onto an electronic platform was a critical accomplishment. The government program called "Health Information Technology for Economic and Clinical Health (HITECH) Act" gave providers cash payments to move onto a digital platform. Between 2010 and 2016 the federal government subsidized EHR installation with over $27 billion dollars.[18] Today the bulk of ambulatory and inpatient information is entered directly into an EHR. The second barrier was due to a lack of data standards. To effectively aggregate information from different sources and contexts, the underlying data must have the same definition. Part of the HITECH Act specifically focused on interoperability and the need to create data standards and definitions so that information could flow from EHR to EHR. The act set out standards for interoperability and data definitions to support data exchange. Leveraging this mechanism, large health entities have used this to bootstrap creation of population-level aggregation of health data.

The ACA also incentivized groups of providers working with health insurance payers to go "at risk" and share care cost and savings. Needing an objective standard, many of these contracts leverage metrics that attempt to quantify compliance with screening programs, vaccination, and preventative health measures. Private insurers and public payers use benchmark performance as a factor in overall reimbursement. To manage this exposure, health organizations have made changes in the EHR to specifically capture these data elements. These data are then rolled up to the plan level to understand overall performance. Providers and payers pool clinical and claims data to round out these efforts.

Population health is an outgrowth from these reporting needs. As compared to the public health efforts, population health approaches this arena from a completely different direction, with the foundation being personally identifiable health information including clinical, demographic, and claims. EHR vendors have responded with software platforms aimed specifically at this market. The large vendors such as Epic or Cerner have built HealthyPlanet and HealthyIntent, respectively. These applications support population health aggregating clinical data, insurance claims, and third party information. Typically based on a data warehouse, the applications create a master patient index. That is, a mapping function that deduplicates patients and creates a patient record that has a unique identifier for each entrant. No matter where or in what organization that patient has been taken care of, the system maps all the data of that patient to a unique patient identifier. Third party data sets are also supported, and geospatial mapping information creates an environment able to address questions that go beyond the clinical or billing context.

Population health differs from public health in that it uses findings or evidence at the population level to impact the care of individual patients within the clinical context. Public health efforts are unable to bridge this divide as they lack personally identifiable health data and a clinical interaction with the patient. The tie back to the patient takes many forms. Commonly, providers are presented with a number of preventative health metrics such as cancer screenings, vaccinations, and other health recommendations in the medical record at the time of the patient visit. The physician is responsible for addressing the list of items presented and many times these items are part of the shared risk insurance plan the provider and patient have entered into, affecting compensation. Physician performance around these items directly drives reimbursements.

Not all applications of this data involve providers. With the third party data gathered that surrounds the patient, the ability to understand the home environment becomes more possible. A recent example involves patients with chronic conditions requiring frequent clinical follow up to optimize their health status. Patients unable to consistently travel to appointments have higher rates of emergency visits and higher cost. Correctly identifying this population is the first step. Using appointment, diagnosis, socioeconomic, and pharmacy data, at-risk members can be segregated. This information bridges all three domains of clinical, reimbursement, and publicly available data sets. Modeling the scope and cost of a mobility program takes place and the targeted population established. This blending of clinical/medicine with social/environmental is still at the early stages; however, companies are stepping up to address this market. Uber and Lyft have both launched programs to address mobility challenges for medical patients. Payers can set up accounts with these companies to assist patients using these services for health-related needs. Travel between health-related activities can be automatically approved with the application geofencing destinations such as provider offices, clinics, pharmacies, or emergency centers. In the correct circumstances, patients have improved access to health services, fewer missed appointments, and a higher level of care at minimal cost.

With the fusion of the data discussed above, much better insight can be derived into individual's lives. The question ultimately becomes one of privacy, autonomy, and personal choice. All of the technologies discussed previously from data warehousing to machine learning, genetic sequencing, and population health stretch the boundaries that health care has traditionally occupied. They represent powerful tools that reveal intimate details of how patients choose to live their lives, choices they make, and how they approach their environment. These are intensely personal. Using the tools currently at our disposal, the health system clearly intends on influencing these choices and bringing our private lives into wider view.

Deep insight can be gleaned from our daily choices and local circumstances. In 2012 the retailer Target used machine learning models to target populations of shoppers with specific coupon offers that those populations would find valuable. The deep learning model used purchasing patterns, demographic information from loyalty cards, and socioeconomic information from store locality. One score attempted to recognize newly pregnant women and capitalize on their specific buying needs. The store would send those women coupons for prenatal vitamins, diapers, cribs, and other items commonly purchased. A father of a Minneapolis teenager was one of the individuals who received these mailings. Confronting his daughter it was revealed she was expecting.[19] These tools are powerful. Focused in the right directions, they have the potential to improve care, survival, and cost; however, tools also have the potential to harm.

Impact on Anesthesia

While the first-order effects of these technologies are currently beginning to be felt in medicine, their impact on anesthesia thus far has been muted.[20] Oftentimes, artificial intelligence is leveraged to enable less skilled individuals to work at higher level guided through decision support or just-in-time learning support structures. Applicability of this type of advanced support to the intraoperative environment demands low false-positive rates coupled with high accuracy. Currently these levels of confidence are difficult to achieve. Within the perioperative space, however, tasks such as booking, scheduling, staffing, and OR utilization modeling are clearly useful and appropriate for this technology. Unused or wasted operative time is expensive. Harnessing historical data and future demand for information to drive higher facility utilization is well within current reach. Machine learning is able to include and integrate variables far removed from the local environment. Accounting for postanesthesia care unit (PACU) space, daily staffing, and procedure-based length of recovery could substantially curtail overloading and cases requiring recovery in the OR. Adding in factors such as hospital bed availability, pending admissions, and discharge patterns could help optimize scheduling well beyond the abilities of the human mind.

Within the clinical realm, NLP coupled with machine learning could cull the EHR and gather relevant historical documents/test results to be used to screen patients in the preoperative period. These screening applications could build a multidimensional risk score and suggest potential follow up assessments to help quantify specific risk. Driven by a machine learning agent, unnecessary testing and inadequate evaluation leading to day of surgery cancellation would be reduced. These types of applications could improve OR performance and reduce day of surgery chaos, favorably impacting patients and providers.

Conclusions

Over the past 50 years there has been a revolution as technology has become an integral part of our human existence. Increasing computational power, ongoing data collection, and innovation in how we view data and information has impacted clinical medicine from workflow to diagnosis and treatment. As this trend continues, it will inevitably continue to change relationships between payers, providers, and patients. The rapid deployment of EHR platforms is forming the basis for a sustainable digital infrastructure in health care. Advances in networking and storage serve to increase the scope and power of computing machinery. Cloud providers offer the ability for organizations to move their focus from infrastructure to application and end-user support. Cloud also enables individuals to use advanced infrastructure for analytic projects in an agile and cost-effective manner.

Scientists continue to unravel the human genome, and as the cellular mechanics become further understood, its impact on how we diagnose and treat disease will increase. This waterfall of knowledge will exceed the ability for even highly functioning human brains to consume, and augmented decision support based on machine learning will become critical to deliver state of the art treatment at the point of care. The use of large data and population health models could improve outcomes, reduce cost, and extend life. Bringing together these sensitive personal attributes of our environment, genetics, and home represent an incredible opportunity to improve the human condition. Change, however, is amoral, and the question becomes how we chose to utilize the tools and opportunities presented in this process. Those choices will drive the impact these forces will have on humanity.

References

1. AQI. National Anesthesia Clinical Registry (NACOR), Anesthesia Quality Institute, March 3, 2020. Available at https://www.aqihq.org/introduction-to-nacor.aspx.
2. Codd EF. A relational model of data for large shared data banks. *Commun ACM*. 1970;13(6):377–387.
3. Donovan F. US Hospitals Increasingly Adopt Radiology 3D Image/Display Tech, HIT Infrastructure, December 27, 2018. Available at https://hitinfrastructure.com/news/us-hospitals-increasingly-adopt-radiology-3d-image-display-tech.
4. Lojek BO. *History of Semiconductor Engineering*: Springer Science & Business Media; 2007:321–323.
5. Sah C-T. Evolution of the MOS transistor-from conception to VLSI (PDF). *Proc IEEE*. 1988;76(10):1280–1326.
6. Moore GE. Cramming more components onto integrated circuits. *Electronics*. 1965;38(8):114–117.
7. Cherry S. Edholm's law of bandwidth. *IEEE Spectrum*. 2004; 41(7):58–60.
8. Analytics. Wikipedia, Feb 4, 2004, November 22, 2021. Available at http://en.wikipedia.org/wiki/Analytics.
9. CMS Staff, Quickstats, HealthIT.gov, October 1, 2019. Available at https://dashboard.healthit.gov/quickstats/quickstats.php.
10. SAS. Machine Learning and Why it Matters, sas.com, September 22, 2019. Available at https://www.sas.com/en_us/insights/analytics/machine-learning.html.
11. Warren A. 3 Voice Recognition Platforms that Integrate with EHRs, InformaConnect, April 3, 2017. Available at https://knect365.com/pharmanext/article/32f56225-6c48-40cc-8f8e-cf710fe4aed0/3-voice-recognition-platforms-that-integrate-with-ehrs.
12. Lakhani P., Sundaram B. Deep learning at chest radiography: automated classification of pulmonary tuberculosis by using convolutional neural networks. *Radiology*. 2017;284: 574–582.
13. Morris D. 6th New York City Cab Driver Takes His Life in Crisis Blamed on Uber, Fortune, June 16, 2018. Available at http://fortune.com/2018/06/16/new-york-cab-driver-suicide-uber.
14. Siemaszko C. In the Shadow of Uber's Rise, Taxi Driver Suicides Leave Cabbies Shaken, NBC News, June 7, 2018, Updated June 8, 2018. Available at https://www.nbcnews.com/news/us-news/shadow-uber-s-rise-taxi-driver-suicides-leave-cabbies-shaken-n879281.
15. Stewart N, Ferré-Sadurn L. Another Taxi Driver in Debt Takes His Life. That's 5 in 5 Months, New York Times, May 27, 2018. Available at https://www.nytimes.com/2018/05/27/nyregion/taxi-driver-suicide-nyc.html.
16. Sanger F, Donelson JE, Coulson AR, Kössel H, Fischer D. Use of DNA polymerase I primed by a synthetic oligonucleotide to determine a nucleotide sequence in phage f1 DNA. *Proc Natl Acad Sci USA*. 1973;70(4):1209–1213.
17. National Human Genome Research Institute. Human Genome Project FAQ, National Genome Research Project, Febuary 24, 2020. Available at https://www.genome.gov/human-genome-project/Completion-FAQ.
18. Schilling B. The Federal Government Has Put Billions into Promoting Electronic Health Record Use: How Is It Going? The Commonwealth Fund, September 11, 2019. Available at https://www.commonwealthfund.org/publications/newsletter-article/federal-government-has-put-billions-promoting-electronic-health.
19. Hill K. How Target Figured Out A Teen Girl Was Pregnant Before Her Father Did. Forbes, Feburary. 2012;16. https://www.forbes.com/sites/kashmirhill/2012/02/16/how-target-figured-out-a-teen-girl-was-pregnant-before-her-father-did/#29f8af1b6668.
20. Connor CW. Artificial intelligence and machine learning in anesthesiology. *Anesthesiology*. 2019;131(6):1346–1359. doi. https://org/10.1097/ALN.0000000000002694.

62

The MD Anderson Cancer Center Moon Shots Program®: A Global Priority

PAMELA C. PAPADOPOULOS, EMILY B. ROARTY, ROSALIND S. BELLO, JOËL FOKOM DOMGUE, SANJAY SHETE, AND ANIRBAN MAITRA

Introduction

The University of Texas MD Anderson Cancer Center's Moon Shots Program® is a collaborative effort to accelerate the development of scientific discoveries into clinical advances that save patients' lives. The program was inspired by President John F. Kennedy's speech in Houston in 1962, where he declared our nation's mission to go to the moon. Launched in 2012, the Moon Shots Program® began under the leadership of then-President of the University of Texas MD Anderson Cancer Center, Dr. Ronald DePinho. During an interview describing the motivation behind the program, he stated, "Humanity urgently needs bold action to defeat cancer. I believe that we have many of the tools we need to pick the fight of the 21st century. Let us focus our energies on approaching cancer comprehensively and systematically, with the precision of an engineer, always asking … *'What can we do to directly impact patients?'*"[1]

Since its inception, the Moon Shots Program® has expanded to 13 multidisciplinary teams of clinicians and researchers tasked with developing comprehensive approaches to advance cancer prevention, early detection, and treatment to improve the lives of patients and reduce cancer mortality. In addition to launching innovative clinical trials and accelerating scientific research, the achievements of the Moon Shots Program® include public awareness campaigns for cancer prevention. These accomplishments include contributing to legislation banning teenage tanning bed use in Texas and other states, expanding a smoking cessation program, and expanding HPV vaccination efforts in the United States and globally. Furthermore, significant efforts have been made to detect cancer early when patient outcomes can be profoundly impacted. In this chapter, we highlight examples of the program's success in reducing global cancer mortality, using three salient examples: promoting smoking cessation as part of the Lung Cancer Moon Shot, enhancing HPV vaccination as part of the HPV Moon Shot, and facilitating early detection of pancreatic cancer as part of the Pancreatic Cancer Moon Shot.

Lung Cancer Moon Shot: Smoking Cessation Initiatives

Smoking is a significant public health problem and is currently responsible for nearly 6 million premature deaths each year worldwide (including 480,000 in the United States alone),[2] with estimates as high as 8 million deaths annually by the year 2030.[3] Tobacco plays a causal role in at least 15 types of cancer[4,5] and accounts for 85% of lung cancer cases[6] and approximately 30% of the attributable risk for overall cancer mortality.[7] While there are several approved smoking cessation medications, including varenicline, bupropion, and several types of nicotine replacement therapy products (NRT), each with demonstrated efficacy against placebo,[8–11] there is considerable heterogeneity in treatment response. Individual variation in response to medication, in particular, suggests that "one size does not fit all" and improving our understanding of individual-level predictors of treatment outcome is critical to the advancement of the field. One of our major challenges lies in determining how to optimize a smoker's chance of achieving initial treatment success and what approaches should be taken at treatment failure. The potential to match smokers to a specific initial treatment based on factors observable prior to quitting (at baseline) has been investigated using a variety of behavioral, genetic, biological, affective, and neurobiological factors[12–16] in an effort to predict the response to pharmacotherapy. However, matching patients to a "rescue" treatment after initial failure remains unclear, and there is little guidance for providers to select the optimal follow up treatment.

A second important challenge is the delivery of the most effective treatment to the largest group of smokers. National surveys show that less than one-third of smokers who attempt to quit actually receive counseling and pharmacotherapy.[17] Traditional state "quitlines," while offering a service to a large number of smokers at any one time, are highly underutilized and, in comparison to the most effective treatment approaches using both counseling and pharmacotherapy, are much less effective.[11]

Smoking Cessation Solutions

To achieve the goal of changing clinical practice for smoking cessation, we initiated a series of prospective clinical trials and conducted an extensive analysis of genetic information from previously completed trials that collectively examined the relationship between specific individual-level predictors (behavioral, affective, neurophysiologic) and response to smoking cessation treatments. While each of these trials individually addressed specific research questions, the collective goal in this effort was to extract critical information from each trial regarding individual differences that can be used to predict, or personalize, response to various treatments, including pharmacotherapy and behavioral treatments. These factors include age, sex, motivation, nicotine dependence, affect, psychiatric comorbidity (depression), neural and behavioral indicators of brain deficits in reward, metabolic (nicotine metabolic ratio), and genetic profiles, and importantly, the specific treatment pathways (which medications or series of medications they use) before they successfully quit. In parallel, we also examined the optimal treatment configuration for delivering smoking cessation in the context of lung cancer screening, focusing on older age, heavy smokers who have not yet quit, and for whom additional genetic data on lung cancer risk will be available. We expect this study to provide additional individual-level information on predictors of treatment outcome for this unique population that can be related to lung cancer risk, and may further the development of a predictive algorithm.

In addition to identifying predictive markers of response, we have also worked to promulgate the basic cessation treatment model developed and refined within the MD Anderson Cancer Center Tobacco Treatment Program (TTP). TTP began modestly in 2006 with clinician referral, later incorporating automated referral using electronic health records. The program currently treats nearly 1200 new patients at MD Anderson and conducts more than 11,000 patient visits per year. The TTP is comprehensive, consisting of individualized smoking cessation counseling, over-the-counter and prescription pharmacotherapy, and the integrated assessment and treatment of mental health conditions and other psychosocial concerns. The TTP plan consists of an initial in-person consultation (60–90 min), plus 6–8 subsequent follow up treatment sessions conducted over an 8- to 12-week period, 95% of which were conducted by telephone. Treatment involves behavioral counseling for smoking cessation and other psychologic or psychiatric interventions, as needed, for related mental health issues. Counseling is based on the principles of motivational interviewing[18] and social cognitive behavioral problem solving.[19] Patients typically receive 10–12 weeks of pharmacotherapy, including nicotine replacement (patch or lozenge), bupropion, and varenicline, either alone or in various combinations. Each treatment plan is personalized in terms of counseling session number, duration, content, and choice of pharmacotherapy, which followed a previously defined protocol[20] consistent with the National Comprehensive Cancer Network guidelines.[21]

To determine the effectiveness of long-term abstinence and evaluate differences between patients with and without cancer, we analyzed data from more than 3000 individuals who received smoking cessation treatment through the MD Anderson TTP.[22] Overall self-reported abstinence rates for the sample were 45.1% at 3 months, 45.8% at 6 months, and 43.7% at 9 months for the multiply imputed data (averaged over 10 imputed data sets), 41.1% at 3 months, 39.5% at 6 months, and 35.6% at 9 months for intention-to-treat (ITT); and 44.5% at 3 months, 45.6% at 6 months, and 43.7% at 9 months for respondents only. We also obtained expired carbon monoxide levels during all in-person visits. Congruence between self-reported, 7-day point prevalence abstinence and expired carbon monoxide was 93% for less than 8 ppm and 87% for carbon monoxide levels of less than 6 ppm. No significant differences in abstinence for the multiply imputed sample were found when comparing no cancer history versus cancer history at the 3-month (relative risk [RR], 1.03; 95% CI, 0.93–1.16; $P = 0.55$), 6-month (RR, 1.05; 95% CI, 0.94–1.18; $P = 0.38$), and 9-month (RR, 1.10; 95% CI, 0.97–1.26; $P = 0.14$) follow ups, as well as in the longitudinal models (RR, 1.06; 95% CI, 0.95–1.18; $P = 0.27$). In addition, no significant differences were noted in the comparisons of no cancer history versus those with and without smoking-related cancer (RR, 1.02; 95% CI, 0.90–1.14; $P = 0.8$) or patients with a history of cancer (RR, 1.04; 95% CI, 0.89–1.20; $P = 0.64$).

TTP dissemination occurs through two major initiatives within our Moon Shots Program®. First, we developed and oversaw the clinical content within an MD Anderson Cancer Center-certified tobacco treatment specialist training program (CTTS). This program successfully disseminates the TTP model to other health care systems and health care providers through direct training and supervision of counselors and providers from around the country. The second initiative provides clinical content and expertise for Project ECHO (Extension for Community Healthcare Outcomes),[23] a telementoring program that provides expert consultation to providers across the country, based on the TTP treatment model.

HPV Cancer Moon Shot: The Global Burden of HPV-Associated Cancers

Human papillomavirus (HPV) infection causes nearly 5% of all new cancer cases globally, affecting the uterine cervix, vulva, vagina, anus, penis, and oropharynx.[24] With

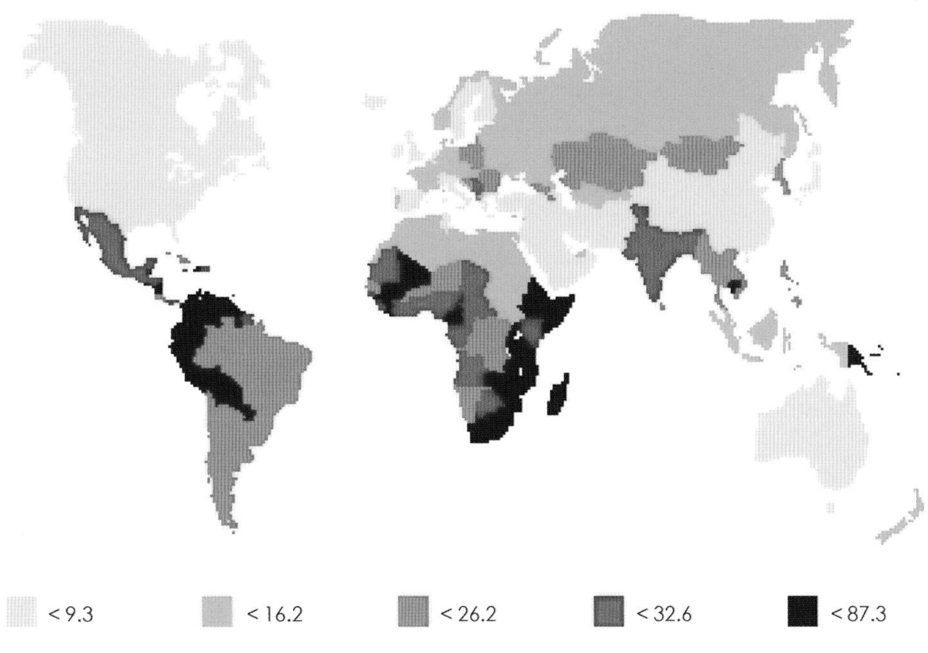

• **Fig. 62.1** Global burden of HPV-related cancers. (From J. Ferlay, F. Bray, P. Pisani, D.M. Parkin, GLOBOCAN 2002 cancer incidence. Mortality and prevalence worldwide. IARC CancerBase No. 5 version 2.0, IARC Press, Lyon (2004)).[68]

approximately 530,000 new cases annually, cervical cancer is the most common HPV-associated cancer worldwide, compared to other HPV-associated cancers (113,000 annual cases).[3] This global picture is driven by low- and middle-income countries (LMICs), where approximately 85% of new cases of cervical cancer occur mainly due to the lack of organized cervical screening and HPV vaccination programs (Fig. 62.1). With the evolution of sexual practices in recent decades, an increasing incidence of HPV-related anal and oropharyngeal cancers has been observed.[25,26]

Unlike LMICs, where cervical cancer is by far the most common HPV-related cancer, widespread screening programs in high-income countries (HICs) have dramatically reduced the burden of cervical cancer.[27] To date, the burden of HPV-associated noncervical cancers outweighs that of cervical cancer in HICs. In the United States, where an average of 44,000 HPV-associated cancers are reported annually, oropharyngeal cancers (12,600) are more common than cervical cancers (9700).[28]

HPV Vaccine Development, Evolution, and Recommendations

The discovery of HPV as the necessary cause of cervical cancer has led to the development of prophylactic HPV vaccines. The HPV vaccine is composed of self-assembled virus-like particles (VLPs) that form when a specific protein (the viral L1 major capsid protein) is produced by microorganisms (yeast for Gardasil, Merck) or insect cells (for Cervarix, GSK) through a fermentation process. These VLPs closely resemble native HPV particles and act as antigens that evoke the production of HPV-neutralizing antibodies in the human body.[29] The vaccine does not contain DNA and is therefore considered noninfectious.

In 2006 the US Food and Drug Administration (FDA) approved the first commercially available prophylactic HPV vaccine, Gardasil (Merck & Co., USA), for the primary prevention of infections by HPV16 and HPV18, as well as HPV6 and HPV11, the two HPV genotypes that cause 90% of genital warts. In 2007 the Centers for Disease Control and Prevention's Advisory Committee for Immunization Practices (ACIP) recommended routine HPV vaccination in women aged 9–26 years.[30] In 2010 a second HPV vaccine for the primary prevention of infections by HPV16 and HPV18, Cervarix (GSK, Belgium), was approved by the FDA and recommended by the ACIP.[31] Further, 4vHPV vaccination of males aged 9–26 years was approved by the US FDA in October 2009 and subsequently recommended by the ACIP in 2010.[32]

In 2014 the FDA approved a second-generation vaccine, Gardasil 9 (9vHPV), which targets five additional HPV genotypes: HPV31, 33, 45, 52, and 58. Following this, the ACIP recommended in 2015 that routine HPV vaccination is initiated at 11 or 12 years of age but can be started as young as 9 years of age for females and males.[33] Vaccination was also recommended for females and males aged 13–21 years and women aged 22–26 years who have not been vaccinated previously or who have not completed the three-dose series, and it was stated that males aged 22–26 years may be vaccinated.[33] Since 2017 Gardasil-9 has been the only HPV vaccine available in the United States. In 2018 the FDA approved the use of the 9vHPV vaccine in adults aged 27–45 years, and in 2019 ACIP expanded its recommendation to this age group based on a shared clinical decision-making procedure.[34]

Until 2016, the ACIP recommended a three-dose regimen for HPV vaccination (at M0, M1, and M6) regardless of age at initiation of HPV vaccination. In 2016 a two-dose (at M0 and M6) schedule was recommended for girls and boys who initiated the vaccination series at ages 9 through 14 years,[35] but three doses remained the recommendation for persons who initiated the vaccination series at age ≥15 years and for immunocompromised persons.

Barriers to Implementation of HPV Vaccination

Despite progress achieved in recent years, HPV vaccination rates in the United States remain suboptimal. In 2018 only 51% of eligible adolescents were up to date on their vaccination schedule,[36] far below the Healthy People 2020 goal of 80%, and below the rates achieved by other HICs, such as Australia, the United Kingdom, and Belgium.[37] Many factors contribute to low HPV vaccination uptake in the United States. At the system or policy level, missed clinical opportunities to recommend and offer HPV vaccines constitute a major limiting factor.[37,38] This suggests the need for (i) health care organizations to use electronic office systems, including electronic health records and immunization information systems; (ii) the CDC to develop, test, disseminate, and evaluate the impact of integrated, comprehensive communication strategies for physicians and other relevant health professionals; (iii) Healthcare Effectiveness Data and Information Set quality measure for HPV vaccination to be expanded to males; and (iv) states to enact laws and implement policies that allow pharmacists to administer vaccines.

At the provider level, lack of high-quality recommendation for HPV vaccine to patients is a strong correlate of underutilization of HPV vaccine in the United States.[39] At the individual or community level, people's knowledge, perception, and acceptance of the HPV vaccine is limited.[40] In a study assessing the reasons for not receiving HPV vaccine among eligible US adults, the most frequently reported reasons were as follows: did not know about the vaccine (18.5% [14.9–22.1]), provider did not recommend (14.1% [10.9–17.4]), vaccine not needed or necessary (13.8% [10.0–17.0]), not sexually active (13.7% [10.5–16.9]), and not required to get the vaccine (11.4% [8.5–14.3]) (Fig. 62.2). In another US study examining beliefs about HPV vaccine effectiveness in preventing cervical cancer, only 29.8% of women believed that HPV vaccine is successful in preventing cervical cancer.[41]

Global Examples of Vaccine Efficacy/Effectiveness and Success in Overcoming Barriers

Of the nearly 100 countries that have introduced HPV vaccination, only a few have achieved vaccination higher than 80% coverage.[37,42] This includes Australia in Oceania, Scotland in Europe, Bhutan in Asia, and Rwanda in Africa. Overall, analysis of the average reported coverage by delivery strategy shows that countries using school-based vaccination had, on average, 20% higher coverage than those providing vaccines through primary care or health centers.[37]

In Australia, parental opinions were key drivers of vaccination, with HPV vaccination associated with the parent being the vaccine decision-maker and with previous completion of the childhood vaccination schedule.[43] In Austria, where males and females are vaccinated, information on the vaccine from physicians was found to strongly influence vaccine uptake.[44] In that country, higher paternal educational status has shown to significantly increase boy's HPV vaccination but did not influence girl's vaccination, suggesting that sex-specific strategies may be required.[44] In 2011, following a national education and awareness campaign, Rwanda was the first LMIC to implement a national HPV vaccination program.[45] Since then, Rwanda has achieved more than 90% coverage with 4vHPV vaccination every year, through school-based vaccination and community outreach to females absent from or not enrolled in school. The roll-out of HPV vaccination nationally through the Merck Donation Program (2011–2013) served as the

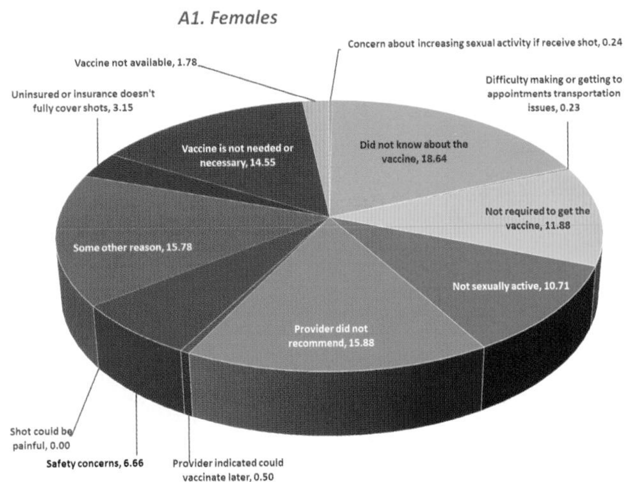

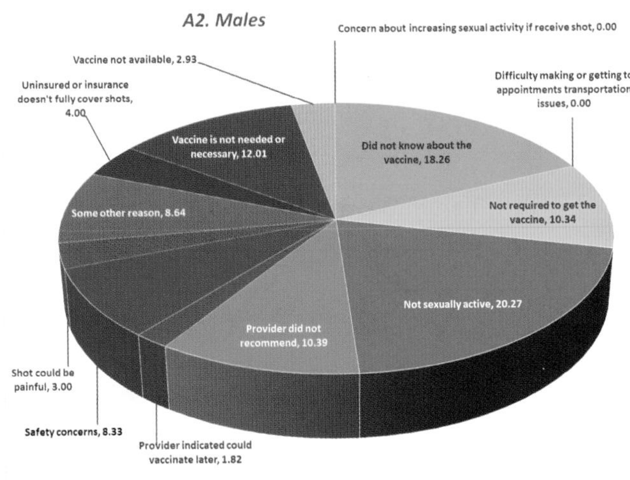

• **Fig. 62.2** Main reasons for not getting the HPV vaccine in the eligible adult US population, by sex.

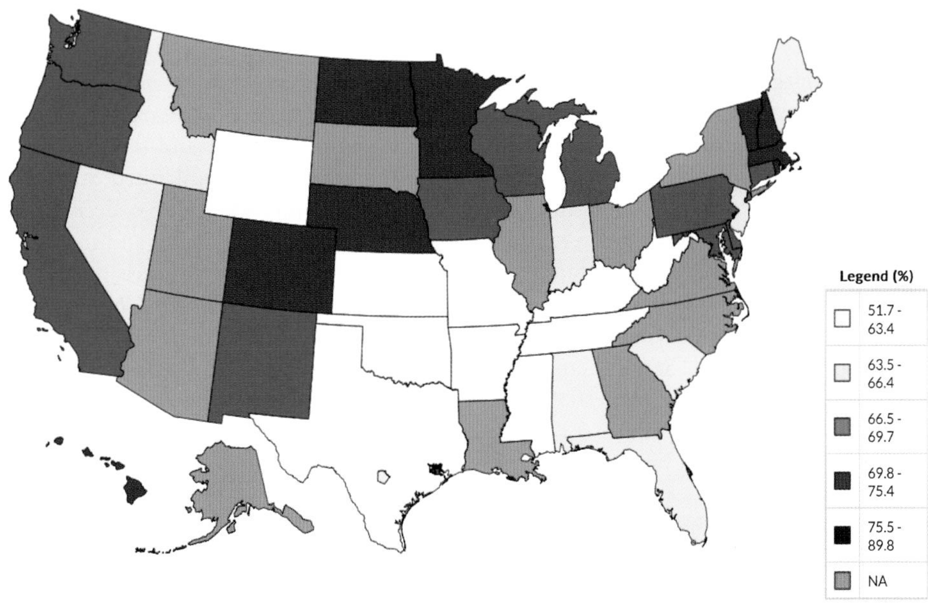

• **Fig. 62.3** HPV vaccination coverage in the United States, by state.

"demonstration" necessary to become a GAVI-supported program in 2013.

In the United States, HPV vaccination rates vary widely across states[36] (Fig. 62.3). The states that have enacted the HPV vaccination mandate have achieved the highest coverage rates (Rhode Island, District of Columbia) and the largest annual increase in HPV vaccination rates (Virginia),[46] and the most conservative and highly religious states (Wyoming, Mississippi, South Carolina, Utah, and Texas) exhibit the lowest HPV vaccination rates and/or a decrease in HPV vaccination uptake.[46]

How the Cancer Moon Shots Program® Has Worked With Policy Makers and Other Stakeholders in Promoting Vaccine Rates in Texas and Around the Nation/World

MD Anderson has almost 10 years of engagement and leadership in cancer prevention and control initiatives to promote awareness of HPV-associated cancers and to provide education about HPV vaccination for public and health care professionals. MD Anderson Cancer Center has relied on partnerships with key stakeholders throughout its history in promoting awareness and utilization of HPV vaccination for cancer prevention. These partnerships informed the formation of MD Anderson's HPV Moon Shot in 2014 and supported efforts in three cancer prevention and control domains: public and professional education, policy, and services.

MD Anderson's efforts in HPV vaccination stemmed from public and professional initiatives focused on cervical cancer prevention. In 2012 and 2013 the MD Anderson Cervical Cancer Workgroup partnered with Cervical Cancer-Free Texas, Houston Community College Coleman College for Health Sciences, and National Cervical Cancer Coalition to host the Houston Cervical Cancer Summit with an overarching aim to reduce the incidence of cervical cancer and improve the quality of life of cancer survivors. In 2014 the partners expanded the scope of the summit to focus on HPV-associated cancers. The summits and the formation of an HPV Moon Shot team in September 2014 allowed MD Anderson to grow and strengthen relationships with professional organizations. The Community Relations and Education (CRE) team at MD Anderson Cancer Center has continuously developed print and integrated media products to enhance community knowledge about HPV vaccination. The CRE team also offers "Prevent Cancer: The HPV Vaccine." It is a program that educates parents and other adults about HPV, related cancers, risk factors, and HPV vaccination. Many CRE products and programs are available in English, Spanish, and Vietnamese.

The HPV Moon Shot commitment to education on HPV-associated cancers and vaccination extended to the completion of an environmental scan, policy forums, and strategic plan development. In September 2014 MD Anderson received a notice from the Cancer Center Support Grant supplement (NCI 3 P30 CA016672–39S4). MD Anderson engaged 46 external partners during the data collection process. The completed scan identified barriers, facilitators, and best practices associated with HPV vaccination uptake in children aged 9–17 years in pediatric care settings.

The James A. Baker III Institute for Public Policy at the Rice University and the University of Texas MD Anderson Cancer Center convened an annual, joint public policy forum consisting of panel discussions to raise awareness about challenges and opportunities in the fields of biomedical science, public health, and health care. The December 3, 2014, forum focused on HPV-related diseases, the HPV vaccine, and the potential impact of broadly disseminated HPV vaccination on public health, resulting in the publication of a policy brief, *Human Papillomavirus Vaccine: A Public Health Opportunity for Texas*. This engagement was followed by an HPV Vaccination Frequently Asked Questions document developed in January 2015. MD Anderson and its partner organizations educated decision-makers about HPV vaccination in advance of the passage of Senate Bill 200, 84th Legislature, Regular Session, 2015. SB200 charged the Health and Human Services Commission (HHSC), developing a strategic plan to significantly reduce morbidity and mortality from HPV-associated cancer. MD Anderson worked with HHSC, the Department of State Health Services, and the Cancer Prevention and Research Institute of Texas (CPRIT) to contribute content to the draft strategic plan.

In 2015 MD Anderson hosted the 2nd National Cancer Institute (NCI) Cancer Centers HPV Vaccination Summit to share findings from all of the environmental scans funded by the 2014 NCI Cancer Center Support Grant supplements. As a result of discussions at this convening, MD Anderson joined 68 other NCI-designated cancer centers in issuing a consensus statement on January 27, 2016 calling for increased HPV vaccination. Two additional statements (January 2017 and June 2018) were issued by cancer centers. The latter statement was also supported by the American Cancer Society, the American Association for Cancer Research, the American Society for Clinical Oncology, the Prevent Cancer Foundation, the American Society for Preventive Oncology and the Association of American Cancer Institutes.

On June 11, 2016 MD Anderson established an HPV vaccination clinic for MD Anderson employees and their children, with MD Anderson Blue Cross Blue Shield insurance. The clinic began as a clinic once a month on the second Saturday of each month at the Cancer Prevention Center and now operates quarterly via the Child and Adolescent Center. MD Anderson continues to support expanded access to HPV vaccination by participating with others in CPRIT-funded projects designed to bring HPV vaccination to school settings via mobile units. MD Anderson also assists in leveraging its relationships with school districts and funded vaccination programs to develop new proposals for expanded vaccine access.

A planning core team was formed in September 2018 to develop an institutional strategic framework (Framework) to increase HPV vaccination in Texas. The planning core team's aim was to develop and propose a framework through a multiphased approach aligned with MD Anderson's Community Outreach and Engagement (COE) model. The COE model highlights key resources, relationships, and evidence-based actions taken in priority areas to reduce the cancer burden and associated risk factors of Texans. Cancer prevention and control leaders have now been charged with building upon the institution's history and relationships with key external stakeholders to activate roles and implement strategies within the framework. The expectation is that the actions taken by the institution will result in a significant increase in HPV vaccination rates in Texas.

Pancreatic Cancer Moon Shot: The Quest for Early Detection

Pancreatic ductal adenocarcinoma (PDAC) is the tenth most common cancer and the third leading cause of death from all cancers in the United States.[47] While many other types of cancers have seen a decrease in mortality due to improvements in screening and treatments, PDAC remains the sole major cancer with a rising mortality rate. The 5-year death rate for PDAC in the United States rose by 0.3% during the 2012–2016 period[48] and is expected to increase. PDAC is projected to become the second leading cause of cancer-related deaths by 2030.[49]

Cancer stage at diagnosis determines treatment options and strongly influences the length of survival.[50,51] Unfortunately, only ~15% of patients with pancreatic cancer are diagnosed when the malignancy is localized to the pancreas and is often asymptomatic at this stage. The overall 5-year survival rate for pancreatic cancer patients is a dismal 9.3%[52] but there is substantial evidence that earlier diagnosis of PDAC impacts survival. It is estimated that increasing the proportion of subjects diagnosed with stage I or stage II PDAC to 50%, from the current 15%, would result in more than doubling of the 5-year survival.[51] Given the development of PDAC through progressive stages, strategies that target the detection of small-volume PDAC or advanced precursor lesions (PanIN-3) are likely to be effective in reducing mortality.[53] Extrapolation from mutational burden in terminal PDAC samples has identified a wide window of opportunity for early detection, justifying the need for the development of reliable blood-based markers to assess the risk of harboring asymptomatic PDAC.[54] Such screening could be applied initially to individuals who are at "high risk" for PDAC (due to an inherited predisposition or other underlying factors), and eventually expanded to the average risk population.

Early detection of PDAC has been at the forefront of the efforts of our Pancreatic Moon Shots Team. We have focused on building tools for assessing patients who are at high risk for developing PDAC, developing blood-based biomarkers to detect abnormalities before the patient experiences symptoms, and constructing processing techniques that enhance computed tomography (CT) and magnetic resonance imaging (MRI) images to reveal lesions in the body that have yet to produce symptoms.

Pancreatic Cancer High-Risk Clinic

Several national and international centers have been screening asymptomatic high-risk patients to diagnose PDAC at the earliest stages before it spreads. Given the low incidence of the disease, screening the entire population would not be cost-effective, which has recently been reiterated by the updated recommendation from the United States Prevention and Screening Task Force[55]. The International Cancer of the Pancreas Screening (CAPS) Consortium, consisting of worldwide experts, has advocated for both establishing guidelines to classify individuals as high risk based on family history and genetic susceptibility and developing screening and surveillance programs for this population.[4–8,56] In order to address the needs of patients at risk for developing the disease, we established our own Pancreatic Cancer High-Risk Clinic at MD Anderson, funded through one of the Moon Shot flagships.

There is no clear consensus on the time at which to start screening, the best method and interval of follow up surveillance following an initial examination, and when to consider surgery. Despite this, endoscopic ultrasound (EUS) and MRI are the preferred modalities for initial screening. The goal of a surveillance program in asymptomatic patients should be the detection of stage I pancreatic cancer, ideally with the goal of detecting advanced ("high-grade") premalignant lesions, as detection would dramatically increase survival rates. Novel imaging methods and biomarkers should evolve together, and the challenge is to increase the sensitivity and specificity of the detection methods to avoid unnecessary overtreatment of patients.

The risk assessment performed individually on these patients is based on individual germline mutational status, family history, personal medical history, and environmental exposures. Based on the relative risk obtained by one of more factors combined, in the past 4 years we have subdivided our patients into three risk categories: (1) mildly elevated risk, (2) moderately elevated risk, and (3) high risk. We only continue prospective screening in patients from the moderately elevated and high-risk categories. Most of these screening criteria are in agreement with the consensus reached by the international CAPS Consortium[57] and are based on several other epidemiologic studies conducted and validated. In the past 4 years, we have seen more than 260 patients at the Pancreatic Cancer High-Risk Clinic, of which ~190 patients qualified for prospective screening and were enrolled into our MD Anderson Pancreatic Cancer High-Risk Cohort. We enrolled more than 150 patients in the cohort and collected and stored biospecimens, including blood, saliva, urine, and stool. This biorepository is fundamental for the validation of early detection biomarkers.

In July 2018 the National Comprehensive Cancer Network (NCCN) guidelines outlined germline testing for all PDAC patients.[58] In addition, these guidelines also include testing for patients with a family history of PDAC, which includes many patients in our high-risk clinic. The NCCN guidelines were followed by those of the American Society of Clinical Oncology (ASCO),[59] which further stratified the importance of germline testing in PDAC patients and their family members. Having an established high-risk clinic made the implementation of these guidelines seamless.

Our team recently published a paper that showed that long-term PDAC survivors exhibited distinct intratumoral microbiome signature.[60] Based on these results, we will investigate whether the microbiome signature (oral/gut) can be used as a biomarker for early detection or risk assessment based on screening of saliva and stool samples collected at our high-risk clinic.

Blood-Based Biomarkers

Developing a blood-based biomarker to detect the presence of pancreatic cancer early, as is available for other major cancers (prostate, ovarian) has been a goal of our Moon Shot team. CA 19-9, currently the only FDA-approved marker for PDAC, is limited by its sensitivity of 70%–90% and specificity of 68%–90% in symptomatic patients with large burden disease. Its diagnostic accuracy diminishes in patients with early stage disease.[61–63] Our goal was to perform a screening blood test for those who are at an elevated risk for developing PDAC. Thus far, we have built a three-protein anchor panel in combination with a plasma metabolite panel.[64,65] We will continue to validate a blood-based biomarker panel indicative of the risk of either harboring or developing early stage PDAC by leveraging access to large numbers of presymptomatic blood samples obtained from multiple longitudinal cohorts in the United States and Europe.

Imaging Tools for Early Detection

While imaging is an integral tool for cancer diagnosis, the resolution of current CT and MRI images is not adequate to reveal small, early lesions. We are leading efforts to develop quantitative imaging processing methods to enable the enhanced detection of small-volume cancers. We have also shown how images with contrast can be processed on a voxel-wise basis to improve the contrast-to-noise ratio, which may improve the detectability of small lesions and provide additional metrics for characterization of tissues.[66,67] This processing technique, called enhancement pattern mapping, improved the contrast-to-noise ratio by a factor of two over gray-scale images. We plan to test how the imaging properties of the pancreas may differ between benign and malignant pancreatic conditions using this technique. Specifically, in collaboration with six other institutions across the United States, we will establish an imaging repository for prediagnostic scans of PDAC. Furthermore, we are collaborating with the pancreatic cyst clinic, working with biostatisticians to integrate radiomics, pathologic, and biomarker data to help differentiate benign from malignant mucinous pancreatic cysts.

Our approach for early detection of PDAC, one of the deadliest forms of cancer, requires interdisciplinary research teams to work together. We do not envision that a single tool will satisfy the criteria of high specificity and sensitivity to diagnose PDAC; however, a combination of patient risk assessment, biomarkers, and imaging advances to reverse the current status where the overwhelming majority of patients are diagnosed with advanced disease.

Conclusion

The Moon Shots Program® has made great strides in transforming cancer prevention, early diagnosis, and treatment to improve the lives of all patients. Although the Moon Shots Program is currently focused on 13 cancers, the lessons learned from our progress will lead to advancements in the prevention, diagnosis, and treatment of all cancers.

The anesthesiology and perioperative community can become involved in the Moon Shots Program® in several ways. For example, perioperative physicians can counsel patients during preoperative visits to cancer prevention strategies. Clinicians can focus on perioperative efforts to minimize preventable complications due to cancer-related illnesses and rapid rescue efforts. The dissemination of core knowledge gained by the Moon Shots Program® can be spread locally and globally to the anesthesiology and perioperative community for cancer prevention programs, novel treatments, and early diagnosis methods.

References

1. MD Anderson Communications Office. UT MD Anderson Cancer Center Launches Unprecented Moon Shots Program, 2012 September 20 (December 4, 2012): p. 2019; Available from: https://www.mdanderson.org/newsroom/ut-md-anderson-cancer-center-launches-unprecedented-moon-shots-p.h00-158753901.html.
2. Jamal A, Phillips E, Gentzke AS, et al. Current cigarette smoking among adults—United States, 2016. *MMWR Morb Mortal Wkly Rep*. 2018;67(2):53–59.
3. World Health Organization, WHO Report on the Global Tobacco Epidemic, 2011: Warning about the Dangers of Tobacco—Executive Summary, 2011. cited: p. 2019; Available from: www.who.int/tobacco/global_report/2011/en/.
4. American Cancer Society. Tobacco Related Cancer Fact Sheet, 2014 [cited. 2019]; Available at www.cancer.org/cancer/cancer-causes/tobaccocancer/tobacco-related-cancer-fact-sheet.
5. American Cancer Society. Cancer Facts and Figures. 2017; Available at www.cancer.org/research/cancer-facts-statistics/all-cancer-facts-figures/cancer-facts-figures-2017.html.
6. Strauss GM. Screening for lung cancer: an evidence-based synthesis. *Surg Oncol Clin N Am*. 1999;8(4):747–774, viii.
7. Jacobs EJ, Newton CC, Carter BD, et al. What proportion of cancer deaths in the contemporary United States is attributable to cigarette smoking? *Ann Epidemiol*. 2015;25(3):179–182.e1.
8. Cahill K, Lindson-Hawley N, Thomas KH, Fanshawe TR, Lancaster T. Nicotine receptor partial agonists for smoking cessation. *Cochrane Database Syst Rev*. 2011;2:CD006103.
9. Hughes JR, Stead LF, Lancaster T, Cahill K, Lancaster T. Antidepressants for smoking cessation. *Cochrane Database Syst Rev*. 2007;1:CD000031.
10. 2008 PHS Guideline Update Panel, Liaisons, and Staff. Treating tobacco use and dependence: 2008 update U.S. Public Health Service Clinical Practice Guideline executive summary. *Respir Care*. 2008;53(9):1217–1222.
11. Stead LF, Perera R, Bullen C, et al. Nicotine replacement therapy for smoking cessation. *Cochrane Database Syst Rev*. 2012;11:CD000146.
12. Allenby CE, Boylan KA, Lerman C, Falcone M. Precision medicine for tobacco dependence: Development and validation of the nicotine metabolite ratio. *J Neuroimmune Pharmacol*. 2016;11(3):471–483.
13. Chen LS, Bloom AJ, Baker TB, et al. Pharmacotherapy effects on smoking cessation vary with nicotine metabolism gene (CYP2A6). *Addiction*. 2014;109(1):128–137.
14. Cinciripini PM, Green CE, Robinson JD, et al. Benefits of varenicline *vs*. bupropion for smoking cessation: a Bayesian analysis of the interaction of reward sensitivity and treatment. *Psychopharmacology*. 2017;234(11):1769–1779.
15. Hymowitz N, Cummings KM, Hyland A, et al. Predictors of smoking cessation in a cohort of adult smokers followed for five years. *Tob Control*. 1997;6 (Suppl 2):S57–S62.
16. King DP, Paciga S, Pickering E, et al. Smoking cessation pharmacogenetics: Analysis of varenicline and bupropion in placebo-controlled clinical trials. *Neuropsychopharmacology*. 2012;37(3):641–650.
17. Babb S, Malarcher A, Schauer G, et al. Quitting smoking among adults—United States, 2000–2015. *MMWR Morb Mortal Wkly Rep*. 2017;65(52):1457–1464.
18. Hurt RD, Krook JE, Croghan IT, et al. Nicotine patch therapy based on smoking rate followed by bupropion for prevention of relapse to smoking. *J Clin Oncol*. 2003;21(5):914–920.
19. Jamerson BD, Nides M, Jorenby DE, et al. Late-term smoking cessation despite initial failure: an evaluation of bupropion sustained release, nicotine patch, combination therapy, and placebo. *Clin Ther*. 2001;23(5):744–752.
20. Karam-Hage, M., P.M. Cinciripini, C.Y. Lam, J.A. Blalock. Increasing Varenicline to 3 Mgs/Day Improves Abstinence Rates: A Preliminary Efficacy Report in Cancer Patients. Paper presented at: Society for Research on Nicotine and Tobacco Annual Meeting; 2019, Baltimore.
21. Rose JE, Behm FM. Adapting smoking cessation treatment according to initial response to precessation nicotine patch. *Am J Psychiatry*. 2013;170(8):860–867.
22. Cinciripini PM, Karam-Hage M, Kypriotakis G, et al. Association of a comprehensive Smoking Cessation program with smoking abstinence among patients with cancer. *JAMA Netw Open*. 2019;2(9):e1912251.
23. Arora S, Thornton K, Murata G, et al. Outcomes of treatment for hepatitis C virus infection by primary care providers. *N Engl J Med*. 2011;364(23):2199–2207.
24. Plummer M, de Martel C, Vignat J, Ferlay J, Bray F, Franceschi S. Global burden of cancers attributable to infections in 2012: a synthetic analysis. *Lancet Glob Health*. 2016;4(9):e609–e616.
25. Islami F, Ferlay J, Lortet-Tieulent J, Bray F, Jemal A. International trends in anal cancer incidence rates. *Int J Epidemiol*. 2017;46(3):924–938.
26. Gillison ML, Chaturvedi AK, Anderson WF, Fakhry C. Epidemiology of human papillomavirus-positive head and neck squamous cell carcinoma. *J Clin Oncol*. 2015;33(29):3235–3242.
27. Gustafsson L, Pontén J, Zack M, Adami HO. International incidence rates of invasive cervical cancer after introduction of cytological screening. *Cancer Causes Control*. 1997;8(5):755–763.
28. Senkomago V, Henley SJ, Thomas CC, Mix JM, Markowitz LE, Saraiya M. Human papillomavirus-attributable cancers—United States, 2012–2016. *MMWR Morb Mortal Wkly Rep*. 2019;68(33):724–728.
29. Kirnbauer R, Booy F, Cheng N, Lowy DR, Schiller JT. Papillomavirus L1 major capsid protein self-assembles into virus-like particles that are highly immunogenic. *Proc Natl Acad Sci USA*. 1992;89(24):12180–12184.
30. Markowitz LE, Dunne EF, Saraiya M, Lawson HW, Chesson H, Unger ER. Quadrivalent human papillomavirus vaccine: Recommendations of the Advisory Committee on Immunization Practices (ACIP). *MMWR Recomm Rep*. 2007;56(RR-2):1–24.

31. Centers for Disease Control and Prevention (CDC). FDA licensure of bivalent human papillomavirus vaccine (HPV2, Cervarix) for use in females and updated HPV vaccination recommendations from the Advisory Committee on Immunization Practices (ACIP). *MMWR Morb Mortal Wkly Rep.* 2010;59(20):626–629.
32. Centers for Disease Control and Prevention (CDC). Recommendations on the use of quadrivalent human papillomavirus vaccine in males—Advisory Committee on Immunization Practices (ACIP), 2011. *MMWR Morb Mortal Wkly Rep.* 2011;60(50):1705–1708.
33. Petrosky E, Bocchini JA Jr, Hariri S. Use of 9-valent human papillomavirus (HPV) vaccine: Updated HPV vaccination recommendations of the Advisory Committee on Immunization Practices. *MMWR Morb Mortal Wkly Rep.* 2015;64(11):300–304.
34. Meites E, Szilagyi PG, Chesson HW, Unger ER, Romero JR, Markowitz LE. Human papillomavirus vaccination for adults: Updated recommendations of the Advisory Committee on Immunization Practices. *MMWR Morb Mortal Wkly Rep.* 2019; 68(32):698–702.
35. Meites E, Kempe A, Markowitz LE. Use of a 2-dose schedule for human papillomavirus vaccination—updated recommendations of the Advisory Committee on Immunization Practices. *MMWR Morb Mortal Wkly Rep.* 2016;65(49): 1405–1408.
36. Walker TY, Elam-Evans LD, Yankey D, et al. National, regional, state, and selected local area vaccination coverage among adolescents aged 13–17 years—United States, 2018. *MMWR Morb Mortal Wkly Rep.* 2019;68(33):718–723.
37. Brotherton JML, Bloem PN. Population-based HPV vaccination programmes are safe and effective: 2017 update and the impetus for achieving better global coverage. *Best Pract Res Clin Obstet Gynaecol.* 2018;47:42–58.
38. Orenstein WA, Gellin BG, Beigi RH, et al. Overcoming barriers to low HPV vaccine uptake in the United States: recommendations from the national vaccine advisory committee: approved by the National Vaccine Advisory Committee on June 9, 2015. *Public Health Rep.* 2016;131(1):17–25.
39. Gilkey MB, Calo WA, Moss JL, Shah PD, Marciniak MW, Brewer NT. Provider communication and HPV vaccination: the impact of recommendation quality. *Vaccine.* 2016;34(9):11871192.
40. Holman DM, Benard V, Roland KB, Watson M, Liddon N, Stokley S. Barriers to human papillomavirus vaccination among US adolescents: a systematic review of the literature. *JAMA Pediatr.* 2014;168(1):76–82.
41. Fokom Domgue J, Chido-Amajuoyi OG, Yu RK, Shete S. Beliefs about HPV vaccine's successfulness at cervical cancer prevention among adult US women. *JNCI Cancer Spec.* 2019;3(4):pkz064.
42. Gallagher KE, LaMontagne DS, Watson-Jones D. Status of HPV vaccine introduction and barriers to country uptake. *Vaccine.* 2018;36(32 Pt A):4761–4767.
43. Tung ILY, Machalek DA, Garland SM. Attitudes, knowledge and factors associated with human papillomavirus (HPV) vaccine uptake in adolescent girls and young women in Victoria, Australia. *PLoS One.* 2016;11(8):e0161846.
44. Borena W, Luckner-Hornischer A, Katzgraber F, Holm-von Laer D, et al. Factors affecting HPV vaccine acceptance in west Austria: Do we need to revise the current immunization scheme? *Papillomavirus Res.* 2016;2:173–177.
45. Gatera M, Bhatt S, Ngabo F, et al. Successive introduction of four new vaccines in Rwanda: high coverage and rapid scale up of Rwanda's expanded immunization program from 2009 to 2013. *Vaccine.* 2016;34(29):3420–3426.
46. Franco M, Mazzucca S, Padek M, Brownson RC. Going beyond the individual: How state-level characteristics relate to HPV vaccine rates in the United States. *BMC Public Health.* 2019;19(1):246.
47. ACS, Key Statistics for Pancreatic Cancer. November 25, 2019; Available from: https://www.cancer.org/cancer/pancreatic-cancer/about/key-statistics.html.
48. NCI, State Cancer Profiles: Death Rate Report for United States. 2012–2016.
49. Rahib L, Smith BD, Aizenberg R, Rosenzweig AB, Fleshman JM, Matrisian LM. Projecting cancer incidence and deaths to 2030: the unexpected burden of thyroid, liver, and pancreas cancers in the United States. *Cancer Res.* 2014;74(11):2913–2921.
50. Ryan DP, Hong TS, Bardeesy N. Pancreatic adenocarcinoma. *N Engl J Med.* 2014;371(11):1039–1049.
51. Chari ST, Kelly K, Hollingsworth MA, et al. Early detection of sporadic pancreatic cancer: summative review. *Pancreas.* 2015;44(5):693–712.
52. NCI, Surveillance, *Epidemiology, and End Results (SEER) Program.*
53. Andea A, Sarkar F, Adsay VN. Clinicopathological correlates of pancreatic intraepithelial neoplasia: A comparative analysis of 82 cases with and 152 cases without pancreatic ductal adenocarcinoma. *Mod Pathol.* 2003;16(10):996–1006.
54. Yachida S, Jones S, Bozic I, et al. Distant metastasis occurs late during the genetic evolution of pancreatic cancer. *Nature.* 2010;467(7319):1114–1117.
55. Owens DK, Davidson KW, Krist AH, et al. US Preventive Services Task Force. Screening for pancreatic cancer: US Preventive Services Task Force reaffirmation recommendation statement. *JAMA.* 2019;322(5):438–444.
56. Goggins M, Overbeek KA, Brand R, et al. Management of patients with increased risk for familial pancreatic cancer: updated recommendations from the International Cancer of the Pancreas Screening (CAPS) Consortium. *Gut.* 2020;69(1):7–17.
57. Canto MI, Harinck F, Hruban RH, et al. International Cancer of the Pancreas Screening (CAPS) Consortium summit on the management of patients with increased risk for familial pancreatic cancer. *Gut.* 2013;62(3):339–347.
58. National Comprehensive Cancer Network (NCCN), Guidelines Version 2.2019 Pancreatic Adenocarcinoma. Accessed November 25, 2019.
59. Stoffel EM, McKernin SE, Brand R, et al. Evaluating susceptibility to pancreatic cancer: ASCO provisional clinical opinion. *J Clin Oncol.* 2019;37(2):153–164.
60. Riquelme E, Zhang Y, Zhang L, et al. Tumor microbiome diversity and composition influence pancreatic cancer outcomes. *Cell.* 2019;178(4):795–806.e12.
61. Scarà S, Bottoni P, Scatena R., CA 19-9: Biochemical and clinical aspects. *Adv Exp Med Biol.* 2015;867:247–260.
62. O'Brien DP, Sandanayake NS, Jenkinson C, et al. Serum CA19-9 is significantly upregulated up to 2 years before diagnosis with pancreatic cancer: implications for early disease detection. *Clin Cancer Res.* 2015;21(3):622–631.
63. Nolen BM, Brand RE, Prosser D, et al. Prediagnostic serum biomarkers as early detection tools for pancreatic cancer in a large prospective cohort study. *PLoS One.* 2014;9 (4):e94928.

64. Capello M, Bantis LE, Scelo G, et al. Sequential validation of blood-based protein biomarker candidates for early-stage pancreatic cancer. *J Natl Cancer Inst*. 2017;109(4):djw266.
65. Fahrmann JF, Bantis LE, Capello M, et al. A plasma-derived protein-metabolite multiplexed panel for early-stage pancreatic cancer. *J Natl Cancer Inst*. 2019;111(4):372–379.
66. Park PC, Choi GW, Koay EJ. Voxel-based enhancement pattern mapping (EPM) improves the contrast-to-noise ratio and detection of abnormalities in multiphase contrast-enhanced CT. *Proceedings of the AAPM Annual Meeting, 2017*, UT MD Anderson Cancer Center: Houston, TX; 2017.
67. Park PC, Choi GW, Zaid MM, et al. Enhancement pattern mapping (EPM) technique for improving contrast-to-noise ratios (CNRs) and detectability of hepatobiliary tumors on multiphase contrast-enhanced CT (MPCT). *Med Phys* 2020;47: 64–74.
68. Parkin DM, Bray F. Chapter 2: The burden of HPV-related cancers. Vaccine. 2006;24(Suppl 3):S11–S25.

Index

Note: Page numbers followed by "*f*" indicate figures, "*t*" indicate tables, and "*b*" indicate boxes.

B

C

F

G

H

S